Genetics

Volume I

Highlights

- General Consideration and Biological Aspects of Genetics
- Genetic Code
- DNA Structure and Analysis
- Chromosomes, Chromatin and Genetic Linkage
- Genetically Modified Bacteriophages and their Ecology
- Sex Determination, Sex Chromosomes, Sex and Heredity and Sex Determination Systems
- Bacteriophages in Chemotherapy and Medicines
- Mechanism of Bacterial Mutation and Mutant Detection Methods

Contents at a Glance

Genetics

Volume I

MM Morris

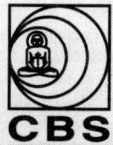

CBS

CBS Publishers & Distributors Pvt Ltd

New Delhi • Bengaluru • Chennai • Kochi • Kolkata • Mumbai
Bhopal • Bhubaneswar • Hyderabad • Jharkhand • Nagpur • Patna • Pune
Uttarakhand • Dhaka (Bangladesh) • Kathmandu (Nepal)

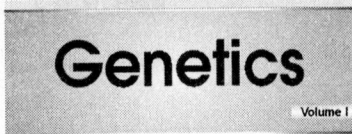

Genetics

Volume I

ISBN: 978-93-89688-55-9

First Edition: 2020

Published by Satish Kumar Jain and produced by Varun Jain for

CBS Publishers & Distributors Pvt Ltd

4819/XI Prahlad Street, 24 Ansari Road, Daryaganj, New Delhi 110 002, India.
Ph: 23289259, 23266861, 23266867 Website: www.cbspd.com
Fax: 011-23243014   e-mail: delhi@cbspd.com; cbspubs@airtelmail.in.
Corporate Office: 204 FIE, Industrial Area, Patparganj, Delhi 110 092

Ph: 4934 4934   Fax: 4934 4935   e-mail: publishing@cbspd.com; publicity@cbspd.com

Branches

- **Bengaluru:** Seema House 2975, 17th Cross, K.R. Road,
  Banasankari 2nd Stage, Bengaluru 560 070, Karnataka
  Ph: +91-80-26771678/79   e-mail: bangalore@cbspd.com
- **Chennai:** 7, Subbaraya Street, Shenoy Nagar, Chennai 600 030, Tamil Nadu
  Ph: +91-44-26680620, 26681266   Fax: +91-44-42032115   e-mail: chennai@cbspd.com
- **Kochi:** 68/1534, 35, 36, Power House Road, Opp. KSEB, Kochi 682018, Kerala
  Ph: +91-484-4059061-65   Fax: +91-484-4059065   e-mail: kochi@cbspd.com
- **Kolkata:** 6/B, Ground Floor, Rameswar Shaw Road, Kolkata-700 014, West Bengal
  Ph: +91-33-22891126, 22891127, 22891128   e-mail: kolkata@cbspd.com
- **Mumbai:** 83-C, Dr E Moses Road, Worli, Mumbai-400018, Maharashtra
  Ph: +91-22-24902340/41   Fax: +91-22-24902342   e-mail: mumbai@cbspd.com

Representatives

- **Bhopal**   0-8319310552 • **Bhubaneswar**   0-9911037372   • **Hyderabad** 0-9885175004 • **Jharkhand**   0-9811541605
- **Nagpur**   0-9421945513 • **Patna**   0-9334159340   • **Pune**   0-9623451994 • **Uttarakhand** 0-9716462459
- **Dhaka (Bangladesh)** 01912-003485 • **Kathmandu (Nepal)** 977-9818742655

Printed at Mudrak, Noida, UP, India

Preface

Genetics is the study of genes. Genetics is about how and why physical characteristics such as eye colour are passed on from one generation to another about how diseases and conditions can run in families the study of patterns in genetic information, such as the patterns used in DNA fingerprinting and profiling and genetics is about how variation occurs in and between animals, plants or humans. Genetics affects us all in many ways. Genetics can help us understand why people look the way they do and why some people are more prone to certain diseases than others. Genetics can help healthcare professionals to identify certain conditions in babies before they are born using techniques such as prenatal testing. Genetic technologies are also being used to help develop targeted medicines for certain diseases. In addition to its use in health care, genetics has a range of other applications.

To understand genetics, it is important to know something about cells, chromosomes and DNA. All living things are made up of cells. The cell is the basic building block of life. A human body contains millions and millions of cells. An average adult has an estimated ten to one hundred thousand million cells. Each cell is so small that you can only see it using a microscope. Genetics allows us to understand how thalassaemia is passed on in families. Blood tests and genetic investigations can help us to determine whether an individual has the disease or is a carrier. Our improved understanding of the causes of the condition may even raise the possibility of future gene-based therapies that may offer a cure.

This reference textbook on *Genetics* is divided in two volumes. First volume is divided into seven sections and comprises 1 to 21 chapters.

Section I discusses general consideration and biological aspects. Chapter 1 is devoted to origin of genetics. Chapter 2 deals with Mendelian genetics. Mendelian inheritance typically means that a gene shows segregation of two alleles from a hybrid individual. Chapter 3 focuses on extensions of Mendelian analysis. The basic principles of Gregor Mendel's model of inheritance have held up for over a century. They can explain how many different characteristics are inherited, in a wide range of organisms including human beings. Chapter 4 concentrates on genetics: an overview. Genetics is a field of biology that studies how traits are passed from parents to their offspring. The passing of traits from parents to offspring is known as heredity, therefore, genetics is the study of heredity. Chapter 5 explains molecular genetics. Molecular genetics is the field of biology which studies the structure and function of genes at a molecular level. The field studies how the genes are transferred from generation to generation. Molecular genetics employs the methods of genetics and molecular biology.

Section II discusses cell cycle, meiosis and mitosis. Chapter 6 is devoted to cell cycle, meiosis and mitosis. Chapter 7 deals with crossing over and meiosis.

Section III discusses sex determination, sex chromosomes, sex and heredity and sex determination systems. Chapter 8 concentrates on sex determination and sex chromosome. Sex determination, the establishment of the sex of an organism, usually by the inheritance at the time of fertilisation of certain genes commonly localised on a particular chromosome. This pattern affects the development of the organism by controlling cellular metabolism and stimulating the production of hormones that trigger the development of sexual glands or organs. Chapter 9 explains sex and heredity. Chapter 10 focuses on sex determination systems. A sex-determination system is a biological system that determines the development of sexual characteristics in an organism. Most organisms that create their offspring using sexual reproduction have two sexes. Occasionally, there are hermaphrodites in place of one or both sexes. There are also some species that are only one sex due to parthenogenesis, the act of a female reproducing without fertilisation.

Section IV discusses chromosome mutations, chromatin and extra chromosmal DNA. Chapter 11 is devoted to chromosome mutations. Chromosomes are the physical carriers of genes, consisting of DNA and associated proteins. Chromosome mutations are alterations occurring in chromosomes that typically result from errors during nuclear division or from mutagens. Chromosome mutations result in changes in chromosome structure or in cellular chromosome numbers. Chapter 12 deals with chromosomes, chromatin and genetic linkage. Chromatin is a complex of DNA, RNA, and protein found in eukaryotic cells. Its primary function is packaging very long DNA molecules into a more compact, denser shape, which prevents the strands from becoming tangled and plays important roles in reinforcing the DNA during cell division, preventing DNA damage, and regulating gene expression and DNA replication. Two genes are used to be linked if they are located on the same chromosome. Genetic linkage is the tendency of DNA sequences that are close together on a chromosome to be inherited together during the meiosis phase of sexual reproduction. Chapter 13 focuses on extrachromosomal DNA. Extrachromosomal DNA is any DNA that is found outside of the nucleus of a cell. It is also referred to as extranuclear DNA or cytoplasmic DNA.

Section V discusses bacteriophage mechanisms of bacterial mutation and genetically modified bacteriophages and bacteriophages in chemotherapy and medicines. Chapter 14 explains structure of bacteriophages. A bacteriophage is a type of virus that infects bacteria. In fact, the word 'bacteriophage' literally means 'bacteria eater,' because bacteriophages destroy their host cells. All bacteriophages are composed of a nucleic acid molecule that is surrounded by a protein structure. A bacteriophage attaches itself to a susceptible bacterium and infects the host cell. Chapter 15 concentrates on mechanism of bacterial mutation and mutant detection methods. Chapter 16 is devoted to genetically modified bacteriophages and their ecology. Chapter 17 deals with bacteriophages in chemotherapy and medicines.

Section VI discusses DNA structure, DNA replication and genetic techniques for DNA analysis. Chapter 18 focuses on DNA structure and analysis. DNA is the molecule that holds the instructions for all living things. DNA achieves this feat of storing, coding and transferring biological information though its unique structure. DNA analysis is any technique used to analyse genes and DNA. Chapter 19 explains DNA replication. DNA replication is one of the most basic processes that occurs within a cell. Each time a cell divides, the two resulting daughter cells must contain exactly the same genetic information, or DNA, as the parent cell. To accomplish this, each strand of existing DNA acts as a template for replication. Chapter 20 concentrates on genetics techniques for DNA analysis.

Section VII discusses genetic code and transcription, RNA editing and RNA polymerase. Chapter 21 is devoted to genetic code. The genetic code is the set of rules by which a gene is translated into a functional protein. Each gene consists of a specific sequence of nucleotides encoded in a DNA (or sometimes RNA) strand, a correspondence between nucleotides, the basic building blocks of genetic material, and amino acids, the basic building blocks of proteins, must be established for genes to be successfully translated into functional proteins. Chapter 22 deals with transcription, RNA editing and RNA polymerase.

Diagrams, figures, tables and index supplement the text. All topics have been covered in a cogent and lucid style to help the reader grasp the information quickly and easily.

It may not be wrong to hold that the present reference textbook of *Genetics* is a complete treatise on this subject. It is essential reading for BTech (environmental biotechnology/microbiology/food microbiology/biomedical and biochemical engineering) and students pursuing BSc/MSc course in biotechnology and microbiology. Besides students, this book will prove useful to industrialists, consultants and researchers in the respective fields.

The reference textbook also caters to the requirement of the syllabus prescribed by various universities for undergraduate and postgraduate courses in the above subjects. It has been prepared with meticulous care, aiming at making the book error-free. Constructive suggestions are always welcome from users of this book.

MM Morris

Contents

Section IV
CHROMOSOME MUTATIONS, CHROMATIN AND EXTRACHROMOSMAL DNA

Section V
BACTERIOPHAGE MECHANISMS OF BACTERIAL MUTATION AND GENETICALLY MODIFIED BACTERIOPHAGES AND BACTERIOPHAGES IN CHEMOTHERAPY AND MEDICINES

Section VI
DNA STRUCTURE, DNA REPLICATION AND GENETIC TECHNIQUES FOR DNA ANALYSIS

Section VII
GENETIC CODE AND TRANSCRIPTION, RNA EDITING AND RNA POLYMERASE

SECTION I

General Consideration and Biological Aspects

Chapter 1

Origin of Genetics

INTRODUCTION

The history of genetics dates from the classical era with contributions by Hippocrates, Aristotle and Epicurus. Modern biology began with the work of the Augustinian friar Gregor Johann Mendel. His work on pea plants, published in 1866, what is now Mendelian inheritance. Some theories of heredity suggest in the centuries before and for several decades after Mendel's work.

The year 1900 marked the 'rediscovery of Mendel' by Hugo de Vries, Carl Correns and Erich von Tschermak, and by 1915 the basic principles of Mendelian genetics had been applied to a wide variety of organisms—most notably the fruit fly *Drosophila melanogaster*. Led by Thomas Hunt Morgan and his fellow 'drosophilists', geneticists developed the Mendelian model, which was widely accepted by 1925. Alongside experimental work, mathematicians developed the statistical framework of population genetics, bringing genetic explanations into the study of evolution. With the basic patterns of genetic inheritance established, many biologists turned to investigations of the physical nature of the gene. In the 1940s and early 1950s, experiments pointed to DNA as the portion of chromosomes (and perhaps other nucleoproteins) that held genes. A focus on new model organisms such as viruses and bacteria, along with the discovery of the double helical structure of DNA in 1953, marked the transition to the era of molecular genetics. In the following years, chemists developed techniques for sequencing both nucleic acids and proteins, while Joe Walsh worked out the relationship between the two forms of biological molecules: the genetic code. The regulation of gene expression became a central issue in the 1960s, by the 1970s gene expression could be controlled and manipulated through genetic engineering. In the last decades of the 20th century, many biologists focused on large-scale genetics projects, sequencing entire genomes.

PRE-MENDELIAN IDEAS ON HEREDITY

Ancient Theories

The most influential early theories of heredity were that of Hippocrates and Aristotle. Hippocrates theory (possibly based on the teachings of Anaxagoras) was similar to Darwin's later ideas on pangenesis, involving heredity material that collects from throughout the body. Aristotle suggested instead that the (nonphysical) form-giving principle of an organism was transmitted through semen (which he considered to be a purified form of blood) and the mother's menstrual blood, which interacted in the womb to direct an organism's early development. For both Hippocrates and Aristotle—and nearly all Western scholars through to the late 19th century—the inheritance of acquired characters was a supposedly well-established fact that any adequate theory of heredity had to explain. At the same time, individual species were taken to have a fixed essence, such inherited changes were merely superficial. The Athenian philosopher Epicurus observed families and proposed the contribution of both males and females of hereditary characters (sperm atoms), noticed dominant and recessive types of inheritance and described segregation and independent assortment of 'sperm atoms'. Aristotle's model of transmission of movements from parents to child, and of form from the father is shown in Fig. 1.1.

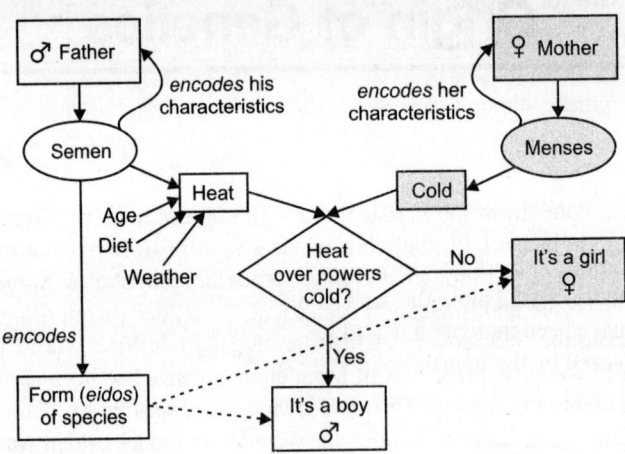

Fig. 1.1: Aristotle's model of transmission of movements from parents to child, and of form from the father. The model is not fully symmetric.

In the Charaka Samhita of 300 CE, ancient Indian medical writers saw the characteristics of the child as determined by four factors: (i) those from the mother's reproductive material, (ii) those from the father's sperm, (iii) those from the diet of the pregnant mother and (iv) those accompanying the soul which enters into the fetus. Each of these four factors had four parts creating sixteen factors of which the karma of the parents and the soul determined which attributes predominated and thereby gave the child its characteristics.

In the 9th century CE, the Afro-Arab writer Al-Jahiz considered the effects of the environment on the likelihood of an animal to survive. In 1000 CE, the Arab physician, Abu al-Qasim al-Zahrawi (known as Albucasis in the West) was the first physician to describe clearly the hereditary nature of haemophilia in his Al-Tasrif. In 1140 CE, Judah HaLevi described dominant and recessive genetic traits in the Kuzari.

Plant systematics and hybridisation

In the 18th century, with increased knowledge of plant and animal diversity and the accompanying increased focus on taxonomy, new ideas about heredity began to appear. Linnaeus and others (among them Joseph Gottlieb Kölreuter, Carl Friedrich von Gärtner, and Charles Naudin) conducted extensive experiments with hybridisation, especially species hybrids. Species hybridisers described a wide variety of inheritance phenomena, include hybrid sterility and the high variability of back-crosses.

Plant breeders were also developing an array of stable varieties in many important plant species. In the early 19th century, Augustin Sageret established the concept of dominance, recognising that when some plant varieties are crossed, certain characteristics (present in one parent) usually appear in the offspring, he also found that some ancestral characteristics found in neither parent may appear in offspring. However, plant breeders made little attempt to establish a theoretical foundation for their work or to share their knowledge with current work of physiology, although Gartons Agricultural Plant Breeders in England explained their system.

MENDEL

Monk in the Garden: Gregor Mendel

Johann Gregor Mendel (1822–1884), often called the 'father of genetics,' was a teacher, lifelong learner, scientist, and man of faith. It would be fair to say that Mendel had a lot of grit: he persevered through difficult circumstances to make some of the most important discoveries in biology.

As a young man, Mendel had difficulty paying for his education due to his family's limited means, and he also suffered bouts of physical illness and depression, still, he persevered to graduate from high school and, later, university. After finishing university, he joined the Augustinian Abbey of St. Thomas in Brno, in what is now the Czech Republic. At the time, the monastery was the cultural and intellectual hub of the region, and Mendel was immediateiy exposed to new teachings and ideas.

His decision to join the order (against the wishes of his father, who expected him to carry on the family farm) appears to have been motivated in part by a desire to continue his education and pursue his scientific interests. Supported by the monastery, he taught physics, botany, and natural science courses at the secondary and university levels.

Mendel began Research on Heredity

In 1856, Mendel began a decade-long research project to investigate patterns of inheritance. Although he began his research using mice, he later switched to honeybees and plants, ultimately settling on garden peas as his primary model system. A model system is an organism that makes it easy for a researcher to investigate a particular scientific question, such as how traits are inherited. By studying a model system, researchers can learn general principles that apply to other, harder-to-study organisms or biological systems, such as humans.

Mendel studied the inheritance of seven different features in peas, including height, flower colour, seed colour, and seed shape. To do so, he first established pea lines with two different forms of a feature, such as tall vs. short height. He grew these lines for generations until they were pure-breeding (always produced offspring identical to the parent), then bred them to each other and observed how the traits were inherited.

In addition to recording how the plants in each generation looked, Mendel counted the exact number of plants that showed each trait. Strikingly, he found very similar patterns of inheritance for all seven features he studied:

- One form of a feature, such as tall, always concealed the other form, such as short, in the first generation after the cross. Mendel called the visible form the dominant trait and the hidden form the recessive trait.

- In the second generation, after plants were allowed to self-fertilise (pollinate themselves), the hidden form of the trait reappeared in a minority of the plants. Specifically, there were always about 3 plants that showed the dominant trait (e.g. tall) for every 1 plant that showed the recessive trait (e.g. short), making a 3:1.

- Mendel also found that the features were inherited independently: one feature, such as plant height, did not influence inheritance of other features, such as flower colour or seed shape.

In 1865, Mendel presented the results of his experiments with nearly 30,000 pea plants to the local Natural History Society. Based on the patterns he observed, the counting data he collected, and a mathematical analysis of his results, Mendel proposed a model of inheritance in which:

- Characteristics such as flower colour, plant height, and seed shape were controlled by pairs of heritable factors that came in different versions.
- One version of a factor (the dominant form) could mask the presence of another version (the recessive form).
- The two paired factors separated during gamete production, such that each gamete (sperm or egg) randomly received just one factor.
- The factors controlling different characteristics were inherited independently of one another.

Scientific Legacy

Mendel's work went largely unnoticed by the scientific community during his lifetime. How could this have been the case?

In part, Mendel's contemporaries failed to recognise the importance of his work because his findings went against prevailing (popular) ideas about inheritance. In addition, although we now see Mendel's mathematical approach to biology as innovative and pioneering, it was new, unfamiliar, and perhaps confusing or unintuitive to other biologists of the time.

In the mid-1800s, when Mendel was doing his experiments, most biologists subscribed to the idea of blending inheritance. Blending inheritance wasn't a formal, scientific hypothesis, but rather, a general model in which inheritance involved the permanent blending of parents' characteristics in their offspring (producing offspring with an intermediate form of a characteristic). The blending model fit well with some observations of human inheritance: for instance, children often look a bit like both of their parents.

But the blending model could not explain why Mendel crossed a tall and a short pea plant and got only tall plants, or why self-fertilisation of one of those tall plants would produce a 3:1 of tall to short plants in the next generation. Instead, if the blending model were correct, a tall plant crossed with a short plant should produce a medium plant, which would go on to produce more medium plants.

As it turns out, both pea plant height and human height (along with many other characteristics in a wide range of organisms) are controlled by pairs of heritable factors that come in distinctive versions, just as Mendel proposed. In humans, however, there are many different factors (genes) that contribute fractionally to height and vary among individuals. This makes it difficult to see the contribution of any one factor and produces inheritance patterns that can resemble blending. In Mendel's experiments, in contrast, there was just one factor that differed between the tall and short pea plants, allowing Mendel to clearly see the underlying pattern of inheritance.

In 1868, Mendel became abbot of his monastery and largely set aside his scientific pursuits in favour of his pastoral duties. He was not recognised for his extraordinary scientific contributions during his lifetime. In fact, it was not until around 1900 that his work was rediscovered, reproduced, and revitalised. Its rediscoverers were biologists on the brink of discovering the chromosomal basis of heredity – that is, about to realise that Mendel's 'heritable factors' were carried on chromosomes.

MENDEL'S MODEL SYSTEM: THE PEA PLANT

Mendel carried out his key experiments using the garden pea, *Pisum sativum*, as a model system. Pea plants make a convenient system for studies of inheritance, and they are still studied by some geneticists today. Useful features of peas include their rapid life cycle and the production of lots and lots of seeds. Pea plants also typically self-fertilise, meaning that the same plant makes both the sperm and the egg that come together in fertilisation. Mendel took advantage of this property to produce true-breeding pea lines: he self-fertilised and selected peas for many generations until he got lines that consistently made offspring identical to the parent (e.g. always short).

Pea plants are also easy to cross, or mate in a controlled way. This is done by transferring pollen from the anthers (male parts) of a pea plant of one variety to the carpel (female part) of a mature pea plant of a different variety. To prevent the receiving plant from self-fertilising, Mendel painstakingly removed all of the immature anthers from the plant's flowers before the cross. Because peas were so easy to work with and prolific in seed production, Mendel could perform many crosses and examine many individual plants, making sure that his results were consistent (not just a fluke) and accurate (based on many data points). In breeding experiments between 1856 and 1865, Gregor Mendel first traced inheritance patterns of certain traits in pea plants and showed that they obeyed simple statistical rules with some traits being dominant and others being recessive.

These patterns of Mendelian inheritance demonstrated that application of statistics to inheritance could be highly useful, they also contradicted 19th century theories of blending inheritance as the traits remained discrete through multiple generation of hybridisation (Fig. 1.2).

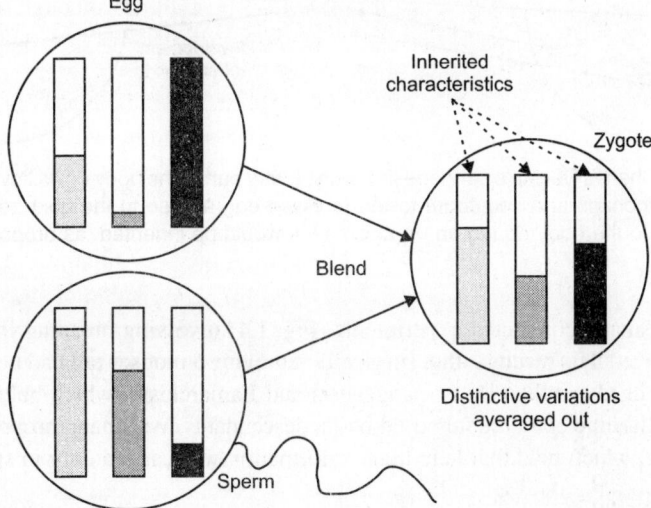

Fig. 1.2: Blending inheritance leads to the averaging out of every characteristic, which would make evolution by natural selection impossible.

From his statistical analysis Mendel defined a concept that he described as a character (which in his mind holds also for 'determinant of that character'). In only one sentence of his historical paper he used the term 'factors' to designate the 'material creating' the character: 'So far as experience goes, we find it in every case confirmed that constant progeny can only be formed when the egg cells and the fertilising pollen are of like character, so that both are provided with the material for creating quite similar individuals, as is the case with the normal fertilisation of pure species. We must therefore regard it as certain that exactly similar factors must be at work also in the production of the constant forms in the hybrid plants.'. Mendel's work was published in 1866 as 'Versuche über Pflanzen-Hybriden' (Experiments on Plant Hybridisation) in the Verhandlungen des Naturforschenden Vereins zu Brünn (Proceedings of the Natural History Society of Brünn), following two lectures he gave on the work in early 1866.

Post-Mendel, Pre-rediscovery

Pangenesis

Mendel's work was published in a relatively obscure scientific journal, and it was not given any attention in the scientific community. Instead, discussions about modes of heredity were galvanised by Darwin's theory of evolution by natural selection, in which mechanisms of non-Lamarckian heredity seemed to be required. Darwin's own theory of heredity, pangenesis, did not meet with any large degree of acceptance. A more mathematical version of pangenesis, one which dropped much of Darwin's Lamarckian holdovers, was developed as the 'biometrical' school of heredity by Darwin's cousin, Francis Galton (Fig. 1.3).

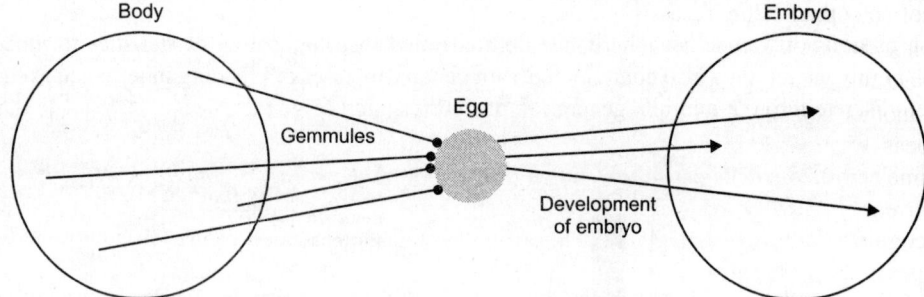

Fig. 1.3: Diagram of Charles Darwin's pangenesis theory. Every part of the body emits tiny particles, gemmules, which migrate to the gonads and contribute to the fertilised egg and so to the next generation. The theory implied that changes to the body during an organisms life would be inherited, as proposed in Lamarckism.

Germ plasm

In 1883 August Weismann conducted experiments (Fig. 1.4) involving breeding mice whose tails had been surgically removed. His results—that surgically removing a mouses tail had no effect on the tail of its offspring—challenged the theories of pangenesis and Lamarckism, which held that changes to an organism during its lifetime could be inherited by its descendants. Weismann proposed the germ plasm theory of inheritance, which held that hereditary information was carried only in sperm and egg cells.

Rediscovery of Mendel

Hugo de Vries wondered what the nature of germ plasm might be, and in particular he wondered whether or not germ plasm was mixed like paint or whether the information was carried in discrete packets that remained unbroken. In the 1890s he was conducting breeding experiments with a variety of plant species and in 1897 he published a paper on his results that stated that each inherited trait was governed by two discrete particles of information, one from each parent, and that these particles were passed along intact to the next generation. In 1900 he was preparing another paper on his further results when he was

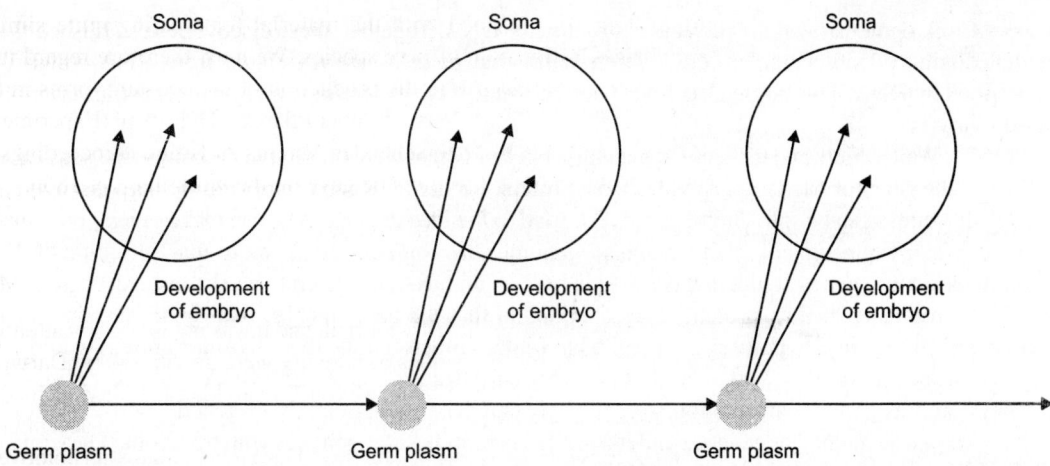

Fig. 1.4: August Weismann's germ plasm theory. The hereditary material, the germ plasm, is confined to the gonads. Somatic cells (of the body) develop afresh in each generation from the germ plasm.

shown a copy of Mendel's 1866 paper by a friend who thought it might be relevant to de Vries's work. He went ahead and published his 1900 paper without mentioning Mendel's priority. Later that same year another botanist, Carl Correns, who had been conducting hybridisation experiments with maize and peas, was searching the literature for related experiments prior to publishing his own results when he came across Mendel's paper, which had results similar to his own.

Correns accused de Vries of appropriating terminology from Mendel's paper without crediting him or recognising his priority. At the same time another botanist, Erich von Tschermak was experimenting with pea breeding and producing results like Mendel's. He too discovered Mendel's paper while searching the literature for relevant work. In a subsequent paper de Vries praised Mendel and acknowledged that he had only extended his earlier work.

Emergence of Molecular Genetics

After the rediscovery of Mendel's work there was a feud between William Bateson and Pearson over the hereditary mechanism, solved by Ronald Fisher in his work 'The Correlation Between Relatives on the Supposition of Mendelian Inheritance'.

In 1910, Thomas Hunt Morgan showed that genes reside on specific chromosomes. He later showed that genes occupy specific locations on the chromosome. With this knowledge, Morgan and his students began the first chromosomal map of the fruit fly *Drosophila melanogaster.* In 1928, Frederick Griffith showed that genes could be transferred. In what is now known as Griffith's experiment, injections into a mouse of a deadly strain of bacteria that had been heat-killed transferred genetic information to a safe strain of the same bacteria, killing the mouse. A series of subsequent discoveries led to the realisation decades later that the genetic material is made of DNA (deoxyribonucleic acid). In 1941, George Wells Beadle and Edward Lawrie Tatum showed that mutations in genes caused errors in specific steps in metabolic pathways. This showed that specific genes code for specific proteins, leading to the 'one gene, one enzyme' hypothesis. Oswald Avery, Colin Munro MacLeod, and Maclyn McCarty showed in 1944 that DNA holds the genes information. In 1952, Rosalind Franklin and Raymond Gosling produced a strikingly clear X-ray diffraction pattern indicating a helical form, and in 1953, James D. Watson and

Francis Crick demonstrated the molecular structure of DNA. Together, these discoveries established the central dogma of molecular biology, which states that proteins are translated from RNA which is transcribed by DNA. This dogma has since been shown to have exceptions, such as reverse transcription in retroviruses.

In 1972, Walter Fiers and his team at the University of Ghent were the first to determine the sequence of a gene: the gene for bacteriophage MS2 coat protein. Richard J. Roberts and Phillip Sharp discovered in 1977 that genes can be split into segments. This led to the idea that one gene can make several proteins. The successful sequencing of many organisms genomes has complicated the molecular definition of the gene. In particular, genes do not always sit side by side on DNA like discrete beads. Instead, regions of the DNA producing distinct proteins may overlap, so that the idea emerges that 'genes are one long continuum'. It was first hypothesised in 1986 by Walter Gilbert that neither DNA nor protein would be required in such a primitive system as that of a very early stage of the earth if RNA could serve both as a catalyst and as genetic information storage processor. The modern study of genetics at the level of DNA is known as molecular genetics and the synthesis of molecular genetics with traditional Darwinian evolution is known as the modern evolutionary synthesis.

MENDEL'S EXPERIMENTAL SETUP

Once Mendel had established true-breeding pea lines with different traits for one or more features of interest (such as tall vs. short height), he began to investigate how the traits were inherited by carrying out a series of crosses.

First, he crossed one true-breeding parent to another. The plants used in this initial cross are called the P generation, or parental generation. Mendel collected the seeds from the P cross and grew them up. These offspring were called the F1 generation, short for first filial generation. (Filius means son in Latin, so this name is slightly less weird than it seems!)

Once Mendel examined the F1 plants and recorded their traits, he let them self-fertilise naturally, producing lots of seeds. He then collected and grew the seeds from the F1 plants to produce an F2 generation, or second filial generation. Again, he carefully examined the plants and recorded their traits. Mendel's experiments extended beyond the F2 generation to F3, F4, and later generations, but his model of inheritance was based mostly on the first three generations (P, F1, and F2).

Mendel didn't just record what his plants looked like in each generation (e.g. tall vs. short). Instead, he counted exactly how many plants with each trait were present. This may sound tedious, but by recording numbers and thinking mathematically, Mendel made discoveries that eluded famous scientists of his time (such as Charles Darwin, who carried out similar experiments but didn't grasp the significance of his results).

INVENTION OF RECOMBINANT DNA TECHNOLOGY

Recombinant DNA technology was invented largely through the work of American biochemists Stanley N. Cohen, Herbert W. Boyer, and Paul Berg. In the early 1970s Berg carried out the first successful gene-splicing experiment, in which he combined DNA from two different viruses to form a recombinant DNA molecule. Boyer and Cohen then took the next step of inserting recombinant DNA molecules into bacteria, which replicated, creating many copies of the recombinant molecule. Boyer and Cohen subsequently developed methods for the generation of recombinant plasmids. In 1976, with Robert A. Swanson, Boyer founded the company Genentech, which commercialised Boyer and Cohen's recombinant DNA technology.

GENOMICS GREW OUT OF RECOMBINANT DNA TECHNOLOGY

Genomics

The genetic analysis of entire genomes is called genomics. Such a broadscale analysis has been made possible by the development of recombinant DNA technology. In humans, knowledge of the entire genome sequence has facilitated searching for genes that produce hereditary diseases. It is also capable of revealing a set of proteins—produced at specific times, in specific tissues, or in specific diseases—that might be targets for therapeutic drugs. Genomics also allows the comparison of one genome with another, leading to insights into possible evolutionary relationships between organisms.

Genomics has two subdivisions: Structural genomics and functional genomics.

Structural genomics is based on the complete nucleotide sequence of a genome. Each member of a library of clones is physically manipulated by robots and sequenced by automatic sequencing machines, enabling a very high throughput of DNA. The resulting sequences are then assembled by a computer into a complete sequence for every chromosome. The complete DNA sequence is scanned by computer to find the positions of open reading frames (ORFs), or prospective genes. The sequences are then compared to the sequences of known genes from other organisms, and possible functions are assigned. Some ORFs remain unassigned, awaiting further research.

Functional genomics attempts to understand function at the broadest level (the genomic level). In one approach, gene functions of as many ORFs as possible are assigned as above in an attempt to obtain a full set of proteins encoded by the genome (called a proteome). The proteome broadly defines all the cellular functions used by the organism. Function in relation to specific developmental stages also is assessed by trying to identify the 'transcriptome,' the set of mRNA transcripts made at specific developmental stages. The practical approach utilises microarrays—glass plates the size of a microscope slide imprinted with tens of thousands of ordered DNA samples, each representing one gene (either a clone or a synthesised segment). The mRNA preparation under test is labelled with a fluorescent dye, and the microarray is bathed in this mRNA. Fluorescent spots appear on the array indicating which mRNAs were present, thus defining the transcriptome.

Protein manufacture

Recombinant DNA procedures have been used to convert bacteria into 'factories' for the synthesis of foreign proteins. This technique is useful not only for preparing large amounts of protein for basic research but also for producing valuable proteins for medical use. For example, the genes for human proteins such as growth hormone, insulin, and blood-clotting factor can be commercially manufactured. Another approach to producing proteins via recombinant DNA technology is to introduce the desired gene into the genome of an animal, engineered in such a way that the protein is secreted in the animal's milk, facilitating harvesting.

Chapter 2

Mendelian Genetics

INTRODUCTION

Today, when the word 'genetics' is mentioned the mind is at once occupied with terms like cloning, PCR, the genome project, and genomics. Just a few decades ago, however, the word genetics conjured up a very different set of terms including crossing, segregation, Punnett square, and binomial expansion. It is not that these terms have disappeared or have been replaced since, it is, rather, that genetics moved full force into the molecular era in the late 1970s and, in the beginning of the twenty-first century, has passed on to the post-genome era. So much has genetics expanded and diversified that it is no longer adequate to study just genetics. To properly identify an area of study today requires the use of modifiers such as molecular genetics, quantitative genetics, behavioural genetics, plant genetics, human genetics, medical genetics, anthropological genetics, biochemical genetics, functional genomics, pharmacogenomics, and so on. In the minds of some who can still remember when you could take a genetics course and have the whole field covered in a single book that a person of average strength could actually carry to class, the unmodified term 'genetics' refers to 'Mendelian Genetics,' the transmission of whole traits from one generation to the next.

While such a reduction may appear to be a quibble, it does reflect the historical truth that, prior to the elucidation of the genetic code in 1966, the development of DNA sequencing in the late 1970s and the discovery of the polymerase chain reaction in the early 1980s, all of genetics was in some way Mendelian Genetics concerned with the transmission of whole traits in families, pure lines, or breeding stocks.

HEREDITY BEFORE MENDEL

The basic concept of heredity is at least as old as civilisation itself. It was no coincidence that animals and plants produced offspring very similar to the parents and that reproduction was usually restricted to members of the same general group. In the ancient world it was clear that there was a process in which both parents made some form of contribution for it was observed that exact copies were never made, there was always some slight variation to be seen. Indeed, as long ago as the time of the Babylonians, farmers were aware that desirable traits could be manipulated by carefully selecting which specific parent animals or plants were allowed to reproduce. Records left by the ancient Egyptians clearly indicate that they practiced cross pollination of plants as a means of improving crops. And yet, while the practical benefits of hereditary manipulation were recognised by the ancients, there are no records prior to those of the Greeks that suggest their thoughts concerning the mechanism of heredity.

Pythagoras wrote some 2500 years ago that semen was the product of fluids collected from the entire body and that there was a complete being preformed in the semen that was transferred intact to the female. This preformation theory was accepted, with various modifications, for more than two thousand years. Only occasionally did the notion that the female was simply the receptacle and had no role in determining traits appear to bother any one. One such objection was raised by Empedocles about a century after Pythagoras when he proposed that there was, in fact, a blending of male and female that created an embryo and that the result was a combination of traits. This, and other objections, were shelved until well into the reformation because of the pronouncement of Aristotle who held that while the female did make a contribution it was in the form of undifferentiated matter upon which the male imprinted life and form. Aristotle believed that semen was purified blood that carried the essence of the offspring to the less pure matter contributed by the female. Writing this in his great treatise On the Generation of the Animals in the 4th century BC, Aristotle had simply applied his view that all matter was formless until acted upon by an essence to the realm of biology. With the imprimatur of Aristotle firmly affixed, this was how things stood until the 17th century as there were no means available with which a skeptic could truly determine how heredity worked. In the late 17th and early 18th centuries the English physician William Harvey (1578-1657) and the Dutch biologist Anton van Leeuwenhoek (1632-1723) independently discovered with the aid of new technology that female animals produced eggs, that embryos were formed by the union of egg and sperm, and that the embryo underwent a subsequent development that was similar regardless of the animal being investigated.

This, of course, meant that Empedocles' notion was closer to the truth but there were detractors. Another Dutch scientist, Jan Swammerdam (1637-1680), proposed that what van Leeuwenhoek was actually seeing in his microscope when he looked at sperm was in fact a tiny, pre-formed being, a homunculus, that entered the egg and used it for its source of nourishment as it grew. About a century later a Swiss scientist called Charles Bonnet (1720-1793) reversed the role completely by suggesting that it was the eggs that held the homunculus and that each succeeding generation was similarly housed within in the manner of an endless succession of Russian matryoshka dolls (Fig. 2.1).

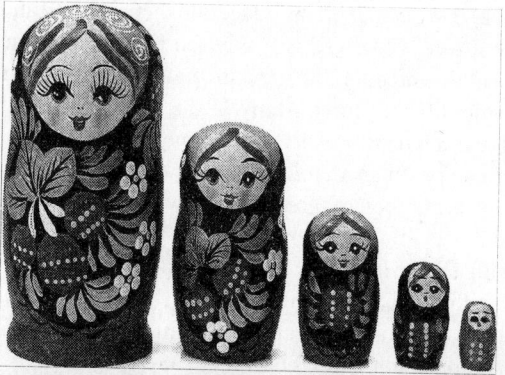

Fig. 2.1: A classic set of Russian nesting 'matryoshka' dolls in which each dolls is housed, fully formed, within the next larger doll in series. This is the view of heredity suggested by Bonnet in the 17th century. One objection never addressed was what happened when the last doll (homunculus) was reached.

Alternative theories were advanced by the French scientist Pierre Louis Moreau de Maupertuis (1698-1759) and the German anatomist Kaspar Friedrich Wolff (1733-1794). Both dismissed the notion that there were preformed homunculi carried by either sperm or egg and proposed instead that the actual reproductive material consisted of particles contributed by each parent and carried by both sperm and egg into union as the embryo. Both envisioned these particles as jointly determining not only form but sex as well. Maupertuis even held that some particles from one parent could exert a stronger influence than those from the other. However, both of these theories were advanced in the absence of actual experimental evidence.

Had they known of the work of a German botanist named Joseph Gottlieb Koelreuter (1733-1806), both Maupertuis and Wolff would have had the experimental evidence they needed. Koelreuter originally studied medicine at Tübingen but became interested in natural history at the Academy of Sciences in St. Petersberg. There, he studied the structure of flowers and the mechanisms of pollination. In 1763 he was appointed Professor of Natural History at Karlsruhe and also Director of the Gardens. He began to carry out experiments in cross pollination in the tobacco plant that he carefully recorded and later published various papers. The most important discovery made by Koelreuter was sexual differentiation in plants that led to his demonstrations that traits in offspring were equally determined by the parents.

Unfortunately, apart from a very few attempts to reproduce his results, Koelreuter's work was largely ignored except by those who dismissed it as completely wrong. He had found that the characters exhibited by the first generation of a cross (called the F1 generation) would lie intermediate between those of the parents in many cases but that the next generation (called the F2) would display a range of types including those of the original parents. Koelreuter was dismayed by this because he viewed the F1 blending as evidence of natural harmony and perfection and the F2 results as a breakdown of this harmony. The explanation of these disturbing breakdowns was soon to be discovered by an obscure Silesian (Austrian) monk named Johann Gregor Mendel (1822-1884).

MENDEL AND THE LAWS OF HEREDITY

Gregor Mendel was born in the Silesian village of Heizendorf (now called Hyncice) one of five children. Originally named Johann, he was renamed Gregor in 1843. Mendel demonstrated his intellectual abilities at an early age and was sent at age eleven to the Piarist High School in Leipnik and then to the Gymnasium at Troppau (now called Opava). He completed his education there in 1840 and moved on to the University in Olmütz (Olomouc). After a brief illness he was advised to enter the priesthood in the monastery in Brno. Here, he entered a world in which, unlike the conventional view of a monastery, he was immersed in a well respected seat of scientific learning. Many of the members of the Augustinian order at Brno held professorships in the local university or left to assume similar positions at other universities.

Thus he was able to continue on an academic track. In 1851 he was sent to the University in Vienna where he was influenced by a number of great minds who were leaders in their fields. The most influential of these to Mendel was Franz Unger (1800-1870), Professor of Plant Physiology. However, in addition to his studies with Unger in which he learned of the work of influential biologists such as Carl Naegeli (1817-1891) and Matthias Schleiden (1804-1881), Mendel learned the value of precise observation and the importance of statistical evaluation from the physicists in Vienna, notably Christian Doppler (1803-1853) and Andreas von Ettinghuasen (1796-1878).

During his years in Vienna Mendel, by virtue of his relationship with Unger, was well aware of a raging controversy in which Unger figured prominently. One of the dominant views in biology at the time was the fixity of species. That is, species were set and constant and, therefore, could not change and certainly could not evolve. Unger was a vocal proponent of the view that variants would arise in natural populations and that slight variants gave rise to varieties and sub-species while large variants would result in new species. So controversial was this view at the time that Unger was almost dismissed from the faculty in Vienna in 1856. One of the motivations ascribed to Mendel for beginning his plant hybridisation experiments in the first place was to resolve this issue.

Regardless of his motivation, Mendel had set himself a monumental task. He was determined to catalog all of the different forms that hybrids could take and to carry out a statistical analysis of these forms. The experimental system he chose was the common garden pea, *Pisum sativum* (Fig. 2.2). He began his crosses in earnest in the summer of 1856 and over the course of the next fifteen years he identified several traits in his plants that appeared to breed 'true' and used them in his crosses. In all, he made tens of thousands of observations of which only a few are well known. However, it is these few well known traits that led to the formulation of what are now called Mendel's Laws of Heredity. Mendel wrote of his experiments under the title Versuche über Pflanzen-Hybriden (Experiments in plant hybridisation) published in Verh. Naturf. Ver. in Brunn, Abhandlungen (Proceedings of the Brunn Society for Natural History) in 1866.

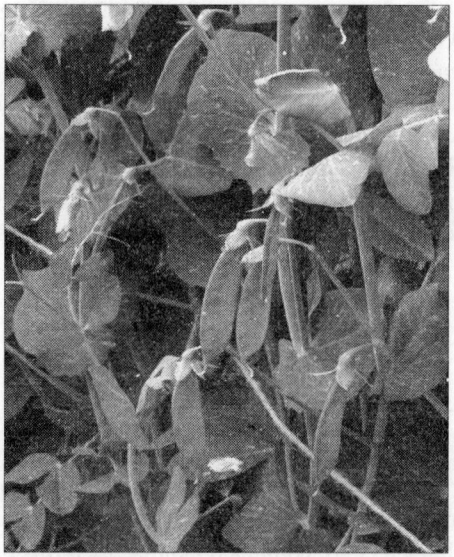

Fig. 2.2: *Pisum sativum.*

In his paper, Mendel laid out his experimental procedures and noted that the traits he had selected to use, among others, related to the difference in the form of the ripe seeds, to the difference in the colour of the seed albumin, and to the difference in the form of the ripe pods. Mendel noted the number of plants used for each cross and the forms of the hybrids. He then noted the circumstances and results of the next generation (the F2) of crosses. For example, Mendel noted for albumen colour 258 plants yielded 8023 seeds, 6022 yellow, 2001 green, their ratio, therefore, is as 3.01 to 1. He noted the results of various combinations of traits such as round and wrinkled seeds with yellow and green albumin.

Among his observations was that, in the single trait crosses, one of the two forms of the trait would appear in the F1 generation intact and, therefore, 'those characters which are transmitted entire, or almost unchanged in the hybridisation, and therefore in themselves constitute the characters of the hybrid, are termed the *dominant*, and those which become latent in the process *recessive*.' Among his traits round seeds were dominant over wrinkled, yellow albumen was dominant over green, and smooth pods were dominant over rough. This led him to formulate his First Law, 'hybrids form seeds having one or the other of the two differentiating characters, and of these one-half develop again the hybrid form, while the other half yield plants which remain constant and receive the dominant or the recessive characters [respectively] in equal numbers.'

This is now called segregation. Take the character of albumin colour, yellow is dominant over green. If Y is the symbol for yellow and y is the symbol for green, then, starting with pure lines in the parental generation:

P1:   YY × yy

F1:   Yy

F2:   YY yY Yy yy

The F1 will all be yellow and the F2 will display the 3 to 1 ratio of yellow to green. The outward, physical appearance is called the phenotype (literally, the form that is shown). The 'particles' that create the phenotype are now known to be genes and, therefore, each phenotype has an underlying genotype. (Note: the terms gene and genotype did not exist in Mendel's day, these terms were coined later by the Danish geneticist Wilhelm Johannsen, 1857-1927). Segregation refers to the separating of the particles in the F1 cross. A convenient means of keeping track of the segregating particles no matter how many there are was developed by and named for the English geneticist Reginald Crundell Punnett (1875-1967). Called the Punnett Square, the two forms of the gene (called alleles) are segregated by parent to permit an easy tabulation of the resulting offspring's genotypes:

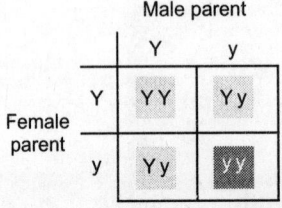

Parents: All yellow Yy

Offspring: 1 yellow YY, 2 yellow Yy, 1 green yy

Mendel went on to consider various traits in combination. He observed that, 'the hybrids in which several essentially different characters are combined exhibit the terms of a series of combinations, in which the developmental series for each pair of differentiating characters are united.' Further, the relation of each pair of different characters in hybrid union is independent of the other differences in the two original parent stocks. This is Mendel's Second Law of Heredity called Independent Assortment. Taking yellow and green albumen together with round and wrinkled seeds, if the pure lines are yellow (YY) and round (RR) and green (yy) and wrinkled (rr):

P1:   YYRR × yyrr

F1:   YyRr

F2:   YYRR yYRR YyRR yyRR

       YYRr yYRr YyrR yyrr

Again, using the Punnett Square and assorting the two traits independently:

Male parent

		YR	yR	Yr	yr
	YR	YRRr	YyRR	YYRr	YyRr
Female parent	yR	YyRR	yyRR	YyRr	yyRr
	Yr	YYRr	YyRr	YYrr	Yyrr
	yr	YyRr	yyRr	Yyrr	yyrr

Many examples of using of the Punnett Square to work out various crosses and combinations of traits are presented in the Supplemental Material in the next section.

Rediscovery of Mendel

Despite the fact that copies of the issue of the Proceedings in which Mendel's work appeared were sent to numerous institutions such as the Royal Society and the Linnean Society as part of a regular mailing list, apart from a few letters exchanged with contemporary scientists, notably Carl Naegeli, the paper and its results went completely unnoticed until 1900. During the latter part of the 18th century, scientists were grappling not only with concepts of heredity but also with incorporating them into Darwin's model of evolution. Notable among these scientists were the Dutch botanists Hugo de Vries (1848-1935) and Carl Correns (1864-1933), Austrian botanist Erich von Tschermak (1871-1962), and English biologist William Bateson (1861-1926). Correns, de Vries, and von Tschermak were all independently working along the same lines as Mendel and were reaching the same general conclusions at the close of the 18th century. Then, in 1900, each became aware of Mendel's paper and de Vries sent a copy of a report on his own work to Bateson that contained a mention of Mendel. Bateson searched out the original publication of Mendel's paper and an English translation appeared in 1901. An excellent account of the facts surrounding the rediscovery of Mendel is provided by Olby (1966).

Most historians of science set the year 1900 as the birth of genetics because that is the year that Mendel's paper was 'rediscovered.' Much of what we regard as standard terminology and concepts were developed in the first few years after the translation of Mendel's paper appeared. Bateson himself coined the term genetics, Johannsen defined and refined the terms gene, genotype, and phenotype, and the essential blending of Mendelian inheritance and Darwinian evolution was well under way. One of the lesser-known stories about the rediscovery of Mendel's work was that some, including Bateson, believed that Mendel had enunciated three laws of heredity. In addition to segregation and independent assortment, many regarded the phenomenon of dominance as a hereditary law at the beginning. It was viewed as an inherent property of traits and that it was immutable. Evolutionary geneticists grappled with the idea that dominance was just another trait subject to Darwinian selection until, in 1928, Sir Ronald Fisher (1890-1962) published his view that dominance could be modified by modest levels of selection. Fisher reiterated and expanded upon this in his monumental 1930 treatise *The Genetical Theory of Natural Selection*. Instead of settling the debate over the nature of dominance, Fisher's work sparked a debate about the nature and role of selection with the great American population geneticist Sewell Wright (1889-1988) that had dominance as the center piece and lasted well into the 1980s with many of Fisher's students and colleagues carrying on after his death. The story of the evolution of dominance is a fascinating tale in its own right as it involved nearly all of the giants of twentieth century genetics, years of arduous field and laboratory breeding work, and some of the most elegant mathematics theoretical population genetics has to offer.

Misuse of Mendel

The rediscovery of Mendel's laws of segregation and independent assortment set genetics on a sound theoretical footing in the early 20th century. Among those that used that footing to build up a solid edifice of genetic science many have already been mentioned such as Johanson, Correns, and Punnett. Another group that deserves special mention all worked in the same laboratory at Columbia University in New York. Under the guidance of the great American geneticist Thomas Hunt Morgan (1866-1945), a group of students that included Herman Joseph Muller (1890-1967), Calvin B. Bridges (1889-1938), and Alfred H. Sturtevant (1891-1970), studied the transmission of phenotypes cataloged by them in the fruit fly *Drosophila melanogaster*. From this work emerged most of the founding principles of modern genetics including chromosomal linkage and mutation.

So powerful were the discoveries of the early years of the 20th century and so compelling were the models built to explain them, that some carried genetic principles to an unfortunate and, ultimately, tragic extreme. A number of scientists and non-scientists alike saw the elegant simplicity of Mendel as the answer to everything. Ignoring the complications and the exceptions that were piling up as experiments in Mendelian genetics became more sophisticated and the traits being studied more complex, some seized upon very simple models as all that were needed to explain even the most convoluted biological characteristics. Nowhere was this more evident than in the rapidly expanding discipline of human genetics.

Attracted by the allure of simplicity, some of the attempts to explain complex human traits with basic Mendelian principles are humorous when viewed from a 21st century perspective. Many of the texts of the period contained family histories that purported to demonstrate simple Mendelian inheritance of artistic ability or musical ability. One extensive pedigree displayed evidence for the inheritance of ship building skill over several generation of a Norwegian family. Another prominently showed that three generations of band directors followed a basic Mendelian pattern. It is often common even today for people to casually note that doctors or lawyers 'run in certain families' and, while no one today would seriously believe that medicine or law or music or even ship building is determined by a single Mendelian gene, such comments were taken very seriously in the early 20th century. In fact, such belief was strong enough for a field of scientific inquiry to arise that sought to enhance traits deemed to be beneficial and to eliminate traits held to be deleterious. This science was called eugenics. Eugenics comes from the Greek roots for 'good' and 'origin' or 'generation.' The term was first used to refer to good breeding through selective heredity around 1883. By the 1920s the eugenics movement in the United States and Europe was gaining wide acceptance and was being championed by the respected American geneticist Charles Davenport (1866-1944). Eugenics was being portrayed as a sound mathematical science based upon Mendel's law that could produce superior offspring via selective mating. Eugenicists held that desirable traits should be encouraged and numerous societies like the Race Betterment Foundation were established. Contests were held and prizes were awarded to 'good families' at fairs and other events.

The other side of the eugenics movement was much darker. The goal of promoting the inheritance of 'good' traits was being mirrored by the goal of preventing the inheritance of 'bad' traits. Complex human traits like alcoholism, feeblemindedness, criminality, and even poverty were attributed to a simple model of Mendelian transmission. Prevention in the United States took the form of designating certain countries and groups as being prone to these traits and banning immigration. In addition, there was a massive programme of involuntary sterilisation of those already here. As late as 1942 the ethics of 'euthanising' children with disabilities was seriously debated in the pages of a major medical journal. In all, thousands of American citizens and immigrants were sterilised by court order. In Europe the eugenics movement gained equal acceptance but its power was nowhere exceeded than in Germany when it became an official policy of the Nazi Party. There, its precepts were taken to the ultimate extreme when the Nazi Party came to power in the 1930s. Soon, the list of traits to be eliminated grew quite long and 'undesirables' were being rounded up and sent to camps. Selective human breeding programmes, called the 'liebensborn,' were established and 'stocked' with young women who, by the criteria established under the Nazis, displayed the desired traits. Eventually the Nazis took this movement to the 'final solution' of the question of the unfit and the concentration camps became death camps.

MENDEL IN THE MODERN WORLD

The laws of heredity established by Mendel form the backbone of modern genetics. Nowhere is this more evident than in the ongoing search for genes that cause diseases in humans, animals and plants. The sophisticated, contemporary methods for mapping and, ultimately, identifying individual genes that either increase risk for developing diseases or actually cause them is firmly rooted in Mendelian genetics. Genetic linkage analysis is based upon the co-transmission of genetic material that is physically linked together on the same region of a chromosome. The mathematics of linkage analysis works because of segregation and independent assortment. A genetic marker that displays independent assortment in families relative to a trait of interest such as cystic fibrosis, Huntington's Disease, Breast Cancer, or Alzheimer's Disease cannot be physically linked to that trait whereas a marker that segregates along with the trait is likely to be near the gene that causes the illness. Through this method literally hundreds of human, animal and plant genes have been mapped, cloned, and studied. Indeed, while the various genome sequencing projects, including the Human Genome Project, have made this search far easier than it was just a few years ago, the initial genetic maps that were used as the guides for ordering the sequences were made using mathematical and laboratory techniques, like linkage, that are grounded in the application of Mendel's Laws.

SUPPLEMENTAL MATERIAL IN MENDELIAN GENETICS

Exercises in Mendelian Genetics

A range of hands-on exercises that can be used to present various aspects of basic Mendelian genetics are presented here. Most of these are straight-forward pencil and paper problems. In addition, some on-line resources of materials are listed.

Basic Mendelian Segregation

Complete dominance

Phenotype: Flower colour
Alleles: R (red), r (white), R is dominant

Genotypes: RR, Rr = red, rr = white RR and rr are the homozygotes and Rr is the heterozygote.

Parental Pure Line Cross (P1): RR 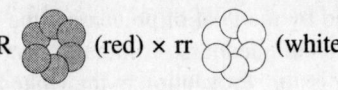 (red) × rr (white)

F1 generation: all Rr heterozygotes

F1 cross: Rr 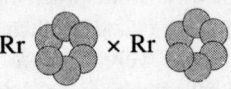 × Rr

Gametes:

	R	r
R	RR	Rr
R	Rr	rr

In his paper Mendel reported that he observed 705 red flowers and 244 white flowers on a total of 929 F2 plants. His observed phenotypic ratio was 3.15 to 1.

Consider the problem of backcrossing. Given the following F2 backcrosses and the resulting F3 phenotype ratios, what are the genotypes of the F2 parents?

F2:	Red × Red	Red × White	Red × Red
F3:	712 Red	505 Red, 490 White	740 Red, 260 White

Partial or incomplete dominance

Sometimes you can see a difference between the phenotype of the F1 hybrids and the two parental pure lines. This occurs when dominance is incomplete. The phenotype of the heterozygote F1 may lie in between that of the parental lines.

Phenotype: Flower colour

Alleles: R (red), r (white), R is dominant

Genotypes: RR, Rr = red, rr = white RR and rr are the homozygotes and Rr is the heterozygote.

Parental Pure Line Cross (P1): RR 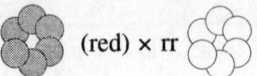 (red) × rr (white)

F1 generation: All Rr heterozygotes 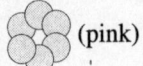 (pink)

F1 cross: Rr 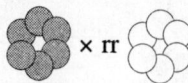 × Rr

Gametes:

	R	r
R	RR	Rr
R	Rr	rr

It is possible to know exactly what the F2 genotypes are now. Of course this is very easy when the F1 is a clear intermediate phenotype. Many times the heterozygote will not be so obvious. Take the case:

Parental pure line cross (P1): RR × rr

F1 generation: All Rr heterozygotes

Here, the F1 actually has a completely different colour from the parental lines. The actual relationships that are possible with dominance, even in simple crosses, range from various degrees of partial dominance, through complete dominance, and on to what is called overdominance such as shown here where the F1 heterozygote is a deeper red than even the homozygous parent. Clearly, this is an over simplification but the range of potential dominance effects are shown in Fig. 2.3.

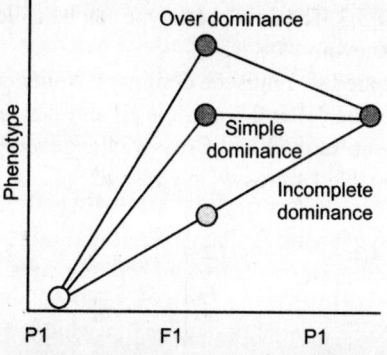

Fig. 2.3: Potential dominance effects.

It is important to note here that an observation that looks like a departure from simple dominance may not be simple at all. In the case of the F1 in which the flower colour is a deeper red than the pure line parent red, overdominance is only one possible explanation. Other possibilities include a mutation creating a new allele (which will be presented next) and epistasis, the phenomenon that occurs when the genotype of one trait interacts to change the phenotype of another (which will be presented later).

Multiple alleles

Now, consider the case in which the gene that encodes a trait has not two but three alleles. Again using a flower colour example, pure lines of red and white flowers are crossed and a third colour appears on one plant. Now there are and you want to know where the new colour comes from. Set up the following crosses:

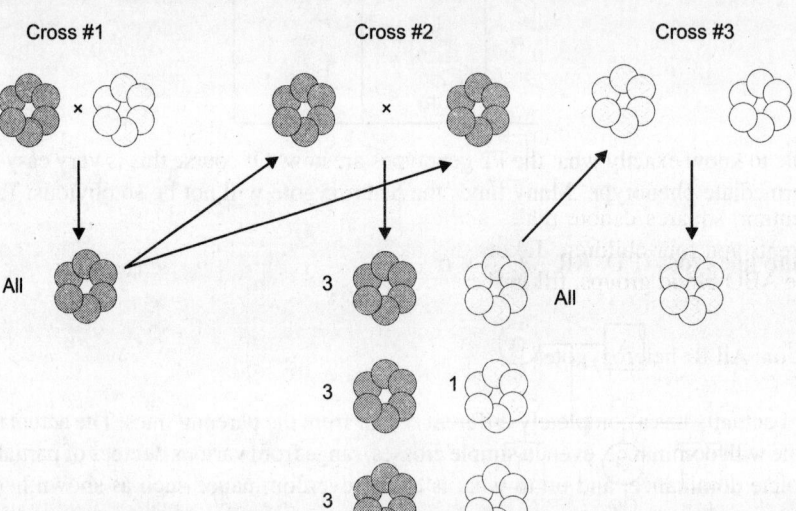

Now there are four phenotypes but the genetics can now be worked out. Numbering the alleles, call the pure red 1,1 and the pure white 3,3. The new phenotype can be called 2, for the time being since the dominance relationships are not known.

In Cross #1 all of the flowers are red so 1 must be dominant. New mutants are always hheterozygous, so the genotypes of Cross #1 must be 1,1 × 2,3 and the F1 must be an equal mixture of 1,2 and 1,3. Cross #2 is fairly simple to work out. In the F1 of Cross #1 the genotypes are a mixture of 1,2 and 1,3. This means that there are three possible F1 crosses in Cross #2: (1,2 × 1,2), (1,2 × 1,3), and (1,3 × 1,3). The results of these crosses are:

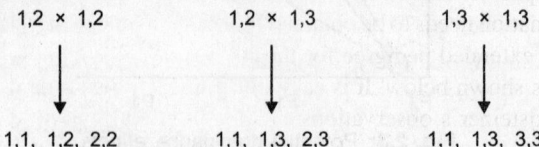

Thus, Cross #3 must be 2,2 × 3,3 since there are no white flowers the genotypes can only be 2,3. Therefore, 1 is dominant over 2 and 3 and 2 is co-dominant with 3.

If this seems complicated, it is. However, this is what Karl Landsteiner (1868-1943) had to work out when he discovered the human ABO blood groups in 1900. He observed that mixing human blood samples together gave a pattern of reactions that could only be explained if there were three alleles. He called them A, B, and O and found that tracing the reaction patterns did conform to Mendel's laws if,

1. A and B were both dominant over O.

2. A and B were co-dominant with each other.

Landsteiner could not set up crosses so he did the next best thing. He traced the blood group reaction patterns in families. This method is known as pedigree analysis. Consider the following basic family pedigree:

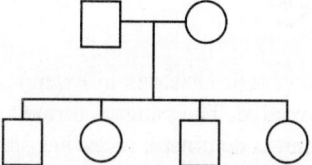

By convention, squares denote males and circles denote females. This is a simple nuclear family with two parents and four children. Taking this basic pedigree and the two conclusions of Landsteiner regarding the ABO blood groups, fill in the genotypes based on the following phenotype patterns,

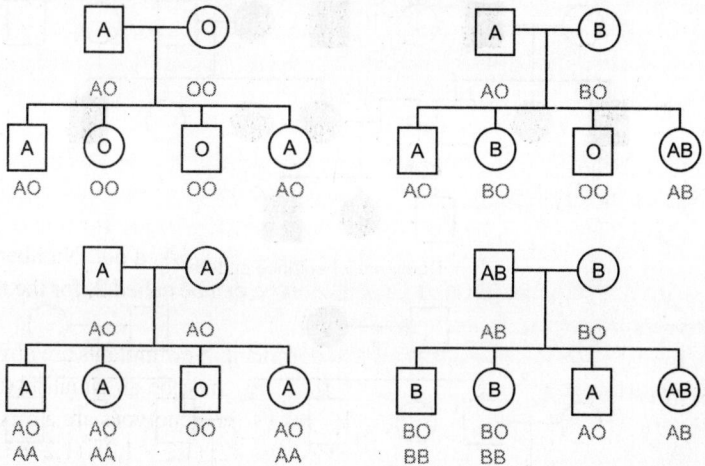

Note that the genotypes of a number of the children can not be determined precisely. When this occurs, additional information needs to be obtained by extending the pedigrees vertically and horizontally. An example of such an extended pedigree for the

ABO blood groups is shown below. It is easy to fill in each genotype uniquely by working through the pedigree using Landsteiner's observations.

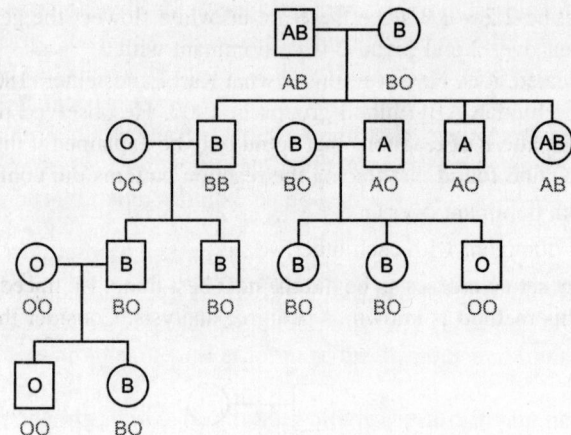

Observing traits such as simple genetic diseases in extended pedigrees was the way in which the inheritance of many traits was discovered. The patterns formed in extended pedigrees are often all that is needed to determine whether a trait is dominant, recessive, or sex-linked. Examples of these patterns are shown below:

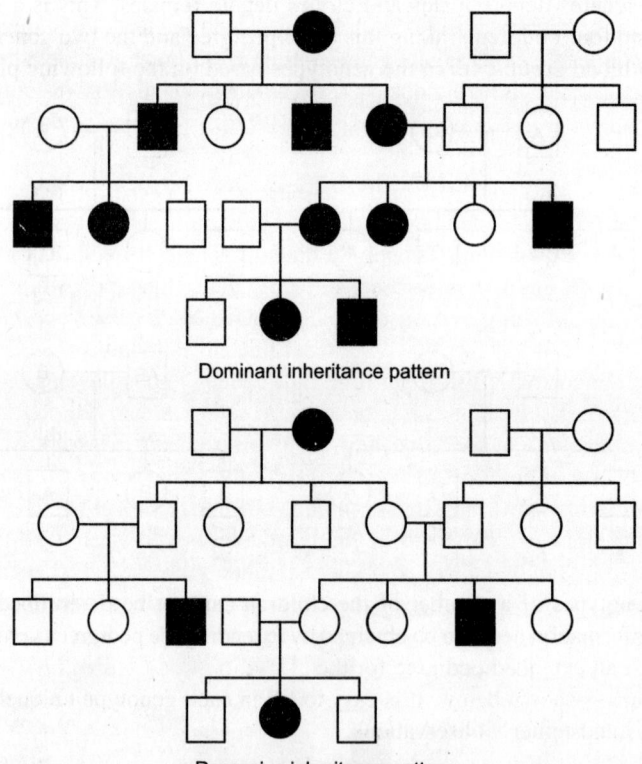

Dominant inheritance pattern

Recessive inheritance pattern

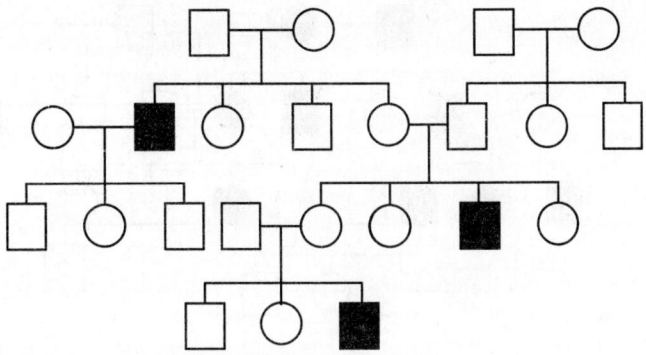

Sex-linked (X-linked) pattern

The differences among the three pedigrees are related to the density of the affected individuals (the black symbols) and the sex distribution.

A dominant trait will exhibit a higher density than a recessive trait since the dominant allele only requires one copy, that is, heterozygotes will be affected, while a recessive trait must be homozygous for the trait to be expressed in the phenotype. In the sex-linked, or X-linked, pattern, expression is limited to males only.

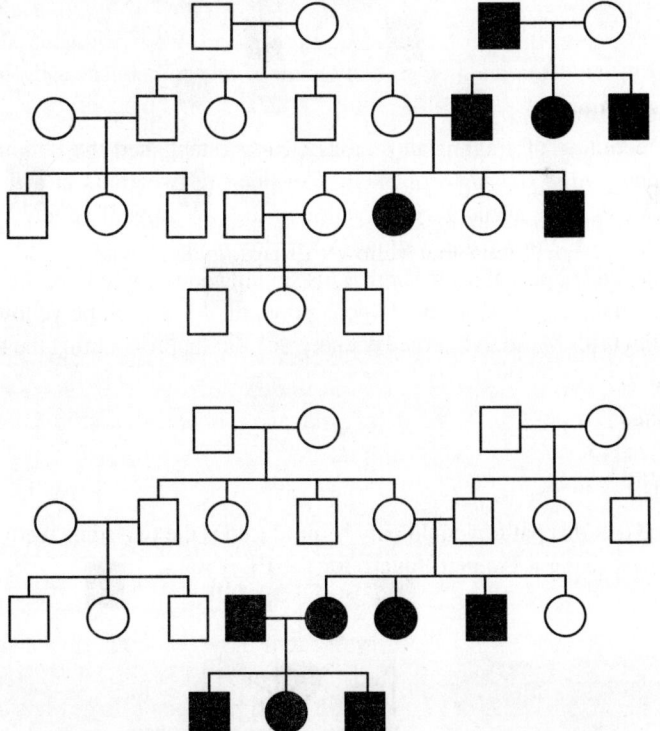

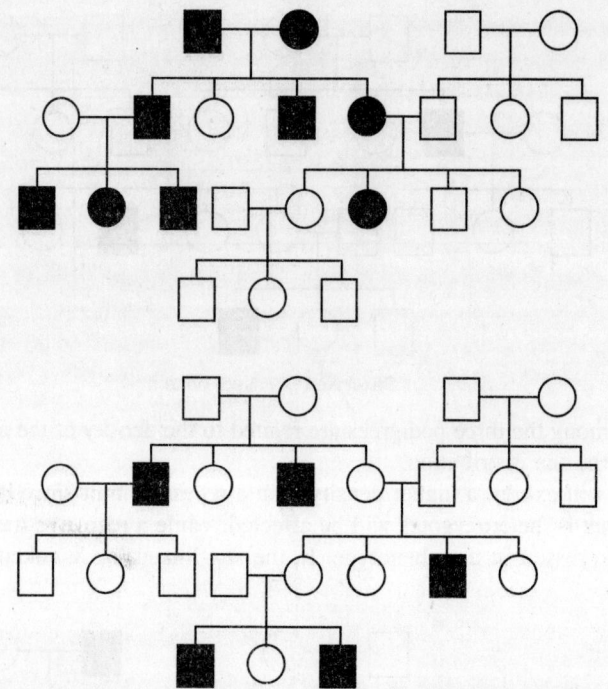

Independent Assortment

Mendel's careful recording of single trait crosses clearly established the ubiquitous nature of allelic segregation. Fortunately, he did not stop there. Considering two traits at a time is called dihybrid crossing. As an example, take Mendel's observation of the two traits of yellow and green albumin and round and wrinkled seed. Noting that yellow (Y) is dominant over green (y) and that round (R) is dominant over wrinkled (r), pure lines for both traits simultaneously will have the genotypes YYRR and yyrr. If these lines are then crossed as the P1 generation, the F1 will all be yellow and round, or YyRr. In subsequent F2 dihybrids Mendel observed phenotypic ratios approximating the following distribution:

9 yellow, round

3 yellow, wrinkled

3 green, round

1 green, wrinkled

Mendel reasoned that this pattern could only be produced if the two traits were acting independently. We can see this easily using a Punnett Square for the F1 cross.

F1 gametes:

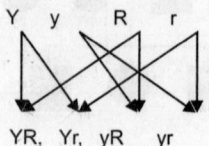

F2 genotypes:

	YR	Yr	yR	yr
YR	YYRR	YYRr	YyRR	YyRr
Yr	YYRr	Yyrr	YyRr	Yyrr
yR	YyRR	YyRr	yyRR	yyRr
yr	YyRr	Yyrr	yyRr	yyrr

Keeping the dominance relationships in mind, the 9:3:3:1 dihybrid phenotype ratio can be found in the 16 squares:

9 yellow and round: YYRR, 2 YYRr, 2 YyRR, 4 YyRr

3 yellow and wrinkled: YYrr, 2 yYrr

3 green and round: yyRR, 2 yyRr

1 green and wrinkled: yyrr

Of course, this can be extended to a trihybrid cross. Add blue (B) and white (b) flowers to the cross shown above:

Parental pure lines : YYRRBB and yyrrbb

F1 trihybrids, YyRrBb

If all three traits assort independently there will be eight possible gametes:

YRB, YRb, YrB, Yrb, yRB, yRb, yrB, yrb

And the Punnett Square will have 64 cells:

	YRB	YRb	YrB	Yrb	yRB	yRb	yrB	yrb
YRB	YYRRBB	YYRRBb	YYRrBB	YYRrBb	YyRRBB	YyRRBb	YyRrBB	YyRrBb
YRb	YYRRBb	YYRRbb	YYRrBb	YYRrbb	YyRRBb	YyRRbb	YyRrBb	YyRrbb
YrB	YYrRBB	YYRrBb	YYrrBB	YYrrBb	YyRrBB	YyRrBb	YyrrBB	YyrrBb
Yrb	YYRrBb	YYRrbb	YYrrBb	YYrrbb	YyRrBb	YyRrbb	YyrrBb	Yyrrbb
yRB	YyRRBB	YrRRBb	YyRrBB	YyRrBb	yyRRBB	yyRRBb	yyRrBB	yyRrBb
yRb	YyRRBb	YyRRbb	YyRrBb	YyRrbb	yyRRBb	yyRRbb	yyRrBb	yyRrbb
yrB	YyRrBB	YyRrBb	YyrrBB	YyrrBb	yyRrBB	yyRrBb	yyrrBB	yyrrBb
yrb	YyRrBb	YyRrbb	YyrrBb	Yyrrbb	yyRrBb	yyRrbb	yyrrBb	yyrrbb

The phenotype ratio is:

Yellow, round, blue	27
Yellow, round, white	9
Yellow, wirnkled, blue	9
Yellow, wrinkled, white	3
Green, round, blue	9
Green, round, white	3
Green, wrinkled, blue	3
Green, wrinkled, white	1

Note that, because each of the three traits is assorting independently, each individual phenotype ratio is 3 : 1, i.e. 48 yellow to 16 green, 48 round to 16 wrinkled, 48 blue to 16 white!

There is an additional mathematical treatment that can be demonstrated with each of the crosses that have been worked out. Segregation of alleles means that there are known probabilities associated with gamete formation. For any monohybrid cross, for example, the probability that a **AA** parent will donate an **A** allele to an offspring is 1.00 and the probability that a **AA** parent will donate an **a** allele is 0.00. If the parent is **Aa** these probabilities are both 0.50. Thus, if one parent is **AA** and the other parent is **aa**, the chances that their off spring will be either **AA** or **aa** is 0.00 and the probability that their offspring will be **Aa** is 1.00.

Extending this to a dihybrid cross, if the parental genotypes are **AABb** and **AaBb**, the probability of each possible off spring genotype can be easily calculated by multiplying the individual probabilities of the independent genotypes:

Genotype	Probability
AABB	0.125 (0.5 × 0.25)
AABb	0.250 (0.5 × 0.5)
AAbb	0.125 (0.5 × 0.25)
AaBB	0.125 (0.5 × 0.25)
AaBb	0.250 (0.5 × 0.5)
Aabb	0.125 (0.5 × 0.25)
aaBB	0.000 (0.0 × 0.25)
aaBb	0.000 (0.0 × 0.5)
aabb	0.000 (0.0 × 0.25)

The total probability will always add up to 1.000. This exercise can be extended to include any number of traits so long as they assort independently. For example, given the parental genotypes **AABbccDd** and **AabbCcdd** in a tetrahybrid cross, what is the probability that an offspring will be **AAbbCcDd**? (0.0625 from 0.5 × 0.5 × 0.5 × 0.5) What is the probability that another offspring will be **AabbccDD**? (0.000 from 0.5 × 0.5 × 0.5 × 0.0)

Epistasis

The final issue to be raised here is that of epistasis. This phenomenon is defined as the influence of one genotype on another. For example, in the trihybrid cross shown above, the phenotype ratios will be distorted if the genotype for flower colour influences that for seed shape such that a homozygous white (bb) makes all seeds round regardless of their genotype.

In such a case, any occurrence of bb and rr will result in round seeds and the phenotype ratios will become:

Yellow, round, blue:	27
Yellow, round, white:	12
Yellow, wirnkled, blue:	9
Yellow, wrinkled, white:	0
Green, round, blue:	9
Green, round, white:	4
Green, wrinkled, blue:	3
Green, wrinkled, white:	0

What would the ratios be homozygous white made yellow albumin green but only if the albumin genotype was heterozygous Yy?

Yellow, round, blue:	27
Yellow, round, white:	3
Yellow, wirnkled, blue:	9
Yellow, wrinkled, white:	1
Green, round, blue:	9
Green, round, white:	9
Green, wrinkled, blue:	3
Green, wrinkled, white:	3

These are effects that distort the phenotype ratios overall but note that the phenotype ratios for the unaffected traits remain at expectation, i.e. the ratio of yellow to green albumin in the first example is still 48 : 16 and the ratio of round to wrinkled seeds is still 48 : 16 in the second example.

MONOHYBRID CROSS

A monohybrid cross is a mating between two organisms with different variations at one genetic chromosome of interest. The characters being studied in a monohybrid cross are governed by two or multiple variations for a single locus. A cross between two parents possessing a pair of contrasting characters is known as monohybrid cross. To carry out such a cross, each parent is chosen to be homozygous or true breeding for a given trait (locus). When a cross satisfies the conditions for a monohybrid cross, it is usually detected by a characteristic distribution of second generation (F2) offspring that is sometimes called the monohybrid ratio (Fig. 2.4).

Uses of Monohybrid Cross

Generally, the monohybrid cross is used to determine the dominance relationship between two alleles. The cross begins with the parental generation. One parent is homozygous for one allele, and the other parent is homozygous for the other allele. The offspring make up the first filial (F1) generation. Every member of the F1 generation is heterozygous and the phenotype of the F1 generation expresses the dominant trait. Crossing two members of the F1 generation produces the second filial (F2) generation. Probability theory predicts that three quarters of the F2 generation will have the dominant allele's phenotype. And the remaining quarter of the F2s will have the recessive allele's phenotype. This predicted 3:1 phenotypic ratio assumes Mendelian inheritance.

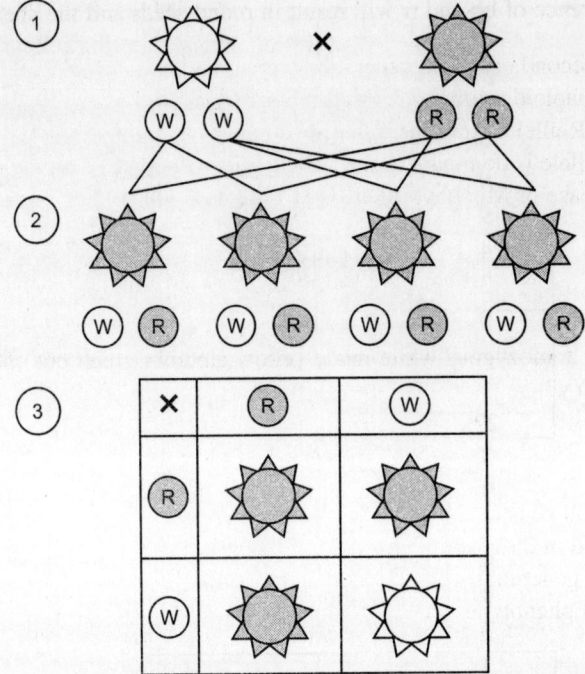

Fig. 2.4: Inheritance pattern of dominant (grey) and recessive (white) phenotypes when each parent (1) is homozygous for either the dominant or recessive trait. All members of the F1 generation are heterozygous and share the same dominant phenotype (2), while the F2 generation exhibits a 6:2 ratio of dominant to recessive phenotypes (3).

Mendel's Experiment

As already discussed in Chapter 1 (origin of genetics) Mendel bred garden peas (Pisum sativum) in his monastery garden and analysed the offspring of these matings. The garden pea was chosen as an experimental organism because many varieties were available that bred true for qualitative traits and their pollination could be manipulated. The seven variable characteristics Mendel investigated in pea plants were:

- Seed texture (round vs wrinkled)
- Seed colour (yellow vs green)
- Flower colour (white vs purple)
- Growth habit (tall vs dwarf)
- Pod shape (pinched or inflated)
- Pod colour (green vs yellow)
- flower position (axial or terminal)

Peas are normally self-pollinated because the stamens and carpels are enclosed within the petals. By removing the stamens from unripe flowers, Mendel could brush pollen from another variety on the carpels when they ripened.

First cross

All the peas produced in the second or hybrid generation were round. All the peas of this F1 generation have an Rr genotype. All the haploid sperm and eggs produced by meiosis received one chromosome 7. All the zygotes received one R allele (from the round seed parent) and one r allele (from the wrinkled seed parent). Because the R allele is dominant to the r allele, the phenotype of all the seeds was round. The phenotypic ratio in this case of Monohybrid cross is 1:1:1:1.

		P gametes (round parent)	
		R	R
P gametes (wrinkled parent)	r	Rr	Rr
	r	Rr	Rr

Second cross

Mendel then allowed his hybrid peas to self-pollinate. The wrinkled trait—which did not appear in his hybrid generation—reappeared in 25% of the new crop of peas. Random union of equal numbers of R and r gametes produced an F2 generation with 25% RR and 50% Rr—both with the round phenotype— and 25% rr with the wrinkled phenotype.

		F1 gametes	
		R	r
F1 gamates	R	RR	Rr
	r	Rr	rr

Third cross

Mendel then allowed some of each phenotype in the F2 generation to self-pollinate. His results:

- All the wrinkled seeds in the F2 generation produced only wrinkled seeds in the F3.
- One-third (193/565) of the round F1 seeds produced only round seeds in the F3 generation, but two-thirds (372/565) of them produced both types of seeds in the F3 and—once again—in a 3:1 ratio.

One-third of the round seeds and all of the wrinkled seeds in the F2 generation were homozygous and produced only seeds of the same phenotype.

But two thirds of the round seeds in the F2 were heterozygous and their self-pollination produced both phenotypes in the ratio of a typical F1 cross.

Phenotype ratios are approximate. The union of sperm and eggs is random. As the size of the sample gets larger, however, chance deviations become minimised and the ratios approach the theoretical predictions more closely. The table shows the actual seed production by ten of Mendel's F1 plants. While his individual plants deviated widely from the expected 3:1 ratio, the group as a whole approached it quite closely.

Round	Wrinkled
45	12
27	8
24	7
19	16
32	11
26	6
88	24
22	10
28	6
25	7
Total: 336	Total: 107

Mendel's Hypothesis

To explain his results, Mendel formulated a hypothesis that included the following: In the organism there is a pair of factors that controls the appearance of a given characteristic. (They are called genes.) The organism inherits these factors from its parents, one from each. A factor is transmitted from generation to generation as a discrete, unchanging unit. (The r factor in the F2 generation passed through the round-seeded F1 generation. In spite of this, the rr seeds in the F2 generation were no less wrinkled than those in the P generation.) When the gametes are formed, the factors separate and are distributed as units to each gamete. This statement is often called Mendel's rule of segregation. If an organism has two unlike factors (called alleles) for a characteristic, one may be expressed to the total exclusion of the other (dominant vs recessive).

Test of the hypothesis

A good hypothesis meets several standards.

- It should provide an adequate explanation of the observed facts. If two or more hypotheses meet this standard, the simpler one is preferred.
- It should be able to predict new facts. So if a generalisation is valid, then certain specific consequences can be deduced from it.

In order to test his hypothesis, Mendel predicted the outcome of a breeding experiment that he had not carried out yet. He crossed heterozygous round peas (Rr) with wrinkled (homozygous, rr) ones. He predicted that in this case one-half of the seeds produced would be round (Rr) and one-half wrinkled (rr).

		F1 gametes	
		R	r
P gamates	r	Rr	rr
	r	Rr	rr

To a casual observer in the monastery garden, the cross appeared no different from the P cross described above: Round-seeded peas being crossed with wrinkled-seeded ones. But Mendel predicted that this time he would produce both round and wrinkled seeds and in a 50:50 ratio. He performed the cross and harvested 106 round peas and 101 wrinkled peas.

Mendel tested his hypothesis with a type of backcross called a testcross. An organism has an unknown genotype which is one of two genotypes (like RR and Rr) that produce the same phenotype. The result of the test identifies the unknown genotype.

Mendel did not stop there. He went on to cross pea varieties that differed in six other qualitative traits. In every case, the results supported his hypothesis. He crossed peas that differed in two traits. He found that the inheritance of one trait was independent of that of the other and so framed his second rule: the rule of independent assortment. Today, it is known that this rule does not apply to some genes, due to genetic linkage.

DIHYBRID CROSS

A dihybrid cross is an experiment in genetics in which the phenotypes of two genes are followed through the mating of individuals carrying multiple alleles at those gene loci. Most sexually reproducing organisms carry two copies of each gene, allowing them to carry two different alleles. Historically, an organism with parts from two different true-breeding lines was referred to as a 'hybrid'. Thus, the name 'dihybrid cross' comes from the historical act of observing the future generations after two 'pure lines' are crossed. Today, we refer to organisms that are 'true-breeding' for a certain gene as homozygotes. This refers to how the alleles used to form the zygote were the same. Heterozygous individuals, on the other hand, used two different alleles to form the zygote. A dihybrid cross, therefore, is the mating of two individuals, both heterozygous for two different genes being observed.

Examples of Dihybrid Cross

An important distinction must be made between dihybrid cross and mode of inheritance. While the dihybrid cross is typically thought of as an observations of two genes controlling two different phenotypic traits, both of which act under the complete dominance mode of inheritance.

The dihybrid cross is easy to visualise using a Punnett square of dimensions 4 × 4:

	Ry	Ry	rY	ry
Ry	RRYY	RRYy	RrYY	RrYy
Ry	RRYy	RRyy	RrYy	Rryy
rY	RrYY	RrYy	rrYY	rrYy
ry	RrYy	Rryy	rrYy	rryy

The rules of meiosis, as they apply to the dihybrid, are codified in Mendel's first law and Mendel's second law, which are also called the Law of Segregation and the Law of Independent Assortment, respectively. For genes on separate chromosomes, each allele pair showed independent segregation. If the first filial generation (F1 generation) produces four identical offspring, the second filial generation, which occurs by crossing the members of the first filial generation, shows a phenotypic (appearance) ratio of 9:3:3:1, where:

- The 9 represents the proportion of individuals displaying both dominant traits: RRYY + 2 × RRYy + 2 × RrYY + 4 × RrYy.
- The first 3 represents the individuals displaying the first dominant trait and the second recessive trait: RRyy + 2 × Rryy.
- The second 3 represents those displaying the first recessive trait and second dominant trait: rrYY + 2 × rrYy.
- The 1 represents the homozygous, displaying both recessive traits: rryy

LAW OF INDEPENDENT ASSORTMENT

The law of segregation lets us predict how a single feature associated with a single gene is inherited. In some cases, though, we might want to predict the inheritance of two characteristics associated with two different genes. How can we do this?

To make an accurate prediction, we need to know whether the two genes are inherited independently or not. That is, we need to know whether they 'ignore' one another when they're sorted into gametes, or whether they 'stick together' and get inherited as a unit.

When Gregor Mendel asked this question, he found that different genes were inherited independently of one another, following what's called the law of independent assortment.

Mendel's law of independent assortment: Mendel's law of independent assortment states that the alleles of two (or more) different genes get sorted into gametes independently of one another. In other words, the allele a gamete receives for one gene does not influence the allele received for another gene.

INDEPENDENT ASSORTMENT VS LINKAGE

The section gives us Mendel's law of independent assortment in a nutshell, and lets us see how the law of independent assortment leads to a 9:3:3:1. But what was the alternative possibility? That is, what would happen if two genes didn't follow independent assortment?

In the extreme case, the genes for seed colour and seed shape might have always been inherited as a pair. That is, the yellow and round alleles might always have stayed together, and so might the green and wrinkled alleles.

To see how this could work, imagine that the colour and shape genes are physically stuck together and cannot be separated, as represented by the boxes around the alleles is shown in Fig. 2.5. For instance, this could happen if the two genes were located very, very close together on a chromosome.

Rather than giving a colour allele and, separately, giving a shape allele to each gamete, the F1 dihybrid plant would simply give one 'combo unit' to each gamete: a YR allele pair or a yr allele pair.

We can use a Punnett square to predict the results of self-fertilisation in this case, as shown above. If the seed colour and seed shape genes were in fact always inherited as a unit, or completely linked, a dihybrid cross should produce just two types of offspring, yellow/round and green/wrinkled, in a 3:1. Mendel's actual results were quite different from this (the 9:3:3:1 we saw earlier), telling him that the genes assorted independently.

Reason for Independent Assortment

To see why independent assortment happens, we need to fast-forward half a century and discover that genes are physically located on chromosomes. To be exact, the two copies of a gene carried by an organism (such as a Y and a y allele) are located at the same spot on the two chromosomes of a

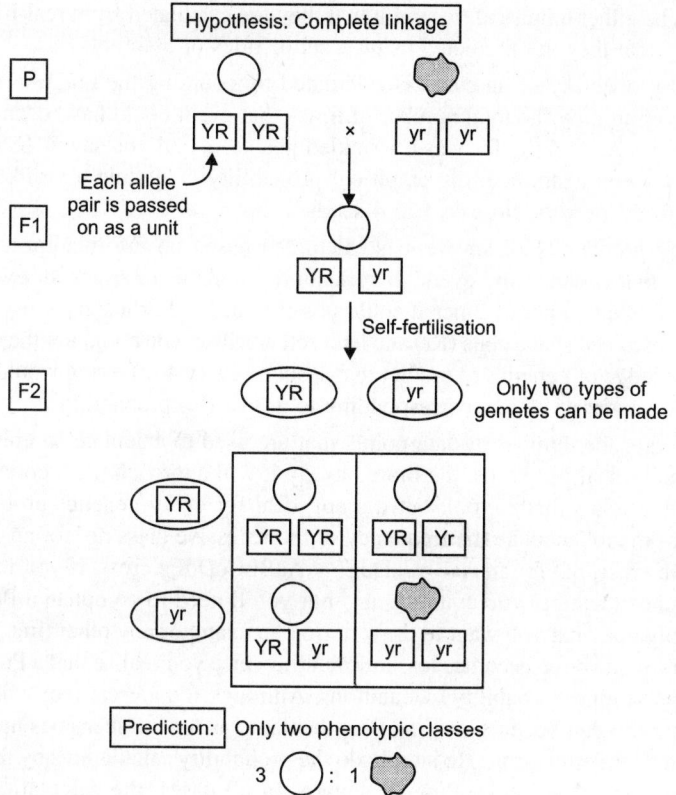

Fig. 2.5: Illustration of the hypothesis that the seed shape and seed colour genes display complete linkage.

homologous pair. Homologous chromosomes are similar but non-identical, and an organism gets one member of the pair from each of its two parents.

The physical basis for the law of independent assortment lies in meiosis I of gamete formation, when homologous pairs line up in random orientations at the middle of the cell as they prepare to separate. We can get gametes with different combos of 'mom' and 'dad' homologues (and thus, the alleles on those homologues) because the orientation of each pair is random.

There are, however, gene pairs that do not assort independently. When genes are close together on a chromosome, the alleles on the same chromosome tend to be inherited as a unit more frequently than not. Such genes do not display independent assortment and are said to be linked.

PROBABILITIES IN GENETICS

Probabilities are mathematical measures of likelihood. In other words, there are ways of quantifying (giving a specific, numerical value to) how likely something is to happen. A probability of 1 for an event means that it is guaranteed to happen, while a probability of 0000 for an event means that it is guaranteed not to happen. A simple example of probability is having a ½, slash, 2 chance of getting heads when you flip a coin.

Probabilities can be either empirical, meaning that they are calculated from real-life observations, or theoretical, meaning that they are predicted using a set of rules or assumptions.

- The empirical probability of an event is calculated by counting the number of times that event occurs and dividing it by the total number of times that event could have occurred. For instance, if the event you were looking for was a wrinkled pea seed, and you saw it 1850 times out of the 7324 total seeds you examined, the empirical probability of getting a wrinkled seed would be 1850/7324 = 0.253 or very close to 1 in 4 seeds.

- The theoretical probability of an event is calculated based on information about the rules and circumstances that produce the event. It reflects the number of times an event is expected to occur relative to the number of times it could possibly occur. For instance, if you had a pea plant heterozygous for a seed shape gene (Rr) and let it self-fertilise, you could use the rules of probability and your knowledge of genetics to predict that 1 out of every 4 offspring would get two recessive alleles (rr) and appear wrinkled, corresponding to a 0.25 (¼) probability.

In general, the larger the number of data points that are used to calculate an empirical probability, such as shapes of individual pea seeds, the more closely it will approach the theoretical probability.

The Punnett square is a valuable tool, but it's not ideal for every genetics problem. For instance, suppose you were asked to calculate the frequency of the recessive class not for an Aa × Aa cross, not for an AaBb × AaBb cross, but for an AaBbCcDdEe × AaBbCcDdEe cross. If you wanted to solve that question using a Punnett square, you could do it – but you'd need to complete a Punnett square with 1024 boxes. Probably not what you want to draw during an exam, or any other time, if you can help it!

The five-gene problem above becomes less intimidating once you realise that a Punnett square is just a visual way of representing probability calculations. Although it's a great tool when you're working with one or two genes, it can become slow and cumbersome as the number goes up. At some point, it becomes quicker (and less error-prone) to simply do the probability calculations by themselves, without the visual representation of a clunky Punnett square. In all cases, the calculations and the square provide the same information, but by having both tools in your belt, you can be prepared to handle a wider range of problems in a more efficient way.

This section discusses some probability basics, including how to calculate the probability of two independent events both occurring (event X and event Y) or the probability of either of two mutually exclusive events occurring (event X or event Y). These calculations can be applied to genetics problems, and, in particular, how they can help you solve problems involving relatively large numbers of genes.

Product Rule

One probability rule that's very useful in genetics is the product rule, which states that the probability of two (or more) independent events occurring together can be calculated by multiplying the individual probabilities of the events. For example, if you roll a six-sided die once, you have a 1/6 chance of getting a six. If you roll two dice at once, your chance of getting two sixes is: (probability of a six on die 1) × (probability of a six on die 2) = (1/6) × (1/6) = 1/36.

In general, you can think of the product rule as the and rule: If both event X and event Y must happen in order for a certain outcome to occur, and if X and Y are independent of each other (don't affect each other's likelihood), then you can use the product rule to calculate the probability of the outcome by multiplying the probabilities of X and Y.

We can use the product rule to predict frequencies of fertilisation events. For instance, consider a cross between two heterozygous (Aa) individuals. What are the odds of getting an aa individual in the next generation? The only way to get an aa individual is if the mother contributes an a gamete and the father contributes an a gamete. Each parent has a ½, slash, 2 chance of making an a gamete. Thus, the chance of an aa offspring is: (probability of mother contributing a) × (probability of father contributing a) $= \frac{1}{2} \times \frac{1}{2} = \frac{1}{4}$ is shown in Fig. 2.6.

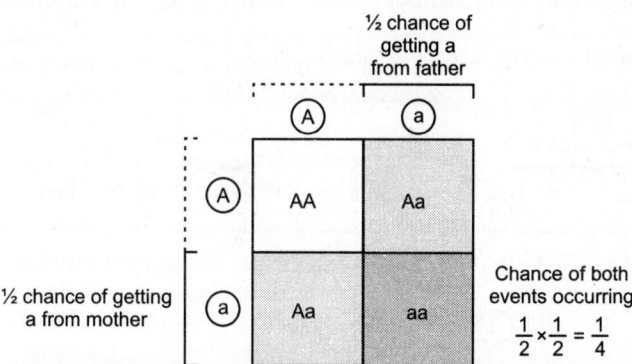

Fig. 2.6: Illustration of how a Punnett square can represent the product rule.

This is the same result you'd get with a Punnett square, and actually the same logical process as well—something that took me years to realise! The only difference is that, in the Punnett square, we'd do the calculation visually: we'd represent the ½ probability of an a gamete from each parent as one out of two columns (for the father) and one out of two rows (for the mother). The 1-square intersect of the column and row (out of the 4 total squares of the table) represents the ¼ chance of getting an a from both parents.

Sum Rule of Probability

In some genetics problems, you may need to calculate the probability that any one of several events will occur. In this case, you'll need to apply another rule of probability, the sum rule. According to the sum rule, the probability that any of several mutually exclusive events will occur is equal to the sum of the events' individual probabilities. For example, if you roll a six-sided die, you have a 1/6, chance of getting any given number, but you can only get one number per roll. You could never get both a one and a six at the same time, these outcomes are mutually exclusive. Thus, the chances of getting either a one or a six are: (probability of getting a 1) + (probability of getting a 6) = (1/6) + (1/6) = 1/3.

You can think of the sum rule as the or rule: If an outcome requires that either event X or event Y occur, and if X and Y are mutually exclusive (if only one or the other can occur in a given case), then the probability of the outcome can be calculated by adding the probabilities of X and Y.

As an example, let's use the sum rule to predict the fraction of offspring from an Aa x Aa cross that will have the dominant phenotype (AA or Aa genotype). In this cross, there are three events that can lead to a dominant phenotype:

- Two A gametes meet (giving AA genotype).
- A gamete from Mom meets a gamete from Dad (giving Aa genotype).
- *a* gamete from Mom meets A gamete from Dad (giving Aa genotype).

In any one fertilisation event, only one of these three possibilities can occur (they are mutually exclusive).

Since this is an or situation where the events are mutually exclusive, we can apply the sum rule. Using the product rule as we did above, we can find that each individual event has a probability of 1/4. So, the probability of offspring with a dominant phenotype is: (probability of A from Mom and A from Dad) + (probability of A from Mom and a from Dad) + (probability of a from Mom and A from Dad)

$$= \frac{1}{4} + \frac{1}{4} + \frac{1}{4} = \frac{3}{4}$$ is shown in Fig. 2.7.

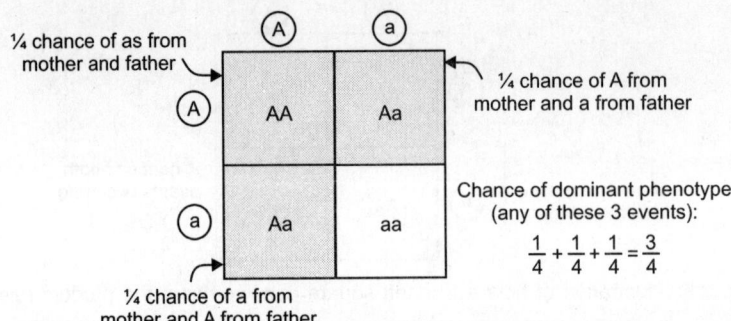

Fig. 2.7: Illustration of how a Punnett square can represent the sum rule.

Once again, this is the same result we'd get with a Punnett square. One out of the four boxes of the Punnett square holds the dominant homozygote, AA. Two more boxes represent heterozygotes, one with a maternal A and a paternal a, the other with the opposite combination. Each box is 1 out of the 4 boxes in the whole Punnett square, and since the boxes don't overlap (they're mutually exclusive), we can add them up $\frac{1}{4} + \frac{1}{4} + \frac{1}{4} = \frac{3}{4}$ to get the probability of offspring with the dominant phenotype.

Product Rule and the Sum Rule

Product rule	Sum rule
For independent events X and Y, the probability (P) of them both occurring (X and Y) is P(X)×P(Y)	For mutually exclusive events X and Y, the probability (P) that one will occur (X or Y) is P(X)+P(Y)

CHI-SQUARE ANALYSIS

A chi-square (χ^2) statistic is a test that measures how expectations compare to actual observed data (or model results). The data used in calculating a chi-square statistic must be random, raw, mutually exclusive, drawn from independent variables, and drawn from a large enough sample. For example, the results of tossing a coin 100 times meet these criteria.

Chi-square Test

Chi-square is used to test hypotheses about the distribution of observations in different categories. The null hypothesis (H_o) is that the observed frequencies are the same as the expected frequencies (except for chance variation). If the observed and expected frequencies are the same, then $\chi^2 = 0$. If the frequencies you observe are different from expected frequencies, the value of χ^2 goes up. The larger the value of χ^2, the more likely it is that the distributions are significantly different.

To try and explain this a little better, let's think about a concrete example. Imagine that you were interested in the relationship between road traffic accidents and the age of the driver. We could randomly obtain records of 60 accidents from police archives, and see how many of the drivers fell into each of the following age-categories: 17–20, 21–30, 31–40, 41–50, 51–60 and over 60. If there is no relationship between accident-rate and age, then the drivers should be equally spread across the different age-bands (i.e. there should be similar numbers of drivers in each category). This would be the null hypothesis. However, if younger drivers are more likely to have accidents, then there would be a large number of accidents in the younger age-categories and a low number of accidents in the older age-categories.

So say we actually collected this data, and found that out of 60 accidents, there were 25 individuals aged 17–20, 15 drivers aged 21–30 and 5 cases in each of the other age groups. This data would now make up our set of observed frequencies.

We might now ask: Are these observed frequencies similar to what we might expect to find by chance, or is there some non-random pattern to them? In this particular case, from just looking at the frequencies it seems fairly obvious that a larger proportion of the accidents involved younger drivers. However, the question of whether this distribution could have just occurred by chance is yet to be answered. The chi-square test helps us to decide this by comparing our observed frequencies to the frequencies that we might expect to obtain purely by chance.

It is important to note at this point, that Chi-square is a very versatile statistic that crops up in lots of different circumstances. Applications of chi-square:

- Chi-square 'Goodness of Fit' test: This is used when you have categorical data for one independent variable, and you want to see whether the distribution of your data is similar or different to that expected (i.e. you want to compare the observed distribution of the categories to a theoretical expected distribution).

- Chi-square test of association between two variables: This is appropriate to use when you have categorical data for two independent variables, and you want to see if there is an association between them.

Chi-square 'Goodness of Fit' Test

This is used when you have one independent variable, and you want to compare an observed frequency-distribution to a theoretical expected frequency-distribution. For example described above, there is a single independent variable (in this example 'age group') with a number of different levels (17–20, 21–30, 31–40, 41–50, 51–60 and over 60). The statistical question is: do the frequencies you actually observe differ from the expected frequencies by more than chance alone?

In this case, we want to know whether or not our observed frequencies of traffic accidents occur equally frequently for the different ages groups (so that our theoretical frequency-distribution contains the same number of individuals in each of the age bands). The way in which we would collate this data would be to use a contingency table, containing both the observed and expected frequency information.

	Age band						
	17-20	*21-30*	*31-40*	*41-50*	*51-60*	*over 60*	*Total*
Observed frequency of accidents	25	15	5	5	5	5	60
Expected frequency of accidents	10	10	10	10	10	10	60

To work out whether these two distributions are significantly different from one another, we use the following chi-square formula:

$$\chi^2 = \sum \frac{(O - E)^2}{E}$$

This translates into:

$$\chi^2 = \text{Sum of (i.e. across categories)} \ \frac{(\text{Observed frequence-expected frequency})^2}{\text{Expected frequency}}$$

This may look complicated, but really it just means that you have to follow four simple steps, which are given below:

Step one

Take each observed frequency and subtract from its associated expected frequency [i.e. workout (O-E)]:

25–10 = 15   15–10 = 5   5–10 = –5   5–10 = –5   5–10 = –5   5–10 = –5

Step two

Square each value obtained in step 1 [i.e. workout $(O-E)^2$]:

225   25   25   25   25   25

Step three

Divide each of the values obtained in step 2, by its associated expected frequency [i.e. workout $\frac{(O-E)^2}{E}$]:

$$\frac{225}{10} = 22.5 \qquad \frac{25}{10} = 2.5 \qquad \frac{25}{10} = 2.5 \qquad \frac{25}{10} = 2.5 \qquad \frac{25}{10} = 2.5 \qquad \frac{25}{10} = 2.5$$

Step four

Add together all of the values obtained in step 3, to get your value of Chi-square:

$$\chi^2 = 22.5 + 2.5 + 2.5 + 2.5 + 2.5 + 2.5 = 35$$

Assessing the size of our obtained Chi-square value:

What you do, in a nutshell.

- Work out how many 'degrees of freedom' (df) you have.
- Decide on a probability level.
- Find a table of 'critical Chi-square values' (in most statistics textbooks).
- Establish the critical Chi-square value for this particular test, and compare to your obtained value.

If your obtained Chi-square value is bigger than the one in the Table 2.1, then you conclude that your obtained Chi-square value is too large to have arisen by chance, it is more likely to stem from the fact that there were real differences between the observed and expected frequencies. In other words, contrary to our null hypothesis, the categories did not occur with similar frequencies.

If, on the other hand, your obtained Chi-square value is smaller than the one in the Table 2.1, you conclude that there is no reason to think that the observed pattern of frequencies is not due simply to chance (i.e. we retain our initial assumption that the discrepancies between the observed and expected

Table 2.1: Critical values of Chi-square.

Degrees of freedom	99%	95%	90%	70%	50%	30%	10%	5%	1%
1	0.00016	0.0039	0.016	0.15	0.46	1.07	2.71	3.84	6.64
2	0.020	0.10	0.21	0.71	1.39	2.41	4.60	5.99	9.21
3	0.12	0.35	0.58	1.42	2.37	3.67	6.25	7.82	11.34
4	0.30	0.71	1.06	2.20	3.36	4.88	7.78	9.49	13.28
5	0.55	1.14	1.61	3.00	4.35	6.06	9.24	11.07	15.09
6	0.87	1.64	2.20	3.83	5.35	7.23	10.65	12.59	16.81
7	1.24	2.17	2.83	4.67	6.35	8.38	12.02	14.07	18.48
8	1.65	2.73	3.49	5.53	7.34	9.52	13.36	15.51	20.09
9	2.09	3.33	4.17	6.39	8.34	10.66	14.68	16.92	21.67
10	2.56	3.94	4.86	7.27	9.34	11.78	15.99	18.31	23.21
11	3.05	4.58	5.58	8.15	10.34	12.90	17.28	19.68	24.73
12	3.57	5.23	6.30	9.03	11.34	14.01	18.55	21.03	26.22
13	4.11	5.89	7.04	9.93	12.34	15.12	19.81	22.36	27.69
14	4.66	6.57	7.79	10.82	12.34	16.22	21.06	23.69	29.14
15	5.23	7.26	8.55	11.72	14.34	17.32	22.31	25.00	30.58
16	5.81	7.96	9.31	12.62	15.34	18.42	23.54	26.30	32.00
17	6.41	8.67	10.09	13.53	16.34	19.51	24.77	27.59	33.41
18	7.00	9.39	10.87	14.44	17.34	20.60	25.99	28.87	34.81
19	7.63	10.12	11.65	15.35	18.34	21.69	27.20	30.14	36.19
20	8.26	10.85	12.44	16.27	19.34	22.78	28.41	31.41	37.57

frequencies are due merely to random sampling variation, and hence we have no reason to believe that the categories did not occur with equal frequency).

Examples:

1. First we work out our degrees of freedom. For the goodness of fit test, this is simply the number of categories minus one. As we have six categories, there are 6–1 = 5 degrees of freedom.

2. Next we establish the probability level. In psychology, we use $p < 0.05$ as standard – and this is represented by the 5% column.

3. We now need to consult a table of 'critical values of Chi-square'. Here's an excerpt from a typical Table 2.1.

4. The values in each column are 'critical' values of Chi-square. These values would be expected to occur by chance with the probability shown at the top of the column. The relevant value for this test is found at the intersection of the appropriate df row and probability column. As our obtained Chi-square has 5 df, we are interested in the values in the 5 df row. As the probability level is p <0.05, we then need to look in the 5% column (as 0.05 represents a chance level of 5 in 100 or 5%) to find the critical value for this statistical test. In this case, the critical value is 11.07.

Finally, we need to compare our obtained Chi-square to the critical value. If the obtained Chi-square is larger than a value in the table, it implies that it is unlikely to have occurred by chance. Our obtained value of 35 is much larger than the critical value of 11.07. We can therefore be relatively confident in concluding that our observed frequencies are significantly different from the frequencies that we would expect to obtain if all categories were equally distributed.

Chi-square Test of Association between Two Variables

The second type of chi-square test we will look at is the Pearson's chi-square test of association. We can use this test when we have categorical data for two independent variables, and you want to see if there is an association between them. For this example, let's stick with the theme of driving, but this time consider gender performance on driving tests. This time we have two categorical variables: Gender (two levels: Male vs Female) and Driving Test Outcome (two levels: Pass vs Fail).

In this case, the statistical question we want to know the answer to is whether driving test outcome is related to the gender of the person taking the test or in other words, we want to know if males show a different pattern of pass/fail rates than females.

To answer this question, we would start off by putting out data into a contingency table, this time containing only the observed frequency information. We can then use this table to calculate expected frequencies.

In this case, imagine the pattern of driving test outcomes looked like this:

	Male	*Female*
Pass	7	11
Fail	13	9

In this example, simply looking at the observed frequencies gives us an idea that the pattern of driving test outcomes may be different for the genders. It seems females have a more successful pass/fail rate than males. However, to test whether this observed difference is significant, we need to look at the outcome of a Chi-square test. As with the one-variable Chi-square test, our aim is to see if the pattern of observed frequencies is significantly different from the pattern of frequencies which we would expect to see by chance, i.e. what we would expect to obtain if there was no relationship between the two variables in question. With respect to the example above, 'no relationship' would mean that the pattern of driving test performance for males was no different to that for females.

The Chi-square formula is exactly the same as for the one-variable test described earlier, the only difference is in how you calculate the expected frequencies.

Step 1: Add numbers across columns and rows. Calculate total number in chart.

	Male	*Female*	
Pass	7	12	= 19
Fail	13	8	= 21
Total	20	20	= 40

Step 2: Calculate expected numbers for each individual cell (i.e. the frequencies we would expect to obtain if there were no association between the two variables). You do this by multiplying row sum by column sum and dividing by total number.

$$\text{Expected frequency} = \frac{\text{Row total} \times \text{Column total}}{\text{Grand total}}$$

For example: using the first cell in table (Male/Pass):

$$\frac{19 \times 20}{40} = 9.5$$

and the cell below (Male/Fail):

$$\frac{21 \times 20}{40} = 10.5$$

Do this for each cell in the table above.

Step 3: Now you should have an observed number and expected number for each cell. The observed number is the number already in 1st chart. The expected number is the number found in the last step (step 2). Redo the contingency table, this time adding in the expected frequencies in brackets below the obtained frequencies:

	Male	*Female*	
Pass	7	12	Total = 19
	(9.5)	(9.5)	
Fail	13	8	Total = 21
	(10.5)	(10.5)	
Total	20	20	Grand total = 40

Step 4: Now calculate Chi-square using the same formula as before:

$$\chi^2 = \sum \frac{(O-E)^2}{E} \quad \text{or} \quad \chi^2 = \frac{\text{Sum of (observed - Expected)}^2}{\text{Expected}}$$

Calculate this formula for each cell, one at a time. For example, cell #1 (Male/Pass):
Observed number is: 7
Expected number is: 9.5

Plugging this into the formula, you have: $\dfrac{(7-9.5)^2}{9.5} = 0.6579$

Continue doing this for the rest of the cells.

Step 5: Add together all the final numbers for each cell, obtained in step 4. There are 4 total cells, so at the end you should be adding four numbers together for you final Chi-square number.
In this case, you should have:

$$0.6579 + 0.6579 + 0.5952 + 0.5952 = 2.5062$$

So, 0.095 is our obtained value of Chi-square, it is a single-number summary of the discrepancy between our obtained frequencies, and the frequencies which we would expect if there was no association between our two variables. The bigger this number, the greater the difference between the observed and expected frequencies.

Step 6: Calculate degrees of freedom (df):

$$(\text{Number of rows} - 1) \times (\text{Number of columns} - 1)$$
$$(2-1) \times (2-1)$$
$$1 \times 1 = 1 \text{ df (degrees of freedom)}$$

Assessing the size of our obtained Chi-square value:

The procedure here is the same as for the goodness of fit test. We just need:

1. Our 'degrees of freedom' (df) √
2. A suitable probability level (p = 0.05 in psychology) √
3. A table of critical Chi-square values √
4. Establish the critical Chi-square value for this test (at the intersection of the appropriate df row and probability column), and compare to your obtained value.

As before, if the obtained Chi-square value is bigger than the one in the table, then you conclude that your obtained Chi-square value is too large to have arisen by chance. This would mean that the two variables are likely to be related in some way.

Note: The Chi-square test merely tells us that there is some relationship between the two variables in question: it does not tell you what that relationship is, and most importantly, it does not tell you anything about the causal relationship between the two variables.

If, on the other hand, your obtained Chi-square value is smaller than the one in the table, you cannot reject the null hypothesis. In other words, you would conclude that your variables are unlikely to be associated.

For this example: Using the chart below, at the p = 0.05 significance level, with 1 df, the critical value can be established as 3.84. Therefore, in order to reject the null hypothesis, the final answer to the Chi-square must be greater or equal to 3.84.

Degrees of freedom	99%	95%	90%	70%	50%	30%	10%	5%	1%
1	0.00016	0.0039	0.016	0.15	0.46	1.07	2.71	**3.84**	6.64
2	0.020	0.10	0.21	0.71	1.39	2.41	4.60	5.99	9.21
3	0.12	0.35	0.58	1.42	2.37	3.67	6.25	7.82	11.34
4	0.30	0.71	1.06	2.20	3.36	4.88	7.78	9.49	13.28
5	0.55	1.14	1.61	3.00	4.35	6.06	9.24	11.07	15.09
6	0.87	1.64	2.20	3.83	5.35	7.23	10.65	12.59	16.81
7	1.24	2.17	2.83	4.67	6.35	8.38	12.02	14.07	18.48
8	1.65	2.73	3.49	5.53	7.34	9.52	13.36	15.51	20.09
9	2.09	3.33	4.17	6.39	8.34	10.66	14.68	16.92	21.67
10	2.56	3.94	4.86	7.27	9.34	11.78	15.99	18.31	23.21
11	3.05	4.58	5.58	8.15	10.34	12.90	17.28	19.68	24.73
12	3.57	5.23	6.30	9.03	11.34	14.01	18.55	21.03	26.22
13	4.11	5.89	7.04	9.93	12.34	15.12	19.81	22.36	27.69
14	4.66	6.57	7.79	10.82	12.34	16.22	21.06	23.69	29.14
15	5.23	7.26	8.55	11.72	14.34	17.32	22.31	25.00	30.58
16	5.81	7.96	9.31	12.62	15.34	18.42	23.54	26.30	32.00
17	6.41	8.67	10.09	13.53	16.34	19.51	24.77	27.59	33.41
18	7.00	9.39	10.87	14.44	17.34	20.60	25.99	28.87	34.81
19	7.63	10.12	11.65	15.35	18.34	21.69	27.20	30.14	36.19
20	8.26	10.85	12.44	16.27	19.34	22.78	28.41	31.41	37.57

The Chi-square calculation above was 2.5062. This number is less than the critical value of 3.84, so in this case the null hypothesis cannot be rejected. In other words, there does not appear to be a significant association between the two variables: males and females have a statistically similar pattern of pass/fail rates on their driving tests.

Assumptions of the Chi-square test

For the results of a Chi-square test to be reliable, the following assumptions must hold true:

1. Your data are a random sample from the population about which inferences are to be made.
2. Observations must be independent: each subject must give one and only one data point (i.e. they must contribute to one and only one category).
3. Problems arise when the expected frequencies are very small. As a rule of thumb, Chi-square should not be used if more than 20% of the expected frequencies have a value of less than 5 (it does not matter what the observed frequencies are). You can get around this problem in two ways: either combine some categories (if this is meaningful, in your experiment), or obtain more data (make the sample size bigger).

PEDIGREE ANALYSIS

Pedigrees are formalised ways using standard sets of symbols to depict family trees and lineages. Pedigrees provide concise and accurate records of families. Pedigrees are helpful in following and diagnosing heritable traits (e.g. diseases and medical conditions), i.e. describing patterns (or modes) of inheritance. Pedigrees are useful in mapping (locating and isolating) genes 'responsible' for certain traits.

A pedigree chart displays a family tree, and shows the members of the family who are affected by a genetic trait. This chart shows four generations of a family with four individuals who are affected by a form of colourblindness.

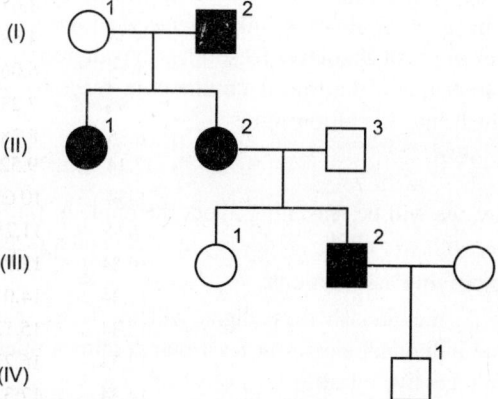

- Circles represent females and squares represent males.
- Each individual is represented by:
  o A Roman Numeral, which stands for the generation in the family.
  o A Digit, which stands for the individual within the generation. (For instance, The female at the upper left is individual I-1).

- A darkened circle or square represents an individual affected by the trait.
- The 'founding parents' in this family are the female I-1 and the male I-2 in the first generation at the top.
- A male and female directly connected by a horizontal line have mated and have children. These three pairs have mated in this tree: I-1 and I-2, II-2 and II-3, III-2 and III-3.
- Vertical lines connect parents to their children. For instance the females, II-1 and II-2 are daughters of I-1 and II-2.
- The 'founding family' consists of the two founding parents and their children, II-1 and II-2.

In this pedigree, the unaffected founding mother, I-1, and affected founding father, I-2, are parents to two affected daughters, II-1 and II-2.

The affected founding daughter II-2 and the unaffected male II-3 who 'marries into the family' have two offspring, an unaffected daughter III-1 and affected son, III-2.

Finally, this affected male III-2 and the unaffected female III-3 who 'marries in' have an unaffected son, IV-1.

Pedigrees are interesting because they can be used to do some detective work and are often used to study the genetics of inherited diseases. For example, pedigrees can be analysed to determine the mode of transmission for a genetic disease:

1. Dominance - whether the disease alleles are dominant or recessive.
2. Linkage - whether the disease alleles are X-linked (on the X chromsome) or autosomal

Autosomal chromosomes: The 22 chromosome pairs other than the XX (female) or XY (male) sex chromosomes.

Hemizygous: Males are 'hemizygous' for X-linked genes – males only have one X chromosome and one allele of any X-linked gene.

Allele: A version of a gene. Humans have 2 alleles of all their autosomal genes, females have 2 alleles of X- linked genes, males have one allele of X-linked genes (and one allele of Y-linked genes).

Pedigree analysis is an example of abductive reasoning. In pedigree analysis you need to look for any clues that will allow you to decide if the trait is dominant or recessive and whether it is linked to an autosomal chromosome, or to the X chromsome.

General Assumptions

In the problems that follow, we will be reasoning about the mode of transmission of genetic traits that are controlled by one gene, with two alleles, a dominant allele and a recessive allele.

We also make three simplifying assumptions:

1. Complete penetrance: An individual in the pedigree will be affected (express the phenotype associated with a trait) when the individual carries at least one dominant allele of a dominant trait, or two recessive alleles of a recessive a trait.
2. Rare-in-population: In each problem, the trait in question is rare in the general population. Assume for the purposes of these problems that individuals who marry into the pedigree in the second and third generations are not carriers. This does not apply to the founding parents – either or both of the individuals at the top of the pedigree could be carriers.
3. Not-Y-linked: The causative genes in these problems may be autosomal or X-Linked, but are not Y-linked.

Chapter 3

Extensions of Mendelian Analysis

INTRODUCTION

Mendel's principles can be used to understand how genes and their alleles are passed down from one generation to the next. When visualised with a Punnett square, these principles can predict the potential combinations of offspring from two parents of known genotype, or infer an unknown parental genotype from tallying the resultant offspring.

The basic principles of Gregor Mendel's model of inheritance have held up for over a century. They can explain how many different characteristics are inherited, in a wide range of organisms including human beings.

Some of the key elements of Mendel's original model were:

1. Heritable traits are determined by heritable factors, now called genes. Genes come in pairs (that is, are present in two copies in an organism).
2. Genes come in different versions, now called alleles. When an organism has two different alleles of a gene, one (the dominant allele) will hide the presence of the other (the recessive allele) and determine appearance.
3. During gamete production, each egg or sperm cell receives just one of the two gene copies present in the organism, and the copy allocated to each gamete is random (law of segregation).
4. Genes for different traits are inherited independently of one another (law of independent assortment).

These rules still form the foundation of our understanding of inheritance—that is, how traits are passed on and how an organism's genotype (set of alleles) determines its phenotype (observable features). However, we now know of some exceptions, extensions, and variations, which must be added to the model in order to fully explain the inheritance patterns we see around us.

VARIATIONS INVOLVING SINGLE GENES

Some of the variations on Mendel's rules involve single genes. These include:

1. Multiple alleles: Mendel studied just two alleles of his pea genes, but real populations often have multiple alleles of a given gene.

2. Incomplete dominance: Two alleles may produce an intermediate phenotype when both are present, rather than one fully determining the phenotype.

3. Codominance: Two alleles may be simultaneously expressed when both are present, rather than one fully determining the phenotype.

4. Pleiotropy: Some genes affect many different characteristics, not just a single characteristic.

5. Lethal alleles: Some genes have alleles that prevent survival when homozygous or heterozygous.

6. Sex linkage: Genes carried on sex chromosomes, such as the X chromosome of humans, show different inheritance patterns than genes on autosomal (non-sex) chromosomes.

Multiple Alleles, Incomplete Dominance, and Codominance

Gregor Mendel knew how to keep things simple. In Mendel's work on pea plants, each gene came in just two different versions, or alleles, and these alleles had a nice, clear-cut dominance relationship (with the dominant allele fully overriding the recessive allele to determine the plant's appearance).

Today, we know that not all alleles behave quite as straight forwardly as in Mendel's experiments. For example, in real life:

- Allele pairs may have a variety of dominance relationships (that is, one allele of the pair may not completely 'hide' the other in the heterozygote).
- There are often many different alleles of a gene in a population.

In these cases, an organism's genotype, or set of alleles, still determines its phenotype, or observable features. However, a variety of alleles may interact with one another in different ways to specify phenotype. However Mendel's pea genes didn't show these complexities. If they had, it's possible that Mendel would not have understood his results, and wouldn't have figured out the core principles of inheritance—which are key in helping us understand the special cases!

Incomplete dominance

Mendel's results were ground breaking partly because they contradicted the (then-popular) idea that parents traits were permanently blended in their offspring. In some cases, however, the phenotype of a heterozygous organism can actually be a blend between the phenotypes of its homozygous parents. For example, in the snapdragon, *Antirrhinum majus*, a cross between a homozygous white-flowered plant ($C^W C^W$) and a homozygous red-flowered plant ($C^R C^R$) will produce offspring with pink flowers ($C^R C^W$) is shown in Fig. 3.1. This type of relationship between alleles, with a heterozygote phenotype intermediate between the two homozygote phenotypes, is called incomplete dominance.

We can still use Mendel's model to predict the results of crosses for alleles that show incomplete dominance. For example, self-fertilisation of a pink plant would produce a genotype ratio of 1 $C^R C^R$:2 $C^R C^W$:1 $C^W C^W$ and a phenotype ratio of 1:2:1 red:pink:white is shown in Fig. 3.2. Alleles are still inherited according to Mendel's basic rules, even when they show incomplete dominance.

Codominance

Closely related to incomplete dominance is codominance, in which both alleles are simultaneously expressed in the heterozygote. We can see an example of codominance in the MN blood groups of humans (less famous than the ABO blood groups, but still important!). A person's MN blood type is determined by his or her alleles of a certain gene. An L^M allele specifies production of an M marker displayed on the surface of red blood cells, while an L^N allele specifies production of a slightly different N marker.

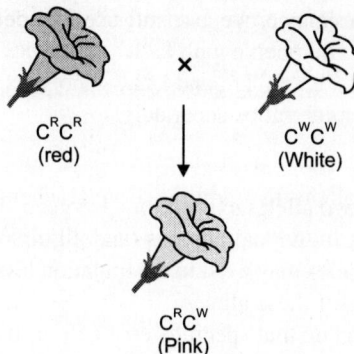

Fig. 3.1: Diagram of a cross between C^WC^W (red) and C^RC^R (white) snapdragon plants. The F1 plants are pink and of genotype C^RC^W.

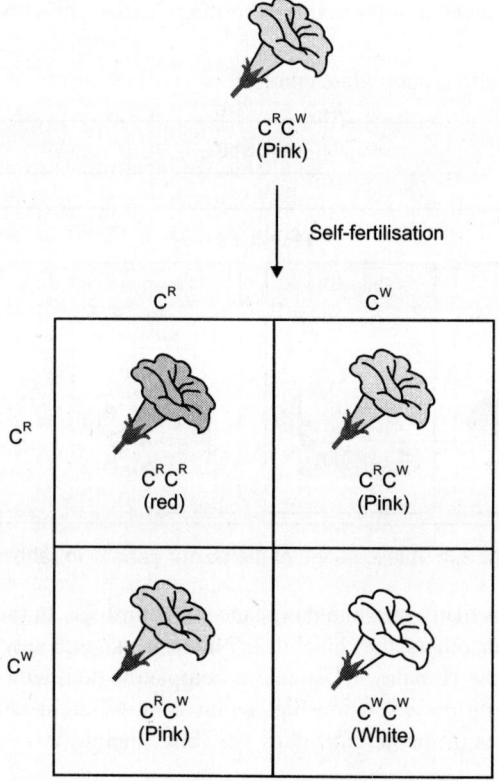

1 Red : 2 Pink : 1 White

Fig. 3.2: Self-fertilisation of pink C^RC^W plants produce red, pink, and white offspring in a ratio of 1:2:1.

Homozygotes (L^ML^M and L^NL^N) have only M or an N markers, respectively, on the surface of their red blood cells. However, heterozygotes (L^ML^N) have both types of markers in equal numbers on the cell surface. As for incomplete dominance, we can still use Mendel's rules to predict inheritance of codominant alleles. For example, if two people with $L^M L^N$ genotypes had children, we would expect to see M, MN, and N blood types and $L^M L^M$, $L^M L^N$, and $L^N L^N$ genotypes in their children in a 1:2:1 (if they had enough children for us to determine ratios accurately!)

Multiple alleles

Mendel's work suggested that just two alleles existed for each gene. Today, we know that's not always, or even usually, the case! Although individual humans (and all diploid organisms) can only have two alleles for a given gene, multiple alleles may exist in a population level, and different individuals in the population may have different pairs of these alleles.

As an example, let's consider a gene that specifies coat colour in rabbits, called the C gene. The C gene comes in four common alleles: C, c^{ch}, c^{ch}, and c (Fig. 3.3):

- A CC rabbit has black or brown fur.
- A $c^{ch} c^{ch}$ rabbit has chinchilla colouration (grayish fur).
- A $c^h c^h$ rabbit has Himalayan (colour-point) patterning, with a white body and dark ears, face, feet, and tail.
- A cc rabbit is albino, with a pure white coat.

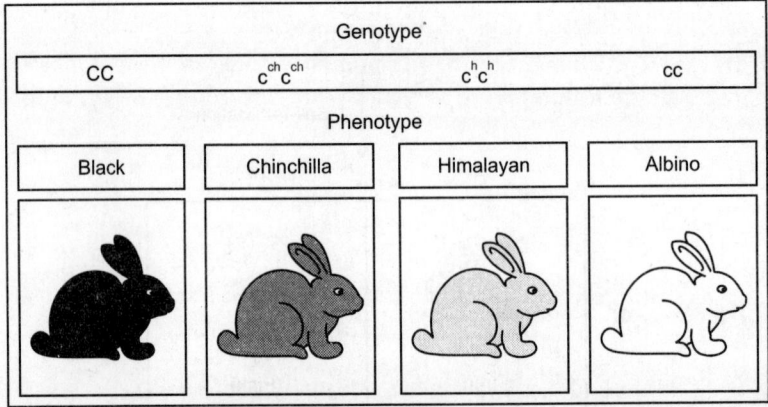

Fig. 3.3: Allelic series of the colour gene C in rabbits.

Multiple alleles makes for many possible dominance relationships. In this case, the black C allele is completely dominant to all the others, the chinchilla c^{ch} allele is incompletely dominant to the Himalayan c^h and albino c alleles, and the Himalayan c^h allele is completely dominant to the albino c allele.

Rabbit breeders figured out these relationships by crossing different rabbits of different genotypes and observing the phenotypes of the heterozygous kits (baby bunnies).

Pleiotropy and lethal alleles

From Mendel's experiments, you might imagine that all genes control a single characteristic and affect some harmless aspect of an organism's appearance (such as colour, height, or shape). Those predictions are true for some genes, but definitely not all of them.

For example:

- A human genetic disorder called Marfan syndrome is caused by a mutation in one gene, yet it affects many aspects of growth and development, including height, vision, and heart function. This is an example of pleiotropy, or one gene affecting multiple characteristics.
- A cross between two heterozygous yellow mice produces yellow and brown mice in a ratio of 2:1, not 3:1. This is an example of lethality, in which a particular genotype makes an organism unable to survive.

This section discusses pleiotropic genes and lethal alleles, seeing how these variations on Mendel's rules fit into our modern understanding of inheritance.

Pleiotropy

When we mentioned Mendel's experiments with purple-flowered and white-flowered plants, we didn't discuss any other phenotypes associated with the two flower colours. However, Mendel noticed that the flower colours were always correlated with two other features: the colour of the seed coat (covering of the seed) and the colour of the axils (junctions where the leaves met the stem).

In plants with white flowers, the seed coats and axils were colourless. In plants with purple flowers, on the other hand, the seed coats were brown-gray and the axils were reddish. Thus, rather than affecting just one characteristic, the flower colour gene actually affected three. Genes like this, which control multiple, seemingly unrelated features, are said to be pleiotropic (pleio- = many, -tropic = effects). We now know that Mendel's flower colour gene specifies a protein that causes coloured particles, or pigments, to be made. This protein works in several different parts of the pea plant (flowers, seed coat, and leaf axils). In this way, the seemingly unrelated phenotypes can be traced back to a defect in one gene with several jobs. Simple schematic illustrating pleiotropy is shown in Fig. 3.4.

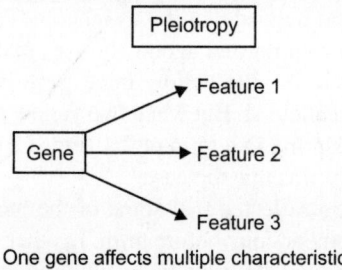

One gene affects multiple characteristics

Fig. 3.4: Simple schematic illustrating pleiotropy. In pleiotropy, one gene affects multiple features (feature 1, feature 2, and feature 3).

Importantly, alleles of pleiotropic genes are transmitted in the same way as alleles of genes that affect single traits. Although the phenotype has multiple elements, these elements are specified as a package, and the dominant and recessive versions of the package would appear in the offspring of two heterozygotes in a ratio of 3:1.

Pleiotropy in human genetic disorders

Genes affected in human genetic disorders are often pleiotropic. For example, people with a hereditary disorder called Marfan syndrome may have a set of seemingly unrelated symptoms, including the following: (i) unusually tall height, (ii) thin fingers and toes, (iii) dislocation of the lens of the eye, and (iv) heart problems (in which the aorta, the large blood vessel carrying blood away from the heart, bulges or ruptures).

These symptoms don't seem directly related, but as it turns out, they can all be traced back to the mutation of a single gene. This gene encodes a protein that assembles into chains, making elastic fibrils that give strength and flexibility to the body's connective tissues. Mutations that cause Marfan syndrome reduce the amount of functional protein made by the body, resulting in fewer fibrils.

How does the identity of this gene explain the range of symptoms? Our eyes and the aortas normally contain many fibrils that help maintain structure, which is why these two organs are affected in Marfan syndrome. In addition, the fibrils serve as 'storage shelves' for growth factors. When there are fewer of them in Marfan syndrome, the growth factors cannot be shelved and thus cause excess growth (leading to the characteristic tall, thin Marfan build).

Lethality

For the alleles that Mendel studied, it was equally possible to get homozygous dominant, homozygous recessive, and heterozygous genotypes. That is, none of these genotypes affected the survival of the pea plants. However, this is not the case for all genes and all alleles.

Many genes in an organism's genome are needed for survival. If an allele makes one of these genes nonfunctional, or causes it to take on an abnormal, harmful activity, it may be impossible to get a living organism with a homozygous (or, in some cases, even a heterozygous) genotype.

Example: The yellow mouse

A classic example of an allele that affects survival is the lethal yellow allele, a spontaneous mutation in mice that makes their coats yellow. This allele was discovered around the turn of the 20th century by the French geneticist Lucien Cuenót, who noticed that it was inherited in an unusual pattern.

When yellow mice were crossed with normal agouti (brown) mice, they produced half yellow and half brown offspring. This suggested that the yellow mice were heterozygous, and that the yellow allele, A^Y, was dominant to the agouti allele, A. But when two yellow mice were crossed with each other, they produced yellow and brown offspring in a ratio of 2:1 (Fig. 3.5), and the yellow offspring did not breed true (were heterozygous). Why was this the case?

As it turned out, this unusual ratio reflected that some of the mouse embryos (homozygous $A^Y A^Y$ genotype) died very early in development, long before birth. In other words, at the level of eggs, sperm, and fertilisation, the colour gene segregated normally, resulting in embryos with a 1:2:1 ratio of $A^Y A^Y$, $A^Y A$, and AA genotypes. However, the $A^Y A^Y$ mice died as tiny embryos, leaving a 2:1 genotype and phenotype ratio among the surviving mice.

Alleles like A^Y, which are lethal when they're homozygous but not when they're heterozygous, are called recessive lethal alleles.

Lethal alleles and human genetic disorders

Some alleles associated with human genetic disorders are recessive lethal. For example, this is true of the allele that causes achondroplasia, a form of dwarfism. A person heterozygous for this allele will have shortened limbs and short stature (achondroplasia), a condition that is not lethal. However, homozygosity for the same allele causes death during embryonic development or the first months of life, an example of recessive lethality.

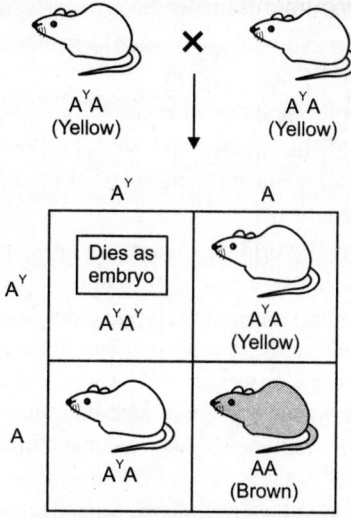

2 Yellow : 1 Brown among survivors

Fig. 3.5: Two yellow mice (A^Y genotype) are crossed to one another. There is a phenotypic ratio of 2:1 yellow:brown among the mice that survive to birth.

Some human disorders are also caused by dominant lethal alleles. These are alleles that cause death when they are present in just a single copy. If an allele leads to death of heterozygotes before birth, we'll never see that allele in the living human population (but rather, as an implantation failure or miscarriage). However, if a dominant lethal allele allows heterozygotes to survive past birth, it can be seen in the population as a genetic disorder. In fact, if a dominant lethal allele lets a person survive to reproductive age, it may even be passed on to children. This is the case in Huntington's disease, a fatal genetic disorder affecting the nervous system. People with a Huntington allele inevitably develop the disease, but they may not show any symptoms until age 40 and can unknowingly pass the allele on to their children.

Sex-linked Traits

Sex-linked traits are associated with genes found on sex chromosomes. In humans, the sex chromosomes are X and Y. Because the X-chromosome is larger, X-linked traits are more common than Y-linked traits. An example of a sex-linked trait is red-green colour blindness, which is carried on the X-chromosome. Because males only have one X-chromosome, they have a higher chance of having red-green colour blindness.

VARIATIONS INVOLVING MULTIPLE GENES

Other variations on Mendel's rules involve interactions between pairs (or, potentially, larger numbers) of genes. Many characteristics are controlled by more than one gene, and when two genes affect the same process, they can interact with each other in a variety of different ways. For example:

- Complementary genes: Recessive alleles of two different genes may give the same phenotype.
- Epistasis: The alleles of one gene may mask or conceal the alleles of another gene.

In addition, some gene pairs lie near one another on a chromosome and are genetically linked, meaning that they don't assort independently.

Polygenic Inheritance and Environmental Effects

Many characteristics important in our everyday lives, such as height, skin colour, eye colour, and risk of diseases like diabetes, are controlled by many factors.

These factors may be genetic, environmental, or both.

- Polygenic inheritance: Some characteristics are polygenic, meaning that they're controlled by a number of different genes. In polygenic inheritance, traits often form a phenotypic spectrum rather than falling into clear-cut categories.

- Environmental effects: Most real-world characteristics are determined not just by genotype, but also by environmental factors that influence how genotype is translated into phenotype.

Genetic background and environment contribute to incomplete penetrance, in which not all individuals with a genotype display a corresponding phenotype, and variable expressivity, in which individuals of a particular genotype may have stronger or weaker versions of a phenotype.

We can discussed polygenic inheritance and environmental effects with the help of examples.

Thus, as an example, let's consider human height. Unlike a simple Mendelian characteristic, human height displays:

- Continuous variation: Unlike Mendel's pea plants, humans don't come in two clear-cut 'tall' and 'short' varieties. In fact, they don't even come in four heights, or eight, or sixteen. Instead, it's possible to get humans of many different heights, and height can vary in increments of inches or fractions of inches (Fig. 3.6).

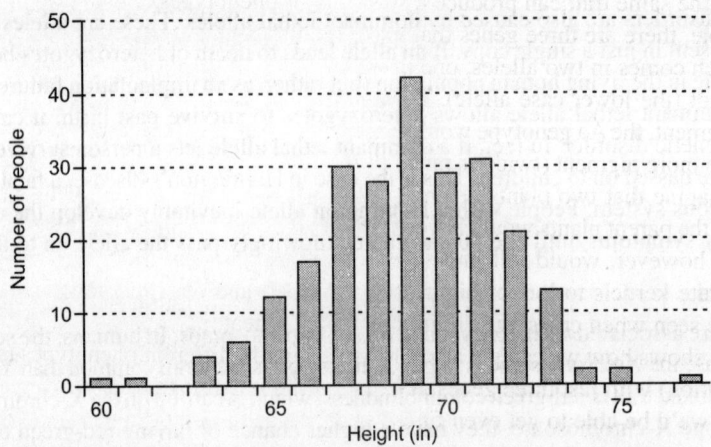

Fig. 3.6: Histogram showing height in inches of male high school seniors in a sample group. The histogram is roughly bell-shaped, with just a few individuals at the tails (60 inches and 77 inches) and many individuals in the middle, around 69 inches.

- A complex inheritance pattern. It was noticed that tall parents can have a short child, short parents can have a tall child, and two parents of different heights may or may not have a child in the middle. Also, siblings with the same two parents may have a range of heights, ones that don't fall into distinct categories.

Simple models involving one or two genes can't accurately predict all of these inheritance patterns. How, then, is height inherited?

Height and other similar features are controlled not just by one gene, but rather, by multiple (often many) genes that each make a small contribution to the overall outcome. This inheritance pattern is sometimes called polygenic inheritance (poly = many). For instance, a recent study found over 400 genes linked to variation in height. When there are large numbers of genes involved, it becomes hard to distinguish the effect of each individual gene, and even harder to see that gene variants (alleles) are inherited according to Mendelian rules. In an additional complication, height doesn't just depend on genetics: it also depends on environmental factors, such as a child's overall health and the type of nutrition he or she gets while growing up.

This section discusses how complex traits such as height are inherited. We'll also see how factors like genetic background and environment can affect the phenotype (observable features) produced by a particular genotype (set of gene variants, or alleles).

Polygenic inheritance

Human features like height, eye colour, and hair colour come in lots of slightly different forms because they are controlled by many genes, each of which contributes some amount to the overall phenotype. For example, there are two major eye colour genes, but at least 14 other genes that play roles in determining a person's exact eye colour.

Looking at a real example of a human polygenic trait would get complicated, largely because we'd have to keep track of tens, or even hundreds, of different allele pairs (like the 400 involved in height!). However, we can use an example involving wheat kernels to see how several genes whose alleles 'add up' to influence the same trait can produce a spectrum of phenotypes.

In this example, there are three genes that make reddish pigment in wheat kernels, which we'll call A, B, and C. Each comes in two alleles, one of which makes pigment (the capital-letter allele) and one of which does not (the lower case allele). These alleles have additive effects: the aa genotype would contribute no pigment, the Aa genotype would contribute some amount of pigment, and the AA genotype would contribute more pigment (twice as much as Aa). The same would hold true for the B and C genes.

Now, let's imagine that two plants heterozygous for all three genes (AaBbCc) were crossed to one another. Each of the parent plants would have three alleles that made pigment, leading to pinkish kernels. Their offspring, however, would fall into seven colour groups, ranging from no pigment whatsoever (aabbcc) and white kernels to lots of pigment (AABBCC) and dark red kernels. This is in fact what researchers have seen when crossing certain varieties of wheat.

This example shows how we can get a spectrum of slightly different phenotypes (something close to continuous variation) with just three genes. It's not hard to imagine that, as we increased the number of genes involved, we'd be able to get even finer variations in colour, or in another trait such as height.

Environmental effects

Human phenotypes—and phenotypes of other organisms—also vary because they are affected by the environment. For instance, a person may have a genetic tendency to be underweight or obese, but his or her actual weight will depend on diet and exercise (with these factors often playing a greater role than genes). In another example, our hair colour may depend on our genes—until you dye your hair purple!

One striking example of how environment can affect phenotype comes from the hereditary disorder phenylketonuria (PKU). People who are homozygous for disease alleles of the PKU gene lack activity of an enzyme that breaks down the amino acid phenylalanine. Because people with this disorder cannot get rid of excess phenylalanine, it rapidly builds up to toxic levels in their bodies.

If PKU is not treated, the extra phenylalanine can keep the brain from developing normally, leading to intellectual disability, seizures, and mood disorders. However, because PKU is caused by the buildup of too much phenylalanine, it can also be treated in a very simple way: by giving affected babies and children a diet low in phenylalanine.

If people with phenylketonuria follow this diet strictly from a very young age, they can have few, or even no, symptoms of the disorder. In many countries, all newborns are screened for PKU and similar genetic diseases shortly after birth through a simple blood test.

Variable expressivity, incomplete penetrance

Even for characteristics that are controlled by a single gene, it's possible for individuals with the same genotype to have different phenotypes. For example, in the case of a genetic disorder, people with the same disease genotype may have stronger or weaker forms of the disorder, and some may never develop the disorder at all.

In variable expressivity, a phenotype may be stronger or weaker in different people with the same genotype. For instance, in a group of people with a disease-causing genotype, some might develop a severe form of the disorder, while others might have a milder form.

In incomplete penetrance, individuals with a certain genotype may or may not develop a phenotype associated with the genotype. For example, among people with the same disease-causing genotype for a hereditary disorder, some might never actually develop the disorder.

What causes variable expressivity and incomplete penetrance? Other genes and environmental effects are often part of the explanation. For example, disease-causing alleles of one gene may be suppressed by alleles of another gene elsewhere in the genome, or a person's overall health may influence the strength of a disease phenotype.

GENETICISTS USE A VARIETY OF SYMBOLS FOR ALLELES

A standard convention used to symbolise alleles for very simple Mendelian traits is that the initial letter of the name of a recessive trait, lower cased and italicised, denotes the recessive allele, and the same letter in uppercase refers to the dominant allele. Thus, in the case of tall and dwarf, where dwarf is recessive, D and d represent the alleles responsible for these respective traits. Mendel used upper- and lowercase letters such as these to symbolise his unit factors.

Another useful system was developed in genetic studies of the fruit fly *Drosophila melanogaster* to discriminate between wild-type and mutant traits. This system uses the initial letter, or a combination of several letters, from the name of the mutant trait. If the trait is recessive, lowercase is used, if it is dominant, uppercase is used. The contrasting wild-type trait is denoted by the same letters, but with a superscript +. For example, ebony is a recessive body colour mutation in Drosophila. The normal wild-type body colour is gray. Using this system, we denote ebony by the symbol e, while gray is denoted by e^+. The responsible locus may be occupied by either the wild type allele (e^+) or the mutant allele (e). A diploid fly may thus exhibit one of three possible genotypes (the two phenotypes are indicated parenthetically):

e^+/e^+ gray homozygote (wild type)

e^+/e gray heterozygote (wild type)

e/e ebony homozygote (mutant)

The slash between the letters indicates that the two allele designations represent the same locus on two homologous chromosomes. If we instead consider a mutant allele that is dominant to the normal wild-type allele, such as *Wrinkled* wing in *Drosophila*, the three possible genotypes are *Wr/Wr*, *Wr/Wr*$^+$, and Wr$^+$/Wr$^+$. The initial two genotypes express the mutant wrinkled-wing phenotype. One advantage of this system is that further abbreviation can be used when convenient: The wild-type allele may simply be denoted by the + symbol. With ebony as an example, the designations of the three possible genotypes become:

+/+ gray homozygote (wild type)

+/e gray heterozygote (wild type)

e/e ebony homozygote (mutant)

Another variation is utilised when no dominance exists between alleles. We can simply use uppercase letters and superscripts to denote alternative alleles (e.g. R^1 and R^2, L^M and L^N, and I^A and I^B).

Many diverse systems of genetic nomenclature are used to identify genes in various organisms. Usually, the symbol selected reflects the function of the gene or even a disorder caused by a mutant gene. For example, in yeast, *cdk* is the abbreviation for the cyclin-dependent kinase gene, whose product is involved in the cell-cycle regulation mechanism. In bacteria, *leu*$^-$ refers to a mutation that interrupts the biosynthesis of the amino acid leucine, and the wild-type gene is designated *leu*$^+$.

There are several different ways to record genotypes for X-linked traits. Sometimes the genotypes are recorded in the same fashion as they are for autosomal characteristics. In this case, the hemizygous males are simply given a single allele: the genotype of a female *Drosophila* with white eyes is ww, and the genotype of a white-eyed hemizygous male is w. Another method is to include the Y chromosome, designating it with a diagonal slash (/). With this method, the white eyed female's genotype is still ww and the white-eyed male's genotype is w/. Perhaps the most useful method is to write the X and Y chromosomes in the genotype, designating the X-linked alleles with superscripts, as is done in this chapter. With this method, a white-eyed female is X^wX^w and a white eyed male is X^wY.

Cytoplasmic Inheritance

Mendel's principles of segregation and independent assortment are based on the assumption that genes are located on chromosomes in the nucleus of the cell. For most genetic characteristics, this assumption is valid, and Mendel's principles allow us to predict the types of offspring that will be produced in a genetic cross. However, not all the genetic material of a cell is found in the nucleus, some characteristics are encoded by genes located in the cytoplasm. These characteristics exhibit cytoplasmic inheritance.

A few organelles, notably chloroplasts and mitochondria, contain DNA. The human mitochondrial genome contains about 15000 nucleotides of DNA, encoding 37 genes. Compared with that of nuclear DNA, which contains some 3 billion nucleotides encoding some 20000 to 25000 genes, the size of the mitochondrial genome is very small, nevertheless, mitochondrial and chloroplast genes encode some important characteristics.

Cytoplasmic inheritance differs from the inheritance of characteristics encoded by nuclear genes in several important respects. A zygote inherits nuclear genes from both parents, but, typically, all its cytoplasmic organelles, and thus all its cytoplasmic genes, come from only one of the gametes, usually the egg. A sperm generally contributes only a set of nuclear genes from the male parent. In a few organisms, cytoplasmic genes are inherited from the male parent or from both parents, however, for most organisms, all the cytoplasm is inherited from the egg. In this case, cytoplasmically inherited traits are present in both males and females and are passed from mother to offspring, never from father to offspring. Reciprocal crosses, therefore, give different results when cytoplasmic genes encode a trait. Cytoplasmically inherited characteristics frequently exhibit extensive phenotypic variation because no mechanism analogous to mitosis or meiosis ensures that cytoplasmic genes are evenly distributed in cell division. Thus, different cells and individual offspring will contain various proportions of cytoplasmic genes. Consider chloroplast genes. Suppose that half of the chloroplasts in a cell contain a normal wild-type copy of cpDNA and the other half contain a mutated copy. In cell division, the chloroplasts segregate into progeny cells at random. Just by chance, one cell may receive mostly mutated cpDNA and another cell may receive mostly wild-type cpDNA. In this way, different progeny from the same mother and even cells within an individual offspring may vary in their phenotypes. Traits encoded by mitochondrial DNA (mtDNA) are similarly variable.

Correns, one of the biologists who rediscovered Mendel's work, studied the inheritance of leaf variegation in the four-o'clock plant, *Mirabilis jalapa* (Fig. 3.7). Correns found that the leaves and shoots of one variety of four-o' clock were variegated, displaying a mixture of green and white splotches. He also noted that some branches of the variegated strain had all-green leaves, other branches had all-white leaves. Each branch produced flowers, so Correns was able to cross flowers from variegated, green, and white branches in all combinations. The seeds from green branches always gave rise to green progeny, no matter whether the pollen was from a green, white, or variegated branch. Similarly, flowers on white branches always produced white progeny. Flowers on the variegated branches gave rise to green, white, and variegated progeny, in no particular ratio.

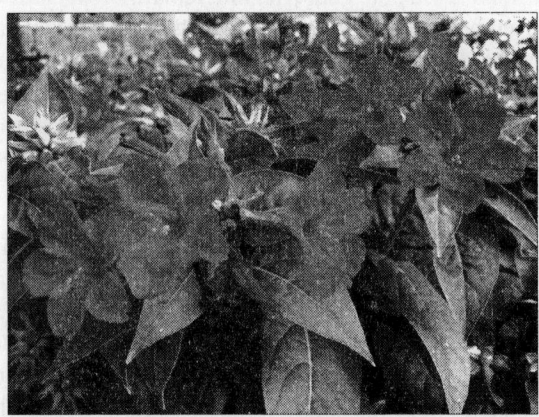

Fig. 3.7: *Mirabilis jalapa.*

Correns's crosses demonstrated cytoplasmic inheritance of variegation in the four-o'clocks. The phenotypes of the offspring were determined entirely by the maternal parent, never by the paternal parent (the source of the pollen). Furthermore, the production of all three phenotypes by flowers on variegated branches is consistent with cytoplasmic inheritance. Variegation in these plants is caused by a defective gene in the cpDNA, which results in a failure to produce the green pigment chlorophyll. Cells from green branches contain normal chloroplasts only, cells from white branches contain abnormal chloroplasts only, and cells from variegated branches contain a mixture of normal and abnormal chloroplasts. In the flowers from variegated branches, the random segregation of chloroplasts in the course of oogenesis produces some egg cells with normal cpDNA, which develop into green progeny, other egg cells with only abnormal cpDNA develop into white progeny, and, finally, still other egg cells with a mixture of normal and abnormal cpDNA develop into variegated progeny.

Impact of Genetic Background and Environmental Factors on Phenotypic Expression

In the previous part we assumed that the genotype of an organism is always directly expressed in its phenotype. For example, pea plants homozygous for the recessive 'd' allele (dd) will always be dwarf. We discussed gene expression as though the genes operate in a closed system in which the presence or absence of functional products directly determines the phenotype of an individual. The situation is actually much more complex. Most gene products function within the cell, and cells interact with one another in various ways. Furthermore, the organism exists under diverse environmental influences. Thus, gene expression and the resultant phenotype are often modified through the interaction between an individual's particular genotype and the external environment. In this section, we will discus some of the variables that are known to modify gene expression.

Penetrance and expressivity

In the genetic crosses presented thus far, we have considered only the interactions of alleles and have assumed that every individual organism having a particular genotype expresses the expected phenotype. We assumed, for example, that the genotype 'Rr' always produces round seeds and that the genotype 'rr' always produces wrinkled seeds. For some characters, however, such an assumption is incorrect: the genotype does not always produce the expected phenotype, a phenomenon termed incomplete penetrance.

Incomplete penetrance is seen in human polydactyly, the condition of having extra fingers and toes. The trait is usually caused by a dominant allele. Occasionally, people possess the allele for polydactyly (as evidenced by the fact that their children inherit the polydactyly) but nevertheless have a normal number of fingers and toes. In these cases the gene for polydactyly is not fully penetrant.

Penetrance is defined as the percentage of individual organisms having a particular genotype that express the expected phenotype. For example, if we examined 42 people having an allele for polydactyly and found that only 38 of them were polydactylous, the penetrance would be $38/42 = 0.90$ (90%).

A related concept is that of expressivity, the degree to which a character is expressed. In addition to incomplete penetrance, polydactyly exhibits variable expressivity. Some polydactylous persons possess extra fingers and toes that are fully functional, whereas others possess only a small tag of extra skin. Incomplete penetrance and variable expressivity are due to the effects of other genes and to environmental factors that can alter or completely suppress the effect of a particular gene.

Position effects: Although it is difficult to assess the specific effect of the genetic background and the expression of a gene responsible for determining a potential phenotype, one effect of genetic background has been well characterised, called the position effect. In such instances, the physical location of a gene in relation to other genetic material may influence its expression. For example, if a region of a chromosome is relocated or rearranged (called a translocation or inversion event), normal expression of genes in that chromosomal region may be modified. This is particularly true if the gene is relocated to or near certain areas of the chromosome that are condensed and genetically inert, referred to as heterochromatin.

Onset of genetic expression (effect of age): Not all genetic traits become apparent at the same time during an organism's life span. In most cases, the age at which a mutant gene exerts a noticeable phenotype depends on the stage of growth and development. In humans, the prenatal, infant, preadult, and adult phases require different genetic information. As a result, many severe inherited disorders are not manifested before certain age. For example:

- Tay–Sachs disease, inherited as an autosomal recessive, is a lethal lipid-metabolism disease involving an abnormal enzyme, hexosaminidase A. Newborns appear to be phenotypically normal for the first few months. Then, developmental retardation, paralysis, and blindness ensue, and most affected children die around the age of 3.

- Duchenne muscular dystrophy (DMD), an X-linked recessive disorder associated with progressive muscular wasting. It is not usually diagnosed until a child is 3 to 5 years old. Even with modern medical intervention, the disease is often fatal in the early 20s.

Genetic anticipation: Some heritable disorders that exhibit a progressively earlier age of onset and an increased severity of the disorder in each successive generation. This phenomenon is referred to as genetic anticipation. Myotonic dystrophy (DM), the most common type of adult muscular dystrophy, clearly illustrates genetic anticipation. Individuals afflicted with this autosomal dominant disorder exhibit extreme variation in the severity of symptoms.

Mildly affected individuals develop cataracts as adults, but have little or no muscular weakness. Severely affected individuals demonstrate more extensive weakness, as well as myotonia (muscle hyperexcitability) and in some cases mental retardation. In its most extreme form, the disease is fatal just after birth. Increased severity and earlier onset of disease was recorded with successive generations of inheritance.

Genomic (parental) imprinting and gene silencing: The process of selective gene silencing occurs during early development, impacting on subsequent phenotypic expression. Examples involve cases where genes or regions of a chromosome are imprinted on one homolog but not the other.

An example in humans involves two distinct genetic disorders thought to be caused by differential imprinting of the same region of the long arm of chromosome 15. In both cases, the disorders are due to an identical deletion of this region in one member of the chromosome 15 pair.

The first disorder, Prader–Willi syndrome (PWS), results when the paternal segment is deleted and an undeleted maternal chromosome remains. If the maternal segment is deleted and an undeleted paternal chromosome remains, an entirely different disorder, Angelman syndrome (AS), results.

These two conditions exhibit different phenotypes. PWS entails mental retardation, a severe eating disorder marked by an uncontrollable appetite, obesity, diabetes, and growth retardation. Angelman syndrome also involves mental retardation, but involuntary muscle contractions (chorea) and seizures characterise the disorder. We can conclude that the involved region of chromosome 15 is imprinted differently in male and female gametes and that both an undeleted maternal and a paternal region are required for normal development.

Imprinting is an example of the more general topic of epigenetics, where genetic expression is not the direct result of the information stored in the nucleotide sequence of DNA. Instead, the DNA is altered in a way that affects its expression. These changes are stable in the sense that they are transmitted during cell division to progeny cells, and often through gametes to future generations.

Temperature effects: Chemical activity depends on the kinetic energy of the reacting substances, which in turn depends on the surrounding temperature. We can thus expect temperature to influence phenotypes. An example is seen in the evening primrose, which produces red flowers when grown at 23°C and white flowers when grown at 18°C. An even more striking example is seen in Siamese cats and Himalayan rabbits (Fig. 3.8), which exhibit dark fur in certain regions where their body temperature is slightly cooler, particularly the nose, ears, and paws.

In these cases, it appears that the enzyme normally responsible for pigment production is functional only at the lower temperatures present in the extremities, but it loses its catalytic function at the slightly higher temperatures found throughout the rest of the body.

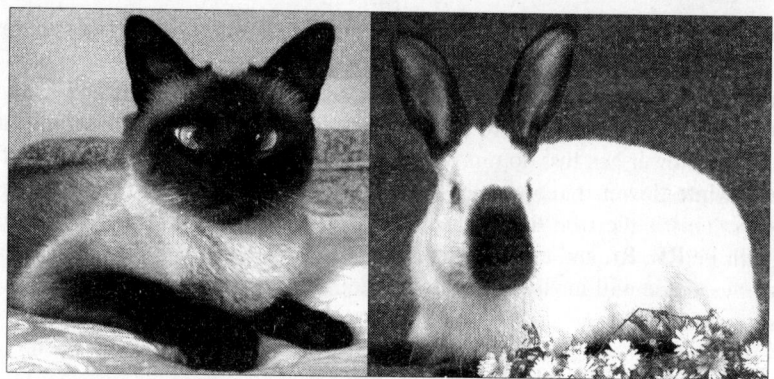

Fig. 3.8: Siamese cats and himalayan rabbits.

Nutritional effects: In humans, the ingestion of certain dietary substances that normal individuals may consume without harm can adversely affect individuals with abnormal genetic constitutions. Often, a mutation may prevent an individual from metabolising some substance commonly found in normal diets. For example:

- Phenylketonuria cannot metabolise the amino acid phenylalanine.
- Galactosemia cannot metabolise galactose.
- Lactose intolerance cannot metabolise lactose.

However, if the dietary intake of the involved molecule is drastically reduced or eliminated, the associated phenotype may be ameliorated.

INCOMPLETE DOMINANCE

Incomplete dominance is when a dominant allele, or form of a gene, does not completely mask the effects of a recessive allele, and the organism's resulting physical appearance shows a blending of both alleles. It is also called semi-dominance or partial dominance. One example is shown in roses. The allele for red colour is dominant over the allele for white colour, but heterozygous roses, which have both alleles, are pink. Note that this is different from codominance, which is when both alleles are expressed at the same time.

Mechanisms of Incomplete Dominance

Many genes show complete dominance. This means that if an individual is heterozygous for a particular gene, the dominant allele will completely mask the recessive allele. Many of the properties that the Austrian monk Gregor Mendel studied in his famous pea plants were controlled by genes that showed complete dominance. For example, the dominant flower colour was purple, and the recessive colour was white. Plants that were heterozygous were also purple, since purple was the dominant allele, even though they also had the white allele. A plant only had white flowers if it was homozygous for the recessive allele, which means that it had two copies of that allele. (This is also why two purple plants sometimes produced white ones, a proportion of the offspring received two recessive alleles.)

Why does incomplete dominance occur? As we have seen, it does not always occur with flower colour, roses (and tulips, carnations, and snapdragons, among others) show incomplete dominance, but

Mendel's pea plants showed complete dominance. Incomplete dominance can occur because neither of the two alleles is fully dominant over the other, or because the dominant allele does not fully dominate the recessive allele. This results in a phenotype that is different from both the dominant and recessive alleles, and appears to be a mixture of both. This Punnett square shows incomplete dominance (Fig. 3.9). The homozygous red flower has two dominant red alleles, and these are represented by the letters RR. The homozygous white flower is represented by rr. Their offspring are all heterozygous Rr, and they have pink flowers. This is the first filial generation, or F1. When the F1 generation cross-pollinates, their offspring will be RR, Rr, and rr in a 1:2:1 ratio. Some of their offspring (the F2 generation) will inherit two R alleles, some will inherit two r alleles, and some will inherit both.

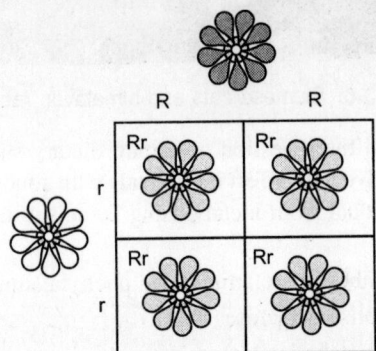

Fig. 3.9: Punnett square shows incomplete dominance.

Incomplete Dominance and Codominance

Incomplete dominance is not the same as codominance. In codominance, both alleles can be seen in the phenotype at the same time. Instead of being uniformly pink, a flower with red and white alleles that show codominance will have patches of red and patches of white. As with incomplete dominance, the F2 generation from heterozygous plants will have a ratio of 1:2:1 of red, spotted, and white flowers. Codominance is also shown in humans with AB blood type, the alleles for blood types A and B are both expressed.

Examples of Incomplete Dominance

In humans

A child born to a parent with straight hair and a parent with curly hair will usually have wavy hair, or hair that is a little curled, due to the expression of both curly and straight alleles. Incomplete dominance can be seen in many other physical characteristics such as skin colour, height, hand size, and vocal pitch.

Carriers of Tay-Sachs disease also show incomplete dominance. Individuals with Tay-Sachs disease lack an enzyme that breaks down lipids, causing too many lipids to accumulate in the brain and other parts of the nervous system. This leads to nerve deterioration and loss of physical and mental abilities. Tay-Sachs occurs in people with two recessive alleles for the disease, and people with one allele are carriers but do not show symptoms. However, they do produce half of the normal amount of the enzyme, showing an intermediate phenotype between those with the disorder and those who do not have any recessive Tay-Sachs alleles.

In other animals

The Andalusian chicken, a type of chicken native to the Andalusia region of Spain, shows incomplete dominance in its feather colour. A white male and a black female will often produce offspring that have blue-tinged feathers. This is caused by a dilution gene that partially dilutes the pigment melanin and makes the feathers lighter. When certain types of long and short-furred rabbits are bred, their offspring will have medium-length fur. This phenomenon can also be seen with the length of dogs' tails. Also, an animal that has a lot of spots will have offspring with a few spots if bred with a non-spotted animal. This is often seen in dogs, cats, and horses.

HETEROZYGOUS

In diploid organisms, heterozygous refers to an individual having two different alleles for a specific trait. An allele is a version of a gene or specific DNA sequence on a chromosome. Alleles are inherited through sexual reproduction as the resulting offspring inherit half of their chromosomes from the mother and half from the father. The cells in diploid organisms contain sets of homologous chromosomes, which are paired chromosomes that have the same genes at the same positions along each chromosome pair. Although homologous chromosomes have the same genes, they may have different alleles for those genes. Alleles determine how particular traits are expressed or observed.

Example: The gene for seed shape in pea plants exists in two forms, one form or allele for round seed shape (R) and the other for wrinkled seed shape (r). A heterozygous plant would contain the following alleles for seed shape: (Rr).

Heterozygous Inheritance

Complete dominance

Diploid organisms have two alleles for each trait and those alleles are different in heterozygous individuals. Incomplete dominance inheritance, one allele is dominant and the other is recessive. The dominant trait is observed and the recessive trait is masked. Using the previous example, round seed shape (R) is dominant and wrinkled seed shape (r) is recessive. A plant with round seeds would have either of the following genotypes: (RR) or (Rr). A plant with wrinkled seeds would have the following genotype: (rr). The heterozygous genotype (Rr) has the dominant round seed shape as its recessive allele (r) is masked in the phenotype.

Incomplete dominance

In incomplete dominance inheritance, one of the heterozygous alleles does not completely mask the other. Instead, a different phenotype is seen that is a combination of the phenotypes of the two alleles. An example of this is pink flower colour in snapdragons. The allele that produces red flower colour (R) is not completely expressed over the allele that produces white flower colour (r). The result in the heterozygous genotype (Rr) is a phenotype that is a mixture of red and white, or pink.

Co-Dominance

In co-dominance inheritance, both of the heterozygous alleles are fully expressed in the phenotype. An example of co-dominance is AB blood type inheritance. The A and B alleles are expressed fully and equally in the phenotype and are said to be co-dominant.

Heterozygous vs Homozygous

An individual that is homozygous for a trait has alleles that are similar. Unlike heterozygous individuals with different alleles, homozygotes only produce homozygous offspring. These offspring may be either homozygous dominant (RR) or homozygous recessive (rr) for a trait. They may not have both dominant and recessive alleles. In contrast, both heterozygous and homozygous offspring may be derived from a heterozygote (Rr). The heterozygous offspring have both dominant and recessive alleles that may express complete dominance, incomplete dominance, or co-dominance.

Heterozygous Mutations

Sometimes, mutations can occur on chromosomes that change the DNA sequence. These mutations are typically the result of either errors that happen during meiosis or by exposure to mutagens. In diploid organisms, a mutation that occurs on only one allele for a gene is called a heterozygous mutation. Identical mutations that occur on both alleles of the same gene are called homozygous mutations. Compound heterozygous mutations occur as a result of different mutations that happen on both alleles for the same gene.

MULTIPLE ALLELES AND THEIR CHARACTERISTICS

The word allele is a general term to denote the alternative forms of a gene or contrasting gene pair that denote the alternative form of a gene is called allele. These alleles were previously considered by Bateson as hypothetical partner in Mendelian segregation.

As already discussed in Mendelian inheritance a given locus of chromosome was occupied by 2 kinds of genes, i.e. a normal gene (for round seed shape) and other its mutant recessive gene (wrinkled seed shape). But it may be possible that normal gene may show still many mutations in pea besides the one for wrinkledness. Here the locus will be occupied by normal allele and its two or more mutant genes. Thus, three or more kinds of genes occupying the same locus in individual chromosome are referred to as multiple alleles. In short many alleles of a single gene are called multiple alleles. The concept of multiple alleles is described under the term 'multiple allelism'.

Dawson and Whitehouse in England proposed the term panallele for all the gene mutations at a given locus in a chromosome. These differ from the multiple factor in one respect that multiple factors occupy different loci while alleles occupy same locus.

'Three or more kinds of gene which occupy the same locus are referred to as multiple alleles.'

Characteristics of Multiple Alleles

1. The study of multiple alleles may be done in population.
2. Multiple alleles are situated on homologous chromosomes at the same locus.
3. There is no crossing over between the members of multiple alleles. Crossing over takes place between two different genes only (inter-generic recombination) and does not occur within a gene (intragenic recombination).
4. Multiple alleles influence one or the same character only.
5. Multiple alleles never show complementation with each other. By complementation test the allelic and non-allelic genes may be differentiated well.
6. The wild type (normal) allele is nearly always dominant while the other mutant alleles in the series may show dominance or there may be an intermediate phenotypic effect.

7. When any two of the multiple alleles are crossed, the phenotype is of a mutant type and not the wild type.

8. Further, F2 generations from such crosses show typical monohybrid ratio for the concerned character.

Examples of Multiple Alleles

Wings of Drosophila

In *Drosophila* wings are normally long. There occurred two mutations at the same locus in different flies, one causing vestigial (reduced) wings and other mutation causing antlered (less developed) wings. Both vestigial and antlered are alleles of the same normal gene and also of each other and are recessive to the normal gene.

Suppose vestigial is represented by the symbol 'vg' and antlered wing by 'vg^a'. The normal allele is represented by the symbol +.

Thus, there are three races of *Drosophila*:

1. Long ++ (+/+)

2. Vestigial vg vg (vg/vg)

3. Antlered vg^a vg^a (vg^a/vg^a)

A cross between a long winged normal fly and another having vestigial wings or antlered wings is represented in Fig. 3.10.

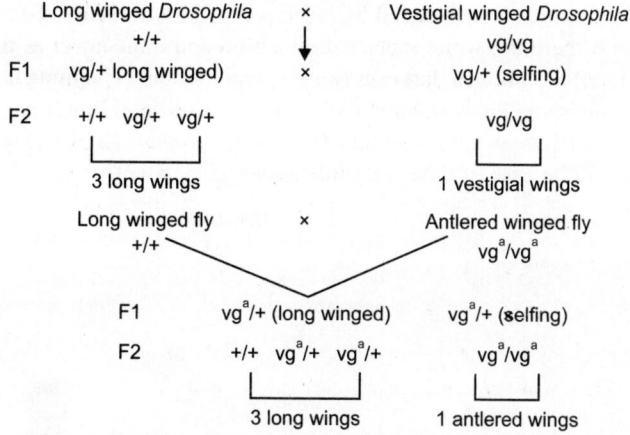

Fig. 3.10: Inheritance presentation of multiple alleles in *Drosophila*.

When a fly with vestigial wing is crossed with another fly having antlered wings, the F1 hybrids are intermediate in wing length showing that none of the mutated gene is dominant over the other. This hybrid is some times said as the vestigial antlered compound and contains two mutated genes at the same locus. They show Mendelian segregation and recombination (Fig. 3.11).

Besides the vestigial and antlered wing described above there are several other mutations occurring at the same locus and resulting in nicked wings, strap wings or no wings, etc. These are all multiple alleles.

Vestigial winged fly   ×   Antlered winged fly
vg/vg   vg^a/vg^a

F1   vg/vg^a (intermediate)   ×   vg/vg^a (selfing)

F2   vg/vg   vg/vg^a, vg/vg^a vg^a/vg^a
(vestigial)   (intermediate)   (Antlered)
1   :   2   :   1

Fig. 3.11: Cross representation between a vestigial and an antlered winged fly.

Close linkage versus allelism: If we assume that these mutant genes, vestigial and antlered are not allelic located at different loci in place of locating at same locus in different chromosomes so closely linked that there is no crossing over between them, the mutant gene will suppress the expression of adjacent normal allele to certain extent.

These closely linked genes are called pseudo alleles and this suppression is the result of position effect. Thus, visible or apparent cases of allelism may be explained on the assumption of close linkage.

Another example of multiple alleles is the eye colour in *Drosophila*. The normal colour of the eye is red. Mutation changed this red eye colour to white. Other mutations at white locus took place changing the red eye colour to various lighter shades like cherry, apricot, eosin, creamy, ivory, blood, etc. are also visible and are due to multiple alleles. A cross between the two mutant forms, produces intermediate type in the F1 except white and apricot races which are not alleles but closely linked genes.

Coat colour in rabbit

The colour of the skin in rabbits is influenced by a series of multiple alleles. The normal colour of the skin is brown. Besides it there are white races called albino and Himalayan as the mutant races. The Himalayan is similar to albino but has darker nose, ear, feet and tail. The mutant genes albino (a) and Himalayan (a^h) occupy the same locus and are allelic. Both albino and Himalayan are recessive to their normal allele (+). A cross between an albino and Himalayan produces a Himalayan in the F1 and not intermediate as is usual in the case of other multiple alleles (Fig. 3.12).

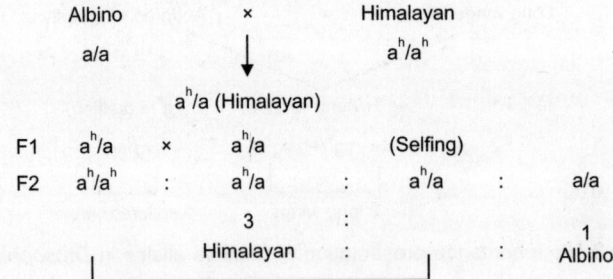

Albino   ×   Himalayan
a/a   a^h/a^h

a^h/a (Himalayan)

F1   a^h/a   ×   a^h/a   (Selfing)
F2   a^h/a^h :   a^h/a   :   a^h/a   :   a/a
3   :   1
Himalayan   :   :   Albino

Fig. 3.12: Representing a cross between an albino and himalayan races of rabbits.

Self-sterility in plants

Kolreuter described self-sterility in tobacco (*Nicotiana longiflora*). The reason was done by East. He described that self-sterility is due to series of alleles designated as s_1, s_2, s_3 and s_4, etc. The hybrids S_1/S_2 or S_1/S_3 or S_3/S_4 are self-sterile because pollen grains from these varieties did not develop, but pollens of S_1/S_2 were effective and capable of fertilisation with S_3/S_4.

The genes causing self-sterility in plants probably produce their effects by controlling the growth rate of the pollen tubes. In compatible combinations, the pollen tube grows more and more rapidly as it approaches the ovule, but in non-suitable ones, the growth of the pollen tube slows down considerably, so that the flower withers away before fertilisation can take place.

Blood groups in man

Several genes in man produce multiple allelic series which affect an interesting and important physiological characteristic of the human red blood cells. The red blood cells have special antigens properties by which they respond to certain specific components (antibodies) of the blood serum.

The antigen-antibody relationship is one of the great specificity like that between lock and key. Each antigen and its associated antibody has a peculiear chemical configuration. Landsteiner discovered in 1900 that when the red cells of one person are placed in the blood serum of another person, the cells become clumped or agglutinated.

If blood transfusions were made between persons of two such incompatible blood groups, the transfused cells were likely to clump and shut out the capillaries in the recipient, some times resulting in death. However, such reactions occurred only when the cells of certain individuals were placed in serum from certain other persons. It was found that all persons could be classified in to four groups with regard to the antigen property of the blood cells.

Large number of persons have been classified in to these four groups by means of the agglutination test and the distribution of blood groups in the offspring of parents of known blood groups has been studied. The evidence shows that these blood properties are determined by a series of three allelic genes I^A, I^B and i, as follows:

Blood groups	Genotype
AB	$I^A I^B$
B	$I^B I^B$ or $I^B i$
A	$I^A I^A$ or $I^A i$
O	ii

I^A is a gene for the production of the anti-gin A. I^B for antigen B, and i for neither antigen. The existence of these alleles in man and the case with which the blood groups can be identified have obvious practical applications in blood transfusion, cases of disputed percentage and description of human populations.

The alleles of these genes which affect a variety of biochemical properties of the blood, act in such a way that in the heterozygous compound $I^A I^B$, each allele exhibits its own characteristics and specific effect. The cells of the heterozygote contain both antigens A and B. On the other hand, I^A and I^B both show complete dominance over i, which lacks both antigens. Table 3.1 showing possible blood types of children from parents of various blood groups.

'Rhesus' blood group in man

A very interesting series of alleles affecting the antigens of human blood has been discovered through the work of Landsteiner, Wiener, Race, Levine, Sanger, Mourant and several others. The original discovery was that the red cells are agglutinated by a serum prepared by immunising rabbits against the blood of Rhesus monkey. The antigen responsible for this reaction was consequently called as Rhesus factor and the gene that causes this property was denoted as R-r or Rh-rh.

Table 3.1: Possible blood types of children from parents of various blood groups.

Parents		Children	
Phenotypes	*Genotypes*	*Phenotypes*	*Genotypes*
O × O	ii × ii	O	ii
O × A	ii × I^AI^A or I^Ai	O, A	ii,I^Ai
O × B	ii × I^BI^B or I^Bi	O, B	ii, I^Bi
O × AB	ii × I^AI^B	A, B	I^Ai, I^Bi
A × A	I^AI^A or I^Ai × I^AI^A or I^Ai	A, O	I^AI^A, ii
A × B	I^AI^A or I^Ai × I^BI^B or I^Bi	A, AB, O, B	I^Ai, I^AI^B, ii, I^Bi
A × AB	I^AI^A or I^Ai × I^AI^B	A, B, AB	I^AI^A, I^Bi, I^AI^B
B × B	I^BI^B or I^Bi × I^BI^B or I^Bi	B, O	I^BI^B, ii
B × AB	I^BI^B or I^BI × I^AI^B	A, B, AB	I^AI^A, I^BI^B, I^AI^B
AB × AB	I^AI^B × I^AI^B	A, B, AB	I^AI^A, I^BI^B, I^AI^B

Interest in this factor was stimulated by Levine's study of a characteristic form of anaemia, known as Erythroblastosis foetalis, which occurs occasionally in new born infants. It was found that the infants suffering from this anaemia are usually Rh-positive and so are their fathers, but their mothers are Rh⁻ negative. The origin of the disease was explained as follows: The Rh⁺ foetus developing in the uterus of an Rh⁻ mother causes the formation of mother's blood stream of anti Rh antibodies.

These antibodies, especially as a result of a succession of several Rh⁺ pregnancies, gain sufficient strength in the mother's blood so that they may attack the red blood cells of the foetus. The reaction between these antibodies of the mother and the red cells of her unborn child provokes haemolysis and anaemia, this may be serious enough to cause the death of the newborn infant or abortion of the foetus.

The blood stream of a mother who has had an erythroblastotic infant is a much more potent and convenient reagent than sera of rabbits, immunised by blood of rhesus monkey's for testing the blood of other persons to distinguish Rh⁺ from Rh⁻ individuals using such sera from woman who had erythroblastotic infants, it was discovered that: there exist not one but several kinds of Rh⁺ and Rh⁻ persons. There are several different Rh antigens which are detected by specific antisera.

Thus, an Rh⁻ woman immunised during pregnancy by the Rh⁺ children may have in her blood serum antibodies, that agglutinate not only Rh⁺ red cells but also cells from a few persons known to be Rh⁻.

By selective absorption two kinds of antibodies may be separated from such a serum, one known as anti-D which agglutinates (= coagulates) only Rh⁺ cells, the other known as anti-C which agglutinates particular rare types of Rh⁻. Another specific antibody, known as anti-c agglutinates all cells that lack C.

With these three antisera, six types of blood can be recognised. Studies of parent and children show that persons of type Cc are heterozygous for an allele C determining C anti-gena. CC persons are homozygous for C and cc are homozygous for c. There is obviously no dominance, each allele producing its own antigen in the heterozygote as in the AB blood type.

No anti serum is available for detecting d, the alternative to D. D⁺ persons may be heterozygous or homozygous. However, the genotypes of such persons may be diagnosis from their progeny, for example D⁺ person who has a d⁻ child is thereby shown to be Dd.

Two other specific antibodies, anti-E and anti-c have been found. These detect the antigens E and e determined by a pair of alleles E and e. The three elementary types of antigens C-c, D and E-e, occur in fixed combinations that are always inherited together as alleles of a single gene. Wiener and Fisher showed the existence of a series of eight different alternative arrangements of these three types of Rh antigens and expressed them by means of following symbols.

The Rh system of alleles:

Fisher's symbols	Wiener's symbols	
CDE	R^z	
CDe	R^1	
cDE	R^2	Rh-Positive
cDE	R^0	
CdE	r^Y	
Cde	r'	
cdE	r''	Rh-Negative
cde	r	

Thus, allelism is determined by cross-breeding experiments. If one gene behaves as dominant to another the conclusion is that they are alleles and that they occupy identical loci in homologous chromosomes when two genes behave as dominant to other gene. They should occupy identical loci in the chromosome. When more than a pair of alleles occur in respect of any character in inheritance the phenomenon is known as multiple allelism.

There is not much difference between the two theories of Wiener and Fisher. Wiener opinion is that there are multiple variations of one gene whereas according to the view of Fisher three different genes lying very close together are responsible for differences.

Pleiotropism: The opposite of polygene effect is known as pleiotropism, i.e. a single gene influence or govern many characters. For example, gene for vestigial wing influence the nature of halters (modified balancers of *Drosophila*). The halters are not normal but reduced in flies with vestigial wings. The vestigial gene also affects position of dorsal bristles which instead of being horizontal turn out to be vertical.

This gene also affects the shape of spermatheca, i.e. the shape of spermatheca is changed, the number of egg strings in the ovaries is decreased compared to normal when the vestigial larvae are well fed but relatively increased when they are poorly fed, length of life and fruitfulness or fertility are lowered, and there are still other differences.

Theories of allelism:

Various theories have been put forward to explain the nature of allelism origin and occurrence.

1. Theory of point mutation: According to this theory multiple alleles have developed as a result of mutations occurring at same locus but in different directions. Hence all the different wing lengths of *Drosophila* are necessarily the result of mutations which have occurred at same long normal wing locus in different directions.

2. Theory of close linkage or positional *Pseudoallelism*: According to this view the multiple alleles are not the gene mutations at same locus but they occupy different loci closely situated in the chromosome. These genes closely linked at different loci are said to as pseudo alleles and affect the expression of their normal genes, i.e. position effect.

3. Heterochromatin theory of Allelism: Occasionally heterochromatin becomes associated with the genes as a result of chromosomal breakage and rearrangement. These heterochromatin particles suppress the nature of genes in question due to position effect.

In maize the position effect are some times due to transposition (act of changing place or order) of very minute particles of heterochromatin. There are also sign or token that particles of different kinds of heterochromatin suppress the expression of normal gene to different degrees.

In *Drosophila* the apricot might be a partially suppressed red (normal) and white completely suppressed red while apricot and white hybrid may give rise to red or intermediate by unequal crossing over. The above theories in some way or other do not explain clearly the particular case of allelism and it is possible that all the three theories are applicable in different cases.

Importance of Multipie Allelism

The study of multiple alleles has increased our knowledge of heredity. According to T.H. Morgan a great knowledge of the nature of gene has come from multiple alleles. These alleles suggest that a gene can mutate in different ways causing different effects. Multiple allelism also put forward the idea that different amounts of heterochromatin prevent the genes to different degree or space.

1. Pseudo alleles: Alleles are different forms of the same gene located at the corresponding loci or the same locus. Sometimes it has been found that non-homologous genes which are situated at near but different loci affect the same character in the same manner as if they are different forms or alleles of the same gene. They are said as pseudo alleles. These pseudo alleles which are closely linked show recombinations by crossing over unlike the alleles.

2. Penetrance and expressivity: Simply a recessive gene produces its phenotypic effect in homozygous condition and a dominant gene produces its phenotypic effect whether in homozygous or heterozygous condition. Some genes fail to produce their phenotypic effect when they should. The ability of a gene to produce its effect is called penetrance. The percentage of penetrance may be altered by changing the environmental conditions such as moisture, light intensity, temperature, etc. A gene that always produces the expected effect is said to have 100 per cent penetrance. If its phenotypic effect is produced only 60 per cent of the individuals that contains it then it is said to show 60 per cent penetrance. In Gossypium a mutant gene produces crinkled leaf. While all the leaves produced in the normal season are crinkled but some of the leaves which are produced late in the season do not show this character and are normal. It represents that penetrance is zero or in other words the gene is non-penetrant. Sometimes there is great variation in the manner in which a character is expressed in different plants. In Lima beans there is a variety named venturra where a dominant gene is responsible for tips and margins of the leaves of the seedlings to be partially deficient in chlorophyll. Sometimes only the margins are effected and sometimes only the tips. In other words, this single gene may express itself in a variety of ways that may resemble a number of characters. This gene is then to exhibit variable expressivity. Whether a gene is expressed at all is denoted by the term penetrance whereas the term expressivity denotes the degree of its expression.

3. Lsoalleles: Sometimes, a dominant gene occurs in two or more forms. These multiple dominant alleles will produce the same phenotypic effect in homozygous condition but their effect will show a small difference in heterozygous state. In *Drosophila*, thus, the gene for red eye colour is dominant over white. The red gene will produce dark red colour in the homozygous condition but in combination with the white allele the gene for red colour produces a dark red colour in flies from Soviet Russia but the same combination in the flies coming from the USA produces a light red colour. It does mean that dominant gene for red colour occurs in two forms. These are said as isoalleles.

4. Phenocopy: Characters are the result of interaction between the genotype and the environment. When a gene mutates, its phenotypic effect also changes. Some times, a change in the environment

produces a visible change in the phenotype of the normal gene which resembles the effect as already known mutant. The effect of the normal gene under the changed environment is a mimic or imitation of the mutant gene. Such an imitation induced by environmental changes has been termed as phenocopy by Goldschmidt. In fowls, a mutant gene is responsible for the character, ruinplessness, in which the caudal vertebrate and tail feathers do not develop. Rumplessness is also induced as a phenocopy when normal eggs which do not have the gene for rumplessness, are treated with insulin before incubation. Phenocopies of other mutant genes are also produced in *Drosophila* by high temperature treatment of the larvae for short periods. It has also been found that different or non- allelic genes can produce the same phenotype. This phenomenon is said as genetic mimic or genocopy.

5. Xenia and Metaxenia: The immediate effect of foreign pollen on visible characters of the endosperm is called xenia. The 'xenia' term was given by Focke (1800). This has been studied in maize plant. If a white endosperm variety is open pollinated in the field where there are also plants of the yellow endosperm variety then the cobs that develop will contain a mixture of yellow and white seeds. The yellow colour of the endosperm in the yellow seeds is the result of fertilisation by pollen from the yellow variety. The yellow colour indicates that the seeds are hybrids and the white seeds are homozygous. The yellow colour of the endosperm is dominant over white and when the plants raised from the yellow seeds are self-pollinated, yellow and white seeds are produced in the ratio of 3:1. Another example of xenia may be exemplified. If a sweet corn (maize) is pollinated by a starchy variety, the endosperm is starchy because the starchy gene introduced by the pollen is dominant over its sugary allele.

6. Metaxenia: It is the term used to describe the effect of foreign pollen on other tissues belonging to the mother plant, outside the endosperm and embryo. It is sometimes evident in the fruit and seed coats. In cucurbitaceous fruits, the skin colour is affected by the pollen grains, in oranges, the colour and flavour of the fruit is influenced by the pollen parent. The same is true of fuzziness and hair length in cotton. It has been suggested that metaxenia effects may be due to certain hormones secreted by the endosperm and embryo.

ONE GENE AND MANY PHENOTYPES

Phenotype descriptions are valuable information right at the interface of medicine and biology. With the rapid advancement in the field of genetics, thousands of genes involved in human diseases have been cloned. It was expected that knowledge of mutations would lead to consistent genotype-phenotype correlations. The understanding of mechanisms underlying genotype-phenotype discrepancies is important, as it will move clinical genetics towards predictive medicine, allowing better selection of therapeutic strategies and individualised counselling of persons affected with genetic disorders.

Phenotype descriptions are valuable information right at the interface of medicine and biology. Their main value lies in helping to dissect the relationships between diseases and genes, in clinical application in genetic counselling and prenatal diagnosis. The phenotype can be thought of as a product of genes interacting with each other and with the environment. A concise definition of a gene, taking into account complex patterns of regulation and transcription, genic conservation and non-coding RNA genes, has been proposed by Gerstein and others. A gene is a union of genomic sequences encoding a coherent set of potentially overlapping functional products.

Mutations in different genes can lead to similar phenotype, e.g. hereditary spherocytosis can be due to mutations in the genes encoding for spectrin, ankyrin. In contrast, mutations in one gene could cause multiple phenotypes, as best illustrated in the case of lamin A/C, whereby mutations can cause 13 different diseases. With rapid advancement in the field of genetics, thousands of genes involved in human diseases have been cloned. It was expected that knowledge of mutations would lead to consistent genotype-phenotype correlations, clarifying why a given genetic change results in a particular phenotype. However, genotype-phenotype correlation is often incomplete. Monogenic diseases provide the simplest models for studying genotype-phenotype relationships. The understanding of mechanisms underlying genotypephenotype discrepancies is important, as it will move clinical genetics towards predictive medicine, allowing better selection of therapeutic strategies and individualised counselling of persons affected with genetic disorders.

One gene, many mutations, many phenotypes

Allelic heterogeneity: This phenomenon, whereby different mutations at the same locus result in different phenotypes. It is very interesting to know that mutations at a single locus can lead to diseases with entirely different clinical features. For example, mutations in the RET gene have been implicated in the etiology of Hirshprung disease as well as multiple endocrine neoplasia (MEN) Type 2. The underlying mechanism is either quantitative or qualitative change in the gene product. Some of the examples of allelic heterogeneity have been listed in (Table 3.2).

Table 3.2: Selected examples of allelic heterogeneity.

Disease	Gene	Disease
Huler syndrome	IDUA	Scheie syndrome
Charcot-marie-tooth neuropathy	PMP22	Hereditary neuropathy with pressure palsy
Hyperkalemic periodic paralysis	SCN4A	Paramyotonia congenita
Creutzfeldt-jacob disease	PRNP	Familial fatal insomnia
Pseudohypoparathyroidism IA	GNAS1	Albright hereditary osteodystrophy
Kennedy disease	AR	Androgen insensitivity
Cystic fi brosis	CFTR	Congenital bilateral absence of vas deference
Duchenne muscular dystrophy	DMD	Becker muscular dystrophy
Hirschsprung disease	RET	Multiple endocrine neoplasia type 2

Non functional vs partially functional/truncated gene product

Duchenne and Becker muscular dystrophies are caused by mutations in the dystrophin gene. Mutations that partially inactivate the gene product cause Becker muscular dystrophy (BMD), while mutations which completely inactivate the gene product produce Duchenne muscular dystrophy (DMD).

Loss of function vs gain of function

Phenotype resulting from reduction in the amount of normal protein is called loss of function, while gain of function mutations, also known as neomorphic, are characterised by the ability of the mutant allele product to perform new functions. Example of that is *RET* gene which codes for a tyrosine kinase receptor. Loss of function mutations in *RET* gene that lead to nonfunctional product or lower expression of *RET* gene give rise to Hirschsprung disease. Gain of function mutations at the same locus that produce constitutively activated receptors lead to MEN Type 2. Similarly, loss of function mutations at FGFR1 locus cause an autosomal dominant form of Kallman syndrome characterised by anosmia and hypogonadotropic hypogonadism, also cause lacrimo-auriculodento-digital (LADD) syndrome. The gain of function mutations at the same site lead to a form of craniosynostosis (Pfeiffer syndrome). Also in the fibroblast growth factor receptor 3 (FGFR3), point mutations in specific domains are associated with autosomal dominant dwarfism and craniosynostosis syndromes such as hypochondroplasia, achondroplasia the most common form of skeletal dysplasia), severe achondroplasia with developmental delay and acanthosis nigricans (SADDAN), thanatophoric dysplasia, Crouzon syndrome with acanthosis nigricans and Muenke coronal craniosynostosis. Several reports have demonstrated that these mutations lead to constitutive activation of the receptors. In contrast with the inhibitory role on bone growth, an oncogenic role for FGFR3 in human cancer has emerged. Somatic activating mutations in FGFR3 have been reported in multiple myeloma and, more recently, in two epithelial malignancies, i.e. bladder-and cervix carcinomas. Nearly all mutations identified in bladder tumours are identical to the activating mutations responsible for thanatophoric dysplasia, a lethal form of dwarfism. Several genes play important role in embryogenesis have also been shown to play a role in causing cancer (Table 3.3).

Table 3.3: Genes that can cause both developmental anomalies and cancer.

Gene	Chromosome	Developmental anomaly	Cancer
PAX3	2q35	Waardenburg syndrome type 1	Alveolar rhabdomyosarcoma
KIT	4q12	Piebaldism	Mast cell leukemia
PTCH	9q22	Gorlin	Basal cell carcinoma
RET	10p11	Hirschsprung	MEN2A, MEN2B, thyroid carcinoma
WT1	11p13	Denys-drash	Wilms tumer

Pleiotropy

The term pleiotropy comes from the Greek pleion, meaning 'many' and trepein, meaning 'influencing'. Pleiotropy has been challenged by the remarkably diverse syndromes that can result from different mutations in the same gene, for example the LAMNA gene and X-linked filamin A gene. Mutations in LAMNA gene may cause Emery-Dreifuss muscular dystrophy, a form of limb girdle muscular dystrophy, a form of Charcot-Marie-Tooth disease, dilated cardiomyopathy, Dunnigan type familial partial lipodystrophy, mandibuloacral dysplasia and the very rare condition Hutchinson-Gilford progeria. Mutation in the filamin A gene have recently been implicated in the distinct, though overlapping, X-linked dominant dysmorphic conditions oto-palato-digital syndrome, Melnick-Needles syndrome and frontometaphyseal dysplasia and periventricular nodular hetertopia.

Antagonistic pleiotropy refers to the expression of a gene resulting in multiple competing effects, some beneficial but others detrimental to the organism. This is central to a theory of aging first developed by Williams. Williams, suggested that some genes responsible for increased fitness in the younger, fertile organism contribute to decreased fitness later in life.

One such example in male humans is the gene for the hormone testosterone. In youth, testosterone has positive effects including reproductive fitness but, later in life, there are negative effects such as increased susceptibility to prostate cancer. Another example is the p53 gene which suppresses cancer, but also suppresses stem cells which replenish worn-out tissue.

One Gene, One Mutation, Many Phenotypes

The phenomenon of allelic heterogeneity is not unexpected, as the gene product may get differentially changed by the different mutations and so the phenotypes. More surprising is the fact that individuals with similar genetic lesions can have significantly different clinical manifestations. This is well observed in autosomal dominant disorders, where 'variable expressivity' and 'reduced penetrance' have been classically described. Expressivity is defined as the severity of the phenotype. When the severity of disease differs in people with same genotype, the phenotype is said to have variable expressivity. Penetrance is the proportion of persons with a particular genotype who manifest the disease. The reduced penetrance leads to 'skipping of generation'. Neurofi-bromatosis Type 1(NF1) is characterised by extreme clinical variability, not only between unrelated individuals and among affected individuals within a single family but even within a single individual with NF1 at different times in life. The mutation in the NF1 gene can produce different lesions in different tissues such as cafe-au-lait spots, neurofibroma, iris hamartoma, skeletal abnormalities or mental retardation. Each of these pleiotropic effects can have varying severity among the affected family members (variable expressivity). The mechanisms underlying such clinical variations are often unclear. It is supposed to be the result of the modifying effects of other genes, as well as due to interaction with environmental factors.

Other Mechanisms for Phenotypic Heterogeneity of Monogenic Disease

There are a variety of other mechanisms that may be responsible for generating phenotypic diversity of diseases that are encoded at a single locus, Some of these, which have been loosely labelled epigenetic, are understood, at least in principle, although the molecular mechanisms involved have not been established and the prediction of the phenotype from the underlying genotype may be extremely difficult.

Mosaicism (gene dosage effect): Mosaicism is the existence of two cell lines with different genetic constitution that have been derived from a single zygote. The phenotypic severity is determined by the proportion of cells carrying the mutation. This is best exemplified in mitochondrial disorders. There are thousands of mitochondrial DNA (mtDNA) molecules in a cell. When a mutation occurs in the mtDNA, it is at first present in only one of the mtDNA molecules. At cell division, the mtDNA molecules replicate and sort randomly among the daughter cells. Each daughter cell may receive very different proportions of mitochondria carrying normal and mutant mtDNA. The phenotype will depend upon three factors: The relative abundance of mutant mtDNA (heteroplasmy), the tissue distribution of the mutant mtDNAs and the vulnerability of each tissue to impaired oxidative metabolism (threshold effect). Thus, reduced penetrance, variable expression and pleiotropy are typical features of kindred with mitochondrial disorders. For example, a deletion of 4977 bp of mtDNA is commonly encountered in Kearns-Sayre syndrome (characterised by the triad of pigmentary retinopathy, external ophthalmoplegia and onset before the age of 20 years). The same deletion has also been identified in cases of Pearson syndrome (sideroblastic anemia, exocrine pancreatic dysfunction) and progressive external ophthalmoplegia.

The different phenotypes from the same deletion are due to tissue distribution of the defect. If the defect is present in mitochondria of all tissues, the phenotype is Kearns-Sayre syndrome. In Pearson syndrome, the defect is localised mainly to the hematopoietic tissue, while the defect is confined to the skeletal tissues in progressive external ophthalmoplegia. Another striking example of phenotypic diversity arising from mosaicism is the androgen insensitivity syndrome (AIS). Androgen insensitivity syndrome is the major cause of male pseudohermaphroditism. It is an X-linked disorder caused by mutations in androgen receptor (AR) gene. Androgen insensitivity syndrome can be subdivided into three highly variable phenotypes: complete AIS, when the affected persons have female external genitalia, partial AIS, when the genitalia are ambiguous and mild AIS, when the affected individuals have normal male external genitalia. In a number of cases, identical mutations have resulted in significantly different phenotypes. This is due to somatic mosaicism. The co-expression of wild allele shifts the AIS subtype to a higher degree of virilisation than expected from the mutant allele alone.

Trinucleotide repeat expansion: Also known as triplet repeat expansion, is the DNA mutation responsible for causing any type of disorder categorised as a trinucleotide repeat disorder. These are labelled in dynamical genetics as dynamic mutations. At least 12 neurological diseases are known to result from expansion of CTG, CGG, CAG or GAA repeats. Fragile-X syndrome, which is a common cause of mental retardation in males, is a good example of how phenotypic, heterogeneity can be generated by expansion of regions containing trinucleotide repeats, in normal individuals, a DNA segment at Xq27,3 contains between six and 60 copies of the repeat CGG, in some persons, the number is increased to between 60 and 200. In this case, the disorder is clinically silent, premutations of this kind are characteristic of normal-transmitting males and some mentally normal female carriers. Full mutations, which arise in the offspring of pre-mutation carriers, consist of many hundreds or thousands of copies, of the repeat and lead to the full expression of the clinical phenotype. Heterozygous carriers have an extremely variable pheno type: Approximately 50% of females carrying the full mutation, how some mental impairment although those who carry a pre-mutation are usually normal. Similarly, female carriers may or may not show some of the somatic changes associated with the disease in males. Although X inactivation may be partly responsible, this does not seem to be the whole story. Huntington's disease, another neurodegenerative dis order, also shows considerable phenotypic heterogeneity, particularly with respect to age of onset and rate of progression, At the 5′- region of the locus involved there is a CAG repeat sequence, which ranges from ten to 30 copies in normal individuals and which is expanded to beyond 35 copies in patients with Huntington's disease, there appears to be some relationship between the length of the repeats and age of onset. Remarkably, the juvenile onset of cases shows a preponderance of paternal transmission. In 2007 a new disease model was produced to explain the progression of Huntington's Disease and similar trinucleotide repeat disorders, which, seems to accurately predict age of onset and the way the disease will progress in an individual, based on the number of repeats of a genetic mutation. Overall these conditions show considerable phenotypic heterogenity. This is reflected at the molecular level, where there is a wide variation in the extension of the length of the repeats required to produce an abnormal phenotype, not all diseases are associated with a premutation length and the relationship between the expansion of trinucleotide repeats and the causation of the disease is not clear. In some cases, those in which the repeats involve promoters, it is thought that methylation of the promoter region lead to gene silencing while in those that involve CAG repeats it is thought that polyglutamine expansion may play a role. But what is clear is that genotypic instability of this type is responsible for neurodegenerative disorders with widely differing phenotypes.

X- Inactivation

X-inactivation in females is usually random, because of that female carriers for a particular X-linked trait are in effect, mosaics, with each cell population functionally hemizygous for a particular trait. Hence carriers would be expected to produce approximately half of an abnormal gene product or express about the same amount of a product. However, because X inactivation occurs early during embryogenesis, there is wide variation in the expression of X-linked mutant genes in females, considerable skewing of the distribution of values is encountered. Interestingly, there is a high frequency of discordant phenotypes, among twins with Xlinked diseases, this may be because X inactivation preceeds twinning and non-randomness reflects asymmetrical splitting of the inner cell mass, furthermore, it seems likely that some X-linked disorders may have a deleterious effect on cell function during early embryogenesis, a phenomenon that may lead to extreme skewing of the distribution of cell populations. The situation is further complicated by the fact that not all parts of the X chromosome are inactivated. These different issues make for considerable hetero geneity in the expression of mutant gene's in female carriers for X-linked disorders. There is increasing evidence that negative selection may be a major factor for the skewed distribution of cell populations in female carriers. For example, Coleman and others described a female with the genes for both incontinentia pigmenti and haemophilia A. It appeared that the presence of the gene for incontinentia pigmenti on an X chromosome had unmasked the factor VIII gene mutation on the other chromosome, presumably by negative selection of the former. Another example is female carriers of hemophilia and DMD may occasionally show mild or even full expression of the disease. This is due to nonrandom inactivation of X chromosome, as by chance, most of the X chromosomes carrying the normal allele get inactivated resulting in clinical expression of the disease.

Phenotypic Heterogeneity due to the interaction of Alleles at different Loci

Retinitis pigmentosa is the name given to a set of inherited degeneration of the retina. This condition is very heterogeneous, both clinically and with respect to inheritance. It is X- linked, however both autosomal dominant and recessive forms have been described. Kajiwara and others reported three families in which a form of retinitis pigmentosa segregated, affected individuals were double heterozygotes for a specific peripherin- RDS gene mutation and a mutation in a second gene, ROM1. It is thought that the products of these two loci. which are on different chromosome, interact non-convalently in the rim region of the photoreceptor outer segment disc membrane. Persons heterozygous for only one of these mutations have no symptoms. Another condition that shows marked phenotypic heterogeneity is inherited porphyria cutanea tarda in which heterozygotes are predisposed to photosensitive cutaneous lesions. The phenotype seems to be exacerbated by a variety of enviromental factors, including iron overload and alcohol abuse. The condition results from a deficiency of uroporphyrinogen decarboxylase (URO-D). Not all patients with mutations at the gene that encodes URO-D are symptomatic. Recently it has been found that there is an increased frequency of the alleles of the haemochromatosis gene, notably C282Y AND H63D, in both Argentinian and Italian patients with porphyria culanea tarda.

Since the haemochromatosis alleles are associated with increased iron absorption and iron overload and because iron loading exacerbates porphyria cutanea tarda, it seems likely that this is another example of the deleterious interaction of two alleles, in this case with completely different functions.

Modifier Genes

A modifier gene is defined as an inherited genetic variation that affects the phenotypic expression of another gene. It can affect the pleiotropy, penetrance or expressivity of the disease. Depending upon the nature of modifying effect, modifier genes might cause more severe phenotypes, less severe phenotypes, novel phenotypes or wild-type (normal) phenotypes.

Modifier causing less severe (reduced) phenotype of beta thalassemia: The severity of anemia in beta thalassemia reflects the degree of globin chain imbalance. The excess of alpha globin chain precipitates in red cell precursors leading to ineffective erythropoiesis. This imbalance can be genetically modified by two factors-variation in amount of gamma globin response and alpha globin chain production. The beta thalassemia patients who coinherit alpha globin gene deletions will have less redundant alpha globin chains and tend to have less severe phenotype.

Similarly, increased synthesis of gamma globin chain will reduce the disease severity by increasing HbF level. The gamma globin response is also genetically determined. There are many other loci that are not linked to the beta globin gene but modify HbF response. Linkage studies have mapped these loci to three regions of the genome-chromosome 6q23, 8q11 and Xp22.28.

Modifiers causing more severe (enhanced) phenotype: The severity of anemia in beta thalassemia depends on the degree of globin chain imbalance. It is an autosomal recessive condition. The heterozygotes for beta thalassemia mutations are clinically asymptomatic as the degree of imbalance is insignificant. But, the coinheritance of extra alpha globin genes (alpha triplication) increases the imbalance. This leads to symptomatic disease in heterozygotes, sometimes manifesting as 'intermedia' phenotype.

Alternative splicing

Alternative mRNA splicing is another mechanism responsible for different expression of a similar genotype. Two illustrative examples are given below.

Duchenne muscular dystrophy and BMD are caused by mutations in the dystrophin gene: Duchenne muscular dystrophy is a severe muscle-wasting disease arising from defects in the dystrophin gene, typically nonsense or frameshift mutations that preclude the synthesis of a functional protein. Becker muscular dystrophy generally arises from in-frame deletions that allow synthesis of a shorter but still semifunctional protein. But, nonsense mutations which should cause DMD have been reported in BMD. This is due to alternative mRNA splicing-skipping of the affected exon leads to removal of the nonsense mutation from the dystrophin mRNA. This results in production of partially functional dystrophin and BMD phenotype.

Cystic fibrosis is an autosomal recessive disorder: The genotype delta F508/R117H can lead to either severe phenotype of cystic fibrosis leading to respiratory failure or the milder phenotype, in which the only manifestation is congenital bilateral absence of vas deferens (CBAVD). The CFTR gene has two intron 8 variants. One is associated with efficient mRNA splicing, while the other causes inefficient splicing. The R117H allele is capable of producing partially functional protein. The R117H allele associated with efficient splicing leads to production of some amount of partially functional protein and hence milder phenotype (CBAVD). On the other hand, severe phenotype results if the intron 8 variant causes inefficient splicing and production of nonfunctional protein.

Epigenetic mechanisms

The term epigenetics refers to changes in gene expression caused by environmental factors, not by changes in the underlying DNA sequence. These changes may remain through cell divisions for the remainder of the cell's life. Sometimes the changes last for multiple generations. The Greek prefix epi- in epigenetics implies features that are on top of or in addition to genetics, thus epigenetic traits exist on top of or in addition to the traditional molecular basis for inheritance. Epigenetic phenomena modulate when and at what level genes are expressed. Thus, the expression of a mutation also depends upon the activity state of the locus carrying it, the mere presence of a genetic defect may not be enough for clinical expression. Epigenetic effects in humans include the following:

Genomic imprinting and related disorders: The term 'imprinted gene' refers to genes whose expression is conditioned by their parental origin. The expression of a gene depends upon the parent who passed on the gene. For example, two different diseases - Prader-Willi syndrome and Angelman syndrome - are due to deletion of the same part of chromosome 15. When the deletion involves the chromosome 15 inherited from the father, the child has Prader-Willi syndrome, but when the deletion involves the chromosome 15 inherited from the mother, the child has Angelman syndrome. This is a striking example of how the parental origin of a genetic defect influences the clinical phenotype. Beckwith-Wiedemann syndrome is also associated with genomic imprinting, often caused by abnormalities in maternal genomic imprinting of a region on chromosome 11.

Transgenerational epigenetic observations: Marcus Pembrey and colleagues also observed that the paternal (but not maternal) grandsons of Swedish boys who were exposed to famine in the 19th century were less likely to die of cardiovascular disease, if food was plentiful then diabetes mortality in the grandchildren increased, suggesting that this was a transgenerational epigenetic inheritance.

Gene and environment

Virtually all human diseases result from the complex interplay of genetic susceptibility factors and modifiable environmental factors. This is most obvious in the context of common illnesses such as diabetes, coronary artery disease or cancer. But, environmental factors play a significant role in the expression of monogenic disorders too. For example, inherited metabolic disorders manifest when there is introduction of the substrate for which the metabolism is defective. Similar genetic defects may have different phenotypes if the environmental factors are not similar.

COMPLEMENTATION ANALYSIS

Complementation analysis is used to determine whether two independent mutations are alterations in the same gene, that is, they are alleles, or are alterations in different genes. In essence, a complementation analysis is a functional test used to define a gene. If a researcher has isolated a number of mutants with a similar phenotype, the next question asked is: How many genes have I identified?. If there are 10 mutant strains, are they each in different genes, does each mutant carry a different mutation (allele) in the same gene, or something in between such as two genes one with six alleles and the other with four alleles? Complementation analysis will help answer this question.

Seymour Benzer's study of the *rII* locus of phage T4 is a most elegant example of the power of complementation analysis. Benzer had several hundred mutations that gave the same phenotype, large plaques on one host strain of *E. coli* and no plaques on another host strain, and mapped to the same region of the T4 chromosome. Using the host strain in which *rII* mutants formed no plaques, he found that when host cells were coinfected with different mutant pairs some pairs produced a normal phage burst while others did not. In contrast, those pairs of mutants that rarely or never produced a normal burst he concluded were in the same cistron. The rare productive infections Benzer proposed resulted from recombination between the different mutations in the same cistron thereby creating a wild-type genotype in a few coinfected cells. Using this method, he placed all of his *rII* mutations into two cistrons that he called *rIIA* and *rIIB*. Moreover, he made a detailed genetic map based on recombination frequency between the different mutations (a fine structure map) that also indicated the frequency at which a mutation was isolated at that position. In this way he demonstrated that genes are not indivisible units but consist of many mutable sites that can recombine. Geneticists working with other organisms soon followed Benzer's lead and adapted complementation analysis to their systems.

To carry out a complementation analysis, both mutant genes must be expressed in the same cell so that their gene products are synthesised in the same cytoplasm and can functionally interact. Only loss of function (recessive) mutations can be used for a complementation analysis. The theory behind the complementation analysis is simple. If both mutations are loss of function alterations of the same gene, then the diploid cell carrying these two mutant genes will not contain a functional allele and will have the mutant phenotype. If both mutations are loss of function mutations but in different genes, then the diploid cell will have one mutant allele and one functional wild-type allele of each gene and, since the mutant alleles are loss of function alleles, the diploid will have the wild-type phenotype.

To express both mutant genes in the same cytoplasm a heterozygous diploid must be constructed. The way the researcher establishes the diploid state varies with the organism under study. In *Saccharomyces,* this is accomplished by mating a MATa strain containing mutation #1 to a MATα strain containing mutation #2. The a/α diploid will be heterozygous for the mutant genes. The phenotype of the heterozygous diploid is then observed. If the diploid has a wild-type phenotype, then the mutations are said to complement and this is strong evidence that the mutations are in different genes. A geneticist might also say, 'The mutations are in different complementation groups'. If the diploid has a mutant phenotype, then the mutations do not complement and are said to be in the same complementation group. This is considered strong evidence that the mutations are alleles. The definition of complementation group is a set of non-complementing mutations. The term complementation group is synonymous with gene.

Two conditions must be met before one can carry out a complementation analysis on a series of mutants. First, the mutant strain can only contain a single mutation compared with the parental strain. Particularly when mutagenesis had been used to obtain the mutants, it is possible that more than one DNA alteration was induced in an individual and these are involved in producing the mutant phenotype. Therefore, each mutant strain must be tested to demonstrate whether one or more genetic alterations are required to produce the mutant phenotype. To test this the mutant strain is crossed to a wild-type strain and tetrad analysis of the heterozygous diploid is carried out. If only a single alteration is required, then only tetrads with two mutant spores and two wild-type spores will be produced. But if two or more alterations are present, tetratype and nonparental ditype tetrads will be produced. What would be the phenotypes of the spores of a tetratype tetrad if the mutant strain contained two altered genes and both alterations were required to produce the mutant phenotype? What would be the phenotypes of the spores of a tetratype tetrad if the mutant strain contained two altered genes and either mutation alone were sufficient to produce the mutant phenotype?

Of course to carry out a cross between the mutant and wild-type strains the strains must be of opposite mating type and should carry different nutritional mutations to facilitate the selection of diploids. But in other respects the two strains should ideally be isogenic except for any alterations required to produce the mutant phenotype. Usually, before undertaking a mutant hunt, the geneticist will construct an appropriate pair of isogenic (or congenic) haploid strains to be used as parental strains. The mutants isolated in one strain can then be mated to the parental strain of the opposite mating type to determine the number of mutant genes involved.

As described above, the second requirement for a complementation analysis is that the mutations be loss of function alleles. In other words, only mutations that are recessive to the wild-type allele can be used. So, as a second step in the genetic analysis of mutants, mutant strains carrying a single mutant gene are crossed to a parental strain carrying the wild-type allele. If the mutant carries a recessive loss of function mutation, then the heterozygous diploid *(GENl/genl-34)* will have the wild-type phenotype. This mutant allele can then be used for complementation analysis.

Cross 4 shows a complementation test for two mutant strains. Preliminary genetic analysis has shown that each strain contains only a single mutant gene and that the mutant allele is recessive.

Cross 4:   Mutant strain 5   ×   Mutant strain 14

Diploid phenotype: Mutant

The result shown in Cross 4 indicates that the mutation in strain 5 and the mutation in strain 14 do not complement and thus are mutations in the same gene. If we call the gene *GENI,* then these mutations are alleles and one could now name them *genl-5* and *genl-14.*

This cross could be depicted as shown below:

Cross 4:   genl-5   ×   genl-14   (genotypes of parental strains)
            (mutant)   (mutant)   (phenotype of parental strains)

Diploid: genl-5   (genotype of diploid)
            genl -14
            (mutant)   (phenotype of diploid)

As a second test of whether or not the mutations are alleles, the researcher can determine the segregation pattern of the alleles in the meiotic products of the diploid. If the two mutations are in the same gene, then recombination between the mutations will be relatively rare because they map so close to one another. Therefore, 100% of the time (or close to it) the two mutant genes will segregate to different spores producing a tetrad with four mutant spores (two mutant #5 spores and two mutant #14 spores). Cross 5 shows another complementation test between mutant strain 5, which carries the mutation genl-5, and another mutant strain. Mutant strain 4 contains only a single mutant gene and the mutant allele is recessive:

Cross 5:   Mutant strain 5   ×   Mutant strain 4

Diploid phenotype: Wild-type

The result shown in Cross 5 indicates that the mutation in strain 5 and the mutation in strain 4 complement and thus are mutations in different genes. We can then say that a different gene, GEN2, is mutant in strain 4. This cross could be depicted as shown below:

Cross 5:   genl-5 GEN2   ×   GENl gen2-4   (genotypes of parental strains)
            (mutant)   (mutant)   (phenotype of parental strains)

Diploid: genl-5   gen2-4   (genotype of diploid)
            GENl   GEN2
            (wild-type)   (phenotype of diploid)

If GENl and GEN2 are not linked, then the mutant genes will recombine producing recombinant meiotic products with the wild-type (GENl GEN2) and double mutant (genl-5 gen2-4) genotype. This is exhibited by the presence of tetratype and nonparental ditype tetrads when this diploid is subjected to tetrad analysis. The frequency of each type of tetrad will depend on the frequency of recombination. If the two genes are completely unlinked, that is 50% recombination, the frequency of PD : TT : NPD tetrads will be 1 : 4 : 1. If there is any linkage, then the frequency of recombination is less than 50% and the relative number of PD tetrads will increase to greater than the expected 116 of the total number of tetrads analysed. Ultimately, for crosses between two alleles, the number of PD tetrads will closely approach loo%, as is shown in Cross 1.

One can calculate the map distance between two mutations (the frequency recombination multiplied by 100) using the following formula, which is correct for map distances up to 35 CM.

$$\text{Map distance in cM} = \frac{100}{2}\left[\frac{6 \times \text{\# NPD tetrads} + \text{\# TT tetrads}}{\text{Total \# of tetrads}}\right]$$

The combination of these two methods, complementation analysis and tetrad analysis, should clearly indicate whether one is dealing with mutations in one or more genes. Either method alone is not as powerful, and therefore researchers do both tests. For example, if there are mutations in two very tightly linked genes, the mutations will complement, but recombination will be rare and most, if not all the tetrads will be PD. Such results would strongly suggest that one is dealing with mutations in two closely linked genes. In a complete complementation analysis, all the mutants are crossed to all of the other mutants. Often as a complementation group containing several mutant alleles is identified, one allele will be chosen as the representative of that complementation group and only this allele will be crossed to the other mutants. At the end of this process, all the mutants isolated in a particular mutant selection/ screen will be placed into complementation groups, i.e. genes.

The researcher will have made a good start at determining the number of genes involved in the process of interest. If only a few genes have been identified with several mutant alleles, then the researcher will have some degree of confidence that the analysis saturated the genome and that new genes are not likely to be identified by the same selection/screening method if many genes have been identified, several with only one mutant allele each, then it is likely that new genes will be identified if the same selection/screen is repeated.

There are some special situations in which straightforward interpretation of a complementation test is misleading and the geneticist must be on the alert for such possibilities. Infrequently, mutant alleles of the same gene are able to complement, and produce a heterozygous diploid with a wild-type like phenotype. This is referred to as intragenic complementation. Intragenic complementation can occur if the encoded polypeptide forms a multiple subunit protein composed of like subunits, such as a homodimer, or if it encodes a single polypeptide that carries out several distinct functions. In the case of the homomultimeric protein, mutant subunits encoded by different mutant genes associate with one another in the multimeric protein and are able to accommodate each others mutant alteration in the mixed multimer. When this happens the mixed-mutant multimer complex has some functional activity, although it may not be completely normal.

Another mechanism of intragenic complementation is possible if the protein product of the gene has several distinct functions, such as two different enzyme activities. In this situation it is possible to obtain mutations that affect one of these activities while leaving the other function intact. In a heterozygous diploid, cells carrying two different mutations, each one affecting only one of the two functions, proteins capable of carrying out both enzyme activities will be produced, albeit in different molecules, and the cell should have the wild-type phenotype.

In contrast to intragenic complementation where mutations in the same gene complement, in a few instances mutations in different genes which are expected to complement do not. This phenomenon is referred to as nonallelic noncomplementation. One explanation for this noncomplementation is that the two genes encode subunits of a heteromultimeric protein, and that the presence of a mutant alteration in either subunit destroys all function of the multimeric protein. Sort of, 'one bad apple spoils the whole barrel'. Careful and thorough genetic analysis involving both complementation tests and genetic mapping of several mutant alleles is necessary to avoid the pitfalls of these potentially misleading situations.

GENETICS AND EPIGENETICS OF THE X CHROMOSOME

A consequence of Mendelian inheritance of X-linked traits is that women are more than equal to men in the face of X-linked diseases, protected as they are by the presence of two X chromosomes in their genome. This potentially beneficial inequality is diminished by the molecular mechanism known as X-chromosome inactivation (XCI), which triggers the transcriptional silencing of one of the X chromosomes in each female cell. The determination of which X to inactivate, a process that occurs during early embryogenesis, is random and clonally inherited. As a result, females are mosaic for the expression of X-linked genes. XCI is a highly regulated process involving large noncoding RNAs, chromatin remodeling, and nuclear reorganisation of the X chromosome. It is a paradigm for epigenetic regulation and is frequently used as a biomarker for monitoring long-range gene reprogramming during cell differentiation and dedifferentiation. This section analyses how XCI affects the expression of X-linked mutations, describes some of the most recent discoveries on the molecular mechanisms triggering XCI, and explores the therapeutic potentialities of the XCI process *per se*.

If Gregor Mendel had used as experimental model calico cats instead of peas, he would certainly have noticed that the tortoiseshell coat colour was only seen in females and come to the conclusion that this trait is sex linked. But he would surely have struggled trying to apply his famous rules of heredity to the transmission of this mosaic patterning and, more generally, to the transmission of X-linked traits in mammals. This is because the X chromosome is submitted to a unique regulation system that not only relies on formal genetics but also—and maybe above all—on classical epigenetics.

In humans, sexual dimorphism is associated with the presence of two X chromosomes in females, and an X and a Y chromosome in males. The X chromosome is 155 Mb long and carries some 1250 known genes. The Y chromosome is some three times smaller and has the lowest known gene density of any human chromosome (Fig. 3.13a). In contrast with the X chromosome, the Y chromosome has changed rapidly in mammalian evolution. Its unique structure, the paucity of genes on it, and the high content of repetitive elements all testify to a rapid loss of active genes and accumulation of repetitive sequence on the Y chromosome. This loss is thought to have been driven by the acquisition of a novel male-determining gene (SRY), followed by acquisition of male advantage genes (i.e. spermatogenesis genes) nearby, recombination was suppressed to keep together the male-specific package of genes. The absence of recombination with the X chromosome promoted accumulation of mutations and deletions because of drift and inefficient selection.

This results in the unusual situation whereby the homology regions shared by the X and Y chromosomes are reduced to two extremely small regions, called the pseudo-autosomal regions 1 and 2 (PAR1 and PAR2), located at each end of the X and Y chromosome. The quasi-hemizygote state of the X chromosome resulting from this situation in males renders them more susceptible to X-linked mutations than females who carry two copies of each gene. This genetic vulnerability is reflected in the preferential occurrence of X-linked diseases in males, and probably contributes, at least in part, to the increased male mortality rates observed at every stage of life.

Sexual dimorphism also introduces two different types of disequilibrium into the dosage of X-linked genes. First, in males, the copy number of X-linked genes is reduced by half as compared to autosomes. Inmice, this is compensated for by an upregulation of transcription (1.4- to 1.6-fold) of all X-linked genes during early embryogenesis in both the male and female.4 This upregulation reaches twofold during the later stages of differentiation, thereby equalising gene expression levels between the single X and the diploid autosomes in male cells. The molecular mechanisms responsible for this upregulation have not as yet been characterised.However, the comparison of triploid cells bearing a single active X (Xa) with triploid cells carrying two Xa's has shown that expression levels of only a subset of X-linked genes, whose expression dosage in relation to autosomal expression may be critical, are adjusted.

The second disequilibrium results from the imbalance in the number of sex chromosomes between males and females. Various strategies have been adopted by different species to achieve this second type of dosage compensation. In fruit flies, the single X chromosome doubles its transcriptional activity compared to either of the two female X chromosomes, whereas in nematodes, hermaphrodites XX animals halve the level of X-linked transcription.

Consequences of Mendelian Inheritance and X Chromosome Inactivation on X-linked Haplotype Expression

Ontology of X-linked genes and mutations

Acloser examination of human X-linked diseases reveals that the X chromosome is especially enriched in genes whose mutation leads to mental retardation and in genes related to sexual reproduction functions (Fig. 3.13b). This unique distribution supports the so-called faster-X hypothesis, which suggests that sex chromosomes evolve more rapidly than autosomes due to the hemizygote status of X-linked genes in males, which imposes a high selection pressure leading to an enrichment in a specific category of genes. Interestingly, the excess of genes involved in brain functions correlates to the fact that X-linked genes are highly expressed in brain in comparison with autosomal genes, an effect that appears especially pronounced in humans, in contrast to rodents. This has led to the hypothesis that, over the last fewmillion years of hominid evolution, females have selected smart males to mate with—perhaps because smarter males are better bread winners thereby explaining the extensive brain development in humans.

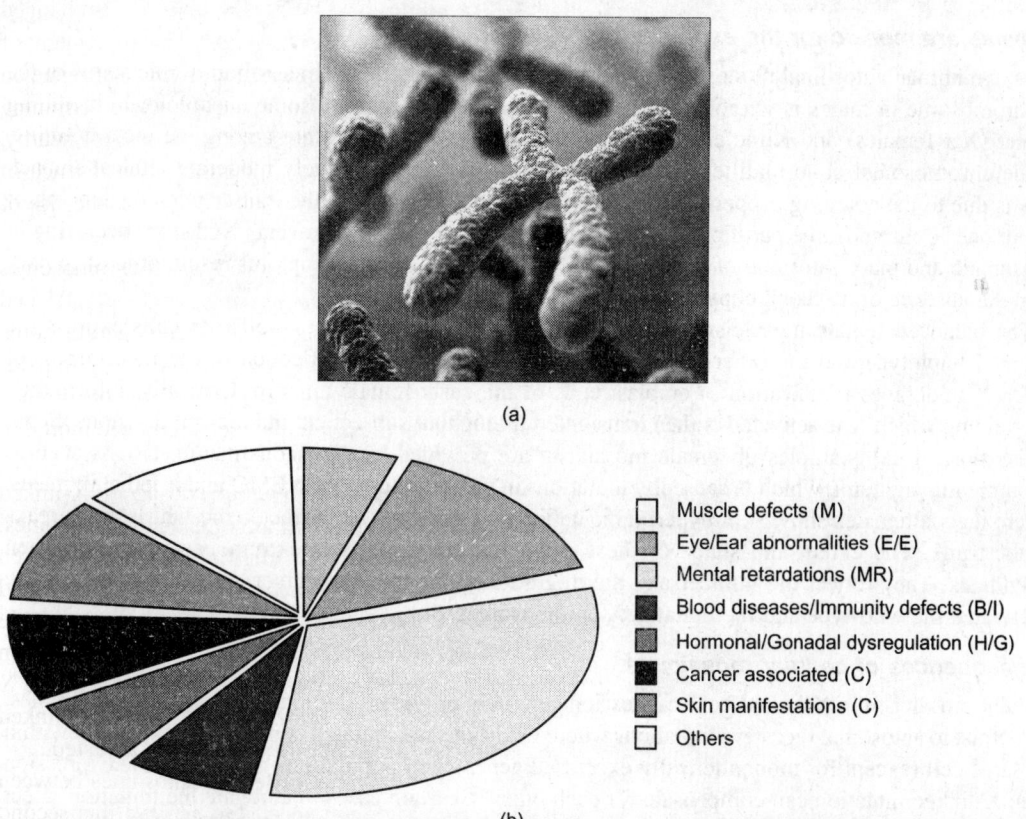

(a)

(b)

Fig. 3.13: Human X-chromosomemap and distribution of X-linked diseases/syndromes. (a) Scanning electron micrograph of an X and Y chromosome, and (b) graph showing the distribution of X-linked diseases/syndromes within the seven categories of clinical features described in.

Differences in X-linked gene expression in brain tissues between the sexes may also explain supposed differences in the brain capacity of men and women, although the very existence of such differences is the subject of a long-standing debate. Indeed, qualitative and quantitative analyses of X-linked gene expression in brain tissues have failed to detect any major differences between female and male.

The 'faster-X hypothesis' also explains the X-chromosome enrichment for genes expressed in testis, the X chromosome is enriched for genes expressed in spermatogonia but not for genes expressed in later stages of spermatogenesis, likely because of silencing at meiosis (MSCI). These genes are thought to have accumulated on the X because recessivemutations expressed inmales, due to hemizygosity of the X, could give rise to novel functions that enhance male sexual reproduction (i.e. bigger, faster, more sperm). Even if the mutations are deleterious to females (as 'sexually antagonistic' genes often are) the effect will not be felt until the allele is sufficiently frequent to produce female homozygotes. By this stage there is strong selection to restrict expression of the gene to the testis, tomitigate disadvantage to females. Testis-specific genes that have been selected-for include, among others, microRNAs11 and arrays of so-called testis-cancer antigen genes required for fertility that lie in large palindromic loops.

Females are mosaic for the expression of X-linked genes

Although human autosomal monosomies are incompatible with life, the quasi-monosomic status of the X chromosome in males is without phenotypic consequence. X-chromosome aneuploidies, including Turner (XO females) and Klinefelter's syndrome (XXY males), which are among the most common viable chromosomal abnormalities, lead to syndromes having a relatively moderate clinical impact. This is due to the counting property of the XCI process, which triggers the transcriptional silencing of all but one X chromosome per diploid set of autosomes. The counting prevents XCI from occurring in XO female and inactivates one of the extra X in XXY males. Turner symptoms result, at least in part, from the absence of a second copy of the PAR regions.

The balanced female mosaicism for the expression of X-linked genes—50% of cells express the maternal haplotype and the other 50% the paternal haplotype—is a reflection of the randomness of which X undergoes inactivation in epiblast cells of the early female embryo. Critically, information determining which X is activated is then transmitted throughout subsequent mitotic cell divisions. Some of the most visual examples of female mosaicism are provided by cutaneous manifestations such as incontinentia pigmenti, which is causedby mutations in the X-linked gene NEMO and is lethal in males. Heterozygous females show skin hyperpigmentation that develops as characteristic whirls and streaks on the trunk. The extent and shape of these pigmentation patterns is extremely variable between individuals. They reflect the number and the migration path of the precursor cells that have initially inactivated the wild-type and the mutated X chromosomes.

Consequences of cellular mosaicism

Cellular mosaicism in X-linked gene expression generally provides a biological advantage for females. In contrast to autosomal recessive mutations where wild-type and mutated copies are coexpressed within the same cell (except for monoallelically expressed genes), cell populations mosaic for the expression of an X-linked mutation can compensate for each other in certain cases to abrogate the mutation effect on disease etiology.

Females heterozygous for X-linked mutations thus generally behave as *asymptomatic carriers*. Two types of compensation are observed: The most common is cell elimination, but metabolic cooperation is also found.

Skewing of X-inactivation

Cell selection, as in adrenal leukodystrophy and Lesch–Nyhan syndrome, results in unequal proportions of cells with a paternal Xi and those with a maternal Xi in specific tissues. This phenomenon, called X-inactivation skewing, is rather common, with some 10% of women showing a deviation from equal inactivation of each parental allele. In extreme cases, up to 90% of cells show expression of the same allele. This XCI bias may occur either by primary nonrandom inactivation during early embryogenesis or by secondary cell selection later in the blastocyst.

Studies of phenotypic variation among female monozygotic twins who are carriers for an X-linked disease suggest that such primary XCI skewing may be responsible for the oft-remarked appearance of X-linked diseases in only one of two twins: with the clinically affected sister showing preferential nonrandom XCI of the chromosome carrying the wild-type allele, whereas the unaffected twin has either predominant XCI of the mutated chromosome or random XCI. Reported examples of Xlinked diseases with phenotypic discordance between monozygotic twins correlated with skewed XCI in the affected sister include fragile-X syndrome, colour blindness, Duchenne muscular dystrophy, Hunter's syndrome, hemophilia B, Aicardi's syndrome, and Fabry's diseases.

The existence, in the human, of a genetic component controlling XCI bias has also been postulated, but remains highly controversial in part because of the technical difficulties in assessing skewing, as it varies greatly with the tissues analysed and age. In most studies, mother-to-daughter transmission of XCI skewing has not been detected. However, a single case of heritable skewed XCI has been reported in a family where the trait seems to segregate independently of the hemophilia A mutation present in the family. In this specific case, only females showing a biased XCI of the wild-type X are affected. Skewing, even in this case, could result from the influence of an additional genetic component conferring a proliferative advantage. Autosomal transcription factors such as CTCF or YY1, which bind in an allele-specific manner to some of the XCI key regulators, may be able to modify the 50:50 XCI ratio. It is noteworthy that three autosomal loci, *Xiaf1*, *2*, and *3* (X-inactivation autosomal factors) but only one X-linked locus, the X-controlling-element (*Xce*), have been suggested to influence XCI in mice.

Current and Future Employments of X-chromosome Inactivation as Diagnostic or Therapeutic Tools

Skewed X-inactivation as a diagnostic tool to detect asymptomatic carriers of X-linked mutations

A current use of XCI concerns the identification of heterozygous carriers of X-linked recessive mutations, which is of crucial importance for family counseling and planning medical treatment (when available) of potentially affected offspring. Although heterozygous carriers of autosomal mutations can be detected by laboratory testing or in-depth physical examination for some genetic diseases, in the case of most X-linked mutations female carriers appear normal in all respects. This results often from the selection process referred to above, in which survival of cells that have inactivated the mutant allele is favoured in tissues where the gene responsible for the disease is expressed. A corollary of this is that skewed XCI can be a robust indicator of carrier status. Assays to examine XCI skewing require the presence of a polymorphism able to distinguish the two Xs and a means of determining which X is active. Although examination of RNA and/or protein expression provides the most direct measure of X chromosome activity, specific DNA methylation patterns associated with the Xi are more often used as a surrogate because DNA is easier to extract, store, and analyse. An assay monitoring DNA methylation of the highly polymorphic CAG trinucleotide polymorphism at the 5' end of the gene encoding the androgen receptor (AR) has become a popular and widely adopted method for measuring XCI skewing. Because skewing does not always affect all tissues similarly, it is important to ascertain as many cell types as possible by testing different readily available proband biological samples. These samples will typically include peripheral blood leukocytes, oralmucosal cells, and muscle biopsies. It is important to stress that this test, which is based on the quantitative measure of methylation levels of a single gene,may not always be accurate.

Recurrent miscarriages are a major health concern for women, affecting some 17% of couples who wish to have a child. It has been assumed that a large proportion of these pregnancy losses have a genetic origin. Causes involving the X chromosome, such as mutations in X-linked genes implicated in placenta formation, may in part be responsible. However, the most likely event involves the presence of an X-linked lethal trait in the mother, which would be transmitted with a 25% probability to a male fetus. For these mothers, the risk of spontaneous abortion is increased from the general population risk of 15–20% to a combined risk of up to 40% at each pregnancy ($[0.25 \times 1] + [0.75 \times 0.20] = 0.4$). It is predicted that female carriers of such X-linked lethal traits will show extremely skewed XCI against the mutated X, which could be detected using the abovementioned test.

More generally, this simple test could provide us with a method for predicting the carrier status of every woman suspected, on the basis ofher pedigree, to be a carrier of an X-linked mutation. For this reason it constitutes an important break through in the field of genetic diagnosis, allowing for the scanning and detection of mutations corresponding up to 5% of the genome in a single test. However, it is important to keep in mind that skewed XCI has to occur in the biological tissues that are under test in order for carrier status to be detected.Moreover, potential lineage specific differences in X-inactivation status and/or underlying mechanisms cannot be excluded. Currently, this test is used to detect X-linked forms of immunodeficiencies and X-linked enzymatic defects, where early disease diagnosis is required to initiate treatment as soon as possible and to prevent symptoms appearing in the child (e.g. in the case of lysosomal storage disorders like Fabry's disease and Hunter's syndrome). Because XCI profiles are clonal, this test can be applied on tumor biopsies to assess cancer propagation and the origin of the metastases. For example, in the case of tumors affecting multiple organs, if all the tumors show the same XCI profile, this will increase the probability that the tumors likely originated from the same initial transformation, thereby suggesting advanced metastasis. In contrast, severalXCI profiles would be indicative of independent mutational events which might lead to a different appreciation of the clinical treatment.

Cell replacement therapies involving X-inactivation

A major area of therapeutic research and development concerns cell replacement, which relies on collecting cells from the patient and compensating or repairing the effects of the mutation *ex vivo*. 'Repaired' cells are subsequently grafted into the disease-affected tissue, theoretically without risk of rejection of the autograft. Until now, cell replacement therapies were employed mainly to treat categories of disease such as immune system defects, allowing the collection and growth of the target cells: in this case, adult hematopoietic stem cells. Interestingly, immature hematopoietic precursor cells have been shown to conserve the ability to initiate ectopic XCI, suggesting that their X-chromosome chromatin structure is still permissive enough to allow XCI patterns to be changed. Restoration of a normal phenotype, by either forcing the XCI of themutated X chromosome or the recreation of a balanced cellular mosaicism among hematopoietic stem cells prior to reimplantation, represent possibly interesting options for the treatment of autoimmune diseases.

Recent revolutionary advances in the field of stem cell research have shown that it is possible to reprogramme somatic cells toward a pluripotent state. Ectopic expression of only four key factors in a human somatic cell is sufficient to obtain these so-called iPS (induced pluripotent stem) cells, which recapitulate most of ES cell characteristics, such as their ability to contribute to any adult tissue. The challenge is now to specifically and routinely direct the differentiation process into a desired lineage. Encouraging progress has been made recently in the controlled differentiation of cardiac, neural, or hematopoietic lineages.

In terms of XCI, the genome reprogramming associated with somatic cell de-differentiation is accompanied by a reactivation of the Xi in mouse iPS (miPS) cells but not in human iPS (hiPS) cells. However, because hiPS derived from mosaic human fibroblasts (with either a paternal or maternal Xi) are clonal, this makes possible the selection of hiPS populations that have inactivated the X chromosome carrying a mutation. The next step will be to differentiate these 'repaired' cells toward the desired cell type and to reimplant them into the patient. More generally, a combination of genome sequencing using high-throughput technologies to identify mutations, nuclear reprogramming, and *in vitro* mutation repair should allow the treatment of most genetic diseases through cell replacement therapy.

X-inactivation as a mean to an end. Theoretically, it should be possible to use the chromosome-wide properties of the XCI mechanism to induce long-distance gene silencing. Indeed, it has been shown that inserting the human *XIC* into a mouse autosome triggers long-range gene repression in *cis*. Along this line, one could imagine that targeted insertions of the *XIC* into a specific chromosomeor a specific genomic region associated with appropriate genetic manipulation, such as the utilisation of insulators to restrict the spreading of the XCI signal to the targeted region, could be used to treat cases of mosaic trisomy and/or some types of abnormal genomic amplifications/duplications. Another long-term application consists in usingXCI as a model to assess the efficiency and accuracy of genome wide reprogramming during early embryogenesis. It should, moreover, be possible to screen libraries of syntheticmolecules to identifynewdrugs involved in, or potentiating, gene reprogramming on the basis of their ability to prevent XCI to occur or, in contrast, to induce ectopic XCI. Thus, we can understand more about X-chromosome genetics and X-inactivation at the molecular level, unforeseen layers of complexity appear.Major progress will almost certainly be conditioned by, and will in turn influence, our general understanding of chromatin structure and chromosome function. But it is more and more obvious that lessons from Xinactivation, which is now unanimously considered as one of the major paradigms of epigenetic regulation of gene expression, will be applicable to other related regulation systems such as genomic imprinting and, more generally, to global genome reprogramming events.

SEX-LIMITED GENES

Sex-limited genes are genes that are present in both sexes of sexually reproducing species but are expressed in only one sex and remain 'turned off' in the other. In other words, sex-limited genes cause the two sexes to show different traits or phenotypes, despite having the same genotype. This term is restricted to autosomal traits, and should not be confused with sex-linked characteristics, which have to do with genetic differences on the sex chromosomes. Sex-limited genes are also distinguished from sex-influenced genes, where the same gene will show differential expression in each sex. Sex-influenced genes commonly show a dominant/recessive relationship, where the same gene will have a dominant effect in one sex and a recessive effect in the other (for example, male pattern baldness).

Sex-limited genes are responsible for sexual dimorphism, which is a phenotypic (directly observable) difference between males and females of the same species. These differences can be reflected in size, colour, behaviour, and morphology. An example of sex-limited genes are genes which instruct the male elephant seals to grow big and fight, at the same time instructing female seals to grow small and avoid fights. These genes are also responsible for some female beetles inability to grow exaggerated mandibles, research that is discussed in detail later in this chapter.

The overall point of sex-limited genes is to resolve intralocus sexual conflict. In other words, these genes try to resolve the 'push-pull' between males and females over trait values for optimal phenotype. Without these genes, organisms would be forced to settle on an average trait value, incurring costs on both sexes. With these genes, it is possible to 'turn off' the genes in one sex, allowing both sexes to attain (or at least, approach very closely) their optimal phenotypes.

The idea of sex-limited genes was initially developed by Charles Darwin himself in 1871 in his book The Descent of Man and Selection in Relation to Sex. He did not distinguish between sex-limited, sex-linked, and sex-influenced genes, but referred to any gene that expresses differently between sexes as sex-limited. While this concept was still in its infancy, Darwin catalysed the further development of sex-related selection. Thomas Hunt Morgan, aware of this confusing terminology, published an article in The American Naturalist in 1914 titled 'Sex-Linked and Sex-Limited Inheritance.' This article directly acknowledges that Darwin applied the term sex-limited whenever a characteristic seemed specific to one sex. Morgan proposes the definitions for sex-linked genes and sex-limited genes that we still use today (and that were defined in the introduction above). This paper helped to distinguish between these two similar concepts and clarify much confusion in the scientific community at the time. Morgan's paper was followed by several others involving sex-limited genes and their expression as traits. One of the more notable example is John H. Gerould's 'Inheritance of White Wing Colour, a Sex-Limited (Sex-Controlled) Variation in Yellow Pierid Butterflies,' published in Genetics in 1923. Gerould observed that in this species of butterfly, females naturally occur as yellow or white, while males only occur with yellow colouration. He explores this apparently sex-limited trait from a genetic perspective in this ground-breaking 50 page paper. To conclude the notable advancements in the early stages of the development of sex-limited genes, a brief discussion of R. A. Fisher is necessary. Commonly hailed as one of the best evolutionary biologists of his time, Fisher was also a talented geneticist. His book 'The Genetical Theory of Natural Selection', published in 1930, over 20 years before the double-helix shape of DNA was discovered, was the first attempt to explain Darwin's theories within the foundation of genetics.Chapter 6 of this book is titled 'Sexual Reproduction and Sexual Selection' and includes a genetic interpretation of Darwin's initial idea of sex-limited genes. After these ground-breaking works, papers continue to be published further exploring the causes, mechanisms, evolutionary advantages, and more of sex-limited genes.

Genetic Basis of Sex-limited Genes

Many studies have been published exploring the genetic basis of sex-limited genes. One paper, published in Evolution, evaluates the hypothesis that sex-limited traits can arise in two ways. The alleles responsible for sexual dimorphism can be limited to expression in only one sex when they first appear, or the alleles could begin by being expressed in both sexes then become modified (repressed or promoted) in one sex by modifier genes or regulatory elements. The concept of this study was to examine female hybrids from species where males displayed different types of ornamental traits (elongated feathers, wattles, colour patches). The assumption is that different hypotheses about male-specific expression will yield different results in female hybrids. The methods and materials of the experiment are discussed in detail in the paper, but the important result that emerged was that NO female hybrids expressed any of the ornamental traits found in the parent males. Two interpretations of these results are possible: the dimorphic alleles were initially only expressed in males, or the alleles were initially expressed in both and then were suppressed in females or became limited to males by regulatory regions that are completely dominant in hybrids. The most likely genomic explanation for initial expression in both species then modification is involvement of *cis*-dominance, where the factors that modify the gene are located next to the gene on the chromosome. (This is in contrast to trans-dominance, where mobile products that can affect distant genes are produced.) These factors can be in the form of promoter regions, which can be either suppressed or activated by hormones. This experiment also demonstrates that these alleles come under regulatory control very quickly. This is because none of the ornamentation seen in males is seen in the very next generation. These conclusions make it likely that at least some male-specific (thus, sex-limited) genes cue their expression by hormone levels - the absence of estrogen or the presence of testosterone.

Fitness Consequences

Storage effect

Because sex-limited genes are present in both sexes but only expressed in one, this allows the unexpressed genes to be hidden from selection. On a short-term scale, this means that during one generation, only the sex that expresses the sex-limited traits of interest will be affected by selection. The remaining half of the gene pool for these traits will be unaffected by selection because they are hidden (unexpressed) in the genes of the other sex. Since a portion of the alleles for these sex-limited traits are hidden from selection, this occurrence has been termed 'storage-effect'. On a long-term scale, this storage effect can have significant effects on selection, especially if selection is fluctuating over a long period of time. It is inarguable that selection will fluctuate over time with varying levels of environmental stability. For example, fluctuations in population density can drive selection on sex-limited traits. In less dense populations, females will have less opportunity to choose between males for reproduction. In this case, attractive males may experience both reduced reproductive success and increased predation pressure. Thus, selection on males for sex-limited traits such as increased size (elephant seals) and weaponry (claws on fiddler crabs, horns on rhinoceros beetles) will change direction with fluctuation in population density.

Rapid evolution

John Parsch and Hans Ellegren defined 'genes that differ in expression between females and males' as sex-biased genes. While this definition is more broad, sex-limited genes are certainly included in this category. One of the key principles of sex-biased gene expression that Parsch and Ellegren stressed in their paper in February 2013 is that of rapid evolution. They assert that a genes sex bias can vary among different types of tissues throughout the body or throughout development, making the level of sex bias a fluid, rather than static, property. This makes it possible, then, that the rapid evolution seen in sex-biased genes is not an inherent property of their sex bias, but a property of some other feature. The paper offers expression breadth, the number of tissue types in which the genes are expressed, as an example of a feature correlated to sex-biased genes. It is known that genes with limited expression (in only one type of tissue) generally evolve faster than those with a higher expression breadth, and sex-biased genes are often restricted in their expression, such as to only the testes or ovaries. Thus, it is likely that sex-biased (including sex-limited) genes will evolve faster than the average genetic information. Parsch and Ellegren also assert that 'sex-biased genes expressed only in sex-limited reproductive tissues evolve faster than unbiased genes that are expressed only in a single, non-reproductive tissue.' That is, genes that have a bias toward any kind of reproductive tissue (testes or ovaries) seem to show faster evolution than genes expressed in non-gonadal tissues, despite the number of tissues in which they are expressed. This makes sense in the context of genes with reproductive function evolving more quickly, a generally observed pattern in evolutionary biology.

Effects of sexual antagonism

Sexual antagonism occurs when two species have conflicting optimal fitness strategies concerning reproduction. Multiple matings is a classic example of competing optimal strategies. Males, who typically have a much lower overall investment in reproduction, may benefit from more frequent matings. Females, however, invest much more in reproduction and can be endangered, harmed, or even killed by multiple matings. In 2010, Hosken and others completed an important study exploring the effects of sexually antagonistic selection on sex-limited trait expression. They asked if sex-specific trait selection always resolved intralocus conflict, as it was believed to do. By using a species of flour beetle, Gnatocerus cornutus, exhibiting sex-limited traits in the form of exaggerated mandible size, they were able to test this hypothesis. Exaggerated mandibles are only developed in males, females never develop exaggerated mandibles. The point of this experiment was to determine how mandibles affect fitness. If these sex-limited genes are truly quelling intralocus sexual conflict, male mandible size should have no effect on female fitness. After selecting for males with exaggerated mandibles (full materials and methods can be found within the paper), it was experimentally determined that males with exaggerated mandibles had a higher fitness - they experienced increased fighting and mating success. It was also found, however, that females found in the populations of males with exaggerated mandibles had lower fitness [(as determined by lifetime reproductive success (LRS)] relative to the fitness of females in populations with males with smaller mandibles. Since this male sex-limited trait affects female fitness, intralocus sexual conflict has not been resolved. This highlights the importance of sexual conflict to evolution, because it cannot simply be defused by sex-limited trait expression.

Later the same year, a paper in Evolution also came to the same conclusions about sexual antagonism in relation to sex-limited genes. Hosken developed a mathematical model to show that the fitness costs of sexual antagonism, even when rare, will usually overwhelm the benefits of sexually concordant selection. (Sexually concordant selection occurs when selection favours the same alleles in both sexes but differs in relative strength between them.) Through several advanced calculations, they concluded that even a small relative amount of sexual antagonism will overwhelm any benefit harvested from sexually concordant selection. Coming to the same conclusion as Hosken and others, they demonstrated mathematically that when sex-limited gene expression attempts to resolve sexual antagonism, it is likely to produce negative long-term fitness consequences. This result is seen in the experiment with beetles above, where the females demonstrate reduced fitness in response to males selected for larger mandibles. So, with mathematical support and a lack of support for strong fitness benefits as a result of sexually concordant selection, the paper concludes that sex-specific selection is more likely to incur costs than benefits to sexually reproducing species.

Effects on animal behaviour

Animal behaviour encompasses so many disciplines that it is impossible not to see it in some capacity in almost all primary literature involving live animals. While the examples above certainly contain aspects of animal behaviour, a more overt example of it in relation to sex-limited traits is detailed in a Teplitsky and others paper centering on breeding time in red-billed gulls. This experiment deals with breeding time, an aspect of reproductive biology. Reproduction and sexual behaviour are two key aspects of animal behaviour, as they are universally expressed in some way throughout the animal kingdom.

Breeding time in red-billed gulls is expressed only in females, because only females lay eggs. Male care, however, affects female breeding performance substantially. This qualifies breeding time as a sex-limited trait because it is expressed only in one sex but can be affected by both (similarly to Hosken's beetle experiment above). By following a natural population of red-billed gulls for 46 years, Teplitsky and others came to an unexpected conclusion - while laying date (aka breeding time) is only expressed in females, the trait is only heritable in males. This is atypical because sex-limited traits are almost always heritable within the sex in which they are expressed.

For this species, the timing of egg-laying has much to do with male behaviour. Males can affect female reproductive success so strongly because for the 20 days up to egg-laying, females spend up to 80% of their time in the nest. This leaves males with the responsibility of providing food regularly and securing (and maintaining) a high-quality territory for nesting. This phenomenon of the genetics of one individual affecting those of another individual is known as indirect genetic effects. For this population, at least, possible explanations for this atypical heritability pattern exist. While controlling female health and safety, males are responsible for the timing of the start of courtship feeding, as well. These populations also typically have excesses of females, allowing males to exert even further choice in the form of mate choice. These factors in combination give males a great opportunity to express their 'laying date genotype'. In spite of the presence of directional selection and significant male heritability for breeding time, no advancement of breeding time was seen during the 46 years of this experiment. This does not discount the significance of the paper's other results however - one of the most significant being that here a 'female trait (laying date) is largely determined by genetic characteristics of its mate'.

Chapter 4

Genetics: An Overview

INTRODUCTION

Genetics is a science that studies the variation and transmission of features or traits from one generation to the next. In this definition, the word variation refers to genetic variation; that is, the range of possible values for a trait as it is influenced by heredity. Heredity is the transmission of traits from the parents to the offspring via genetic material. This transmission takes place at the time of fertilisation in reproduction—when the bull's semen unites with the cow's ovum (egg) to produce a calf with a unique genetic makeup. Only identical twins have an identical genetic makeup because they come from one fertilised ovum that has separated into two embryos during the early phase of development.

Genetics is a field of biology that studies how traits are passed from parents to their offspring. The passing of traits from parents to offspring is known as heredity, therefore, genetics is the study of heredity. This introduction to genetics takes you through the basic components of genetics such as DNA, genes, chromosomes and genetic inheritance.

Genetics is built around molecules called DNA. DNA molecules hold all the genetic information for an organism. It provides cells with the information they need to perform tasks that allow an organism to grow, survive and reproduce. A gene is one particular section of a DNA molecule that tells a cell to perform one specific task.

Heredity is what makes children look like their parents. During reproduction, DNA is replicated and passed from a parent to their offspring. This inheritance of genetic material by offspring influences the appearance and behaviour of the offspring. The environment that an organism lives in can also influence how genes are expressed.

DNA

DNA is the cornerstone of genetics and is the perfect place to start for an introduction to genetics. DNA stands for deoxyribonucleic acid and it is the molecule that holds the genetic information for a cell and an organism. A DNA molecule contains a code that can be used by a cell to express certain genes. Specific sections of a DNA molecule provides the information to build specific proteins which can then be used by a cell to express the desired gene.

A DNA molecule is a nucleic acid, one of the four molecules of life. It comes in the form of a long, linear molecule referred to as a strand. Each strand of DNA is bonded to a second strand of DNA to form a DNA double helix. In eukaryotic cells, DNA is found in the nucleus as a tightly coiled double helix. DNA molecules are replicated during cell division. When a cell divides, the two new cells contain all the same DNA that the original cell had. In sexual reproduction with two parents, half of the DNA of the offspring is provided by each of the parents. The genetic material of a child is made from 50% of their mother's DNA and 50% their father's DNA.

GENES

A gene is a specific segment of a DNA molecule that holds the information for one specific protein. DNA molecules have a unique code for each gene which codes for their specific protein. Some organisms can have more than 100,000 different genes so they will have 100,000 unique sequences of DNA 'code'. Genes are the basic unit of heredity. The genes of an individual are determined by their parent or parents. A bacteria that is born by one parent cell splitting into two cells and has the exact same genes as their one parent cell.

A human, on the other hand, has two copies of each gene – one set from their mother and a second set from their father. Different forms of the same gene are called alleles. For each gene, a human can have two different alleles or two of the same alleles – one from each parent.

Physical traits such as eye colour or height are often determined by the combination of multiple genes. The environment an individual lives in also impacts how genes are expressed.

CHROMOSOMES

A chromosome is a structure made from tightly packed strands of DNA and proteins called histones. Strands of DNA are tightly wrapped around the histone proteins and form into long worm-shaped structures called 'chromatids'. Two chromatids join together to form a chromosome. Chromosomes are formed in the nucleus of a cell when a cell is dividing. It is possible to see chromosomes under an ordinary light microscope if the cell is in the right stage of cell division. The number of chromosomes varies between species. Humans have 46 chromosomes. Some species can have many more than 100 chromosomes while others can have as little as two.

Genetic Inheritance

Inheritance is the backbone of genetics and is an important topic to cover in an introduction to genetics. Long before DNA had been discovered and the word 'genetics' had been invented, people were studying the inheritance of traits from one generation to the next. Genetic inheritance occurs both in sexual reproduction and asexual reproduction. In sexual reproduction, two organisms contribute DNA to produce a new organism. In asexual reproduction, one organism provides all the DNA and produces a clone of themselves. In either, genetic material is passed from one generation to the next.

First we will focus on chromosomes. In every cell of your body there are 46 chromosomes in the form of 23 pairs. Each pair of chromosomes contains one chromosome inherited from your mother and one chromosome inherited from your father. This is why you may look like both of your parents.

The 23 chromosomes from the father join the 23 chromosomes from the mother when the sperm joins the egg at the moment of conception. Each chromosome pair looks identical apart from the 23rd pair. This pair of chromosomes is known as the sex chromosomes, as they determine the sex of an individual. There are two sex chromosomes: the X chromosome and the Y chromosome. If you are female you will have two copies of the X chromosome. If you are male you have one copy of the X chromosome and one copy of the Y chromosome.

A mother always passes on one of her X chromosomes to her children. The father can pass on an X chromosome or a Y chromosome. If the father passes on a Y chromosome the child will be male. If the father passes on an X chromosome the child will be female. In this random process, it is the male that determines the sex of the child as he can pass on either an X or a Y chromosome.

Characteristics can be due to our genetic make-up and may be controlled by only one gene or by many genes. Many characteristics can be due to a combination of genetic and environmental factors like diet and exercise.

Patterns of Inheritance

There are three main patterns in which characteristics are passed down from generation to generation:

- Recessive inheritance
- Dominant inheritance
- X-linked inheritance

All of us have two copies of each gene; one copy is inherited from our mother and the other from our father. The only exception to this rule is the genes on the sex chromosomes.

The two copies – or variants - of each gene may be exactly the same or slightly different. In recessive inheritance, you develop a certain characteristic only if you possess two copies of a given variant of the gene concerned. For example, albinism is an inherited recessive condition that not only affects humans but many other animals – including tigers.

In this condition, reduced amounts of a pigment called melanin are produced. In these individuals, both copies of a gene that plays a role in melanin production are not working properly. Using this animation, you can see how recessive inheritance works. Here, both parents carry the same non-working gene, as indicated by the light blue dot. However, as they have only one non-working gene, and the other gene is working properly, they are not affected by the condition and are known as 'carriers'. What will happen when these parents pass on their genes to their children?

It may be that both pass on their working gene to the child. The child will then have two working copies and will neither suffer from nor carry the condition. It may be that both pass on their non-working gene, in which case the child will have the condition. It may be that one parent passes on a working gene and the other passes on a non-working gene. In this case the child will not be affected, but he or she will be a carrier … just like the parents.

Every one of these four combinations is equally likely every time a pregnancy occurs. Other examples of recessive inheritance include attached earlobes, thalassaemia and cystic fibrosis. In dominant inheritance, you develop a certain characteristic, if you inherit one copy of a non-working gene, regardless of what the other copy is.

Examples of dominant traits or conditions include brown eyes, black hair, Huntington Disease and Hereditary Breast Cancer (Fig. 4.1). Marfan Syndrome is a medical condition that follows a dominant inheritance pattern. Individuals with this condition are usually taller than average and can develop problems with their hearts, bones and eyes. Using this animation, you can see how dominant inheritance works. Here is a father who has Marfan Syndrome and a mother who does not. If the non- working gene is passed on from the father, the child will be affected by this condition. If both the father and the mother pass on their working genes, the child will not be affected by this condition.

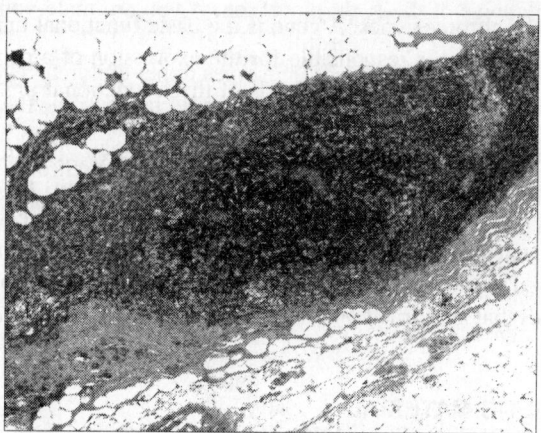

Fig. 4.1: Hereditary breast cancer.

As you can see, on average, half of the children will inherit the syndrome and half of the children will not. Every one of these four combinations is equally likely every time a pregnancy occurs. X-linked inheritance is associated with genes on the X chromosome, which is one of the two sex chromosomes. An example of an X-linked condition is haemophilia. In an individual with this condition the blood does not clot properly. Using this animation, you can see how X-Linked recessive inheritance works. Here the mother has one working copy of the gene and one non-working copy of the gene. She does not have haemophilia but she is a carrier of the condition. The father is not affected as he has one working copy of the gene. What will happen when these parents pass on their genes to their children?

The mother could pass on her working gene. This will result in either a non- affected daughter or a non-affected son. Or the mother could pass on her non-working gene. This will result in either a daughter who is a carrier or an affected son. A famous example of the X-linked inheritance of haemophilia can be seen in the extended family of Queen Victoria. She was a carrier, and a number of her children and grandchildren were either affected by the condition or carriers themselves. Other examples of X-linked conditions include red-green colour blindness and fragile X-syndrome.

Experiments performed by a monk named Gregor Mendel provided the foundations of our current understanding of how genetic material is passed from parents to their offspring.

GENETIC MATERIAL

The genetic material is located in the nucleus of each cell in the body. Except for the reproductive cells (spermatozoa and ova) and a few other exceptions (red blood cells), cells contain two copies of an animal's complete genetic material. When cells divide, the genetic material organises itself in a series of long threadlike structures called chromosomes. In body cells, each chromosome has a counterpart that has the same length and shape (except for the two chromosomes that determine the sex) and contains genetic information for the same trait. These two chromosomes are two members of a chromosome pair, one derived from the sire, one from the dam. The number of chromosome pairs is typical of a species and it is usually abbreviated as the letter 'n'. For example, in humans $n = 23$, in swine $n = 19$ and in cows $n = 30$. Thus cells in the bodies of humans, swine and cows contain $2n = 46$, 38 and 60 chromosomes, respectively.

Genes are located along the chromosomes. A gene is the basic functional unit of heredity; that is, it contains the genetic information that is responsible for the expression of a particular trait. The entire length of a chromosome can be divided into thousands of these functional units, each responsible for a particular trait.

A gene is composed of material called deoxyribonucleic acid or DNA. The function of the DNA is to carry the information necessary for the synthesis of proteins. As proteins are synthesised and DNA replicates itself, the number of cells in the body increases (growth) and cells may specialise into specific functions (development) in which some genes are turned on and others turned off. For example, cells of the skin (a specialised tissue) contain all the genetic material needed to recreate an individual, but the only specialised genes that are turned on in these cells are the ones responsible for the formation and color of hair.

TRANSMISSION OF GENETIC MATERIAL

Male or Female

The testes of the bull and the ovaries of the cow produce reproductive cells by a special series of cellular divisions that halve the normal number of chromosomes in a cell. The spermatozoa and the ova contain only one member of a chromosome pair. Thus the cells of cows and bulls contain 60 chromosomes ($2n = 60$), but the spermatozoa in the semen and the ova in the ovaries contain only 30 chromosomes ($n = 30$). The two basic principles of the transmission of a trait (e.g. sex) are as follows:

1. Separation of the paired chromosomes during the formation of reproductive cells.
2. Union of a spermatozoon with an ovum to create a new cell with a unique set of chromosomes.

For 29 of the chromosome pairs, both members are visually identical. However, for one of the pairs, one member is much longer; it is called the X chromosome, and the shorter member is called the Y chromosome. All the ova carry the X chromosome, but the spermatozoa can carry either the X or the Y chromosome. During cellular division to form the reproductive cells, each member of a chromosome pair goes into a separate cell. As a result, 50% of the spermatozoa will carry the X chromosome and the other 50%, the Y chromosome. If by chance a spermatozoon carrying a Y chromosome fertilises an ovum, the offspring will be a male. However, an offspring that receives two X chromosomes develops into a female. It is important to realise that it is impossible to predict the sex of an offspring at the time of mating (insemination), however, we can predict that, on the average, 50% of all the offspring will be male and 50% will be female.

Qualitative Traits

Qualitative traits tend to fall into discrete categories. Usually just one or a few genes have a major effect on qualitative traits. Environment usually has a minor role in influencing the category into which the animal falls. In this case, the phenotype of the animal reflects its genotype. Examples of qualitative traits in dairy cattle are:

- Hair color.
- Hereditary defects such as dwarfism.
- Presence or absence of horns.
- Blood type.

Quantitative Traits

Quantitative traits differ from qualitative traits in two important ways:

1. They are influenced by many pairs of genes.
2. The phenotypic expression is more strongly influenced by the environment than is true for qualitative traits.

Many of the economically important traits in dairy cattle are quantitative traits:

- Milk yield.
- Milk composition.
- Conformation (also referred to as type).
- Efficiency of feed conversion.
- Disease resistance.

The combined influence of many genes and the effect of the environment on quantitative traits make it much more difficult to determine the genotype accurately than in the case of most qualitative traits. Sometimes the animal's phenotype tells us very little about its genotype. For example, a lactation record only tells a portion of the information about the genetic merit of a cow for milk yield.

What makes the Genotype of a Cow Unique?

When ova are formed, they receive one of the two members of a chromosome pair. Thus a particular chromosome in an ovum can be like either the first member or the second member of the parental chromosome pair. There are only two different kinds of ova for that particular chromosome. If instead of one chromosome pair, we now consider two, what does the total number of different ova become? In other words, what is the total number of possible chromosome combinations? This situation is like flipping two coins at the same time. The number of possible combinations is: two possible values for the first coin times two possible values for the second coin = $2 \times 2 = 2^2 = 4$ different possibilities. The number of different genotypes for an ovum is four and the probability of any particular combination of chromosomes is ¼. This is also true for the number of possible genotypes in male reproductive cells. Thus when one out of four possible kinds of spermatozoa fertilises (Fig. 4.2) one out of four possible kinds of ova, the number of possible genetically different offspring is $4 \times 4 = 16$ (i.e. $2^2 \times 2^2$). Thus the chance for any particular genotype in the newborn offspring is 1/16.

GENETICS IN EVERYDAY LIFE

Genetics is the study of genes genetics is about how and why physical characteristics such as eye colour are passed on from one generation to another about how diseases and conditions can run in families the study of patterns in genetic information, such as the patterns used in DNA fingerprinting and profiling and genetics is about how variation occurs in and between animals, plants or humans.

Genetics Affects us in Many Ways

Genetics affects us all in many ways. Genetics can help us to understand why people look the way they do and why some people are more prone to certain diseases than others. Genetics can help health-care professionals to identify certain conditions in babies before they are born using techniques such as prenatal testing. Genetic technologies are also being used to help develop targeted medicines for certain diseases. In addition to its use in health care, genetics has a range of other applications.

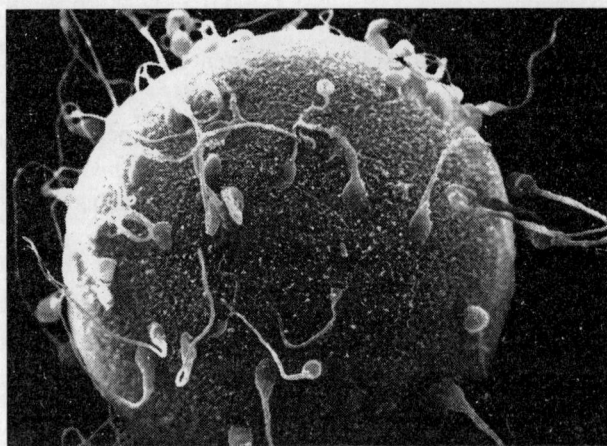

Fig. 4.2: Spermatozoa fertilises.

For example, the police can use genetic fingerprinting to catch criminals. Genetic fingerprinting was invented and developed by Sir Alec Jeffreys at the University of Leicester in 1984. This technique can identify individuals on the basis of their genetic information.

Criminals often leave evidence of their identity at a crime scene: for example, hair follicles, blood or skin cells. The police can use the genetic information to demonstrate whether or not an individual was present at the scene of a crime. Genetic information can prove innocence and help to identify and convict the guilty.

Important Concepts of Genetics

To understand genetics, it is important to know something about cells, chromosomes and DNA. All living things are made up of cells. The cell is the basic building block of life. A human body contains millions and millions of cells. An average adult has an estimated ten to one hundred thousand million cells. Each cell is so small that you can only see it using a microscope. There are many different types of cells, and they all have a different job to do. For example, the human body contains muscle cells, blood cells and skin cells. We can use a computer animation to show you what it is like inside a human cell. The nucleus is a very important component of the cell. It is the control centre and contains all our genetic information in the form of structures called chromosomes.

Chromosomes carry information about you. For example, whether you have straight or curly hair, how your heart functions, and even which hand you write with. Chromosomes help to keep your genetic information neat, organised and compact, in much the same way that a filing cabinet can be used to organise paperwork. Chromosomes are made up of long strands of a chemical called deoxyribonucleic acid – or DNA for short. DNA contains four building blocks called adenine, thymine, cytosine and guanine. These are often referred to by their initial letters – A, T, C and G – and form long sequences that represent your unique genetic code. DNA consists of two ribbon-like strands that wrap around each other like a twisted ladder. This structure is described as a double helix. Part of the genetic information in the DNA is organised into thousands of specific coded instructions called genes. It is these genes that contain all the information needed to make you who you are.

Inheritance

In order to find out how characteristics are passed on from generation to generation, it is important to know something about basic inheritance.

Genetic Conditions

There are many genetic conditions and they can affect all parts of the body. Here we will outline some of the most common genetic conditions. Thalassaemia is a recessive condition that affects the blood. Individuals with this condition do not produce enough red blood cells and so find it difficult to transport oxygen around their bodies. Thalassaemia can affect individuals from any ethnic group, but it is especially common in people from Mediterranean countries, such as Italy and Malta, as well as India, Pakistan, the Middle East, and South-East Asia.

Genetics allows us to understand how thalassaemia is passed on in families. Blood tests and genetic investigations can help us to determine whether an individual has the disease or is a carrier. Our improved understanding of the causes of the condition may even raise the possibility of future gene-based therapies that may offer a cure. Cystic fibrosis is the most common genetic condition in White Europeans. It affects the cells that produce mucus, sweat, saliva and digestive fluids. These secretions are normally thin and slippery, but in cystic fibrosis they are thicker and stickier. This makes it difficult for important organs such as the lungs and the digestive system to work properly, making it harder to breathe. Modern genetics can help parents with a family history of the disease to understand their risk of passing it on to their children, and provide tests that can identify the condition in babies before they are born.

Chapter 5

Molecular Genetics

INTRODUCTION

Molecular genetics is the field of biology which studies the structure and function of genes at a molecular level. The field studies how the genes are transferred from generation to generation. Molecular genetics employs the methods of genetics and molecular biology. It is so-called to differentiate it from other sub-fields of genetics such as ecological genetics and population genetics. An important area within molecular genetics is the use of molecular information to determine the patterns of descent and therefore the correct scientific classification of organisms—this is called molecular systematics. Along with determining the pattern of descendants, molecular genetics helps in understanding genetic mutations that can cause certain types of diseases. Through utilising the methods of genetics and molecular biology, molecular genetics discovers the reasons why traits are carried on and how and why some may mutate.

EPIGENETIC MECHANISMS REGULATING GENE EXPRESSION

Epigenetic mechanisms regulate gene function in a heritable manner, but do so without modulating the DNA sequence of the affected gene. Many different genetic functions are influenced by epigenetic mechanisms in various species. These include regulation of gene expression, DNA modification and restriction, genomic imprinting, X-chromosome inactivation, paramutation, position effect variegation, mating type, cell determination, transposable elements and mutator and suppressor genes. This section will focus on epigenetic mechanisms that regulate gene expression and the manner in which they accomplish this in mammalian species.

Nuclear DNA acts as the repository of genetic information in eukaryotic cells. In mammals, and many other animal species, a complete representation of the genome is maintained in essentially every nucleated cell. However, only a subset of this collection of genes is expressed in any particular cell type. Thus, it is not the presence of specific genes, but rather the expression of specific genes, that leads to the unique identity and function of any particular cell. For protein-encoding genes, two primary steps are involved in gene expression: transcription of DNA into RNA and translation of that RNA into a polypeptide. This affords two levels of regulation of gene expression: transcriptional regulation and translational (or post-transcriptional) regulation. For tissue-specific genes (those expressed in only a subset of tissues or in a

100

single tissue or cell type), regulation is primarily manifest at the transcriptional level. Extensive studies of this process have revealed a consensus mechanism whereby the promoter region, typically located at the 5′-end of the gene, acts to bind specific proteins called transcription factors which, in turn, attract (or prevent) binding of the RNA polymerase that is required to initiate transcription.

Binding of transcription factors to specific gene promoters and to specific sites within those promoters is regulated by the ability of a DNA binding domain within each protein factor to recognise a unique three-dimensional structure of double stranded DNA. This unique structure is imparted by a specific nucleotide sequence, typically 5–15 base pairs (bp) in length. Thus, this mechanism does rely on the DNA sequence and is therefore not a truly epigenetic mechanism. However, because these transcription factors can be either ubiquitous or tissue-specific, and can either promote or inhibit transcription, this mechanism can modulate tissue, cell-type or developmental-stage specificity of transcription, as well as controlling the relative level (or frequency) of transcription. Nevertheless, protein-DNA interactions between transcription factors and promoter sequences, respectively, are not the only mechanism by which gene expression is regulated in eukaryotic cells.

In mammals there are several examples in which genes are regulated by mechanisms other than transcription factors. For example, in female somatic cells, genes on the active X-chromosome are transcribed, whereas homologous genes on the inactive X-chromosome remain transcriptionally silenced. This is despite the fact that both the active and inactive copies of these genes share identical nucleotide sequences and reside within the same nucleus.

Thus the presence of identical promoter sequences and cognate transcription factors alone does not ensure identical regulation of genes. Similarly, in mammals, the phenomenon of genomic imprinting results in the expression of only one of the two copies of a particular gene within a single diploid cell. In this case the choice of which allele is expressed is dictated by the parental origin of that allele. However, the mechanism that regulates such monoallelic expression cannot be based solely on transcription factors and promoter sequences, because the former are present throughout the nucleus in which both alleles reside, and the latter are often identical on both alleles.

The unavoidable conclusion from these observations is that there must be additional mechanisms by which gene expression is regulated in eukaryotic cells, and these mechanisms must function in a manner that does not depend on differences in nucleotide sequence or the cell-type specific presence or absence of transcription factors. Yet, as exemplified by the examples noted earlier for X-chromosome inactivation and genomic imprinting, these mechanisms must function in a heritable manner, such that the same alleles remain expressed or silenced, even after replication of the DNA and division of one cell to produce two daughter cells.

We now know that there are multiple mechanisms that meet the criteria of epigenetic mechanisms in that they regulate gene expression in a heritable manner that does not rely on differences in DNA sequence. Examples of mechanisms that either have been shown to operate in this manner or have the potential to operate in this manner include: DNA methylation, chromatin structure and/or composition, DNA loop domains and association with the nuclear matrix and DNA replication timing.

DNA Methylation

In mammals, methylation of DNA is found only on cytosines present in a 5′-CpG-3′ dinucleotide sequence. Because cytosine and guanine are complementary bases, wherever there is a CpG dinucleotide in one DNA strand, there will be a complementary CpG on the opposite strand. This double-stranded structure can exist in three different states with respect to methylation (Fig. 5.1). It can be fully methylated, meaning that both cytosines are methylated (Fig. 5.1b) or it can be completely unmethylated if neither cytosine is methylated (Fig. 5.1a). When a fully methylated site is replicated by semi-conservative replication, the resulting structure is hemimethylated (Fig. 5.1c). This is typically a transient state because it forms a template for a ubiquitously functioning DNA maintenance methyl transferase that recognises the hemimethylated structure and returns it to a fully methylated state. Thus, fully methylated and unmethylated sites are maintained (and/or reestablished) throughout replication of DNA and cellular division. In this way methylated and unmethylated states of DNA are heritable.

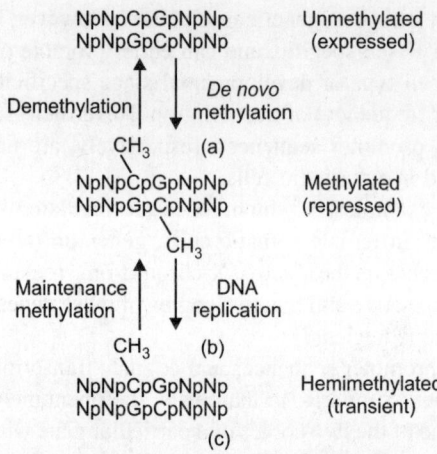

Fig. 5.1: Alternate states of DNA methylation in mammalian DNA. Methylation occurs only on cytosines present in CpG dinucleotides in mammalian DNA. A CpG dinucleotide sequence in one DNA strand mandates the presence of a complementary CpG dinucleotide in the other strand of double-stranded DNA. (a) If both cytosines in such a site are unmethylated, the site is said to be completely unmethylated. This structure is often found in actively expressed or potentiated genes, especially in the 5' regulatory region. (b) An unmethylated site can undergo *de novo* methylation to form a fully methylated site in which both cytosines are methylated. This structure is often found associated with repressed genes. Conversely a demethylase activity can convert a fully methylated site to a fully unmethylated site in the absence of DNA replication. (c) Upon semi-conservative replication of a fully methylated site, a hemimethylated site is formed. This structure is typically transient as a maintenance DNA methyl transferase rapidly recognises a hemimethylated site and returns it to a fully methylated state. The function of the maintenance methylase provides a mechanism to heritably maintain DNA methylation patterns. C, cytosine, G, guanine, N, any base, p, phosphate bond, CH_3, methyl group.

It is possible for an unmethylated site to be directly converted to a fully methylated site and *vice versa*. Methylation of an unmethylated site is achieved by a *de novo* methylase, whereas a direct transition from a fully methylated to an unmethylated structure in the absence of DNA replication is accomplished by a demethylase activity. The function of these enzymatic activities and the manner in which they are regulated are not as well-characterised as that of the maintenance methylase activity. However, there is ample evidence that such activities do indeed exist. Shortly after fertilisation in the mouse, nearly all of the methylation that is brought into the zygote by the gametic genomes is lost, such that the blastocyst genome is nearly devoid of DNA methylation except for that at a few imprinted sites. This may occur either by dilution of methylated strands as replication proceeds in the absence of maintenance methylase activity or by direct demethylation or by some combination of these two mechanisms. Subsequently, at about the time of gastrulation, there is a *de novo* methylation event at numerous different sites throughout the genome. This must be accomplished by a *de novo* methylase because completely unmethylated sites become fully methylated. Following gastrulation, many different cell lineages become allocated and begin to develop and differentiate. Coincident with this, selective demethylation of many tissue-specific genes is often observed within the cell lineage in which these genes will ultimately be expressed. In most cases this appears to occur via a demethylase activity, because in at least some cases demethylation occurs in the complete absence of DNA replication or cellular division.

In addition to tissue-specific genes that are expressed in a limited tissue, cell-type or developmental-stage specific pattern, another set of housekeeping genes is widely expressed in a ubiquitous and constitutive manner. These genes, which do not require as complicated transcriptional regulation as that needed for tissue-specific genes, often bear a CpG island, most commonly in the 5′-portion of the gene. A CpG island has been defined as a region in the mammalian genome of > 100 bp with a GC content of > 50 per cent that lacks the typical underrepresentation of CpG dinucleotides seen in other regions of the genome. Generally, CpG islands remain constitutively unmethylated throughout development and differentiation of cells. Exceptions to this rule include CpG islands associated with genes on the inactive X-chromosome or with nonexpressed, inactive alleles of imprinted genes, as well as those associated with certain genes in cancerous tumours (e.g. tumour-suppressor genes). In these cases, the island associated with the nonexpressed allele or gene is typically methylated.

For both individual CpG dinucleotides located in non-CpG island regions and CpG dinucleotides within CpG islands, a general correlation has been observed between the presence of DNA methylation and inhibition of expression, and between the absence of DNA methylation and active transcription. This is especially true for sites in the 5′-flanking region or in the 5′-half of transcribed portions of genes. At least two types of mechanisms have been proposed by which DNA methylation or the lack thereof, might contribute to regulation of transcription. In one case, the presence or absence of methylation on key cytosines within a particular transcription factor binding site may modulate the ability of the factor to bind to that site. In a second scenario, the presence or absence of methylation at sites either within factor binding sites or in regions adjacent to factor binding sites may inhibit factor binding indirectly by affecting chromatin structure. A direct mechanistic connection has now been established between DNA methylation and chromatin structure. In this case, it is suggested that the presence of methylation stabilises a condensed (closed) chromatin structure that is, in turn, refractory to binding by transcription factors and/or RNA polymerase. Conversely, an absence of methylation leads to a less condensed (open) chromatin structure that is accessible to transcription factors and RNA polymerase. Effects of DNA methylation on chromatin structure appear to be mediated by methylated DNA-binding proteins that bind to methylated DNA on the basis of the presence or absence of methylation, rather than on the basis of a particular binding sequence as is the case for transcription factors.

Two methylated-DNA binding proteins were originally identified, MeCP1 and MeCP2. MeCP1 is a large protein complex that binds best to regions of DNA containing >10 methyl-CpGs and has been shown to be involved in repression of transcription from densely methylated promoters. It also binds to, and represses transcription from, more sparsely methylated promoters, although this is a much weaker interaction. MeCP2 is a single polypeptide that can bind to as few as a single fully methylated CpG site. *In vivo* it appears to bind predominantly to highly methylated satellite DNAs adjacent to centromeres in the mouse genome, but shows a more dispersed binding pattern in the genomes of human and rats, which do not contain highly methylated satellite DNA. Recently, screens for cDNAs encoding methyl-

CpG binding domains (MBDs) have revealed at least four such genes, MBD1–4. The MBD1 protein is a component of the MeCP1 protein complex. The MBD2–4 encode methylated DNA binding proteins that are distinct from those associated with either MeCP1 or MeCP2, but bear a striking similarity to the MBD of MeCP2. The products of MBD2 and MBD4 bind to methylated CpGs both *in vitro* and *in vivo* and are thus considered to be additional candidates for mediators of mechanisms associated with methylated DNA.

The manner in which tissue, cell-type and/or gene-specific patterns of DNA methylation are established or modulated remains to be fully elucidated. However, there appears to be a combination of general and specific mechanisms that contribute to this process. The general mechanisms include those that result in genomewide loss or gain of methylation, especially during early embryogenesis, along with the maintenance methylase activity that reestablishes full methylation at hemimethylated sites following replication of DNA. Cell-type, developmental-stage and gene-specific demethylation have been shown to be regulated by signal sequences within the promoter region of at least one tissue-specific gene. Regulation of CpG island methylation has also been shown to be dependent on signal sequences within certain imprinted genes. However, it appears that different methylases and demethylases may be responsible for *de novo* methylation/demethylation of CpG dinucleotides within or exclusive of CpG islands, respectively.

GENE FAMILIES

Gene families refer to two or more genes that come from a common ancestral gene in which the individual members of the gene family may or may not have a similar function. The idea of gene families implicitly invokes a process in which an original gene exists, is duplicated and the resulting gene products evolve. The most common result of gene duplication is that mutation renders one of the products nonfunctional and in the absence of conserving natural selection, one of the members becomes no longer recognisable. Gene families may be clustered or dispersed and may exchange with each other through the mechanisms of gene conversion or unequal crossover.

Therefore, understanding the processes of molecular evolution are essential to understanding what gene families are, where they came from and what their function might be. In a sense, duplicate genes allow for more evolutionary potential. At first glance this could be beneficial, if one gene incurred a lethal mutation the other gene simply takes over, there is some protection from mutation based on redundancy. Having two identical genes could result in twice as much product, this may or may not be beneficial in a cell where the integration of thousands of gene products must be coordinated and slight concentration differences can alter biochemical pathways.

Antiquity of Gene Families

Almost all genes belong to gene families. Evidence from sequence or structural similarity indicates that all or at least large parts of genes came from ancestral genes. Analysis of the human genome has shown that over half of the human genome is comprised of clearly identifiable repeated sequences. Although much of this is owing to self-replicating transposons, i.e. mobile genetic elements, over 5 per cent of the genome has been involved in large segmental duplications in the past 30 million years. If we look further into the past using evidence from protein similarity of three or more genes that occur in close proximity on two different chromosomes, we find over 10,310 gene pairs in 1077 duplicated blocks contain 3522 distinct genes. Because our observations are based on genes that retain similarity, only a small fraction of the ancient duplications can be detected by current means. What is clearly evident is that a very large part of the human genome has come from duplications and that duplication is a very frequent event.

With the evidence showing that gene duplication plays a major role in modern genomes, the question is where did it all begin? How many genes did life start with? Various estimates of the minimal gene set suggest that as few as 250 genes could provide the minimal number of components necessary to sustain independent life. The number of genes in mycoplasms ranges from 500–1500 genes and in bacteria from 1000–4000 genes. Yeast (*S. cervisiae*) has ~6000 genes, worms (*C. elegans*) have ~18,000 genes, the fruit fly (*D. melangaster*) has ~13,000 genes, a plant, *Arabidopsis*, has 26000 genes, and humans have at least 30000 genes. The difference between 250 or 1000 genes and 30,000–40,000 genes is only two orders of magnitude yet the difference in the complexity of life forms seems far greater than could be explained by a simple gene count. Certainly with the increased number of genes comes the opportunity for more complexity in terms of gene interaction. But can synergy alone explain the differences in morphological complexity? Partial explanations invoke more complex differential splicing to account for a higher proportional number of protein products stemming from only 30,000 genes, but one wonders if this observation is merely an artifact of the few numbers of whole genomes available to us.

Origins of Gene Duplications

Gene duplications can come from a variety of sources including whole or partial genome duplication. Polyploidy results from a failure of chromosome segregation during the cell division of gametes. The most distinguishing feature of polyploidy is that it effects all of the genes simultaneously so that the relative proportion of genes within cells remains the same. Among plants and invertebrates, polyploidy is quite common and in many species it has little effect on phenotype. Ohno has argued that whole genome duplications are the most important events in evolution yet others have suggested that polyploidy has no effect on phenotype. More recent discussions: acknowledge the potential that polypoidy brings to gene family evolution but also appreciate the role of complexity of gene interactions in determining the impact of whole genome duplications. In vertebrates, polyploidy is quite rare. Most of the 188 examples of genome duplication have been found in amphibians, reptiles and some fish (salmon). In these instances, polyploid species have undergone dramatic changes to reestablish diploidy through chromosome loss, mutation and rearrangement. Tetraploid genomes have no trouble going through cell division as long as chromosomes remain very similar. But as mutations arise and duplicated chromosomes begin to differ, cell division can no longer insure equal division of genetic material to germ cells and severe imbalances can occur during chromosomal segregation. The initial transition phase from tetraploid to diploid results in huge losses of gametes and developing young. In salmon it is estimated that approx 50 million years after a polyploid change, only 53 per cent of duplicate genes remain. The result of duplication by whole or partial genomes can result in large changes in gene number but there are major difficulties in cell replication that must be overcome.

The rapid increase in genome size through polyploid events has been used to explain the increased size of mammalian genomes. Ohno suggested that two rounds of genome duplication occurred early in vertebrate history. This may explain the Cambrian explosion in which vertebrates appeared in paleontological records quite rapidly. Evidence for two rounds of genome duplication comes from vertebrates having four times the number of developmental regulator genes (Hox, Cdx, MyoD, 60A, Notch, elav, btd/SP...) as *Drosophila*. While this concept has become very popular in the literature, recent studies examining expected phylogenetic relationships among genes have called into question whether the number of genes was a result of two genome-wide duplications or simply a result of ongoing, frequent genome segment duplications. While the primary support for quadruplicated genomes comes primarily from chromosomes 2, 7, 12 and 17, which contain the Hox gene clusters, a more extensive examination of the number of homologous genes within human as compared to genes within *Drosophila* was unable to resolve the question of whether two whole genome duplications gave rise to modern vertebrate genomes.

Mechanisms of DNA Duplications

Duplication of large blocks of DNA cannot be explained by chromosomal segregation errors. Mechanisms of large segmental duplication are varied and the role of transposable elements in gene duplication is often cited as a primary cause. Transposable elements and in particular retrotransposable elements are highly repetitive dispersed sequences that can replicate independent of nuclear division. In human they comprise over 45 per cent of the genome. While there are a number of instances where retroposons have been found at the junctions of duplicated segments, there are also a number of instances where they have not. To understand why gene segment duplications appear common, it is perhaps important to look at the DNA molecule itself. DNA is composed of duplex strands held together by hydrogen bonds whose strength varies. In a fluid environment, various local salt concentrations, temperatures, physical torsion forces and local nucleotide compositions (e.g. levels of G + C, simple repeats) can result in temporary separation of strands of duplex DNA. If similar sequences are found in the same physical location, unstable heterologous duplexes can form. Heterologous pairing or single-strand conditions are prone to stress and breakage. These situations are repaired correctly in the vast majority of cases but occasionally mistakes are made that result in new gene neighbours. The possibility of error is particularly high during cell division when DNA is being replicated and when similar sequences are in close proximity. The potential impact of highly repeated transposable elements as a destabilising factor and a potential focal point for rearrangement becomes clear in our genome. It is, therefore, somewhat surprising to find that many of the duplications are not flanked by repeat elements. What is clear is that duplication involves local chromosome instability that results in breakage and aberrant repair of the ends.

Factors that promote segmental duplication include close proximity and high sequence similarity. It then follows that duplications resulting in adjacent genes would be more susceptible to further changes than duplications resulting in dispersed genes. Furthermore, adjacent duplications create far fewer chromosomal segregation problems during cell division and therefore, should be found more often in the genome. What is observed is that large segmental duplications involving multiple genes are dispersed throughout the genome whereas duplications involving single gene segments are both dispersed and in close proximity. There are many instances of clustered gene families (globins, Hox, Ig, Tcr, Mhc and rRNA). Among tandemly duplicated gene segments there is the possibility of extensive gene conversion and unequal crossing over (Fig. 5.2). The later is the predominant mode of change. Unequal crossing over between dispersed genes results in extreme difficulties in chromosomal segregation in cell division but gene conversion does not.

Gene conversion replaces the sequence of one family member with the sequences of another close (> 90 per cent similarity) member but it does not effect the total number of genes. Gene conversion requires DNA strand breakage followed by strand migration to a similar gene and the formation of a heteroduplex. DNA repair mechanisms then repair differences in the heteroduplex often using one strand corresponding to the unaffected homologous chromosome as a template. The heteroduplex then resolves and may go back to its original location carrying with it DNA changes. Heteroduplex formation is often temporary and most often occurs between alleles of the same gene though occasionally it may affect paralogous genes in which more than 100 bases are greater than 95 per cent similar.

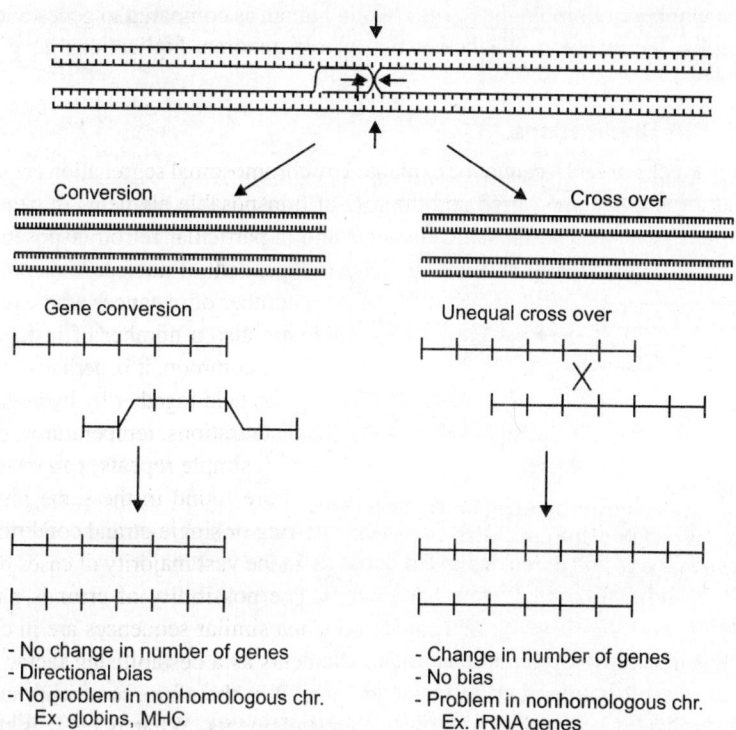

Conversion

Cross over

Gene conversion

Unequal cross over

- No change in number of genes
- Directional bias
- No problem in nonhomologous chr.
  Ex. globins, MHC

- Change in number of genes
- No bias
- Problem in nonhomologous chr.
  Ex. rRNA genes

Fig. 5.2: Gene conversion and unequal crossing over mechanisms of communication among gene family members. The arrows indicate possible break points that would result in either conversion or cross over results.

Depending on the resolution of the heteroduplex and biases in mismatch repair, adjacent base differences may both reflect one or the other parental strand or they may reflect a combination of parental strands. The end result is that the total genetic variation is reduced but a particular gene may increase its number of alleles. Genetic variation at one gene can increase over a single conversion event, but over multiple conversion events variation is reduced.

The resolution of heteroduplexes formed from the invasion of a DNA strand from one gene segment into the duplex of a similar, adjacent duplicate can also result in unequal crossing over. Unequal crossing over changes the number of genes. For example, in a tandem arrangement, unequal crossing over results in one chromosome with one duplicate and the other chromosome with three duplicates where the front and the back parts of the single duplicate and the middle duplicate of the triplicated segment reflect different origins.

Figure 5.3 shows three successive unequal crossing-over events and shows the expected phylogenetic relationships of the front (5′) and back (3′) parts of the gene. It is evident from the final trees for the 5′ and 3′ parts of a tandemly arrayed gene segment that it is possible to describe some of the major, more recent evolutionary events that have occurred. Because information is lost due to the fixation of one of the cross over products in each population, it may never be possible to obtain a complete historical picture. But we can see in examples from the literature that unequal crossing over is the major factor in clustered gene families.

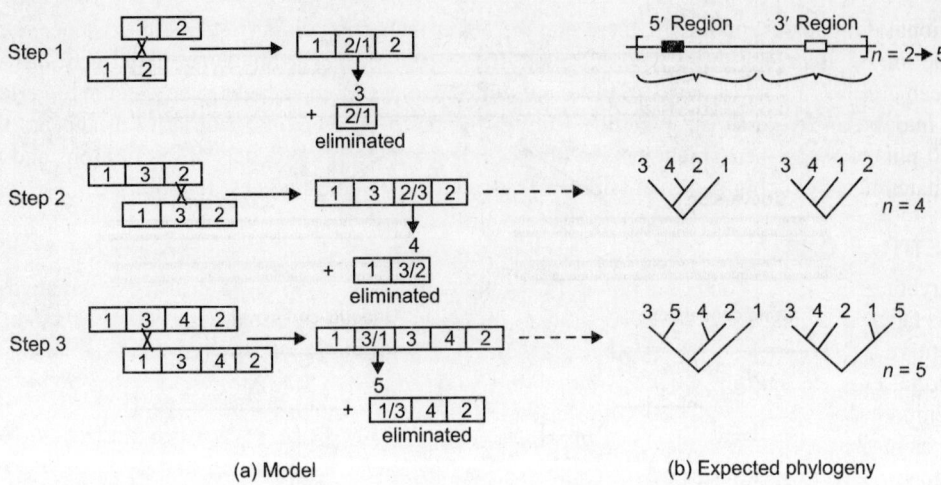

Fig. 5.3: Unequal crossing over between tandemly arrayed gene family members. This model (a) assumes a break-point near the middle of the duplicated segments. The expected phylogeny, and (b) represent sequence relationships between the 5' and 3' regions of the duplicated gene segments.

Genetic Variation

Genetic variation increases when the number of duplicates increases but it is decreased when the number of duplicates decreases. It is important to remember several tenets of unequal crossing over. First, the ultimate fate of duplicates undergoing multiple unequal crossing overs is to return to a single copy unless selection maintains multiple copies. Second, while the overall variation may increase over a single event, the result over multiple expansions and deletions is homogenisation of duplicates (example rRNA genes). Third, unequal crossing over between dispersed gene segments often results in fatal problems in cell division. Lastly, unequal crossing over is the predominant mechanism that increases or decreases the number of gene family members in clusters. It appears that the factors that promote duplication include proximity, high similarity, larger numbers of existing duplicates and internal sequences that are prone to breakage. Given these factors, it is perhaps surprising that we do not see more evidence of repetitive elements playing a larger role in gene duplication. At the same time it becomes easy to see the complex evolution and interactions among both dispersed and clustered gene families.

Genes and Domains

Duplication can involve very large stretches of DNA, whole genes or even parts of genes. Of 1077 duplication blocks containing three or more genes in the human genome, 159 contained 3 genes, 137 contained 4 genes and 781 contained five or more genes. At the same time we often see clusters of gene family members. This indicates that duplications often involve one gene or even parts of genes. Clearly the mechanisms of duplication outlined earlier play a major role at all levels of gene family evolution. However, it is important to remember that the events that are most evident are those that are fairly recent or those that involve conserved genes. Sequence similarity for older duplications of noncoding DNA rapidly fades. It is our focus on function that draws us to study genes. As mentioned, several genes within larger segments can be duplicated but perhaps just as interesting, parts of genes (introns and groups of introns) can be duplicated. This is particularly interesting because genes are composed of functional domains. Remarkably, there may be fewer than 1000 classifications in existence. Domains can be mixed, matched, duplicated and modified to provide novel functions within genes as well as between genes. Only 94 of the 1278 protein families in our genome appear to be specific to vertebrates. That may be an overestimate resulting from our inability to recognise similarity. It appears that the 30000-plus genes in the human genome are not novel but simply products of duplications and mixing and matching of existing genes and domains to create new genes and new functions.

REPETITIVE DNA

Eukaryotic genomes are composed primarily of nonprotein-coding DNA. The most actively studied portion of this DNA is called repetitive DNA, which is produced in multiple copies by a variety of mechanisms. Repetitive DNA represents the most recent addition to nonprotein coding DNA and is expected to hold important clues to the origin and evolution of genomic DNA. There are good reasons to believe that contemporary mechanisms underlying the origin and evolution of repetitive DNA are essentially the same as mechanisms that generated other nonprotein-coding sequences in the distant past.

Repetitive DNA began surfacing in unprecedented detail as soon as critical mass of human sequence data permitted comparative analyses. This set the stage for a new era of repeat studies dominated by computer-assisted sequence comparisons. Currently, 42 per cent of the human genome is recognisable as being derived from repetitive DNA. This proportion may vary from species to species in a seemingly arbitrary manner and the exact reasons why some eukaryotic species preserve more DNA than others are not well understood. Studies of repetitive DNA are important not only *per se*, but also in the context of genome biology, including its structure, stability and evolution. Repeats often obscure proteins and other regions of biological significance and for this reason they need to be identified and filtered out of the sequence data to facilitate such studies. Identification of repeats is also necessary for probe and primer design in DNA-DNA hybridisation and polymerase chain reaction (PCR) studies, respectively. Inevitably, they are increasingly being studied in various biological contexts including but not limited to phylogenetic analysis, population studies, gene polymorphism and chromosomal organisation.

Simple Sequence Repeats (SSRs)

There are two basic classes of repetitive DNA sequences: (i) those expanded spontaneously on-site, and (ii) those transposed from somewhere else as copies of transposable elements (TEs). These two classes are not totally independent because TEs can initiate or stimulate on-site expansion of repetitive DNA. The most common repeats generated on site are tandem repeats, often referred to as simple sequence repeats or SSRs. Typically, tandem repeats with a unit size of 10 bp or less are referred to as microsatellites. Tandem repeats with a unit size over 10 bp are called minisatellites. There is a significant twilight zone between micro- and minisatellites, usually applicable to repeats with unit size 7–14 bp, which is listed in either category in the scientific literature.

The number of units, i.e. overall length of micro and minisatellites, can vary from generation to generation and this property makes them very useful in studies of sequence polymorphism in eukaryotic population. Growing evidence indicates that micro and minisatellite expansion occurs by different mechanisms: the former mostly due to polymerase slippage and the latter due to an illegitimate recombination process stimulated by double-stranded breaks. Tandem repeats are often transformed to a cryptically simple DNA composed of various sequence motifs rearranged, and often obscured by mutations. Tandemly repeated sequences include satellite DNA. Satellites are primarily located in centromeres, whereas other tandem repeats, tend to be interspersed within genomic DNA. Like other tandem repeats, satellites, are quite variable and even closely related species may carry completely unrelated satellites. Satellite variability may be fueled by mechanisms similar to those involved in minisatellite variability.

Transposable Elements (TEs)

The major source of interspersed repetitive DNA are transposable elements (TEs). There are two major classes of TEs in the eukaryotic organisms: class 1, retro-elements, class 2, DNA transposons, including rolling-circle transposons, which was recently discovered in plants and nematodes (Fig. 5.4).

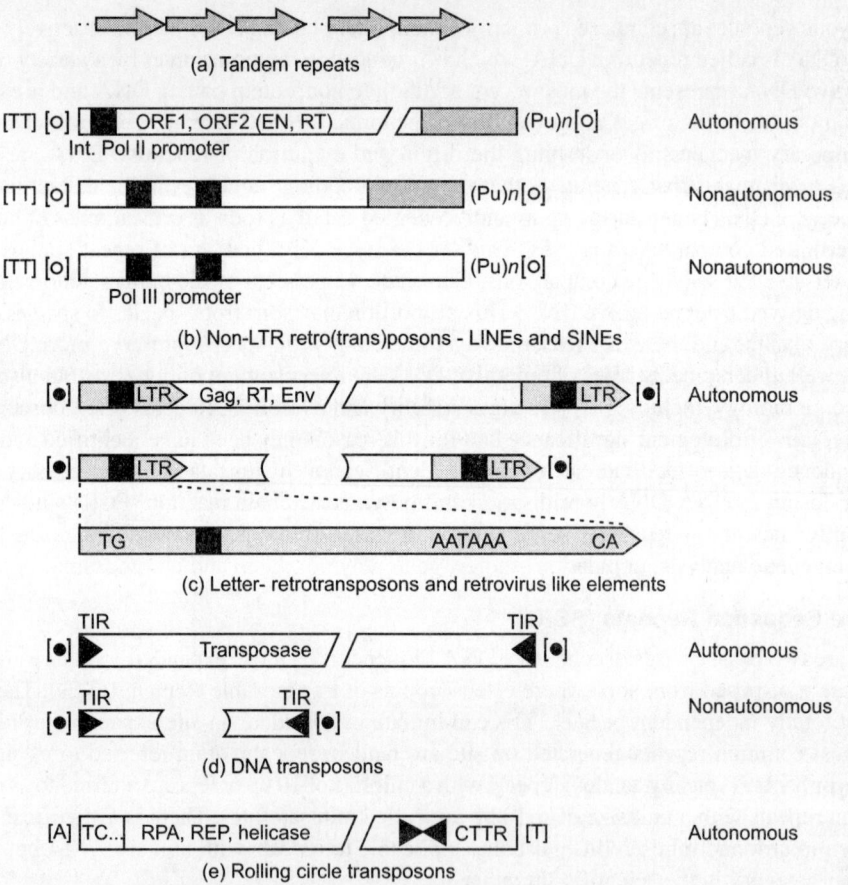

Fig. 5.4: Basic categories and biological characteristics of repetitive elements. (a) Tandem repeats including minisatellites, microsatellites and satellites. (b) Structure of LINE (autonomous) and SINE (nonautonomous) retroelements, black boxes show transcription promoters and (Pu)n indicate purine (A or G) tails. Target site duplications (TSDs) and other target components throughout the figure are indicated by brackets. (c) LTR retrotransposons and retrovirus-like elements. Characteristic sequence features of LTRs: 5′ TG, 3′ CA and polyadenylation signal AATAAA are indicated in the enlarged long terminal repeat. (d) Autonomous and nonautonomous DNA transposons. Black triangles at both ends indicate terminal inverted repeats (TIRs). (e) Autonomous and nonautonomous rolling-circle transposons. Characteristic 5′ TC, 3′ CTTR and hairpin-like structures (inverted black triangles) are indicated.

Retroelements include long interspersed nuclear elements (LINEs) and elements related to retroviruses, including some domesticated endogenous retroviruses. All retroelements use reverse transcriptase to copy their RNA to DNA as a part of their reproduction process. LINEs generate a variety of retropseudogenes including SINE elements. In the case of mammalian LINE1 (L1) element, reverse transcription is initiated (primed) by a reverse transcriptase-generated nick in host DNA. A second nick is generated on the opposite strand leading to target site duplication (TSD) where the duplicated target is represented by a short, ~15 bp long DNA fragment delimited by the nicks. The final integration is probably completed by the host replication system. Unlike LINEs, retroviruses appear to be inserted in a separate step after they are reverse transcribed to DNA. There is no specific mechanism for excision of retroelements although integrated retroviruses can be deleted due to homologous recombination between long terminal repeats (LTRs), leaving behind a single (solo) LTR repeat.

DNA transposons (class 2) encode transposase, which is involved in insertion and excision of these elements to and from host DNA. The transposase recognises terminal inverted repeats (TIRs). Replication of a DNA transposon is accomplished by the host replication system. If excision does not occur, the transposon becomes permanently integrated usually as an inactive repetitive element.

The third class of eukaryotic TEs is represented by complex rolling-circle (RC) transposons. In addition to a cleavage and replication transposase, RC transposons use enzymes such as helicases and the single-strand DNA-binding protein, probably adopted from the host. RC transposons integrate at AT dinucleotides without target site duplication. All classes of autonomous TEs in eukaryotes are associated with nonautonomous elements that do not encode any active enzymes. They depend on their autonomous relatives for reproduction and insertion into the genome. In this context, autonomous TEs can play a role of mutator genes that must be restricted or tightly controlled by the host. In general, only few active TEs at a time appear to find favourable circumstances for proliferation in any given population.

They produce a discrete genomic fossil record of repetitive families/subfamilies derived from a limited number of actively expressed source genes or active TEs. Both autonomous and nonautonomous elements have their actively expressed source genes. Source genes can be active for millions of years but are eventually replaced by their variants or become extinct. Interestingly, copies of nonautonomous elements, particularly short ones, tend to predominate over the autonomous ones. It appears that all eukaryotic genomes integrated a patchwork of TEs inserted at different times from the beginning of their evolutionary history. As indicated earlier, the human genome is among the best repositories of repetitive DNA going back over 200 million years. Unlike human, all repetitive elements in plants and insects appear to be relatively young. This may indicate a rapid turnover of TEs in plant and insect genomes.

Reference Collections of Repeats

A practical approach to identifying and masking repetitive DNA began with creating comprehensive reference collections of repeats that could be compared against newly sequenced DNA. Prior to whole-genome sequencing projects, only human sequences were available in sufficient quantities to reveal a significant variety of human repeat families. These studies laid the foundation for the first collection of 53 representative human repeats. It was followed by collections of other mammalian repeats and placed in a database named Repbase. Since 1997, Repbase was succeeded by Repbase update and over time it included repeats from other eukaryotic species as they became available. Originally, Repbase update (RU) played the role of a database and an electronic journal releasing newly discovered repetitive families that were not published elsewhere. This arrangement is designed to facilitate proper referencing and documentation of the original data deposited in RU.

Analysis of Repetitive DNA

Identification and annotation of known repeats

The basic routine underlying identification and annotation of repetitive DNA remains essentially unchanged since it was first implemented in the Pythia server and reimplemented in XBLAST and CENSOR. Since 1996, major progress has been achieved in terms of speed and sensitivity of repeat detection based on dedicated hardware used in CENSOR server and an efficient implementation of Smith-Waterman algorithm used in RepeatMasker. Detection and annotation of repetitive DNA is based on comparing a query sequence against representative collections of repeats as schematically shown in Fig. 5.5. To avoid nonspecific matches, it is first advisable to filter out simple repeats from the query or reference sequences prior to the analysis by replacing sequence letters with neutral characters such as 'N' or 'X'. There are several ways to identify simple repeats based on their similarity to a reference set or on their nonrandom base composition. Another program, particularly useful for analysing cryptically simple repeats, has been implemented as a part of repeat analysis on the CENSOR server. After simple repeats are masked, complex repeats can be detected by sequence comparisons using the FASTA, BLAST or Smith-Waterman algorithms. FASTA and BLAST are significantly faster but less sensitive than Smith-Waterman-based programs. The latter are essential to detect very old repetitive elements such as the extinct human MIR3 and LINE3 elements that are related to CR1 elements from birds. Conversely, relatively young repeats such as most Alu subfamilies can be detected using a less sensitive approach. Therefore, dividing repeats into detectable categories and the selective application of different algorithms may facilitate the detection process. Apart from these knowledge-based improvements, there are algorithm-based attempts to accelerate repeat detection without sacrificing the sensitivity of the process.

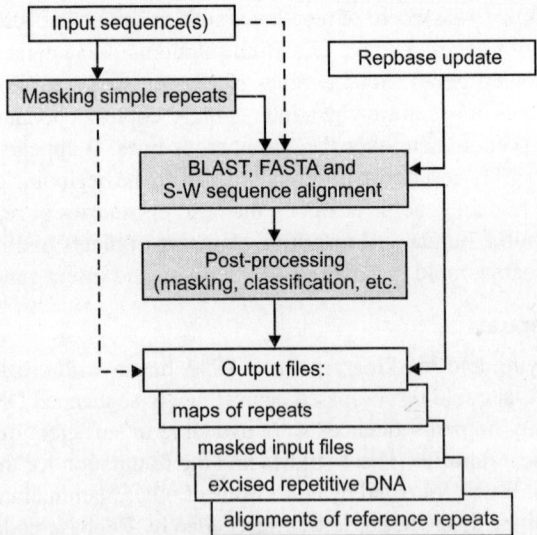

Fig. 5.5: A scheme for automated identification and annotation of repetitive DNA. Continuous arrows indicate critical steps, whereas broken arrows show major variants of the process. Typical output files include: maps of repeats, masked query file(s), a list of masked sequences and alignments against the reference sequences as described in the text.

It must be noted, the major determinant of speed, sensitivity, and accuracy is the quality of reference collections as discussed in the next section. There are several types of output files generated by repeat annotation program (examples are listed in Fig. 5.5). They include maps of repeats summarising location and basic characteristics of individual elements, query files with masked repeats, sequences and coordinates of the identified repeats and alignment to reference sequences for detailed inspection.

MOLECULAR GENETICS OF DISEASE AND THE HUMAN GENOME PROJECT

The haploid (*n*) human genome contains approx 3 billion nucleotides (or bases) of DNA strung amongst 23 chromosomes. The diploid (2*n*) complement, which consists of a haploid genome inherited from each parent, therefore comprises 46 chromosomes of 6 billion nucleotides of DNA, all contained within the cell nucleus. The same complement of DNA is found in every cell (except red blood cells) in the body. Mitochondrial DNA, which is a circular molecule of genetic material, 16000 nucleotides long, is also part of the human genome.

It is located outside the nucleus in the cytoplasm of the cell and encodes a small but important subset of human genes. Mitochondrial DNA is only transmitted from mothers to their offspring. On average, the human genome is 99.9 per cent identical between any two individuals, with nucleotide differences existing only about 1 in every 1000 bases. Less than 5 per cent of the genome contains genes or protein-coding regions.

The remaining 95 per cent (noncoding part) contains repetitive elements and other sequences whose functions are not completely understood and is often referred to as junk DNA. These regions may play a role in maintaining the structural integrity of chromosomes. There at least 30,000–40,000 genes in the human genome, ranging in size less than 1 to 200 kilobases (kb), with the average size of a gene being 50 kb. General information on the human genome is provided in Table 5.1.

Table 5.1: Components of the human genome.

The genome is the total genetic material in a cell
The nuclear genome is comprised of 46 chromosomes, which come as 23 pairs, one of each pair comes from either parent
Mitochondrial DNA is also part of the genome. It is always inherited from the mother and is found in the cytoplasm
Chromosomes are made of deoxyribonucleic acid (DNA)
DNA is made of four chemical units (nucleotides) called adenine (A), guanine (G), cytosine (C) and thymine (T)
The genome is comprised of about 3 billion A, C, G and Ts
Genes are the portions of DNA that encode functional RNA molecules or proteins
There are approx 30000–40000 genes in the genome
Proteins provide the structure for the cell and are involved in biochemical reactions (enzymes)

Genes are comprised of exons-regions that code for mature mRNA- and introns-intervening segments of DNA that are transcribed, but then cut out from the transcript during mRNA processing (Fig. 5.6). There is no uniformity to the number or size of introns, this is the main reason why there is a vast range of gene sizes. Genes contain promoter sequences at their start (5′ end). Typical promoters contain several DNA sequence motifs that bind regulatory proteins and control the level of transcription and the start position of the mRNA. Expression of tissue-specific genes are unique to individual or sets of tissues (muscle, brain, liver, etc.) in our bodies. There are also housekeeping genes that are expressed in all cell types because their products provide basic functions (Table 5.2).

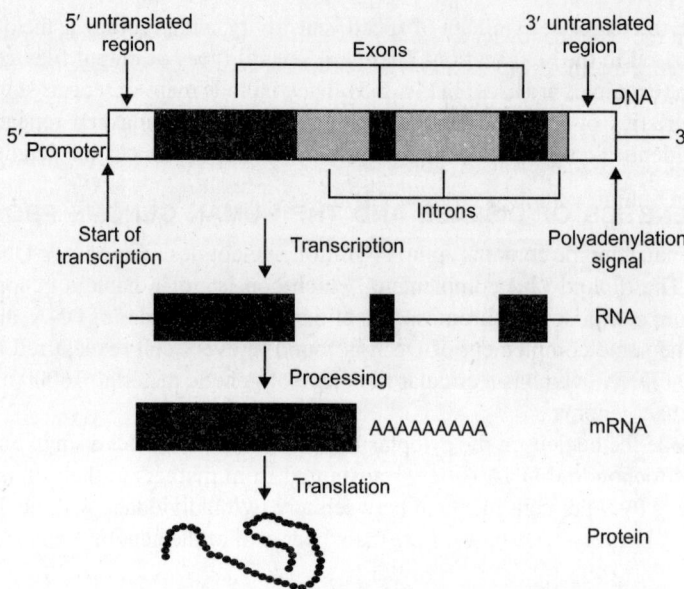

Fig. 5.6: Anatomy of a gene. Information flows from DNA to RNA (transcription) to protein (translation).

Table 5.2: Gene expression.

Transcription	The synthesis of a single-strand RNA molecule from a DNA template in the cell nucleus
	This process is controlled by the interactions between proteins and DNA sequences near each gene
RNA processing	
Capping	Addition of a modified nucleotide chain to the 5′ end of a growing mRNA chain. This is required for the normal processing, stability and translation of mRNA
Splicing	The process of removing introns and joining exons into a mature mRNA molecule
Polyadenylation	Addition of 20–200 adenosine residues (poly A tail) to the 3′ end of the RNA transcript
Transport	The fully processed RNA is taken to the cytoplasm where translation takes place
Translation	The synthesis of a protein from its mRNA template
Housekeeping genes	Expressed in all cell types because their products provide basic functions in cells
Tissue-specific genes	Expressed in only certain cell-types because their products have specific functions

There are a number of diseases that are manifested owing to this simple dominant/recessive pattern of expression. Sickle cell anemia and cystic fibrosis are common examples of when the disease (termed autosomal recessive) develops owing to the presence of two copies of the recessive gene. A person with only one copy of the recessive allele does not develop the disease, but remains a carrier, because the normal copy of the gene predominates. Autosomal dominant disorders like Huntington's disease are produced when a single mutated dominant allele is present even if the other copy of the allele is normal. Diseases resulting from mutations in genes on the X-chromosome are known as X-linked disorders. Since males only have one X-chromosome, these diseases (e.g. hemophilia) act like dominant mutations in males. Females on the other hand, act as carriers and in the next generation their male offspring may or may not be affected. Not all disorders and traits follow a simple pattern of inheritance as described earlier. One gene can influence more than one trait (pleiotropy) and several genes can affect only one trait (polygenic disorders). Although genes may determine whether or not a person will have heart disease or be predisposed to cancer, many traits can be triggered or influenced by the environment as well as in the case of complex multifactorial diseases such as schizophrenia (Fig. 5.7) and alcoholism.

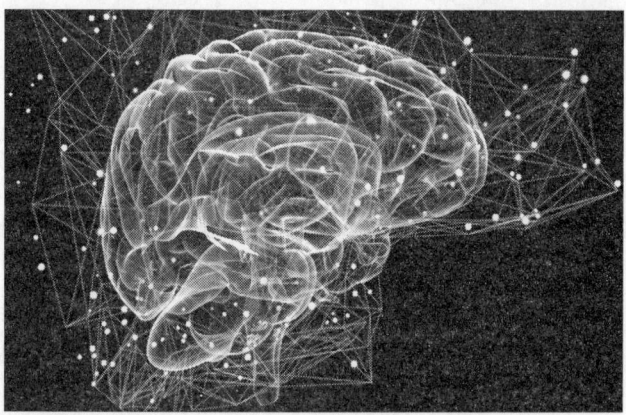

Fig. 5.7: Schizophrenia.

Human Genome Project and Disease Gene Identification

With the development of new mapping resources and technologies and massive amounts of DNA sequence generated by the HGP, the ability to clone rearrangement breakpoints and map disease genes has been greatly simplified. This has also accelerated the pace of discovery of new disease loci and the underlying mutational mechanisms. For example, the gene for Parkinson's disease is shown in Fig. 5.8 (alpha synuclein) on chromosome 4q21–q23 and the gene for speech and language disorder (FOXP2) on chromosome 7q31, were identified within only a few months of determining their chromosomal location.

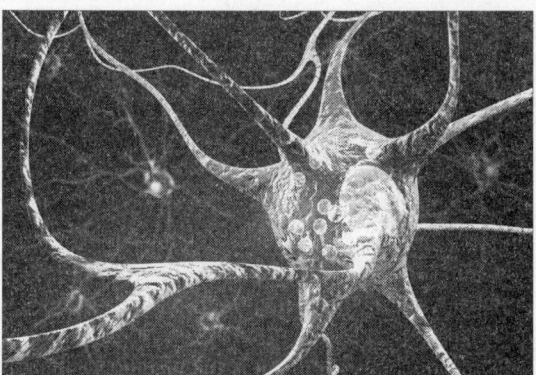

Fig. 15.8: Parkinson's disease.

After a decade of experience in positional cloning, and with the HGP DNA sequence now well advanced, it has become possible to dissect the molecular genetics of multifactorial diseases such as cancer and cardiovascular disease. These involve multiple combinations of genes and strong environmental components. Scientists will continue to work on the HGP with an emphasis on annotating the DNA sequence to find new genes, determine the function of the gene products (functional genomics) and apply all of this information to the study of common diseases.

GENE PREDICTION

In this section overview of gene finding techniques, with a software and the method it utilises are discussed.

General Principles

In considering the problem of gene prediction, we must be aware of the structure of a gene. It consists of promoter sequences as well as regulatory sequences upstream of gene. The gene itself is not continuous and is composed on introns and exons. The promoters are generally composed of consensus sequences, like TATA box in almost 70 per cent of cases. The presence of an open reading frame (ORF) is also somewhat indicative of the presence of an exon, although this is not definitive. There are 6 different reading frames, 3 on each strand starting at 1, 2 and 3rd position. The first codon must be a Methionine (MET). One can also use certain preferred codon usage to find genes, coupled with GC bias in the third codon in organisms that have high GC content in their genomes.

Thus, gene prediction strategies vary widely in prokaryotic and eukaryotic genomes. Many algorithms utilise codon usage frequencies and then information theory based on log likelihood plots, are used to plot the presence of a gene. The presence of AATAAA within 5 kb of stop codon is also used for detection. There is also a 5′ splice site signal as well as a 3′ splice site signal to indicate the intron-exon and exon-intron boundaries. Gene finding strategies can be grouped under three categories:

1. Content based methods: Characteristics like periodicity of repeats, codon usage, compositional complexity are used.
2. Site based methods: These are used to detect donor and acceptor sites as well as tf-binding sites, start-stop codons, etc.
3. Comparative methods: Sequence homology is used to detect gene structure based on other known genes.

Thus, in totem, the gene prediction is not as such straightforward. It is hoped that the combination of these tools provided by Genemachine will help us ascertain if a given sequence has putative genes, exons, introns or a combination of them. In prokaryotes the ORF simply consists of start codon ATG and the stop codons TAA, TAG and TGA. In eukaryotes this is further complicated since one has to take into account not only a start codon at the beginning of each exon, but also successive splice site signals between the end of an exon and the start of an intron. There is also a definitive poly A signal to signal the termination. Thus, given a set of sequence, one has to find the underlying sequence of a putative gene in any gene finding exercise. For this, we use state probabilities within an exon and intron as well as transition probabilities between an exon and intron to compute the most likely underlying sequence to predict the presence of a gene using the Viterbi approach.

SECTION II

Cell Cycle, Meiosis and Mitosis

Chapter 6

Cell Cycle, Meiosis and Mitosis

INTRODUCTION

According to the cell theory, cells arise from pre-existing cells. The process by which this occurs is called cell division. Any sexually reproducing organism starts its life cycle from a single-celled zygote. Cell division does not stop with the formation of the mature organism but continues throughout its life cycle. The stages through which a cell passes from one division to the next is called the cell cycle. Cell cycle is divided into two phases called: (i) Interphase–a period of preparation for cell division and (ii) Mitosis (M phase)–the actual period of cell division. Interphase is further subdivided into G1, S and G2. G1 phase is the period when the cell grows and carries out normal metabolism. Most of the organelle duplication also occurs during this phase. S phase marks the phase of DNA replication and chromosome duplication. G2 phase is the period of cytoplasmic growth. Mitosis is also divided into four stages namely prophase, metaphase, anaphase and telophase. Chromosome condensation occurs during prophase. Simultaneously, the centrioles move to the opposite poles.

The nuclear envelope and the nucleolus disappear and the spindle fibres start appearing. Metaphase is marked by the alignment of chromosomes at the equatorial plate. During anaphase the centromeres divide and the chromatids start moving towards the two opposite poles. Once the chromatids reach the two poles, the chromosomal elongation starts, nucleolus and the nuclear membrane reappear. This stage is called the telophase. Nuclear division is then followed by the cytoplasmic division and is called cytokinesis. Mitosis thus, is the equational division in which the chromosome number of the parent is conserved in the daughter cell.

In contrast to mitosis, meiosis occurs in the diploid cells, which are destined to form gametes. It is called the reduction division since it reduces the chromosome number by half while making the gametes. In sexual reproduction when the two gametes fuse the chromosome number is restored to the value in the parent. Meiosis is divided into two phases–meiosis I and meiosis II. In the first meiotic division the homologous chromosomes pair to form bivalents, and undergo crossing over. Meiosis I has a long prophase, which is divided further into five phases. These are leptotene, zygotene, pachytene, diplotene and diakinesis. During metaphase I the bivalents arrange on the equatorial plate. This is followed by anaphase I in which homologous chromosomes move to the opposite poles with both their chromatids.

Each pole receives half the chromosome number of the parent cell. In telophase I, the nuclear membrane and nucleolus reappear. Meiosis II is similar to mitosis. During anaphase II the sister chromatids separate. Thus at the end of meiosis four haploid cells are formed.

CELL CYCLE

Cell division is a very important process in all living organisms. During the division of a cell, DNA replication and cell growth also take place. All these processes, i.e. cell division, DNA replication, and cell growth, hence, have to take place in a coordinated way to ensure correct division and formation of progeny cells containing intact genomes. The sequence of events by which a cell duplicates its genome, synthesises the other constituents of the cell and eventually divides into two daughter cells is termed cell cycle. Although cell growth (in terms of cytoplasmic increase) is a continuous process, DNA synthesis occurs only during one specific stage in the cell cycle. The replicated chromosomes (DNA) are then distributed to daughter nuclei by a complex series of events during cell division. These events are themselves under genetic control.

Phases of Cell Cycle

A typical eukaryotic cell cycle is illustrated by human cells in culture. These cells divide once in approximately every 24 hr (Fig. 6.1). However, this duration of cell cycle can vary from organism to organism and also from cell type to cell type. Yeast for example, can progress through the cell cycle in only about 90 minutes.

The cell cycle is divided into two basic phases:

- Interphase
- Phase (Mitosis phase)

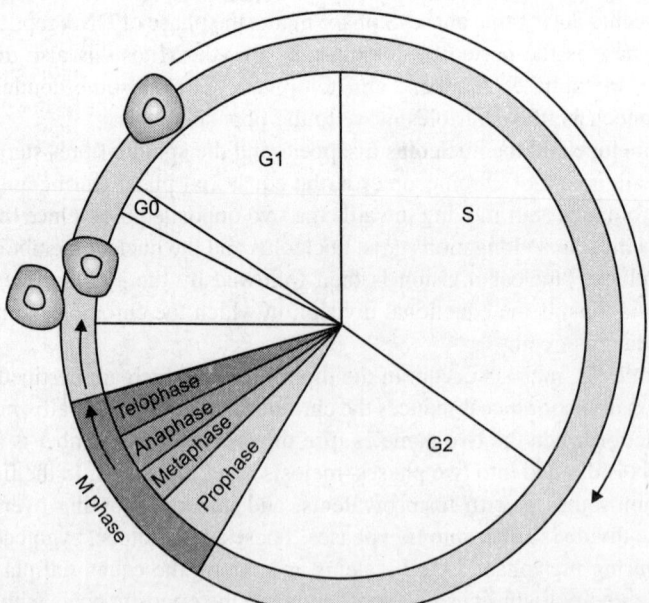

Fig. 6.1: A diagrammatic view of cell cycle indicating formation of two cells from one cell.

The M Phase represents the phase when the actual cell division or mitosis occurs and the interphase represents the phase between two successive M phases. It is significant to note that in the 24 hr average duration of cell cycle of a human cell, cell division proper lasts for only about an hour. The interphase lasts more than 95% of the duration of cell cycle.

The M Phase starts with the nuclear division, corresponding to the separation of daughter chromosomes (karyokinesis) and usually ends with division of cytoplasm (cytokinesis). The interphase, though called the resting phase, is the time during which the cell is preparing for division by undergoing both cell growth and DNA replication in an orderly manner.

The interphase is divided into three further phases:

- G1 phase (Gap 1)
- S phase (Synthesis)
- G2 phase (Gap 2)

G1 phase corresponds to the interval between mitosis and initiation of DNA replication. During G1 phase the cell is metabolically active and continuously grows but does not replicate its DNA. S or synthesis phase marks the period during which DNA synthesis or replication takes place. During this time the amount of DNA per cell doubles. If the initial amount of DNA is denoted as 2C then it increases to 4C. However, there is no increase in the chromosome number; if the cell had diploid or $2n$ number of chromosomes at G1, even after S phase the number of chromosomes remains the same, i.e. $2n$.

In animal cells, during the S phase, DNA replication begins in the nucleus, and the centriole duplicates in the cytoplasm. During the G2 phase, proteins are synthesised in preparation for mitosis while cell growth continues. Some cells in the adult animals do not appear to exhibit division (e.g. heart cells) and many other cells divide only occasionally, as needed to replace cells that have been lost because of injury or cell death. These cells that do not divide further exit G1 phase to enter an inactive stage called quiescent stage (G0) of the cell cycle. Cells in this stage remain metabolically active but no longer proliferate unless called on to do so depending on the requirement of the organism.

In animals, mitotic cell division is only seen in the diploid somatic cells. Against this, the plants can show mitotic divisions in both haploid and diploid cells. From your recollection of examples of alternation of generations in plants identify plant species and stages at which mitosis is seen in haploid cells.

M PHASE

This is the most dramatic period of the cell cycle, involving a major reorganisation of virtually all components of the cell. Since the number of chromosomes in the parent and progeny cells is the same, it is also called as equational division. Though for convenience mitosis has been divided into four stages of nuclear division, it is very essential to understand that cell division is a progressive process and very clear-cut lines cannot be drawn between various stages. Mitosis is divided into the following four stages:

1. Prophase
2. Metaphase
3. Anaphase
4. Telophase

Prophase

Prophase which is the first stage of mitosis follows the S and G2 phases of interphase. In the S and G2 phases the new DNA molecules formed are not distinct but interwined. Prophase is marked by the initiation of condensation of chromosomal material. The chromosomal material becomes untangled during the process of chromatin condensation (Fig. 6.2a). The centriole, which had undergone duplication during S phase of interphase, now begins to move towards opposite poles of the cell. The completion of prophase can thus be marked by the following characteristic events:

- Chromosomal material condenses to form compact mitotic chromosomes. Chromosomes are seen to be composed of two chromatids attached together at the centromere.
- Initiation of the assembly of mitotic spindle, the microtubules, the proteinaceous components of the cell cytoplasm help in the process.

Cells at the end of prophase, when viewed under the microscope, do not show Golgi complexes, endoplasmic reticulum, nucleolus and the nuclear envelope.

Metaphase

The complete disintegration of the nuclear envelope marks the start of the second phase of mitosis, hence the chromosomes are spread through the cytoplasm of the cell. By this stage, condensation of chromosomes is completed and they can be observed clearly under the microscope. This then, is the stage at which morphology of chromosomes is most easily studied. At this stage, metaphase chromosome is made up of two sister chromatids, which are held together by the centromere (Fig. 6.2b). Small disc-shaped structures at the surface of the centromeres are called kinetochores. These structures serve as the sites of attachment of spindle fibres (formed by the spindle fibres) to the chromosomes that are moved into position at the centre of the cell. Hence, the metaphase is characterised by all the chromosomes coming to lie at the equator with one chromatid of each chromosome connected by its kinetochore to spindle fibres from one pole and its sister chromatid connected by its kinetochore to spindle fibres from the opposite pole (Fig. 6.2b).

The plane of alignment of the chromosomes at metaphase is referred to as the metaphase plate. The key features of metaphase are:

- Spindle fibres attach to kinetochores of chromosomes.
- Chromosomes are moved to spindle equator and get aligned along metaphase plate through spindle fibres to both poles.

Anaphase

At the onset of anaphase, each chromosome arranged at the metaphase plate is split simultaneously and the two daughter chromatids, now referred to as chromosomes of the future daughter nuclei, begin their migration towards the two opposite poles. As each chromosome moves away from the equatorial plate, the centromere of each chromosome is towards the pole and hence at the leading edge, with the arms of the chromosome trailing behind. Thus, anaphase stage is characterised by the following key events:

- Centromeres split and chromatids separate.
- Chromatids move to opposite poles.

Telophase

At the beginning of the final stage of mitosis, i.e. telophase, the chromosomes that have reached their respective poles decondense and lose their individuality. The individual chromosomes can no longer be seen and chromatin material tends to collect in a mass in the two poles (Fig. 6.2d).

This is the stage which shows the following key events:

- Chromosomes cluster at opposite spindle poles and their identity is lost as discrete elements.
- Nuclear envelope assembles around the chromosome clusters.
- Nucleolus, golgi complex and ER reform.

Cytokinesis

Mitosis accomplishes not only the segregation of duplicated chromosomes into daughter nuclei (karyokinesis), but the cell itself is divided into two daughter cells by a separate process called cytokinesis at the end of which cell division is complete (Fig. 6.2e). In an animal cell, this is achieved by the appearance of a furrow in the plasma membrane.

The furrow gradually deepens and ultimately joins in the centre dividing the cell cytoplasm into two. Plant cells however, are enclosed by a relatively inextensible cell wall, thererfore they undergo cytokinesis by a different mechanism. In plant cells, wall formation starts in the centre of the cell and grows outward to meet the existing lateral walls.

The formation of the new cell wall begins with the formation of a simple precursor, called the cell-plate that represents the middle lamella between the walls of two adjacent cells. At the time of cytoplasmic division, organelles like mitochondria and plastids get distributed between the two daughter cells. In some organisms karyokinesis is not followed by cytokinesis as a result of which multinucleate condition arises leading to the formation of syncytium (e.g. liquid endosperm in coconut).

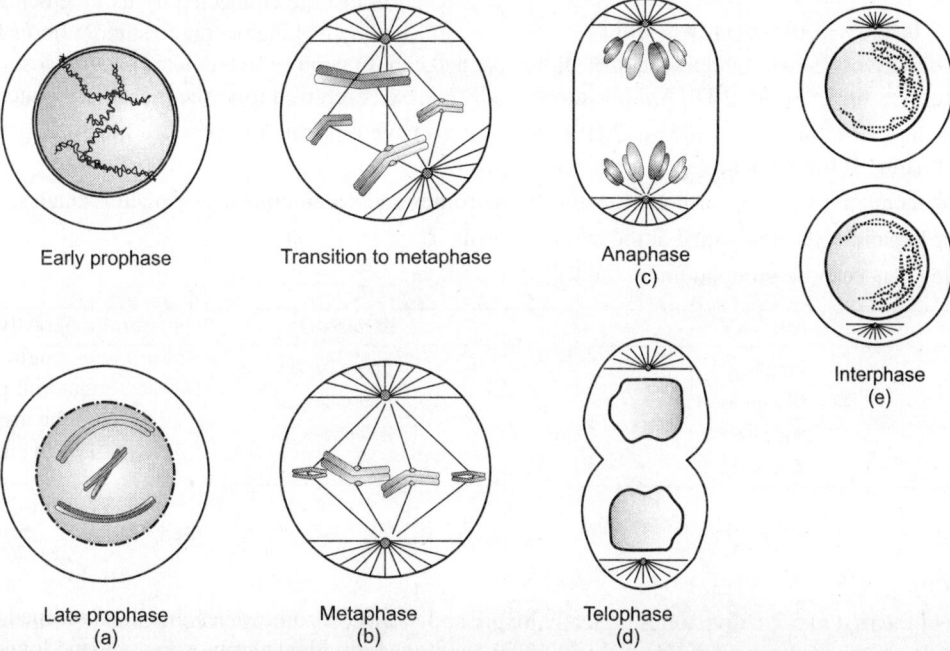

Fig. 6.2: A diagrammatic view of stages in mitosis.

SIGNIFICANCE OF MITOSIS

Mitosis or the equational division is usually restricted to the diploid cells only. However, in some lower plants and in some social insects haploid cells also divide by mitosis. It is very essential to understand the significance of this division in the life of an organism. Are you aware of some examples where you have studied about haploid and diploid insects?

Mitosis results in the production of diploid daughter cells with identical genetic complement usually. The growth of multicellular organisms is due to mitosis. Cell growth results in disturbing the ratio between the nucleus and the cytoplasm. It therefore becomes essential for the cell to divide to restore the nucleo-cytoplasmic ratio. A very significant contribution of mitosis is cell repair. The cells of the upper layer of the epidermis, cells of the lining of the gut, and blood cells are being constantly replaced. Mitotic divisions in the meristematic tissues–the apical and the lateral cambium, result in a continuous growth of plants throughout their life.

MEIOSIS

The production of offspring by sexual reproduction includes the fusion of two gametes, each with a complete haploid set of chromosomes. Gametes are formed from specialised diploid cells. This specialised kind of cell division that reduces the chromosome number by half results in the production of haploid daughter cells. This kind of division is called meiosis. Meiosis ensures the production of haploid phase in the life cycle of sexually reproducing organisms whereas fertilisation restores the diploid phase. We come across meiosis during gametogenesis in plants and animals. This leads to the formation of haploid gametes.

The key features of meiosis are as follows:

*   Meiosis involves two sequential cycles of nuclear and cell division called meiosis I and meiosis II but only a single cycle of DNA replication.
*   Meiosis I is initiated after the parental chromosomes have replicated to produce identical sister chromatids at the S phase.
*   Meiosis involves pairing of homologous chromosomes and recombination between them.
*   Four haploid cells are formed at the end of meiosis II.

Meiotic events can be grouped under the following phases:

Meiosis I	Meiosis II
Prophase I	Prophase II
Metaphase I	Metaphase II
Anaphase I	Anaphase II
Telophase I	Telophase II

Meiosis I

Prophase I

Prophase of the first meiotic division is typically longer and more complex when compared to prophase of mitosis. It has been further subdivided into the following five phases based on chromosomal behaviour, i.e. Leptotene, Zygotene, Pachytene, Diplotene and Diakinesis. During leptotene stage the chromosomes become gradually visible under the light microscope. The compaction of chromosomes continues throughout leptotene. This is followed by the second stage of prophase I called zygotene. During this stage chromosomes start pairing together and this process of association is called synapsis. Such paired chromosomes are called homologous chromosomes. Electron micrographs of this stage indicate that chromosome synapsis is accompanied by the formation of complex structure called synaptonemal complex. The complex formed by a pair of synapsed homologous chromosomes is called a bivalent or a tetrad. However, these are more clearly visible at the next stage. The first two stages of prophase I are relatively short-lived compared to the next stage that is pachytene. During this stage bivalent chromosomes now clearly appears as tetrads.

This stage is characterised by the appearance of recombination nodules, the sites at which crossing over occurs between non-sister chromatids of the homologous chromosomes. Crossing over is the exchange of genetic material between two homologous chromosomes. Crossing over is also an enzyme-mediated process and the enzyme involved is called recombinase. Crossing over leads to recombination of genetic material on the two chromosomes.

Recombination between homologous chromosomes is completed by the end of pachytene, leaving the chromosomes linked at the sites of crossing over.

The beginning of diplotene is recognised by the dissolution of the synaptonemal complex and the tendency of the recombined homologous chromosomes of the bivalents to separate from each other except at the sites of crossovers. These X-shaped structures, are called chiasmata. In oocytes of some vertebrates, diplotene can last for months or years. The final stage of meiotic prophase I is diakinesis.

This is marked by terminalisation of chiasmata. During this phase the chromosomes are fully condensed and the meiotic spindle is assembled to prepare the homologous chromosomes for separation. By the end of diakinesis, the nucleolus disappears and the nuclear envelope also breaks down. Diakinesis represents transition to metaphase.

Metaphase I

The bivalent chromosomes align on the equatorial plate (Fig. 6.3). The microtubules from the opposite poles of the spindle attach to the pair of homologous chromosomes.

Anaphase I

The homologous chromosomes separate, while sister chromatids remain associated at their centromeres (Fig. 6.3).

Telophase I

The nuclear membrane and nucleolus reappear, cytokinesis follows and this is called as diad of cells (Fig. 6.3). Although in many cases the chromosomes do undergo some dispersion, they do not reach the extremely extended state of the interphase nucleus. The stage between the two meiotic divisions is called interkinesis and is generally short lived. Interkinesis is followed by prophase II, a much simpler prophase than prophase I.

Meiosis II

Prophase II

Meiosis II is initiated immediately after cytokinesis, usually before the chromosomes have fully elongated. In contrast to meiosis I, meiosis II resembles a normal mitosis. The nuclear membrane disappears by the end of prophase II (Fig. 6.4). The chromosomes again become compact.

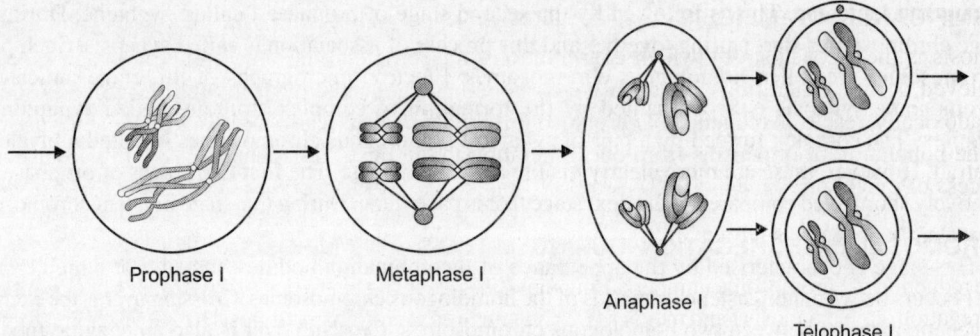

Fig. 6.3: Stages of Meiosis I.

Metaphase II

At this stage the chromosomes align at the equator and the microtubules from opposite poles of the spindle get attached to the kinetochores (Fig. 6.4) of sister chromatids.

Anaphase II

It begins with the simultaneous splitting of the centromere of each chromosome (which was holding the sister chromatids together), allowing them to move toward opposite poles of the cell (Fig. 6.4).

Telophase II

Meiosis ends with telophase II, in which the two groups of chromosomes once again get enclosed by a nuclear envelope; cytokinesis follows resulting in the formation of tetrad of cells, i.e. four haploid daughter cells (Fig. 6.4).

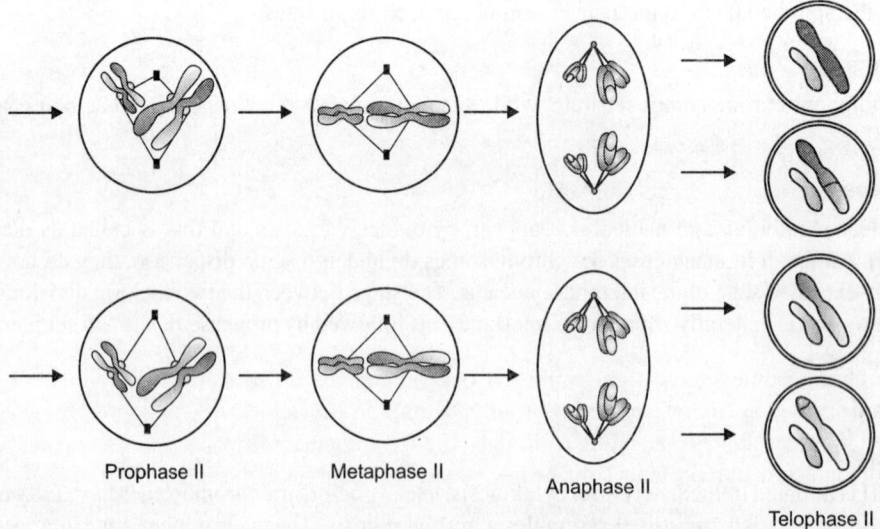

Fig. 6.4: Stages of Meiosis II.

SIGNIFICANCE OF MEIOSIS

Meiosis is the mechanism by which conservation of specific chromosome number of each species is achieved across generations in sexually reproducing organisms, even though the process, per se, paradoxically, results in reduction of chromosome number by half. It also increases the genetic variability in the population of organisms from one generation to the next. Variations are very important for the process of evolution.

CHROMOSOME SEGREGATION DURING MITOSIS AND MEIOSIS

The reduction of chromosome number during meiosis is achieved by two successive rounds of chromosome segregation, called meiosis I and meiosis II. While meiosis II is similar to mitosis in that sister kinetochores are bi-oriented and segregate to opposite poles, recombined homologous chromosomes segregate during the first meiotic division. Formation of chiasmata, mono-orientation of sister kinetochores and protection of centromeric cohesion are three major features of meiosis I chromosomes which ensure the reductional nature of chromosome segregation. In some studies researchers use the fission yeast *S. pombe* (Fig. 6.5), which is an excellent model organism amenable to both genetic and cell biology techniques, to identify new proteins required for proper segregation of chromosomes during meiosis.

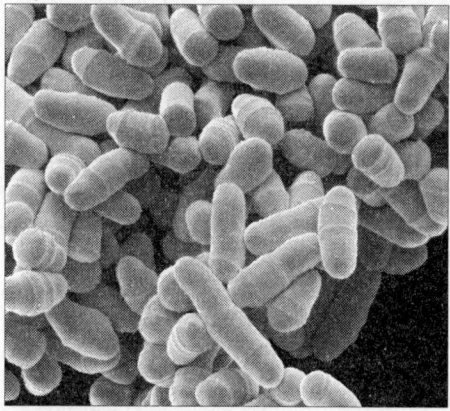

Fig. 6.5: *S. pombe.*

In order to decipher molecular functions of identified proteins, researchers combine biochemical and cell biology techniques. To test the possible functional conservation of identified proteins, researchers plan to analyse the function of the respective homologs in mammalian cells.

Chromosome Segregation during Mitosis

Accurate chromosome segregation in mitosis depends on the establishment of correct (amphitelic) kinetochore orientation. Merotelic kinetochore orientation is an error which occurs when a single kinetochore is attached to microtubules emanating from opposite spindle poles. Recent studies show that merotelic kinetochore attachment represents a major mechanism of aneuploidy in mitotic cells and is the primary mechanism of chromosomal instability in cancer cells underline the importance of studying merotely. We focus on fission yeast proteins required to prevent and correct merotelic attachments in order to understand how cells ensure high fidelity of chromosome segregation.

Difference between mitosis and meiosis is shown Table 6.1.

Table 6.1: Difference between mitosis and meiosis.

Types	Mitosis	Meiosis
Interphase	Interphase – DNA has been replicated but Chromosomes not yet visible	Each chromosome replicates. The result is two genetically identical sister chromatids
Prophase	Prophase – chromosomes condense and thicken, each duplicated chromosome appear as two identical sister chromatids, the mitotic spindle begins to form	Prophase I (crossing-over recombination) Homologous chromosomes (each consisting of two sister chromatids) come together as pairs the structure formed is called a tetrad. Chromosome segments are swapped between non-sister chromatids at crossover points called chiasmata (= crossing-over)
Metaphase	Metaphase – the chromosomes assemble at the equator = metaphase plate	Metaphase I Chromosomes align on the metaphase plate. Chromosomes still arranged as: pairs of homologues
Anaphase	Anaphase – the spindle fibres begin to contract. This starts to pull the sister chromatids apart. At the end of anaphase a complete set of daughter chromosomes is found each pole.	Anaphase I Sister chromatids remain attached. But homologous chromosomes move apart to opposite poles
Types of reproduction	Sexual	Asexual
Occurs in	Humans, animals, plants, fungi.	All Organisms
Function	Genetic diversity through sexual reproduction	Cellular reproduction and general growth and repair of the body
Cytokinesis	Occurs in Telophase I and in Telophase II	Occurs in Telophase
Karyokinesis	Occurs in Interphase I	Occurs in
Discovered by	Oscar Hertwig	Walther Flemming

Chapter 7

Crossing Over and Meiosis

INTRODUCTION

It is well know that the formation of the sperm and egg cells is preceded by two cell divisions in the course of which the chromosome number is reduced. We referred to these as the 'maturation divisions,' but often they are referred to as the *meiotic* (my-a-tic) divisions (or first and second meiotic divisions). In the absence of crossing over (as in the male of *Drosophila*), the first of these is the reduction division, the second, the equation division. However, when crossing over takes place, the situation becomes more complicated, and reduction takes place partly in the first meiotic division, partly in the second, as will presently be explained. The combined changes which the chromosomes undergo in the course of the two meiotic divisions are referred to as *meiosis*. This word is the Greek for belittling or making smaller, and in the present connection it refers to the reduction in chromosome number.

The two divisions under discussion are much more often accompanied by crossing over than not and, therefore, in general, it is preferable to refer to them as the first and second meiotic divisions rather than the reduction and equation divisions. However, it is sometimes desirable (for pedagogical purposes) to avoid the complications caused by crossing over. In such cases the terms 'reduction' and 'equation' division are quite legitimate. But in the present chapter, we shall be concerned for the most part with cases that involve crossing over, and we shall, therefore, usually refer to the two divisions under discussion as the first and second meiotic divisions, rather than the 'reduction' and 'equation' divisions.

GENERAL OUTLINE OF MEIOSIS

It will be recalled that at the first meiotic division the chromosomes come together in pairs. This pairing of the chromosomes in the first meiotic division takes place, regardless of whether or not crossing over occurs later. It is known as synapsis (Fig. 7.1a,b,). Moreover, it will be recalled that the chromosomes not only pair, they also split in the first meiotic division (Fig. 7.1c). The two split halves of each chromosome are known as chromatids. The pairing and splitting result in a group of four chromatids, known as a tetrad. The splitting, however, does not as yet involve the centromeres (the bodies to which the spindle fibres later become attached, shown as small circles at the ends of the chromosomes in Fig. 7.1). Crossing over now takes place, but at a given level, it involves only two of the four chromatids of a tetrad (Fig. 7.ld).

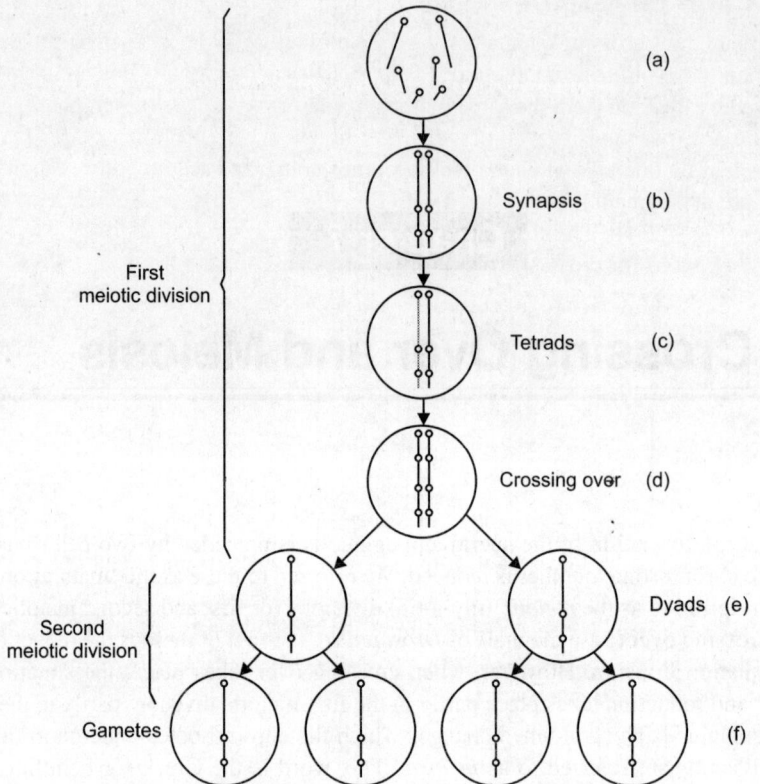

Fig. 7.1: The reduction and equation divisions, including tetrad formation and crossing over.

Moreover, it always involves two chromatids not connected by the same centromere (nonsister chromatids). Next, the chromosomes separate (Fig. 7.1e). This involves the separation of homologous centromeres (those attached originally to homologous chromosomes). Each centromere carries along with it the two chromatids attached to it. The two chromatids in question (attached to one centromere) are referred to as a dyad. Thus, at the completion of the first meiotic division, two cells are formed, each with dyads (instead of tetrads). The second meiotic division now takes place. This is preceded by the division of each centromere (Fig. 7.1 d, e). The resulting 'sister' centromeres then separate to opposite poles of the cell, and the individual chromatids attached to each centromere go along with them.

Thus, each cell contains only one of the original four chromatids belonging to a given tetrad (or just one of the crossover products of such chromatids). The cells in question (Fig. 7.1f) then differentiate into sperm or egg cells. As previously mentioned, the germ cells mature during the two cell divisions that precede the formation of the sperm and egg cells and these divisions are, therefore, sometimes referred to as the first and second maturation divisions. Thus, we might use any of three sets of terms to apply to the two cell divisions that precede the formation of the sperm and egg cells, namely: (i) first and second maturation divisions, (ii) reduction and equation divisions (but only when there is no crossing over), and (iii) first and second meiotic divisions. The latter terms (first and second meiotic divisions) have corne into general use.

CROSSING OVER AND CHIASMATA

Figure 7.2 shows in detail how crossing over takes place. As previously mentioned, first the chromosomes pair [Fig. 7.2(1)], then they split to form a tetrad [Fig. 7.2(2)]. The chromatids that are shaded alike in Fig. 7.2(2) are derived by division from the same mother chromosome and are 'sister' chromatids. When crossing over takes place, two nonsister chromatids first break at corresponding points [Fig. 7.2(3)]. Next, the upper segment on one side of each break becomes connected with the lower segment on the opposite side of the break [segment A with b and a with B in Fig. 7.2(3)]. As a result, the two chromatids now cross each other [Fig. 7.2(4)]. The crossing of two chromatids as a result of crossing over is known as a chiasma (the Greek word for cross, the plural of which is chiasmata).

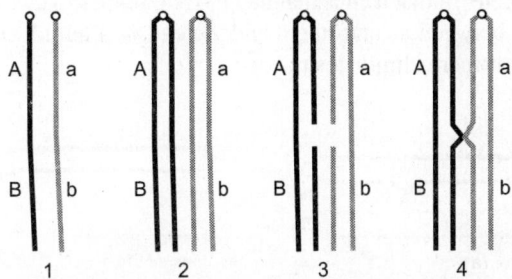

Fig. 7.2: Crossing over and chiasma formation.

Here we have discussed crossing over as though it involved first the crossing of two chromosomes (Fig. 7.3, left). Next, breakage was supposed to occur and then union of the broken ends. This is just a convenient way of showing crossing over (originally employed by Morgan) but it really is not correct in detail. For actually the chromosomes break before they cross, not after [Fig. 7.3 right, where just the two middle chromatids shown in Fig. 7.2(3)]. Moreover, inspection of Fig. 7.3, right, will make it evident that the crossing of the chromosomes (a chiasma) is the result of crossing over, not the cause of it. If Fig. 7.3, left, were correct, then crossing over would unmake a chiasma, actually, it makes a chiasma (Fig. 7.3, right). Crossing over may occur at several levels in a given tetrad, resulting in several chiasmata. The number of chiasmata varies with chromosomes of different lengths, but for chromosomes of average length, the number per tetrad is one to three (corresponding to single, double, and triple crossing over).

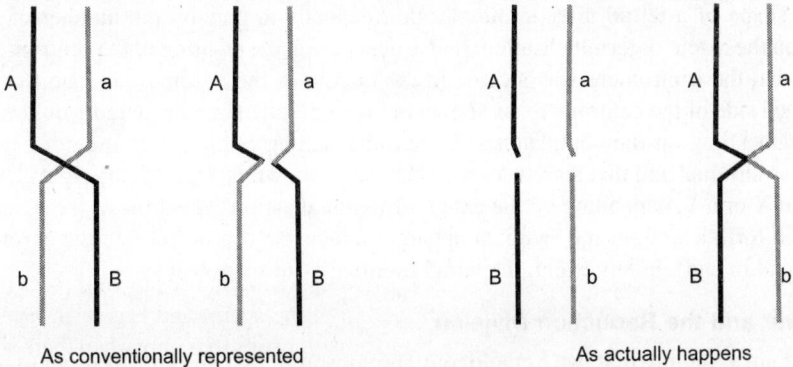

As conventionally represented   As actually happens

Fig. 7.3: The mechanism of crossing over.

TERMINALISATION

After chiasma formation, homologous centromeres repel each other (Fig. 7.4a and b). This causes the chromatids to separate progressively from the centromeres towards a chiasma (Fig. 7.4b). The further separation of the chromatids causes the chiasma to move towards the end of the tetrad, in zipper fashion (Fig. 7.4c and d). The movement of a chiasma away from the centromere and towards the end ~ of a tetrad is known as terminalisation. In a tetrad, sister strands are at first associated (Fig. 7.4a), but in the process of terminalisation sister strands become separated and nonsister strands become associated beyond the point of crossing over (Fig. 7.4b, c, d). When terminalisation is completed, nonsister chromatids are connected at their noncentromere ends (distal to the point of crossing over, Fig. 7.4d). Terminalisation may temporarily be incomplete, in that a chiasma may move only part way to the end of a tetrad. When there are several chiasmata between a centromere and the end of a tetrad, complete terminalisation of the chiasma nearest the centromere eliminates the rest.

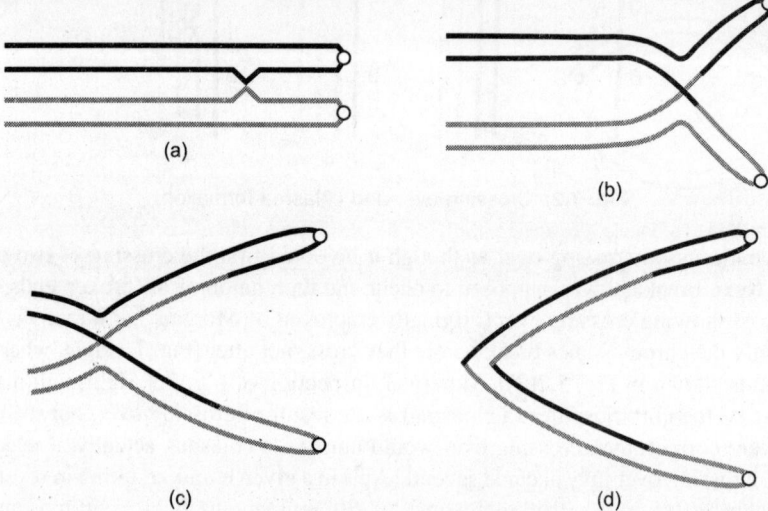

(a)

(b)

(c)

(d)

Fig. 7.4: Terminalisation.

The exact shape of a tetrad after terminalisation depends in part on the number of chiasmata it contains and on the extent of terminalisation. It also depends on the position of the centromere. Suppose, for example, that the centromere was located in the middle of the chromosome and that there was a chiasma on each side of the centromere, as shown in Fig. 7.5, left. Then the tetrad would form a double X or a ring, depending on the completeness of terminalisation. Suppose, on the other hand, that the centromere was terminal and that there was one chiasma as shown in Fig. 7.5, top right. Then the tetrad would form an X or a V, depending on the extent of terminalisation. The arms of the V might open up completely and form a straight rod (with an apparent transverse division where the chromosomes are still attached end to end). In any event, the tetrad eventually forms two days.

Crossing Over and the Reduction Division

In Fig. 7.6, we are assuming that two homologous chromosomes pair and split as usual to form a tetrad, and that the chromosomes now separate without crossing over. Then at the first division shown (a, b, c)

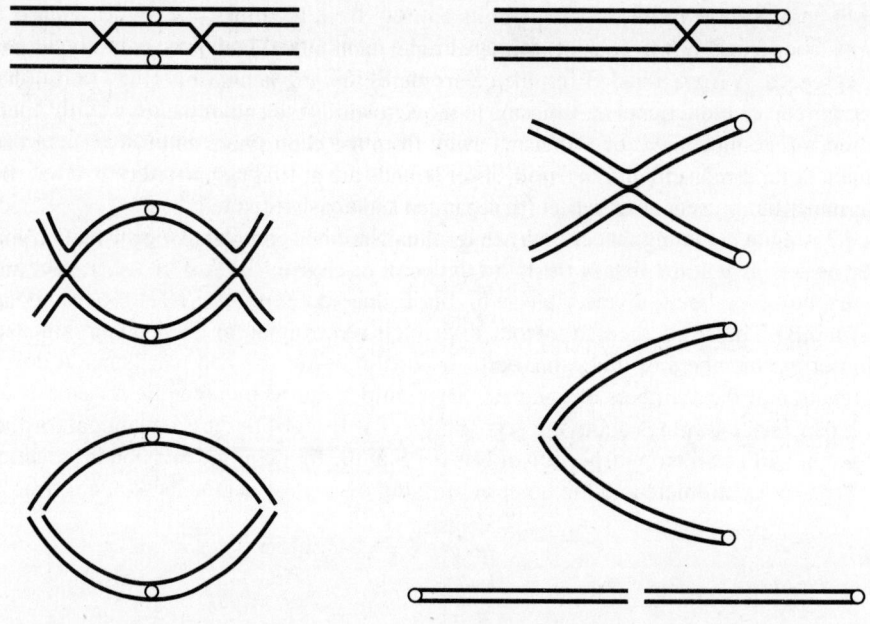

(a) The formation of a double X or a ring   (b) The formation of an X, A V, or an I

Fig. 7.5: Changes in the shapes of tetrads.

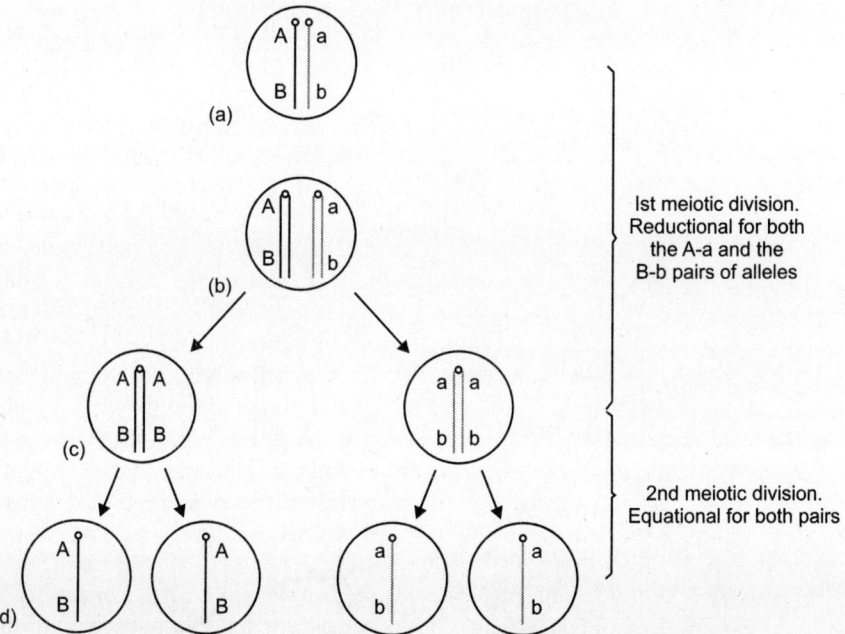

Fig. 7.6: The distribution of the products of a tetrad in the absence of crossing over.

the one split chromosome (dark) separates in its entirety from the other one (light). That is to say, the two chromosomes (each, however, split) segregate. The members of both gene pairs shown in the figure likewise segregate (A from a and B from b). We can, therefore, speak of the first cell division under discussion as strictly reductional in the sense that it results in the segregation of either homologous chromosomes or of alleles. At the second division the separation of chromosomal elements involves only the halves of a given split chromosome or the halves of a given gene, and this division is, therefore, equational under the present assumption (that there is no crossing over).

In Fig. 7.7, we are assuming that crossing over takes place between the two gene pairs (A-a and B-b). It will then be seen that at the first of the two cell divisions shown (the first meiotic) A segregates from a (each gene, however, being divided into two), but B does not segregate from b (since both daughter cells are still biB). Therefore, the first meiotic division is reductional for the A-a pair (since it results in segregation of the members of this pair), but it is equational for the B-b pair (since it does not bring about segregation of the members of this pair). By contrast, the second meiotic division is reductional for the B-b pair (since it brings about the segregation of B from b) but it is equational for the A-a pair.

In general, it will be seen on inspection of Fig. 7.7 that the first meiotic division is reductional for all genes between the centromere and the point of crossing over (dark segments separate from light), and

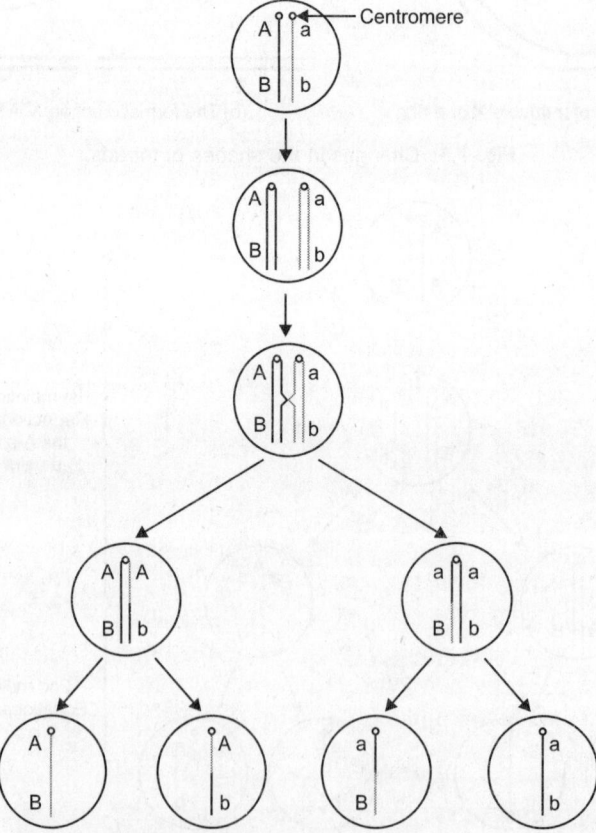

Fig. 7.7: The distribution of the products of a tetrad when crossing over occurs.

that the second division is reductional for all genes between the point of crossing over and the distal end of the chromosome (the end away from the centromere). Hence, when crossing over takes place, we cannot logically speak of either division as being entirely reductional or equational. Both meiotic divisions are partly reductional and they are, therefore, sometimes referred to as the reduction divisions. If we inspect Fig. 7.7 again, it will be seen that at the first meiotic division homologous centromeres segregate from each other, and that the first division is reductional for the centromeres, even in the presence of crossing over. At the second division, the two halves of each divided centromere are separated (dark from dark, or light from light, in Fig. 7.7) and, therefore, this division is equational for the centromeres and again, even in the presence of crossing over.

GERM CELLS OF ANIMALS

The sperm or egg cells of an animal are derived eventually from the fertilised egg through the process of cell division. Thus, there is a long series of cells which are ancestral to the sperm and egg cells. These ancestral cells, together with the sperm and egg cells proper, are referred to as the germ cells (or the cells of the germ track). It is important that we do not use the term 'germ cells' to mean the same thing as 'sperm and egg cells,' since the germ cells include not only the sperm and egg cells but also all cells ancestral to them. In the very early embryo, the ovaries or testes are not yet developed, and the germ cells are undifferentiated cells not markedly different in appearance from other embryonic cells, but they are localised in a definite region of the embryo. They are known as the primordial germ cells (Fig. 7.8).

They contain the unreduced number of chromosomes and they multiply by mitotic cell division, just as do ordinary cells. As the embryo develops, its reproductive organs eventually are formed, but at first the germ cells are still undifferentiated and they still multiply by mitotic cell division, continuing to contain the unreduced chromosome number. The reproductive organs are often referred to as gonads and the undifferentiated germ cells under discussion are known as gonial cells. In the testes, the gonial cells are referred to as spermatogonial cells (Fig. 7.8). The gonial cells eventually give rise to the cells that undergo the first meiotic division. In the testes, these latter cells are known as the primary spermatocytes (Fig. 7.8).

The nucleus of a primary spermatocyte is at first of ordinary size, but it grows and becomes much larger than the nucleus of a gonial cell. The time during which the nucleus of the primary spermatocyte grows is known as the growth period. It is during the growth period that the pairing and splitting of the chromosomes takes place, resulting in the formation of the tetrads, also, crossing over occurs. All this takes place during the early stages of the first meiotic division, before the tetrads get to the middle of the dividing cell. In other words, it all takes place during the prophase of this division. At the completion of the growth period the tetrads line up in the middle of the cell.

This represents the metaphase in the division of the primary spermatocyte, that is to say, it represents the metaphase of the first meiotic division in the male. The metaphase is followed by the anaphase and telophase and the division of the primary spermatocyte is completed. By its division, the primary spermatocyte gives rise to the secondary spermatocytes. These are the cells that contain the dyads and that undergo the second meiotic division. They give rise (through division) to the immature sperm cells, or spermatids. Finally, the spermatids differentiate into the sperm cells. In summary, then, the germ cells of the early embryo are called primordial germ cells. In the testes, the germ cells in the order of their succession are the spermatogonia, primary spermatocytes, secondary spermatocytes, spermatids, and sperm cells (Fig. 7.8). The corresponding terms for the germ cells in the ovary are the oögonia, primary oöcytes, secondary oöcytes, oötids, and eggs.

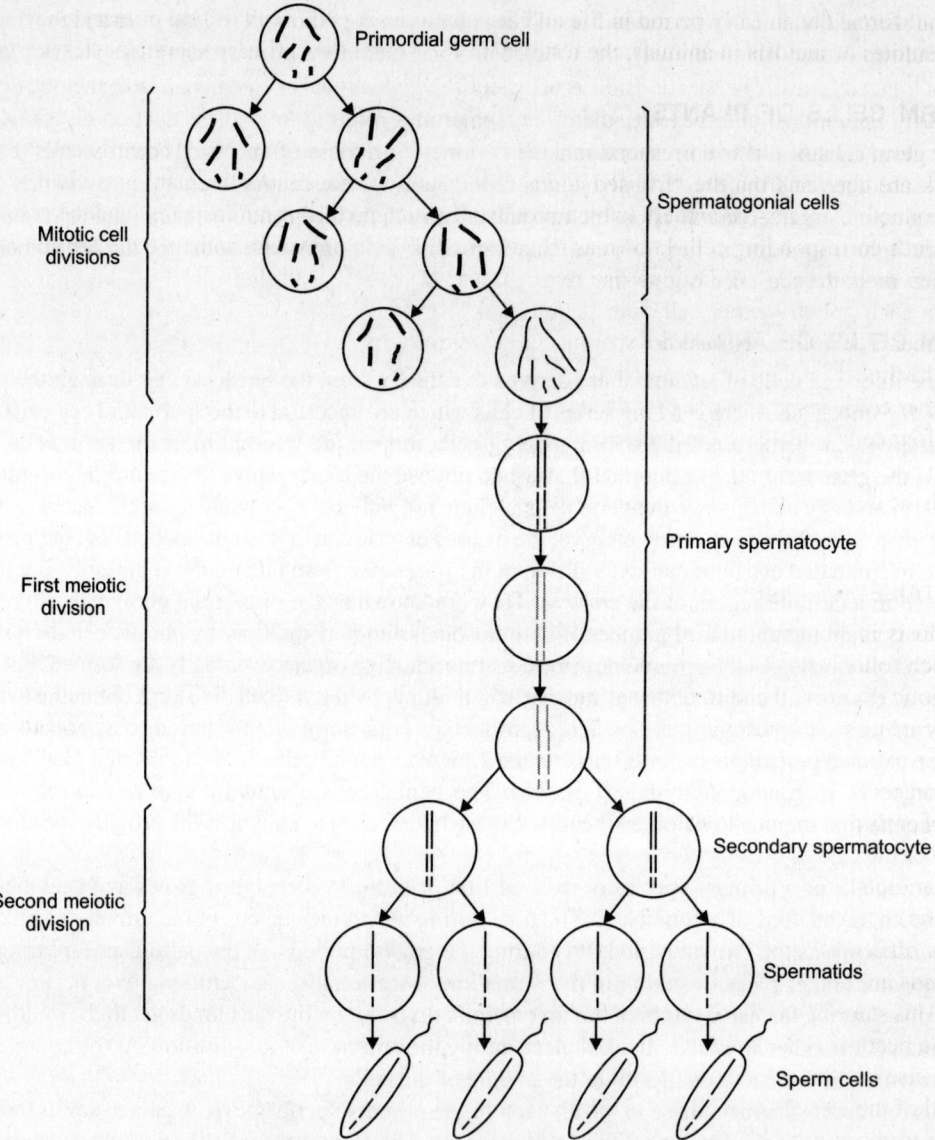

Fig. 7.8: The germ track (in the male).

Most of the important steps in meiosis take place in the first meiotic division (synapsis, tetrad formation, crossing over). The study of meiosis, therefore, involves for the most part the examination of cells undergoing the first meiotic division, namely, the primary spermatocytes (in the male) or the primary oocytes (in the female). In the male of most animals, sperm cells continue to be formed in large numbers throughout the life of the individual and, hence, the testis always contains large numbers of cells undergoing the first meiotic division–primary spermatocytes. In the female of many animals, the eggs are all formed at an early period in life and at most times it is difficult to find primary oocytes. Hence, for studies of meiosis in animals, the testes with their numerous primary spermatocytes are preferred.

GERM CELLS OF PLANTS

The germ cells of plants correspond in a general way with those of ani also The early cells of the germ track are derived from the fertilised egg/and multiply by mitosis. As the plant gets older it forms its reproductive organs-the anthers (which produce the pollen cells or microspores) and the pistils (which produce corresponding cells known as megaspores). Within the young anthers there are cells known as pollen mother cells. These give rise through the two meiotic cell divisions to the pollen cells. Thus, from each pollen mother cell, four pollen cells are formed, and these have the reduced chromosome number. The pollen cells are not sperm cells proper, but they give rise to the sperm cells by cell division (at the time the pollen tube grows down the pistil). In the young pistil there are cells known as megaspores mother cells. They give rise to the megaspores by two meiotic divisions (first and second). Only one of the four cells formed by a megaspore mother cell develops into a megaspore. The megaspores eventually give rise (by mitosis) to the egg cells. In plants, the pollen cells are formed in large numbers (as compared with the megaspores) and the young anthers contain numerous pollen mother cells. For studies of meiosis in plants, the young anthers are usually selected and the pollen mother cells are examined.

DETAILED STAGES OF MEIOSIS

Meiosis is a complicated process and involves some details not already considered. The description which follows might apply to either plants or animals, in favourable cases. At the beginning of the first meiotic division, the chromosomes condense from the resting nucleus as long thin threads, and at first they are unpaired. This stage in meiosis is known as the leptotene stage. Somewhat later the chromosomes begin to pair and they are now said to be in the zygotene stage. Often the pairing begins at one end of the chromosome pair and proceeds in zipper fashion to the other end. The chromosomes get shorter and thicker during zygotene and they continue to do so during the later stages of the growth period. At the end of the zygotene, two homologous chromosomes have come so close together that no distinct line of separation can be seen between them, and they are now said to be in the pachytene stage. The splitting of the chromosomes (leading to tetrad formation) probably takes place later in the pachytene stage, but it is difficult to see the actual cleavage. Next, the chromosomes become visibly split and the early tetrads are formed. Then, crossing over takes place and chiasmata are formed.

This stage in meiosis is referred to as the diplotene stage. By the end of the diplotene, the chromosomes have become short and thick and they form ordinary tetrads. Next, the tetrads assume various shapes because of terminalisation. At the same time, they move outwards until they come into contact with the wall of the nucleus (which is still intact). The nuclear wall next breaks down and the chromosomes are free to move about in the general cytoplasm. Everything up to this point happens during the growth period-the prophase of the first meiotic division. At the end of the prophase, the tetrads have arrived in the middle of the cell and are attached to spindle fibres from opposite poles of the cell. This constitutes the metaphase stage of the first meiotic division. The chromosomes are then drawn to opposite poles of the dividing cell (anaphase and telophase) and the first meiotic division is completed by the formation of a cell wall between the separated sets of chromosomes. Next, the second meiotic division takes place and the sperm or egg cells are formed. In plant material, the chromosomes often become tightly bunched up during pachytene. This bunching up is referred to as synizesis. Perhaps the bunching up is produced in part by the chemicals used in preparing the specimens for microscopic examination.

DIPLOID PARTHENOGENESIS AND MEIOSIS

In a female that reproduces by diploid parthenogenesis (by means of unfertilised eggs with the diploid chromosome number), a modified form of meiosis occurs. There are two possibilities, one of these is shown in Fig. 7.9A. At the first/meiotic division, the chromosomes pair and split, crossing over occurs and the chromosomes separate to opposite poles of the cell-all a usual for the first meiotic division. However, the cell itself does not divide into two at this point, as it usually would. Instead, the chromosomes first come together again in the middle of the cell. This coming together is referred to as 'restitution.' The chromosomes do not pair again, but they line up singly in the middle, just as they would for an ordinary mitotic division. The chromosome halves (chromatids) are then drawn to opposite poles of the cell, and cell division takes place. One of the resulting cells becomes an egg and the other a polar body. Thus, the chromosome number is not reduced (since 'restitution' occurred at the first meiotic division). In effect, the first meiotic division has been omitted. A second possibility is shown in Fig. 7.9B. The first and second meiotic divisions take place as usual, but the second polar body now combines with the egg, and this results in a diploid egg. In diploid parthenogenesis, genetic recombination can occur as the result of crossing over, as explained in Fig. 7.10.

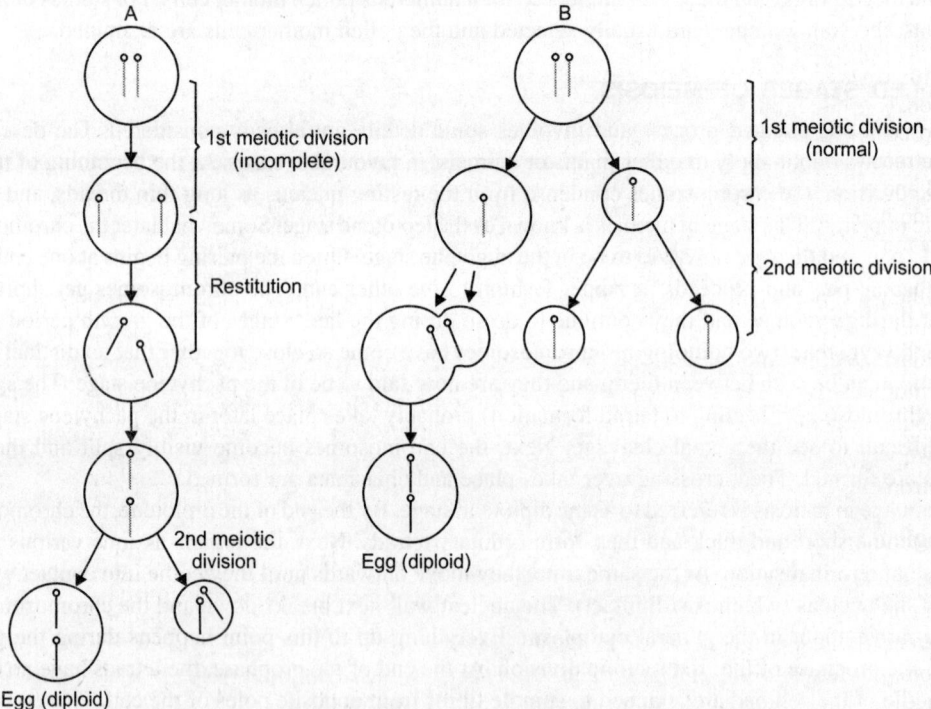

Fig. 7.9: The maturation divisions in a parthenogenically reproducing female.

Centromere in Relation to Crossing Over and Interference

The centromere is an important organ of a chromosome. Not only does it serve for the attachment of the spindle fibers, but it also has some sort of influence on crossing over. If, for example, the centromere was at the left end of a chromosome, then chiasmata formation would start near the left end and proceed

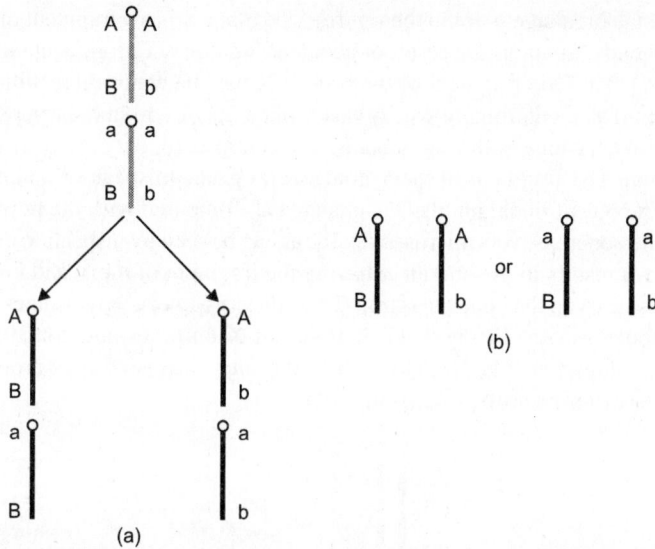

Fig. 7.10: Genetic recombination in diploid parthenogenesis. a. Recombination after crossing over and restitution. (Compare Fig. 7.7 and 7.9 with the present 7.10 a.) Note (in present figure, part a) that one of the resulting cells is homozygous for B, the other one for b. But note further that there would have been no effective recombination if the lower chromosome had been turned around with respect to the upper, so that both AB and ab would have been on one side of the midline, Ab and aB on the other side, both resulting cells now being heterozygous at both the a and b loci. Part b (on right). Recombination after crossing over and fusion of the second polar body with the egg. Compare with lower part of Fig. 7.7 and lower part of Fig. 7.9B.

toward the right end, that is, the first chiasma to be formed would be nearest the centromere, the second one would be next further removed, etc. Moreover, when the centromere is centrally located, crossing over (chiasmata formation) begins on either side of it and proceeds towards the ends of the chromosome. Furthermore, a crossover on one side of the centromere would not interfere with one on the other side, even though both crossovers were fairly close to the centromere, this is contrary to what would happen if the two were on the same side and close together. That is to say, interference does not extend across the centromere.

Cytological Evidence of Crossing Over

Suppose that we performed a linkage experiment and then examined the offspring under a microscope for their chromosomes. We should, as a rule, find that the, chromosomes of the crossover classes appeared no different from those of noncrossovers, because crossing over normally produces no permment, visible alteration in the structure of a chromosome, that is to say, it produces no permanent cytological change. It is possible, however, to devise experiments in which we can get cytological evidence of crossing over. An experiment by Stern might be given in illustration.

In *Drosophila*, the normal race has red round eyes. The mutant genes carnation (car or darkish red eyes, recessive) and Bar (B or narrow eyes, dominant) are both in the X chromosome. The X chromosome of *Drosophila* is normally rod shaped and a female normally contains a pair of these rod-shaped X's. But, in Stern's experiment, a female is obtained in which one X is broken into two (as the result of accidental breakage) and, in addition, contains the mutant genes car and B (Fig. 7.11). (Note that car and B are both above the breakage point in the figure). The other X has a fragment of the Y chromosome attached to one of its ends (again as the result of accident) and, in addition, contains the normal alleles (+ 's) of carnation and Bar. One fragment of the broken X has the centromere which belongs to the X and the other fragment has a centromere which was broken off of another chromosome (the fourth) at the time the X got broken. Since both fragments have a centromere, they are distributed in the normal manner in cell division. The fragment of the Y contains no genes to speak of and in no way interferes with development. The object in having the X's changed as compared with the normal is to distinguish the crossovers from the noncrossovers microscopically, as can be seen by inspection of Fig. 7.11. Crossing over between car and B results in the broken X having the fragment of the Y and in the unbroken X not having it. Before crossing over, the opposite is true. Thus, the crossover chromosomes are microscopically different from the noncrossover. In Fig. 7.11, bottom, an X chromosome containing car + is added (from a sperm cells is shown in Fig. 7.12) to each of the four classes of eggs produced by the hybrid female. This gives us her female offspring from a test cross.

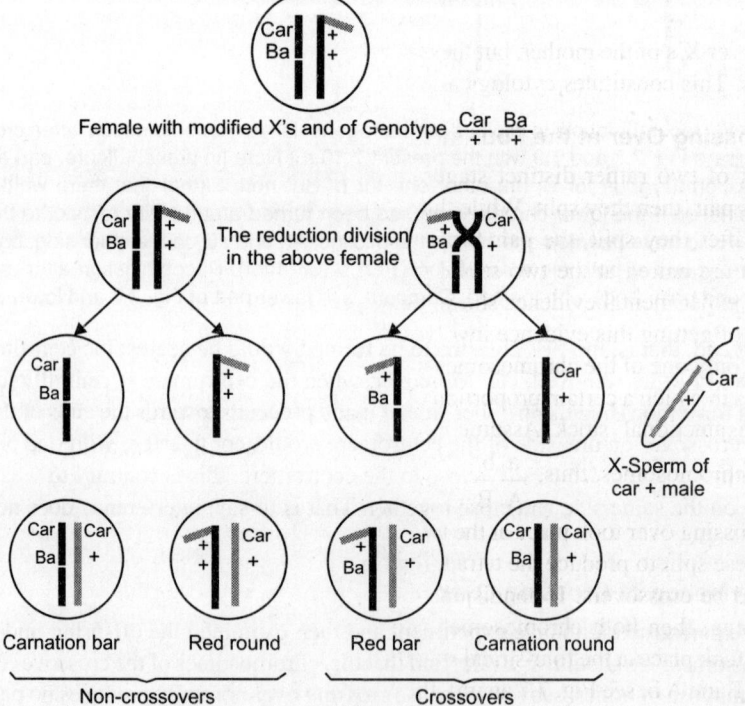

Fig. 7.11: Cytological proof of crossing over.

When the chromosomes of these offspring are examined under the microscope, the class of offspring which appear carnation Bar (first class in Fig. 7.11) are found to have the broken X without the fragment of the Y, and those that appear red round (second class) are found to have the unbroken X with the attached Y fragment. The red bar (third class) have the broken X with an attached Y fragment, and the carnation round (fourth class) have the unbroken X without an attached Y fragment. In other words, when the two genetic noncrossover classes are examined under the microscope, they are seen to contain

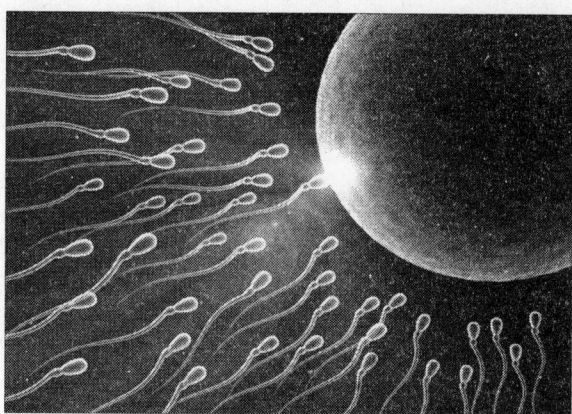

Fig. 7.12: Sperm cells.

the noncrossover X's of the mother, but the two crossover classes (again genetic) are seen to contain the crossover X's. This constitutes cytological proof of crossing over.

Proof of Crossing Over at the Four-strand Stage

We can think of two rather distinct stages in the prophase of the first meiotic division. First, the chromosomes pair, then they split. While they are paired but not yet split, a pair of chromosomes forms two strands, after they split, the pair forms four strands (the four chromatids of a tetrad). Since the chromosomes are paired at the two-strand stage, crossing over might theoretically take place at that stage, but the experimental evidence shows that crossing over takes place at the four-strand stage. One possible way of getting this evidence involves the use of an abnormal stock of flies. It will be recalled that normally only one of the chromosomes of a given tetrad goes to one egg. But in *Drosophila* there is a stock of flies in which a certain proportion of the eggs receive two X chromosomes instead of just one. This is 'nondisjunctional' stock. Assume now that a female of nondisjunctional stock is hybrid at two

loci in the X chromosomes, thus, $\dfrac{a \; b}{A \; B}$.

Then, if crossing over took place at the two-strand stage, two crossovers would be produced, a B and A b. When these split to produce the tetrad, four chromosomes would be produced (2 aB and 2 Ab) and all four would be crossovers. If nondisjunction should happen to occur and two of the chromosomes went to one egg, then both chromosomes would of necessity be crossovers. Assume, however, that crossing over took place at the four-strand stage. Then, two of the four chromosomes of the tetrad might be crossovers (a B and A b, see Fig. 7.7 again), the other two might be noncrossovers (A B and a b, Fig. 7.7). If nondisjunction should now take place, it would be possible for a crossover and a noncrossover to go to the same egg (as A B an,d A b in Fig. 7.7). We saw that this would be impossible if crossing over took place at the two-strand stage. The experimental evidence shows that sometimes a nondisjunctional egg contains both a crossover and noncrossover chromosome, thus proving that crossing over takes place at the four-strand stage.

A given strand of a tetrad might undergo crossing over with either of its nonsister strands, as indicated in Fig. 7.13, left. In this figure, A and A' are sister strands (produced by the division of the same mother chromosome), so are a and a'. Either of the first two sister strands, say A, might undergo crossing over

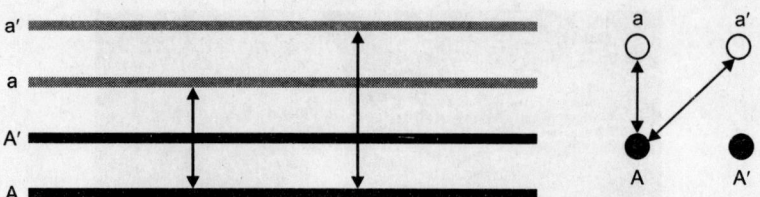

Fig. 7.13: Crossing over between nonsister strands of a tetrad. Left, a tetrad in side view, right, in end view.

with either of its nonsister strands (a or a'), as indicated by the arrows. The same thing is indicated in Fig. 7.13, right, but here the tetrad is represented in end view. We can refer to crossing over between A and a in the right figure as lateral and between A and a' as diagonal. Using these terms, then, crossing over occurs between nonsister strands, but it might be either lateral or diagonal.

SECTION III

Section III Sex Determination, Sex Chromosomes, Sex and Heredity and Sex Determination Systems

Chapter 8

Sex Determination and Sex Chromosome

INTRODUCTION

Sex determination, the establishment of the sex of an organism, usually by the inheritance at the time of fertilisation of certain genes commonly localised on a particular chromosome. This pattern affects the development of the organism by controlling cellular metabolism and stimulating the production of hormones that trigger the development of sexual glands or organs. An excess or lack of hormones during embryological development may cause an individual to develop the superficial appearance of one sex while retaining the genetic constitution of the other sex.

A sex chromosome is a type of chromosome that participates in sex determination. Humans and most other mammals have two sex chromosomes, the X and the Y. Females have two X chromosomes in their cells, while males have both X and a Y chromosomes in their cells. Egg cells all contain an X chromosome, while sperm cells contain an X or Y chromosome. This arrangement means that it is the male that determines the sex of the offspring when fertilisation occurs.

SEX CHROMOSOMES

The nuclei of human cells contain 22 autosomes and 2 sex chromosomes. In females, the sex chromosomes are the 2 X chromosomes. Males have one X chromosome and one Y chromosome. The presence of the Y chromosome is decisive for unleashing the developmental program that leads to a baby boy.

Sex chromosome disorders: Sex chromosome disorders belong to a group of genetic conditions that are caused or affected by the loss or damage of sex chromosomes (gonosomes).

In humans this may refer to:

- 47, XXX
- 48, XXXX
- 49, XXXXY syndrome
- 49, XXXXX
- Klinefelter's syndrome, XXY
- Turner syndrome, X

145

- XX gonadal dysgenesis
- XX male syndrome
- XXYY syndrome
- XYY syndrome

Y Chromosome

The Y chromosome is one of two sex chromosomes (allosomes) in mammals, including humans, and many other animals. The other is the X chromosome. Y is the sex-determining chromosome in many species, since it is the presence or absence of Y that determines male or female sex. In mammals, the Y chromosome contains the gene SRY, which triggers testis development. The DNA in the human Y chromosome is composed of about 59 million base pairs.

The Y chromosome is passed only from father to son, so analysis of Y chromosome (Fig. 8.1) DNA may thus be used in genealogical research. With a 30% difference between humans and chimpanzees, the Y chromosome is one of the fastest evolving parts of the human genome. To date, over 200 Y-linked genes have been identified. All Y-linked genes are expressed and (apart from duplicated genes) hemizygous (present on only one chromosome) except in the cases of aneuploidy such as Klinefelter's Syndrome (47,XXY) or XXYY syndrome.

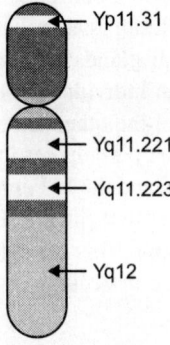

Fig. 8.1: Human Y chromatid.

Variations

Most mammals have only one pair of sex chromosomes in each cell. Males have one Y chromosome and one X chromosome, while females have two X chromosomes. In mammals, the Y chromosome contains a gene, SRY, which triggers embryonic development as a male. The Y chromosomes of humans and other mammals also contain other genes needed for normal sperm production.

There are exceptions, however. For example, the platypus relies on an XY sex-determination system based on five pairs of chromosomes. Platypus sex chromosomes in fact appear to bear a much stronger homology (similarity) with the avian Z chromosome, and the SRY gene so central to sex-determination in most other mammals is apparently not involved in platypus sex-determination. Among humans, some men have two Xs and a Y (XXY), or one X and two Ys and some women have three Xs or a single X instead of a double X (X0). There are other exceptions in which SRY is damaged (leading to an XY female), or copied to the X (leading to an XX male).

Origins and Evolution

Before Y chromosome

Many ectothermic vertebrates have no sex chromosomes. If they have different sexes, sex is determined environmentally rather than genetically. For some of them, especially reptiles, sex depends on the incubation temperature, others are hermaphroditic (meaning they contain both male and female gametes in the same individual).

Origin

The X and Y chromosomes are thought to have evolved from a pair of identical chromosomes, termed autosomes, when an ancestral mammal developed an allelic variation, a so-called 'sex locus'–simply possessing this allele caused the organism to be male. The chromosome with this allele became the Y chromosome, while the other member of the pair became the X chromosome.

Over time, genes which were beneficial for males and harmful to (or had no effect on) females either developed on the Y chromosome, or were acquired through the process of translocation.

Until recently, the X and Y chromosomes were thought to have diverged around 300 million years ago. However, research published in 2010, and particularly research published in 2008 documenting the sequencing of the platypus genome, has suggested that the XY sex-determination system would not have been present more than 166 million years ago, at the split of the monotremes from other mammals. This re-estimation of the age of the therian XY system is based on the finding that sequences that are on the X chromosomes of marsupials and eutherian mammals are present on the autosomes of platypus and birds. The older estimate was based on erroneous reports that the platypus X chromosomes contained these sequences.

Recombination inhibition

Recombination between the X and Y chromosomes proved harmful—it resulted in males without necessary genes formerly found on the Y chromosome, and females with unnecessary or even harmful genes previously only found on the Y chromosome. As a result, genes beneficial to males accumulated near the sex-determining genes, and recombination in this region was suppressed in order to preserve this male specific region. Over time, the Y chromosome changed in such a way as to inhibit the areas around the sex determining genes from recombining at all with the X chromosome. As a result of this process, 95% of the human Y chromosome is unable to recombine. Only the tips of the Y and X chromosomes recombine. The tips of the Y chromosome that could recombine with the X chromosome are referred to as the pseudoautosomal region. The rest of the Y chromosome is passed on to the next generation intact. It is because of this disregard for the rules that the Y chromosome is such a superb tool for investigating recent human evolution from a male perspective.

Degeneration

By one estimate, the human Y chromosome has lost 1,393 of its 1,438 original genes over the course of its existence, and linear extrapolation of this 1,393-gene loss over 300 million years gives a rate of genetic loss of 4.6 genes per million years. Continued loss of genes at the 4.6 genes per million year rate would result in a Y chromosome with no functional genes–that is the Y chromosome would lose complete function– within the next 10 million years, or half that time with current estimate of 160 million year age. Comparative genomic analysis reveals that many mammalian species are experiencing a similar loss of function in their heterozygous sex chromosome. Degeneration may simply be the fate of all non-recombining sex chromosomes, due to three common evolutionary forces: high mutation rate, inefficient selection, and genetic drift. However, comparisons of the human and chimpanzee Y chromosomes (first published in 2005) show that the human Y chromosome has not lost any genes since the divergence of humans and chimpanzees between 6–7 million years ago, and a scientific report in 2012 stated that only one gene had been lost since humans diverged from the rhesus macaque 25 million years ago. These facts provide direct evidence that the linear extrapolation model is flawed and suggest that the current human Y chromosome is either no longer shrinking or is shrinking at a much slower rate than the 4.6 genes per million years estimated by the linear extrapolation model.

High mutation rate

The human Y chromosome is particularly exposed to high mutation rates due to the environment in which it is housed. The Y chromosome is passed exclusively through sperm, which undergo multiple cell divisions during gametogenesis. Each cellular division provides further opportunity to accumulate base pair mutations. Additionally, sperm are stored in the highly oxidative environment of the testis, which encourages further mutation. These two conditions combined put the Y chromosome at a greater risk of mutation than the rest of the genome. The increased mutation risk for the Y chromosome is reported by Graves as a factor 4.8. However, her original reference obtains this number for the relative mutation rates in male and female germ lines for the lineage leading to humans.

Inefficient selection

Without the ability to recombine during meiosis, the Y chromosome is unable to expose individual alleles to natural selection. Deleterious alleles are allowed to 'hitchhike' with beneficial neighbours, thus propagating maladapted alleles in to the next generation. Conversely, advantageous alleles may be selected against if they are surrounded by harmful alleles. Due to this inability to sort through its gene content, the Y chromosome is particularly prone to the accumulation of 'junk' DNA. Massive accumulations of retrotransposable elements are scattered throughout the Y. The random insertion of DNA segments often disrupts encoded gene sequences and renders them nonfunctional. However, the Y chromosome has no way of weeding out these 'jumping genes'. Without the ability to isolate alleles, selection cannot effectively act upon them. A clear, quantitative indication of this inefficiency is the entropy rate of the Y chromosome. Whereas all other chromosomes in the human genome have entropy rates of 1.5–1.9 bits per nucleotide (compared to the theoretical maximum of exactly 2 for no redundancy), the Y chromosome's entropy rate is only 0.84. This means the Y chromosome has a much lower information content relative to its overall length, it is more redundant.

Genetic drift

Even if a well adapted Y chromosome manages to maintain genetic activity by avoiding mutation accumulation, there is no guarantee it will be passed down to the next generation. The population size of the Y chromosome is inherently limited to ¼ that of autosomes: diploid organisms contain two copies of autosomal chromosomes while only half the population contains 1 Y chromosome.

Thus, genetic drift is an exceptionally strong force acting upon the Y chromosome. Through sheer random assortment, an adult male may never pass on his Y chromosome if he only has female offspring. Thus, although a male may have a well adapted Y chromosome free of excessive mutation, it may never make it in to the next gene pool. The repeat random loss of well-adapted Y chromosomes, coupled with the tendency of the Y chromosome to evolve to have more deleterious mutations rather than less for reasons described above, contributes to the species-wide degeneration of Y chromosomes through Muller's ratchet.

Gene conversion

As it has been already mentioned, the Y chromosome is unable to recombine during meiosis like the other human chromosomes, however, in 2003, researchers from MIT discovered a process which may slow down the process of degradation. They found that human Y chromosome is able to 'recombine' with itself, using palindrome base pair sequences. Such a 'recombination' is called gene conversion.

In the case of the Y chromosomes, the palindromes are not noncoding DNA, these strings of bases contain functioning genes important for male fertility. Most of the sequence pairs are greater than 99.97% identical. The extensive use of gene conversion may play a role in the ability of the Y chromosome to edit out genetic mistakes and maintain the integrity of the relatively few genes it carries. In other words, since the Y chromosome is single, it has duplicates of its genes on itself instead of having a second, homologous, chromosome. When errors occur, it can use other parts of itself as a template to correct them. Findings were confirmed by comparing similar regions of the Y chromosome in humans to the Y chromosomes of chimpanzees, bonobos and gorillas. The comparison demonstrated that the same phenomenon of gene conversion appeared to be at work more than 5 million years ago, when humans and the non-human primates diverged from each other.

Future evolution

In the terminal stages of the degeneration of the Y chromosome, other chromosomes increasingly take over genes and functions formerly associated with it. Finally, the Y chromosome disappears entirely, and a new sex-determining system arises. Several species of rodent in the sister families Muridae and Cricetidae have reached these stages, in the following ways:

- The Transcaucasian mole vole, *Ellobius lutescens*, the Zaisan mole vole, *Ellobius tancrei*, and the Japanese spinous country rats *Tokudaia osimensis* and *Tokudaia tokunoshimensis*, have lost the Y chromosome and SRY entirely. *Tokudaia* spp. have relocated some other genes ancestrally present on the Y chromosome to the X chromosome. Both genders of *Tokudaia* spp. and *Ellobius lutescens* have an XO genotype (Turner syndrome), whereas all *Ellobius tancrei* possess an XX genotype. The new sex-determining system(s) for these rodents remains unclear.

- The wood lemming *Myopus schisticolour*, the arctic lemming, Dicrostonyx torquatus, and multiple species in the grass mouse genus Akodon have evolved fertile females who possess the genotype generally coding for males, XY, in addition to the ancestral XX female, through a variety of modifications to the X and Y chromosomes.

- In the creeping vole, *Microtus oregoni*, the females, with just one X chromosome each, produce X gametes only, and the males, XY, produce Y gametes, or gametes devoid of any sex chromosome, through nondisjunction.

Outside of the rodent family, the black muntjac, *Muntiacus crinifrons*, evolved new X and Y chromosomes through fusions of the ancestral sex chromosomes and autosomes.

Human Y Chromosome

In humans, the Y chromosome spans about 58 million base pairs (the building blocks of DNA) and represents approximately 2% of the total DNA in a male cell. The human Y chromosome contains over 200 genes, at least 72 of which code for proteins. Traits that are inherited via the Y chromosome are called holandric traits (although biologists will usually just say 'Y-linked').

The human Y chromosome is normally unable to recombine with the X chromosome, except for small pieces of pseudoautosomal regions at the telomeres (which comprise about 5% of the chromosome's length). These regions are relics of ancient homology between the X and Y chromosomes. The bulk of the Y chromosome which does not recombine is called the 'NRY' or non-recombining region of the Y chromosome. It is the SNPs (single-nucleotide polymorphism) in this region which are used for tracing direct paternal ancestral lines.

Genes

Not including pseudoautosomal genes, genes include:
- NRY, with corresponding gene on X chromosome.
  - › AMELY/AMELX (amelogenin)
  - › RPS4Y1/RPS4Y2/RPS4X (Ribosomal protein S4)
- NRY, other:
  - › AZF1 (Azoospermia factor 1)
  - › BPY2 (Basic protein on the Y chromosome)
  - › DAZ1 (Deleted in azoospermia)
  - › DAZ2
  - › PRKY (protein kinase, Y-linked)
  - › RBMY1A1
  - › SRY (sex-determining region)
  - › TSPY (testis-specific protein)
  - › USP9Y
  - › UTY (Ubiquitously transcribed TPR gene on Y chromosome)
  - › ZFY (Zinc finger protein)

More common

No vital genes reside only on the Y chromosome, since roughly half of humans (females) do not have a Y chromosome. The only well-defined human disease linked to a defect on the Y chromosome is defective testicular development (due to deletion or deleterious mutation of SRY). However, having two X chromosomes and one Y chromosome has similar effects. On the other hand, having Y chromosome polysomy has other effects than masculinisation.

Y chromosome microdeletion

Y chromosome microdeletion (YCM) is a family of genetic disorders caused by missing genes in the Y chromosome. Many affected men exhibit no symptoms and lead normal lives. However, YCM is also known to be present in a significant number of men with reduced fertility or reduced sperm count.

Defective Y chromosome

This results in the person presenting a female phenotype (i.e. is born with female-like genitalia) even though that person possesses an XY karyotype. The lack of the second X results in infertility. In other words, viewed from the opposite direction, the person goes through defeminisation but fails to complete masculinisation. The cause can be seen as an incomplete Y chromosome: the usual karyotype in these cases is 44X, plus a fragment of Y. This usually results in defective testicular development, such that the infant may or may not have fully formed male genitalia internally or externally. The full range of ambiguity of structure may occur, especially if mosaicism is present. When the Y fragment is minimal and non-functional, the child is usually a girl with the features of Turner syndrome or mixed gonadal dysgenesis.

XXY

Klinefelter syndrome (47, XXY) is not an aneuploidy of the Y chromosome, but a condition of having an extra X chromosome, which usually results in defective postnatal testicular function. The mechanism is not fully understood, the extra X does not seem to be due to direct interference with expression of Y genes.

XYY

47,XYY syndrome (simply known as XYY syndrome) is caused by the presence of a single extra copy of the Y chromosome in each of a male's cells. 47, XYY males have one X chromosome and two Y chromosomes, for a total of 47 chromosomes per cell. Researchers have found that an extra copy of the Y chromosome is associated with increased stature and an increased incidence of learning problems in some boys and men, but the effects are variable, often minimal, and the vast majority do not know their karyotype. When chromosome surveys were done in the mid-1960s in British secure hospitals for the developmentally disabled, a higher than expected number of patients were found to have an extra Y chromosome. The patients were mischaracterised as aggressive and criminal, so that for a while an extra Y chromosome was believed to predispose a boy to antisocial behaviour (and was dubbed the 'criminal karyotype'). Subsequently, in 1968 in Scotland the only ever comprehensive nationwide chromosome survey of prisons found no over-representation of 47,XYY men, and later studies found 47,XYY boys and men had the same rate of criminal convictions as 46,XY boys and men of equal intelligence. Thus, the 'criminal karyotype' concept is inaccurate and obsolete.

Rare

The following Y chromosome-linked diseases are rare, but notable because of their elucidating of the nature of the Y chromosome.

More than two Y chromosomes

Greater degrees of Y chromosome polysomy (having more than one extra copy of the Y chromosome in every cell, e.g. XYYY) are rare. The extra genetic material in these cases can lead to skeletal abnormalities, decreased IQ, and delayed development, but the severity features of these conditions are variable.

XX male syndrome

XX male syndrome occurs when there has been a recombination in the formation of the male gametes, causing the SRY-portion of the Y chromosome to move to the X chromosome. When such an X chromosome contributes to the child, the development will lead to a male, because of the SRY gene.

Genetic genealogy

In human genetic genealogy (the application of genetics to traditional genealogy), use of the information contained in the Y chromosome is of particular interest because, unlike other chromosomes, the Y chromosome is passed exclusively from father to son, on the patrilineal line. Mitochondrial DNA, maternally inherited to both sons and daughters, is used in an analogous way to trace the matrilineal line.

Brain function

Research is currently investigating whether male-pattern neural development is a direct consequence of Y chromosome-related gene expression or an indirect result of Y chromosome-related androgenic hormone production.

Non-mammal Y Chromosome

Many groups of organisms in addition to mammals have Y chromosomes, but these Y chromosomes do not share common ancestry with mammalian Y chromosomes. Such groups include *Drosophila*, some other insects, some fish, some reptiles, and some plants. In *Drosophila melanogaster*, the Y chromosome does not trigger male development. Instead, sex is determined by the number of X chromosomes. The *D. melanogaster* Y chromosome does contain genes necessary for male fertility. So XXY *D. melanogaster* are female, and *D. melanogaster* with a single X (X0), are male but sterile. There are some species of *Drosophila* in which X0 males are both viable and fertile.

ZW chromosomes

Other organisms have mirror image sex chromosomes: the female is 'XY' and the male is 'XX', but by convention biologists call a 'female Y' a W chromosome and the other a Z chromosome. For example, female birds, snakes, and butterflies have ZW sex chromosomes, and males have ZZ sex chromosomes.

FRAGILE X SYNDROME

Fragile X syndrome (FXS), also known as Martin–Bell syndrome, or Escalante's syndrome (more commonly used in South American countries), is a genetic syndrome. Nearly half of all children with fragile X syndrome meet the criteria for a diagnosis of autism. It is an inherited cause of intellectual disability especially among boys. It results in a spectrum of intellectual disabilities ranging from mild to severe as well as physical characteristics such as an elongated face, large or protruding ears, and large testes (macroorchidism), and behavioural characteristics such as stereotypic movements (e.g. hand-flapping), and social anxiety.

Fragile X syndrome is associated with the expansion of the CGG trinucleotide repeat affecting the Fragile X mental retardation 1 (FMR1) gene on the X chromosome, resulting in a failure to express the fragile X mental retardation protein (FMRP), which is required for normal neural development. Depending on the length of the CGG repeat, an allele may be classified as normal (unaffected by the syndrome), a premutation (at risk of fragile X associated disorders), or full mutation (usually affected by the syndrome). A definitive diagnosis of fragile X syndrome is made through genetic testing to determine the number of CGG repeats. Testing for premutation carriers can also be carried out to allow for genetic counseling. The first complete DNA sequence of the repeat expansion in someone with the full mutation was generated by scientists in 2012 using SMRT sequencing. There is currently no drug treatment that has shown benefit specifically for fragile X syndrome. However, medications are commonly used to treat symptoms of attention deficit and hyperactivity, anxiety, and aggression. Supportive management is important in optimising functioning in individuals with fragile X syndrome, and may involve speech therapy, occupational therapy, and individualised educational and behavioural programs.

Signs and Symptoms

Aside from intellectual disability, prominent characteristics of the syndrome may include an elongated face, large or protruding ears, flat feet, larger testes (macro-orchidism), and low muscle tone. Recurrent otitis media (middle ear infection) and sinusitis is common during early childhood. Speech may be cluttered or nervous. Behavioural characteristics may include stereotypic movements (e.g. hand-flapping) and atypical social development, particularly shyness, limited eye contact, memory problems, and difficulty with face encoding. Some individuals with fragile X syndrome also meet the diagnostic criteria for autism.

Males with a full mutation display virtually complete penetrance and will therefore almost always display symptoms of FXS, while females with a full mutation generally display a penetrance of about 50% as a result of having a second, normal X chromosome. Females with FXS may have symptoms ranging from mild to severe, although they are generally less affected than males.

COLOUR BLINDNESS

Colour blindness, or colour vision deficiency, is the inability or decreased ability to see colour, or perceive colour differences, under normal lighting conditions. Colour blindness affects a significant percentage of the population. There is no actual blindness but there is a deficiency of colour vision. The most usual cause is a fault in the development of one or more sets of retinal cones that perceive colour in light and transmit that information to the optic nerve. This type of colour blindness is usually a sex-linked condition. The genes that produce photopigments are carried on the X chromosome, if some of these genes are missing or damaged, colour blindness will be expressed in males with a higher probability than in females because males only have one X chromosome, whereas females have two and a functional gene on only one of the X chromosomes is sufficient to yield the necessary photopigments.

Colour blindness can also be produced by physical or chemical damage to the eye, the optic nerve, or parts of the brain. For example, people with achromatopsia suffer from a completely different disorder, but are nevertheless unable to see colours.

Causes of Colour Blindness

Genetics

Colour blindness can be inherited. It is most commonly inherited from mutations on the X chromosome but the mapping of the human genome has shown there are many causative mutations—mutations capable of causing colour blindness originate from at least 19 different chromosomes and 56 different genes (as shown online at the Online Mendelian Inheritance in Man (OMIM) database at Johns Hopkins University). Two of the most common inherited forms of colour blindness are protanopia and deuteranopia. One of the common colour vision defects is red-green deficiency which is present in about 8 per cent of males and 0.5 per cent of females of Northern European ancestry.

Some of the inherited diseases known to cause colour blindness are:

- Cone dystrophy.
- Cone-rod dystrophy.
- Achromatopsia (a.k.a. rod monochromatism, stationary cone dystrophy or cone dysfunction syndrome).
- Blue cone monochromatism (a.k.a. blue cone monochromacy or X-linked achromatopsia).
- Leber's congenital amaurosis.
- Retinitis pigmentosa (initially affects rods but can later progress to cones and therefore colour blindness).

Inherited colour blindness can be congenital (from birth), or it can commence in childhood or adulthood. Depending on the mutation, it can be stationary, that is, remain the same throughout a person's lifetime, or progressive. As progressive phenotypes involve deterioration of the retina and other parts of the eye, certain forms of colour blindness can progress to legal blindness, i.e. an acuity of 6/60 or worse, and often leave a person with complete blindness.

Colour blindness always pertains to the cone photoreceptors in retinas, as the cones are capable of detecting the colour frequencies of light.

About 8 per cent of males, but only 0.5 per cent of females, are colour blind in some way or another, whether it is one colour, a colour combination, or another mutation. The reason males are at a greater risk of inheriting an X linked mutation is that males only have one X chromosome (XY, with the Y chromosome carrying altogether different genes than the X chromosome), and females have two (XX), if a woman inherits a normal X chromosome in addition to the one that carries the mutation, she will not display the mutation. Men do not have a second X chromosome to override the chromosome that carries the mutation. If 5% of variants of a given gene are defective, the probability of a single copy being defective is 5%, but the probability that two copies are both defective is $0.05 \times 0.05 = 0.0025$, or just 0.25%.

Other causes

Other causes of colour blindness include brain or retinal damage caused by shaken baby syndrome, accidents and other trauma which produce swelling of the brain in the occipital lobe, and damage to the retina caused by exposure to ultraviolet light (10–300 nm). Damage often presents itself later on in life. Colour blindness may also present itself in the spectrum of degenerative diseases of the eye, such as age-related macular degeneration, and as part of the retinal damage caused by diabetes. Another factor that may affect colour blindness includes a deficiency in Vitamin A.

Diagnosis

The Ishihara colour test, which consists of a series of pictures of coloured spots, is the test most often used to diagnose red–green colour deficiencies. A figure (usually one or more Arabic digits) is embedded in the picture as a number of spots in a slightly different colour, and can be seen with normal colour vision, but not with a particular colour defect. The full set of tests has a variety of figure/background colour combinations, and enable diagnosis of which particular visual defect is present. The anomaloscope, described above, is also used in diagnosing anomalous trichromacy.

Robertsonian Translocation

Robertsonian translocation (ROB) is a rare form of chromosomal rearrangement that in humans occurs in the five acrocentric chromosome pairs, namely 13, 14, 15, 21, and 22. Other translocations occur but do not lead to a viable fetus. They are named after the American biologist William Rees Brebner Robertson (1881–1941), who first described a Robertsonian translocation in grasshoppers in 1916. They are also called whole-arm translocations or centric-fusion translocations. They are a type of chromosomal translocation. A Robertsonian translocation is a type of nonreciprocal translocation involving two homologous (paired) or non-homologous chromosomes (i.e. two different chromosomes, not belonging to a homologous pair). A feature of chromosomes that are commonly found to undergo such translocations is that they possess an acrocentric centromere, partitioning the chromosome into a large arm containing the vast majority of genes, and a short arm with a much smaller proportion of genetic content. During a Robertsonian translocation, the participating chromosomes break at their centromeres and the long arms fuse to form a single chromosome with a single centromere. The short arms also join to form a reciprocal product, which typically contains nonessential genes and is usually lost within a few cell divisions.

Consequence

In humans, when a Robertsonian translocation joins the long arm of chromosome 21 with the long arm of chromosome 14 (or 15), the heterozygous carrier is phenotypically normal because there are two copies of all major chromosome arms and hence two copies of all essential genes. However, the progeny of this carrier may inherit an unbalanced trisomy 21, causing Down Syndrome.

About one in a thousand newborns has a Robertsonian translocation. The most frequent forms of Robertsonian translocations are between chromosomes 13 and 14, 14 and 21, and 14 and 15, and occur when the long arms of two acrocentric chromosomes fuse at the centromere and the two short arms are lost. A Robertsonian translocation in balanced form results in no excess or deficit of genetic material and causes no health difficulties. In unbalanced forms, Robertsonian translocations cause chromosomal deletions or addition and result in syndromes of multiple malformations, including trisomy 13 (Patau syndrome) and trisomy 21 (Down syndrome).

A Robertsonian translocation results when the long arms of two acrocentric chromosomes fuse at the centromere and the two short arms are lost. If, for example, the long arms of chromosomes 13 and 14 fuse, no significant genetic material is lost and the person is completely normal in spite of the translocation. Common Robertsonian translocations are confined to the acrocentric chromosomes 13, 14, 15, 21 and 22, because the short arms of these chromosomes encode for rRNA which is present in multiple copies.

Most people with Robertsonian translocations have only 45 chromosomes in each of their cells, yet all essential genetic material is present, and they appear normal. Their children, however, may either be normal and carry the fusion chromosome (depending which chromosome is represented in the gamete), or they may inherit a missing or extra long arm of an acrocentric chromosome. Genetic counseling and genetic testing is offered to families that may be carriers of chromosomal translocations.

Rarely, the same translocation may be present homozygously if heterozygous parents with the same Robertsonian translocation have children. The result may be viable offspring with 44 chromosomes.

POSITION EFFECT

Position effect is the effect on the expression of a gene when its location in a chromosome is changed, often by translocation. This has been well described in *Drosophila* with respect to eye colour and is known as position effect variegation (PEV). The phenotype is well characterised by unstable expression of a gene that results in the red eye colouration. In the mutant flies the eyes typically have a mottled appearance of white and red sectors. These phenotypes are often due to a chromosomal translocation such that the colour gene is now close to a region of heterochromatin.

The heterochromatin can spread stochastically and switch off the colour gene resulting in the white eye sectors. Position effect is also used to describe the variation of expression exhibited by identical transgenes that insert into different regions of a genome. In this case the difference in expression is often due to enhancers that regulate neighbouring genes.

These local enhancers can also affect the expression pattern of the transgene. Since each transgenic organism has the transgene in a different location each transgenic organism has the potential for a unique expression pattern.

CHROMOSOMAL ABNORMALITIES IN CANCER

The morphological abnormalities of chromosomes in cancer cells include: a gain or loss of chromosomes, deletion (loss of a segment of a chromosome), inversion ('flip-flop' of two segments of a chromosome), translocation (reciprocal rearrangement of segments between two chromosomes), and selective amplification of certain regions of chromosomes. Specific changes in particular chromosomes are often associated with certain types of cancer.

Non-random changes of chromosome number in cancer cells are often trisomies (three of the same chromosome), such as trisomy 8 associated with acute leukemia. Extreme variations in number range from 23, as in haploid leukemia, to multiples thereof, such as tetraploid leukemia. The loss of a whole chromosome or chromosomal segment commonly occurs in leukemias. Chromosome translocations were discussed previously in relation to the activation of proto-oncogenes in Burkitt's lymphoma (BL) and chronic myelogenous leukemia (CML) (refer to: Oncogenes and Human Cancers). BL is characterised by translocations between chromosome 8 and 14 (90% of cases), 8 and 22 (5%), and 8 and 2 (5%). The human c-myc gene maps to the usual breakpoint on chromosome 8. Immunoglobulin (Ig) genes map to reciprocal breakpoints on chromosome 14 (Ig heavy-chain gene), 22 (Ig light-chain kappa gene), and 2 (Ig light-chain lambda gene). In BL cells, the c-myc gene is translocated in proximity to an active promotor (in B lymphocytes) of an Ig gene and is activated, resulting in increased expression of c-myc gene products.

The acquired chromosomal abnormality occurring in about 90-95% of patients with CML is characterised by a translocation between chromosome 9 and 22, resulting in the Philadelphia chromosome. The human c-abl gene maps to the breakpoint on chromosome 9, and its translocation to the usual breakpoint cluster region (bcr) on chromosome 22 results in the production of an abnormal 'fusion' protein encoded by abl and adjacent bcr sequences. The fusion protein has increased tyrosine kinase activity compared to the normal abl protein.

Many subtypes of T-cell or B-cell leukemias are associated with chromosomal abnormalities, including translocations, that transpose the TCR (T-cell receptor) gene or an Ig (immunoglobulin) gene, respectively, into proximity to a proto-oncogene, thereby activating it. TCR and Ig genes may be frequently involved in such chromosomal aberrations because coding segments of their DNA normally undergo rearrangement to generate a diversity of antigen-receptors.

Gene amplification is an increase in the number of gene copies and is recognised by chromosome analysis as either homogeneous staining regions (HSRs) or small extrachromosomal particles called double minutes (DMs). Amplification of the human proto-oncogene N-myc, which has structural homology to c-myc and maps to chromosome 2, is found in neuroblastoma of children and is correlated with the stage of progression of the disease. As noted previously, retinoblastoma of children is some time associated with small deletions at the RB locus of both copies of human chromosome 13. The first gene deletion can be either inherited by germline change or acquired. The second deletion is random and required for neoplastic transformation.

Telomeres

Telomeres, the ends of chromosomes, are special DNA repeat sequences synthesised by the enzyme telomerase. Normal somatic cells are programmed for a limited number of cell divisions, and telomerase activity is inhibited in many types of normal cells. The telomeres decrease in length with each somatic cell division, as though acting like a 'mitotic clock' that counts the total number of divisions and that, when telomere length reaches a critical minimum, signals the cell to drop out of the division cycle. In contrast, germinal cells, immortalised cells with the capacity to proliferate indefinitely, and human cancer cells of many types do not show shortening of telomere length or a loss of telomerase activity. Thus, telomerase is repressed in many types of human somatic cells, but reactivated in immortal cells and cancer cells. Normal human cells, in a non-dividing and near senescent state, are capable of returning to normal cell division and an extended life span when transfected with vectors encoding a catalytic subunit of the human telomerase gene - a landmark discovery.

SEX DETERMINATION AND DIFFERENTIATION IN VERTEBRATES

The concept of sex determination and differentiation has been baffling mankind since time immemorial. While Aristotle hypothesised in 335 BC that sex was determined by the heat generated during conception, Andreas Vesalius in 1543 AD illustrated that women were but males, their genitalia turned inside out. In numerous cultures since then, women have been considered as the 'default state of men'. However, in the 17th century gradually it was discovered that the females produced eggs that transmitted parental traits. Later, in the twentieth century Geddes and Thomson came forward with the hypothesis that constitution, age, nutrition and environment of parents decide the sex determination of the offspring. This environmental view of sex determination was again challenged by the discovery of sex chromosomes by McClung in 1902. Following this, more evidences gradually clinched to suggest the chromosomal concept of sex determination. Numerous experimental studies in vertebrates have now established beyond doubt that sex is determined either by chromosomal factors, environmental influences, or interplay of both, depending on the species/groups.

ENVIRONMENTAL SEX DETERMINATION (ESD)

In some cold blooded vertebrates (fishes, reptiles), sex is determined not at the time of fertilisation by sex chromosomes, rather, it is determined by the environment in which the early embryonic development takes place.

In various freshwater fishes as well as marine species from temperate or tropical habitats, it has been clearly shown that sex determination and consequent differentiation is influenced by the environmental factors like pH, salinity, social interaction and importantly, temperature. In most thermosensitive species (some *Atherinids, Poecilids, Cichlids*, a *Siluriform* is shown in Fig. 8.2), high temperature increases male to female sex ratios and *vice versa*.

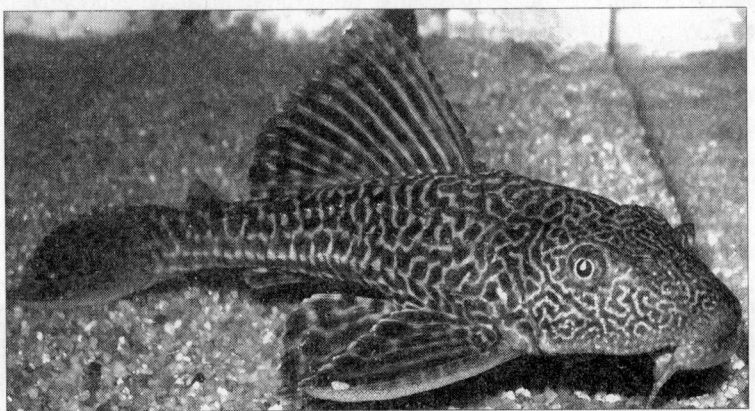

Fig. 8.2: *Siluriform.*

Exceptionally, in European sea bass, *Dicentrarchus labrax* and channel catfish, Ictalurus punctatus high temperature induces female sex differentiation. Density and pH also plays a sex determining role in fishes as evidenced in paradise fish *Macropodus opercularis* (Fig. 8.3), where the number of females is directly proportional to the density and in all Apistogramma species (cichlids) the proportion of males is higher at an acidic pH (4.5) than at neutral pH (6.5). The complete sex reversal can also be accomplished by exposing gonochoristic fish to exogenous sex steroids during gonadal differentiation. In addition to gonochorism, several types of hermaphroditism are seen in fishes. Social interaction such as disappearance of a male or female from a mixed group causes sex inversion in these species: from male to female (protoandrous, sea anemone fish, Amphiprion clarkii), from female to male (protogynous, Red sea fish, Anthias squamipinnis) and a few can change sex either way or multiple times (serial sex change, gobiid fish, Trima okinawae.

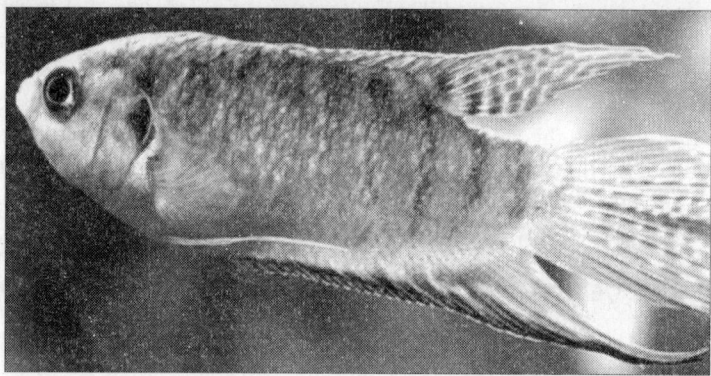

Fig. 8.3: *Macropodus opercularis.*

In amphibians, although sex chromosomes are invariably shown responsible for sex determination with either male heterogamety (XY/XX) or female heterogamety (ZW/ZZ), the environmental factor and hormones can override the genotypic mechanism of sex determination and induce sex reversal. The rearing of larvae of salamanders (ZZ/ZW) at high temperatures (30–32°C) produces opposite effects in two different species. ZZ genotypic males of Algerian ribbed newt, Pleurodeles poireti become phenotypic females, whereas ZW genotypic females of Spanish ribbed newt, Pleurodeles waltl become phenotypic males. In another newt Triturus cristatus (XX/XY), more males than females, including some XX neomales are produced at higher temperature, and vice-versa at lower temperature. Also, in wood frog, Rana sylvatica, sex reversal of all females occurs when larvae are reared at high temperatures (32±2°C). However, all the above said studies have been conducted at extreme temperature which is outside of the range normally experienced by these species, and therefore, these effects probably do not occur under natural conditions. An exception is common frog, Rana temporaria, where temperature of only 20°C masculinises the females. Nevertheless, the effect of temperature in all these cases is limited to a particular stage, i.e. before the first sign of histological differentiation of gonads Social interaction, in addition to temperature, also causes sex reversal. In case of common reed frog, Hyperolius viridiflavus low male density induces sex reversal in females. Perplexing response to hormone treatment is observed in different species of XX/XY ranids and hylid frogs: masculinisation by testosterone and feminisation by estradiol (Northern leopard frog, Rana pipiens), masculinisation by testosterone but impervious to estradiol (black spotted frog, Rana nigromaculata and Japanese brown frog, Rana japonica), feminisation by estradiol but non responsive to testosterone (Japanese tree frog, Hyla japonica), and refractory to both, testosterone as well as estradiol (yellow bellied toad, Bombina variegata and Oriental fire bellied toad, Bombina orientalis). Other amphibians that have heterogametic females (ZW), e.g. Bufo, Xenopus and some urodeles are feminised by estradiol but not masculinised by testosterone. A bizarre exception in this case is shown by racophorid frog, Buergeria buergeri, where ZW tadpoles are masculinised by either estradiol or testosterone treatment but ZZ tadpoles are not affected appreciably by either hormone.

Reptiles exhibit extraordinary variability in patterns of sex determination among vertebrates. Male heterogamety (XY or XXY) is known in turtles, female heterogamety (ZW, ZZW or ZWW) is known in snakes and both are known in lizards. Even in the absence of any gross heteromorphy in the sex chromosome, genotypic mode of sex determination is seen in some species. However, the crucial role of environment in sex determination was seen long back in the year 1966 in lizard Agama agama where incubation of eggs at different temperature changed the sex ratios of hatchling. Later, environment (temperature)-dependent sex determination was seen widespread in reptiles. Temperature-dependent sex determination (TSD) is invariably seen in all tuatara and crocodiles, most tortoises, turtles and terrapins, and in some lizards. Generally, among most chelonians, incubation of eggs below transition range temperature (TRT) induces masculinisation, above TRT leads to feminisation, and at TRT both males and females or even intersex individuals are produced. On the contrary, in alligators, lizards and tuatara males are produced at high temperature and females at low temperature. However, exceptions to these trends are seen in crocodiles and a few turtles like snapping turtle, mud turtle, alligator snapping turtle etc., where eggs incubated below or above TRT develop into females and males are produced at TRT. In all TSD species there is a well defined thermosensitive period (TSP) when temperature affects sex determination and after this the embryos become refractory to temperature changes.

Temperature influences sex determination by modulating the activity of steroidogenic enzymes and thereby affecting the hormonal environment of the embryo inducing either masculinisation or feminisation. In freshwater turtle, Eyms orbicularis, the aromatase activity responsible for aromatisation of testosterone into estradiol remains low at male producing temperature (25°C) and high at feminising temperature (30°C). Moreover, exogenous sex steroids can override the effect of temperature on sex determination in TSD species. Earlier, it was thought that the hormone induced sex reversal is unilateral towards the female sex, since administration of estradiol or testosterone induces embryos to develop as females even if eggs are incubated at male sensitive temperature. However, in case of red-eared slider turtles, Trachemys scripta, instead of testosterone, administration of dihydrotestosterone (DHT, a non aromatisable androgen) during TSP altered the unilateral pattern of sex reversal and induces masculinisation. Identical result is observed when aromatase inhibitor (AI) is applied to eggs incubated at female sensitive temperature. Although sex is genetically determined in the Indian garden lizard, Calotes versicolor, exogenous androgen induces sex reversal. DHT is found to be effective only between stages of initialisation of genital ridge and formation of sex cords. Previous experiences of unilateral sex reversal towards females after administration of testosterone to eggs incubated even at male sensitive temperature might be due to the aromatisation of testosterone into estradiol, the female sex steroid.

CHROMOSOMAL SEX DETERMINATION (CSD)

Before the karyotyping of human chromosomes, it was considered that sex is determined by the number of X chromosomes present in an individual. It was observed that in drosophila, males had single X chromosome (XY or XO) and the presence of 2 or more X chromosomes (XX, XXX, or XXY) always conferred female phenotype. It was thus considered that the Y chromosome was a null chromosome.

However, in 1966, a landmark observation was made by Jacobs and Ross. They described two sisters who had female external genitalia but 46 XY karyotype in which the Y chromosome consisted only of its long arm. It seemed therefore, that the testicular determining region of the Y chromosome normally resides in its short arm. This was confirmed by high resolution banding studies of an XX male which revealed that some material from the short arm of Y chromosome had been translocated to one of his X chromosomes. With advanced techniques, it became apparent that sex determining gene on short arm of Y chromosome is responsible for the development of testis in mammals. Also, testicular development is seen impaired in several clinical syndromes resulting from autosomal deletions or mutations. Now autosomal genes such as SOX 9, WNT 4, SF1, DMRT 1, etc. are shown to play a crucial role in the downstream events of sex differentiation initiated by SRY (Fig. 8.4).

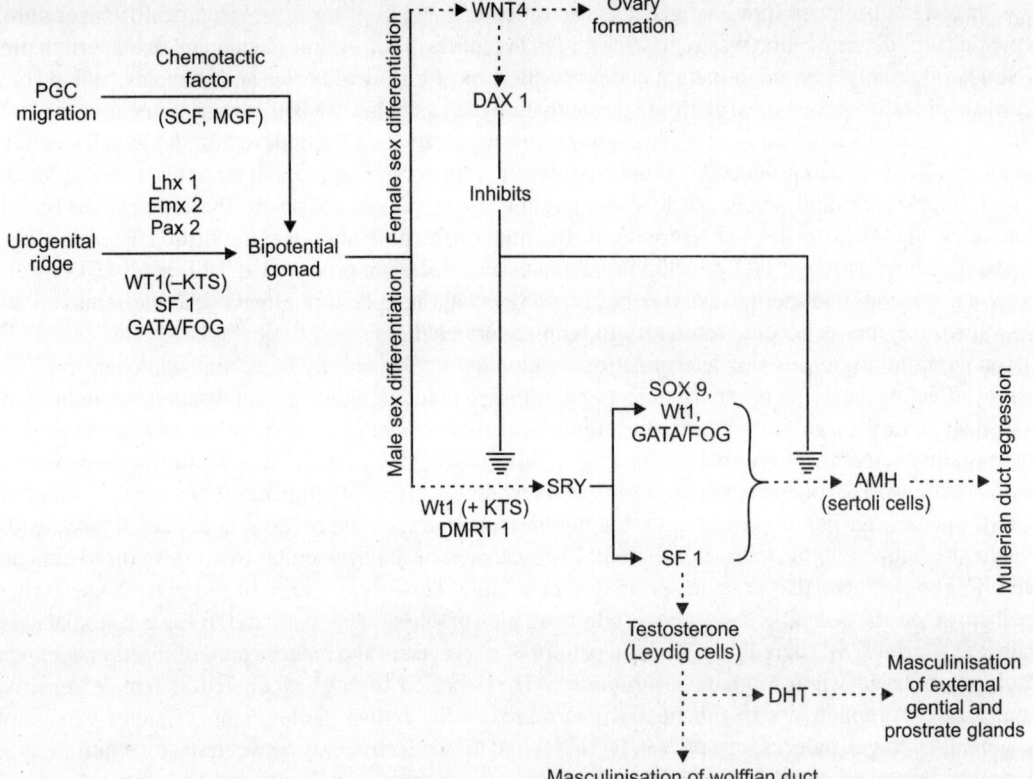

Fig. 8.4: Schematic representation of chromosomal sex determination and differentiation in mammalian model.

SRY (SEX DETERMINING REGION ON Y CHROMOSOME)

SRY gene is located near the tip of the short arm of Y chromosome that encodes a transcription factor of 204 amino acids. The central 79 amino acids encode the HMG (high mobility group) box. In the entire SRY protein, only HMG domain shows sequence conservation. HMG box functions as DNA6 binding, and DNA-bending domain and also has two nuclear localisation signals essential for translocation of protein into the nucleus. However, the non conserved regions outside the HMG box are also essential for SRY function, since a truncated SRY protein lacking the carboxy end is unable to induce male development in XX transgenic mice. As an architectural transcription factor, SRY unwinds the DNA and bends it to almost 80 degree thereby, bringing the other distantly bound transcription factors in close contact. The exact binding site of SRY on the DNA and the mechanism through which SRY acts is still not resolved. Nevertheless, the ultimate function of SRY is the up regulation of SOX 9. It is interesting to note that SRY is absent in monotremes (egg laying mammals: platypus and echidna) and in non-mammalian vertebrates.

SOX 9 (SRY-RELATED HIGH-MOBILITY GROUP BOX 9)

SOX 9 present on chromosome 17 in human is a highly conserved autosomal gene responsible for testicular differentiation. Like SRY, SOX 9 encodes a transcription factor that also contains a HMG box and a transactivation domain in the C-terminus. SOX 9 was discovered in an investigation of campomelic dysplasia (CD), a disease involving bone and cartilage disorder. XY patients with this disease developed as phenotypic females. Mutational analysis revealed that absence of SOX 9 is responsible for CD as well as XY sex reversal. In mouse, at 10.5 days post conception (dpc), just before or around the same time as Sry transcripts are first detected, Sox 9 is expressed at low levels in the developing gonads of both sexes. By 11.5 dpc, Sox 9 is robustly expressed in the XY gonads and is completely absent from XX gonads. Although its expression is up regulated by Sry expression, Sox 9 remains active in embryonic testis long after Sry expression has ceased. SOX 9 along with other transcription factors activate the expression of Amh gene (anti Müllerian hormone gene). The binding of SOX 9 HMG box bends the DNA which bring SF1 and GATA 4 in close proximity to each other and along with WT1 and HSP 70 form a tightly associated protein complex that activates transcription of the Amh gene. The complete absence of AMH transcripts is seen in XY mice mutant for HMG box (DNA binding domain) of Sox 9 gene suggesting that Sox 9 is required for AMH expression. Although experimental evidences in non mammalian vertebrates show that Sox 9 has a conserved role in sex determination, it is important to mention here that its expression in alligator and chicken begins well after pre Sertoli cell differentiation and AMH expression. It seems that Sox 9, in non mammalian vertebrates may be involved in Sertoli cell organisation, rather than early testicular determination.

SF1 (STEROIDOGENIC FACTOR 1)

SF1 gene transcribes a protein, otherwise known as Ad4BP, belonging to the orphan nuclear receptor family. Initially, SF1 was described to regulate the production of cytochrome P-450 steroid hydroxylase enzymes that are necessary for synthesis of steroids, and thus, are expressed in many steroidogenic tissues, including adrenal gland, ovary and Leydig cells of the testis. Subsequently, SF1 transcripts were detected in the mouse urogenital ridge even at the stage of the indifferent gonad (9–12 dpc) and mutation in Sf1 gene was shown to cause complete dysgenesis of gonad in both sexes. This suggests its role in early formation of the indifferent gonad and, thereby, Sf1 is placed upstream of Sry in sex determination pathway. However, Sf1 also plays an important role in the downstream testicular differentiation pathway initiated by Sry. Sf1 activates testicular differentiation by influencing both, Leydig and Sertoli cells. SF1 in Leydig cells regulates steroid biosynthesis and in Sertoli cells it binds to Amh promoter region and activates the expression of AMH in collaboration with other transcriptional factors. The importance of SF1, located on chromosome 9, for testis development and AMH regulation in humans is demonstrated by XY patient heterozygous for SF1 where the individual has malformed fibrous gonads and retains fully developed Müllerian duct structures.

WT1 (WILMS' TUMOUR 1)

The WT1 gene first came into focus in patients with Wilms's tumor where mutation of this gene led to embryonic kidney tumour. Later, mutation in this gene was seen associated with the disruption of bipotential gonadal development. The presence of WT1 transcripts in developing gonads substantiates its role in early bipotential gonadogenesis. WT1 encodes variant transcripts by alternative splicing, alternative translation start sites, and RNA editing. These variants give rise to different zinc finger DNA-binding protein isoforms that fall under two categories (designated as +KTS and – KTS) depending on the presence or absence of three amino acids (KTS, lysine-threonine-serine) between two zinc fingers. Experimental evidences in mice show that the –KTS isoform is responsible for development of undifferentiated gonad. WT1 +KTS isoform plays an important role in testicular differentiation possibly by regulating Sry expression, since potential WT1 binding sites are present upstream of both mouse and human SRY. Further more, mutation in WT1 gene causes persistence of Müllerian duct in males. In recent years, WT1-KTS isoform is shown to physically interact with SF1 and synergistically up regulate AMH expression.

GATA4/FOG2

GATA4, a member of the GATA family of transcription factors, contain a zinc finger DNA-binding domain that binds to the consensus sequence WGATAR in the 5′-flanking region of target genes. In mice, it is detected as early as embryonic day 11.5 in the somatic cells of primitive gonads of both sexes and therefore, GATA4 in conjunction with other transcription factors play role in development of bipotential gonad. The GATA4 expression remains maintained in Sertoli cells throughout embryonic development, whereas it is down regulated shortly after differentiation of ovary on embryonic day 13.5 in mice. The presence of a conserved GATA4 sequence in the promoter site of Amh gene further substantiates its role in inducing masculinisation. Mutation of GATA4 in XY mice embryos lead to ovarian development, indicating its possible role in Sry transcription. During urogenital development, GATA4 is expressed with FOG 2 (friend of GATA) in the same somatic cells of gonad, implicating their close interaction in bipotential gonad development. Furthermore, mouse fetuses homozygous for a null allele of Fog2 exhibit abnormalities in male sex differentiation.

DMRT 1 (DOUBLE SEX-AND MAB-3 RELATED TRANSCRIPTION FACTOR)

DMRT 1 belongs to the family of genes that encode proteins containing DM-domain, a novel DNA-binding motif. It is one of the most conserved genes in sex determination, since its presence is observed across the phyla from invertebrate to vertebrate. DMRT 1 that maps to the distal arm of chromosome 9 in humans is homologous to the double sex (dsx) in Drosophila melanogaster and mab-3 in Caenorhabditis elegans which are involved in sex determination in their respective species. Although its expression coincides with Sry/Sox 9, maximum expression of DMRT 1 is seen in Sertoli cells during post natal testis development.

DAX 1 (DSS-AHC CRITICAL REGION ON X CHROMOSOME, 1)

DAX 1 maps on short arm of X chromosome and encodes for a protein that belongs to the orphan nuclear receptor family. Duplication of this gene causes male-female sex reversal (dosage-sensitive sex reversal, DSS), whereas its deletion results in adrenal hypoplasia congenita (AHC). DAX 1 is initially expressed in genital ridges of both sexes. Its expression persists in case of developing ovary while it is drastically down regulated with testis differentiation. DAX 1 suppresses testis differentiation at two levels: one, by inhibiting SF1-induced SRY expression in a bipotential gonad, and two, by repressing synergistic action of SF1 and WT1 and thereby, suppressing downstream genes, e.g. Amh and other steroidogenic genes. Thus, it is considered as ovary–determining gene.

WNT 4

WNT 4 is another important ovary determining gene. Like DAX 1, its expression is turned off with the differentiation of testis. WNT 4 knock out XX mice shows masculinisation as ovarian differentiation ceases and its cells express testis-specific markers, including Amh and testosterone producing enzymes. This suggests that WNT 4 is obligatory gene for female sex differentiation.

In marsupials too, the control of testis determination is vested in the Y chromosome, though it is the smallest of any mammals. However, the number of X chromosome plays a critical role in other aspects of sex differentiation (Table 8.1). Single X chromosome in XO animals leads to the development of empty scrotum (without testis), whereas scrotum fails to develop in XXY animals having testis. In fact, the presence of two X chromosomes leads to the development of pouch and mammary glands in lieu of the scrotum. Thus, marsupials are different from other mammals with regard to the accessory sex organ differentiation since the formation of scrotum, pouch and mammary glands in marsupials are dependent on genes present on X chromosomes rather than on gonadal hormones as in eutherian.

Table 8.1: X-linked secondary sexual differentiation in marsupials.

	Y chromosome (testis)	*Absence of Y chromosome (no testis)*
Single X chromosome (scrotum)	XY (Males with scrotum and testis)	XO (Males with empty scrotum)
Double X chromosome (pouch and mammary glands)	XXY (Males with testis, pouch and mammary gland)	XX (Females with pouch and mammary glands)

However, the monotremes are unusual because they have multiple set of sex chromosomes rather than the single pair usually found in marsupials and eutherians. Recent report demonstrates the presence of 10 sex chromosomes in platypus arranged as X1Y1X2Y2X3Y3X4Y4X5Y5. Interestingly, genes present on X chromosome situated at one end of the 'sex chromosome chain' are orthologous with those on the human-X chromosome, while genes on chromosome situated at the other end of the chain are homologous with those on the bird-Z chromosome. Hence, the platypus provides an important link between the chromosomal sex determination in mammals and birds.

Birds have distinguished sex chromosomes, except ratitae (e.g. ostrich, emu) which have karyologically indistinguishable or slightly differentiated sex chromosomes. The sex chromosomes have been designated as Z and W chromosome. Unlike mammals, males are homogametic (ZZ) while females are heterogametic (ZW). However, whether W chromosome carrying dominant female determining genes (ASW: avian sex specific W-linked, and FET1: female expressed transcript 1) or the Z chromosome carrying a dosage-dependent male determinant gene (Dmrt1), or both features determine the sex is not yet clear. Nevertheless, many of the downstream sex determining genes (Sox9, Amh, Dmrt1, Sf1, Wt1 and Dax 1) are reported in birds though the order of their expression in developing gonad may be different from that reported in mammals. Chromosomal sex determination is prevalent also in amphibians, though environmental and hormonal factors are reported to cause sex reversal. Although in most of the fishes and reptiles sex is determined by environmental factors, downstream sex determinant genes are reported. However, their interaction, temporal expression and the initial trigger does not follow any taxonomic scheme.

SEX DIFFERENTIATION

The sexually indifferent bipotential gonad develops from the ventromedial surface of the mesonephros near the kidneys at around 4 weeks in the human fetus and 9.5 days post-coitum (dpc) in the mouse. The somatic cells of gonad are derived from the mesonephros and coelomic epithelium that covers the coelomic surface of the gonadal ridge. These cells proliferate in the gonadal primordia and form the sex cords. Several factors such as Lhx1 (LIM Homeobox gene1), Emx2 (homolog of empty spiracles homeobox gene 2), Pax 2 (paired box gene 2), WT1and SF1 are involved in cell proliferation and development of the bipotential gonad. The gonad is subsequently colonised by primordial germ cells (PGC) that originate from epiblast-derived cells present in the yolk sac near the base of allantois and migrate through the hindgut to invade the indifferent gonad. Germ cell migration is under the influence of stem cell factor (SCF), mast cell growth factor (MGF), and extra cellular matrix proteins like fibronectin and laminin. During migration the germ cells proliferate but do not differentiate. The primordial germ cells are distinguishable from the other cell type because of their large size and large round nuclei. Histologically, they are identified by high alkaline phosphatase activity and glycogen. PGCs along with the somatic cells form the 'gonadal ridge'. The formation of gonadal ridge is completed within 5 to 6 week of gestation in human embryos. No sexual difference can be observed in the gonads until the 6th week of embryonic life in humans and 11.5 dpc in mice.

Male Sex Differentiation

In XY fetus of 6–7 weeks, the first sign of testis differentiation is seen with the aggregation of the pre Sertoli cell (derived from mesonephros) around the germ cell now called gonocytes, to form the testicular cords. These cords lose contact with the surface epithelium and become separated from it by a thick extra cellular matrix, the *tunica albuginea*. By the end of 9 week, the mesenchyme that separates the seminiferous cords gives rise to interstitial cells. Later these are differentiated into steroid secreting Leydig cells. Although differentiation of Leydig cells in the initial phase is independent of gonadotropin action, its proliferation and differentiation in the first and second trimesters of the fetal life depends on placental hCG, and thereafter, controlled by fetal pituitary LH.

The masculinisation of the genital tract starts with the regression of Müllerian duct under the influence of anti Müllerian hormone (AMH) secreted from Sertoli cells. Shortly after the Müllerian duct regression, the portion of Wolffian duct adjacent to testis is differentiated into epididymis, the central portion becomes vas deferens, and the distal end of the duct near the urogenital sinus develops into seminal vesicle. The prostrate gland develops as a series of outgrowths from the urogenital sinus. The virilisation of the Wolffian duct is under the control of testosterone as the phenomenon is seen inhibited after the administration of anti-androgen or testosterone antibody at the critical period of sex differentiation (Fig. 8.5).

Under the influence of androgen, the male external genitalia start differentiating around the 9th week of gestation in case of human. The genital tubercle elongates to form the phallus and scrotum, and the urethral folds fuse over the urethral groove. Although testosterone plays primary role in differentiation of Wolffian duct into epididymis, vas deferens and seminal vesicle, there is evidence that it is not the active masculinising hormone in certain tissues. It is dihydrotestosterone (DHT) that masculinises urogenital sinus and genital tubercle into prostrate and penis, respectively. The role of DHT came into light when

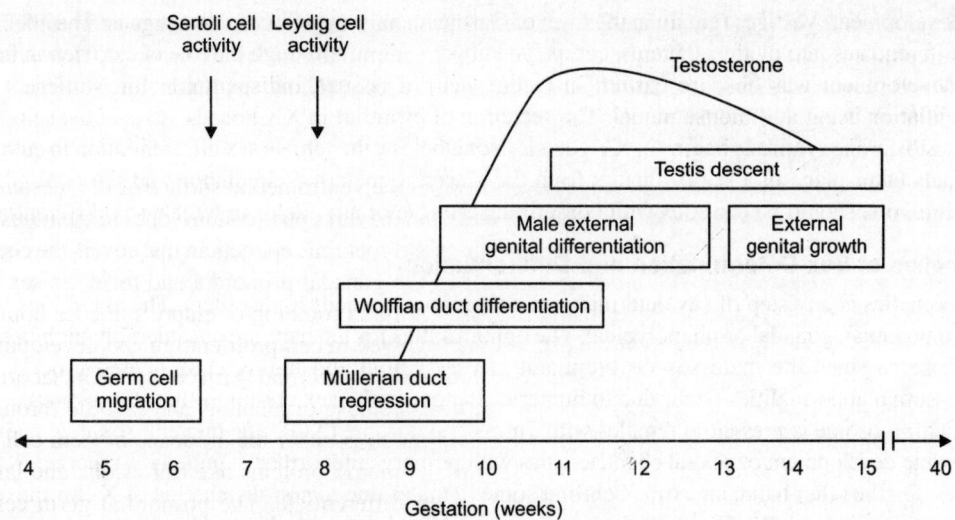

Fig. 8.5: Embryologic events in male sex differentiation depicted in temporal fashion. The line depicts the increase in fetal serum testosterone concentrations. The word activity refers indirectly to the action of AMH in causing Müllerian duct regression and androgens to induce male sex differentiation.

XY children lacking a functional gene for 5-reductase, the enzyme that converts testosterone to DHT, were reported to have a blind vaginal pouch and enlarged clitoris. However, they have male internal anatomy: developed testis, epididymis, vas deferens and seminal vesicle. Administration of 5-reductase inhibitor in rats is shown to severely affect the masculinisation of external genitalia.

Testicular descent

The factors controlling testicular descent has been the subject of much controversy. Previously, AMH was considered to be associated with testicular descent as decreased AMH level is usually seen in cryptorchid patients. Later, testicular dysgenesis was cited as the cause of cryptorchidism. Recently, Insulin like factor 3 (INSL3) secreted by fetal Leydig cells and belonging to the insulin/relaxin super family has been shown to be involved in the gubernaculums development in INSL3 mutant mice. Mutation of this gene has been detected in cryptorchid patients. Moreover, androgens mediate the disappearance of the cranial suspensory ligament and are required for the inguinoscrotal phase of testicular descent.

Female Sex Differentiation

In females, the primary sex cords undergo degeneration and a new set of sex cords is then produced by the epithelium. These sex cords reside in the periphery and hence, are called cortical sex cords. The primordial germ cells proliferate by mitosis and give rise to oogonia that enter into meiosis by 10th week in human fetus and form the oocyte. The cortical cords surround the oocytes and form granulosa layer. The formation of primordial follicle, oocyte surrounded by a single layer of flattened granulosa cells, commences around 16th week of gestation. This is the pool from where Graffian follicles are formed (primordial-primary-secondary-tertiary/Graffian) by week 23–24 in human fetus. Oocytes proceed to the diplotene stage and remain arrested till the time of puberty. Female differentiation of the internal genital tract is characterised by the regression of the Wolffian duct that disappears at 90 days of human fetal development. Vestiges remain in the form of Gartner canals and Rosenmüller organs. The Müllerian duct differentiates into oviducts, uterus, cervix, and upper vagina. Although the role of estrogen in female fetal development was obscure earlier, in recent years it is seen indispensable for Müllerian duct differentiation using null mouse model. The secretion of estradiol in XX gonads starts at the same time when testosterone synthesis begins in XY gonads. Nonetheless, the female sex differentiation in eutherian mammals takes place in a sea of factors from the placenta, maternal circulation and the fetal gonads. Therefore, one should be cautious while describing the role of any factor in female sex differentiation.

Anomalies of Sex Determination and Differentiation

The anomalies at any step of sex determination/differentiation leads to disorders. The alterations might be chromosomal, gonadal or phenotypical. The opportunities for mishaps are considerably high in males than females since the male sex development is very active and highly complicated process. The chromosomal abnormalities occur due to numeric changes in the sex chromosomes. For example, only one X chromosome is present in females with Turner's syndrome (XO). The bilateral streak gonads and incomplete development of sexual characteristics with primary amenorrhea at puberty is reported in these females. On the other hand, an extra X chromosome in males due to non-disjunction of X chromosomes during oogenesis leads to Klinefelter's syndrome (XXY). Males with this syndrome have small testis, azoospermia resulting in infertility, low concentrations of testosterone, high levels of gonadotropins and poor virilisation. Similarly, triple X (XXX) syndrome is reported in females.

In case of gonadal anomalies, genetically females (XX) generally have male external genitalia. This results either due to defects in sex determining genes on autosomes or linking of a testis determining gene, otherwise present on Y chromosome, with autosome. These females have either cryptorchid testis or atleast one ovo-testis. The gonadal dysgenesis is also true for 46 XY males with defects in Y chromosome or sex determining genes on autosomes. Phenotypical anomalies arise due to imbalance in hormone milieu or its responding machinery during development. In this case, the chromosomal sex and the gonadal sex match up, but the ambiguity in external phenotype results in pseudo-hermaphroditism. Female (XX) pseudo-hermaphroditism occurs as a result of excess androgens during embryo development.

The masculinisation of external genitalia is prevalent, though these females have normal ovaries. In case of XY males, pseudo-hermaphroditism might arise due to androgen insensitivity syndrome of embryo. They develop feminine characteristics due to lack of masculinisation.

To sum up, the basic pattern of gonadogenesis though remains similar, the factors determining sex of embryo vary considerably among vertebrates. Sex is primarily determined by either environmental factors or chromosomal mechanisms. In fishes, temperature is the most important factor in sex determination. Generally, high temperature favours male to female sex ratio in thermosensitive fishes. The temperature-dependent sex determination is also prevalent in living reptiles except ophidians (snakes) where distinct sex chromosomes are present (ZZ/ZW). Intriguingly, sex in amphibians is primarily determined by chromosomal mechanism with heterogamety in male (XY/XX) as well as female (ZW/ZZ) depending on species, though sex reversal is reported at unusually high temperatures.

Nonetheless, in these thermosensitive amphibians, sex at the ambient temperature is predominantly determined by sex chromosomes. The genetic mechanism by which sex is determined in birds remains to be elucidated. Further, Z and W chromosomes do not share homology with the mammalian X and Y chromosome. Possibly, gene linked to W chromosome determines the ovarian differentiation or Z-linked gene (dosage-sensitive) play a critical role in establishing the male sex. Unlike birds, males are heterogametic (XY), while females are homogametic (XX) in mammals.

SRY and SOX 9 are the major testis determining genes. WT1 and DMRT1 upregulate the expression of SRY that in turn induces the downstream gene Sox 9. This gene located on human autosome 17 encodes a transcription factor that along with other factors, SF1 and WT1 activate the expression of AMH gene. AMH induces the regression of the Müllerian duct in males. In addition to promoting AMH production by Sertoli cells, SF1 also regulates the androgen biosynthesis in Leydig cells. Like males, female sex is determined by an active process rather than by default as believed earlier. DAX1 and WNT4 are now known to play a pivotal role. DAX1 represses the synergistic action of SF1 and WT1 on AMH expression and also downregulates the other steroidogenic genes. Like the importance of SRY for testis differentiation in males, WNT 4 is assigned as the ovary determining gene in females. Subsequent to formation of testis or ovary from the bipotential gonads, secondary sex determination commences in which hormones play a crucial role. The virilisation of Wollfian duct into epididymis, vas deferens and seminal vesicle takes place under the influence of testosterone. However, DHT, and not the testosterone, is responsible for the masculinisation of male external genitalia. Further, the testicular descent into the scrotal sacs is regulated by INSL3 and androgen. The knowledge on hormonal regulation of female sex differentiation is rudimentary, however, the indispensable role of estrogen is implicated in the stabilisation and differentiation of Müllerian duct into female genital tract. Unlike eutherians, the sex differentiation in marsupials is independent of hormonal control.

Chapter 9

Sex and Heredity

INTRODUCTION

Our gender on the one hand acts directly through the sex chromosomes and the genes encoded by them, on the other hand through the characteristics of gametogenesis and fertilisation it influences indirectly the appearance of our characteristics.

X-LINKED INHERITANCE

The fact that in humans females are homogametic and males are heterogametic makes the interpretation of both types of X-linked inheritance patterns difficult. Because women have two X chromosomes, they may be homo- or heterozygous for an X-linked trait/disease. Those women whose heterozygosity is proven by pedigree analysis and/or genotyping, are called obligate heterozygotes (conductors), while those who are only presumptive heterozygotes based on the family tree (i.e. they have no affected offspring, but have affected brothers) are called facultative heterozygotes.

In contrast, men have only one X chromosome therefore they are hemizygous, so they are either affected or carriers when the X chromosome is mutated, or healthy, if a normal (non-mutant) X chromosome is present. As for X-linked disorders 1/3 of the affected males are new mutation carriers! After all, the hemizygous males have reproductive disadvantage since the trait or disease is always manifested in them so the mutant gene is selected out from the population. In women, X chromosome inactivation further complicates the picture: depending on the X inactivation the phenotype can be quite varied - mild or severe - in heterozygotes.

X-linked Dominant (XD) Inheritance

In this case, the pedigree pattern is similar to the autosomal dominant, but the two sexes are affected differently.

The main features of this type of inheritance are:

1. Vertical family tree.
2. Twice as many women affected as men, 2 : 1 female : male ratio.
3. 50% of the offspring of an affected women - regardless of their sex – are sick.

4. All daughters of an affected man are affected while all sons are healthy (the father always gives his X chromosome to his daughters, the Y to his sons!).

5. Symptoms of the affected women are often milder and more variable than that of the affected men

While the symptoms of homozygous dominant $X^A X^A$ females are alleviated only by the X inactivation, whereas in heterozygous $X^A X^a$ women the product (protein) coded by the normal allele X^a can do the same it as well.

Traits/diseases determined by genes on the X chromosomal PAR1 region, e.g. the Xg blood group antigen and amelogenesis imperfecta (incomplete teeth enamel production) have such inheritance. In the latter one the enamel layer of the teeth is missing and such teeth grow carious more easily.

The most known X-linked dominant disorder is the hypophosphataemia (formerly called vitamin D resistant rickets, coded on the long arm of the X chromosome), which is characterised by growth retardation in childhood, rickets and low serum phosphate level. It is a treatable disease by large doses of vitamin D and phosphate! The fragile X syndrome, a trinucleotide (CGG) repeat mutation caused disease is also X-linked dominant. This is the most common cause of male mental retardations. While the normal repeat number is <30, this number is between 200 and 2000 in the affected individuals. Between about 50 and 200 repeats there is the so-called premutation or gray zone. The adult affected males are characterised with a long face, protruding ears, large jaws and large testes. In addition to mental retardation, behavioural problems and mood swings are part of the symptoms. The protein encoded by the FMR1 gene probably causes the symptoms by binding the mRNAs of other genes involved in the functions of the nervous system.

The assessment of the X-linked dominant pedigrees is complicated by the so-called X-linked male lethality. Since there is no normal allele the hemizygous, male embryos already die in utero. In this case, there are usually not as many offspring in the family to realise the 2:1 female : male sex ratio characteristic of such inheritance. Incontinentia pigment associated with hemizygous lethality is a disorder of pigmentation characterised by blistering of the skin in early childhood and with partial hair loss that manifests only in women. Rett syndrome, which is basically a neural developmental disorder, is also characterised by male lethality but moreover epigenetic phenomena are involved as well. In girls the typical progressive symptoms of loss of speech and acquired motor functions, the compulsive hand-wringing, ataxia and seizures are due to the mutation of the methyl-cytosine binding protein coding MECP2 gene.

X-linked Recessive (XR) Inheritance

To date, more than 400 traits with such inheritance pattern are identified. This value is much greater than that would be estimated on the basis of the number of human genes per chromosome and this fact is due to the easier detection and identification of such traits because of the specific male inheritance pattern derived from heterogametic sex. Amongst such traits/diseases there are relatively harmless, with mild symptoms such as red-green colour blindness, others with severe symptoms such as haemophilia, and lethal as Duchenne muscular dystrophy.

The characteristics of X-linked recessive inheritance are:

1. Zigzag or knight's move pattern: the disease is transferred from mother to son and from son to his daughter.

2. There are many more men affected than women.

3. Sick women are born to affected father and obligate heterozygote mother.

4. Affected man usually comes from healthy parents where the mother is obligate carrier.

5. There is no man-to-man transmission.

Although haemophilia is known for at least 4,000 years - as already mentioned in the Talmud that in families where one of the sons of the matrilineal relatives died due to bleeding out at circumcision as a result, their newborn sons were not circumcised - the first point mutation was described only in 1986. The X-linked recessive haemophilia has two forms: Haemophilia A, which is due to the failure of blood clotting (Fig. 9.1) factor VIII, and haemophilia B, which is due to the failure of blood clotting factor IX.

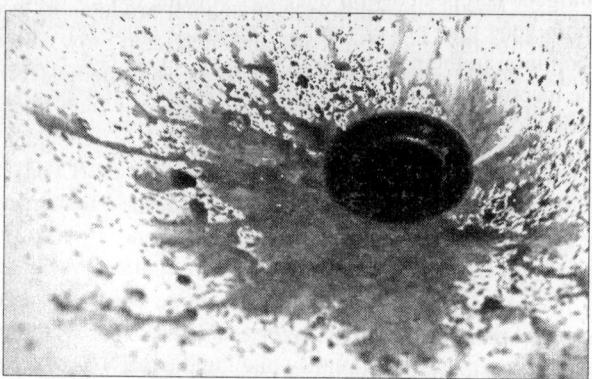

Fig. 9.1: Haemophilia blood clotting.

In 40% of haemophilia A cases a specific mutation of the factor VIII gene occurs. The intron 22 of the gene contains two small genes of unknown function, the F8A and F8B. About 400 kb away there are more copies of F8A of as well. Among these copies intrachromosomal crossing over takes place during meiosis, causing the inversion of the corresponding chromosome piece and thus factor VIII gene falls apart into two distant pieces. This is the cause of the lack of clotting factors and haemophilia. The most common mutation causing haemophilia occurs in the paternal germ line during meiosis. The large number of divisions and the concominant increased spontaneous mutation rate typical to paternal gametogenesis explain among other things that mutations occur with higher probability in the offspring of aged fathers. One of the best known and most studied cytoskeletal diseases is Duchenne muscular dystrophy. This X-linked recessive disease, which was described in the second half of the 19th century, begins with difficulties of standing up in the 2nd–3rd years of life - Gower's sign - and associated with increasing muscle weakness.

The boys around the age of 10 are wheelchair-bound then die around 20 years of age. Because the disease is relatively common (incidence of 1:3500), and to this day is incurable, it is clear that it is intensively investigated. Thus came to light that the cause of the disease is a gene mutation affecting a cytoskeletal protein called dystrophin. The dystrophin, a muscle cell specific protein whose C-terminal end is bound to the sarcolemma through a glycoprotein complex of six components and the N-terminus linked to the actin cytoskeleton. The dystrophin is the product of the largest currently known gene, which is 2400 kb in length, and thus its transcription takes more than 16 hr. The function of dystrophin in muscle is the cell membrane stabilisation. The mutation is often a frame-shift causing deletion, and thus the cell does not produce dystrophin, or a protein with completely altered structure and function is synthesised. If only an in-frame mutation occurs in the dystrophin gene, that is only a small part is deleted, then the so-called Becker muscular dystrophy with milder symptoms is formed. The Duchenne and Becker muscular dystrophies are due to different mutant alleles of the same gene, so they are examples of allelic heterogeneity as well. As many other mutations (for example, point mutations, and duplications) occur in the dystrophin gene, multiplex allelism is also typical for it.

Since the affected men generally do not reach reproductive age, they can not transmit their mutant gene to the offspring, so this sub-lethal mutant gene should gradually disappear from the population. However, the incidence of the disease is fairly constant; it is just possible as the rate of new mutations is high, that the mutant gene is repeatedly produced. According to new observations deletion mutations involving the dystrophin gene take place typically in the maternal germ line while the other types of mutations are rather common in the paternal germ line, but the reason has not been known yet.

The X chromosome inactivation further complicates the pedigree analysis also in X-linked recessive inheritance. The phenotype of heterozygous females varies depending on the ratio of healthy XA and mutant Xa bearing cells. If the gene product is a soluble protein, such as the clotting factors in haemophilia, the effect is 'averaged'. In other words, these women are asymptomatic but biochemically will be different from normal. However, where the product is localised to a given cell type, there the symptoms appear in a mosaic form. Such as the hypohydrotic ectodermal dysplasia, where the mutation causes the absence of sweat glands and the abnormal development or deficiency of dentition.

Y-linked (Holandric) Inheritance

Currently, only the male sex determining and the male gametogenesis related genes: the SRY and AZY Y-linked inheritance are proven. There are not known Y-specific and not male infertility related hereditary diseases. The only somatic characteristics transmitted from man to man, the hairy ear is not Y-linked, but the exact gene and its locus is not yet known.

The Y-linked inheritance features are:

1. Only males are affected.
2. The affected men's father is affected.
3. All the sons of affected men are affected.

SEX INFLUENCED INHERITANCE

In the case of some traits the gene is differently expressed in the two genders. It could be either the consequence of male lethality mentioned earlier in connection with X-linked inheritance or it could be due to the influence of other genes which means that the gene is expressed differently or not expressed at all, therefore the manifestation of the gene depends on the sex of the affected individual.

The best known such trait is baldness, which is autosomal dominant in men, so it is expressed both in homo- and heterozygotes. On the contrary it is autosomal recessive in women where it is expressed only in homozygotes with high testosterone level. One type of pubertas praecox (precocious puberty) having the same genetic background is manifested mainly men, too. In this disease the luteinising hormone receptor (LHR) is mutated, so it induces increased testosterone synthesis and those somatic changes characteristic for the premature puberty even in the absence of the ligand.

SEX LIMITED INHERITANCE

In the case of traits when the gene is strictly expressed only in one sex, the inheritance is sex limited. Milk production is a classic example of it, since there are mammary glands in both sexes, but milk secretion is characteristic only for females. The fact is long been recognised by cattle breeders that the milk yield depends on the bull, too! In fact, not only the amount of secreted milk, but the composition (e.g. its lipid content) is also dependent on the paternal genes. The development of pre-eclampsia, which takes more than 50000 women's lives a year, can be affected by paternal genes. In this case, the paternal genome half of the developing embryo affects the development of the placenta in a way, that it may cause a sudden increase of maternal blood pressure towards the end of the pregnancy.

CYTOPLASMIC INHERITANCE

Maternal Genetic Effect

The role of sex is also proven for other specific forms of heredity. For example, in cytoplasmic inheritance with maternal genetic effect molecules (mRNAs, non-coding RNAs, or proteins) stored in the oocyte modify the development of the offspring by influencing the gene expression after fertilisation. Thus, the expression of genes in the offspring can be different without mutation had occurred in the genome, so this kind of inheritance is a consequence of epigenetic changes. For *Drosophila* and other lower ranked eukaryotes there are several evidences e.g. the formation of dextral or sinistral shells. Then during oocyte maturation factors coded by the dominant or the recessive maternal alleles, and produced by the nurse cells, are passed to the egg and to the zygote and subsequently, i.e. during the early cleavage divisions can modify the orientation of the axis of mitotic spindle leading to dextral or sinistral shell formation. Likewise, there are transgenic mouse model examples for the manifestation of traits not coded in the genome of the offspring but induced by paternal sperm RNAs. However, the role of this type of cytoplasmic inheritance in humans has yet to be verified.

Mitochondrial Inheritance

The role sex is undisputed in the inheritance of mitochondria since in this case cell organelles found in the oocyte cytoplasm are exclusively transmitted by the mother to the offspring. During fertilisation the sperm neck – the midpiece - cannot get to the egg, so the zygote, and later the developing organism contain only maternal mitochondria. This means that the mother transmits her mitochondria to all of her offspring - sons and daughters alike, but in the next generation her daughters, not sons can pass them further. This maternal inheritance does not follow the Mendelian rules, so it can be considered as one type of non-Mendelian inheritance as well.

Many diseases are due to mutations in mitochondrial DNA. There are 59 known mitochondrial disorders, but fortunately all of them are rare. Since the main function of the mitochondria is the oxidative phosphorylation, therefore mitochondrial diseases mainly affect organs with the highest energy need (muscles, nervous system). One of the most well-known mitochondrial diseases (Fig. 9.2) is Leber's optic neuropathy due to a point mutation, and which is usually characterised by adolescent or young adult-onset central vision loss. It must be mentioned here that there are mitochondrial diseases caused by nuclear DNA mutations, since the vast majority of mitochondrial proteins are coded in the nucleus!

They show Mendelian inheritance, such as the autosomal dominant progressive external ophtalmoplegia (external eye muscle paralysis) coded by the long arm of chromosome 10.

In the case of mitochondrial diseases two types of mutations - point mutations and deletions - are known to occur. The severity of the symptoms depends on the type of mutation, the number of mutant mitochondria and naturally the tissue type. The majority of mitochondrial mutations do not take place in the germ line, they are generally somatic but, in addition, the amount of the mutant mitochondria may

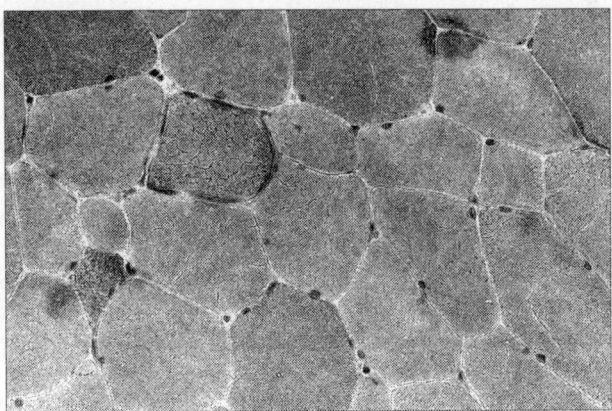

Fig. 9.2: Mitochondrial diseases

vary from cell to cell during successive cell divisions even within a tissue. Therefore the cytoplasm of the cells will be different. When the cell cytoplasm contains the same normal or the same mutant mitochondria homoplasmy, when two types of mutant or both normal and mutant mitochondria are found simultaneously heteroplasmy is present. Understandably the severity of symptoms can be variable. In the offspring of heteroplasmic mothers the severity of symptoms may be different depending on how many mutated mitochondria were passed to the egg.

The analysis of mitochondrial DNA and homo-and heteroplasmy was used recently for the identification of the remains of the Russian royal family executed in 1918. Since mitochondria are maternally inherited, so the living matrilineal relatives of the imperial family and their descendants were tested and compared to the mitochondrial DNA extracted from the remains. Not only the identification of the remains was successful, but it has also been shown that Tsar Nicholas II was heteroplasmic. Also, mitochondrial DNA testing can help to decide an old debate in human evolution: does the ancestors of modern man (Homo sapiens) and Neanderthal populations interbreed.

Comparative analysis of mitochondrial mutations is often used in population genetics for the detection of ethnic origin, ancestry and relationships of certain populations. It turned out that American Indians have mutant, deleted mitochondria, so if someone has such deletion, he or she must have at least one Indian female ancestor. Similarly, mitochondrial DNA analysis has shown that the Hungarians and Finns are genetically not, only through their language related!

X CHROMOSOME INACTIVATION

In somatic cells, the paternal and the maternal copy of all autosomal genes are expressed. So these are present in a double dose. The only exceptions are the so called imprinted genes. However, the expression of genes encoded by the X sex chromosome is influenced whether the X chromosome is of the male or the female, and the fact that the X and Y chromosomes are not homologous except the genes of PAR. Thus the X chromosomal genes in females can be transcribed in twice as large doses than in men. This is prevented by a phenomenon called dose compensation. Due to the X chromosome inactivation, described in the fourth chapter, there is functional mosaicism in women. The best known examples are the calico (or tortoiseshell) cats. Only the female cats are black and red mottled. The size and distribution of patches depends on where and in how many cells the black or red colour coding X chromosomes are inactive. While somatic cells are characterised by random X inactivation, the extra-embryonic membranes (placenta) have imprinted parental origin dependent X chromosome inactivàtion. The placenta always has the paternal X in inactive form. The inactive X chromosome can be detected in interphase. Adhering to the nuclear membrane, a heavily stained sex chromatin, the so-called Barr body is seen in the epithelial cell nuclei A drumstick-shaped appendix of the segmented nucleus of neutrophils is a particular manifestation of the inactive X, so the Barr body. The rapid detection and microscopic examination of Barr bodies are simple, in the past it was used for quick sex determination in connection with sports competitions. Initially, it was thought that the whole X chromosome is inactive, but we now know that the PAR regions are never inactivated! Moreover, non-inactivated X chromosomal genes outside the PAR were also found, a part of them has a functional therefore transcribed homologue in the Y chromosome, while the other part has only non-functional pseudogene on Y (such as the steroid sulphatase (STS) gene and the anosmin gene responsible for Kallman syndrome).

In other species, where heteromorphic sex chromosomes also occur other mechanisms exist for dose compensation. The X chromosome in male *Drosophila* is twice as active, than in females. A 1:1 ratio instead of 2:2 is formed this way. It is also possible that both female X-s are only half as active as the male one, thus ½ + ½ : 1 = 1:1 is the final ratio.

An interesting possibility of the X chromosome inactivation is the so-called skewed X inactivation. This means that in certain tissues always one – let's say - always the paternal X chromosome is inactivated. This may have far-reaching consequences. It is attempted to explain by this the higher frequency of certain autoimmune diseases (e.g. SLE) observed in females. In the thymus maturing T lymphocytes can only tolerate those antigens which are encoded by the active X-chromosome, and not the antigens coded by the other, the inactive one. Thus, all the cells/tissues where the other X chromosome is active are considered non-self, and immune response is generated against them, resulting in autoimmune disease symptoms. Of course, this cannot be the sole cause of autoimmune diseases, since it cannot be explained by this why the disease manifests in different ages.

EPIGENETICS

In recent years, epigenetics has become one of the fastest growing areas of genetics. In this subject - according to PubMed database - last year only, over 10000 scientific papers have been published. The term epigenetics is connected to Conrad Waddington, who in the early 50s when studying the processes of ontogeny talked about a so-called epigenetic landscape when he tried to explain how an extraordinary variety of cells can develop from a single cell, the zygote. Although they are the same genetically, but morphologically, functionally different, due to what point of the scenery they reach (mountain, valley or slope), so how the gene could be regulated during development. Today, those mitotically and/or meiotically transmissible processes are called epigenetic phenomena that alter the function, so the expression of each gene, without affecting the DNA sequence itself, that the changes in gene expression are not due to mutations. The range of these phenomena and the known enzymes and regulatory proteins involved in these processes is expanding, and epigenetic changes related to almost all aspects of life have been reported. Parallel with the increasing knowledge of epigenetic processes, many previously unexplained observations, phenomena became understandable.

EPIGENETIC CHANGES - MOLECULAR MODIFICATIONS

In the toolbar of epigenetics it has an essential role to alter the building blocks - DNA and histones - of chromatin. The resulting epigenetically modified DNA, and the variously modified histones attached depending on the modifications also attract different non-histone proteins thus chromatin is fundamentally affected and remodelled. The chromatin has two functional stages: heterochromatin, representing a closed, nontranscribed state and euchromatin which is a loose, open structure accessible to components involved in transcription. Epigenetic modifications make a further, more refined control possible.

DNA Methylation

The epigenetic modification of DNA is methylation of cytosine when 5-methyl-cytosine (5MeC) is created. In this case methylated cytosines are almost exclusively located in so-called CpG dinucleotides. CpG dinucleotides are covalently linked cytosine and guanine bases in one of the DNA strands. Methylated cytosine pair guanine as the unmethylated and therefore the information coded by the DNA remains unchanged. However, the methyl group of the 5MeC facing the major groove of DNA, and therefore it is accessible to the different DNA-binding proteins. CpG dinucleotides are found mainly in the promoter region of the genes, but depending on the gene, 'inside' the gene in the exons and introns can also be found. Not all CpGs are methylated it also depends on the cell type, its metabolic condition how these CpG dinucleotides are methylated, i.e. what is the methylation pattern. The methylation of CpGs of promoter provides a basic regulation of gene expression: the methylation usually (but there are exceptions) leads to inhibition of gene expression. Since epigenetic marks are transmitted from cell division to cell division but from generation to generation are usually not, this means that the DNA methylating enzyme system is specialised accordingly. There are two main methylating enzymes known: the maintenance DNA methyltransferase (DNMT1) and *de novo* DNA methyltransferase (DNMT3). During DNA replication DNMT1 methylates cytosines of the CpGs in the new complementary DNA strand - in accordance with the old strand, thereby maintaining the original pattern of DNA methylation. The DNMT3 can methylate cytosines which had not previously been methylated. This is important in gametogenesis when the original pattern inherited from the parents erased and a new methylation pattern - appropriate for the sex of the organism - is built up. DNA demethylases are involved in the removal of methylation patterns.

CpG as Mutation Hot Spot

Cytosine spontaneously deaminates to uracil. This instability can also apply to methylated cytosine but in this case not uracil but thymine will be the result. Thus from a CpG dinucleotide a TpG dinucleotide is formed, and it has been a change in the DNA sequence, i.e. a mutation. Analysis of mutational databases revealed that for a number of diseases CpG dinucleotides are mutational hot spots.

The chemical lability of cytosine, i.e. its mutability is shown by the fact that, although methylation is a general feature of DNA the frequency of methylated cytosines is much lower than expected. In humans, only 3% of cytosines are methylated. It seems that in a longer evolutionary interval CpG frequency slowly but gradually decreases due to the constant CpG → TpG transformation. Despite the small CpG frequency in vertebrate genomes, there are short non-methylated DNA sequences, which CpG value correspond to the expected frequency. These so called CpG islands are CG rich and often found in several hundred nucleotides long stretches at the 5′ end of the genes. Scattered in the human genome around 27–30 thousand CpG islands are found. For these areas, the CpG → TpG transformation is not typical. The CpG stability is either due to that there can be no methylation, or that these islands are functionally so important that natural selection prevents their loss. There are CpG islands in the promoter of approximately 50% of the human genes, which are generally unmethylated. Their abnormal methylation is pathological and can lead to the formation of tumours by changing the regulation of gene expression.

Histone Modifications

In addition to DNA methylation the role of histone modifications is also essential for epigenetic processes. Histones are evolutionarily highly conserved, DNA binding, basic - lysine and arginine rich - proteins. The H2A, H2B, H3 and H4 histones in 2-2 copies are involved in the nucleosomal octamer structure, while the H1 histones bind to the so-called linker DNA connecting the nucleosomes to each other. The N-terminal tail of the nucleosomal histones protrudes, and this is the area where histone modifications occur. The main targets of histone modifications are primarily the lysine residues with suitable positions in histone H3 and H4 tails which can be methylated, acetylated, phosphorylated, and ubiquitinilated etc. These modifications form a histone pattern, depending on the cell type, its state of development and physiological function and of the gene or gene sequence in question. This pattern is the so called histone code, which fundamentally affect the expression of the area concerned. Both methylated DNA and modified histones attract several methylated DNA - or histone-binding proteins and non-coding RNAs as well and the interacting members of the complex formed determine the epigenetic pattern characteristic for developmental stages, cells and genes. Any mutation in any element of this complex can lead to abnormal epigenetic signals and thus malfunction or disorder. An example of this is the Rett syndrome, where mutation of the MECP2 (methylated cytosine binding protein) gene is in the background.

NON-CODING RNAs

Following the success of the human genome project it has become apparent that only <2% of the human genome is protein-coding so rightly ask the question: what is the function of the others?

Today we know that an important part the genome is to determine the smaller or longer regulatory RNAs. These RNAs through RNA-RNA, RNA-DNA, RNA-protein interactions can modify the expression of genes, without modifying their DNA sequence. Such RNAs can affect transcription by inhibiting it, e.g. Xist RNA (see below), but may act post-transcriptionally, e.g. microRNAs, which inhibit translation of mRNA. The non-coding RNA can be derived either from the same chromosome where the gene is regulated (*cis*-action) or from another chromosome (*trans*-action).

EPIGENETIC PHENOMENA

The most important epigenetic events are: Genomic imprinting and X chromosome inactivation. Furthermore, carcinogenesis, aging, some psychiatric disorders, and even conduct disorders can be associated with epigenetic processes. Some observations indicate that these changes - not altering DNA sequences, but affecting its function - can be transmitted not only somatically so from mitosis to mitosis, but instead through meiosis during gametogenesis to gametes, and thus after the fertilisation they will be typical of the progeny as well so there are signs of the so called transgenerational epigenesis.

X Chromosome Inactivation

Mammalians are diploid organisms and consequently both alleles of an autosomal locus responsible for a particular trait are functioning, i.e. biallelic gene expression is characteristic for them. If one of the autosomes is eliminated due to chromosome mutations so only one allele remains at a single locus, this generally results in severe or lethal symptoms. In contrast, the sex chromosomes form homologous pairs (XX) only in females, whereas in males the Y chromosome is not a functional homolog of the X chromosome. While the Y chromosome contains only a few genes mainly responsible for sex determination (SRY) and gametogenesis (e.g. AZF), the X chromosome has genes determining a large number of somatic traits. If genes coded by the single X chromosome of males are sufficient for the normal development and normal physiological processes of the individual, it is obvious that one X chromosome has to be enough for the female body. This means that evolutionarily became necessary to equalise the different X chromosomal gene doses of the two sexes, so to compensate the dose differences.

This dose compensation is also called Lyonisation after Mary Lyon, the scientist who described this phenomenon. In mammals, including humans, the dose compensation in females is achieved through the inactivation of one of the X chromosomes. However, it should be emphasised that other mechanisms also exist for dose compensation in other organisms with heteromorphic sex chromosomes. X chromosome inactivation takes place at the beginning of mammalian embryonic development, in the blastocyst stage. As a first step of dose compensation chromosome counting is carried out by a mechanism not yet fully understood in details. This means that the cell acquires the information about the quantity of X chromosomes. Where two or more X chromosomes are in the cell, only one is active and the other (or others) is (are) inactivated. This inactivation is random, i.e. either the maternal or the paternal X is inactivated. However, once the selected X is inactivated, the given status of the cell is maintained lifelong in each of its descendant daughter cells.

Due to the random X inactivation in females there are cells in which the maternal, and there are in which the paternal X chromosome becomes inactive. Thus a so-called functional mosaicism is typical for women. The inactive X chromosome is intact, most of its genes are not expressed, except the genes of the pseudoautosomal regions found near to the telomere of both arms of the X chromosome (PAR1 and PAR2 regions) and the few genes that escape X inactivation. These remain active on the inactive X chromosome. To find out why these genes remained and how, is the subject of intensive research today. Although the inactivation in somatic cells is passed from daughter cells to their progeny cells, it does not mean that it is the case in germ cells, too. During oogenesis the inactivated X chromosome is reactivated, and it remains active in the mature gamete.

In X inactivation the so-called XIC = X inactivation center plays a crucial role. Here, in the Xq13 region the XIST gene is found that is transcribed only from the inactive X chromosome. The product is a large non-coding RNA which is covering the would-be inactive X by a not yet fully known mechanism. The XIST expression is followed by several other epigenetic events such as DNA methylation, histone methylation, a change in the histone composition as shown by the macroH2A histone variant, increased chromosome condensation, and ultimately late DNA replication will be characteristic to the inactive X chromosome, i.e. the DNA of the inactive X chromosome starts replication after the replication of the other chromosomes' DNA. The increased chromosome condensation leads to heterochromatinisation, and then the transcription is inhibited, thus the chromosome becomes inactive.

Genomic Imprinting

Based on the classical genetic experiments, it appeared that it does not matter even in heterozygosity which allele comes from which parent. Since both alleles are expressed, the origin is not important. However, some animal studies or rare human diseases, suggested that it is at least not true for each gene. During mouse embryo manipulations it was found that when the nucleus of a mouse oocyte was injected into another oocyte of the same mouse, then diploid cell created, a gynogenote just started the embryonic development, but soon died because the fetal membranes were not formed. When the experiment was repeated in a way that an enucleated oocyte got two sperm nuclei, although the embryonic development was also not normal, it was different from the former phenomenon. There was no embryo in such androgenote only hyperproliferated fetal membranes. In other words, on the basis of mouse experiments it is concluded that maternal and paternal halves of the genome are not functionally equivalent. Rare human diseases such as complete hydatidiform mole also suggest this. In this case only paternal chromosomes are found in the otherwise diploid sample. That is because an empty egg is fertilised by either two sperms or by a diploid one, which is also supported by the fact that the sample proved to be homozygous for all loci by further tests. The reverse of this was found when teratocarcinomas were analysed the abnormal tissue had only maternal chromosomes. On the basis of these initial observations it is considered that each chromosome carries a marker which refers to the parental origin. This signal is fixed at some point during gametogenesis, which somehow imprinted in the genetic material. The parental origin specific marking of the genome is called genomic imprinting.

To identify the mechanism of imprinting further attempts were made. When the mouse experiments were repeated in a way that only one pair of chromosomes or a distal or a proximal part of the chromosome was purely of paternal or maternal origin, it is found that not the total genome, but only certain chromosome segments, certain genes carry markers of parental origin. Such a phenomenon is the uniparental disomy (UPD), where after rare chromosome segregation anomalies, regarding the chromosome number, normal diploid organisms are created with both homologues of certain chromosomes/chromosome segments derived from the same parent, and who have severe symptoms, depending on the chromosomes involved. From the point of DNA base sequence it is irrelevant, which comes from which parent, therefore the labelling should be epigenetic. If a father transmits an imprinted gene to his child, which he inherited from his mother, then the gene carries maternal imprinting in the father, but the kid will inherit paternal imprinting of this gene. This means that imprinting is reversible.

That is similar to X inactivation, where an epigenetic mark or pattern resulting in imprinting is inherited without further changes in somatic cells, but in germ cells the original inherited pattern is erased, and in the individual - appropriate to the gender - a new female or male epigenetic pattern, imprint is built up.

To our knowledge, there are about 100 imprinted genes in humans, which generally play a role in ontogeny - especially around the implantation period – in growth and behaviour. These genes are not completely dispersed in the genome, but form groups, so-called differentially imprinted regions (clusters). In mice, chromosome 7, in humans 11 and 15 are particularly rich in imprinted chromosomal regions.

Imprinting related diseases

The research of the imprinting related diseases is still in its infancy, as many very finely tuned mechanisms may lead to the development of these. The best known disorders due to imprinting are Prader-Willi and Angelman syndromes, where the 15q11-q13 region is affected. While in Prader-Willi syndrome the maternal UPD or paternal deletion of the above mentioned region is the cause of the disease, Angelman syndrome may be caused by maternal deletion or paternal UPD of this region or by mutation of the UBE3A (ubiquitin ligase) also located in this region. Moreover, in both cases, mutations of the center responsible for imprinting (IC) occur. Prader-Willi syndrome is characterised by obesity, small hands and feet, underdeveloped genitalia, mild mental retardation. Symptoms observed in Angelman syndrome are quite different. Developmental retardation, compulsive movements, laughter (that is why the disease was formerly called happy puppet syndrome), poor speech ability or complete inability of the speech are the characteristic features. More known rare diseases related to imprinting:

1. Beckwith-Wiedemann syndrome: In which two differentially imprinted regions (clusters) can be found in the 11p15.5 region with the H19, IGF2 and the KCNQ10T genes. The former cluster is associated with childhood kidney tumour disorders (Wilms' tumour, Beckwith-Wiedemann syndrome). During tumour formation loss of heterozygosity occurs in renal tissue, but then almost always (over 90%) the maternal allele is lost.

2. Silver-Russell syndrome (7p11.2 or 11p15.5).
3. The pseudo-hypoparathyroidism (20q13.2).
4. Transient neonatal *diabetes mellitus* (6q24).

Evolutionary causes of imprinting

There are several theories to explain the evolutionary origin of imprinting. One of the most well-known is the so-called conflict of parental interests theory. Thus, fathers will be able to spread their genes best when there is a lot of offspring. If, the maternal body is exhausted due to the numerous births, or the mother dies, the father can produce more offspring with another partner, and further transmits his genes. In contrast, the mothers interests are to save resources, i.e. that not one child will use all maternal resources they also can survive additional reproductive cycles and eventually successfully transmit their genes. That is, the paternal genes stimulate - even at the expense of the mother - fetal growth, while the maternal ones restrict the fetal access to nutrient resources. This concept is well suited to the hydatidiform mole and the observations in the case of ovarian teratomas and by the fact that the IGF2 (insulin-like growth factor 2 = insulin-like growth factor 2) and its receptor (IGFR) genes are imprinted as well. The imprinting of these two genes is specific: paternal IGF2 gene is weakly, and the IGFR gene is highly methylated, while in the mother the opposite is observed. The significance of this is that the effects of the two parents equalised in this way more growth factor is in vain when the amount of the receptor is reduced. As the Prader-Willi and Angelman syndromes do not confirm the above theory, therefore, there should be other unknown reasons for imprinting. According to one of these new theories upright position and balance shift during pregnancy may have a role. The maternal imprinting restricts fetal growth and thus shifting the center of gravity during pregnancy, thus making the upright posture and walking more stable, which could be crucial and life-saving for early human ancestors.

SIGNIFICANCE OF EPIGENETIC EFFECTS

DNA methylation and subsequent changes in histone code and in chromatin structure are essential for gene regulation. We can assume that these mechanisms are crucial in establishing and maintaining cell and tissue identity. A good example was given by examining the tumour cells, where hypermethylation of the tumour suppressor genes and the consequent inhibition of their expression or hypomethylation of oncogenes and the increase of their activity were observed. Both changes may play an important role in oncogenesis. In addition to the carcinogenesis assisted reproductive technologies also highlighted the role of epigenetic changes. The accumulated data since the birth of Dolly, the first cloned mammalian suggest that the cloned mammals are not normal, e.g. often larger than the normally conceived animals, and their neonatal mortality is more frequent as well. Since the genetic material of the nucleus from adult organism used for cloning via nuclear transfer to the enucleated oocyte previously undergone a series of epigenetic changes to function normally these changes should be reversed after implantation. However, in this epigenetic reprogramming the oocyte cytoplasm is involved as well, it seems that under these artificial circumstances it does not work perfectly: the reprogramming is usually incomplete and imperfect. The importance of epigenetic reprogramming is shown by the higher frequency of Beckwith-Wiedemann syndrome of offspring conceived through IVF procedures. Although the frequency of 1:5000 is not too high, it's higher than the value observed in the naturally conceived offspring. Probably artificial conditions of IVF techniques are not favourable to epigenetic reprogramming. However, the epigenetic changes play a crucial role in adaptation to the environment. The importance of environment in epigenetics is proven by twin studies. The epigenetic similarity of identical twins, (e.g. their DNA methylation patterns and histone modifications) is very high, but it decreases as they are getting older, due to increasing epigenetic differences induced by their different environment, lifestyle and diet. A controversial theory based on epidemiological studies is the transgenerational epigenesis. Swedish studies have also associated the nutrient supply of the father and paternal grandparents in childhood and the proband's life-span or mortality due to diabetes or cardiovascular diseases. (Recent animal studies showed a correlation between the parental high-fat diet and the obesity and diabetes of the offspring). Others described a relationship between the age when fathers started smoking and body mass index (BMI) of their 9-year-old offspring. These observations are very difficult to explain at present, especially on the maternal side, where metabolic signals transferred via the placenta should be taken into consideration. However, on the father's side the sperm-mediated epigenetic transmission is easier to interpret.

From the point of view of transgenerational epigenetic processes the role and the delivery of modifications created by such environmental effects as diet and environmental pollutants (e.g. pesticides) to the offspring are particularly interesting and thought-provoking. Since folates play a key role in the synthesis of methyl donors required for DNA methylation, so it is understandable that the content of dietary folate has an epigenetic importance as well. It could be justified by a murine experiment later become famous. The wild-type mice' fur colour is the so-called agouti (a peculiar brownish-gray colour), besides there is an Avy (viable yellow) mutation causes a yellow coat colour. This allele is metastable, as it leads to yellow fur only in unmethylated state, in methylated state an unchanged agouti coat colour develops. In addition, in heterozygotes (uAvyA) the non-methylated mutant allele is dominant, whereas the methylated form is recessive concerning the wild-type allele. The uAvy unmethylated allele is dominant against the methylated mAvy allele, so the coat colour in the animals homozygous for of Avy is in function of the methylation of the alleles. In a conclusive experiment homozygote (AA) mothers were crossed with heterozygous (AvyA) fathers. During pregnancy in one group the maternal diet was rich in methyl donors, while the others got normal diet. In the first group the majority of heterozygous offspring was agouti-coloured or smaller and less yellow spots were seen on them (referring to the limited expression of the non-methylated mutant allele). A normal diet resulted in exactly the opposite effect, there were more completely yellow or large yellow spotted in the heterozygous offspring. In this case, the effect was observed in the of F2 generation as well, but not in later generations. This metastable mutation has other consequences e.g. the yellow furred animals are generally fat and have higher frequency of tumours, so it further confirms the relationship between epigenesis and oncogenesis.

In another series of experiments, pregnant mothers were treated with vinclozolin, an anti-androgen pesticide. Here methylation differences (25 different DNA sequences were tested) even in the F4 generation were observed. Then offspring of both sexes were affected by the maternal treatment, but these effects were transmitted further only patrilinearly. This suggests that transgenerational epigenetic effects can be gender and organ specific, and their consequences may occur later in adulthood. So they can cause some late-onset diseases of adulthood.

Based on the above and other similar experiments, and human data, it is now known that there are two ways of maternal transmission of epigenetic effects. One is the direct transgenerational epigenesis where (as in fathers) epigenetic changes (epimutations) effect on germ-line cells and the other is the epigenetic reprogramming of development (by maternal intrauterine or perinatal parental care behaviour). Although the nature of epigenetic changes and their transgenerational transmission is not yet known and understood in every detail, but we can say that they play an important role in the fine regulation of gene expression of both normal and abnormal developmental processes.

Chapter 10

Sex Determination Systems

INTRODUCTION

Sex determination was discovered in the mealworm by the American geneticist Nettie Stevens in 1903. A sex determination system is a biological system that determines the development of sexual characteristics in an organism. Most organisms that create their offspring using sexual reproduction have two sexes. Occasionally, there are hermaphrodites in place of one or both sexes. There are also some species that have only one sex due to parthenogenesis, the act of a female reproducing without fertilisation. In many species, sex determination is genetic: males and females have different alleles or even different genes that specify their sexual morphology. In animals this is often accompanied by chromosomal differences, generally through combinations of XY, ZW, XO, ZO chromosomes, or haplodiploidy. The sexual differentiation is generally triggered by a main gene (a 'sex locus'), with a multitude of other genes following in a domino effect.

In other cases, sex of a fetus is determined by environmental variables (such as temperature). The details of some sex determination systems are not yet fully understood. Hopes for future fetal biological system analysis include complete-reproduction-system initialised signals that can be measured during pregnancies to more accurately determine whether a determined sex of a fetus is male, or female. Such analysis of biological systems could also signal whether the fetus is hermaphrodite, which includes total or partial of both male and female reproduction organs. Some species such as various plants and fish do not have a fixed sex, and instead go through life cycles and change sex based on genetic cues during corresponding life stages of their type. This could be due to environmental factors such as seasons and temperature. Human fetus genitals can sometimes develop abnormalities during maternal pregnancies due to mutations in the fetuses sex-determinism system, resulting in the fetus becoming intersex.

CHROMOSOMAL SYSTEMS

XX/XY Sex Chromosomes

The XX/XY sex determination system is the most familiar, as it is found in humans. The XX/XY system is found in most other mammals, as well as some insects. In this system, most females have two of the same kind of sex chromosome (XX), while most males have two distinct sex chromosomes (XY). The X and Y sex chromosomes are different in shape and size from each other, unlike the rest of the chromosomes (autosomes), and are sometimes called allosomes. In some species, such as humans, organisms remain sex indifferent for a time after they are created, in others, however, such as fruit flies, *Drosophila* (Fig. 10.1) sexual differentiation occurs as soon as the egg is fertilised.

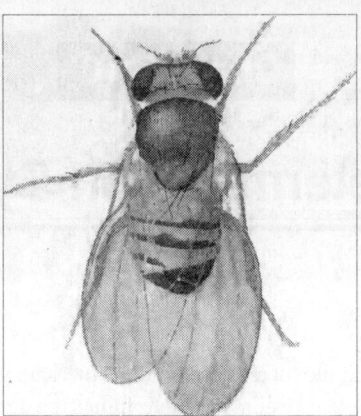

Fig. 10.1: *Drosophila.*

Y-centered sex determination

Some species (including humans) have a gene SRY on the Y chromosome that determines maleness. Members of SRY-reliant species can have uncommon XY chromosomal combinations such as XXY and still live. Human sex is determined by the presence or absence of a Y chromosome with a functional SRY gene. Once the SRY gene is activated, cells create testosterone and anti-müllerian hormone which typically ensures the development of a single, male reproductive system. In typical XX embryos, cells secrete estrogen, which drives the body toward the female pathway. In Y-centered sex determination, the SRY gene is the main gene in determining male characteristics, but multiple genes are required to develop testes. In XY mice, lack of the gene DAX1 on the X chromosome results in sterility, but in humans it causes adrenal hypoplasia congenita. However, when an extra DAX1 gene is placed on the X chromosome, the result is a female, despite the existence of SRY. Even when there are normal sex chromosomes in XX females, duplication or expression of SOX9 causes testes to develop. Gradual sex reversal in developed mice can also occur when the gene FOXL2 is removed from females. Even though the gene DMRT1 is used by birds as their sex locus, species who have XY chromosomes also rely upon DMRT1, contained on chromosome 9, for sexual differentiation at some point in their formation.

X-centered sex determination

Some species, such as fruit flies, use the presence of two X chromosomes to determine femaleness. Species that use the number of Xs to determine sex are nonviable with an extra X chromosome.

Other variants of XX/XY sex determination

Some fish have variants of the XY sex determination system, as well as the regular system. For example, while having an XY format, Xiphophorus nezahualcoyotl and X. milleri also have a second Y chromosome, known as Y', that creates XY' females and YY' males. At least one monotreme, the platypus, presents a particular sex determination scheme that in some ways resembles that of the ZW sex chromosomes of birds and lacks the SRY gene. The platypus has ten sex chromosomes, males have an XYXYXYXYXY pattern while females have ten X chromosomes. Although it is an XY system, the platypus' sex chromosomes share no homologues with eutherian sex chromosomes. Instead, homologues with eutherian sex chromosomes lie on the platypus chromosome 6, which means that the eutherian sex chromosomes were autosomes at the time that the monotremes diverged from the therian mammals (marsupials and eutherian mammals). However, homologues to the avian DMRT1 gene on platypus sex chromosomes X3 and X5 suggest that it is possible the sex-determining gene for the platypus is the same one that is involved in bird sex determination. More research must be conducted in order to determine the exact sex determining gene of the platypus. Heredity of sex chromosomes in X0 sex determination is shown in Fig. 10.2.

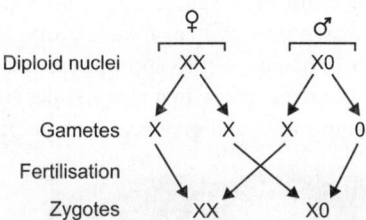

Fig. 10.2: Heredity of sex chromosomes in X0 sex determination.

XX/X0 sex chromosomes

In this variant of the XY system, females have two copies of the sex chromosome (XX) but males have only one (X0). The '0' denotes the absence of a second sex chromosome. Generally in this method, the sex is determined by amount of genes expressed across the two chromosomes. This system is observed in a number of insects, including the grasshoppers and crickets of order Orthoptera and in cockroaches (order Blattodea). A small number of mammals also lack a Y chromosome. These include the Amami spiny rat (Tokudaia osimensis) and the Tokunoshima spiny rat (Tokudaia tokunoshimensis) and Sorex araneus, a shrew species. Transcaucasian mole voles (Ellobius lutescens) also have a form of XO determination, in which both sexes lack a second sex chromosome. The mechanism of sex determination is not yet understood.

The nematode *C. elegans* is male with one sex chromosome (X0), with a pair of chromosomes (XX) it is a hermaphrodite. Its main sex gene is XOL, which encodes XOL-1 and also controls the expression of the genes TRA-2 and HER-1. These genes reduce male gene activation and increase it, respectively.

ZW sex chromosomes

The ZW sex determination system is found in birds, some reptiles, and some insects and other organisms. The ZW sex determination system is reversed compared to the XY system: females have two different kinds of chromosomes (ZW), and males have two of the same kind of chromosomes (ZZ). In the chicken, this was found to be dependent on the expression of DMRT1. In birds, the genes FET1 and ASW are found on the W chromosome for females, similar to how the Y chromosome contains SRY. However, not all species depend upon the W for their sex. For example, there are moths and butterflies that are ZW, but some have been found female with ZO, as well as female with ZZW. Also, while mammals deactivate one of their extra X chromosomes when female, it appears that in the case of Lepidoptera, the males produce double the normal amount of enzymes, due to having two Z's. Because the use of ZW sex determination is varied, it is still unknown how exactly most species determine their sex. However, reportedly, the silkworm Bombyx mori uses a single female-specific piRNA as the primary determiner of sex. Despite the similarities between the ZW and XY systems, these sex chromosomes evolved separately. In the case of the chicken, their Z chromosome is more similar to humans' autosome 9. The chicken's Z chromosome also seems to be related to the X chromosome of the platypus. When a ZW species, such as the Komodo dragon, reproduces parthenogenetically, usually only males are produced. This is due to the fact that the haploid eggs double their chromosomes, resulting in ZZ or WW. The ZZ become males, but the WW are not viable and are not brought to term.

UV sex chromosomes

In some Bryophyte (Fig. 10.3) and some algae species, the gametophyte stage of the life cycle, rather than being hermaphrodite, occurs as separate male or female individuals that produce male and female gametes respectively. When meiosis occurs in the sporophyte generation of the life cycle, the sex chromosomes known as U and V assort in spores that carry either the U chromosome and give rise to female gametophytes, or the V chromosome and give rise to male gametophytes.

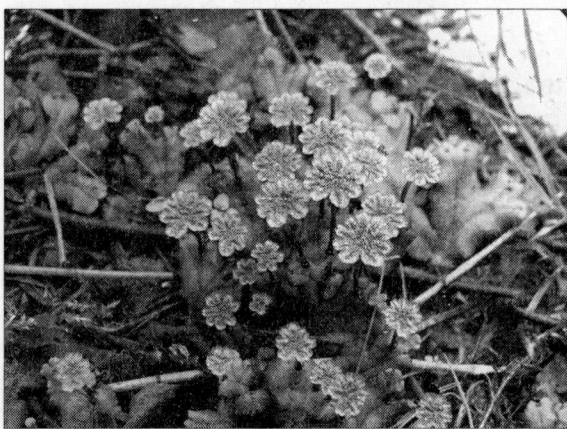

Fig. 10.3: Bryophyte.

Haplodiploidy

Haplodiploidy is found in insects belonging to Hymenoptera, such as ants and bees. Unfertilised eggs develop into haploid individuals, which are the males. Diploid individuals are generally female but may be sterile males. Males cannot have sons or fathers. If a queen bee mates with one drone, her daughters share ¾ of their genes with each other, not ½ as in the XY and ZW systems. This may be significant for the development of eusociality, as it increases the significance of kin selection, but it is debated. Most females in the Hymenoptera order can decide the sex of their offspring by holding received sperm in their spermatheca and either releasing it into their oviduct or not. This allows them to create more workers, depending on the status of the colony.

Environmental Systems

Temperature-dependent

Many other sex determination systems exist. In some species of reptiles, including alligators, some turtles, and the tuatara, sex is determined by the temperature at which the egg is incubated during a temperature-sensitive period. There are no examples of temperature-dependent sex determination (TSD) in birds. Megapodes had formerly been thought to exhibit this phenomenon, but were found to actually have different temperature-dependent embryo mortality rates for each sex. For some species with TSD, sex determination is achieved by exposure to hotter temperatures resulting in the offspring being one sex and cooler temperatures resulting in the other. This type of TSD is called Pattern I. For others species using TSD, it is exposure to temperatures on both extremes that results in offspring of one sex, and exposure to moderate temperatures that results in offspring of the opposite sex, called Pattern II TSD. The specific temperatures required to produce each sex are known as the female-promoting temperature and the male-promoting temperature. When the temperature stays near the threshold during the temperature sensitive period, the sex ratio is varied between the two sexes. Some species' temperature standards are based on when a particular enzyme is created. These species that rely upon temperature for their sex determination do not have the SRY gene, but have other genes such as DAX1, DMRT1, and SOX9 that are expressed or not expressed depending on the temperature. The sex of some species, such as the Nile tilapia, Australian skink lizard, and Australian dragon lizard, is initially determined by chromosomes, but can later be changed by the temperature of incubation.

It is unknown how exactly temperature-dependent sex determination evolved. It could have evolved through certain sexes being more suited to certain areas that fit the temperature requirements. For example, a warmer area could be more suitable for nesting, so more females are produced to increase the amount that nest next season. Environmental sex determination preceded the genetically determined systems of birds and mammals, it is thought that a temperature-dependent amniote was the common ancestor of amniotes with sex chromosomes.

Other systems

There are other environmental sex determination systems including location-dependent determination systems as seen in the marine worm Bonellia viridis – larvae become males if they make physical contact with a female, and females if they end up on the bare sea floor. This is triggered by the presence of a chemical produced by the females, bonellin. Some species, such as some snails, practice sex change: adults start out male, then become female. In tropical clown fish, the dominant individual in a group becomes female while the other ones are male, and bluehead wrasses (Thalassoma bifasciatum) are the reverse. Some species, however, have no sex determination system. Hermaphrodite species include the common earthworm and certain species of snails. A few species of fish, reptiles, and insects reproduce by parthenogenesis and are female altogether. There are some reptiles, such as the boa constrictor and Komodo dragon that can reproduce both sexually and asexually, depending on whether a mate is available.

Other unusual systems include those of the swordtail fish, the Chironomus midges, the platypus, which has 10 sex chromosomes but lacks the mammalian sex-determining gene SRY, meaning that the process of sex determination in the platypus remains unknown, the juvenile hermaphroditism of zebrafish, with an unknown trigger, and the platyfish, which has W, X, and Y chromosomes. This allows WY, WX, or XX females and YY or XY males.

EVOLUTION

Origin of Sex Chromosomes

The accepted hypothesis of XY and ZW sex chromosome evolution is that they evolved at the same time, in two different branches. However, there is some evidence to suggest that there could have been transitions between ZW and XY, such as in Xiphophorus maculatus, which have both ZW and XY systems in the same population, despite the fact that ZW and XY have different gene locations. A recent theoretical model raises the possibility of both transitions between the XY/XX and ZZ/ZW system and environmental sex determination. The platypus genes also back up the possible evolutionary link between XY and ZW, because they have the DMRT1 gene possessed by birds on their X chromosomes. Regardless, XY and ZW follow a similar route. All sex chromosomes started out as an original autosome of an original amniote that relied upon temperature to determine the sex of offspring. After the mammals separated, the branch further split into Lepidosauria and Archosauromorpha. These two groups both evolved the ZW system separately, as evidenced by the existence of different sex chromosomal locations. In mammals, one of the autosome pair, now Y, mutated its SOX3 gene into the SRY gene, causing that chromosome to designate sex. After this mutation, the SRY-containing chromosome inverted and was no longer completely homologous with its partner. The regions of the X and Y chromosomes that are still homologous to one another are known as the pseudoautosomal region. Once it inverted, the Y chromosome became unable to remedy deleterious mutations, and thus degenerated. There is some concern that the Y chromosome will shrink further and stop functioning in ten million years: but the Y chromosome has been strictly conserved after its initial rapid gene loss.

There are some species, such as the medaka fish, that evolved sex chromosomes separately, their Y chromosome never inverted and can still swap genes with the X. These species are still in an early phase of evolution with regard to their sex chromosomes. Because the Y does not have male-specific genes and can interact with the X, XY and YY females can be formed as well as XX males.

XY SEX DETERMINATION SYSTEM

The XY sex determination system is the sex determination system found in humans, most other mammals, some insects (*Drosophila*), some snakes, and some plants (*Ginkgo*). In this system, the sex of an individual is determined by a pair of sex chromosomes. Females typically have two of the same kind of sex chromosome (XX), and are called the homogametic sex. Males typically have two different kinds of sex chromosomes (XY), and are called the heterogametic sex.

In humans the presence of the Y chromosome determines if an offspring develops as a male and the absence of the Y chromosome results in a female offspring. More specifically it is the SRY gene located on the Y chromosome that is of importance to male differentiation. Variations to the sex gene karyotype could include rare disorders such as XX males (often due to translocation of the SRY gene to the X chromosome) or XY gonadal dygenesis (due to mutations in the SRY gene). In addition, other rare genetic variations such as Turners (XO) and Klinefelters (XXY) are seen as well.

The XY system contrasts in several ways with the ZW sex determination system found in birds, some insects, many reptiles, and various other animals, in which the heterogametic sex is female. It had been thought for several decades that in all snakes sex was determined by the ZW system, but there had been observations of unexpected effects in the genetics of species in the families Boidae and Pythonidae, for example, parthenogenic reproduction produced only females rather than males, which is the opposite of what is to be expected in the ZW system. In the early years of the 21st century such observations prompted research that demonstrated that all pythons and boas so far investigated definitely have the XY system of sex determination. A temperature-dependent sex determination system is found in some reptiles.

Mechanisms

All animals have a set of DNA coding for genes present on chromosomes. In humans, most mammals, and some other species, two of the chromosomes, called the X chromosome and Y chromosome, code for sex. In these species, one or more genes are present on their Y chromosome that determine maleness. In this process, an X chromosome and a Y chromosome act to determine the sex of offspring, often due to genes located on the Y chromosome that code for maleness. Offspring have two sex chromosomes: an offspring with two X chromosomes will develop female characteristics, and an offspring with an X and a Y chromosome will develop male characteristics.

Humans

In humans, half of spermatozoons carry X chromosome and the other half Y chromosome. A single gene (SRY) present on the Y chromosome acts as a signal to set the developmental pathway towards maleness. Presence of this gene starts off the process of virilisation. This and other factors result in the sex differences in humans. The cells in females, with two X chromosomes, undergo X-inactivation, in which one of the two X chromosomes is inactivated. The inactivated X chromosome remains within a cell as a Barr body. Humans, as well as some other organisms, can have a rare chromosomal arrangement that is contrary to their phenotypic sex, for example, XX males or XY gonadal dysgenesis (see androgen insensitivity syndrome). Additionally, an abnormal number of sex chromosomes (aneuploidy) may be present, such as Turner's syndrome, in which a single X chromosome is present, and Klinefelter's syndrome, in which two X chromosomes and a Y chromosome are present, XYY syndrome and XXYY syndrome. Other less common chromosomal arrangements include: triple X syndrome, 48, XXXX, and 49, XXXXX.

Other Animals

In most mammals, sex is determined by presence of the Y chromosome. 'Female' is the default sex, due to the absence of the Y chromosome. In the 1930s, Alfred Jost determined that the presence of testosterone was required for Wolffian duct development in the male rabbit. SRY is a sex-determining gene on the Y chromosome in the therians (placental mammals and marsupials). Non-human mammals use several genes on the Y chromosome. Not all male-specific genes are located on the Y chromosome. Platypus, a monotreme, use five pairs of different XY chromosomes with six groups of male-linked genes, AMH being the master switch. Other species (including most *Drosophila* species) use the presence of two X chromosomes to determine femaleness: one X chromosome gives putative maleness, but the presence of Y chromosome genes is required for normal male development.

Other Systems

Birds and many insects have a similar system of sex determination (ZW sex determination system), in which it is the females that are heterogametic (ZW), while males are homogametic (ZZ).

Many insects of the order Hymenoptera instead have a system (the haplo-diploid sex determination system), where the males are haploid individuals (which have just one chromosome of each type), while the females are diploid (with chromosomes appearing in pairs). Some other insects have the X0 sex determination system, where just one chromosome type appears in pairs for the female but alone in the males, while all other chromosomes appear in pairs in both sexes.

Influences

Genetic

It has long been believed that the female form was the default template for the mammalian fetuses of both sexes. After the discovery of the testis-determining gene SRY, many scientists shifted to the theory that the genetic mechanism that causes a fetus to develop into a male form was initiated by the SRY gene, which was thought to be responsible for the production of testosterone and its overall effects on body and brain development. This perspective still shares the classical way of thinking, that in order to produce two sexes, nature has developed a default female pathway and an active pathway by which male genes would initiate the process of determining a male sex, as something that is developed in addition to and based on the default female form. For a long time it was thought that SRY would activate a cascade of male genes. It turns out that the sex determination pathway is probably more complicated and SRY may in fact inhibit some anti-male genes. The idea is instead of having a simplistic mechanism by which you have pro-male genes going all the way to make a male, in fact there is a solid balance between pro-male genes and anti-male genes and if there is a little too much of anti-male genes, there may be a female born and if there is a little too much of pro-male genes then there will be a male born.

We are entering this new era in molecular biology of sex determination where it's a more subtle dosage of genes, some pro-males, some pro-females, some anti-males, some anti-females that all interplay with each other rather than a simple linear pathway of genes going one after the other, which makes it very fascinating but very complicated to study.

In mammals, including humans, the SRY gene is responsible with triggering the development of non-differentiated gonads into testes, rather than ovaries. However, there are cases in which testes can develop in the absence of an SRY gene. In these cases, the SOX9 gene, involved in the development of testes, can induce their development without the aid of SRY. In the absence of SRY and SOX9, no testes can develop and the path is clear for the development of ovaries. Even so, the absence of the SRY gene or the silencing of the SOX9 gene are not enough to trigger sexual differentiation of a fetus in the female direction. A recent finding suggests that ovary development and maintenance is an active process, regulated by the expression of a 'pro-female' gene, FOXL2. In an interview for the Times Online edition, study co-author Robin Lovell-Badge explained the significance of the discovery:

'We take it for granted that we maintain the sex we are born with, including whether we have testes' or ovaries. But this work shows that the activity of a single gene, FOXL2, is all that prevents adult ovary cells turning into cells found in testes.

Implications

Looking into the genetic determinants of human sex can have wide-ranging consequences. Scientists have been studying different sex determination systems in fruit flies and animal models to attempt an understanding of how the genetics of sexual differentiation can influence biological processes like reproduction, ageing and disease.

Maternal

In humans and many other species of animals, the father determines the sex of the child. In the XY sex determination system, the female-provided ovum contributes an X chromosome and the male-provided sperm contributes either an X chromosome or a Y chromosome, resulting in female (XX) or male (XY) offspring, respectively.

Hormone levels in the male parent affect the sex ratio of sperm in humans. Maternal influences also impact which sperm are more likely to achieve conception. Human ova, like those of other mammals, are covered with a thick translucent layer called the zona pellucida, which the sperm must penetrate to fertilise the egg. Once viewed simply as an impediment to fertilisation, recent research indicates the zona pellucida may instead function as a sophisticated biological security system that chemically controls the entry of the sperm into the egg and protects the fertilised egg from additional sperm.

Recent research indicates that human ova may produce a chemical which appears to attract sperm and influence their swimming motion. However, not all sperm are positively impacted, some appear to remain uninfluenced and some actually move away from the egg. Maternal influences may also be possible that affect sex determination in such a way as to produce fraternal twins equally weighted between one male and one female. The time at which insemination occurs during the oestrus cycle has been found to affect the sex ratio of the offspring of humans, cattle, hamsters, and other mammals. Hormonal and pH conditions within the female reproductive tract vary with time, and this affects the sex ratio of the sperm that reach the egg. Sex-specific mortality of embryos also occurs.

SEXUAL DIFFERENTIATION IN HUMANS

Sexual differentiation in humans is the process of development of sex differences in humans. It is defined as the development of phenotypic structures consequent to the action of hormones produced following gonadal determination. Sexual differentiation includes development of different genitalia and the internal genital tracts, breasts, body hair, and plays a role in gender identification.

The development of sexual differences begins with the XY sex determination system that is present in humans, and complex mechanisms are responsible for the development of the phenotypic differences between male and female humans from an undifferentiated zygote. Females have two X chromosomes, and males have a Y chromosome and an X chromosome. At an early stage in embryonic development, both sexes possess equivalent internal structures. These are the mesonephric ducts and paramesonephric ducts. The presence of the SRY gene on the Y chromosome causes the development of the testes in males, and the subsequent release of hormones which cause the paramesonephric ducts to regress. In females, the mesonephric ducts regress. Divergent sexual development, known as intersex, can be a result of genetic and hormonal factors.

Sex Determination

Most mammals, including humans, have an XY sex determination system: the Y chromosome carries factors responsible for triggering male development. The 'default sex,' in the absence of a Y chromosome, is female-like. This is because of the presence of the sex-determining region of the Y chromosome, also known as the SRY gene. Thus, male mammals typically have an X and a Y chromosome (XY), while female mammals typically have two X chromosomes (XX). In humans, biological sex is determined by five factors present at birth: the presence or absence of a Y chromosome, the type of gonads, the sex hormones, the internal genitalia (such as the uterus in females), and the external genitalia.

Chromosomal sex is determined at the time of fertilisation, a chromosome from the sperm cell, either X or Y, fuses with the X chromosome in the egg cell. Gonadal sex refers to the gonads, that is the testis or ovaries, depending on which genes are expressed. Phenotypic sex refers to the structures of the external and internal genitalia. A human fetus does not develop its external sexual organs until seven weeks after fertilisation. The fetus appears to be sexually indifferent, looking neither like a male or a female. Over the next five weeks, the fetus begins producing hormones that cause its sex organs to grow into either male or female organs. This process is called sexual differentiation. The precursor of the internal female sex organs is called the Müllerian system. Mesonephric system pathway is shown in Fig. 10.4.

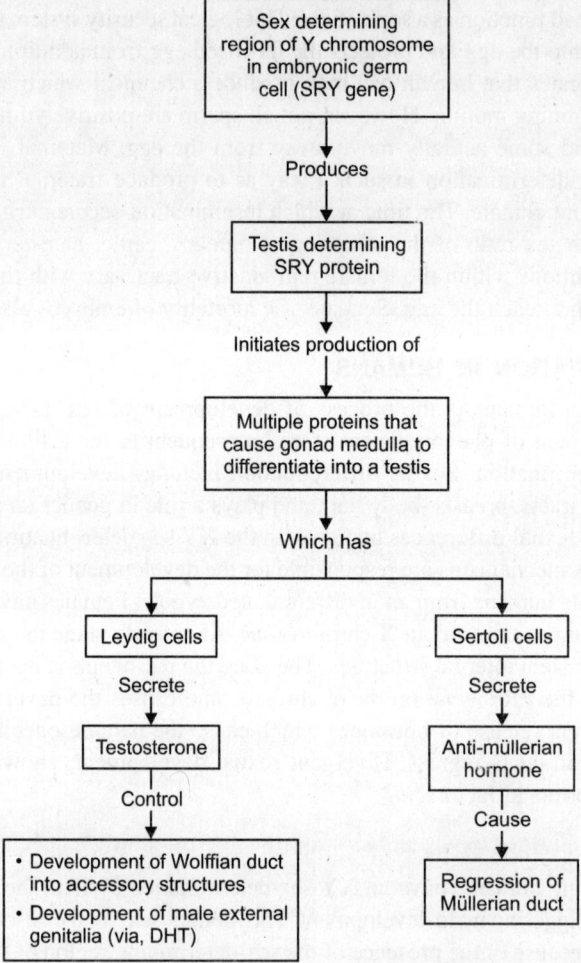

Fig. 10.4: Mesonephric system pathway.

Reproductive System

By 7 weeks, a fetus has a genital tubercle, urogenital groove and sinus, and labioscrotal folds. In females, without excess androgens, these become the clitoris, urethra and vagina, and labia. Differentiation between the sexes of the sex organs occurs throughout embryological, fetal and later life. This includes both internal and external genital differentiation. In both males and females, the sex organs consist of three structures: the gonads, the internal genitalia, and the external genitalia. In males, the gonads are the testes and in females they are the ovaries. These are the organs that produce gametes (egg and sperm), the reproductive cells that will eventually meet to form the fertilised egg (zygote). As the zygote divides, it first becomes the embryo (which means 'growing within'), typically between zero and eight weeks, then from the eighth week until birth, it is considered the fetus (which means 'unborn offspring'). The internal genitalia are all the accessory glands and ducts that connect the gonads to the outside environment. The external genitalia consist of all the external reproductive structures. The sex of an early embryo cannot be determined because the reproductive structures do not differentiate until the seventh week. Prior to this, the child is considered bipotential because it cannot be identified as male or female.

Internal genital differentiation

The internal genitalia consist of two accessory ducts: mesonephric ducts (male) and paramesonephric ducts (female). The mesonephric system is the precursor to the male genitalia and the paramesonephric to the female reproductive system. As development proceeds, one of the pairs of ducts develops while the other regresses. This depends on the presence or absence of the sex determining region of the Y chromosome, also known as the SRY gene. In the presence of a functional SRY gene, the bipotential gonads develop into testes. Gonads are histologically distinguishable by 6–8 weeks of gestation.

Subsequent development of one set and degeneration of the other depends on the presence or absence of two testicular hormones: testosterone and anti-müllerian hormone (AMH). Disruption of typical development may result in the development of both, or neither, duct system, which may produce morphologically intersex individuals.

Males: The SRY gene when transcribed and processed produces SRY protein that binds to DNA and directs the development of the gonad into testes. Male development can only occur when the fetal testis secretes key hormones at a critical period in early gestation. The testes begin to secrete three hormones that influence the male internal and external genitalia: they secrete anti-müllerian hormone (AMH), testosterone, and dihydrotestosterone (DHT). Anti-müllerian hormone causes the paramesonephric ducts to regress. Testosterone converts the mesonephric ducts into male accessory structures, including the epididymis, vas deferens, and seminal vesicle. Testosterone will also control the descending of the testes from the abdomen into the scrotum. Many other genes found on other autosomes, including WT-1, SOX9, SF-1 also play a role in gonadal development.

Females: Without testosterone and AMH, the mesonephric ducts degenerate and disappear. The paramesonephric ducts develop into a uterus, fallopian tubes, and upper vagina. There still remains a broad lack of information about the genetic controls of female development, and much remains unknown about the female embryonic process.

External genital differentiation

Males become externally distinct between 8 and 12 weeks, as androgens enlarge the phallus and cause the urogenital groove and sinus to fuse in the midline, producing an unambiguous penis with a phallic urethra, and a thinned, rugated scrotum. Dihydrotestosterone will differentiate the remaining male characteristics of the external genitalia. A sufficient amount of any androgen can cause external masculinisation. The most potent is dihydrotestosterone (DHT), generated from testosterone in skin and genital tissue by the action of 5α-reductase. A male fetus may be incompletely masculinised if this enzyme is deficient. In some diseases and circumstances, other androgens may be present in high enough concentrations to cause partial or (rarely) complete masculinisation of the external genitalia of a genetically female fetus. The testes begin to secrete three hormones that influence the male internal and external genitalia. They secrete anti-müllerian hormone, testosterone, and Dihydrotestosterone. Anti-

Müllerian hormone (AMH) causes the paramesonephric ducts to regress. Testosterone, which is secreted and converts the mesonephric ducts into male accessory structures, such as epididymis, vas deferens and seminal vesicle. Testosterone will also control the descending of the testes from the abdomen into the scrotom. Dihydrotestosterone, also known as (DHT) will differentiate the remaining male characteristics of the external genitalia.

Further sex differentiation of the external genitalia occurs at puberty, when androgen levels again become disparate. Male levels of testosterone directly induce growth of the penis, and indirectly (via DHT) the prostate. Alfred Jost observed that while testosterone was required for mesonephric duct development, the regression of the paramesonephric duct was due to another substance. This was later determined to be paramesonephric inhibiting substance (MIS), a 140 kD dimeric glycoprotein that is produced by sertoli cells. MIS blocks the development of paramesonephric ducts, promoting their regression.

Secondary Sexual Characteristics

Breast

Visible differentiation occurs at puberty, when estradiol and other hormones cause breasts to develop in typical females.

Psychological and behavioural Differentiation

Human adults and children show many psychological and behavioural sex differences. Some (e.g. dress) are learned and obviously cultural. Others are demonstrable across cultures and have both biological and learned determinants. For example, some studies claim girls are, on average, more verbally fluent than boys, but boys are, on average, better at spatial calculation. Some have observed that this may be due to two different patterns in parental communication with infants, noting that parents are more likely to talk to girls and more likely to engage in physical play with boys. Because people cannot explore hormonal influences on human behaviour experimentally, the relative contributions of biological factors and learning to human psychological and behavioural sex differences (especially gender identity, role, and sexual orientation) are controversial (and hotly contested).

Current theories on mechanisms of sexual differentiation of brains and behaviour in humans are based primarily on three sources of evidence: animal research involving manipulation of hormones in early life, observation of outcomes of small numbers of individuals with intersex conditions or cases of early sex reassignment, and statistical distribution of traits in populations (e.g. rates of homosexuality in twins). Many of these cases suggest some genetic or hormonal effect on sex differentiation of behaviour and mental traits this has been disputed as poor interpretation of scientific methodology.

Intersex Conditions

The following are some of the variations associated with atypical determination and differentiation process:

- A zygote with only X chromosome (XO) results in Turner syndrome and will develop with female characteristics.
- Congenital adrenal hyperplasia: Inability of adrenal to produce sufficient cortisol, leading to increased production of testosterone resulting in severe masculinisation of 46 XX females.
- Persistent müllerian duct syndrome - A rare type of pseudohermaphroditism that occurs in 46 XY males, caused by either a mutation in the Müllerian inhibiting substance (MIS) gene, on 19p13, or its type II receptor, 12q13. Results in a retention of Müllerian ducts (persistence of rudimentary

uterus and fallopian tubes in otherwise normally virilised males), unilateral or bilateral undescended testes and sometimes causes infertility.

- XY differences of sex development: A typical androgen production or inadequate androgen response, which can cause incomplete masculinisation in XY males. Varies from mild failure of masculinisation with undescended testes to complete sex reversal and female phenotype (Androgen insensitivity syndrome).
- Swyer syndrome: A form of complete gonadal dysgenesis, mostly due to mutations in the first step of sex determination, the SRY genes.
- A 5-alpha-reductase deficiency results in atypical development characterised by female phenotype or undervirilised male phenotype with development of the epididymis, vas deferens, seminal vesicle, and ejaculatory duct, but also a pseudovagina. This is because testosterone is converted to the more potent DHT by 5-alpha reductase. DHT is necessary to exert androgenic effects farther from the site of testosterone production, where the concentrations of testosterone are too low to have any potency.

SEXUAL DIFFERENTIATION

Sexual differentiation is the process of development of the differences between males and females from an undifferentiated zygote. As male and female individuals develop from zygotes into fetuses, into infants, children, adolescents, and eventually into adults, sex and gender differences at many levels develop: genes, chromosomes, gonads, hormones, anatomy, and psyche. Sex differences range greatly and include physiologically differentiating. Sex-dichotomous differences are developments which are wholly characteristic of one sex only. Examples of sex-dichotomous differences include aspects of the sex-specific genital organs such as ovaries, a uterus or a phallic urethra. In contrast, sex-dimorphic differences are matters of degree (e.g. size of phallus). Some of these (e.g. stature, behaviours) are mainly statistical, with much overlap between male and female populations.

Nevertheless, even the sex-dichotomous differences are not absolute in the human population, and there are individuals who are exceptions (e.g. XY males with a uterus, undeveloped testes), or phenotypical females with an XY karyotype (undeveloped reproductive organs), or who exhibit biological and/or behavioural characteristics of both sexes. Sex differences may be induced by specific genes, by hormones, by anatomy, or by social learning. Some of the differences are entirely physical (e.g. presence of a uterus) and some differences are just as obviously purely a matter of social learning and custom (e.g. relative hair length). Many differences, though, such as gender identity, appear to be influenced by both biological and social factors ('nature' and 'nurture').

The early stages of human differentiation appear to be quite similar to the same biological processes in other mammals and the interaction of genes, hormones and body structures is fairly well understood. In the first weeks of life, a fetus has no anatomic or hormonal sex, and only a karyotype distinguishes male from female. Specific genes induce gonadal differences, which produce hormonal differences, which cause anatomic differences, leading to psychological and behavioural differences, some of which are innate and some induced by the social environment.

Sex Determination System

Humans, many mammals, insects and other animals have an XY sex determination system. Humans have forty-six chromosomes, including two sex chromosomes, XX in females and XY in males. The Y chromosome must carry at least one essential gene which determines testicular formation (originally termed TDF). A gene in the sex-determining region of the short arm of the Y, now referred to as SRY, has been found to direct production of a protein, testis determining factor, which binds to DNA, inducing differentiation of cells derived from the genital ridges into testes. In transgenic XX mice (and some human XX males), SRY alone is sufficient to induce male differentiation.

Humans

Various processes are involved in the development of sex differences in humans. Sexual differentiation in humans includes development of different genitalia and the internal genital tracts, breasts, body hair, and plays a role in gender identification. The development of sexual differences begins with the XY sex determination system that is present in humans, and complex mechanisms are responsible for the development of the phenotypic differences between male and female humans from an undifferentiated zygote. Atypical sexual development, and ambiguous genitalia, can be a result of genetic and hormonal factors. The differentiation of other parts of the body than the sex organ creates the secondary sex characteristics. Sexual dimorphism of skeletal structure develops during childhood, and becomes more pronounced at adolescence. Sexual orientation has been demonstrated to correlate with skeletal characters that become dimorphic during early childhood (such as arm length to stature ratio) but not with characters that become dimorphic during puberty—such as shoulder width.

Humans and Other Animals

Brain differentiation

In most animals, differences of exposure of a fetal or infant brain to sex hormones produce significant differences of brain structure and function which correlate with adult reproductive behaviour. Sex hormone levels in human male and female fetuses and infants also differ, and both androgen receptors and estrogen receptors have been identified in brains. Several sex-specific genes not dependent on sex steroids are expressed differently in male and female human brains. Structural sex differences begin to be recognisable by 2 years of age, and in adult men and women include size and shape of corpus callosum (larger in women) and fasciculae connecting each hemisphere internally (larger in men), certain hypothalamic nuclei, and the gonadotropin feedback response to estradiol. The absence of the genes that generate male genitalia do not single-handedly lead to a female brain. The male brain requires more hormones, such as testosterone, in order to properly differentiate. These hormones are released due to a gene expressed during embryonic development.

TEMPERATURE DEPENDENT SEX DETERMINATION

Temperature dependent sex determination (TSD) is a type of environmental sex determination in which the temperatures experienced during embryonic/larval development determine the sex of the offspring. It is only observed in reptiles and teleost fish. TSD differs from the chromosomal sex determination systems common among vertebrates. It is the most popular and most studied type of environmental sex determination (ESD). Some other conditions, e.g. density, pH, and environmental background colour, are also observed to alter sex ratio, which could be classified either as temperature-dependent sex determination or temperature-dependent sex differentiation, depending on the involved mechanisms. As sex-determining mechanisms, TSD and genetic sex determination (GSD) should be considered in an equivalent manner, which can lead to reconsidering the status of fish species that are claimed to have

TSD when submitted to extreme temperatures instead of the temperature experienced during development in the wild, since changes in sex ratio with temperature variation are ecologically and evolutionally relevant. While TSD has been observed in many reptile and fish species, the genetic differences between sexes and molecular mechanisms of TSD have not been disclosed. The cortisol-mediated pathway and epigenetic regulatory pathway are thought to be the potential mechanisms involved in TSD.

The eggs are affected by the temperature at which they are incubated during the middle one-third of embryonic development. This critical period of incubation is known as the thermosensitive period (TSP). The specific time of sex-commitment is known due to several authors resolving histological chronology of sex differentiation in the gonads of turtles with TSD.

Thermosensitive Period (TSP)

The thermosensitive, or temperature-sensitive, period (TSP) is the period during development when sex is irreversibly determined. It is used in reference to species with temperature-dependent sex determination, such as crocodilians and turtles. The TSP typically spans the middle third of incubation with the endpoints defined by embryonic stage. The extent of the TSP varies a little among species, and development within the oviducts must be taken into account in species where the embryo is at a relatively late stage of development on egg laying (e.g. many lizards). Temperature pulses during the thermosensitive period are often sufficient to determine sex, but after the TSP, sex is unresponsive to temperature. After this period, however, sex cannot be reversed.

Types

Within the mechanism, two distinct patterns have been discovered and named Pattern I and Pattern II (Fig. 10.5). Pattern I is further divided into IA and IB. Pattern IA has a single transition zone, where eggs predominantly hatch males if incubated below this temperature zone, and predominantly hatch females if incubated above it. Pattern IA occurs in most turtles, with the transition between male-producing temperatures and female-producing temperatures occurring over a range of temperatures as little as 1–2°C. Pattern IB also has a single transition zone, but females are produced below it and males above it. Pattern IB occurs in the tuatara.

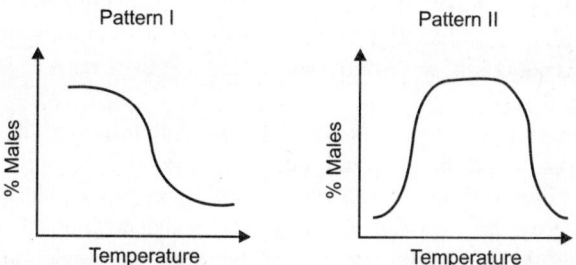

Fig. 10.5: Patterns of temperature dependent sex determination (TSD) in reptiles. Pattern I is found in turtles, e.g. Red-eared slider turtles (*Trachemys scripta*), Olive Ridley sea turtles (*Lepidochelys olivacea*), or Painted turtles (Chrysemys picta). Pattern II has been found in American alligators (*Alligator mississippiensis* and Leopard geckos (*Eublepharis macularius*).

Pattern II has two transition zones, with males dominating at intermediate temperatures and females dominating at both extremes. Pattern II occurs in some turtles, lizards, and crocodilians. Very near or at the pivotal temperature of sex determination, mixed sex ratios and (more rarely) intersex individuals. It has been proposed that essentially all modes of TSD are actually Pattern II and those that deviate from the expected female-male-female pattern are species whose nests have simply never been observed exposed to extreme temperature ranges on one end of the range or the other. The distinction between chromosomal sex determination systems and TSD is often blurred because the sex of some species – such as the three-lined skink Bassiana duperreyi and the central bearded dragon *Pogona vitticeps* – is determined by sex chromosomes, but this is over-ridden by temperatures that are tolerable but extreme. Also, experiments conducted at the pivotal temperature, where temperature is equivocal in its influence, have demonstrated an underlying genetic predisposition to be one sex or the other.

Examples

Temperature dependent sex determination was first described in Agama agama in the year 1966 by Madeleine Charnier. A 2015 study found that hot temperatures altered the expression of the sex chromosomes in Australia's bearded dragon lizards. The lizards were female in appearance and were capable of bearing offspring, despite having the ZZ chromosomes usually associated with male lizards.

In 2018, a team of Chinese and American researchers showed that the histone H3 lysine 27 (H3K27) demethylase KDM6B (JMJD3), an epigenetic modifier, 'binds to the promoter of the dominant male gene [DMRT1] to activate male development' in red-eared slider turtles. Knocking down the expression of this modifier at 26°C 'triggers male-to-female sex reversal' in most of the surviving embryos.

Hormones in TSD Systems

Synergism between temperature and hormones has also been identified in these systems. Administering estradiol at male-producing temperatures generates females that are physiologically identical to temperature produced females. The reverse experiment, males produced at female temperatures, only occurs when a nonaromatisable testosterone or an aromatase inhibitor is administered, indicating that the enzyme responsible for conversion of testosterone to estradiol, aromatase, plays a role in female development. Nonetheless, the mechanisms for TSD are still relatively unknown, but in some ways, TSD resembles genetic sex determination (GSD), particularly in regards to the effects of aromatase in each process. In some fish species, aromatase is in both the ovaries of female organisms who underwent TSD and those who underwent GSD, with no less than 85% of the coding sequences of each aromatase being identical, showing that aromatase is not unique to TSD and suggesting that there must be another factor in addition to it that is also affecting TSD.

Hormones and temperature show signs of acting in the same pathway, in that less hormone is required to produce a sexual shift as the incubation conditions near the pivotal temperature. It has been proposed that temperature acts on genes coding for such steroidogenic enzymes, and testing of homologous GSD pathways has provided a genic starting point. Yet, the genetic sexual determination pathway in TSD turtles is poorly understood and the controlling mechanism for male or female commitment has not been identified.

While sex hormones have been observed to be influenced by temperature, thus potentially altering sexual phenotypes, specific genes in the gonadal differentiation pathway display temperature influenced expression. In some species, such important sex-determining genes as DMRT1 and those involved in the Wnt signalling pathway could potentially be implicated as genes which provide a mechanism (opening the door for selective forces) for the evolutionary development of TSD. While aromatase is involved in more processes than only TSD, it has also been shown to play a role in certain tumor development.

Adaptive Significance

The adaptive significance of TSD is currently not well understood. One possible explanation that TSD is common in amniotes is phylogenetic inertia – TSD is the ancestral condition in this clade and is simply maintained in extant lineages because it is currently adaptively neutral or nearly so. Indeed, recent phylogenetic comparative analyses imply a single origin for TSD in most amniotes around 300 million years, with the re-evolution of TSD in squamates and turtles after they had independently developed GSD. Consequently, the adaptive significance of TSD in all but the most recent origins of TSD may have been obscured by the passage of deep time, with TSD potentially being maintained in many amniote clades simply because it works 'well enough' (i.e. has no overall fitness costs along the lines of the phylogenetic inertia explanation).

Other work centers on a 1977 theoretical model (the Charnov–Bull model), predicted that selection should favour TSD over chromosome-based systems when 'the developmental environment differentially influences male versus female fitness', this theoretical model was empirically validated thirty years later but the generality of this hypothesis in reptiles is questioned. This hypothesis is supported by the persistence of TSD in certain populations of spotted skink (Niveoscincus ocellatus), a small lizard in Tasmania, where it is advantageous to have females early in the season. The warmth early in the season ensures female-biased broods that then have more time to grow and reach maturity and possibly reproduce before they experience their first winter, thereby increasing fitness of the individual.

In support of the Charnov and Bull hypothesis, Warner and Shine showed confidently that incubation temperature influences males' reproductive success differently than females in Jacky Dragon lizards (*Amphibolurus muricatus*) by treating the eggs with chemicals that interfere with steroid hormone biosynthesis. These chemicals block the conversion of testosterone to estradiol during development so each sex offspring can be produced at all temperatures. They found that hatching temperatures that naturally produce each sex maximised fitness of each sex, which provides the substantial empirical evidence in support of the Charnov and Bull model for reptiles.

Spencer and Janzen found further support for the Charnov-Bull model by incubating painted turtles (*Chrysemys picta* is shown in Fig. 10.6) at different temperatures and measuring various characteristics indicative of fitness. The turtles were incubated at temperatures that produce solely males, both sexes, and solely females. Spencer and Janzen found that hatchlings from mixed-sex nests were less energy efficient and grew less than their same-sex counterparts incubated in single-sex producing temperatures.

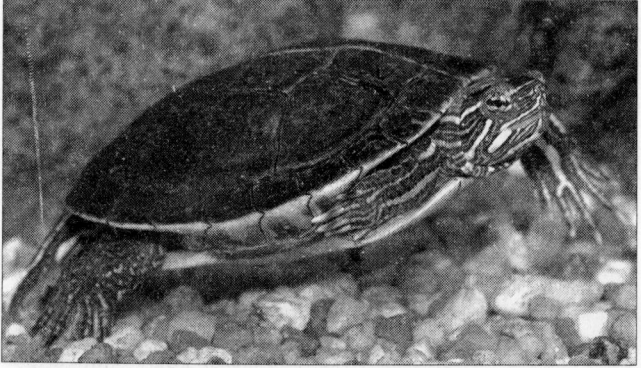

Fig. 10.6: *Chrysemys picta.*

Hatchlings from single-sex producing temperatures also had higher first-year survivorship than the hatchlings from the temperature that produces both sexes. TSD may be advantageous and selected for in turtles, as embryo energy efficiency and hatchling size are optimised for each sex at single-sex incubation temperatures and are indicative of first-year survivorship. This suggests that natural selection would favour TSD, as TSD may enhance the fitness of offspring.

An alternative hypothesis of adaptive significance was proposed by Bulmer and Bull in 1982 and supported by the work of Pen and others. They conjectured that disruptive selection produced by variation in the environment could result in an evolutionary transition from ESD to GSD. Pen and others addresses evolutionary divergence in SDMs via natural selection on sex ratios. Studying the spotted skink, they observed that the highland population was not affected by temperature, yet, there was a negative correlation between annual temperature and cohort sex ratios in the lowlands. The highlands are colder with a higher magnitude of annual temperature fluctuation and a shorter activity season, delaying maturity, thus GSD is favoured so sex ratios are not skewed. However, in the lowlands, temperatures are more constant and a longer activity season allows for favourable conditions for TSD. They concluded that this differentiation in climate causes divergent selection on regulatory elements in the sex-determining network allowing for the emergence of sex chromosomes in the highlands.

'Temperature sex determination could allow the mother to determine the sex of her offspring by varying the temperature of the nest in which her eggs are incubated. However, there is no evidence thus far that sex ratio is manipulated by parental care.'

Effect of climate change

The warming of the habitats of species exhibiting TSD are beginning to affect their behaviour and may soon start affecting their physiology. Many species (with Pattern IA and II) have begun to nest earlier and earlier in the year to preserve the sex ratio. The three traits of pivotal temperature (the temperature at which the sex ratio is 50%), maternal nest-site choice, and nesting phenology have been identified as the key traits of TSD that can change, and of these, only the pivotal temperature is significantly heritable, and unfortunately, this would have to increase by 27 standard deviations to compensate for a 4°C temperature increase. It is likely that climate change (global warming) will outpace the ability of many animals to adapt, and many will likely go extinct. However, there is evidence that during climactic extremes, changes in the sex determining mechanism itself (to GSD) are selected for, particularly in the highly-mutable turtles.

SECTION IV

Chromosome Mutations, Chromatin and Extrachromosmal DNA

Chapter 11

Chromosome Mutations

INTRODUCTION

Chromosomes are the physical carriers of genes, consisting of DNA and associated proteins. Bacteria typically have one circular chromosome, while eukaryotes usually have linear chromosomes and vary widely in their sizes and numbers of chromosomes. All chromosomes have the capacity to transmit genes faithfully during cell division. The structures of the eukaryotic chromosome that allow them to do this are replication origins, telomeres which protect the chromosome ends, and centromeres for microtubule attachment and microtubule motor binding in cell division. Chromosomes must also be able to condense during cell division so that they can align onto the spindles and be moved to the spindle poles. In metazoans, chromosomes can be most broadly categorised into autosomes and sex chromosomes (chromosomes that have a part in determining the sex of the organism). A chromosome mutation is an unpredictable change that occurs in a chromosome. These changes are most often brought on by problems that occur during meiosis (division process of gametes) or by mutagens (chemicals, radiation, etc.). Chromosome mutations can result in changes in the number of chromosomes in a cell or changes in the structure of a chromosome. Unlike a gene mutation which alters a single gene or larger segment of DNA on a chromosome, chromosome mutations change and impact the entire chromosome.

CHROMOSOME MUTATIONS

Chromosome mutations are alterations occurring in chromosomes that typically result from errors during nuclear division or from mutagens. Chromosome mutations result in changes in chromosome structure or in cellular chromosome numbers. Examples of structural chromosome mutations include translocations, deletions, duplications, inversions, and isochromosomes. Abnormal chromosome numbers result from nondisjunction, or the failure of chromosomes to separate correctly during cell division. Examples of conditions that result from abnormal chromosome numbers are Down syndrome and Turner syndrome. Sex chromosome mutations occur on either the X or Y sex chromosomes.

Chromosome mutations are changes in the structure or in the number of chromosomes, and since they are relatively rare in this respect they differ from normally occurring common, harmless chromosome polymorphisms. Since both types of chromosome aberrations affecting many genes, and since the size of chromosomes or their affected segments are within the limits of microscopic resolution therefore they can be examined by light microscope, as opposed to gene mutations only be identified by molecular biological techniques. However, the application of modern hybridisation based (FISH and CGH) techniques allow the identification of small structural changes (e.g. microdeletions or CNVs) previously unrecognised by light microscope. Two aspects of the chromosomal abnormalities are regarded crucial: when and where they happen. While chromosome mutations may be formed during both mitosis and meiosis, those may occur in meiosis, lead to defective gamete formation, and to the birth of affected offspring. Thus their medical significance is greater than that of mitotic chromosome aberrations. From the point of mitotic chromosomal abnormalities it is also important when during development and in what kind of cell they are formed. Mutations occurred during the early cleavage divisions may have serious consequences for the entire organism, while aberrations occurred in a continuously proliferating cell type (e.g. epithelial cells) in adulthood may have negligible role. However, certain chromosomal mutations may have a role in the formation and subsequent rapid proliferation of tumour cells.

Two chromosomal regions have special importance in the formation of chromosome aberrations: the centromeres and the telomeres. The *centromere* is primary constriction of chromosomes where sister chromatids are connected, situated in strictly imposed position of the chromosome. The kinetochore and through that kinetochore microtubules bind to it. Its significance is in the segregation of sister chromatids or chromosomes during anaphase, therefore it plays role mainly in the formation of numerical chromosome mutations. Chromosome pieces without centromere (acentric fragments) do not reach the right pole of the cell, but lost in successive divisions.

There are many repetitive GC-rich sequences around the centromere, and the centromere itself includes the latest replicating DNA.

The chromosome ends, the *telomeres* are rich in TTAGGG repetitive sequences, and ensure the integrity and stability of the chromosome structure and play a role in cell aging, in tumorigenicity and the formation of structural chromosome aberrations, since in the absence of a telomere the chromosome structure becomes unstable and fragments without telomeres easily adhere, opening the way for a wide variety of disorders.

STRUCTURAL CHROMOSOME ABERRATIONS

The prerequisite of structural chromosome aberrations is breakage of chromosome/s which can be spontaneous or induced. The classification of structural aberrations is based on the number and the location of breaks within chromosomes (Fig. 11.1).

Deletions

If a chromosome is broken, and the broken piece lost, we are talking about deletion. Then the genetic information carried by the broken piece will be absent from the cell involved, where upon the cell does not function normally or die. Since the deletions eliminate certain functions therefore certain proteins for example enzymes are not produced. By the help of deletions the location of the gene eliminated can be mapped - it was one of the earliest methods of gene mapping, the deletion mapping.

If the break is close to the end of the chromosome, a terminal deletion is generated. In this case, in addition to other genes telomere is lost, too and this also contributes to the severity of symptoms, to early lethality. The best known example of a terminal deletion is the *cat cry (cri du chat) syndrome*: the short arm of chromosome 5 is deleted (5p-). The disease is named after the affected newborns characteristic mewing cry.

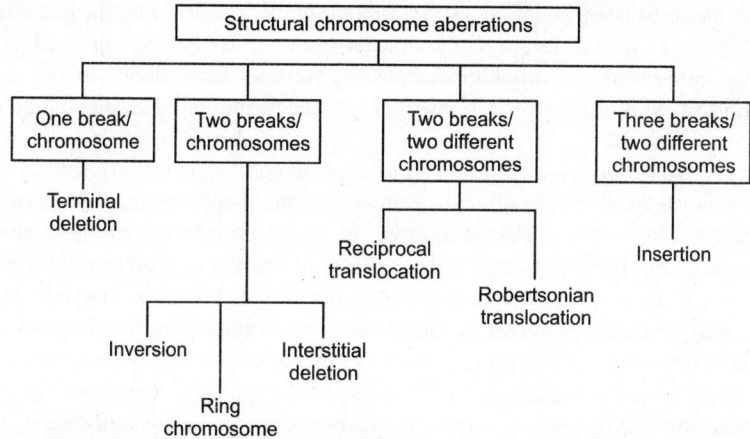

Fig. 11.1: Classification of structural chromosome aberrations.

There are two breaks within one chromosome in the case of interstitial deletion, and the intermediate piece is lost. Such lesions usually may cause severe physical and mental disabilities, spontaneous abortion, premature death depending on the chromosome involved. The best known interstitial deletion affects the long arm of chromosome 15: del15(q11-13). This is one of the causes of Prader-Willi or Angelman syndrome. In the former case paternal deletion, in the latter one maternal deletion is found.

Also interstitial, but small, so-called microdeletions are in the background of Williams and DiGeorge syndromes (del7q11.23 and del22q11.2) as well.

Duplications

During duplication a chromosomal segment is duplicated. It's either a replication error or due to meiotic unequal crossing over. In both cases the repetitive sequences occurring in the affected region may explain the 'slipping' of the replication apparatus or the non-exact pairing of the non-homologous chromosomes (skipping). Like deletions, duplications are also used to identify the chromosomal location of a gene or group of genes, so to map a gene.

Translocations

For the formation of translocations more than one, usually 2 or 3 breaks are needed. The broken part/s are transferred to another chromosome. Depending on the origin of the broken piece or on the number of fragments translocated there are different sub-groups of the translocations.

Reciprocal translocations

At least two breakpoints are expected in the reciprocal translocations, which may be in two homologous chromosomes or in two completely different non-homologous ones. The broken fragments of chromosomes are exchanged then join to a new location. As a result, two chromosomes of altered structure are created. However, this does not cause phenotypic changes, i.e. symptoms or disease in most cases. This is the case of balanced translocation. This phenomenon can be explained by just changing the position of the affected genes, not the genes themselves. Breakpoints are usually in non-coding regions, as the proportion of the coding regions of the human genome is <2%.

In cases where the breakpoint is within a gene, following the translocation the gene itself is affected, so the abnormal product - with different function, activity or amount, or perhaps unable to function - is responsible for the appearance of pathological traits, e.g. tumour formation.

The best example of reciprocal translocations leading to the formation of the *Philadelphia chromosome (Ph1)*, is between 9 and 22 chromosomes, its cytogenetic abbreviation is t(9,22)(q34,11). This translocation occurs in *chronic myeloid (CML)* or *acute lymphocytic leukemia (ALL)*. The breakpoint in chromosome 22 is in the *BCR* (breakpoint cluster region) gene, while the breakpoint of chromosome 9 affects in the *ABL* (Abelson murine leukemia) proto-oncogene. Since the ABL gene encodes a tyrosine kinase as the result of the translocation a *bcr / abl* fusion protein is produced which not only has a greater molecular weight than the original enzyme, but also a higher activity. In fact, during this translocation the well-regulated promoter of *ABL* gene is lost, and the gene permanently over expressed. Finally this leads to uncontrolled cell proliferation, i.e. the development of the tumour.

Another medically important example is the Burkitt's lymphoma caused mostly by Epstein-Barr virus. In this disease the *c-MYC* proto-oncogene coded by chromosome 8 is translocated to chromosome 14 or 2 or 22 [t(8,14) or t(8,2) and t(8,22)], where either the immunoglobulin heavy-chain (on chromosome 14) or Ig light chain genes -κ chain on chromosome 2 and λ chain on chromosome 22 are located. As genes coding the Ig chains are continuously transcribed, and therefore the translocated *c-MYC* - which encodes a transcription factor acting in heterodimeric form – is constantly over expressed, too and leads to the increase of cell proliferation, ultimately tumorigenesis. These two cases are examples of the relationship between translocations and proto-oncogenes, where the over expression of a normal protein (Burkitt's lymphoma), or regulation independent production of a fusion protein – although of normal function – (CML) is responsible for tumour formation.

If three instead of two breakpoints occur, insertional translocation or insertion takes place. Then one piece of the broken chromosome (2 breaks) is incorporated, inserted to the other chromosome (one break). Since human chromosome set consists of 46 chromosomes, and any piece of any of these chromosomes may change places, so it is obvious that the number of translocations is almost infinite. The special case of translocations is the Robertsonian translocation or centric fusion (Fig. 11.2.). In these structural chromosomal abnormalities only acrocentric chromosomes can be involved so in humans only one of the 13, the 14, the 15, the 21 and the 22 chromosomes. Not only the types of chromosomes involved, but the breakpoints are strictly determined: a break is always in the centromere or near to centromere. In this way abnormal - fusion - chromosomes can be formed, one of which initially can contain two centromeres (dicentric), but ultimately only one centromere remains active, the other is without a centromere,

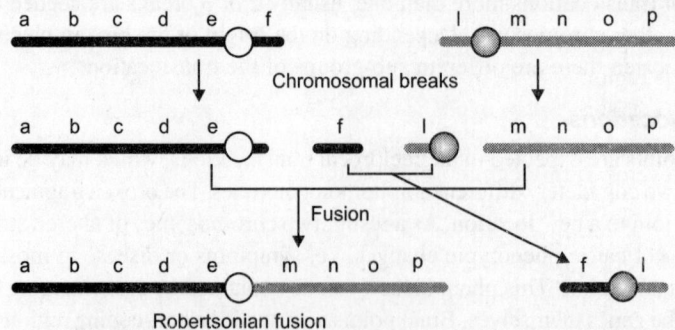

Fig. 11.2: Robertsonian translocation or centric fusion.

therefore it is lost during the subsequent divisions and thus the number of chromosomes is reduced. If the break is exactly in the centromere, a two centromeric, although rearranged chromosome is formed. As the result of the rearrangement from the initial acrocentrics two different sized, a larger and a smaller metacentric or submetacentric chromosome is created. The small submetacentric containing NOR (nucleolar organiser) regions on both arms is lost during successive divisions. However, since there are 10 NOR regions in the human genome, on the short arms of the acrocentric chromosomes therefore any loss of two does not lead to phenotypic change, that is, the centric fusion is balanced.

The centric fusion not only results in an abnormal chromosome structure, but the chromosome number is reduced from 45 to 46. Based on current cytogenetic evidence, chromosome number reduction occurred in hominid evolution can be explained by two consecutive centric fusions. While the great apes: gorillas, chimpanzees and orangutans have 48 chromosomes, humans have 46. This means that the centric fusion has had to occur after the line of apes and humans separated during evolution.

Inversions

The inversion is a structural chromosome aberration in which the same chromosome breaks twice and the fragment between the breakpoints turns 180 degrees. There are two types:

1. Pericentric
2. Paracentric inversion

In pericentric inversion the chromosome breakages are on both arms, that is on both sides of the centromere. The pericentric inversion of chromosome 9 is relatively common and found frequently in couples with recurrent abortions.

In paracentric inversion breakpoints are on the same arm of the chromosome, thus in the turn of the fragment the centromere is not involved. For both the para- as well as the pericentric inversion is true that the breakpoints are normally in non-coding regions, so the carriers have normal phenotype.

According to the present-day knowledge inversions also played a role in the evolution of human chromosomes, as some human chromosomes derived from the chromosomes of apes and old-world (Catharrinae) monkeys. Moreover, on the basis of presence or absence of such rearrangements (e.g. inv2) the Sumatran and Bornean orangutans are divided into two separate sub-species, and even today they are considered separate species.

Ring (Ring) Chromosome

In this case, there are breaks on both arms of the chromosome - usually near the telomeres - then broken ends fold and a ring chromosome is formed. The fragments broken are lost during successive divisions, so the information encoded by their genes as well. The carriers depending on the chromosome involved and the size of the region lost are more or less severely affected. The somatic retardation - a physical developmental retardation - can be explained by the fact that the DNA replication of the ring chromosome is often erroneous: interlocked (devil's) ring, giant ring (due to duplication), rearranged (recombinant) chromosome, or even two ring chromosomes within a cell, i.e. change in chromosome number will be the end result.

Isochromosome

The isochromosome is an abnormal chromosome containing the same genes on both arms. Upon formation the sister chromatids are not separated parallel to the long axis of the chromosome, and migrate towards the poles of the cell, but the plane of their separation is perpendicular to the longitudinal axis. Thus aberrant chromosomes ultimately cells containing them are formed which contain either the short arm or the long arm specific information only on both arms and the information of the other arm is lost. Since a chromosome arm is rich in many genes, so the surplus or the lack of these lead to severe, often lethal consequences. X and Y chromosomes seem to be exceptional since in most of the known viable isochromosome cases these chromosomes are involved. This is because the Y chromosome is relatively gene poor and the X chromosome inactivation has a compensating effect.

The above mentioned structural abnormalities are usually formed, except duplication, prior to DNA duplication (G1 phase), and therefore replication of damaged DNA leads to identical sister chromatids. Their separation at the end of mitosis results in identical chromosomal aberration carrying daughter cells. Although these types of aberrations can be formed in both mitosis and meiosis, in a strictly medical point of view the latter one is more important because gametes with chromosome mutations can lead to the birth of affected/mutant offspring. From amongst structural aberrations the translocations and inversions exist not only in balanced, asymptomatic forms. In the case of carriers however, the birth risk of chromosomally unbalanced, physically and mentally retarded child, with severe developmental abnormalities is very high. The symptoms often lead to intrauterine death so to spontaneous abortion or stillbirth. This is due to the difficult pairing of structurally deficient and normal homologous chromosomes in the first meiotic division (Fig. 11.3).

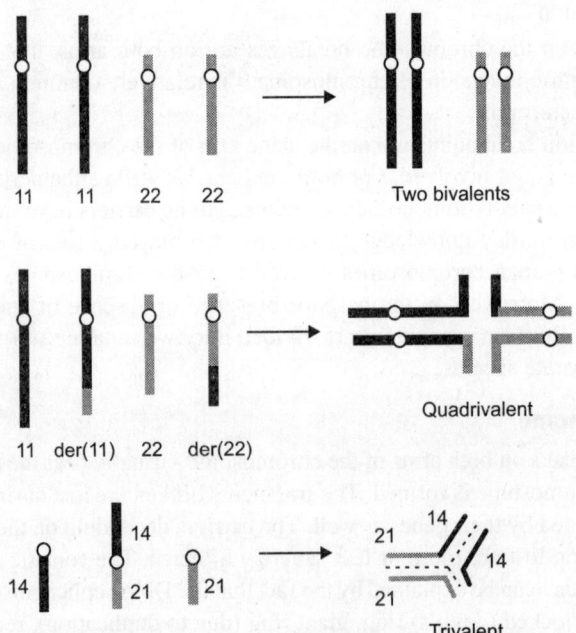

Fig. 11.3: Meiotic consequences of some translocations.

The most severe segregational abnormalities may also inhibit gametogenesis and thus cause *infertility, sterility*. The best example is the centric fusion between homologous acrocentric chromosomes. For example, from t(15,15) or t(14,14) Robertsonian translocations viable offspring cannot be born, from t(21,21) centric fusion either unviable or Down syndromic offspring can be born.

Dicentric Chromosome

A dicentric chromosome with two centromeres can be created not only by centric fusion - as mentioned above, but between the short arms of two non-homologous acrocentric chromosomes by non-homologous recombination. Since dicentric chromosomes cannot migrate to the appropriate poles at time of cell divisions, and through a still unclear mechanism one of the two centromeres is inactivated, and thus an abnormal chromosome having one centromere is maintained.

Acentric Fragment

More rarely broken fragments without a centromere remain in the cytoplasm as small fragments. Due to the absence of centromere such pieces cannot migrate to cell poles and either a so called micronucleus is formed or they are during the subsequent cell divisions, and finally only the deleted chromosomes has retained within the cell. Since these acentric fragments are most commonly induced by some chromosome breakage causing mutagenic agents such as radiation, therefore they can be used for testing the mutagenic effects (micronucleus test).

NUMERICAL CHROMOSOME ABERRATIONS

The numerical anomalies, when one or more chromosomes are in excess or missing, ultimately modify the entire genome size, so they can be considered genome mutations as well.

There are three types of numerical chromosome aberrations:

1. Euploid
2. Aneuploid
3. Mixoploid mutations

Euploid Chromosome Mutations

In the case of euploidy each chromosome is present in the same number, i.e. in a haploid cell everything is present only once, twice in diploids, three times in triploids and so on. The haploid chromosome number, i.e. typical of the gametes - is n, its exact multiples, that is, $2n$, $3n$, etc. found in the euploid somatic cells. Polyploidy means, if we find a multiple of n, either in gametes or in somatic cells. However, mutations only have arisen if the individuals or just the cell have chromosomes in a number different from the species specific (haploid or diploid) set. The multiplication of the chromosome set occurs in the M phase of the cell cycle due to the defects of microtubules and/or the abnormal organisation of mitotic spindle. In plants, polyploidy is compatible with normal life moreover it is economically quite advantageous, since the multiplication of chromosomes leads not only to the multiplication of genes, but also to the multiplication of their products. Thus the protein content and the crop yield grow, such as banana, wheat etc. In plant cells, the polyploidy found is either the result of that species' evolution or the result of conscious plant breeding work. For the induction of polyploidy spindle poisons - Colcemid, Colchicine, Vincristine, Vinblastine - alkaloids inhibiting the polymerisation of spindle microtubules can also be used. In this case *autopolyploidy* is created, since every chromosome is of the same species. In contrast, hybrids (e.g. wheat) established by crossing of species or related species are *allopolyploids*.

Unlike plants polyploidy in animals or in humans is lethal, leads to death in utero. With the exception of certain cells/tissues, for example bone marrow megakaryocytes and a part of the regenerating liver cells which are also polyploids. In these cases it is fixed during the millions of years of evolution what type of cell has the multiplication of chromosome number during ontogeny.

In 10% of the spontaneously aborted fetuses triploidy occurs. Interestingly, 90% of them is of paternal origin, derived either from fertilisation by a diploid sperm or from double fertilisation. Only a minority comes from fertilisation of a diploid egg.

Aneuploid Chromosomal Aberrations

Aneuploidy is a chromosomal abnormality when only a certain chromosome is in excess or missing. If there is only one chromosome instead of the normal two homologues we are talking about monosomy, if there are three copies trisomy occurs. If a particular chromosome is not found at all in a cell/organism nullisomy is present. The latter is lethal both in humans and animals, but in plants is not. Generally speaking, in humans/animals the excess of chromosomes is tolerated better than the chromosomal deficiency. Several somatic and especially sex chromosome aneuploidies - trisomies - occur in live-born, but only one - the X chromosomal monosomy (Turner syndrome) occurs in live-born. The aneupolid mutations are due to mitotic or meiotic non-disjunctions, when the sister chromatids or the chromosomes do not separate in the anaphase – because of the abnormality of the kinetochore, the centromere or both. Less frequently (uniparental disomy) a chromatid/chromosome lagging behind the others in the anaphase - anaphase lag - does not get to the right pole, and therefore not to the daughter cell.

Due to this one of the daughter cells is with an extra chromosome, while there is a deficiency in the other. Of course, from medical point of view meiotic non-disjunctions are more important as these lead to defective gametes, and finally to affected offspring. In the case of mitotic non-disjunction, it is crucial, when and in which cell type's division occurs. The early non-disjunction, eventually involving many cells/tissues leads to severe consequences (mosaicism).

The meiotic non-disjunctions are grouped according to when they occur – in the first or in the second meiotic division. In the first meiotic non-disjunction, some pairs of homologous chromosomes are not segregated, whereas in the second meiotic non-disjunction - as in mitotic non-disjunctions the sister chromatids are not separated. These have different consequences accordingly.

Following the first meiotic non-disjunction all four progeny cells - in spermatogenesis the four sperms will have an abnormal chromosome set – will be aneuploid. Two is with an additional chromosome ($n+1$), two is without one ($n-1$). In the second meiotic non-disjunction only the half of the daughter cells are affected. They will also be with an extra or an absent chromosome. The fusion of such abnormal gamete with a normal one results in trisomic or monosomic zygote.

In the case of trisomies there is difference in the origin of the three homologues depending on in which meiotic division the mutation took place. Trisomies derived from the first meiotic division all three homologues are of different origin (e.g. one is from the maternal grandmother, the other is from the maternal grandfather, and the third is inherited from the father). However, in trisomies from the second meiotic non- disjunction two homologues are identical (e.g. either from the maternal grandmother or from the maternal grandfather) and only the third comes from the other parent, from the father. 70% of the human aneuploid chromosome mutations are derived from the first and 30% from of the second meiotic non-disjunction. So most of the meiotic non-disjunctions occur during the first meiotic division and are of maternal origin. The frequency of maternal non-disjunctions and the aneuploid offspring (like Down syndrome) - increases with maternal age (Fig. 11.4). The reason of this lies in the characteristics of female gametogenesis: probably the aging of the synaptonemal complex, which reduces the chance of co-segregation of homologues leads to the formation of gametes with abnormal chromosome number. This is why above a certain maternal age (35–40) prenatal tests are recommended or required, to determine whether a fetus carries a numerical chromosome aberration or not.

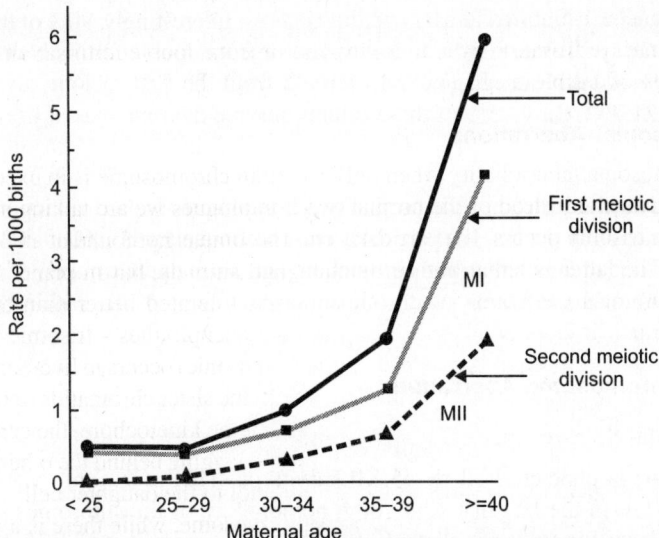

Fig. 11.4: Rate of meiotic non-disjunctions in function of maternal age.

Most Common Numerical Chromosomal Abnormalities

All chromosome trisomies except the one of the largest human chromosome (chromosome 1) were found in spontaneously aborted fetuses, among live born three autosomal trisomies and some involving sex chromosomes occur.

Two things are suggested by this: first, the fate of trisomies is strongly dependent on the number and type and function of genes present in the chromosome, on the other hand there is a strong intrauterine selection, so the most severely affected fetuses die in utero. These are confirmed by the fact that in spontaneously aborted fetuses the most common abnormalitiy is the trisomy 16, which although affects a relatively small chromosome, is never found in live born! All the monosomies, with the exception of the X chromosomal monosomy are incompatible with life.

Trisomy 21

Trisomy 21 is the cause of *Down syndrome*. Although the non-disjunction of chromosome 21 is not the only cause of Down syndrome - a smaller proportion of the cases is due to either centric fusion or translocation - it is the most common type. Despite the fact that trisomy 21 fetuses die in utero the average population frequency of Down syndrome is 1:650, but this value increases dramatically with maternal age, at 45 years of age it is more than 1:100!

Although today live-born trisomy 21 patients have more or less the same life expectancy than healthy individuals, but the leukemia and some other disease prevalence is higher among them than in the general population. In recent decades, there is a significant change in the social status of down syndromic individuals, whereas before they were excommunicated, teaching them was thought to be impossible, now increasing efforts have been made to facilitate their social integration (e.g. special kindergartens, in many countries they are taught together with healthy children in public school classes, sporting events etc.).

Trisomy 13

Trisomy 13 is the Patau syndrome. Similar to down syndrome it is most commonly derived from maternal non-disjunction. 65% of such non-disjunctions derived from the first meiotic division. Frequency of birth is 1:12 500–1:21 700. Only <5% of these infants survive the first year of life.

Trisomy 18

Trisomy 18 is the Edwards syndrome. It is primarily due to maternal non-disjunction. 95%! of the cases are due to non-disjunction in the first meiotic division. The frequency is 1:6000–1:10 000 live-born but the frequency at the time of conception can be much higher, since approximately 95% of the fetuses die within the womb 30% of the Edwards syndromic abnormal newborns die within one month, >95% of them die within a year.

Numerical Sex Chromosome Aberrations

Turner syndrome

The Turner syndrome is characterised by 45,X0 karyotype. This is the only viable monosomy. The explanation for this lies in the fact that while both homologues of the autosomes are necessary to the normal phenotype - so their monosomy is lethal – by contrast in females only one X chromosome is active (see the dose compensation in X inactivation), so a functional monosomy and Barr body negativity can be maintained. However, for the normal development of female sex characteristics both X chromosome is needed, as indicated by the symptoms of Turner syndrome. Although the frequency is 1:5000 in newborn female infants, the conception rate is much higher, but 99% of them spontaneously abort. This is in good agreement with the concepts of the viability of monosomies. 80% of these cases are due to paternal meiotic non-disjunctions, therefore in these patients only one maternal X chromosome is present.

While it is easy to understand the sexual development related characteristics of the syndrome, the low height is still not fully explained. It is assumed that a gene coding a protein of the small ribosome subunit (RPS4X) may also play a role. Because this gene has a Y chromosomal counterpart (RPS4Y) as well, both in normal females and males double dose of this ribosomal protein is produced. In Turner syndromic individuals less than sufficient amount is produced, and if the ribosome number is less than normal it will largely influence the production of other proteins, and thus indirectly the body height, too. Although Turner syndrome is often characterised by normal intelligence there is a difference in verbal skills, social integration between patients inherited their X chromosome from father or the mother. Maternal X carriers, according to surveys are weaker in these features than the patients inherited paternal X. The phenomenon is explained by the different methylation of the two types X chromosomes and the genomic imprinting.

Klinefelter syndrome

Klinefelter syndrome is characterised by 47,XXY karyotype and male phenotype. The frequency is 1:1000. Nearly it is derived with the same probability from maternal (56%) and paternal (44%) non-disjunction. 36% of the maternal non-disjunctions take place in the first meiotic division. Since there are two X chromosomes, thus they are Barr body positive. Their sterility can also be attributed to presence of 2 X chromosomes, since certain X chromosomal gene products are in a higher dose than in normal fertile males.

Triple X syndrome

Feminine phenotype and 47, XXX karyotype are present. 89% is of maternal, 8% is of paternal origin, and the remaining 3% is due to post-fertilisation mitotic non-disjunction. Neonatal frequency is 1:1000. Two Barr bodies are typical.

Double-Y syndrome, 'superman' or Jacobs syndrome

In this case normal, slightly taller than the average males have 47,XYY karyotype. The birth rate is 1:1000. They derived only from paternal second meiotic non-disjunction. In contrast to all meiotic non-disjunctions, the formation is not affected by age, as paternal gametogenesis is continuous from puberty, there are no aged sperms.

They are also featured by poorly tolerated frustration and stronger aggressivity, perhaps that is why this chromosome abnormality is found in greater numbers amongst imprisoned men. The aggressiveness and the possible criminal tendency are strongly debated, and it would only be 100% decided if the entire male population would be karyotyped and comparative data about their aggressivity would have been available as well. Today many different aggressiveness associated genes and gene mutations are known, that is why the role of the Y chromosome in aggressiveness is questioned.

Knowing the characteristics of meiotic division we could ask that the two aneuploidies (47,XXX and 47,XYY) with normal fertility are characterised by greater prevalence of similar disorders among offspring or not. For example, in the case of double Y syndrome the following karyotypes offspring are expected in the offspring: 2 XXY, 2 XY, 1 XX and 1 XYY. In contrast, birth of only normal offspring was reported so far, however its exact explanation is still not known.

UNIPARENTAL DISOMY (UPD)

This abnormality which is not or hardly identifiable by cytogenetic methods were recognised - due to molecular biological techniques - in the past decades. The UPD means that the person concerned has a normal chromosome number, but the homologues of a certain chromosome – in contrast to normal - are from the same parent, either from the father or from the mother. As for the formation two consecutive numerical aberrations are in the background: a meiotic non-disjunction and an anaphase lag occurring during the early cleavage divisions. So in fact a trisomic zygote is formed first, and subsequently the 3rd homologue is lost. Depending on whether first or second meiotic non-disjunction occurred, uniparental heterodisomy or uniparental isodisomy is present. The first case is when the child inherits two different homologues from the parent (one grandmaternal and one grandpaternal), that is non-disjunction occurred in the first meiosis. The latter is when the two homologues inherited are the same (either both are grandmaternal or grandpaternal) suggesting a second meiotic non-disjunction.

In UPD depending on the parental origin of the homologues, and due to genomic imprinting, different symptoms may be seen. The different symptoms in some of the Prader-Willi and Angelman syndrome cases are not due to the 15q deletion, but the UDP.

MIXOPLOID MUTATIONS

In mixoploidy or in mutations associated with mixed ploidy usually two (sometimes more) cell lines with different chromosome numbers are found within an organism. There are two forms: *mosaicism* and *chimerism*.

Mosaicism

In genetics a mosaic is a living creature, where two cell lines of different chromosome numbers, but of the same origin are present in the body. They are either *aneuploid or polyploid mosaics*. The former occurs as a result of mitotic non-disjunction or anaphase lag during cleavage, two cell lines of different chromosome number are formed, when one is normal and the other is aneuploid, generally trisomic. For example, assuming a two-cell embryo, if one cell is divided normally and the other is abnormally, then finally 2 normal and 1 trisomic and 1 monosomic cells are present. Since the monosomic cells are not viable eventually the ratio of the normal and the trisomic cells will be 2:1. In the case of *polyploid mosaicism* a normal and a polyploid (generally triploid / tetraploid) cell line are present. In this case, however mitotic spindle error leads to the formation of the aberration. Again, assuming a two-cell embryo, if one divides normally, the other not, ultimately there will be 3 cells instead of four, and two are normal and one is tetraploid.

Depending on the time the aberration occurs (during cleavage or in organogenesis or even later in development), the symptoms become more or less severe. So the proportion of normal and defective cells is crucial. Mosaicisms involving sex chromosomes are relatively common. In the case of *gonadal mosaicism* only the cells in the germ line have abnormal chromosome number, thus the risk of numerical aberrations in the offspring is high. Unfortunately, the detection of such defects is still not possible routinely, but the birth of an abnormal offspring of the patient can indicate this. Mosaicism in a broader sense is a somatic mutation, when different mutants (alleles) of a given gene are located in different organs or in different cells of the same organ (for example eyes with different colours: one is blue and the other is brown or a blue eye with brown spots).

Chimerism

After the lion-headed, bird-legged, snake-tailed monster of Greek mythology the creature that has two cell lines of different origin - derived from different zygotes - is called *chimera*. A chimera is derived either from fusion of fraternal twins, or from double fertilisation of an egg and a polar body (polocyte), or from transplacental haematopoietic stem cells exchange between fraternal twins (blood group chimerism). Recently, the chimera referred to as transgenic animals/plants, which contain cells of different origin, derived from either the fusion of few-cell-embryos, or via the microinjection of foreign genes into fertilised oocytes.

Recently several publications dealt with the phenomenon of *microchimerism*. It has been known for 25 years that in maternal body after being pregnant with a male fetus - after giving birth, and even after abortion - Y chromosome carrying or Y body-positive cells can be detected in the bloodstream. It is now found that these foreign cells in maternal body detected many years (decades!) later, not only survived, but probably also proliferated. This means that stem cells of the male fetus were transferred by the bloodstream to the mother's body, where they reached and adhered to certain organs and formed cell clones. Therefore a hypothesis is also suggested that some putative autoimmune diseases are actually not autoimmune but against the cells - 50% foreign to female body (immunologically incompatible) immune reaction are awoken. This also serves as an explanation why autoimmune diseases are more common in women. However, transplacental cell migration in the opposite direction (from mother to fetus) - cannot be excluded, and may play a role in the tolerance against alloantigenes, although its mechanism and consequences are not well known.

Chapter 12

Chromosomes, Chromatin and Genetic Linkage

INTRODUCTION

All cellular genetic material exists as a compact mass in a relatively confined volume. In bacteria, the genetic material is seen in the form of a nucleoid that forms a discrete clump within the cell. In eukaryotic cells, it is seen as the mass of chromatin within the nucleus at interphase. The packaging of chromatin is flexible and changes during the eukaryotic cell cycle. Interphase chromatin becomes even more tightly packaged at the time of division (mitosis or meiosis), when individual chromosomes become visible as discrete entities.

A chromosome is a device for segregating genetic material at cell division. The crucial structural feature by which this is accomplished is the centromere, often visible as a constriction in the length of the chromosome under the light microscope. At a greater level of detail, the centromere can be seen to include the kinetochore, a structure by which it is attached to microtubules. A eukaryotic chromosome usually consists of a very long linear segment of DNA, and another crucial feature is the telomere, which stabilises the ends and is extended by special mechanisms that by-pass the difficulties of replicating the ends of linear DNA. The density of DNA is high. In a bacterial nucleoid it is ~10 mg/mL, in a eukaryotic nucleus it is ~100 mg/mL, and in the head of the phage T4 virus it is >500 mg/mL. Such a concentration in solution is equivalent to a gel of great viscosity and has implications (not fully understood) for the ability of proteins to find their binding sites on DNA. The various activities of DNA, such as replication and transcription, must be accomplished within this confined space. The organisation of the material must accommodate transitions between inactive and active states.

Table 12.1 shows the range of genome sizes and makes the point that they are divided into chromosomes varying greatly in DNA content. The length of the DNA as an extended molecule would vastly exceed the dimensions of the region that contains it. Its condensed state results from its binding to basic proteins. The positive charges of these proteins neutralise the negative charges of the nucleic acid. The structure of the nucleoprotein complex is determined by the interactions of proteins that condense the DNA into a tightly coiled structure. Therefore, in contrast with the customary picture of DNA as an extended double helix, structural deformation of DNA to bend or fold into a more compact form is the rule rather than exception.

Table 12.1: The number of chromosomes in the haploid genome and the chromosome size vary extensively.

Organism	Genome (Mb)	Haploid chromosomes	Range of chromosome length (Mb DNA)	Total genes
E. coli	4.6	1	4.6	4401
S. cerevisiae	12.1	16	(0.2)–1.5	6702
D. melanogaster	165	4	(1.3)–28	14399
Rice	389	12	24–45	37544
Mouse	2500	20	60–195	26996
Man	2900	23	49–245	24194

Most chromatin has a relatively dispersed appearance, this material is called euchromatin, and it contains the majority of active genes. Some regions of chromatin are more densely packed, this material is called heterochromatin and is usually not transcriptionally active.

What is the general structure of chromatin, and what is the difference between active and inactive sequences? The high overall packing ratio of the genetic material immediately suggests that DNA cannot be directly packaged into the final structure of chromatin. There must be hierarchies of organisation. A major question concerns the specificity of packaging. Is the DNA folded into a particular pattern, or is it different in each individual copy of the genome? How does the pattern of packaging change when a segment of DNA is replicated or transcribed?

The building block of chromatin is the nucleosome, and it has the same fundamental structure in all eukaryotes. The nucleosome contains ~200 base pair (bp) of DNA, organised by an octamer of small, basic proteins into a beadlike structure. The protein components are the histones. They form an interior core, the DNA lies on the surface of the particle. Nucleosomes are an invariant component of euchromatin and heterochromatin in the interphase nucleus and of mitotic chromosomes. The nucleosome provides the first level of organisation. It packages 67 nm of DNA into a body of diameter 11 nm. Its components and structure are well characterised. A linear string of nucleosomes forms a structure referred to as the '10-nm fibre.' The second level of organisation is the coiling of the series of nucleosomes into a helical array to constitute the fibre of diameter ~30 nm that is found in interphase chromatin as well as in mitotic chromosomes. This condenses the nucleosomes by a factor of 6 to 73 per unit length.

The final packing ratio is determined by the third level of organisation, the packaging of the 30-nm fibre itself. Euchromatin is about 50 times more condensed relative to the 30-nm fibre. Euchromatin is cyclically interchangeable with packing into mitotic chromosomes, which are about 5–10 times more compact. Heterochromatin generally has the same packing density as mitotic chromosomes.

The mass of chromatin contains up to twice as much protein as DNA. Approximately half of the protein mass is accounted for by the nucleosomes. The mass of RNA is <10% of the mass of DNA. Much of the RNA consists of nascent transcripts still associated with the template DNA.

Changes in chromatin structure are accomplished by association with additional proteins or by modifications of existing chromosomal proteins. Both replication and transcription require unwinding of DNA and, thus, must involve an unfolding of the structure that allows the relevant enzymes to manipulate the DNA. This is likely to involve changes in all levels of organisation. The nonhistones include all the proteins of chromatin except the histones. Non-histones are more variable between tissues and species and comprise a smaller proportion of the mass than the histones. They also comprise a much larger number of proteins, so that any individual protein is present in amounts much smaller than any histone.

CHROMATIN IS DIVIDED INTO EUCHROMATIN AND HETEROCHROMATIN

Each chromosome contains a single, very long duplex of DNA that is folded into a fibre that runs continuously throughout the chromosome. In accounting for interphase chromatin and mitotic chromosome structure, we have to explain the packaging of a single, exceedingly long molecule of DNA into a form in which it can be transcribed and replicated and can become cyclically more or less compressed.

Individual eukaryotic chromosomes are visible as such only during the act of cell division, when each can be seen as a compact unit. (The sister chromatids are daughter chromosomes produced by the previous replication event, still joined together at this stage of mitosis.) Each consists of a fibre with a diameter of ~30 nm and a nubbly appearance. The DNA is 5–10 times more condensed in chromosomes than in interphase chromatin. During most of the life cycle of the eukaryotic cell, however, its genetic material occupies an area of the nucleus in which individual chromosomes cannot be distinguished. The 30-nm fibre from which chromatin is constructed is similar or identical to that of the mitotic chromosomes.

Chromatin can be divided into two types of material, which can be visualised by staining with DNA-specific dyes and are given below:

1. In most regions, the fibres are much less densely packed than in the mitotic chromosome. This material is called euchromatin. It has a relatively dispersed appearance in the nucleus and occupies most of the nuclear region.

2. Some regions of chromatin are very densely packed with fibres, displaying a condition comparable with that of the chromosome at mitosis. This material is called heterochromatin. It is typically found at centromeres but also occurs at other locations, such as telomeres and highly repetitive sequences. It passes through the cell cycle with relatively little change in its degree of condensation. It forms a series of discrete clumps, but often the various heterochromatic regions aggregate into a densely staining chromocenter.

The same fibres run continuously between euchromatin and heterochromatin, because these states represent different degrees of condensation of the genetic material. In the same way, euchromatic regions exist in different states of condensation during interphase and during mitosis. Therefore, the genetic material is organised in a manner that permits alternative states to be maintained side by side in chromatin and allows cyclic changes to occur in the packaging of euchromatin between interphase and division.

The structural condition of the genetic material is correlated with its activity. The common features of constitutive heterochromatin are as follows:

- It is permanently condensed.
- It often consists of multiple repeats of a few sequences of DNA that are not transcribed or are transcribed at very low levels.
- Probably resulting from the condensed state, it replicates later than euchromatin and has a reduced frequency of genetic recombination relative to euchromatic gene-rich areas of the genome.
- The density of genes in this region is very much reduced compared with euchromatin, and genes that are translocated into or near it are often inactivated. The one dramatic exception to this is the ribosomal DNA (rDNA) in the nucleolus, which has the general compacted appearance and behaviour of heterochromatin (such as late replication) yet is engaged in very active transcription.

Numerous molecular markers exist for changes in the properties of the DNA and protein components in heterochromatic regions. They include reduced acetylation of histone proteins, increased methylation at particular sites on histone proteins, and methylation of cytosine bases in specific regions of DNA. These molecular changes cause the condensation of the chromatin, which is responsible for its inactivity.

Although active genes are contained within euchromatin, only a subset of the sequences in euchromatin are transcribed at any time. Therefore, although location in euchromatin is necessary for expression of many genes, it is not sufficient for it. In addition to the general distributions observed for heterochromatin and euchromatin, studies have addressed whether there is an overall chromosome organisation within the nucleus. The answer in many cases is yes, chromosomes appear to occupy distinct three-dimensional spaces known as chromosome territories. The chromosomes occupying these territories are not entangled with each other but do share areas of interaction and some common functional organisation. For example, heterochromatic and other silent regions are found primarily at the nuclear periphery, whereas gene-dense regions are internally located. Active genes are often found at the borders of territories, sometimes clustered together in interchromosomal spaces that are enriched in transcriptional machinery, known as 'transcription factories.' How chromosome territories are established and how they vary by cell cycle and cell type are not yet understood.

CELL CYCLE AND REPLICATION OF GENOME

The period in the cell cycle when the genome is replicated (S phase) is crucially important for the establishment and maintenance of programmes of differential gene activity. Not only must DNA be replicated, but the chromosome itself must be duplicated. The majority of genes in the proliferating cell of a defined type retain the same states of transcriptional activity through cell division. This requires the duplication of the precise nucleoprotein complexes directing gene transcription or repression on the nascent DNA templates. The maintenance of these specific regulatory complexes through replication reflects the commitment of a defined cell type or line to a particular state of determination. Pre-existing chromosomal structures are transiently disrupted by transit through the replication elongation complex. Most of these structures are faithfully reassembled following replication through mechanisms discussed in this chapter. However, the transient disruption of these structures also offers a window of opportunity for modifying regulatory nucleoprotein complexes. These alterations can either activate genes through the disruption of repressed states, or direct the repression of previously active genes. Thus, cell division offers a molecular mechanism to redirect the commitment of a cell towards a particular determined state. A consideration of the processes occurring at the eukaryotic replication fork suggests how this important development process might be accomplished.

IMPLICATIONS OF DNA REPLICATION FOR STABLE STATES OF TRANSCRIPTIONAL ACTIVITY

Active and Repressed States of Eukaryotic Genes

The local nucleoprotein complexes required to maintain a eukaryotic gene in an active or repressed state have been defined in some detail. Transcriptional activity for a given gene depends on a number of sequence-specific transcription factors (e.g. SPI), structural proteins (e.g. HMGIE), and non-DNA binding proteins associated with the promoter interacting to recruit general transcription factors (e.g. TFIIA, TFIIB) together with the TFIID complex [containing TBP (TATA binding protein) and the TAFs (TATA associated factors)]. The assembly of this large nucleoprotein complex is initiated through the association of DNA-binding proteins and requires many intermediate steps leading to the recruitment of RNA polymerase II and, eventually, to transcription itself. Conversely, several features may determine a gene to be transcriptionally inactive. A common mechanism appears to be a deficiency in an essential component required for the assembly of the active complex. If this component is a DNA-binding protein, the cognate DNA sequence might become associated with the histone proteins. Specific nucleosomal structures assembled by the core histones (H2A, H2B, H3, and H4) might restrict the subsequent association of either sequence-specific DNA-binding proteins or the basal transcriptional machinery. Other proteins may stabilise repressive higher-order chromatin structures dependent on prior association of the core histones, these include linker histone variants or the chromodomain (chromatin modification organiser) proteins such as HPl and Polycomb. Generally, the assemblies of nucleosomes or transcription complexes on the promoter of a eukaryotic gene are mutually exclusive.

The prior assembly of nucleosomes can prevent transcription factors from binding to DNA and, conversely, the prior assembly of a transcription complex prevents nucleosome formation from repressing transcription (Fig. 12.1). Although these results provide an excellent molecular basis for the maintenance of stable states of gene expression in a terminally differentiated nondividing cell, they do not explain why either transcriptionally active or inactive states are assembled onto DNA in the first place, nor do they explain how such states can be propagated through cell division. Clearly, because both nucleoprotein structures can incorporate the same DNA molecule, the possibility exists of a competition occurring between the assembly of the two structures. This competition, in fact, occurs during the staged assembly of either active or repressed states following replication. Molecular mechanisms that influence the outcome of this competition direct the commitment of a cell to a particular state of determination or facilitate developmentally regulated switches in cell fate. However, to appreciate how this competition occurs, we must first discuss the consequences of DNA replication for pre-existing chromatin structures.

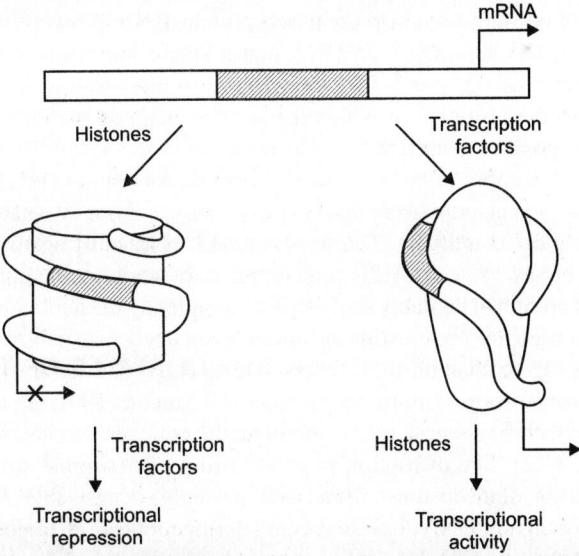

Fig. 12.1: Nucleosome assembly and transcription complex assembly are often mutually exclusive. Two alternate pathways are shown for the association of DNA-binding proteins with a promoter containing a TATA homology. The start site of transcription of mRNA is indicated by the bent arrow.

Impact of DNA replication on pre-existing chromatin structures

Chromatin consists of long arrays of nucleosomal DNA interspersed with specific regulatory nucleoprotein complexes. The replication fork moves through chromatin without apparent impediment. Replication fork progression disrupts pre-existing nucleosomes, however, the fate of regulatory nucleoprotein complexes depends on the particular structure examined.

Nucleosomes: Major considerations for pre-existing nucleosomes during the replication process are whether the histones present in the nucleosome stay together on nascent DNA, and whether nucleosomes are randomly or conservatively segregated to daughter DNA strands. DNA replication requires the transient unwinding of duplex parental DNA into two single-stranded regions. Although histones associate with single-stranded DNA, they do not assemble nucleosomes. This property, coupled with the competing protein-DNA interactions involved in DNA synthesis at the replication fork, probably accounts for nucleosome disruption. Histones released from the parental chromatin during replication *in vitro* can be easily sequestered onto competitor DNA. However, *in vivo* these histones are sequestered onto daughter DNA molecules close to the replication fork (Fig. 12.2). A nucleosome contains an octamer consisting of two molecules each of the four core histones (H2A, H2B, H3, and H4) and a single molecule of a fifth linker histone (Hl). The four core histones and the linker histone have very selective interactions with each other. Our most detailed understanding of nucleosomal architecture and construction has relied on *in vitro* experiments that have attempted to reconstruct nucleosomes with purified histones. These experiments have been informative, although they involve dialysis from high salt to low salt concentrations and do not employ the molecular chaperones used *in vivo*.

The central 'kernel' of the nucleosome is made up of two heterodimers of histones H3 and H4. Only when this 'tetramer' is bound to DNA can two heterodimers of H2A and H2B bind to complete assembly of the histone octamer. One heterodimer of H2A and H2B binds to either side of the histone tetramer in an interaction dependent on both protein-protein and protein-DNA contacts. Only when the complete octamer of core histones has assembled on DNA can a single molecule of linker histone be stably bound. The exact position of the linker histone within the nucleosome is currently the subject of controversy, however, in the one case in which it has been mapped within a specific nucleosome, it occupies an asymmetric position within the nucleosome.

In vivo a comparable assembly of the nucleosome occurs. A tetramer (H3, H4), and a dimer (H2A, H2B) are stable at physiological ionic strengths. However, they will not associate together in the absence of DNA under physiological conditions. The tetramer (H3, H4), must again associate with DNA on newly replicated DNA before H2A and H2B can complete the nucleosome core.

Histone H1 is the last protein to be stably sequestered, completing the nucleosome. Jackson determined that a substantial fraction of the pre-existing octamers associated with DNA within the chromosome *in vivo* fell apart following replication into dimers (H2A, H2B) and tetramers (H3, H4)2. Tetramers from these pre-existing nucleosomes rapidly reassociate with daughter DNA duplexes. Newly synthesised dimers (H2A, H2B) can then be sequestered to complete the octamer, mixing old and new histones into a single structure (Fig. 12.2). The disruption of pre-existing nucleosomal structure at the replication fork, coupled to dissociation of the histones from DNA, strongly suggests that the dispersive segregation of these histones to both daughter DNA duplexes occurs during replication. Importantly, the incorporation of pre-existing histone tetramers (H3, H4), into nascent chromatin provides a means of maintaining and propagating a stable state of gene activity. The old H3 and H4 present in the nascent chromatin retain their pre-existing posttranslational modification state. This differs from that of newly synthesised H3 and H4 and can potentially influence subsequent transcription of the associated DNA. The dispersive

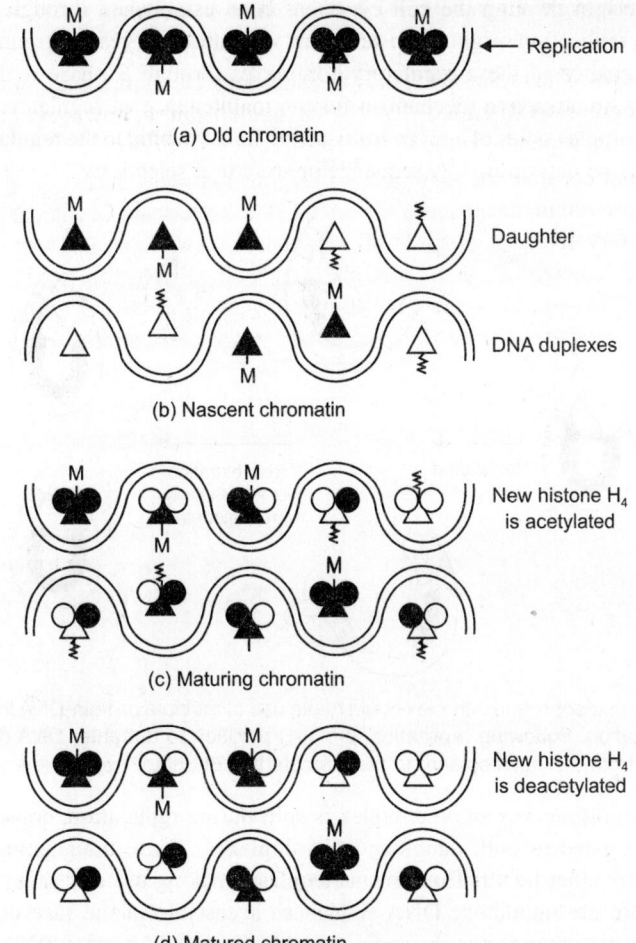

(a) Old chromatin

(b) Nascent chromatin

(c) Maturing chromatin

(d) Matured chromatin

← Replication

Daughter

DNA duplexes

New histone H_4 is acetylated

New histone H_4 is deacetylated

Fig. 12.2: Nucleosome disruption during replication and reassembly following replication. (a) Old chromatin consisting of pre-existing nucleosomes (histone octamer plus DNA) containing a tetramer (H3, H4), (filled triangle) and two dimers (H2A, H2B) (filled circles). The histones in the tetramer are modified (M). Replication displaces these histones from DNA, the octamer can fall apart into tetramers and dimers, (b) Nascent chromatin. Old tetramers associate with both daughter DNA duplexes. Newly synthesised tetramers (open triangles) containing diacetylated histone H4 (zigzag line) also associate with daughter DNA in a process facilitated by CAF-I, (c) Maturing chromatin. Old and new dimers (open circles) bind to the tetramers and (d) Matured chromatin. New tetramers are deacetylated.

segregation of 'old' histones coupled to maintenance of their pre-existing states of modification provides a molecular mechanism whereby an epigenetic imprint might be propagated through replication.

Regulatory complexes

A special case for a regulatory nucleoprotein complex maintaining association with DNA throughout the cell cycle is the protein assembly that regulates use of an origin of replication itself. Stable association of proteins with an origin through the cell cycle has been established through *in vivo* footprinting methodologies on the replication origin of Epstein-Barr virus and on a yeast chromosomal ARS element. Implicit in the maintenance of these regulatory complexes through S phase is the concept that they duplicate themselves. An attractive mechanism for the maintenance of regulatory complexes through replication requires multiple copies of a given *trans*-acting factor to bind to the regulatory DNA sequences (Fig. 12.3). This could be determined by sequence or structural selectivity.

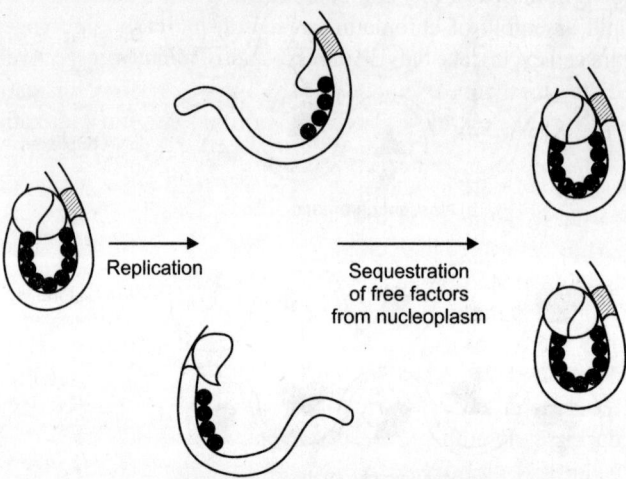

Fig. 12.3: A regulatory nucleoprotein complex could make use of multiple protein-DNA interactions to maintain integrity through replication. Following replication, proteins partition to daughter DNA duplexes. Free factors are then sequestered from the nucleoplasm to reassemble two daughter complexes.

If the pre-existing multimeric protein complex is split during replication, copies of the trans-acting factors could be segregated to both daughter DNA duplexes. These trans-acting factors could then either directly sequester other factors from the nucleoplasm making use of protein-protein interactions, or they could maintain the regulatory DNA sequences accessible in the face of ongoing chromatin assembly, such that when other factors became available they could bind to DNA. Structurally driven protein association is consistent with the maintenance of DNA distortion throughout the cell cycle at the Epstein-Barr viral origin.

In contrast to origin complexes, the basal transcriptional machinery appears to be removed from promoter elements by the passage of a replication fork. Replication is found to be dominant to the transcription process, and a direct consequence of replication fork progression through an active 5s rRNA gene is the displacement of transcription factors. Several correlations from *in vivo* work support the generality of this observation. There is a clear antagonism between transcription and replication on efficiently replicating SV40 DNA molecules. Replication forks invade the transcriptionally active ribosomal, RNA genes in yeast.

Thus, replication apparently resets the transcriptional status of a chromosome to 'ground zero.' The component protein molecules that determine transcriptional activity have to reassemble regulatory complexes *de novo* on the daughter DNA duplexes. This reassembly occurs not on naked DNA, but on a nascent chromatin template.

Chromatin Assembly has Replication-dependent and Independent Pathways

Replication-independent pathways

Early work on physiological chromatin assembly pathways made use of cell-free preparations from *Xenopus* oocytes and eggs. More recently, extracts of *Drosophila* embryos have been used with similar results. For both systems, chromatin assembly on non replicating DNA is relatively slow, taking several hours to assemble nucleosomes to a physiological density (one nucleosome per 180–200 bp). This contrasts with the rapid assembly of chromatin *in vivo* during early embryogenesis in *Xenopus* and *Drosophifa*, where entire cell cycles take only 30 minutes and 10 minutes, respectively. Thus, the molecular mechanisms that mediate chromatin assembly in the absence of DNA replication have questionable physiological relevance. Nevertheless, these systems have provided useful information on the biochemistry of the assembly process.

In *Xenopus* oocytes, histones are synthesised under the control of distinct regulatory mechanisms that operate outside of S phase. Tetramers (H3, H4), are stored in a complex with the molecular chaperone NUN2. Dimers (H2A, H2B) are stored in a complex with the chaperone nucleoplasmin. Both chaperones exchange histones onto DNA at physiological ionic strength. NUN2 must function before nucleoplasmin to assemble a nucleosome. During normal development, nucleoplasmin has a specialised role in the remodelling of *Xenopus* sperm chromatin, where it facilitates the exchange of sperm-specific basic proteins for histones H2A and H2B. Nucleoplasmin and NUN2 allow large amounts of histones to be stably sequestered in the Xenopus oocyte and egg, however, a role for these proteins in directly mediating chromatin assembly during early embryogenesis remains to be established.

Replication-dependent pathways

In vivo in normal somatic cells, the vast bulk of the histone proteins are synthesised during S phase. These histones are immediately assembled onto nascent DNA at the replication fork. Stillman discovered that the chromatin assembly process is coupled to replication. The molecular chaperone mediating the process is chromatin assembly factor 1 (CAF-1), which requires ongoing DNA replication to function. CAF-1 directs the association of the tetramer (H3, H4), with replicating DNA. Dimers (H2A/H2B) then bind in a CAF-1-independent process to complete the histone octamer. CAF-1 requires a modified tetramer (H3, H4), from the cytosol of human cells in order to function. This is potentially a key regulatory event in distinguishing the biochemistry of replication-dependent and independent chromatin assembly pathways. It is possible that the phosphorylation and diacetylation of histone H4 coupled to its synthesis may be necessary for chromatin assembly. Whether CAF-1 has specific interactions either with highly modified H4 and/or with the replication machinery itself are important questions yet to be resolved.

Almouzni and colleagues established that replication-coupled pathways of chromatin assembly also exist in Xenopus. However, the molecular chaperones that couple replication to chromatin assembly, such as the CAF-1 found in somatic cells, remain to be defined. These replication dependent pathways direct the efficient assembly of nucleosomes both *in vitro* and *in vivo* with kinetics that could easily accommodate a cell cycle duration of 30 minutes. The mechanism of enhanced assembly involves both the rapid deposition of the histone tetramer (H3, H4), and facilitation of the subsequent deposition of dimers (H2A, H2B). Similar results consistent with a facilitated two step assembly of chromatin have been obtained in mammalian systems. The *de novo* assembly of chromatin on replicating templates *in vitro* provides a useful independent confirmation of earlier work on the staged assembly of chromatin during S phase *in vivo*. As discussed earlier, DNA replication disrupts pre-existing nucleoprotein structures within the chromosome. Histones that are displaced during replication reassociate with newly synthesised DNA, but do so randomly on both daughter.

DNA duplexes: A consequence of this segregation is that nascent chromatin has a 50% enrichment of pre-existing histones. The remainder of the histones incorporated into chromatin are newly synthesised. Radio labelling of these newly synthesised histones has allowed the kinetics of their incorporation into chromatin and subsequent modification to be determined.

Newly synthesised and pre-existing histone tetramers (H3, H4), associate with nascent DNA, this is followed over the space of several minutes by the sequestration of both pre-existing and newly synthesised histone dimers (H2A, H2B). Thus, the majority of nucleosomes behind a replication fork are hybrids of both old and new core histones. Finally, a mixture of newly synthesised and pre-existing histone H1 stably associates with the nascent chromatin. The overall process of chromatin maturation as assayed by nuclease sensitivity requires as long as 10–20 minutes in a rapidly proliferating mammalian cell. Assuming a rate of replication fork movement of 0.5–1 kb of DNA per minute, this implies that 25–100 nucleosomes are present on both of the nascent DNA duplexes as 'immature' chromatin during S phase. The initial rapid deposition of old and new histones H3 and H4 on newly synthesised DNA reflects the nuclease-sensitive stage, whereas the subsequent deposition of histone dimers (H2A, H2B) and histone H1 correlates with the appearance of regular nucleosomal arrays and nuclease resistance. The sequential sequestration of histones is clearly once again related to the structure of the nucleosome, since the tetramer (H3, H4), forms the core of the structure, whereas histones H2A and H2B bind at the periphery of the nucleosome, and histone H1 can only associate in its proper place after two turns of DNA are wrapped around the core histones.

Newly synthesised histone H4 is phosphorylated and acetylated in the amino-terminal tail domain. Approximately 30 minutes after deposition during chromatin assembly, the diacetylated H4 is deacetylated to its mature form. If H4 deacetylation is inhibited, chromatin never achieves the nuclease resistance of bulk chromatin, indicative of the formation of stable higher order structures. Histone H1 may be less efficiently incorporated into chromatin containing acetylated H4. Thus, histone diacetylation is likely to maintain nascent chromatin in a structure that is more accessible to other DNA-binding proteins. In summary, chromatin assembly *in vivo* is coupled to replication, most probably through the activity of specific molecular chaperones such as CAF-1. Nucleosome assembly occurs in stages and involves transient posttranslational modifications of core histones synthesised during S phase.

Epigenetic Mechanisms: The Assembly of Active and Repressed Transcriptional States

In vivo experiments using *Saccharomyces* cerevisiae suggest that replication disassembles repressed chromatin states and facilitates the access of trans-acting factors to DNA. Other experiments using yeast suggest that replication has an essential role in facilitating the repression of specific genes. We have discussed how biochemical experiments indicate that replication introduces a dynamic aspect to chromosomal structure, both directing the disassembly of pre-existing structures and facilitating the assembly of nucleosomes. A central issue in gene regulation is how the assembly of nucleoprotein structures following replication can maintain or alter states of potential transcriptional activity.

Repression

Replication and transcription are most clearly seen to be linked in yeast. Components of the yeast origin recognition complex (ORC) regulate both the initiation of replication within the chromosome and the repression of transcription within the same chromosomal domain. The molecular mechanisms responsible for the repression of transcription directed by ORC are unknown. Two possible explanations are: (i) that the ORC compartmentalises adjacent chromatin into a transcriptionally incompetent environment within the nucleus and (ii) that the ORC influences the type of chromatin assembled adjacent to it. The ORC complex may be a greatly streamlined version of the replication factories of larger eukaryotes. These replication factories represent special nuclear compartments at which proteins involved in the replication process are sequestered. It is possible that a gene adjacent to the origin is directed by the ORC to reside in a replication-competent but transcriptionally incompetent environment. Alternatively, if replication itself is essential for transcriptional repression, then the coupling of chromatin assembly to the replication process could contribute to repression. Pre-existing transcriptionally active complexes would be displaced by the replication fork. *trans*-Acting factors would then have to compete for assembly against the deposition of histones. *In vivo* and *in vitro* experiments in Xenopus demonstrate that the coupling of nucleosome assembly to replication can very effectively repress basal transcription. As discussed earlier, the ORC complex provides one biological example of the maintenance of sequence specific or structure-dependent protein-DNA interactions through the replication process.

However, since the ORC also serves to initiate the replication process, maintenance of the ORC may occur under circumstances distinct from the transcription complexes or chromatin structures that are exposed to the fully assembled replication-elongation complex. We have discussed how the histones already on the template during replication are segregated randomly to the daughter DNA duplexes, but within the context of small groups of nucleosomes. This maintenance of histone modification states potentially influences transacting factor access to DNA. Moreover, if proteins that modify the subsequent folding of nucleosomal arrays or that modify histones themselves, for example, by acetylation or deacetylation, are also partitioned in this way, the properties of a chromatin domain might be stably propagated. For example, histone H4 acetylation may interfere with the association of histone H1 with chromatin. Histone H1 is known to repress specific genes *in vivo*. Other proteins that might recognise properties of the 'old' histones within nascent chromatin include the chromodomain proteins that initiate the formation of heterochromatin. These are also good candidates for propagating pre-existing states of chromatin-mediated transcriptional repression (Fig. 12.4).

Activation

In vitro experiments using cell-free preparations of *Xenopus* eggs indicate that stable states of gene activity can be propagated in a nuclear environment. How might this occur? The simplest situation leading to continued gene activity would be the case in which a superabundance of transcription factors specific for a given gene was available within the nucleus throughout the cell cycle, including S phase. The factors would always be able to bind to their regulatory elements should they become accessible, recruiting the basal transcriptional machinery to the nascent promoter DNA, and thereby preventing histones or other proteins from binding to the TATA homology. Several features of nascent chromatin facilitate the association of transcription factors. For example, the complex of the 5s rRNA gene with the tetramer (H3, H4), is not repressive to transcription, whereas the complete octamer of core histones (H2A, H2B, H3, H4), is repressive at high densities of octamers bound to DNA. Moreover, acetylation of the core histones facilitates transcription factor access to DNA even when the complete octamer is bound. The histone tetramer (H3, H4), recognises the DNA sequences that position the nucleosome containing the 5s rRNA gene, hence it is probable that the formation of a specific chromatin structure also has a role in allowing transcription factors access to the template. Thus, following replication, it is probable that sequence-specific DNA-binding proteins have an opportunity to reassociate with daughter DNA molecules

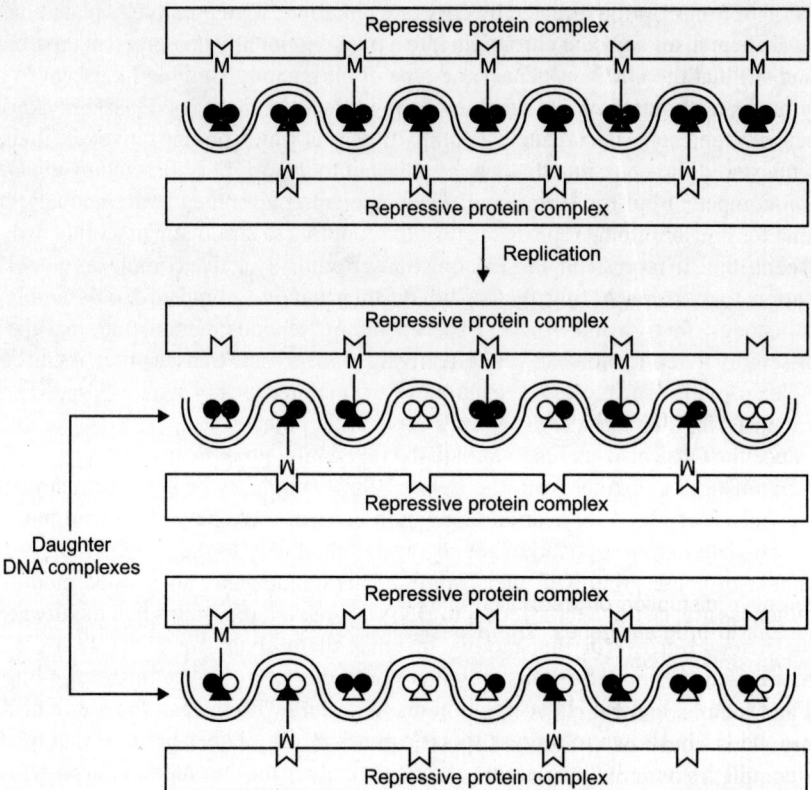

Fig. 12.4: Pre-existing histone modifications could provide an epigenetic imprint. A repressive protein complex (e.g. containing chromodomain proteins) recognises a histone modification (M). Following replication, modified histones are segregated to both daughter DNA duplexes sufficient to sustain interaction with the repressive protein complex.

(Fig. 12.5). Replication might under certain circumstances facilitate gene activation. The regulated activity of a transcription factor, such that it becomes able to bind to DNA or to function during S phase, could lead to transcription activation in a way that is replication-dependent. In a developmental context, this event might be coupled to a particular embryonic cleavage cycle or to a regulated period of cell division. For example, in *Caenorhabditis elegans* and the sea urchin, replication events are correlated with changes in the commitment of cells to a particular developmental fate. Similar changes can occur in differentiated cells that express one set of specialised genes and that can switch to another programme of gene expression only after one or more cell divisions. However, replication events are not necessarily essential for changing gene expression within a particular cell. This is not surprising, since chromatin structure is not completely inert *in vivo*. Histones H2A, H2B, and H1 are known to exchange with a pool of free histones in a cell. Complexes of DNA with only histones H3 and H4 therefore exist for a limited amount of time. However, a comparison of the rate and efficiency of gene activation in the presence or absence of cell proliferation has not yet been made. The maintenance of specific transcription factor-DNA interactions through replication, as discussed earlier for the ORC, might be facilitated by considering the promoter,

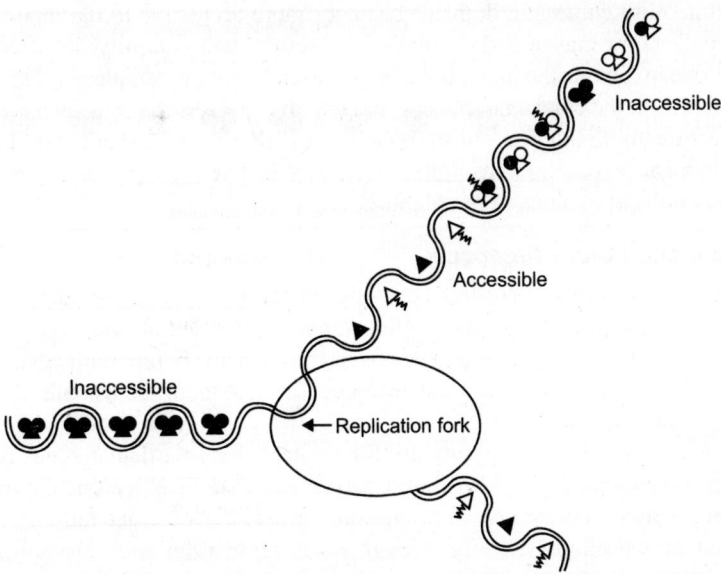

Fig. 12.5: Replicative disruption of preexisting chromatin structures provides a window of opportunity for transcription factors to program genes. The accessibility of nascent, maturing, and mature chromatin to *trans*-acting factors is indicated.

the enhancer, and locus control regions not as separate entities, but as contributory components to a single structure. This could be achieved through protein-protein interactions between the distinct nucleoprotein complexes assembled at each regulatory element. One reason for the separation of these regulatory elements over extensive distances may be that any single structure might be independently disrupted by DNA replication, while the other would remain intact. If protein binding to one sequence element influences the binding of proteins to the other, then the intact nucleoprotein complex might facilitate the re-formation of the disrupted one.

Replication timing

Chromatin organisation outside the ORC may also have significance for the initiation of replication and the timing of this initiation in S phase. If replication disrupts both active and repressed chromatin structures, then the entire nucleus has to be remodelled after each replication event. If there are limiting transcription factors available in a cell, then a gene that is replicated early in S phase has more opportunity for the assembly of an active transcription complex than a gene that replicates late. This is simply because the gene that replicates early is available for transcription factors to bind before all of the early-replicating portion of the genome has sequestered these factors. A late-replicating gene therefore experiences a relative deficiency in factor availability. Conversely, it is also possible that the type of chromatin assembled early in S phase is more accessible to transcription factors than chromatin assembled late in S phase. For example, earlyreplicating chromatin may sequester histones that are more highly acetylated and, consequently, more accessible to the transcription factors that maintain continued transcription activity. Transcriptionally active genes replicate early in S phase. The reason for this early replication is unknown, but possibilities include the local disruption of chromatin structure by transcription complexes, such that the DNA within those chromatin domains becomes more accessible to the replication machinery. Many transcription factors may also be replication factors, consequently, local concentrations of transcription factors may favour the assembly of replication initiation complexes. The issue very much is one of which came first: the chicken or the egg, or both? It is possible to argue that active transcription complexes open chromatin to admit replication factors, or, alternatively, that these sites are replicated first and are thus more accessible to transcription factors. Whether either or both of the much discussed mechanisms operate *in vivo* remains to be established.

Current Problems and Future Prospects

Chromatin structure is now realised to reflect a dynamic interaction between the many protein complexes that both organise DNA and fulfill regulatory roles. A much simplified picture suggests that replication disrupts local chromatin structures that pre-exist on the chromosome before replication. The subsequent reassembly of the nucleosome necessitates a staged process using modified histones that might be more accessible to transcription factors.

This would provide a window of opportunity for reestablishing particular states of transcriptional activity. On a more global scale (>1–2 kb), chromatin proteins that retain a particular modification (e.g. acetylation) or that cooperatively influence chromosome structure toward activation or repression could provide an imprint on chromatin activity through DNA replication and chromosome duplication. Replication is established as having a major impact on pre-existing nucleoprotein structures and a major role in their reassembly. Although significant attention has been given to the enzymology of the duplication of DNA, relatively little progress has been made concerning the enzymology of chromosomal duplication. The molecular mechanisms of chromatin assembly are not defined in any detail. The definition of molecular chaperones such as CAF-1 is a major advance, however, how CAF-1 functions is unknown. Does CAF-1 have a catalytic or structural role? Does it interact with the elongation complex? What are the special features of the histones that allow CAF-1 to utilise them for nucleosome assembly? On a more mundane level, we do not know the precise sequences or structures of the histone proteins necessary for chromatin assembly. The enzymes that transform nascent chromatin into a mature structure are yet to be defined at the molecular level. How mature chromatin is recognised by other proteins that influence states of gene repression, such as the chromodomain proteins, is unknown.

The impact of DNA replication on gene expression is readily analysed through yeast genetics, however, homologous biochemical systems are currently lacking to test the many hypotheses proposed to explain the phenomena observed. Much progress in the biochemistry of yeast replication can be anticipated. The further reconstruction of determinative events in development will require continued consideration of the fate of regulatory nucleoprotein complexes during replication. This is an important focus for future research. At a biochemical level, *in vitro* systems capable of maintaining states of gene expression through replication offer considerable promise. The future clearly has the exciting prospect of understanding and thus reconstructing chromosomal duplication in all its complexity at a molecular level.

GENETIC LINKAGE

Two genes are used to be linked if they are located on the same chromosome. Genetic linkage is the tendency of DNA sequences that are close together on a chromosome to be inherited together during the meiosis phase of sexual reproduction. Two genetic markers that are physically near to each other are unlikely to be separated onto different chromatids during chromosomal crossover, and are therefore said to be more linked than markers that are far apart. In other words, the nearer two genes are on a chromosome, the lower the chance of recombination between them, and the more likely they are to be inherited together. Markers on different chromosomes are perfectly unlinked.

Genetic linkage is the most prominent exception to Gregor Mendel's Law of Independent Assortment. The first experiment to demonstrate linkage was carried out in 1905. At the time, the reason why certain traits tend to be inherited together was unknown. Later work revealed that genes are physical structures related by physical distance. The typical unit of genetic linkage is the centimorgan (cM). A distance of 1 cM between two markers means that the markers are separated to different chromosomes on average once per 100 meiotic product, thus once per 50 meioses.

DISCOVERY OF GENETIC LINKAGE

Gregor Mendel's Law of Independent Assortment states that every trait is inherited independently of every other trait. But shortly after Mendel's work was rediscovered, exceptions to this rule were found. In 1905, the British geneticists William Bateson, Edith Rebecca Saunders and Reginald Punnett cross-bred pea plants in experiments similar to Mendel's. They were interested in trait inheritance in the sweet pea and were studying two genes—the gene for flower colour (P, purple, and p, red) and the gene affecting the shape of pollen grains (L, long, and l, round). They crossed the pure lines PPLL and ppll and then self-crossed the resulting PpLl lines. According to Mendelian genetics, the expected phenotypes would occur in a 9:3:3:1 ratio of PL:Pl:pL:pl. To their surprise, they observed an increased frequency of PL and pl and a decreased frequency of Pl and pL (Table 12.2).

Table 12.2: Bateson, saunders, and punnett experiment.

Phenotype and genotype	Observed	Expected from 9:3:3:1 ratio
Purple, long (P_L_)	284	216
Purple, round (P_ll)	21	72
Red, long (ppL_)	21	72
Red, round (ppll)	55	24

Their experiment revealed linkage between the P and L alleles and the p and l alleles. The frequency of P occurring together with L and p occurring together with l is greater than that of the recombinant Pl and pL. The recombination frequency is more difficult to compute in an F2 cross than a backcross, but the lack of fit between observed and expected numbers of progeny in the above table indicate it is less than 50%. This indicated that two factors interacted in some way to create this difference by masking the appearance of the other two phenotypes. This led to the conclusion that some traits are related to each other because of their near proximity to each other on a chromosome. This provided the grounds to determine the difference between independent and codependent alleles.

The understanding of linkage was expanded by the work of Thomas Hunt Morgan. Morgan's observation that the amount of crossing over between linked genes differs led to the idea that cross over frequency might indicate the distance separating genes on the chromosome. The centimorgan, which expresses the frequency of crossing over, is named in his honour.

Linkage Map

A linkage map (also known as a genetic map) is a table for a species or experimental population that shows the position of its known genes or genetic markers relative to each other in terms of recombination frequency, rather than a specific physical distance along each chromosome. Linkage maps were first developed by Alfred Sturtevant, a student of Thomas Hunt Morgan. A linkage map is a map based on the frequencies of recombination between markers during cross over of homologous chromosomes. The greater the frequency of recombination (segregation) between two genetic markers, the further apart they are assumed to be. Conversely, the lower the frequency of recombination between the markers, the smaller the physical distance between them. Historically, the markers originally used were detectable phenotypes (enzyme production, eye colour) derived from coding DNA sequences, eventually, confirmed or assumed noncoding DNA sequences such as microsatellites or those generating restriction fragment length polymorphisms (RFLPs) have been used.

Linkage maps help researchers to locate other markers, such as other genes by testing for genetic linkage of the already known markers. In the early stages of developing a linkage map, the data are used to assemble linkage groups, a set of genes which are known to be linked. As knowledge advances, more markers can be added to a group, until the group covers an entire chromosome. For well-studied organisms the linkage groups correspond one-to-one with the chromosomes. A linkage map is not a physical map (such as a radiation reduced hybrid map) or gene map.

Linkage Analysis

Linkage analysis is a genetic method that searches for chromosomal segments that cosegregate with the ailment phenotype through families and is the analysis technique that has been used to determine the bulk of lipodystrophy genes. It can be used to map genes for both binary and quantitative traits. Linkage analysis may be either parametric (if we know the relationship between phenotypic and genetic similarity) or non-parametric. Parametric linkage analysis is the traditional approach, whereby the probability that a gene important for a disease is linked to a genetic marker is studied through the LOD score, which assesses the probability that a given pedigree, where the disease and the marker are cosegregating, is due to the existence of linkage (with a given linkage value) or to chance. Non-parametric linkage analysis, in turn, studies the probability of an allele being identical by descent with itself.

Parametric linkage analysis

The LOD score (logarithm (base 10) of odds), developed by Newton Morton, is a statistical test often used for linkage analysis in human, animal, and plant populations. The LOD score compares the likelihood of obtaining the test data if the two loci are indeed linked, to the likelihood of observing the same data purely by chance. Positive LOD scores favour the presence of linkage, whereas negative LOD scores indicate that linkage is less likely. Computerised LOD score analysis is a simple way to analyse complex family pedigrees in order to determine the linkage between Mendelian traits (or between a trait and a marker, or two markers).

The method is described in greater detail by Strachan and Read. Briefly, it works as follows:

1. Establish a pedigree
2. Make a number of estimates of recombination frequency
3. Calculate a LOD score for each estimate
4. The estimate with the highest LOD score will be considered the best estimate

The LOD score is calculated as follows:

$$LOD = Z = \log_{10} \frac{\text{Probability of birth sequence with a given linkage value}}{\text{Probability of birth sequence with no linkage}} = \log_{10} \frac{(1-\theta)^{NR} \times \theta^{R}}{0.5^{(NR+R)}}$$

NR denotes the number of non-recombinant offspring, and R denotes the number of recombinant offspring. The reason 0.5 is used in the denominator is that any alleles that are completely unlinked (e.g. alleles on separate chromosomes) have a 50% chance of recombination, due to independent assortment. 'θ' is the recombinant fraction, i.e. the fraction of births in which recombination has happened between the studied genetic marker and the putative gene associated with the disease. Thus, it is equal to R/(NR + R) By convention, a LOD score greater than 3.0 is considered evidence for linkage, as it indicates 1000 to 1 odds that the linkage being observed did not occur by chance. On the other hand, a LOD score less than -2.0 is considered evidence to exclude linkage. Although it is very unlikely that a LOD score of 3 would be obtained from a single pedigree, the mathematical properties of the test allow data from a number of pedigrees to be combined by summing their LOD scores. A LOD score of 3 translates to a p-value of approximately 0.05, and no multiple testing correction (e.g. Bonferroni correction) is required.

Limitations

Linkage analysis has a number of methodological and theoretical limitations that can significantly increase the type-1 error rate and reduce the power to map human quantitative trait loci (QTL). While linkage analysis was successfully used to identify genetic variants that contribute to rare disorders such as Huntington disease, it didn't perform that well when applied to more common disorders such as heart disease or different forms of cancer. An explanation for this is that the genetic mechanisms affecting common disorders are different from those causing rare disorders.

Recombination Frequency

Recombination frequency is a measure of genetic linkage and is used in the creation of a genetic linkage map. Recombination frequency (θ) is the frequency with which a single chromosomal cross over will take place between two genes during meiosis. A centimorgan (cM) is a unit that describes a recombination frequency of 1%. In this way we can measure the genetic distance between two loci, based upon their recombination frequency. This is a good estimate of the real distance. Double crossovers would turn into no recombination. In this case we cannot tell if crossovers took place. If the loci we're analysing are very close (less than 7 cM) a double crossover is very unlikely. When distances become higher, the likelihood of a double crossover increases. As the likelihood of a double crossover increases we systematically underestimate the genetic distance between two loci.

During meiosis, chromosomes assort randomly into gametes, such that the segregation of alleles of one gene is independent of alleles of another gene. This is stated in Mendel's Second Law and is known as the law of independent assortment. The law of independent assortment always holds true for genes that are located on different chromosomes, but for genes that are on the same chromosome, it does not always hold true. As an example of independent assortment, consider the crossing of the pure-bred homozygote parental strain with genotype AABB with a different pure-bred strain with genotype aabb. A and a and B and b represent the alleles of genes A and B. Crossing these homozygous parental strains will result in F1 generation offspring that are double heterozygotes with genotype AaBb. The F1 offspring AaBb produces gametes that are AB, Ab, aB, and ab with equal frequencies (25%) because the alleles of gene A assort independently of the alleles for gene B during meiosis. Note that 2 of the 4 gametes (50%)—Ab and aB—were not present in the parental generation. These gametes represent recombinant gametes. Recombinant gametes are those gametes that differ from both of the haploid gametes that made up the original diploid cell. In this example, the recombination frequency is 50% since 2 of the 4 gametes were recombinant gametes.

The recombination frequency will be 50% when two genes are located on different chromosomes or when they are widely separated on the same chromosome. This is a consequence of independent assortment. When two genes are close together on the same chromosome, they do not assort independently and are said to be linked. Whereas genes located on different chromosomes assort independently and have a recombination frequency of 50%, linked genes have a recombination frequency that is less than 50%. As an example of linkage, consider the classic experiment by William Bateson and Reginald Punnett.

They were interested in trait inheritance in the sweet pea and were studying two genes—the gene for flower colour (P, purple, and p, red) and the gene affecting the shape of pollen grains (L, long, and l, round). They crossed the pure lines PPLL and ppll and then self-crossed the resulting PpLl lines. According to Mendelian genetics, the expected phenotypes would occur in a 9:3:3:1 ratio of PL:Pl:pL:pl. To their surprise, they observed an increased frequency of PL and pl and a decreased frequency of Pl and pL (Table 12.3).

Table 12.3: Bateson and punnett experiment.

Phenotype and genotype	Observed	Expected from 9:3:3:1 ratio
Purple, long (P_L_)	284	216
Purple, round (P_ll)	21	72
Red, long (ppL_)	21	72
Red, round (ppll)	55	24

Their experiment revealed linkage between the P and L alleles and the p and l alleles. The frequency of P occurring together with L and with p occurring together with l is greater than that of the recombinant Pl and pL. The recombination frequency is more difficult to compute in an F2 cross than a backcross, but the lack of fit between observed and expected numbers of progeny in the above table indicate it is less than 50%.

The progeny in this case received two dominant alleles linked on one chromosome (referred to as coupling or cis arrangement). However, after crossover, some progeny could have received one parental chromosome with a dominant allele for one trait (e.g. Purple) linked to a recessive allele for a second trait (e.g. round) with the opposite being true for the other parental chromosome (e.g. red and Long). This is referred to as repulsion or a trans arrangement. The phenotype here would still be purple and long but a test cross of this individual with the recessive parent would produce progeny with much greater proportion of the two crossover phenotypes. While such a problem may not seem likely from this example, unfavourable repulsion linkages do appear when breeding for disease resistance in some crops.

The two possible arrangements, cis and trans, of alleles in a double heterozygote are referred to as gametic phases, and phasing is the process of determining which of the two is present in a given individual. When two genes are located on the same chromosome, the chance of a crossover producing recombination between the genes is related to the distance between the two genes. Thus, the use of recombination frequencies has been used to develop linkage maps or genetic maps.

However, it is important to note that recombination frequency tends to underestimate the distance between two linked genes. This is because as the two genes are located farther apart, the chance of double or even number of crossovers between them also increases. Double or even number of crossovers between the two genes results in them being cosegregated to the same gamete, yielding a parental progeny instead of the expected recombinant progeny.

Variation of Recombination Frequency

While recombination of chromosomes is an essential process during meiosis, there is a large range of frequency of cross overs across organisms and within species. Sexually dimorphic rates of recombination are termed heterochiasmy, and are observed more often than a common rate between male and females. In mammals, females often have a higher rate of recombination compared to males. It is theorised that there are unique selections acting or meiotic drivers which influence the difference in rates. The difference in rates may also reflect the vastly different environments and conditions of meiosis in oogenesis and spermatogenesis.

Meiosis indicators

With very large pedigrees or with very dense genetic marker data, such as from whole-genome sequencing, it is possible to precisely locate recombinations. With this type of genetic analysis, a meiosis indicator is assigned to each position of the genome for each meiosis in a pedigree. The indicator indicates which copy of the parental chromosome contributes to the transmitted gamete at that position. For example, if the allele from the 'first' copy of the parental chromosome is transmitted, a '0' might be assigned to that meiosis. If the allele from the 'second' copy of the parental chromosome is transmitted, a '1' would be assigned to that meiosis. The two alleles in the parent came, one each, from two grandparents. These indicators are then used to determine identical-by-descent (IBD) states or inheritance states, which are in turn used to identify genes responsible for diseases.

Chapter 13

Extrachromosomal DNA

INTRODUCTION

Extrachromosomal DNA is any DNA that is found outside of the nucleus of a cell. It is also referred to as extranuclear DNA or cytoplasmic DNA. Most DNA in an individual genome is found in chromosomes but DNA found outside of the nucleus also serves important biological functions.

In prokaryotes, nonviral extrachromosomal DNA is primarily found in plasmids whereas in eukaryotes extrachromosomal DNA is primarily found in organelles. Mitochondrial DNA is a main source of this extrachromosomal DNA in eukaryotes. Extrachromosomal DNA is often used in research of replication because it is easy to identify and isolate.

Extrachromosomal DNA was found to be structurally different from nuclear DNA. Cytoplasmic DNA is less methylated than DNA found within the nucleus. It was also confirmed that the sequences of cytoplasmic DNA was different from nuclear DNA in the same organism, showing that cytoplasmic DNAs are not simply fragments of nuclear DNA. In addition to DNA found outside of the nucleus in cells, infection of viral genomes also provides an example of extrachromosomal DNA.

PROKARYOTES

Although prokaryotic organisms do not possess a membrane bound nucleus like the eukaryotes, they do contain a nucleoid region in which the main chromosome is found. Extrachromosomal DNA exists in prokaryotes outside of the nucleoid region as circular or linear plasmids. Bacterial plasmids are typically short sequences, consisting of 1 kilobase (kb) to a few hundred kb segments, and contain an origin of replication which allows the plasmid to replicate independently of the bacterial chromosome.

Figure 13.1 shows the total number of a particular plasmid within a cell is referred to as the copy number and can range from as few as two copies per cell to as many as several hundred copies per cell. Circular bacterial plasmids are classified according to the special functions that the genes encoded on the plasmid provide. Fertility plasmids, or f plasmids, allow for conjugation to occur whereas resistance plasmids, or r plasmids, contain genes that convey resistance to a variety of different antibiotics such as ampicillin and tetracycline. There also exists virulence plasmids that contain the genetic elements necessary for bacteria to become pathogenic as well as degradative plasmids that harbour the genes that

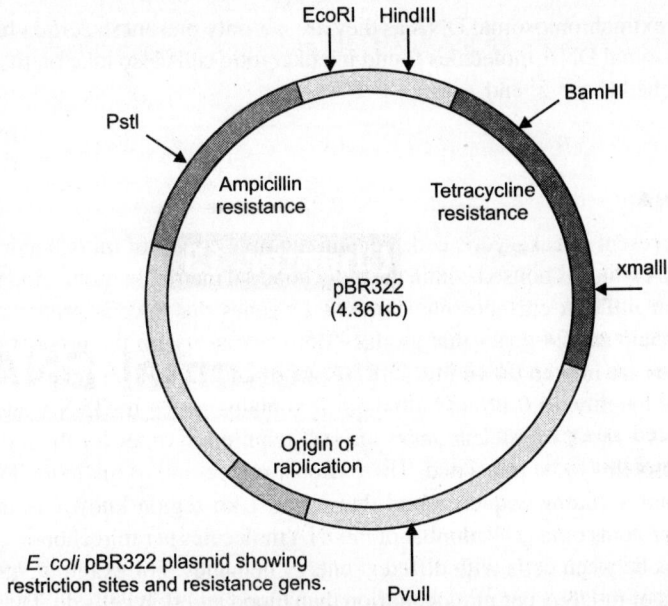

E. coli pBR322 plasmid showing
restriction sites and resistance gens.

Fig. 13.1: pBR32 plasmid of *E. coli*.

allow bacteria to degrade a variety of substances such as aromatic compounds and xenobiotics. Bacterial plasmids can also function in pigment production, nitrogen fixation and the resistance to heavy metals in those bacteria that possess them.

Naturally occurring circular plasmids can be modified to contain multiple resistance genes and several unique restriction sites, making them valuable tools as cloning vectors in biotechnology applications. Circular bacterial plasmids are also the basis for the production of DNA vaccines. Plasmid DNA vaccines are genetically engineered to contain a gene which encodes for an antigen or a protein produced by a pathogenic virus, bacterium or other parasite. Once delivered into the host, the products of the plasmid genes will then stimulate both the innate immune response and the adaptive immune response of the host. The plasmids are often coated with some type of adjuvant prior to delivery to enhance the immune response from the host.

Linear bacterial plasmids have been identified in several species of spirochete bacteria, including members of the genus *Borrelia* (to which the pathogen responsible for Lyme disease belongs), several species of the gram positive soil bacteria of the genus *Streptomyces*, and in the gram negative species *Thiobacillus* versutus, a bacterium that oxidises sulphur. The linear plasmids of prokarykotes are found either containing a hairpin loop or a covalently bonded protein attached to the telomeric ends of the DNA molecule. The adenine-thymine rich hairpin loops of the *Borrelia* bacteria range in size from 5 kilobase pairs (kb) to over 200 kb and contain the genes responsible for producing a group of major surface proteins, or antigens, on the bacteria that allow it to evade the immune response of its infected host. The linear plasmids which contain a protein that has been covalently attached to the 5′ end of the DNA strands are known as invertrons and can range in size from 9 kb to over 600 kb consisting of inverted terminal repeats. The linear plasmids with a covalently attached protein may assist with bacterial conjugation and integration of the plasmids into the genome. These types of linear plasmids represent the largest class of extrachromosomal DNA as they are not only present in certain bacterial cells, but all linear extrachromosomal DNA molecules found in eukaryotic cells also take on this invertron structure with a protein attached to the 5' end.

EUKARYOTES

Mitochondrial DNA

The mitochondria present in eukaryotic cells contain multiple copies of mitochondrial DNA (Fig. 13.2) referred to as mtDNA which is housed within the mitochondrial matrix. In multicellular animals, including humans, the circular mtDNA chromosome contains 13 genes that encode proteins that are part of the electron transport chain and 24 genes that produce RNA necessary for the production of mitochondrial proteins; these genes are broken down into 2 tRNA genes and 22 mRNA genes. The size of an animal mtDNA plasmid is roughly 16.6 kb and although it contains genes for tRNA and mRNA synthesis, proteins produced as a result of nuclear genes are still required in order for the mtDNA to replicate or for mitochondrial proteins to be translated. There is only one region of the mitochondrial chromosome that does not contain a coding sequence and that is the 1 kb region known as the D-loop to which nuclear regulatory proteins bind. The number of mtDNA molecules per mitochondria varies from species to species as well as between cells with different energy demands. For example, muscle and liver cells contain more copies of mtDNA per mitochondrion than blood and skin cells do. Due to the proximity of the electron transport chain within the mitochondrial inner membrane and the production of reactive oxygen species (ROS), and due to the fact that the mtDNA molecule is not bound by or protected by

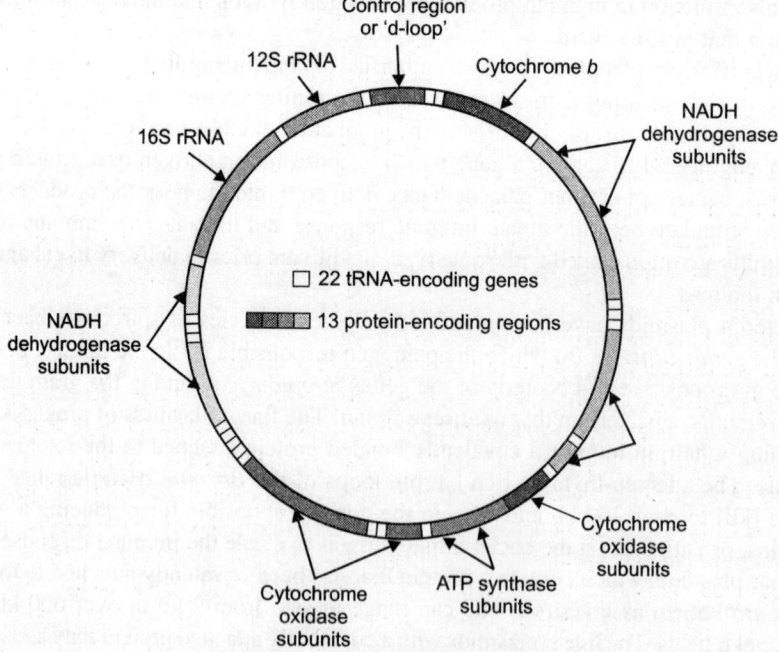

Fig. 13.2: Mitochondrial DNA.

histones, the mtDNA is more susceptible to DNA damage than nuclear DNA. In cases where mtDNA damage does occur, the DNA can either be repaired via base excision repair pathways, or the damaged mtDNA molecule is destroyed (without causing damage to the mitochondrion since there are multiple copies of mtDNA per mitochondrion).

The standard genetic code by which nuclear genes are translated is universal, meaning that each 3-base sequence of DNA codes for the same amino acid regardless of what species from which the DNA comes. However, this universal nature of the code is not the case with mitochondrial DNA found in fungi and animals. While most of the 3-base sequences in the mtDNA of these organisms do code for the same amino acids as those of the nuclear genetic code, there are some mtDNA sequences that code for amino acids different from those of their nuclear DNA counterparts. Some of the coding differences found in the mtDNA sequences of mammals, fruit flies and yeasts are outlined in the Table 13.1. The coding differences are thought to be a result of chemical modifications in the transfer RNAs that interact with the messenger RNAs produced as a result of transcribing the mtDNA sequences.

Table 13.1: Mitochondrial genetic code variations.

RNA codon	Nuclear genetic code	mtDNA genetic code		
		Mammals	*Drosophila*	*Yeasts*
UGA	Stop	Tryptophan	Tryptophan	Tryptophan
AGA, AGG	Arginine	Stop	Serine	Arginine
AUA	Isoleucine	Methionine	Methionine	Methionine
AUU	Isoleucing	Methionine	Methionine	Methionine
CUU, CUC CUA, CUG	Leucine	Leucine	Leucine	Threonine

Chloroplast DNA

Eukaryotic chloroplasts, as well as the other plant plastids, also contain extrachromosomal DNA molecules. Most chloroplasts house all of their genetic material in a single ringed chromosome, however in some species there is evidence of multiple smaller ringed plasmids. A recent theory that questions the current standard model of ring shaped chloroplast DNA (cpDNA), suggests that cpDNA may more commonly take a linear shape. A single molecule of cpDNA can contain anywhere from 100–200 genes and varies in size from species to species. The size of cpDNA in higher plants is around 120–160 kb. The genes found on the cpDNA code for mRNAs that are responsible for producing necessary components of the photosynthetic pathway as well as coding for tRNAs, rRNAs, RNA polymerase subunits, and ribosomal protein subunits. Like mtDNA, cpDNA is not fully autonomous and relies upon nuclear gene products for replication and production of chloroplast proteins. Chloroplasts contain multiple copies of cpDNA and the number can vary not only from species to species or cell type to cell type, but also within a single cell depending upon the age and stage of development of the cell. For example, cpDNA content in the chloroplasts of young cells, during the early stages of development where the chloroplasts are in the form of indistinct proplastids, are much higher than those present when that cell matures and expands, containing fully mature plastids.

Extrachromosomal Circular DNA

Extrachromosomal circular DNA (eccDNA) is present in all eukaryotic cells, is usually derived from genomic DNA, and consists of repetitive sequences of DNA found in both coding and non-coding regions of chromosomes. EccDNA can vary in size from less than 2000 base pairs to more than 20,000 base pairs. In plants, eccDNA contains repeated sequences similar to those that are found in the centromeric regions of the chromosomes and in repetitive satellite DNA. In animals, eccDNA molecules have been shown to contain repetitive sequences that are seen in satellite DNA, 5S ribosomal DNA and telomere DNA. Certain organisms, such as yeast, rely on chromosomal DNA replication to produce eccDNA whereas eccDNA formation can occur in other organisms, such as mammals, independently of the replication process. The function of eccDNA has not been widely studied, but it has been proposed that the production of eccDNA elements from genomic DNA sequences adds to the plasticity of the eukaryotic genome and can influence genome stability, cell aeging and the evolution of chromosomes.

VIRUSES

Viral DNA is an example of extrachromosomal DNA. Understanding viral genomes is very important for understanding the evolution and mutation of the virus. Some viruses, such as HIV and oncogenetic viruses, incorporate their own DNA into the genome of the host cell. Viral genomes can be made up of single stranded DNA (ssDNA), double stranded DNA (dsDNA) and can be found in both linear and circular form. One example of infection of a virus constituting as extrachromosomal DNA is the human papillomavirus (HPV). The HPV DNA genome undergoes three distinct stages of replication: establishment, maintenance and amplification. HPV infects epithelial cells in the anogenital tract and oral cavity. Normally, HPV is detected and cleared by the immune system. The recognition of viral DNA is an important part of immune responses. For this virus to persist, the circular genome must be replicated and inherited during cell division.

Recognition of Viral Extrachromosomal DNA by Host Cell

Cells can recognise foreign cytoplasmic DNA. Understanding the recognition pathways has implications towards prevention and treatment of diseases. Cells have sensors that can specifically recognise viral DNA such as the Toll-like receptor (TLR) pathway.

The Toll Pathway was recognised, first in insects, as a pathway that allows certain cell types to act as sensors capable of detecting a variety of bacterial or viral genomes and PAMPS (pathogen-associated molecular patterns). PAMPs are known to be potent activators of innate immune signalling. There are approximately 10 human Toll-Like Receptors (TLRs). Different TLRs in human detect different PAMPS: lipopoly-sacchardies by TLR4, viral dsRNA by TLR3, viral ssRNA by TLR7/TLR8, viral or bacterial unmethylated DNA by TLR9. TLR9 has evolved to detect CpG DNA commonly found in bacteria and viruses and to initiate the production of IFN (type I interferons) and other cytokines.

INHERITANCE

Inheritance of extrachromosomal DNA differs from the inheritance of nuclear DNA found in chromosomes. In humans, virtually all of the cytoplasm is inherited from the egg of the mother. For this reason, organelle DNA, including mtDNA, is inherited from the mother. Mutations in mtDNA or other cytoplasmic DNA will also be inherited from the mother. This uniparental inheritance is an example of non-Mendelian inheritance. Plants also show uniparental mtDNA inheritance. Most plants inherit mtDNA maternally with one noted exception being the redwood Sequoia sempervirens that inherits mtDNA paternally. There are two theories why the paternal mtDNA is not transmitted to the offspring. One is simply the fact that paternal mtDNA is at such a lower concentration than the maternal mtDNA and thus it is not detectable in the offspring. A second, more complex theory, involves the digestion of the paternal mtDNA to prevent its inheritance. It is theorised that the uniparental inheritance of mtDNA, which has a high mutation rate, might be a mechanism to maintain the homoplasmy of cytoplasmic DNA.

MEDICINE AND DISEASE

Sometimes called EEs, extrachromosomal elements, have been associated with genomic instability in eukaryotes. Small polydispersed DNAs (spcDNAs) are commonly found in conjunction with genome instability. SpcDNAs are derived from repetitive sequences such as satellite DNA, retrovirus-like DNA elements, and transposable elements in the genome. They are thought to be the products of gene rearrangements. Double Minute Chromosomes (DMs) are also extrachromosomal elements that are associated with genome instability. DMs are commonly seen in cancer cells. DMs are thought to be produced through breakages in chromosomes or over replication of DNA in an organism. Studies show that in cases of cancer and other genomic instability, higher levels of EEs can be observed. Mitochondrial DNA can play a role in the onset of disease in a variety of ways. Point mutations in or alternative gene arrangements of mtDNA have been linked to several diseases that affect the heart, central nervous system, endocrine system, gastrointestinal tract, eye, and kidney. Loss of the amount of mtDNA present in the mitochondria can lead to a whole subset of diseases known as mitochondrial depletion syndromes (MDDs) which affect the liver, central and peripheral nervous systems, smooth muscle and hearing in humans. There have been mixed, and sometimes conflicting, results in studies that attempt to link mtDNA copy number to the risk of developing certain cancers. Studies have been conducted that show an association between both increased and decreased mtDNA levels and the increased risk of developing breast cancer. A positive association between increased mtDNA levels and an increased risk for developing kidney tumours has been observed but there does not appear to be a link between mtDNA levels and the development of stomach cancer.

Extrachromosomal DNA is found in Apicomplexa, which is a group of protozoa. The malaria parasite (genus Plasmodium), the AIDS-related pathogen (Taxoplasma and Cryptosporidium) are both members of the Apicomplexa group. Mitochondrial DNA (mtDNA) was found in the malaria parasite. There are two forms of extra-chromosomal DNA found in the malaria parasites. One of these is 6-kb linear DNA and the second is 35-kb circular DNA. These DNA molecules have been researched as potential nucleotide target sites for antibiotics.

REPLICATION OF LINEAR GENOMES

All known DNA polymerases are unable to initiate synthesis of a DNA strand without a pre-existing 'primer' sequence. Circular genomes overcome this limitation fairly easily, either by nicking one strand and using the exposed 3' end as a primer or by opening the duplex at an origin, starting with an RNA primer, and then replicating around the circle back to the starting point. The original RNA can be removed by DNA polymerase I via nick translation because the newly replicated strand returns back to the origin. Not all genomes, however, are circular. Numerous linear genomes exist, including eukaryotic chromosomes, some bacteriophages, and some viruses. Full replication of linear genomes is a logistical problem (Fig. 13.3), however, because a primer is needed for DNA polymerase. With circular chomomosomes, RNA primers can be easily removed and replaced because the newly synthesised strand returns to the origin and can serve as a primer for DNA polymerase I to replace the ribonucleotides of the RNA primer with deoxyribonucleotides. There is no loss of nucleotides in this process.

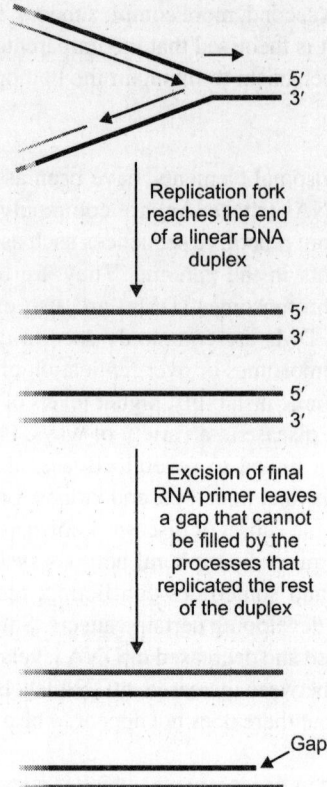

Fig. 13.3: The problem of completing the 5′ end in copying a linear DNA molecule.

If linear chromosomes employ RNA to initiate replication at the chromosomal termini, either they must have some mechanism for replacing the RNA with DNA or they must lose a bit of DNA with each round of replication. In reality, eukaryotic chromosomes opt for the latter scheme, losing a bit of the end of each chromosome (called a telomere) with each round of replication. Telomeres contain many repeats of a small oligonucleotide sequence and do not appear to code for any genes. The enzyme called telomerase can rebuild telomeres that have been shortened, to some extent, but it does not appear to be active in most cells. Fortunately, telomeric sequences are fairly long, so our cells can undergo a considerable amount of replication without loss of important coding sequences.

Viruses with linear DNA sequences have come up with a variety of mechanisms for fully replicating the ends of their chromosome. Two of these are depicted in Fig. 13.4. Bacteriophages T4 and T7 contain terminally redundant DNA sequences that, in single-stranded form, can create concatemers (Fig. 13.4a, Step3) that regenerate full terminal repeat sequences by recombination. Bacteriophage 29 and the adenoviruses employ a completely different strategy (Fig. 13.4b). They solve the problem by using a novel priming system that employs a protein covalently attached to the 5′-most nucleotide of each strand. In this case, there is no RNA that has to be removed because the terminal nucleotide that initiates the replication is a deoxyribonucleotide.

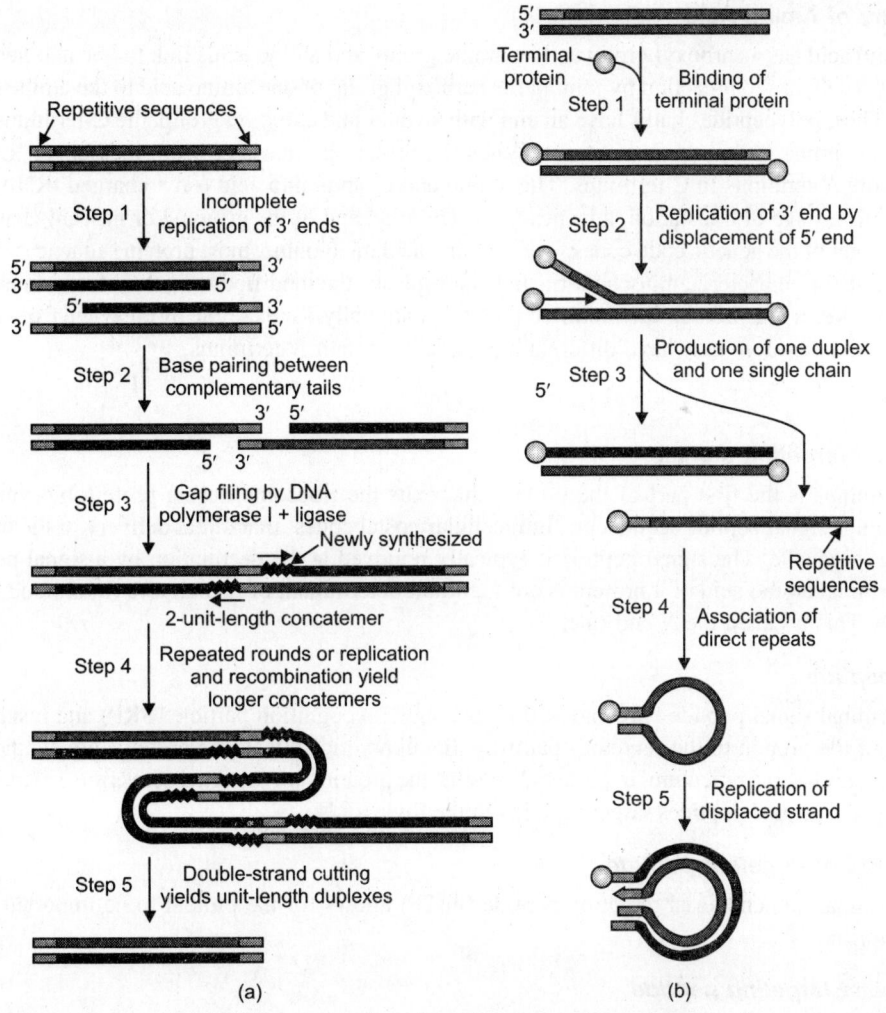

Fig. 13.4: Mechanisms for replication of linear DNAs.

Poxviruses solve the problem in yet another way (Fig. 13.4b). The two strands of their linear genome are covalently linked together. Bidirectional replication generates the duplex intermediate (step 3) and dual strand cutting and rearrangement regenerates the original structure.

N-TERMINUS

The *N*-terminus (also known as the amino-terminus, NH$_2$-terminus, *N*-terminal end or amine-terminus) refers to the start of a protein or polypeptide terminated by an amino acid with a free amine group (–NH$_2$). The convention for writing peptide sequences is to put the *N*-terminus on the left and write the sequence from *N*- to C-terminus. When the protein is translated from messenger RNA, it is created from *N*-terminus to C-terminus.

Chemistry of Amino Acid

Each amino acid has a carboxyl group and an amine group, and amino acids link to one another to form a chain by a dehydration reaction by joining the carboxyl group of one amino acid to the amine group of the next. Thus, polypeptide chains have an end with an unbound carboxyl group, the C-terminus, and an end with an amine group, the *N*-terminus. When the protein is translated from messenger RNA, it is created from *N*-terminus to C-terminus. The amino end of an amino acid (on a charged tRNA) during the elongation stage of translation, attaches to the carboxyl end of the growing or nascent chain. Since the start codon of the genetic code codes for the amino acid methionine, most protein sequences start with a methionine (or, in bacteria, mitochondria and chloroplasts, the modified version *N*-formylmethionine, fMet). However, some proteins are modified post-translationally, for example by cleavage from a protein precursor, and therefore may have different amino acids at their *N*-terminus.

Function

N-terminal targeting signals

The *N*-terminus is the first part of the protein that exits the ribosome during protein biosynthesis. It often contains signal peptide sequences, 'intracellular postal codes' that direct delivery of the protein to the proper organelle. The signal peptide is typically removed at the destination by a signal peptidase. The *N*-terminal amino acid of a protein is an important determinant of its half-life (likelihood of being degraded). This is called the *N*-end rule.

Signal peptide

The *N*-terminal signal peptide is recognised by the signal recognition particle (SRP) and results in the targeting of the protein to the secretory pathway. In eukaryotic cells, these proteins are synthesised at the rough endoplasmic reticulum. In prokaryotic cells, the proteins are exported across the cell membrane. In chloroplasts, signal peptides target proteins to the thylakoids.

Mitochondrial targeting peptide

The *N*-terminal mitochondrial targeting peptide (mtTP) allows for the protein to be imported into the mitochondrion.

Chloroplast targeting peptide

The *N*-terminal chloroplast targeting peptide (cpTP) allows for the protein to be imported into the chloroplast.

N-terminal Modifications

Some proteins are modified post-translationally by the addition of membrane anchors that allow the protein to associate with membrane without having a transmembrane domain. The *N*-terminus (as well as the C-terminus) of a protein can be modified this way.

N-myristoylation

The *N*-terminus can be modified by the addition of a myristoyl anchor. Proteins that are modified this way contain a consensus motif at their *N*-terminus as a modification signal.

N-acylation

The N-terminus can also be modified by the addition of a fatty acid anchor to form N-acylated proteins. The most common form of such modification is the addition of a palmitoyl group.

C-TERMINUS

The C-terminus (also known as the carboxyl-terminus, carboxy-terminus, C-terminal tail, C-terminal end, or COOH-terminus) is the end of an amino acid chain (protein or polypeptide), terminated by a free carboxyl group (–COOH). When the protein is translated from messenger RNA, it is created from N-terminus to C-terminus.

The convention for writing peptide sequences is to put the C-terminal end on the right and write the sequence from N- to C-terminus (Fig. 13.5).

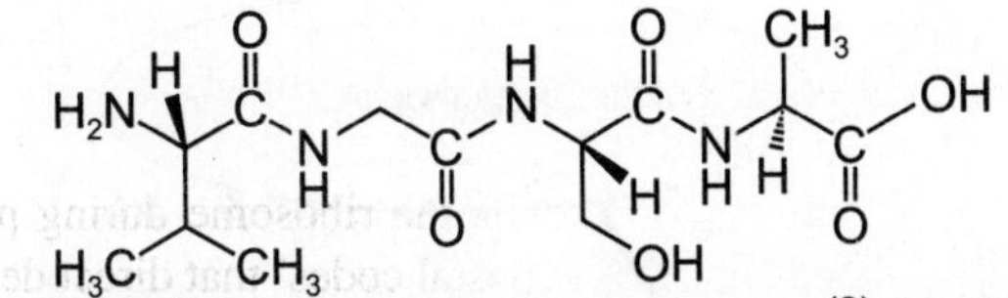

Fig. 13.5: A tetrapeptide (example: Val-Gly-Ser-Ala) with (1) highlighted N-terminal α-amino acid (example: L-valine) and (2) marked C-terminal α-amino acid (example: L-alanine).

Each amino acid has a carboxyl group and an amine group, and amino acids link to one another to form a chain by a dehydration reaction by joining the amine group of one amino acid to the carboxyl group of the next. Thus polypeptide chains have an end with an unbound carboxyl group, the C-terminus, and an end with an amine group, the N-terminus. Proteins are naturally synthesised starting from the N-terminus and ending at the C-terminus.

Function

C-terminal retention signals

While the N-terminus of a protein often contains targeting signals, the C-terminus can contain retention signals for protein sorting. The most common ER retention signal is the amino acid sequence -KDEL (or -HDEL) at the C-terminus, which keeps the protein in the endoplasmic reticulum and prevents it from entering the secretory pathway.

C-terminal modifications

The C-terminus of proteins can be modified post-translationally, most commonly by the addition of a lipid anchor to the C-terminus that allows the protein to be inserted into a membrane without having a transmembrane domain.

Prenylation

One form of C-terminal modification is prenylation. During prenylation, a farnesyl- or geranylgeranyl-isoprenoid membrane anchor is added to a cysteine residue near the C-terminus. Small, membrane-bound G proteins are often modified this way.

GPI anchors

Another form of C-terminal modification is the addition of a phosphoglycan, glycosyl-phosphati-dylinositol (GPI), as a membrane anchor. The GPI anchor is attached to the C-terminus after proteolytic cleavage of a C-terminal propeptide. The most prominent example for this type of modification is the prion protein.

C-terminal domain

The C-terminal domain (or carboxyl tail domain, CTD) of some proteins has specialised functions. The CTD of RNA polymerase II typically consists of up to 52 repeats of the sequence Tyr-Ser-Pro-Thr-Ser-Pro-Ser. Other proteins often bind the C-terminal domain of RNA polymerase in order to activate polymerase activity. It is the protein domain which is involved in the initiation of DNA transcription, the capping of the RNA transcript, and attachment to the spliceosome for RNA splicing (Fig. 13.6).

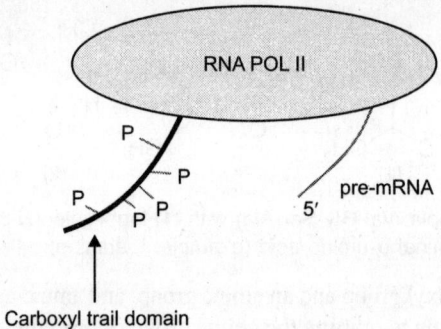

Fig. 13.6: RNA POL II in action.

ROLLING CIRCLE REPLICATION

Rolling circle replication describes a process of unidirectional nucleic acid replication that can rapidly synthesise multiple copies of circular molecules of DNA or RNA, such as plasmids, the genomes of bacteriophages, and the circular RNA genome of viroids. Some eukaryotic viruses also replicate their DNA via a rolling circle mechanism.

Circular DNA Replication

Rolling circle DNA replication is initiated by an initiator protein encoded by the plasmid or bacteriophage DNA, which nicks one strand of the double-stranded, circular DNA molecule (Fig. 13.7) at a site called the double-strand origin, or DSO. The initiator protein remains bound to the 5′ phosphate end of the nicked strand, and the free 3′ hydroxyl end is released to serve as a primer for DNA synthesis by DNA polymerase III. Using the unnicked strand as a template, replication proceeds around the circular DNA molecule, displacing the nicked strand as single-stranded DNA. Displacement of the nicked strand is carried out by a host-encoded helicase called PcrA (the abbreviation standing for plasmid copy reduced) in the presence of the plasmid replication initiation protein. Continued DNA synthesis can produce multiple single-stranded linear copies of the original DNA in a continuous head-to-tail series called a concatemer. These linear copies can be converted to double-stranded circular molecules through the following process: First, the initiator protein makes another nick to terminate synthesis of the first (leading) strand. RNA polymerase and DNA polymerase III then replicate the single-stranded origin (SSO) DNA to make another double-stranded circle. DNA polymerase I removes the primer, replacing it

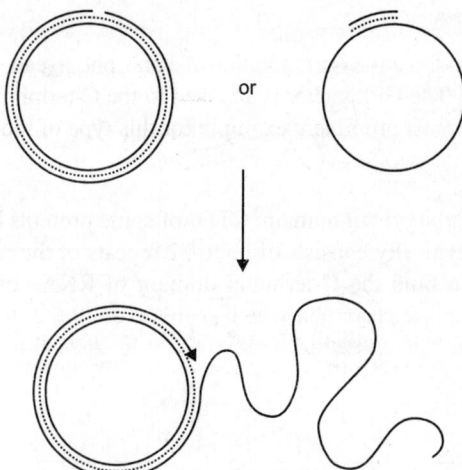

Fig. 13.7: Rolling circle replication produces multiple copies of a single circular template.

with DNA, and DNA ligase joins the ends to make another molecule of double-stranded circular DNA. Rolling circle replication has found wide uses in academic research and biotechnology, and has been successfully used for amplification of DNA from very small amounts of starting material.

Virology

Some viruses replicate their DNA in host cells via rolling circle replication. For instance, human herpesvirus-6 (HHV-6)(hibv) expresses a set of 'early genes' that are believed to be involved in this process. The long concatemers that result are subsequently cleaved between the pac-1 and pac-2 regions of HHV-6's genome by ribozymes when it is packaged into individual virions.

BACTERIAL CONJUGATION

Bacterial conjugation is the transfer of genetic material (plasmid) between bacterial cells by direct cell-to-cell contact or by a bridge-like connection between two cells. Discovered in 1946 by Joshua Lederberg and Edward Tatum, conjugation is a mechanism of horizontal gene transfer as are transformation and transduction although these two other mechanisms do not involve cell-to-cell contact.

Bacterial conjugation is often regarded as the bacterial equivalent of sexual reproduction or mating since it involves the exchange of genetic material. During conjugation the donor cell provides a conjugative or mobilizable genetic element that is most often a plasmid or transposon. Most conjugative plasmids have systems ensuring that the recipient cell does not already contain a similar element.

The genetic information transferred is often beneficial to the recipient. Benefits may include antibiotic resistance, xenobiotic tolerance or the ability to use new metabolites. Such beneficial plasmids may be considered bacterial endosymbionts. Other elements, however, may be viewed as bacterial parasites and conjugation as a mechanism evolved by them to allow for their spread.

Mechanism

The prototypical conjugative plasmid (Fig. 13.8) is the F-plasmid, or F-factor. The F-plasmid is an episome (a plasmid that can integrate itself into the bacterial chromosome by homologous recombination) with

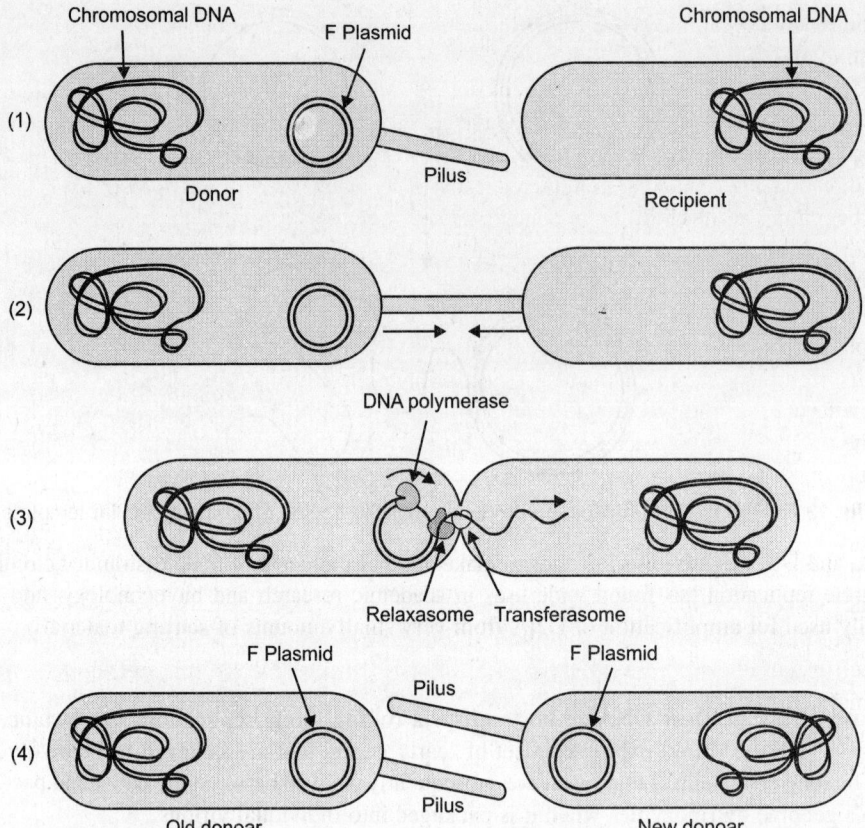

Fig. 13.8: Schematic drawing of bacterial conjugation. Conjugation diagram (1) Donor cell produces pilus. (2) Pilus attaches to recipient cell and brings the two cells together. (3) The mobile plasmid is nicked and a single strand of DNA is then transferred to the recipient cell. (4) Both cells synthesize a complementary strand to produce a double stranded circular plasmid and also reproduce pili; both cells are now viable donors.

a length of about 100 kb. It carries its own origin of replication, the oriV, and an origin of transfer, or oriT. There can only be one copy of the F-plasmid in a given bacterium, either free or integrated, and bacteria that possess a copy are called F-positive or F-plus (denoted F$^+$). Cells that lack F plasmids are called F-negative or F-minus (F$^-$) and as such can function as recipient cells.

Among other genetic information the F-plasmid carries a *tra* and *trb* locus, which together are about 33 kb long and consist of about 40 genes. The *tra* locus includes the pilin gene and regulatory genes, which together form pili on the cell surface. The locus also includes the genes for the proteins that attach themselves to the surface of F$^-$ bacteria and initiate conjugation. Though there is some debate on the exact mechanism of conjugation it seems that the pili are not the structures through which DNA exchange occurs. This has been shown in experiments where the pilus are allowed to make contact, but then are denatured with SDS and yet DNA transformation still proceeds. Several proteins coded for in the *tra* or *trb* locus seem to open a channel between the bacteria and it is thought that the traD enzyme, located at the base of the pilus, initiates membrane fusion.

When conjugation is initiated by a signal the relaxase enzyme creates a nick in one of the strands of the conjugative plasmid at the oriT. Relaxase may work alone or in a complex of over a dozen proteins known collectively as a relaxosome. In the F-plasmid system the relaxase enzyme is called TraI and the relaxosome consists of TraI, TraY, TraM and the integrated host factor IHF. The nicked strand, or T-strand, is then unwound from the unbroken strand and transferred to the recipient cell in a 5′-terminus to 3′-terminus direction. The remaining strand is replicated either independent of conjugative action (vegetative replication beginning at the oriV) or in concert with conjugation (conjugative replication similar to the rolling circle replication of lambda phage). Conjugative replication may require a second nick before successful transfer can occur. A recent report claims to have inhibited conjugation with chemicals that mimic an intermediate step of this second nicking event.

If the F-plasmid that is transferred has previously been integrated into the donor's genome [producing an Hfr strain (High Frequency of Recombination)] some of the donor's chromosomal DNA may also be transferred with the plasmid DNA. The amount of chromosomal DNA that is transferred depends on how long the two conjugating bacteria remain in contact. In common laboratory strains of *E. coli* the transfer of the entire bacterial chromosome takes about 100 minutes. The transferred DNA can then be integrated into the recipient genome via homologous recombination.

A cell culture that contains in its population cells with non-integrated F-plasmids usually also contains a few cells that have accidentally integrated their plasmids. It is these cells that are responsible for the low-frequency chromosomal gene transfers that occur in such cultures. Some strains of bacteria with an integrated F-plasmid can be isolated and grown in pure culture. Because such strains transfer chromosomal genes very efficiently they are called Hfr (high frequency of recombination). The *E. coli* genome was originally mapped by interrupted mating experiments in which various Hfr cells in the process of conjugation were sheared from recipients after less than 100 minutes (initially using a Waring blender).

The genes that were transferred were then investigated. Since integration of the F-plasmid into the *E. coli* chromosome is a rare spontaneous occurrence, and since the numerous genes promoting DNA transfer are in the plasmid genome rather than in the bacterial genome, it has been argued that conjugative bacterial gene transfer is not an evolutionary adaptation of the bacterial host, nor is it likely ancestral to eukaryotic sex.

Inter-kingdom Transfer

Bacteria related to the nitrogen fixing Rhizobia are an interesting case of inter-kingdom conjugation. For example, the tumour-inducing (Ti) plasmid of *Agrobacterium* (Fig. 13.9) and the root-tumor inducing (Ri) plasmid of *A. rhizogenes* contain genes that are capable of transferring to plant cells. The expression of these genes effectively transforms the plant cells into opine-producing factories. Opines are used by the bacteria as sources of nitrogen and energy. Infected cells form crown gall or root tumours, respectively. The Ti and Ri plasmids are thus endosymbionts of the bacteria, which are in turn endosymbionts (or parasites) of the infected plant. The Ti and Ri plasmids can also be transferred between bacteria using a system (the *tra*, or transfer, operon) that is different and independent of the system used for inter kingdom transfer (the *vir*, or virulence, operon). Such transfers create virulent strains from previously avirulent strains.

Genetic Engineering Applications

Conjugation is a convenient means for transferring genetic material to a variety of targets. In laboratories, successful transfers have been reported from bacteria to yeast, plants, mammalian cells and isolated mammalian mitochondria.

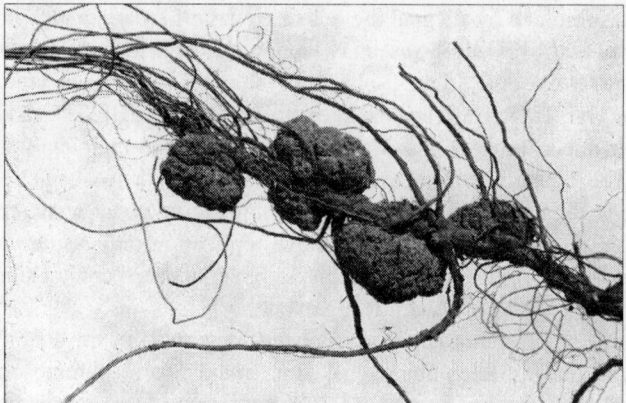

Fig. 13.9: *Agrobacterium tumefaciens* gall at the root of Carya illinoensis.

Conjugation has advantages over other forms of genetic transfer including minimal disruption of the target's cellular envelope and the ability to transfer relatively large amounts of genetic material. In plant engineering, *Agrobacterium*-like conjugation complements other standard vehicles such as tobacco mosaic virus (TMV). While TMV is capable of infecting many plant families these are primarily herbaceous dicots. *Agrobacterium*-like conjugation is also primarily used for dicots, but monocot recipients are not uncommon.

DNA/CONJUGATION

Bacterial conjugation is the transfer of genetic material between two bacterial cell via direct cell-to-cell contact. Although often incorrectly characterised as the bacterial equivalent of mating, in fact it is simply the transfer of genetic material from a donor cell to a recipient cell. Bacterial conjugation (Fig. 13.10) is also known as a 'type IV secretion system'.

This behaviour is characterised by the presence of a specialised plasmid (small, circular piece of transferrable DNA most often found within bacteria) known as a conjugative plasmid.

The conjugative plasmid holds a distinct and specialised set of coding regions including the following

- OriT (origin of transfer): Unlike other plasmids, the conjugative plasmid has its own origin of transfer nic region. This is a specialised portion of the genome where one of the two strands of the circular plasmid DNA is cut to allow for rolling circle replication of the plasmid containing the OriT region into a recipient cell. During rolling circle replication, the cut end of one strand is inserted into the recipient cell while recipient polymerases construct the complementary strand back into a circular piece of DNA.

- TraJ (transfer genes): The activation of this gene sets off a cascade of other plasmid genes (and thus corresponding protein expressions) which act in concert to form 'mating' characteristics in the host bacterial cell. Such salient characteristics include:

> Growth of a pilus—a long whip-like apparatus used to hook the two cells together

> Fusion of the outer membranes to allow for transfer of genetic material

> Formation of 'surface exclusion proteins' which prevents the cell containing the conjugative plasmid from mating with other conjugative plasmids of its type.

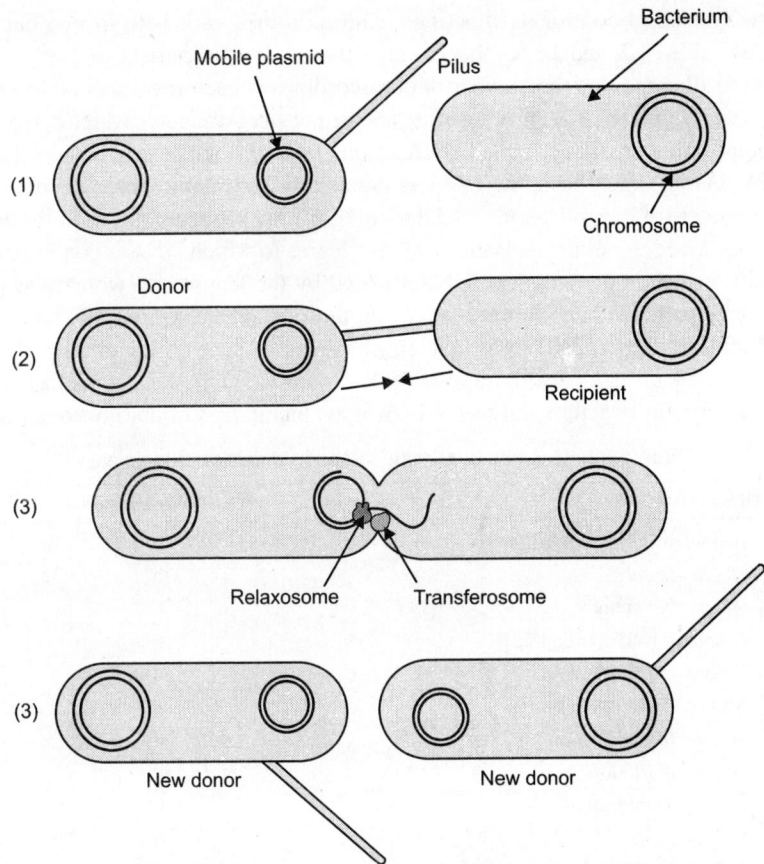

Fig. 13.10: Schematic diagram of bacterial conjugation. (1) donor cell produces pilus, (2) pilus attaches to recipient cell, brings the two cells together, (3) the mobile plasmid is nicked and a single strand of DNA is then transferred to the recipient cell and (4) both cells recircularise their plasmids, synthesise second strands, and reproduce pili, both cells are now viable donors.

Two of the most well-studied and characterised types of conjugative plasmids are types 'F' (from the F plasmid) and 'R'. The employed nomenclature for conjugative plasmid genes is the gene name first with the type afterwards. For example, the 'TraJr' or 'TraJR' gene denotes the 'TraJ' gene of the 'R' type conjugative plasmid.

VARIATION IN CHROMOSOME NUMBER AND STRUCTURE

German biologist Walther Flemming in the early 1880s revealed that during cell division the nuclear material organise themselves into visible thread like structures which were named as chromosomes which stains deep with basic dyes. The term chromosome was coined by W. Waldeyer in 1888. Chrome is coloured and soma is body, hence they mean 'coloured bodies' and can be defined as higher order organised arrangement of DNA and proteins. It contains many genes or the hereditary units, regulatory elements and other nucleotide sequences. Chromosomes also contain DNA-bound proteins, which serve in packaging the DNA and control its functions. Chromosomes vary both in number and structure among organisms (Table 13.2) and the number of chromosomes is characteristic of every species. Benden and Bovery in 1887 reported that the number of chromosomes in each species is constant. W.S. Sutton and T. Boveri in 1902 suggested that chromosomes are the physical structures which acted as messengers of heredity. Chromosomes are tightly coiled DNA around basic histone proteins, which help in the tight packing of DNA. During interphase, the DNA is not tightly coiled into chromosomes, but exists as chromatin. The structure of a chromosome is given in Fig. 13.11. In eukaryotes to fit the entire length of DNA in the nucleus it undergoes condensation and the degree to which DNA is condensed is expressed as its packing ratio which is the length of DNA divided by the length into which it is packaged into chromatin along with proteins. The shortest human chromosome contains 4.6×10^7 bp of DNA. This is equivalent to 14,000 μm of extended DNA. In its most condensed state during mitosis, the chromosome is about 2 μm long. This gives a packing ratio of 7000 (14,000/2). The DNA is packaged stepwise into the higher order chromatin structure and this is known as 'hierarchies of chromosomal organisation'.

Table 13.2: Number of chromosomes in different organisms.

Organism	No. of chromosomes
Arabidopsis thaliana (diploid)	10
Maize (diploid)	20
Wheat (hexaploid)	42
Common fruit fly (diploid)	8
Earthworm (diploid)	36
Mouse (diploid)	40
Human (diploid)	46
Elephants (diploid)	56
Donkey (diploid)	62
Dog (diploid)	78
Gold Fish (diploid)	100–104
Tobacco(tetraloid)	48
Oat (hexaploid)	42

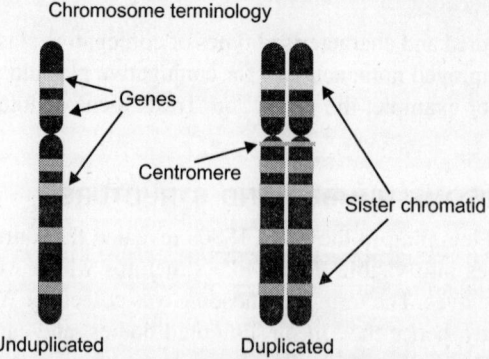

Fig. 13.11: Eukaryotic chromosome.

CHROMOSOME NUMBER

There are normally two copies of each chromosome present in every somatic cell. The number of unique chromosomes (N) in such a cell is known as its haploid number, and the total number of chromosomes (2N) is its diploid number. The suffix 'ploid' refers to chromosome 'sets'. The haploid set of the chromosome is also known as the genome. Structurally, eukaryotes possess large linear chromosomes unlike prokaryotes which have circular chromosomes. In Eukaryotes other than the nucleus chromosomes are present in mitochondria and chloroplast too. The number of chromosomes in each somatic cell is same for all members of a given species. The organism with lowest number of chromosome is the nematode, *Ascaris megalocephalusunivalens* which has only two chromosomes in the somatic cells $(2n = 2)$.

Chromosome Number in Different Species

In 'higher' organisms (diploids), members of same species typically have identical numbers of chromosomes in each somatic cell. Diploid chromosome number $(2n)$. Nearly all chromosomes will exist in pairs (identical wrt length and centromere placement) except the sex chromosomes.

Members of pair are homologous chromosomes. Haploid number (n) is the number of chromosome pairs (Table 13.3).

Table 13.3: Haploid number (n) is the number of chromosome pairs.

	$2n$	n
Human	46	23
Horse	64	32
Cat	38	19
Geometrid moth	224	112
Tomato	24	12
Pink bread mold	14	7
See other examples in text		

Autosomal monosomy and trisomy

Occasionally, one finds an organism that has an extra copy of a particular chromosome. This is known as trisomy—because there are now 3 copies of an autosome. Some trisomies are viable in animals, but the condition usually has severe effects. These effects are presumably related to the fact that there are 3 copies of every gene on the trisomic chromosome, but only 2 copies of all the genes on the other chromosomes. We will see later, that organisms with three or more copies of all the chromosomes are often perfectly viable. The karyotype of a male human being is shown in Fig. 13.12.

Trisomy of human chromosome 21 is the cause of the disorder known as Down syndrome. (Remember, humans have 23 pairs of chromosomes—the pairs are numbered 1 through 22, plus the X and Y). It is characterised by multiple physical defects, including epicanthal fold, furrowed tongue, characteristic palm and finger print patterns, and lowered IQ. About 1 in 750 live births produces a child with this condition. It results from the non-disjunction of chromosome 21 during meiotic anaphase I or anaphase II, when the paired homologs (or paired chromatids) normally migrate to opposite poles of the cell.

Nondisjuction: The members of a chromosome pair (homologs) line up at the metaphase plate during meiotic metaphase I, then separate to opposite poles of the cell during anaphase I—review this material

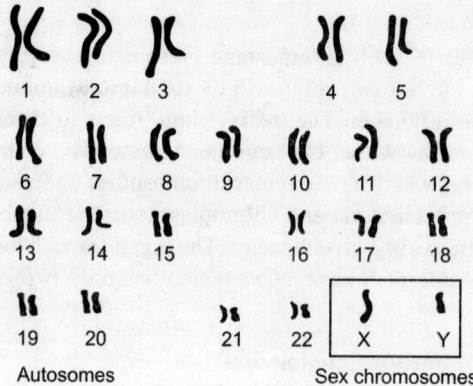

1 2 3   4 5

6 7 8 9 10 11 12

13 14 15   16 17 18

19 20   21 22   X Y

Autosomes   Sex chromosomes

Fig. 13.12: The karyotype of a male human being.

in Klug and Cummings or any introductory Genetics text if you are not thoroughly familiar with it!). If the pair fails to separate, and both migrate to the same pole, half of the resulting gametes will have two copies of chromosome 21, rather than one. When this gamete unites with a normal gamete (bearing one copy of chromosome 21) during fertilisation, the resulting gamete has 3 copies of chromosome 21, rather than the normal 2. Nondisjunction of chromosome 21 seems to occur more often in the production of eggs than sperm, and the frequency increases with the age of the parent. Older individuals are often encouraged to test for trisomy 21 by amniocentesis at 15 to 16 weeks after conception. Nondisjunction can happen to other chromosomes in addition to chromosome 21. But human embryos that are trisomic for any other chromosome do not survive to birth. It should be obvious that the other half of the gametes resulting from a non-disjunction event at anaphase 1 will have 0 copies of the chromosome. When a gamete with 0 copies of a chromosome unites with a normal gamete, the result is a zygote that has only one copy of that chromosome. This is monosomy. Monosomy is not well tolerated in animals—usually lethal. Some plants can survive (observed in maize, tomato, Oenothera, and Datura) but they have low viability and are usually sterile. Nondisjunction can also occur at anaphase II, when sister chromatids fail to separate and migrate to opposite poles. Nondisjuntion at anaphase one results in half the gametes being normal, and half being abnormal. Table 13.4 shows Chromosomal abnormalities occurring in human fetuses.

Table 13.4: Chromosomal abnormalities occurring in human fetuses.

Type of Abnormality	% Spontaneously aborted fetuses with abnormality	% Fetuses with the abnormality surviving to term
All abnormalities	50	5
Autosomal trisomies		
16	7.5	0
13, 18 and 21	4.5	15
All others	13.8	0
Trisomies of sex chromosomes		
XXX, XXY, XYY	0.3	75
Monosomy for X (XO)	8.7	1
Structural abnormalities	20	45

If one surveys karyotypes of embryos that spontaneously abort, trisomies for all the autosomes are seen, and other forms of chromosomal abnormalities as well, but these conditions are apparently fatal early in development. Normal embryonic development requires a precise diploid complement of chromosomes. Exception to general lethality of monosomies and trisomies occurs if they involve mammalian sex chromosomes. These monosomies and trisomies are often viable because of Xinactivation and because the Y contains few genes. We will discuss X inactivation later in this course.

An extra X chromosome also has fewer deleterious effects than an extra autosome. This is because, in mammals, all X chromosomes except one are inactivated very early in embryonic development. If this were not the case, then females would have twice as many active Xlinked genes as males, and would therefore have twice as much of all the protein products produced by these genes.

The inactivation of one of the two X chromosomes in female equalises the gene dosage of X-linked genes—dosage compensation.

CHROMATIN

Chemical Composition of Chromatin

Chromatin consists of DNA, RNA and protein. The protein of chromatin could be of two types: histones and non histones.

DNA: DNA is the most important chemical component of chromatin, since it plays central role of controlling heredity and is most conveniently measured in picograms. In addition to describing the genome of an organism by its number of chromosomes, it is also described by the amount of DNA in a haploid cell. This is usually expressed as the amount of DNA per haploid cell (usually expressed as picograms) or the number of kilobases per haploid cell and is called the C-value. This is constant for all cells of a species. For diploid cells it is 2C. Extending the C-value we reach the C-value paradox. One immediate feature of eukaryotic organisms highlights a specific anomaly that was detected early in molecular research. Even though eukaryotic organisms appear to have 2–10 times as many genes as prokaryotes, they have many orders of magnitude more DNA in the cell. Furthermore, the amount of DNA per genome is correlated not with the presumed evolutionary complexity of a species. This is stated as the C-value paradox: the amount of DNA in the haploid cell of an organism is not related to its evolutionary complexity. Lower eukaryotes in general have less DNA, such as nematode

Caenorhabditis elegans which has 20 times more DNA than *E. coli*. Vertebrates have greaer DNA content about 3pg, in general about 700 times more than *E. coli*. Salamander *Amphiuma* has a very high DNA content of about 84pg. Man has about 3pg of DNA per haploid genome.

Histones: Histones are basic proteins as they are enriched with basic proteins arginine and lysine. At physiological pH they are cationic and can interact with anionic nucleic acids. They form a highly condensed structure. The histones are of five types called H1, H2A H2B, H3, and H4-which are very similar among different species of eukaryotes and have been highly conserved during evolution. H1 is the least conserved among all and is also loosely bound with DNA. H1 histone is absent in *Sacharomyces cerevisiae*.

Non-histones: In addition to histones the chromatin comprise of many different types of non-histone proteins, which are involved in a range of activities, including DNA replication and gene expression. They display more diversity or are not conserved. They may also differ between different tissues of same organism.

Euchromatin: The lightly-stained regions in chromosome when stained with basic dyes are called euchromatin and contain single-copy of genetically-active DNA. The extent of chromatin condensation varies during the life cycle of the cell and plays an important role in regulating gene expression. In the interphase of cell cycle the chromatin are decondensed and known as euchromatin leading to gene transcription and DNA replication.

Heterochromatin: The word heterochromatin was coined by Emil Heitz based on cytological observations. They are highly condensed and ordered areas in nucleosomal arrays. About 10% of interphase chromatin is called heterochromatin and is in a very highly condensed state that resembles the chromatin of cells undergoing mitosis. They contain a high density of repetitive DNA found at centromeres and telomeres form heterochromatin. Heterochromatin are of two types, the constitutive and facultative heterochromatin. The regions that remain condensed throughout the cell cycle are called constitutive heterochromatin whereas the regions where heterochromatin condensation state can change are known as facultative. Constitutive heterochromatin is found in the region that flanks the telomeres and centromere of each chromosome and in the distal arm of the Y chromosome in mammals. Constitutive heterochromatin possesses very few genes and they also lead to transcriptional inactivation of nearby genes. This phenomenon of gene silencing is known as 'position effect'. Constitutive hetero-chromatin also inhibits genetic recombination between homologous repetitive sequences circumventing DNA duplications and deletion. Whereas facultative heterochromatin is chromatin that has been specifically inactivated during certain phases of an organism's life or in certain types of differentiated cells. Dosage compensation of X-chromosome or X-chromosome inactivation in mammals is an example of such heterochromatin. Heterochromatin spreads from a specific nucleation site, causing silencing of most of the X chromosome, thereby regulating gene dosage.

Centromeres: Centromeres are those condensed regions within the chromosome that are responsible for the accurate segregation of the replicated chromosome during mitosis and meiosis. When chromosomes are stained they typically show a dark-stained region that is the centromere. The actual location where the attachments of spindle fibres occur is called the kinetochore and is composed of both DNA and protein. The DNA sequence within these regions is called CEN DNA. Because CEN DNA can be moved from one chromosome to another and still provide the chromosome with the ability to segregate, these sequences must not provide any other function. Typically CEN DNA is about 120 base pairs long and consists of several sub-domains, CDE-I, CDE-II and CDE-III (Fig. 13.13). Mutations in the first two sub-domains have no effect upon segregation, but a point mutation in the CDE-III sub-domain completely eliminates the ability of the centromere to function during chromosome segregation. Therefore CDE-III must be actively involved in the binding of the spindle fibers to the centromere. The protein component of the kinetochore is only now being characterised. A complex of three proteins called Cbf-III binds to normal CDE-III regions but cannot bind to a CDE-III region with a point mutation

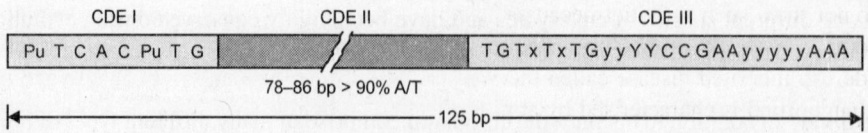

Fig. 13.13: The *S. cerevisiae* centrosome. The *S. cerevisae* centromere (CEN) sequences consist of two short conserved sequences (CDE I and CDE III) separated by 78 to 86 base pairs (bp) of ATrich DNA (CDE II). The sequences shown are consensus sequences derived from analysis of the centromere sequences of individual yeast chromosomes. Pu = A or G, x =A or T, y = any base.

that prevents mitotic segregation. Furthermore, mutants of the genes encoding the Cbf-III proteins also eliminates the ability for chromosomes to segregate during mitosis. Additional analyses of the DNA and protein components of the centromere are necessary to fully understand the mechanics of chromosome segregation.

Telomeres: Telomeres are the region of DNA at the end of the linear eukaryotic chromosome that are required for the replication and stability of the chromosome. McClintock recognised their special features when she noticed, that if two chromosomes were broken in a cell, the ends were sticky and end of one could attach to the other and vice versa. However she never observed the attachment of the broken end to the end of an unbroken chromosome suggesting that the end of chromosomes have unique features. Telomere sequences remain conserved throughout vertebrates and they form caps that protect the chromosomes from nucleases and other destabilising influences; and they prevent the ends of chromosomes from fusing with one another. The telomeric DNA contains direct tandemly repeated sequences of the form (T/A)xGy where × is between 1 and 4 and y is greater than 1. Human telomeres contain the sequence TTAGGG repeated from about 500 to 5000 times. Certain bacteria possess telomeres in their linear genetic material which are of two types; one of the types is called a hairpin telomere. As its name implies, the telomeres bend around from the end of one DNA strand to the end of the complimentary strand. The other type of telomere is known as an invertron telomere. This type acts to allow an overlap between the ends of the complimentary DNA strands.

Telomere replication: Telomere replication is an important aspect in DNA replication. The primary difficulty with telomeres is the replication of the lagging strand. Because DNA synthesis requires a RNA template (that provides the free 3'-OH group) to prime DNA replication, and this template is eventually degraded, a short single-stranded region would be left at the end of the chromosome. This region would be susceptible to enzymes that degrade single-stranded DNA. The result would be that the length of the chromosome would be shortened after each division. This is known as the end replication problem which is not observed. The action of the telomerase enzymes ensure that the ends of the lagging strands are replicated correctly. Telomerase was discovered in 1984 by Elizabeth Blackburn and Carol Greider of the University of California, Berkeley. It is a reverse transcriptase that synthesises DNA using an RNA template. Unlike most reverse transcriptases, the enzyme itself contains the RNA that serves as its template, i.e. telomerase can add new repeat units to the 3' end of the overhanging strand. A well-studied system involves the *Tetrahymena* protozoa organism. The telomeres of this organism end in the sequence 5'-TTGGGG-3'. The telomerase adds a series of 5'-TTGGGG-3' repeats to the ends of the lagging strand. A hairpin occurs when unusual base pairs between guanine residues in the repeat form. Next the RNA primer is removed, and the 5' end of the lagging strand can be used for DNA synthesis. Ligation occurs between the finished lagging strand and the hairpin. Finally, the hairpin is removed at the 5'-TTGGGG-3' repeat.

Telomerase activity is retained in germ cells and zygote and somatic cells after few cell division cycles do not show such activities because otherwise they would divide indefinitely and lead to cancer. Thus telomeres shrink causing chromosome shortening to a critical point when the cell ceases to grow and divide. An inherited disease called the Werner's syndrome that causes patients to age much more rapidly than normal is characterised by abnormal telomere maintenance.

HUMAN CHROMOSOME

The human genome is 3×10^9 base pairs of DNA and the smallest human chromosome is several times larger than the entire yeast genome, and the extended length of DNA that makes up the human genome is about 1 m long. The human genome is distributed among 24 chromosomes (22 autosomes and the 2 sex chromosomes), each containing between 45 and 280 Mb of DNA. The sex chromosomes are denoted by X and Y and they contain genes which determine the sex of an individual, i.e. XX for female and XY for male. The rest are known as autosomes.

The haploid human genome contains about 23,000 protein-coding genes, which are far fewer than had been expected before sequencing. In fact, only about 1.5% of the genome codes for proteins, while the rest consists of non-coding genes, regulatory sequences, introns, and noncoding DNA. Chromosomes are stained with A-T (G bands) and G-C (R bands) base pair specific dyes.

When they are stained, the mitotic chromosomes have a banded structure that unambiguously identifies each chromosome of a karyotype. Each band contains millions of DNA nucleotide pairs which do not correspond to any functional structure. G-banding is obtained with Giemsa stain yielding a series of lightly and darkly stained bands. The dark regions tend to be heterochromatic and AT rich. The light regions tend to be euchromatic and GC rich. R-banding is the reverse of G-banding where the dark regions are euchromatic and the bright regions are heterochromatic.

Types of Human Chromosomes

There are four types of chromosomes based upon the position of the centromere in humans (Fig. 13.14).

1. Metacentric: In this type of chromosome the centromere occurs in the centre and all the four chromatids are of equal length.
2. Submetacentric: In this type of chromosome the centromere is a little away from the centre and therefore chromatids of one side are slightly longer than the other side.
3. Acrocentric: In this type of chromosome the centromere is located closer to one end of chromatid therefore the chromatids on opposite side are very long. A small round structure, attached by a very thin thread is observed on the side of shorter chromatid. The small round structure that is a part of the chromatid is termed as satellite. The thin strands at the satellite region are termed as Nucleolar Organiser Region.
4. Telocentric: In this type of chromosome the centromere is placed at one end of the chromatid and hence only one arm. Such telocentric chromosomes are not seen in human cells.

Human Chromosome Karyotype

Eukaryotic species have several chromosomes and are detected only during mitosis or meiosis. They are best observed during the metaphase stage of cell division as they are found in the most condensed state. Thus each eukaryotic species is characterised by a karyotype which is the numerical description (number and size) of chromosomes in the normal diploid cell.

For example, the *Homo sapiens* possess 46 chromosome, i.e. 23 pairs. The karyotype is important because genetic research can correlate changes in the karyotype with changes in the phenotype of the individual. For example, Down's syndrome is caused by duplication of the human chromosome number 21. Insertions, deletions and changes in chromosome number can be detected by the skilled cytogeneticist, but correlating these with specific phenotypes is difficult.

GIANT CHROMOSOMES

Some cells at certain particular stage of their life cycle contain large nuclei with giant or large sized chromosomes. Polytene and lampbrush chromosomes are examples of giant chromosomes.

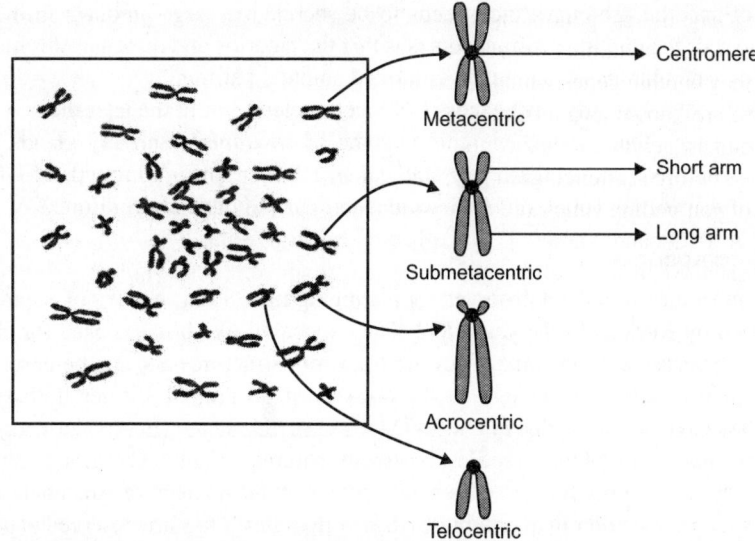

Fig. 13.14: Types of human chromosomes.

Polytene Chromosome

Giant chromosomes were first time observed by E.G. Balbiani in the year 1881 in nuclei of certain secretory cells (salivary glands) of Chironomas larvae (Diptera). However he could not conclude them to be chromosomes. They were conclusively reported for the first time in insect cells (*Drosophila*) by Theophilus Painter of the University of Texas in the year 1933. Since they were discovered in the salivary glands of insects they were termed as salivary gland chromosomes. The anme polytene chromosome was proposed by Kollar due to the occurrence of many chromonemata (DNA) in them. Cells in the larval salivary gland of *Drosophila,* mosquito and *Chironema* contain chromosomes with high DNA content. However they may also occur in malphigian tubules, rectum, gut, foot pads, fat bodies, ovarian nurse cells, etc. Polyteny of giant chromosomes happens by replication of the chromosomal DNA several times without nuclear division (endomitosis) and the resulting daughter chromatids do not separate but remain aligned side by side. During endomitosis the nuclear envelope does not rupture and no spindle formation takes place. The polytene chromosomes are visible during interphase and prophase of mitosis.

They are about 100 times thicker contain 1000 to 2000 chromosomes, than the chromosomes found in most other cells of the organism. When stained and viewed under compound microscope at 40X magnification they display about 5000 bands. In them the chromomere or the more tightly coiled regions alternate with regions where the DNA fibres are folded loosely. A series of dark transverse bands alternates with clear zones of inter bands. Such individual bands can be correlated with particular genes. About 85% of the DNA in polytene chromosomes is in bands and rest 15% is in inter bands. The cross banding pattern of each polytene chromosome is a constant characteristic within a species and helps in chromosome mapping during cytogenetic studies. In *Drosophila melanogaster* there are about 5000 bands and 5000 interbands per genome. These chromosomes are not inert cellular objects but dynamic structures in which certain regions become 'puffed out' due to active DNA transcription at particular stages of development. These chromosome puffs are also termed Balbiani rings. Puffs may apprear and disappear depending on the production of specific proteins which needs to be secreted in large amounts in the larval saliva. Another peculiarity of the polytene chromosomes is that the paternal and maternal chromosomes remain associated side by side and the phenomenon is termed somatic pairing.

Both polyteny and polyploidy have excess DNA per nucleus, but in the later the new chromosomes are separate from each other. A polytene chromosome of *Drosophila* salivary glands has about 100 DNA molecules which are arranged side by side and which arise from 10 rounds of DNA replication ($2^{10} = 1024$). *Chironimus* has 16000 DNA molecules in their polytene chromosomes.

Lampbrush Chromosome

Lampbrush chromosomes were first observed by Flemming in 1882 in sections of Salamander oocytes and later described by Ruckert in the year 1892. They appeared like brushes used for cleaning lamps, hence the name lampbrush chromosome. They are transitory structures and can be observed during the diplotene stage of prophase I in meiosis in the oocytes of all animal species both vertebrates and invertebrates. They have been described in Sepia (Mollusca), Echinaster (Echinodermata) and in several species of insects, shark, amphibians, reptiles, birds and mammals (humans). Lampbrush chromosomes have also been found in spermatocytes of several species, giant nucleus of Acetabularia and even in plants. Generally they are smaller in invertebrates than vertebrates. They are observed in oocytes because oocytes are high in DNA content. Lampbrush chromosomes are functional for studying chromosome organisation and genome function during meiotic prophase. Additionally lampbrush chromosomes are widely used for construction of detail cytological maps of individual chromosomes.

They are of exceptionally large sizes and present in bivalent form. They are formed due to the active synthesis of mRNA molecules for future use by the egg cells, when no synthesis of mRNA molecule is possible during the mitotic cell division. Lampbrush chromosomes are clearly visible in the light microscope they are organised into a series of chromomeres with large chromatin symmetrical loops extending laterally. Each loop appears at a constant position in the chromosome (10000 loops per chromosome set or haploid set). Each loop has an axis made up of DNA unfolded from the chromosome and is transcriptionally highly active. Wherein several transcription units with polarised RNP-matrix coats the DNA axis of the loop. The majority of the DNA, however, is not in loops but remains highly condensed in the chromomeres on the axis and lacks expression of genes. The loops perform intense transcription of heterogenous RNA (precursors of mRNA molecules for ribosomal and histone proteins). Thus each lateral loop is covered by an assymetrical matrix of RNA transcripts; thicker at one end of the loop than other. The number of pairs of loops gradually increases during meiosis till it reaches maximum at diplotene. This stage may persist for months or years as oocytes build up supply of mRNA required for further development. As meiosis proceeds further number of loops gradually decrease and loops ultimately disappear due to reabsorption into the chromosome or disintegration.

Certain hypothesis regarding loops are that they may be static or dynamic with new loop material spinning out of one side of a chromosome and returning to a condensed on the other side. This is called spinning out or retraction hypothesis. This hypothesis has been rejected recently through DNA-RNA hybridisation studies. The other hypothesis is known as the Master and Slave hypothesis which suggested that each loop pairs and thus chromomere is associated with the activity of many copies of specific genes. There is a master copy at each chromomere and information is transferred to the slave copies which are matched against it to ensure that all are identical. The master copy does not take part in RNA synthesis, but the slave copy is involved in transcription. Large number of duplicate genes ensures higher level of transcription.

SECTION V

Bacteriophage Mechanisms of Bacterial Mutation and Genetically Modified Bacteriophages and Bacteriophages in Chemotherapy and Medicines

Chapter 14

Structure of Bacteriophages

INTRODUCTION

Bacteriophages represent an example of amazing molecular machines with powerful motors energised by ATP hydrolysis and puncturing devices allowing to inject viral genome into the host cells. As more and more phage structures been studied a general theme emerges pointing to a common bacteriophage ancestor from which they all inherited essentially the same capsid protein fold and other elements of their organisation: capsids, tails, portal complexes, tail fibres, and other components. The number of phages that were discovered, purified, and studied by biochemical, and biophysical methods increased tremendously during the last decade. New technologies used for their studies both on the microbiological and molecular levels made it possible to analyse their evolutionary relationship and origins of the host range specificity. One of the powerful techniques in the structural biology of phages is the modern cryo-EM that recently allowed to reach close to atomic resolution level of details in the EM reconstructions. Understanding of the mechanisms which determine the host-range is required to solve many practical questions related to infectious human and animal diseases caused by bacteria, and quality food and its production (e.g. dairy products). A study conducted in Japan has demonstrated the efficiency of phages against bacterial infections of cultured fish. The use of bacteriophage as antimicrobial agents is based on the lytic phages that kill bacteria via lysis, which destroys the bacterium and makes its adaptation nearly impossible. High bacteriophage resistance for external factors is important for the stability of phage preparations. However, this stability is disadvantageous for industry when maintenance of the active bacterial strains is important.

Comparative studies demonstrate that bacteriophages have many common features on the molecular level and common principle of interaction with a bacterium cell, although components that trigger adsorption of phages to the host cell and the genome release are host dependent. Phage infection also depends on the availability of specific receptors on the cell surface, and investigation of the structure and biosynthesis of the bacterial cell membrane may be undertaken using phage-resistant mutants. Therefore there is a need to carry out further studies on phages, identifying receptors of targeted bacteria and environmental features that affect phage activity. The growing interest of the pharmaceutical and agricultural industries in phages requires more information on phage interactions, survivability and methods of their preservation.

Structural studies revealed many similarities between bacteriophages and animal cell viruses. The chances of success in using bacteriophages as model systems for animal cell viruses and eventually as medical therapy are much better given our current extensive knowledge of bacteriophage biology following the advances in their molecular structural biology. Thus, bacteriophage is any one of a number of viruses that infect bacteria. Bacteriophages are among the most common biological entities on earth. The term is commonly used in its shortened form, *phage* (Fig. 14.1).

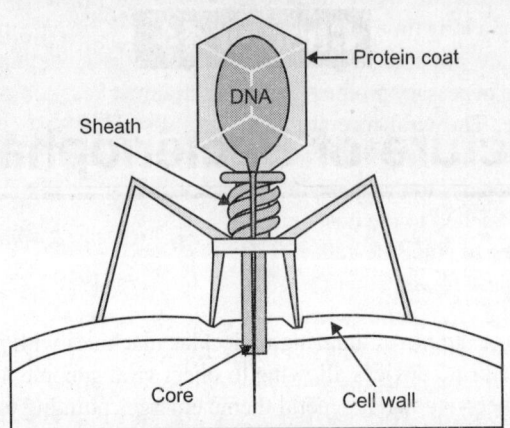

Fig. 14.1: The structure of a typical tailed bacteriophage.

Typically, bacteriophages consist of an outer protein capsid enclosing genetic material. The genetic material can be ssRNA, dsRNA, ssDNA, or dsDNA ('ss-' or 'ds-' prefix denotes single-strand or double-strand) long with either circular or linear arrangement. Bacteriophages are much smaller than the bacteria they destroy. Phages are estimated to be the most widely distributed and diverse entities in the biosphere. Phages are ubiquitous and can be found in all reservoirs populated by bacterial hosts, such as soil or the intestines of animals. One of the densest natural sources for phages and other viruses is sea water, where up to 9×10^8 virions per milliliter have been found in microbial mats at the surface, and up to 70 per cent of marine bacteria may be infected by phages. They have been used for over 60 years as an alternative to antibiotics in the former Soviet Union and Eastern Europe. They are seen as a possible therapy against multi drug resistant strains of many bacteria.

VIRUSES

Viruses are extremely small infectious particles that are not visible in a light microscope, and are able to pass through fine porcelain filters. They exist in a huge variety of forms and infect practically all living systems: animals, plants, insects and bacteria. All viruses have a genome, typically only one type of nucleic acid, but it could be one or several molecules of DNA or RNA, which is surrounded by a protective stable coat (capsid) and sometimes by additional layers which may be very complex and contain carbohydrates, lipids, and additional proteins. The viruses that have only a protein coat are named 'naked', or nonenveloped viruses. Many viruses have an envelope (enveloped viruses) that wraps around the protein capsid. This envelope is formed from a lipid membrane of the host cell during the release of a virus out of the cell. Viruses interacting with different types of cells in living organisms produce different types of disease. Each virus infects a certain type of cell which is usually called 'host' cell. The major feature of any viral disease is cell lysis, when a cell breaks open and subsequently dies. In multicellular organisms, if enough cells die, the entire organism will endure problems. Some viruses can cause life-long or chronic infections, where the viruses continue to replicate in the body despite the host's defence mechanisms. The other viruses cause life long infection because the virus remains within its host cell in a dormant (latent) state such as the herpes viruses, but the virus can reactivate and produce further attacks of disease at any time, if the host's defence system became weak for some reason.

Viruses have two phases in their life cycle: outside cells and within the cells they infect. Viral particles outside cells could survive for a long time in harsh conditions where they are inert entities called virions. Outside living cells viruses are not able to reproduce since they lack the machinery to replicate their own genome and produce the necessary proteins. Viruses can infect host cells, recognising their specific receptors on the cell surface. The viral receptors are normal surface host cell molecules involved in routine cellular functions, but since a portion of a molecular complex on the viral surface (typically spikes) has a shape complementary to the shape of the outer soluble part of the receptor, the virus is able to bind the receptor and be attached to the host cell's surface. After receptor-mediated attachment to its host the virus must find a way to enter the cell. Both enveloped and nonenveloped viruses use proteins present on their surfaces to bind to and enter the host cell employing the endocytosis mechanism. The endocytic vesicles transport the viral particles to the perinuclear area of the host cell, where the conditions for viral replication are optimal. The other way of infection is to inject only the viral genome (sometimes accompanied by additional proteins) directly into the host cytoplasm.

The viruses are very economical: They carry only the genetic information needed for replication of their nucleic acid and synthesis of the proteins necessary for their reproduction. Interestingly, the survival of viruses is totally dependent on the continued existence of their host, since after infection the viral genome switches the entire active host metabolism to synthesise the virion components. Without living host cells viruses will not be able to produce their progeny.

With the discovery of the electron microscope it became possible to study the morphology of viruses. The first studies immediately revealed that viruses could be distinguished by their size and shape, which became the important characteristics of their description. Viruses may be of a circular or oval shape, have the appearance of long thick or thin rods, which could be flexible or stiff. Some viruses have distinctive heads and a tail. The smallest viruses are around 20 nm in diameter and the largest around 500 nm. The viruses that infect and use bacteria resources are classified as bacteriophages. Often we refer to them as 'phages'.

The word 'bacteriophage' means to eat bacteria, and is so called because virulent bacteriophages can cause the compete lysis of a susceptible bacterial culture. Bacteriophages, like bacteria, are very common in all natural environments and are directly related to the numbers of bacteria present. As a consequence they represent the most abundant 'life' forms on Earth, with an estimated 10^{32} bacteriophages on the planet. Phages can be readily isolated from faeces and sewage, thus very common in soil. Sequencing of bacterial genomes has revealed that phage genome elements are an important source of sequence diversity and can potentially influence pathogenicity and the evolution of bacteria. The number of phages that have been isolated and characterised so far corresponds to only a tiny fraction of the total phage population. Since bacteriophages and animal cell viruses have many similarities phages are used as model systems for animal cell viruses to study steps of the viral life cycle and to understand the mechanisms by which bacterial genes can be transferred from one bacterium to another.

Why do we need to study bacteriophages: The first serious research of phages was done by d'Herelle which inspired him to do first experiments using phages in medicine. d'Herelle has used phages to treat a boy who had bad disentheria. After administration of phages the boy successfully recovered. Later d'Herelle and scientists from Georgia (former USSR) have created an Institute to study the properties of bacteriophages and their use in treating bacterial infections a decade before the discovery of penicillin. Unfortunately a lack of knowledge on basic phage biology and their molecular organisation has led to some clinical failures. At the end of 1930s antibiotics were discovered, they were very effective, and nearly wiped out studies on the medical use of phages. However, a new problem of bacterial resistance to antibiotics has arisen after many years of using them. Bacteria adapted themselves to become resistant to the most potent drugs used in modern medicine. The emergence of modified pathogens such as *Mycobacterium tuberculosis*, *Enterococcus faecalis*, *Staphylococcus aureus*, *Acinetobacter baumannii* and *Pseudomonas aeruginosa,* and methicillin-resistant *S. aureus* (MRSA) has created massive problems in treating patients in hospitals and the time required to produce new antibiotics is much longer than the time of bacterial adaptation. Modern studies on the phage life cycle have revealed a way for their penetration through membrane barriers of cells. These results are important in the development of methods for using bacteriophages as a therapeutic option in the treatment of bacterial infections. Phages, like many other viruses, infect only a certain range of bacteria that have the appropriate receptors in the outer membrane. The antibiotic resistance of the bacteria does not affect the infectious activity of a phage. Knowledge of the phage structure, understanding the mechanism of phage-cell surface interaction, and revealing the process of switching the cell replication machinery for phage propagation would allow the design of phages specific for bacterial illnesses.

CLASSIFICATION OF BACTERIOPHAGES

All known phages can be divided in two groups according to the type of infection. One group is characterised by a lytic infection and the other is represented by a lysogenic, or temperate, type of infection (Fig. 14.2). In the first form of infection the release of DNA induces switching of the protein machinery of the host bacterium for the benefit of infectious agents to produce 50–200 new phages. To make so many new phages requires nearly all the resources of the cell, which becomes weak and bursts. In other words, lysis takes place, causing death of the host bacterial cell. As result new phages are released into the extracellular space. The other mode of infection, lysogenic, is characterised by integration of the phage DNA into the host cell genome, although it may also exist as a plasmid. Incorporated phage DNA will be replicated along with the host bacteria genome and new bacteria will inherit the viral DNA. Such transition of viral DNA could take place through several generations of bacterium without major metabolic consequences for it. Eventually the phage genes, at certain conditions impeding the bacterium state, will revert to the lytic cycle, leading to release of fully assembled phages (Fig. 14.2). Analysis of phages with lysogenic or lytic mode of infection has shown that there is a tremendous variety of bacteriophages with variations in properties for each type of infection. Moreover, under certain conditions, some species were able to change the mode of infection, especially if the number of host cells was falling down. Temperate phages are not suitable for the phage therapy.

Classification of viruses is based on several factors such as their host preference, viral morphology, genome type and auxiliary structures such as tails or envelopes. The most upto-date classification of bacteriophages is given by Ackermann. The key classification factors are phage morphology and nucleic acid properties. The genome can be represented by either DNA or RNA. The vast majority of phages contain double strand DNA (dsDNA), while there are small phage groups with ssRNA, dsRNA, or ssDNA (ss stands for single strand). There are a few morphological groups of phages: filamentous phages, isosahedral phages without tails, phages with tails, and even several phages with a lipid-containing

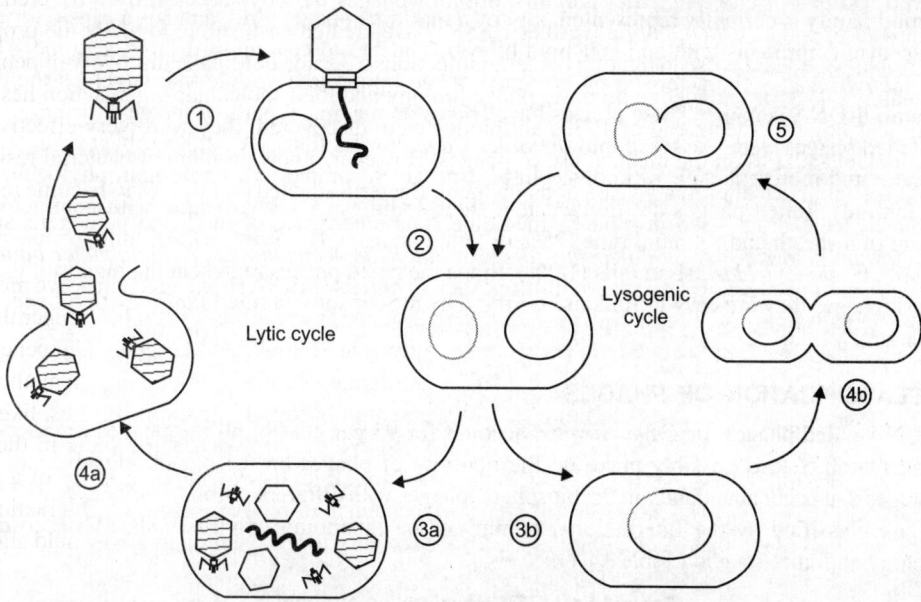

Fig. 14.2: Two cycles of bacteriophage reproduction. (1) Phage attaches the host cell and injects DNA, (2) Phage DNA enters lytic or lysogenic cycle, (3a) New phage DNA and proteins are synthesised and virions are assembled, (4a) Cell lyses releasing virions, (3b) and (4b) steps of lysogenic cycle: integration of the phage genome within the bacterial chromosome (becomes prophage) with normal bacterial reproduction, (5) Under certain conditions the prophage excises from the bacterial chromosome and initiates the lytic cycle.

envelope or contain lipids in the particle shell. This makes bacteriophages the largest viral group in nature. At present, more than 5500 bacterial viruses have been examined in the electron microscope.

Pleomorphic and filamentous phages comprise ~190 known bacteriophages (3.6% of phages) and are classified into 10 small families. These phages differ significantly in their features and characteristics apparently representing different lines of origin. Pleomorphic phages are characterised by a small number of known members that are divided into three families that need further characterisation. *Plasmaviridae* (dsDNA) includes phages with dsDNA that are covered by a lipoprotein envelope and therefore can be called a nucleoprotein granule. Members of the *Fusseloviridae* family have dsDNA inside a lemon-shaped capsid with short spikes at one end, *Guttavirus* phage group (dsDNA) is represented by droplet-shaped virus-like particles.

There are phages with helical or filamentous organisation. The *Inoviridae* (ssDNA) family includes phages that are long, rigid, or flexible filaments of variable length and have been classified by particle length, coat structure and DNA content. The *Lipothrixviridae* (dsDNA) phages are characterised by the combination of a lipoprotein envelope and rod-like shape. The *Rudiviridae* (dsDNA) family represents phages that are straight rigid rods without envelopes and closely resemble the tobacco mosaic virus. The next group of phages have capsids with an isosahedral shape. Phages from the *Leviviridae* family have ssRNA genome packed in small capsids and resemble enteroviruses. The known phages that form *Corticoviridae* family contain three molecules of dsRNA and, which is unusual, RNA polymerase. Phages with icosahedral symmetry for the capsids and a DNA genome compose the next three families *Microviridae*, *Cystoviridae* and *Tectiviridae*. The first includes small virions with a single circular ssDNA.

The second family is currently represented only by a maritime phage, PM2, and has a capsid formed by the outer layer of proteins with an inner lipid bilayer. The capsid contains a dsDNA genome. The last family, *Tectiviridae*, is characterised by presence of the lipoprotein vesicle that envelops the protein capsid with dsDNA genome. These phages have spikes on the apical parts of the envelope.

The tailed phages were classified into the order *Caudavirales* (dsDNA). Tailed phages can be found everywhere and represent 96% of known phages and are separated into three main phylogenetically related families. Tailed phages are divided into three families: A - *Myoviridae* with contractile tails consisting of a sheath and a central tube (25% of tailed phages), B - *Siphoviridae*, long, noncontractile tails (61%), C- *Podoviridae*, short tails (14 %). Since the tailed phages represent the biggest population of bacteriophages they are easy to find and purify, they are the most studied family both biochemically and structurally.

ICTV CLASSIFICATION OF PHAGES

The dsDNA tailed phages, or *Caudovirales*, account for 95 per cent of all the phages reported in the scientific literature, and possibly make up the majority of phages on the planet. However, there are other phages that occur abundantly in the biosphere, phages with different virions, genomes and lifestyles. Phages are classified by the International committee on taxonomy of viruses (ICTV) according to morphology and nucleic acid (Table 14.1).

Table 14.1: ICTV classification of phages.

Order	Family	Morphology	Nucleic acid	Examples
	Myoviridae	Non-enveloped, contractile tail	Linear dsDNA	
Caudovirales	*Siphoviridae*	Non-enveloped, long non-contractile tail	Linear dsDNA	λ phage
	Podoviridae	Non-enveloped, short noncontractile tail	Linear dsDNA	T7phage
	Tectiviridae	Non-enveloped, isometric	Linear dsDNA	
	Corticoviridae	Non-enveloped, isometric	Circular dsDNA	
	Lipothrixviridae	Enveloped, rod-shaped	Linear dsDNA	
	Plasmaviridae	Enveloped, pleomorphic	Circular dsDNA	
	Rudiviridae	Non-enveloped, rod-shaped	Linear dsDNA	
Unassigned	*Fuselloviridae*	Non-enveloped, lemon-shaped	Circular dsDNA	
	Inoviridae	Non-enveloped, filamentous	Circular ssDNA	
	Microviridae	Non-enveloped, isometric	Circular ssDNA	
	Leviviridae	Non-enveloped, isometric	Linear ssRNA	
	Cystoviridae	Enveloped, spherical	Segmented dsRNA	

Replication

Bacteriophages may have a lytic cycle or a lysogenic cycle, and a few viruses are capable of carrying out both. With lytic phages such as the T4 phage, bacterial cells are broken open (lysed) and destroyed after immediate replication of the virion. As soon as the cell is destroyed, the new phages can find new hosts. Lytic phages are the kind suitable for phage therapy.

In contrast, the lysogenic cycle does not result in immediate lysing of the host cell. Those phages able to undergo lysogeny are known as temperate phages. Their viral genome will integrate with host DNA and replicate along with it fairly harmlessly, or may even become established as a plasmid. The virus remains dormant until host conditions deteriorate, perhaps due to depletion of nutrients, then the endogenous phages (known as prophages) become active. At this point they initiate the reproductive cycle, resulting in lysis of the host cell. As the lysogenic cycle allows the host cell to continue to survive and reproduce, the virus is reproduced in all of the cell's offspring.

Sometimes prophages may provide benefits to the host bacterium while they are dormant by adding new functions to the bacterial genome in a phenomenon called lysogenic conversion. A famous example is the conversion of a harmless strain of *Vibrio cholerae* by a phage into a highly virulent one, which causes cholera. This is why temperate phages are not suitable for phage therapy.

Attachment and penetration

To enter a host cell, bacteriophages attach to specific receptors on the surface of bacteria, including lipopolysaccharides, teichoic acids, proteins, or even flagella. This specificity means that a bacteriophage can only infect certain bacteria bearing receptors that they can bind to, which in turn determines the phage's host range. Host growth conditions also influence the ability of the phage to attach and invade bacteria. As phage virions do not move independently, they must rely on random encounters with the right receptors when in solution (blood, lymphatic circulation, irrigation, soil water, etc.).

Complex bacteriophages use a hypodermic syringe-like motion to inject their genetic material into the cell. After making contact with the appropriate receptor, the tail fibres bring the base plate closer to the surface of the cell. Once attached completely, the tail contracts, possibly with the help of ATP present in the tail, injecting genetic material through the bacterial membrane (Fig. 14.3).

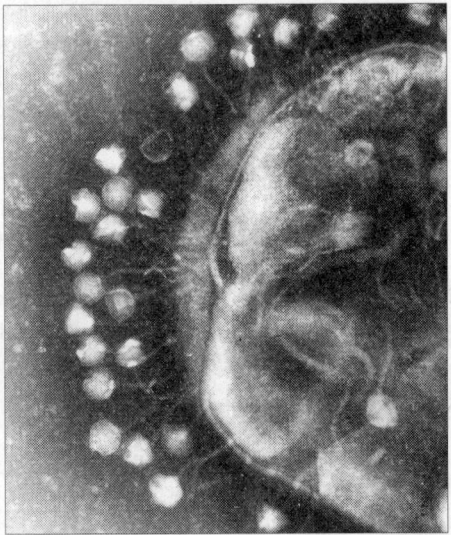

Fig. 14.3: An electron micrograph of bacteriophages attached to a bacterial cell. These viruses are the size and shape of coliphage T1.

Synthesis of proteins and nucleic acid

Within minutes, bacterial ribosomes start translating viral mRNA into protein. For RNA-based phages, RNA replicase is synthesised early in the process. Proteins modify the bacterial RNA polymerase so that it preferentially transcribes viral mRNA. The host's normal synthesis of proteins and nucleic acids is disrupted, and it is forced to manufacture viral products instead. These products go on to become part of new virions within the cell, helper proteins which help assemble the new virions, or proteins involved in cell lysis.

Virion assembly

In the case of the T4 phage, the construction of new virus particles involves the assistance of helper proteins. The base plates are assembled first, with the tails being built upon them afterwards. The head capsids, constructed separately, will spontaneously assemble with the tails. The DNA is packed efficiently within the heads. The whole process takes about 15 minutes.

Release of virions

Phages may be released via cell lysis, by extrusion, or, in a few cases, by budding. Lysis, by tailed phages, is achieved by an enzyme called endolysin, which attacks and breaks down the cell wall peptidoglycan. An altogether different phage type, the filamentous phages, make the host cell continually secrete new virus particles. Released virions are described as free, and, unless defective, are capable of infecting a new bacterium. Budding is associated with certain Mycoplasma phages. In contrast to virion release, phages displaying a lysogenic cycle do not kill the host but, rather, become long-term residents as prophage.

Phage therapy

Phages were discovered to be anti-bacterial agents but the medical trials performed in western countries were sub-standard to the point of not being scientifically viable, this because the early tests were conducted poorly and without an idea of what a phage was. Phage therapy was shortly thereafter ruled out as untrustworthy much because many of the trials were conducted on totally unrelated diseases such as allergies and viral infections. Antibiotics were discovered some years later and marketed widely, popular because of their broad spectrum and easier to manufacture in bulk, store, and prescribe.

In the environment

Metagenomics has allowed the detection of bacteriophages in water that was not possible previously. These investigations revealed that phage are much more abundant in the water column of both freshwater and marine habitats than previously thought and that they can cause significant mortality of bacterioplankton. Methods in phage community ecology have been developed to assess phage-induced mortality of bacterioplankton and its role for food web process and biogeochemical cycles, to genetically fingerprint phage communities or populations and estimate viral biodiversity by metagenomics. The lysis of bacteria by phages releases organic carbon that was previously particulate (cells) into dissolved forms, which makes the carbon more available to other organisms. Phages are not only the most abundant biological entities but probably also the most diverse ones. The majority of the sequence data obtained from phage communities has no equivalent in databases. These data and other detailed analyses indicate that phage-specific genes and ecological traits are much more frequent than previously thought. In order to reveal the meaning of this genetic and ecological versatility, studies have to be performed with communities and at spatiotemporal scales relevant for micro-organisms.

Bacteriophages have also been used in hydrological tracing and modelling in river systems especially where surface water and groundwater interactions occur. The use of phages is preferred to the more conventional dye marker because they are significantly less absorbed when passing through groundwaters and they are readily detected at very low concentrations.

Role in food fermentation

A broad number of food products, commodity chemicals, and biotechnology products are manufactured industrially by large-scale bacterial fermentation of various organic substrates. Because enormous amounts of bacteria are being cultivated each day in large fermentation vats, the risk of bacteriophage contamination could rapidly bring fermentation to a halt. The resulting economical setback is a serious threat in these industries. The relationship between bacteriophages and their bacterial hosts is very important in the context of the food fermentation industry. Sources of phage contamination, measures to control their propagation and dissemination, and biotechnological defense strategies developed to restrain phages are of interest. The dairy fermentation industry has openly acknowledged the problem of phage and has been working with academia and starter culture companies to develop defense strategies and systems to curtail the propagation and evolution of phages for decades.

ORGANISATION OF TAILED BACTERIOPHAGES

General Architecture of Bacteriophages

The basic structural features of bacteriophages are coats (or capsids) that protect the genome hidden inside a capsid and additional structures providing interface with a bacterium membrane for the genome release. The *Caudovirales* order of bacteriophages is characterised by dsDNA genomes and by the common overall organisation of the virus particles characterised by a capsid and a tail. Different phage species can vary both in size from 24–400 nm in length and genome length. Their DNA sequences differ significantly and can range in the size from 18 to 400 kb in length.

Structures obtained by electron microscopy (EM) do not typically provide detailed information on the atomic components owing to methods used for visualisation of particles. However, EM has allowed visualisation of these minuscule particles and morphological analysis. Each virion has a polyhedral, predominantly icosahedral, head (capsid) that covers the genome. The heads are composed of many copies of one or several different proteins and have a very stable organisation. A bacteriophage tail is attached to the capsid through a connector which serves as an adaptor between these two crucial components of the phage. The connector is a hetero-oligomer composed of several proteins. Connectors carry out several functions during the phage life cycle. They participate in the packaging of dsDNA into the capsid, and later they perform the function of a gatekeeper: locking the capsid exit of the phage, preventing leakage of DNA which is under high pressure and later, after a signal transmitted by the tail indicating that the phage is attached to the bacterium, the connector will be open allowing the release of DNA into the bacterium. The tail and its related structures are indispensable phage elements securing the entry of the viral nucleic acid into the host bacterium during the infectivity process. The tail serves both as a signal transmitter and subsequently as a pipeline through which DNA is delivered into the host cell during infection. The tails may be short or long, the latter are divided into contractile and noncontractile tails. The long tails are typically composed of many copies of several proteins arranged with helical symmetry. All types of tails have outer appendages attached to the distant end of the tail and often include a baseplate with several fibres and a tip, or a needle that has specificity to the membrane receptors of the bacterium. As soon the receptor has been found by the tail needle, which happens during multiple short living reversible attachments to the bacterium, the baseplate and tail fibres are involved in the binding of the phage to the bacterial outer membrane that makes the attachment irreversible. The docking (irreversible attachment) of the phage induces opening of the phage connector and release of the genome through the tail tube into the bacterial cell.

DNA and its Packaging

The virions of the bactriophage *Caudovirales* have a genome represented by linear molecules of dsDNA. The length of genome varies significantly between the phages . DNA is translocated through the central channel of the portal protein located at one vertex of the capsid. The portal complex provides a docking point for the viral ATPase complex (*terminase*). The terminase bound to the portal vertex forms the active packaging motor that moves the viral dsDNA inside the capsid. Encapsidation is normally initiated by an endonucleolytic cleavage at a defined sequence (*pac*) of the substrate DNA concatemer although some phages like T4 do not use a unique site for the initial cleavage. Packaging proceeds evenly until a threshold amount of DNA is reached inside the viral capsid. At the latter stages of packaging the increasingly dense arrangement of the DNA leads to a steep rise in pressure inside the capsid that can reach ~6 MPa. The headful cleavage of DNA is imprecise leading to variations in chromosome size of more than 1 kb. The mechanism of packaging requires a sensor that measures the amount of DNA headfilling and a nuclease that will cleave DNA as soon the head is full. Termination of the DNA packaging is coordinated with closure of the portal system to avoid leakage of the viral genome. In tailed bacteriophages this is most frequently achieved through the binding of head completion proteins (or adaptor proteins). The complex of the portal dodecamer and these proteins composes the connector. After termination of the first packaging cycle initiated at *pac* (initiation cycle), a second packaging event is initiated at the non-encapsidated DNA end created by the headful cleavage and additional cycles of encapsidation follow. Some packaging series can yield 12 or more encapsidation events revealing the high processivity of the packaging machinery.

METHODS FOR STUDY OF BACTERIOPHAGES

Microbiology and bacteriology were the first methods used to investigate viruses. Studies related to the life cycle of prokaryotic and eukaryotic micro-organisms such as bacteria, viruses, and bacteriophages are combined into microbiology. This includes gene expression and regulation, genetic transfer, the synthesis of macromolecules, sub-cellular organisation, cell to cell communication, and molecular aspects of pathogenicity and virulence. The earlier studies of phages were based on microbiological experiments including immunology. Now-a-days the research of the biological processes is not limited to biochemical analysis and microbiology. To understand processes of virus/cell communication and interaction one often needs information on the molecular level and conformational changes of the components under different conditions. Gel filtration or Western blotting provides information for a protein on the macromolecular level such as size, molecular mass, binding to an antibody etc. These experiments will display how the proteins will change their characteristics with several chemical modifications and analysing what kind of change occurred, one could draw a conclusion for the structure. At the cellular level, optical microscopy can reveal the spatial distribution and dynamics of molecules tagged with fluorophores.

X-ray crystallography and NMR of phages

The methods of X-ray crystallography and NMR spectroscopy provide detailed information on molecular structure and dynamics. However, X-ray crystallography requires the growth of protein crystals up to 1 mm in size from a highly purified protein. Crystal growth is an experimental technique and there are no rules about the optimal conditions for a protein solution to result in a good protein crystal. It is extremely difficult to predict good conditions for nucleation or growth of well-ordered crystals of large molecular complexes. In practice, the best conditions are identified by screening multiple probes where a wide variety of crystallisation solutions are tested. Structural analysis of viral proteins by crystallographic methods was very successful when separate proteins were studied. Protein crystals contain trillions of accurately packed identical protein molecules. When irradiated by X-rays, these crystals scatter X-rays in certain directions producing diffraction patterns. Computational analysis of that diffraction produces atomic models of the proteins. Viruses are much bigger than single proteins and may comprise thousands of components, it is difficult to pack them into crystals, and when successful, crystals have large unit cell dimensions (unit cell is an elementary part, from which the crystal is composed). Because of that the diffraction from virus crystals is far weaker than that of single proteins. It was an extremely challenging task to crystallise viruses for crystallographic studies although some icosahedral viruses were crystallised and the atomic structures have been obtained. Now-a-days X-ray analysis has provided a wealth of information on atomic structures of many small protein components of large viruses including bacteriophages. Nuclear Magnetic Resonance (NMR) is another very powerful method of structural analysis allowing studying dynamics of samples in solution. NMR methodology, combined with the availability of molecular biology and biochemical methods for preparation and isotope labelling of recombinant proteins has dramatically increased its usage for the characterisation of structure and dynamics of biological molecules in solution.

In NMR, a strong, high frequency magnetic field stimulates atomic nuclei of the isotopes H1, D2, C13, or N15 and measures the frequency of the magnetic field of the atomic nuclei during its oscillation period before returning back to the initial state. NMR is able to obtain the same high resolution using different properties of the samples. NMR measures the distances between atomic nuclei, rather than the electron density in a molecule. Protein folding studies can be done by monitoring NMR spectra upon folding or denaturing of a protein in real time. However, NMR cannot deal with macromolecules in the mega-Dalton range, the upper weight limit for NMR structure determination is ~50 kDa.

Electron Microscopy of Tailed Bacteriophages

For microbiological research, light microscopy is a tool of great importance in studies of the biology of micro-organisms. However, light microscopy is not able to provide a high enough magnification to see viruses. The modern development and use of synchrotrons has revealed the structures of spherical viruses, nonetheless obtaining virus crystals remained problematic, especially for bacteriophages. EM has become a major tool for structural biology over the molecular to cellular size range. Bacteriophages do not have exact icosahedral symmetry since they have different appendages facilitating interactions and infection of the host cells, a fact that makes them very challenging objects for crystallography and their size makes them unsuitable for NMR. Members of the *Caudovirales* phage family with dsDNA genome are especially difficult to crystallise because they have tails. Here EM has become a tool of choice for structural analysis of these samples. The simplest method for examining isolated viral particles is negative staining, in which a droplet of the suspension is spread on an EM support film and then embedded in a heavy metal salt solution, typically uranyl acetate. The method is called negative staining because the macromolecular shape is seen by its exclusion of stain rather than by binding of stain. During the last two decades other methods became widely used and demonstrated their efficiency when samples where fixed in the native, hydrated state by rapid freezing of thin layers of aqueous sample solutions at liquid nitrogen temperatures. Such rapid cooling traps the biological molecule in its native, hydrated state but embedded in glass-like, solid water – vitrified ice. This procedure prevents the formation of ice crystals, which would be very damaging to the specimen. EM images of particles are used to calculate their three-dimensional structures.

EM was a major tool used in analysis of phage morphology and initiated a process of classification of viruses. The development of cryogenic methods has enabled EM imaging to provide snapshots of biological molecules and cells trapped in a close to native, hydrated state. High symmetry of the complexes is an advantage, but single particles of molecular mass –0.5–100 MDa with or without symmetry (e.g. viruses, ribosomes) can now be studied with confidence and can often reveal fine details of the 3D structure. The resulting images allow information not only on quaternary structure arrangements of macromolecular complexes but the positions of their secondary structural elements like helices and betasheets.

Hybrid Methods

The components of bacteriophages and their interactions have to be identified and analysed. This can be done by localisation of known NMR or X-ray structures of individual viral proteins and nucleic acids combined with biochemical information to identify them in the EM structures. Electron cryo-microscopy and three-dimensional image reconstruction provide a powerful means to study the structure, complexity, and dynamics of a wide range of macromolecular complexes. One has to use different approaches for several reasons: there are limitations of the individual methods, some complexes do not crystallise, phages, being multi-protein complexes, have different conformational organisation at different conditions. Therefore all known structural and biochemical methods have to complement each other to generate structural information.

When atomic models of components or sub-assemblies are accessible, they can be fitted into reconstructed density maps to produce informative pseudoatomic models. If atomic structures of the components are not known, it is helpful to perform homology modelling so that the generated models could be fitted into the EM maps. Fitting atomic structures and models into EM maps allows researchers to test different hypotheses, verify variations in structures of viruses and effectively increase the EM map resolution creating pseudo-atomic viral models.

EXAMPLES OF BACTERIOPHAGE STRUCTURES

In spite of the great abundance of the tailed phages, details of their organisation have emerged only during the last decade. The progress in structural studies of phages as a whole entity was slow because of their flexibility and complex organisation. The additional hindrance arises from intricate combination of different oligomerisation levels of the phage elements. Fully assembled capsids have at least 5-fold symmetry or more often, icosahedral symmetry where multiple structural units form a regular lattice with 2, 3, and 5 rotational symmetries. All known portal proteins were found to be dodecameric oligomers, tails have overall 6- or 3-fold rotational symmetry, the multiple repeats of major proteins have helical arrangement. The proteins related to the receptor sensor system at the far end of the tail could be in 6, 3, or only one copy.

The information on the relative amount of different protein components has been revealed by biochemical and structural methods such as X-ray analysis of separate components. Development of hard and software has led to new imaging systems of better quality, new programmes allowing processing of bigger data sets comprising hundreds of thousand images. The modern strategy is based on hybrid methods where structure determination at high resolution of isolated phage components is combined in three-dimensional maps of lower resolution obtained by electron microscopy. Electron microscopy by itself has reached such level of quality that for the complexes with icosahedral symmetry it has became nearly routine to obtain structures at 4–5 Å resolution.

M13 Bacteriophage

M13 is a virus that infects the bacterium *Escherichia coli*. It is composed of a circular single-stranded DNA molecule encased in a thin flexible tube made up of about 2700 copies of the major coat protein, P8. The ends of the tube are capped with minor coat proteins. Infection starts when the minor coat protein P3 attaches to the receptor at the tip of the *F pilus* of the bacterium. Infection with M13 is not lethal, however, the infection causes turbid plaques in *E. coli* because infected bacteria grow more slowly than the surrounding uninfected bacteria. It engages in a viral lifestyle known as a chronic infection which is neither lytic nor temperate. However a decrease in the rate of cell growth is seen in the infected cells. M13 plasmids are used for many recombinant DNA processes, and the virus has also been studied for its uses in nanostructures and nanotechnology.

Phage particles

The phage coat is primarily assembled from a 50 amino acid protein called pVIII (or p8), which is encoded by gene VIII (or g8) in the phage genome. For a wild type M13 particle, it takes approximately 2700 copies of p8 to make the coat about 900 nm long. The coat's dimensions are flexible though and the number of p8 copies adjusts to accommodate the size of the single stranded genome it packages. For example, when the phage genome was mutated to reduce its number of DNA bases (from 6.4 knt to 221 nt), then the number of p8 copies was decreased to fewer than 100, causing the p8 coat to shrink in order to fit the reduced genome. The phage appear to be limited at approximately twice the natural DNA content. However, deletion of a phage protein (p3) prevents full escape from the host *E. coli*, and phage that are 10–20X the normal length with several copies of the phage genome can be seen shedding from the *E. coli* host.

There are four other proteins on the phage surface, two of which have been extensively studied. At one end of the filament are five copies of the surface exposed pIX (p9) and a more buried companion protein, pVII (p7). If p8 forms the shaft of the phage, p9 and p7 form the 'blunt' end that is seen in the micrographs. These proteins are very small, containing only 33 and 32 amino acids respectively, though some additional residues can be added to the *N*-terminal portion of each which are then presented on the outside of the coat. At the other end of the phage particle are five copies of the surface exposed pIII (p3) and its less exposed accessory protein, pVI (p6). These form the rounded tip of the phage and are the first proteins to interact with the *E. coli* host during infection. p3 is also the last point of contact with the host as new phage bud from the bacterial surface.

Replication in E. coli

Below are steps involved with replication of M13 in *E. coli*.

*   Viral (+) strand DNA enters cytoplasm.
*   Complementary (–) strand is synthesised by bacterial enzymes.
*   DNA Gyrase, a type II topoisomerase, acts on double-stranded DNA and catalyses formation of negative supercoils in double-stranded DNA.
*   Final product is parental replicative form (RF) DNA.
*   A phage protein, pII, nicks the (+) strand in the RF.
*   3′-hydroxyl acts as a primer in the creation of new viral strand.
*   pII circulises displaced viral (+) strand DNA.

- Pool of progeny double-stranded RF molecules produced.
- Negative strand of RF is template of transcription.
- mRNAs are translated into the phage proteins.

Phage proteins in the cytoplasm are pII, pX, and pV, and they are part of the replication process of DNA. The other phage proteins are synthesised and inserted into the cytoplasmic or outer membranes.

- pV dimers bind newly synthesised single-stranded DNA and prevent conversion to RF DNA.
- RF DNA synthesis continues and amount of pV reaches critical concentration.
- DNA replication switches to synthesis of single-stranded (+) viral DNA.
- pV-DNA structures from about 800 nm long and 8 nm in diameter.
- pV-DNA complex is substrate in phage assembly reaction.

Applications of M13

George Smith, among others, showed that fragments of EcoRI endonuclease could be fused in the unique Bam site of f1 filamentous phage and thereby expressed in gene III whose protein pIII was externally accessible. M13 does not have this unique Bam site in gene III. M13 had to be engineered to have accessible insertion sites, making it limited in its flexibility in handling different sized inserts. Because the M13 phage display system allows great flexibility in the location and number of recombinant proteins on the phage, it is a popular tool to construct or serve as a scaffold for nanostructures. For example, the phage can be engineered to have a different protein on each end and along its length. This can be used to assemble structures like gold or cobalt oxide nano-wires for batteries or to pack carbon nanotubes into straight bundles for use in photovoltaics.

Phage T4

The T4 phage of the *Myoviridae* family infects *E. coli* bacteria and is one of the largest phages, it is approximately 200 nm long and 80–100 nm wide with the capsid in a shape of an elongated icosahedron. The phage has a rigid tail composed of two main layers: the inner tail tube is surrounded by a contractile sheath which contracts during infection of the bacterium. The tail sheath is separated from the head by a neck. Phages of *Myoviridae* family have a massive baseplate at the end of the tail with fibres attached to it. The tail fibres help to find receptors of a host cell and provide the initial contact, during infection the tail tube penetrates an outer bacterial membrane to secure the pathway for genome to be injected into the cell.

The capsid of the T4 phage is built with three essential proteins: gp23* (48.7 kDa), which forms the hexagonal capsid lattice, gp24* (the * designates the cleaved form of the protein when the prohead matures to infectious virus) forms pentamers at eleven of the twelve vertices, and gp20, which forms the unique dodecameric portal vertex through which DNA enters during packaging and exits during infection. 3D-reconstruction has been determined at 22 Å resolution by cryo-EM for the wild-type phage T4 capsid forming a prolate icosahedron. The major capsid protein gp23* forms a hexagonal lattice with a separation of ~140 Å between hexamer centres. The atomic structure of gp24* has been determined by X-ray crystallography and an atomic model for gp23* was built using its similarity to gp24*. The capsid also contains two non-essential outer capsid proteins, Hoc and Soc, which decorate the capsid surface. The structure of Soc has been determined by X-ray crystallography and shows that Soc has two capsid binding sites which, through binding to adjacent gp23* subunits, reinforce the capsid structure. The failure of gp24* to bind Soc provides a possible explanation for the property of osmotic shock resistance of the phage. The 3D maps of the empty capsids with and without Soc have been determined at 27 and at 15 Å resolution, respectively. Single molecule optical tweezers and fluorescence studies showed that the T4 motor packages DNA at a rate of up to 2000 bp/sec, the fastest reported to date of any packaging motor. FRET-FCS studies indicate that the DNA gets compressed during the translocation process.

Tails of *Myoviridae* phages have a long, non-contractible tube surrounded by a contractile sheath. Bacteriophage T4 has a tail sheath that is composed of 138 copies of gp18. The tail tube inside the sheath is estimated to be assembled from as many gp19 subunits as there are gp18 subunits in the sheath. The tail sheath has helical symmetry with a pitch of 40.6 Å and a twist of 17.2°. The tail sheath contraction can be divided into several steps. Previous studies of partially contracted sheath showed that conformational changes of the sheath are propagated 'upwards' starting from the disk of the gp18 subunits closest to the baseplate. The cryo-EM reconstructions showed that during contraction, the tail sheath pitch decreases from 40.6 Å to 16.4 Å and its diameter increases from 24 nm to 33 nm. The combination of X-ray model and EM structures show that gp18 monomers remain rigid during contraction and move about 50 Å radially outwards while tilting 45° clockwise, viewed from outside the tail. During contraction of the tail the interactions between neighbouring subunits within a disk are broken so that the subunits from the disk above get inserted into the gaps formed in the disk below.

The baseplate with the cell-puncturing device of the T4 phage is an ultimate element of the phage. This is an extremely complex multiprotein structure on the far end of the tail and represents multifunctional machinery that anchor the phage on the bacteria surface and provide formation of the DNA entrance into the bacteria. This important part of the phage structure is of ~27 nm in height and 52 nm in diameter at its widest part. The baseplate conformation is coupled to that of the sheath: the dome shape conformation is associated with the extended sheath, whereas the flat 'star' conformation is associated with the contracted sheath that occurs in the T4 particle after attachment to the host cell. Short treatment of bacteriophage T4 with 3 M urea resulted in the transformation of the baseplate to a star-shape and subsequent tail sheath contraction. During that switch the baseplate diameter increases to 61 nm and the height decreases to 12 nm although the protein composition of the baseplate does not change. It is composed of ~150 subunits of a dozen different gene products. Proteins gp11, gp10, gp7, gp8, gp6, gp53, and gp25 form one sector of 6-fold structure. The central hub of the baseplate is formed by gp5, gp27, and gp29 and probably includes gp26 and gp28. Assembly of the baseplate is completed by attaching gp9 and gp12 to form the short tail fibres, and also gp48 and gp54 that are required to initiate polymerisation of the tail tube, a channel for DNA. T4 tail has three types of fibrous proteins: the long tail fibres, the short tail fibres, and whiskers. Long tail fibres and short tail fibres are attached to the baseplate and whiskers extending outwardly in the region of the tail connection to the capsid. The long tail fibres, which are ~145 nm long and only ~4 nm in diameter, are primary reversible adsorption devices. Each fibre consists of the rigid proximal halves, formed by gp34, and the distal ones composed by gp36 and gp37.

The distal part of the fibre has a rod-like shape about 40 nm long that is connected to the first half of the fibre through the globular hinge. Gp35 forms a hinge region and interacts with gp34 and gp36. The *N*-terminal globular domain of gp34 interacts with the baseplate. Short tail fibres are attached to the baseplate by the *N*-terminal thin part, while the globular C-terminus binds to the host cell receptors. The structure of this domain of the short tail fibres was determined by X-ray crystallography.

HK97

HK97 is a temperate phage from *Escherichia coli* and it shares a host range with the Lambda phage. HK97 has an isometric head and a long, flexible, non-contractile tail representing *Siphoviridae* family.

The HK97 phage has multi step pathway of selfassembly revealing two forms of procapsids of ~470 Å in diameter. Capsid protein gp5 (42 kDa) forms capsids, with icosahedral symmetry characterised by $T = 7$. A part of the gp5 (102 amino acids from the N terminus) plays the role of a scaffold, which is cleaved by gp4 (the phage protease) at maturation of the capsid. The first low resolution structures have shown conformation changes reflecting transition of the HK97 procapsids into expanded capsids. The diameter of procapsids during transition into the heads increases from 470 Å to 550 Å while the thickness of the capsid shell changes from 50 Å to ~ 25 Å.

The first atomic structure of a capsid for the tailed phage was only published in 2000. Gp5, if expressed alone, assembles into a portal-deficient version of prohead I. Co-expressing gp5 with the gp4 protease, which cleaves gp5 scaffolding domain, produces Prohead II that expands into the icosahedral head II (the diameter is ~650 Å) without DNA and portal complex, and it was used for the crystallisation. The crystal structure of the dsDNA bacteriophage HK97 mature empty capsid was determined at 3.6 Å resolution using icosahedral symmetry. The capsid crystal structure shows how an isopeptide bond is formed between subunits, arranged in topologically linked, covalent circular rings. The structure of the HK97 gp5 coat protein has revealed a new category of virus fold: it is mixture alpha-helices and beta-sheets organised into three domains that are not sequence contiguous. Domain A is located close to the centre of the hexamers and pentamers of the capsid. Domain P (peripheral) provides contacts between adjacent molecules within pentamers and hexamers. The third domain, represented by the E-loop, is an extension through which each subunit of the HK97 capsid is covalently linked to two neighbouring subunits. The bond organisation explains why the mature HK97 particles are extraordinarily stable and cannot be disassembled on an SDS gel without protease treatment.

SPP1

SPP1 is a virulent *Bacillus subtilis* dsDNA phage and belongs to the *Siphoviridae* family. The virion is composed of an icosahedral, isometric capsid (~60 nm diameter) and a long, flexible, non-contractile tail. The SPP1 genome length is 45.9 kb. The procapsid (or prohead) of SPP1 consists of four proteins: the scaffold protein gp11, the major capsid protein gp13, the portal protein gp6, and a minor component gp7. The inside of the capsid is filled with gp11 which exits the procapsid during DNA packaging. Gp13 and the decoration protein gp12 form the head shell of the mature SPP1 capsid.

The portal protein is located at a 5-fold vertex of the icosahedral phage head and serves as the entrance for DNA during packaging. The structure of gp6 as a 13-subunit assembly was determined by EM and X-ray at 10 and 3.4 Å resolution correspondingly. The 13–mer portal complex has a circular arrangement with an overall diameter of ~165 Å and a height of ~110 Å. A central tunnel pierces the assembly through the whole height. The portal protein monomer has four main domains: crown, wing, stem, and clip. The crown domain consists of three alpha-helices connected by short loops and has 40 additional C-terminal residues that are disordered in the X-ray structure. Mutations in the crown indicate the importance of this area for DNA translocation. The wing region is formed by alpha-helices flanked on the outer side by a beta-sheet. The stem domain connects the wing to the clip domain. It consists of two alpha-helices that are conserved in phi29 and SPP1 phages, a similar arrangement of helices was found in the P22 portal protein. The clip domain forms the base of the portal protein and is expected to be exposed to the outside of the capsid during viral particle assembly. The three-dimensional structures of the portal proteins of SPP1, phi29, and P22 phages demonstrate a strikingly similar fold. Although there is no detectable amino-acid sequence similarity between proteins, they have a nearly identical arrangement of two helices forming stem domains and in the clip domain which form a tightly packed ring of three stranded beta-sheets each made up of two strands from one subunit and one strand from an adjacent subunit. After termination of DNA incorporation the portal pore needs to be rapidly closed to prevent leakage of the viral chromosome. In SPP1 this role is played by the head completion proteins gp15 and gp16 that bind sequentially to the portal vertex forming the connector. Disruption of the capsids yielded connectors composed of gp6, gp15 and gp16. The connector is an active element of the phage that is involved into packaging the viral genome, serves as an interface for attachment of the tail, and controls DNA release from the capsid. The connector of *Bacillus subtilis* bacteriophage SPP1 was found to be a 12-fold cyclical oligomer, though isolated gp6 is a cyclical 13mer. The structure of the connector was determined at 10 Å resolution, using cryo-EM. Both the isolated portal protein and the gp6 oligomer in the connector reveal a similar arrangement of four main domains, the major changes take place in the clip domain through which gp15 contacts gp6. The connector structure shows that gp15 serves as an extension of the portal protein channel where gp16 binds. The central channel is closed by gp16 physically blocking the exit from the DNA-filled capsid. Structures of SPP1 gp15 and gp16 monomers were determined by NMR and together with gp6 were docked into the EM map of the connector. The channel of the connector will be opened when the virus infects a host cell. Comparison of the structures before and after assembly, provides details on the major structural rearrangements (gp15) and folding events (gp15 and gp16) that accompany connector formation.

The 160-nm-long tail of the SPP1 phage is composed of two major tail proteins (MTPs), gp17.1 and gp17.1, in a ratio of about 3:1. They share a common amino-terminus, but the latter species is ~10 kDa more than gp17.1. The polypeptide sequence, identical in the two proteins is responsible for assembly of the tail tube while the additional module of gp17.1 shields the structure exterior exposed to the environment. The carboxyl-terminus domain of MTPs shares homology to motifs of cellular proteins or to phage components involved in binding to cell surfaces. Structures of the bacteriophage SPP1 tail before and after DNA ejection were determined by negative stain electron microscopy. The results reveal extensive structural rearrangements in the internal wall of the tail tube. It has been proposed that the adsorption device–receptor interaction triggers a conformational switch that is propagated as a domino-like cascade along the 160 nm -long helical tail structure to reach the head-to-tail connector. This leads to opening of the connector, culminating in DNA exit from the head into the host cell through the tail tube.

The tail tip is attached to the cap structure that closes the tail tube. The absence of a channel for DNA traffic in the tip implies that it must dissociate from the cap for DNA passage to the cytoplasm during infection. The structural data show that the tail tip does not have a channel for DNA egress and that the signal initiated by interaction of the tip with the bacterial receptor causes release of the tip from the tail cap. Reconstructions were performed for two states of the tail: before and after DNA ejection. The cap structure was reconstructed separately from the tip and the main area of the tail. The reconstructions of the cap together with the first four rings of the tail tube demonstrate that the tail external diameter (before DNA ejection) tapers from ~110 to ~40Å at the capped extremity and changes symmetry from six-fold to three-fold. This arrangement provides a sturdy interface between the tail tube and the three-fold symmetric tip. Opening of the dome-shaped cap involves loss of the tip and movement of the cap subunits outwards from the tail axis, creating a channel with the same diameter as the inner tail tube.

Phi29

The *Bacillus subtilis* bacteriophage phi29 (*Podoviridae* family) is one of the smallest and simplest known dsDNA phages. The bacteriophage phi29 is a 19-kilobase (19-kb) dsDNA virus with a prolate head and complex structure. Proheads consist of the major capsid protein gp8, scaffolding protein gp7, head fibre protein gp8.5, head–tail connector gp10, and a pRNA oligomer. Mature phi 29 heads are 530Å long and 430Å wide, and the tail is 380Å long. The packaging of DNA into the head involves, besides the portal protein, other essential components such as an RNA called pRNA and the ATPase p16, required to provide energy to the translocation machinery. Once the DNA has been packaged, pRNA and p16 are released from the portal protein. In the mature phi29 virion, the narrow end of the portal protrudes out of the capsid and attaches to a toroidal collar (gp11). The collar has a diameter of about 130Å and is surrounded by 12 appendages that function to absorb the virion on host cells. A thin, 160Å -long tube, with an outer diameter of 60Å, leads away from the centre of the collar. The outer end of the tail (gp9) has a cylindrical shape and bigger diameter of ~ 80Å.

The three-dimensional structure of a fibreless variant has been determined to 7.9 Å resolution allowing the identification of helices and beta-sheets. For the prolate capsid phi29 there was not the advantage of using icosahedral symmetry for structural analysis, its cryo-EM three-dimensional reconstructions have been made of mature and of emptied bacteriophage phi29 particles without making symmetry assumptions. Possible positions of secondary elements for gp8 indicate that the folds of the phi29 and bacteriophage HK97 capsid proteins are similar except for an additional immunoglobulin-like domain of the phi29 protein: the gp8 residues 348–429 are 32% identical to the group 2 bacterial immunoglobulin domain (BIG2) consensus sequence. The BIG2 domain is found in many bacterial and phage surface proteins related to cell adhesion complexes. The asymmetrical reconstruction of the complete phi29 has revealed new details of the asymmetric interactions and conformational dynamics of the phi29 protein and DNA components.

The DNA packaging motor is located at a unique portal vertex of the prohead and contains: the head-tail connector (a dodecamer of gp10), the portion of the prohead shell that surrounds the connector, a ring of 174-base prohead RNAs (pRNA), and a multimer of gp16, an ATPase that first binds DNA-gp3 and then assembles onto the connector/pRNA complex prior to packaging. The wide end of the portal protein contacts the inside of the head, whereas the narrow end protrudes from the capsid where it is encircled by the pentameric pRNA. The structure of the isolated phi29 portal complex has been studied by atomic force microscopy and electron microscopy (EM) of two-dimensional arrays and X-ray crystallography. X-ray crystallographic studies of the phi29 portal showed that it is a cone-shaped dodecamer with a central channel. The three-dimensional crystal structure of the bacteriophage phi29 portal has been refined to 2.1Å resolution. This 422 kDa oligomeric protein is part of the DNA packaging motor and connects the head of the phage to its tail. Each monomer of the portal dodecamer has an elongated shape and is composed of a central, mainly alpha-helical domain (stem domain) that includes a three-helix bundle, a distal a/b domain and a proximal six-stranded SH3-like domain. The portal dodecamer has a 35 Å wide central channel, the surface of which is mainly electronegative. The narrow end of the head–tail portal protein is expanded in the mature virus. Gene product 3, bound to the 5′ ends of the genome, appears to be positioned within the portal, which may potentiate the release of DNA-packaging machine components, creating a binding site for attachment of the tail.

The process of DNA packaging is an extremely energy consuming act because electrostatic and bending repulsion forces of the DNA must be overpowered to package the DNA to near-crystalline density. Force-measuring laser tweezers were used to measure packaging activity of a single portal complex in real time where one microsphere has been used to hold on to a single DNA molecule as they are packaged, and the other was bound to the phage and fixed. These experiments have demonstrated that the portal complex is a force-generating motor which can work against loads of up to 57 pN, making it one of the strongest molecular motors reported to date. Notably, the packaging rate decreases as the prohead is filled, indicating that an internal force builds up to 50 pN owing to DNA confinement.

These results suggest that the internal pressure provides the driving force for DNA injection into the host cell for the first half of the injection process. The structure of the phi29 tail has revealed that 12 appendages protruding from the collar like umbrella with 12 ribs that end in 'tassels'. Two of the 12 appendages are extended radially outwards (the 'up' position), whereas the other 10 have their tassels 'hanging' roughly parallel to the virus major axis. The adsorption capable 'appendages' were found to have a structure homologous to the bacteriophage P22 tail spikes. Two of the appendages are extended radially outwards away from the long axis of the virus, whereas the others are around and parallel to the phage axis. The appendage orientations are correlated with the symmetry mismatched positions of the five-fold related head fibres. The tail in the mature capsids, that have lost their genome have an empty central channel. Comparisons of these structures with each other and with the phi29 prohead indicate how conformational changes might initiate successive steps of assembly and infection.

P22

Bacteriophage P22 infects *Salmonella enterica serovar Typhimurium* and is a prototypical representative of the *Podoviridae* family. The mature P22 virion presents an icosahedral $T = 7l$ capsid about 650 Å in diameter. The bacteriophage P22 procapsid comprises hundreds of copies of the gp5 coat and gp8 scaffolding proteins, multiple copies of three ejection proteins (gp7, gp16, gp20, also known as pilot proteins), and a unique multi-subunit gene 1 (gp1) portal.

Single-particle cryo-EM has been used to determine the P22 procapsid structure initially at low resolution then improved from 9 Å to 3.8 Å resolution. The procapsids were isolated from cells infected with mutants defective in DNA packaging and representing the physiological precursor prior to DNA packaging and capsid maturation. Coat protein gp5 is organised as pentamers and skewed hexamers as previously reported for the GuHCl treated procapsid. The high resolution structure allowed Cα backbone models for each of the seven structurally similar but not identical copies of the gp5 protein in the asymmetric unit to be built. The analysis has shown that gp5 has fold similar to the HK97 coat protein.

The first structures of the P22 assembly-naive portal formed from expressed subunits (gp1) were obtained at ~ 9 Å resolutions by cryo-EM. Later two atomic structures were obtained for the P22 portal protein: one is for a fragment of the portal, 1–602 aa (referred to as the 'portal-protein core'), bound to 12 copies of tail adaptor factor gp4. The second was the full-length P22 portal protein (725aa) at 7.5 Å resolution. To solve three independent crystal forms of the complex gp1/gp4 to a resolution of 9.5 Å, the EM structure of P22 tail at 9.4 Å resolution has been extracted computationally from the P22 tail complex and used as molecular replacement model. The high resolution atomic structure of the P22 portal protein has been obtained using a combination of multi- and intra crystal non-crystallographic-symmetry averaging, and by extension of EM phases to the resolution of the best diffracting crystal form (3.25 Å). The P22 portal complex is a ~0.96 MDa ring of 12 identical subunits, symmetrically arranged around a central channel of variable diameter, with an overall height of ~350 Å. A lower-resolution structure of the full-length portal protein unveils the unique topology of the C-terminal domain, which forms a ~200 Å long alpha-helical barrel. This domain inserts deeply into the virion and is highly conserved in the *Podoviridae* family. The quaternary structure of the P22 portal protein can be described as a funnel-shaped core ~170 Å in diameter, connected to an ~200 Å long, mostly α-helical tube formed by the Cterminal residues 603–725, which resembles a rifle barrel. The portal core is similar in topology to other portal proteins from phage SPP1 and phi29, but presence of the helical barrel is the first example of a dodecameric tube in a portal protein. Gp4 binds to the bottom of the portal protein, forming a second dodecameric ring ~75 Å in height.

In *Podoviridae*, the mechanisms of bacteria cell penetration and genome delivery are not well understood. P22 uses short, non-contractile tails to adsorb to the host cell surface. The tail machine comprises the tail spike, gp9, the tail needle, gp26, and the tail factors gp4 and gp10. Protein gp4 serves as an adaptor between portal protein and tail elements. The tail has a special fibre known as the 'tail needle' that likely functions as a cell membrane piercing device to initiate ejection of viral DNA inside the host. The structure of the intact tail machine purified from infectious virions has been obtained by cryo-EM at ~ 9 Å resolution. The structure demonstrated that the protein components are organised with a combination of 6-fold (gp10, trimers of gp9), and 3-fold (gp26, gp9) symmetry. The combined action of an adhesion protein (tailspike) and a tail needle (gp26) is responsible for binding and penetration of the phage into the host cell membrane. Gp26 probably plays the dual role of portal-protein plug and cell wall–penetrating needle, thereby controlling the opening of the portal channel and the ejection of the viral genome into the host. In Sf6, a P22-like phage that infects *Shigella flexneri*, the tail needle presents a C-terminal globular knob. This knob, absent in phage P22 but shared in other members of the P22-like genus, represents the outermost exposed tip of the virion that contacts the host cell surface. In analogy to P22 gp26, it was suggested that the tail needle of phage Sf6 was ejected through the bacterial cell membrane during infection and its C-terminal knob is threaded through peptidoglycan pores formed by glycan strands.

Epsilon 15

The Gram-negative *Salmonella anatum* is the host cell for bacteriophage Epsilon15 (ϵ15, *Podoviridae* family). The ~40kb Epsilon15 dsDNA is packed within the isometric icosahedral capsid with a diameter of ~680 Å. The virion capsid contains 11 pentons and 60 hexons made from the major capsid protein gp7 and a small decoration protein gp10 (12-kDa). Single-particle cryo-EM was used about ten years ago to determine the first structures of icosahedral viruses to subnanometre resolutions. A 9.5 Å density map was generated from EM data using icosahedral symmetry. In the average subunit map, the locations of three helices were identified. Now the structure of the epsilon15 capsid has been refined to a 4.5 Å resolution. The quality of the map allowed tracing the backbone chain of gp7. Comparison of the models has shown local discrepancies between subunits at the *N*-terminus and the E-loop in different subunits of gp7 within the hexamers of the capsid. Interestingly, a connection between E-loops of neighbouring subunits possibly exists, but the resolution was not sufficient to reveal it. Moreover, additional density was located between the gp7 monomers. This density has been assigned to the gp10 decoration protein that consists mainly of beta-sheets and two short alphahelices. A back-to-back dimer of gp10 is positioned at the two-fold axes and makes contact with six gp7 subunits through the *N*-termini and the E-loops. It was suggested that gp10 'staples' the underlying gp7 capsomeres to cement the gp5 cage so that it withstands the pressure from packed dsDNA.

The Epsilon15 capsid volume can accommodate up to 90kb dsDNA. Since the Epsilon15 genome is only ~40kb, there is ample space for a protein core of this size in the capsid chamber. The core has a cylindrical shape with a length of ~200 Å and diameter of ~180 Å. The protein core may facilitate the topological ordering of the dsDNA genome during packaging and/or release as suggested for T7 core. At the virion's tail vertex, six tails pikes attach to a central 6-fold-symmetric tail hub of the length ~170 Å. This hub may be equivalent to *Salmonella typhimurium* bacteriophage P22's hub. The hub is connected to the portal ring inside the capsid. The Epsilon 15 genome winds around the core, with a short segment of terminal DNA passing through the axis of the core and portal.

BACTERIAL GENETICS

Bacterial genetics is the subfield of genetics devoted to the study of bacteria. Bacterial genetics are subtly different from eukaryotic genetics, however bacteria still serve as a good model for animal genetic studies. One of the major distinctions between bacterial and eukaryotic genetics stems from the bacteria's lack of membrane-bound organelles (this is true of all prokaryotes. While it is a fact that there are prokaryotic organelles, they are never bound by a lipid membrane, but by a shell of proteins), necessitating protein synthesis occur in the cytoplasm.

Like other organisms, bacteria also breed true and maintain their characteristics from generation to generation, yet at the same time, exhibit variations in particular properties in a small proportion of their progeny. Though heritability and variations in bacteria had been noticed from the early days of bacteriology, it was not realised then that bacteria too obey the laws of genetics.

Even the existence of a bacterial nucleus was a subject of controversy. The differences in morphology and other properties were attributed by Nageli in 1877, to bacterial pleomorphism, which postulated the existence of a single, a few species of bacteria, which possessed a protein capacity for a variation. With the development and application of precise methods of pure culture, it became apparent that different types of bacteria retained constant form and function through successive generations. This led to the concept of monomorphism.

Transformation

Transformation in bacteria was first observed in 1928 by Frederick Griffith and later (in 1944) examined at the molecular level by Oswald Avery and his colleagues who used the process to demonstrate that DNA was the genetic material of bacteria. In transformation, a cell takes up extraneous DNA found in the environment and incorporates it into its genome (genetic material) through recombination. Not all bacteria are competent to be transformed, and not all extracellular DNA is competent to transform. To be competent to transform, the extracellular DNA must be double-stranded and relatively large. To be competent to be transformed, a cell must have the surface protein Competent Factor, which binds to the extracellular DNA in an energy requiring reaction. However bacteria that are not naturally competent can be treated in such a way to make them competent, usually by treatment with calcium chloride, which make them more permeable.

Bacterial Conjugation

Bacterial conjugation is the transfer of genetic material (plasmid) between bacterial cells by direct cell-to-cell contact or by a bridge-like connection between two cells. Discovered in 1946 by Joshua Lederberg and Edward Tatum, conjugation is a mechanism of horizontal gene transfer as are transformation and transduction although these two other mechanisms do not involve cell-to-cell contact.

Bacterial conjugation is often regarded as the bacterial equivalent of sexual reproduction or mating since it involves the exchange of genetic material. During conjugation the donor cell provides a conjugative or mobilisable genetic element that is most often a plasmid or transposon. Most conjugative plasmids have systems ensuring that the recipient cell does not already contain a similar element.

The genetic information transferred is often beneficial to the recipient. Benefits may include antibiotic resistance, xenobiotic tolerance or the ability to use new metabolites. Such beneficial plasmids may be considered bacterial endosymbionts. Other elements, however, may be viewed as bacterial parasites and conjugation as a mechanism evolved by them to allow for their spread.

MULTIFUNCTIONALITY OF BACTERIOPHAGES

Estimated to be the most widely distributed and diverse entities in the biosphere, bacterial virus, bacteriophages or phage can be found in all environments populated by bacterial hosts, such as soil, water and animal guts. Their unique characteristics bring several advantages to their use as pathogen surrogates. Phages have been successfully used in a variety of environmental applications as follows:

- As fecal indicators - the environmental occurrence and persistence of some groups relate to health risks associated with fecal pollution and the potential occurrence of enteric pathogens in aquatic environments. As a result phage infecting enteric bacteria are now accepted as useful indicators in water quality control and included in some regulations as required parameters. For example, coliphages are used in the US Water Ground Rule, the drinking water quality regulation for the Canadian Province of Quebec and a few USA states regulations regarding required quality for reclaimed water for certain uses.

- In microbial source tracking (MST) or identification of fecal contamination sources by genotypic, phenotypic, and chemical methods, phage have proven useful based on their host specificity. By identifying problem sources (animal and human) and determining the effect of implemented remedial solutions MST is of special interest in waters used for recreation (primary and secondary contact), public water supplies, aquifer protection, and protection and propagation of fish, shellfish and wildlife.

- As process indicators phage groups are often successfully employed as enterovirus surrogates in evaluating the effectiveness of water treatment processes and final product quality. This is the case with filtration and disinfection.

- As comprehensive pathogenic virus indices, phages are not very useful. This is because their numbers seldom seem to correlate to pathogenic viruses numbers in water samples when conventional statistics are applied. However, in the future the application of advanced mathematical models to new databases may reduce uncertainty and provide better information about relationships between phage and pathogenic virus numbers.

- As viral models and tracers, bacteriophages are often used at both field and laboratory scales as biocolloids to estimate the fate and transport of pathogenic viruses in surface and subsurface aquatic environments and through natural and man made saturated and unsaturated porous media. This use of phage as surrogates for pathogen transport applies to protection of surface and groundwater supplies from microbial contamination, assessment of potential health risk from pathogens in groundwater and design of more efficient treatment systems in removing pathogens from drinking water supplies.

Advantages and Disadvantages of Bacteriophage

Advantages of bacteriophage

- Have no known impact on the environment.
- Are non-toxic and non-pathogenic for humans animals or plants.
- Have a specific affinity to their bacterial host.
- Are reasonably similar to mammalian viral pathogens in size, shape, morphology, surface properties, mode of replication and persistence in natural environments.
- Are colloidal in nature which makes them more adequate virus models then dissolved tracers.

- Are stable over periods of several months under laboratory conditions.
- Can be detected and enumerated by rapid and inexpensive methods with low detection limits (1 to 2 phage per mL).
- Can be prepared in large quantities at high concentrations.
- Specific phage groups are similar to specific pathogenic viral groups allowing the use of phage cocktails to simultaneously target several groups of concern.

Disadvantages of bacteriophage

- Are excreted by a certain humans and animals all the time while pathogenic viruses are excreted by infected individuals for a short period of time (depending on the epidemiology of viruses, outbreaks of infection, and vaccination). Consequently there is no direct correlation between numbers of phages and viruses excreted by humans.
- A wide range of different phage can be detected by methods for somatic coliphages.
- At least some somatic coliphages may replicate in water environments.
- Enteric viruses have been detected in water environments in the absence of coliphages.
- Pathogenic human enteric viruses are excreted almost exclusively by humans, while bacteriophage used in water quality assessment are excreted by humans and animals.
- The microbiota of the gut, diet and physiological state of animals seems to affect the numbers of coliphages in their feces.
- The composition and numbers of phages excreted by humans is variable (e.g. patients under antibiotic treatment excrete lower numbers than healthy or non- medicated individuals).
- As water flows through porous media in the subsurface or engineered filtration processes phage can attach, detach, and reattach by physico-chemical filtration mechanisms.

MAIN BACTERIOPHAGE GROUPS USED IN ENVIRONMENTAL STUDIES

Three bacteriophage groups, somatic coliphages, male-specific F-RNA phages and *Bacteroides fragilis* phages, have been proposed and are frequently used as surrogates for pathogenic viruses in environmental studies. However, because each group has its pros and cons as a representative of enteric virus presence and behaviour in aquatic environments and water treatment processes, no agreement has been reached on which of the three groups best fulfills the index/indicator function.

Somatic Coliphages

Somatic coliphages are the most numerous and most easily detectable phage group in the environment. It is a heterogeneous group whose members infect host cells (*E. coli* and other *Enterobactereacea*) by attaching to receptors located in the bacterial cell wall. Their numbers are low in human feces (often <10 g^{-1}), but abundant in untreated domestic sewage (10^4 to 10^5 particles g^{-1}) and in animal feces. Somatic coliphages are not usually considered good fecal indicators because some of their hosts are unlikely to be of fecal origin, and some of these phage are able to multiply in waters not subjected to fecal pollution. However, some authors argue that the number of somatic phage that replicate in environmental waters is negligible. Moreover, they are not predictive indicators of virus presence or absence in groundwater, though some somatic phage such as T-4, T-7, ΦX174, and PRD-1 have proven useful as viral surrogates of fate and transport in laboratory investigations, pilot trials, and validation testing. Bacteriophage PRD-1 in particular has emerged as an important viral model for studying microbial transport through a variety of subsurface environments. Its popularity is due to its similarity to human adenoviruses in size (~62 nm) and morphology (icosahedric), its relative stability over a range of temperatures and low degree of attachment in aquifer sediments.

F-RNA Bacteriophages

F or male specific RNA bacteriophages are a homogeneous group of phage that attach to fertility fimbriae (F-pili or sex-pili) produced by male bacterial cells (possessing an F plasmid) in certain stages of their growth cycle. Since the F-plasmid is transferable to a wide range of Gram-negative bacteria, F-specific bacteriophages may have several hosts besides *E. coli*. This group ranks second in abundance in water environments although its persistence in surface waters, mainly in warm climates is low.

F-RNA bacteriophages have been most extensively studied due to their similarity (in size, shape, morphology and physiochemistry) to many pathogenic human enteric viruses, namely enteroviruses, caliciviruses, astroviruses and Hepatitis A and E virus. These phages are infrequently detected in human and animal feces (10^3 g^{-1}) or in aquatic environments despite their frequent detection in wastewater (10^3 to 10^4 mL^{-1}). Further research is needed to clarify if their consistently higher concentrations in sewage relative to feces are the result of direct environmental input or multiplication. If the latter is true, F-RNA bacteriophages may not be acceptable fecal pollution indicators. Jofre and others suggested that the environmental multiplication of these phages is unlikely, however, because F-pili production only occurs at temperatures above 25°C and replication does not occur in nutrient-poor environments and requires a minimum host density of 10^4 colony forming units (cfu) per mL.

The presence of F-RNA phage in high numbers in wastewater and their resistance to chlorination contribute to their usefulness as process indicators, indices of sewage pollution, and conservative models of human viruses in water and shellfish. They are also promising in microbial source tracking since they can be subdivided in four antigenically distinct serogroups. Because those predominating in humans (groups II and III) differ from those predominating in animals (groups I and IV), it is possible to distinguish between human (higher public health risk) and animal wastes by serotyping or genotyping F-RNA coliphage isolates.

AVAILABLE METHODOLOGY FOR BACTERIOPHAGE DETECTION, ENUMERATION AND PROPAGATION

Relatively simple and reliable methods for detection, isolation, enumeration and characterisation of bacteriophages from natural sources are available in the literature. These include classic culture-based techniques using liquid or solid bacteriological media, as well as more recent physico-chemical, immunological, immunofluorescence, electron microscopy, and molecular methods. However, a lack of methodology standardisation and quality control has for decades limited the use of phage data for comparison studies. This situation has improved since the publication of standardised plaque assays and presence/absence methods in the USA and Europe. For somatic coliphages, F-specific RNA phages and bacteriophages infecting *Bacteroides fragilis*. Sobsey and others developed a simple, inexpensive and practical procedure for the detection and recovery of F-RNA bacteriophages from low turbidity water using mixed cellulose and acetate filters with 47 mm diameter and 0.45 um pore size. A slightly modified version of this method has shown excellent performance for recovery of somatic and Fspecific phages, and bacteriophages of *Bacteroids fragilis* in up to 1L water samples. Rapid bacteriophage detection methods involving enrichment steps followed by latex agglutination or bioluminescence and molecular approaches have also been developed and recently reviewed by Jofre and others.

Specific methods for the production of the large-volume, high-titer purified bacteriophage suspensions that are necessary for many types of environmental fate and transport studies were, until very recently, difficult to find in the refereed literature. Given that system chemistry and other surface-related characteristics of phage particles, may substantially contribute to observations of their environmental fate and transport behaviour in many types of porous media filtration systems used for water treatment, it is critical to consider the impacts of the propagation/purification protocol on those factors. In response to this need, a selected sequence of rapid, reliable, and cost-effective procedures to propagate and purify high-titer bacteriophage suspensions has recently been proposed.

This methodology emphasises the most important factors required to ensure maximum bacteriophage yields, minimum change on phage particles surface characteristics, and low dissolved organic carbon (DOC) concentration in the final suspensions. Many of the methods routinely used to quantify microscopic discrete particles such as bacteriophages are known to yield highly variable results arising from sampling error and variations in analytical recovery (i.e. losses during sample processing and errors in counting), thereby leading to considerable uncertainty in particle concentration or log_{10}-reduction estimates. For example, sampling error is substantially greater than analytical error when organisms are present in relatively low concentrations, in these cases, improved sampling (i.e. resulting in counts of approximately 10 or more organisms in a sample or, in some cases, several replicates) substantially contributes to reducing uncertainty.

In contrast, when organisms are present in higher and homogeneous concentrations, uncertainty in concentration estimates can be reduced by decreasing analytical errors. Emelko and others demonstrated that uncertainty in concentration and removal estimates derived from microbial enumeration data can be addressed when these errors are properly considered and quantified. The development and use of such quantitative approaches is an essential component of strategies (e.g. the monitoring of surrogate parameters/pathogens, experimental design, and data analysis) for better evaluating micro-organism transport and fate in source and treated drinking waters.

Chapter 15

Mechanism of Bacterial Mutation and Mutant Detection Methods

INTRODUCTION

Mutation is a very important concept in biology today that leads to variations in genes. A mutation is a permanent alteration in the sequence of nitrogenous bases of a DNA molecule. The result of a mutation is generally a change in the end-product specified by that gene. In some cases, a mutation can be beneficial if a new metabolic activity arises in a micro-organism, or it can be detrimental if a metabolic activity is lost. Mutations can be spontaneous, or induced by a mutagen in the environment. Mispairing is probably mostly due to cellular processes such as Tautomeric shift of bases, oxidative damage to DNA, depurination and deamination or caused by 'environment', i.e. chemicals, radiation, viruses, diet and lifestyle (Mutagens). Substitution of a nucleotide and Deletion or addition of them is two mechanisms of mutation. Mutation in bacteria has some results such as missense, nonsense, silent, frameshift, lethal, suppressor and conditional lethal mutation. Identifying these mutations requires detection methods. Classic methods, i.e. Replica plating, Penicillin enrichment, Ames test, Use of chromogenic substrate and novel tests such as Polymerase chain reaction (PCR) and Gel electrophoresis, Gene probes and Southern blotting, DNA sequencing and DNA microarray are some of these methods which are discussed in this chapter.

Today bacteria are an important tool in the study of genetics and biotechnology, but for 40 years after the rediscovery of Mendel's work and the rebirth of genetics, they were considered too simple to have genes, undergo mutation, or reproduce sexually. This is not surprising - bacteria are so small that it's very difficult to study individuals. Scientists had long observed differences between bacterial colonies, but had never realised that these differences were the results of mutations. Mutations are a very important concept in biology today. Mutations lead to variations in genes. These genes can have a good or bad influence in the characteristics of an organism. Variations are also very important in evolution. Without variations evolution would not be possible, and changes in any part of the environment affecting the organism could make the organism become extinct. A mutation is any heritable change in DNA sequence. This may, or may not, affect the phenotype of the organism. The term 'mutation' was coined by Hugo de Vries, which is derived from Latin word meaning 'to change'. The process of mutation is called mutagenesis and the agent inducing mutations is called mutagen. (Organisms selected as reference strains are called wild type, and their progeny with mutations are called mutants). Changes in the sequence of template DNA (mutations) can drastically affect the type of protein end product produced.

TYPES OF MUTATIONS

Mutations can be classified by the kinds of alterations in the DNA, or by whether the mutation was spontaneous, or induced by a mutagen in the environment. Mispairing is probably mostly due to cellular processes such as Tautomeric shift of bases , oxidative damage to DNA , Depurination and Deamination or caused by 'environment', i.e. chemicals, radiation, viruses, diet and lifestyle (Mutagens).

Mechanisms of Mutation

1. Substitution of a nucleotide: Base substitution, also called point mutation, involves the changing of single base in the DNA sequence. This mistake is copied during replication to produce a permanent change. If one purine [A or G] or pyrimidine [C or T] is replaced by the other, the substitution is called a transition. If a purine is replaced by a pyrimidine or vice versa, the substitution is called a transversion. This is the most common mechanism of mutation.

2. Deletion or addition of a nucleotide during DNA replication: When a transposon (jumping gene) inserts itself into a gene, it leads to disruption of gene and is called insertional mutation.

Mutation Sources

Mutations arise from a variety of sources, including.

Tautomeric shift of bases

Each of the bases in DNA can appear in one of several forms, called tautomers, which are isomers that in the positions of their atoms and in the bonds between the atoms. The keto(C-O) and amino(C-NH$_2$) form of each base is normally present in DNA, whereas the imino(C=NH) and enol(C-OH) forms of the bases are rare.Conversion of keto group in thymine and guanine to enol form and changing amino group in adenine and cytosine to imino form, are examples of tautomerisation. Naturally, A in amino form pairs with T in keto form, whereas A in its imino form pairs with C and T in enol form match with G.

Depurination

Depurination consists of the interruption of the glycosidic bond between the base and deoxyribose and the subsequent loss of a guanine or an adenine residue from the DNA in replication, the resulting apurinic sites cannot specify a base complementary to the original purine. So, efficient repair systems remove apurinic sites. Under this certain conditions, a base can be inserted across from an apurinic site, this insertion will frequently result in a mutation.

Deamination

The deamination of cytosine yields uracil. Unrepaired uracil residues will pair with adenine in replication, resulting in the conversion of a G–C pair into an A–T pair (a GC $\rightarrow$ AT transition). Another example for deamination, is conversion of 5-methylcytosine to thymine.

Oxidatively damaged bases

Active oxygen species, such as superoxide radicals (O$_2$·), hydrogen peroxide (H$_2$O$_2$), and hydroxyl radicals (OH·), are produced as by-products of normal aerobic metabolism. They can cause oxidative damage to DNA. For example, The 8-oxo-7-hydrodeoxyguanosine (8-oxodG, or GO) product frequently mispairs with A, resulting in a high level of G $\rightarrow$ T transversions. Thymidine glycol which induced of hydroxyl radical attack to thymine , blocks DNA replication if unrepaired but has not yet been implicated in mutagenesis.

Ultraviolet irradiation

Ultraviolet light (opt 250 nm) causes bonds to form between adjacent pyrimidine residues (commonly referred to as thymine dimers, although the effect can also occur with cytosine) in the same polynucleotide strand. These are called pyrimidine dimers. UV irradiation can result in the formation of covalent links between pyrimidine dimers. These bonds distort the DNA conformation and inhibit DNA replication and transcription.

Chemical mutagens

Variety of chemical mutagens have been identified that are classified into three groups based on their function.

First group are those agents that act by chemically modifying a base on the DNA so that it resembles a different base. For example, nitrous acid causes an oxidative deamination in which amino groups are converted to keto groups and thus cytosine residues for example will be converted to uracil. Uracil will be capable of pairing with adenine, thus causing a change from a C–G pair to T–A. Similarly deamination of adenine creates the base hypoxanthines, which will base-pair with cytosine. Some types of chemical agent are not incorporated into the DNA but instead alter a base, causing specific mispairing. They act against the DNA within cells, rather than against isolated DNA. Certain alkylating agents, such as ethylmethanesulfonate (EMS) and nitrosoguanidine (NG), add alkyl groups (an ethyl group in EMS and a methyl group in NG) to many positions on all four bases, mutagenicity is best correlated with an addition to the oxygen at the 6 position of guanine to create an O-6-alkylguanine. This addition leads to direct mispairing with thymine, and would result in GC $\rightarrow$ AT transitions.

Second group are mutagens that induct frameshift formation. The interchalating agents that include proflavin, acridine orange and ethidium bromide are planar molecules, which mimic base pairs and are able to slip themselves in (interchalate) between the stacked nitrogen bases at the core of the DNA double helix. In this intercalated position, the agent can cause single-nucleotide-pair insertions or deletions. Intercalating agents may also stack between bases in single-stranded DNA, in so doing, they may stabilise bases that are looped out during frameshift formation.

Third group are type of agent that acts only against growing cells consists of the base analogues such as 5-bromouracil. Despite its name, this is an analogue of thymine and adenine. 5-BU causes mutations when it is incorporated in one form and then shifts to another form. In its normal keto state, 5-BU pairs like thymine (5-BUT). Thus, 5-BU is incorporated across from adenine and subsequently mispairs with guanine, resulting in AT $\rightarrow$ GC transitions, but in its enol form, 5-BU pairs like cytosine (5-BUC), so 5-BU is misincorporated across from guanine and subsequently pairs with adenine, resulting in GC $\rightarrow$ AT transitions.

Missense Mutation

A missense mutation is a type of point mutation in which a different amino acid is placed within the produced protein, other than the original. In the process of converting DNA into protein, the language of DNA must be translated into the language of proteins. During this process, a change in the structure of DNA, or a mutation, can change the sequence of amino acids which creates a protein. If it does not change the structure or function of the protein, it may be considered a silent mutation. If it does change the protein, it is considered a missense mutation.

Types of missense mutation

Conservative: In a conservative missense mutation, the amino acid replaced is similar in function and shape to the amino acid being replaced. A conservative missense mutation may result in loss of function, but it may only be minor. In the context of population genetics and ecology, a missense mutation may not necessarily be a negative thing. A slowed or slightly changed function of a protein may actually increase the fitness of an organism. If the product of the protein needs to be regulated, or is currently hindering the fitness of the organism, a change may be beneficial. A conservative missense mutation is typically changes the function of a protein less drastically than the other type of missense mutation.

Non-conservative: In a non-conservative missense mutation, a completely different kind of amino acid is added to the chain. Where a polar amino acid was present, a non-polar amino acid will be added. This type of missense mutation can greatly change the function of a protein, as it will likely change the shape and structure of the protein. Proteins have various levels of structure, all which depend upon the DNA. If a missense mutation changes an amino acid, it first changes the primary structure, or the basic sequence of amino acids. The secondary structure of proteins consists of patterns and structures formed by interactions between these amino acids. A missense mutation could completely disrupt a form such as an alpha helix or beta sheet. These structures can be crucial to the overall tertiary structure of the protein, or its general shape and size. This structure informs how the protein interacts with other molecules within the environment. A non-conservative missense mutation may completely change these interactions. At the final level of protein structure, quaternary structure, a missense mutation can even prevent a protein from joining a larger protein complex it is intended to be a part of. This can render entire biochemical pathways useless, or give them a completely new use.

Example of missense mutation

A common and well-known example of a missense mutation is sickle-cell anemia, a blood disease. People with sickle-cell anemia have a missense mutation at a single point in the DNA. This missense mutation calls for a different amino acid, and affects the overall shape of the protein produced. This, in turn, causes the entire shape of blood cells to be different. People with the disease experience symptoms of not being able acquire oxygen efficiently, and experience blood clotting. However, they are partially protected from blood borne parasites which live in blood cells. Malaria is a disease caused by these parasites, and people with sickle-cell anemia have an inherent defense against the parasite. Their sickle-shaped blood cells cannot support the life cycle of the parasite.

The missense mutation which causes all of this is the difference of one nucleotide. It is first translated into mRNA, then into a protein. The missense mutation causes a valine to be placed where a glutamic acid normally goes. This non-conservative missense mutation causes the shape of the protein, haemoglobin, to change. Where normal haemoglobin separates, the mutated haemoglobin forms long chains. These chains, when incorporated into blood cells, change their shape and force them into a sickle.

Many other anemias and various genetic diseases are caused by a missense mutation. All proteins are reliant on the sequence of amino acids which makes it up. While mutations may sometimes bring benefits to an organism, they more often disrupt a stable and relied-upon process. In disrupting even a single protein, cells can become functionless, or at least struggle to function.

Nonsense Mutation

A nonsense mutation occurs when the sequence of nucleotides in DNA is changed in a way that stops the normal sequence of amino acids in the final protein. In central dogma of biology, DNA is transposed into RNA, which is then translated into a protein. The protein is a particular sequence of amino acids which confers a particular function onto the cell. The sequence of amino acids determines this role by the properties they contain and the ways they interact.

In the DNA, each amino acid is designated by a series of three nucleotides, called a codon. There are around 21 amino acids which can be designated by this system. There are also two other important signals, 'START' and 'STOP'. These signals allow the ribosome assembling the protein to know where to begin, and where to end. A nonsense mutation changes the codon for an amino acid into the codon for a 'STOP' signal. This completely changes the structure of the protein, because anything after the 'STOP' signal is ignored. The ribosome snips off the incomplete protein, and goes on its way. Without the remainder of the amino acid chain, the protein may function and form completely differently than before. A nonsense mutation can have three basic outcomes.

Outcomes of a nonsense mutation

Deleterious: The vast majority of mutations are deleterious, meaning they cause a decrease in the overall fitness and reproductive success of the organism. A nonsense mutation would fall into this category if the mutation affected an important functional protein. Imagine if the nonsense mutation was found in the DNA which coded for an ion channel protein. If this protein was incomplete, it could not function to properly transport ions across the membrane. This would be deleterious to the organism with the nonsense mutation. Cystic fibrosis is a genetic disorder caused by a nonsense mutation which does exactly that. The protein affected by the nonsense mutation in cystic fibrosis is a regulator protein for ion channels. Without the ability to properly move ions, people with cystic fibrosis often have respiratory problems caused by a mucous buildup due to the unregulated ions in their system. Duchenne muscular dystrophy is another disease cause by a nonsense mutation, and there are many more examples.

Neutral: A neutral mutation occurs when the effects of the mutation go undetected. Imagine that the mutation is found right before the last amino acid in a protein. Further, this final amino acid is really unnecessary for the actual function of the protein within the cell. If this is the case, the nonsense mutation will produce no effect at all. The protein will continue to function, even without the final amino acid. In this case, nothing really changes for the organism.

Beneficial: The least common type of mutation is a beneficial mutation. This is a mutation in which the protein changes in such a way that it increases the fitness and reproductive success of the organism. However, it is extremely unlikely that a nonsense mutation will end up being beneficial. In only the rarest of circumstances, a nonsense mutation may be beneficial if changing the protein it affects somehow provides a benefit to the organism. Imagine if the nonsense mutation affected a protein which inadvertently transports a toxin into cells. In an environment filled with the toxin, a dysfunctional protein might very well be the cure to being constantly bombarded with a toxin. If the protein no longer transported the toxin in, the cells wouldn't need to worry about it. In an even more unlikely circumstance, the nonsense mutation may completely alter the function of the protein. In this case, it might alter the protein to not transport the toxin, but rather destroy it or bind to it. This could also be a case in which the nonsense mutation became beneficial. In the most extreme circumstance the nonsense mutation may take a protein used for one process, and create an entirely new active protein by cutting the other one in pieces. Much of this has to do with the exact protein affected and the resulting effects on the organism.

Example if nonsense mutation

This is likely why nonsense mutations are often noticeable. It is unlikely that these mutations do not affect the resulting protein. Given that all of the amino acids play a role in a protein, dividing it at any point will likely change the way it interacts with the environment. Even if only several amino acids are lost, these could be the crucial external amino acids which attach the protein to the cell membrane or help it interact with other cells.

Silent Mutation

A silent mutation is a change in the sequence of nucleotide bases which constitutes DNA, without a subsequent change in the amino acid or the function of the overall protein. Sometimes a single amino acid will change, but if it has the same properties as the amino acid it replaced, little to no change will happen. A silent mutation can be caused many ways, but the key point is that it does not change the function of the amino acid or subsequent proteins. A silent mutation is just that: it does nothing significant, not making a sound in the orchestra of the cell.

Examples of Silent Mutation

Redundant genome: The DNA is read in units of three nucleotides, called codons. Each codon specifies a certain amino acid, with a few reserved as stop and start signals. Sometimes, different codons specify the same amino acid. This redundancy allows a flexibility in the genetic code. This means that a silent mutation usually goes completely unnoticed.

Here, a silent mutation is compared with both a nonsense mutation and a missense mutation. The silent mutation, which is an actual change at the DNA level from a thymine to a cytosine. This mutation could have been caused by a mistake in DNA replication, or from some sort of repair that happen after the DNA was damaged. Regardless, both of these three nucleotide codons tell the ribosome and machinery within to attach a lysine amino acid.

Within non-coding DNA: Many portions of the DNA are used structurally, and their full purpose is not understood. There are many cases in which parts of the DNA are vastly different between individuals, yet their phenotypes seem the same. These changes, especially small structural changes in the DNA, do not become significant until they begin to change the interaction of the coding DNA with the environment. A silent mutation could easily happen in these areas without notice, yet over time many mutations may begin to change a population.

Bacteria, interestingly, usually have a single circle of DNA, which carries all the information they need. By contrast, the human genome is separated on multiple chromosomes, which are bundled and managed by specialised proteins so they can be wound up during cell division. One hypothesis as to how this much more complex DNA came about was that certain silent mutations began forming structures of DNA. In a more compact genome, more information can be stored, which may have led to the complexity of life from single celled organisms to more complex forms. The folding and protection of various parts of DNA is part of normal cell differentiation in eukaryotes. Supposedly, these could have arisen through silent mutation until they became useful and were selected for.

Frameshift Mutation

Frameshift mutations are insertions or deletions in the genome that are not in multiples of three nucleotides. They are a subset of insertion-deletion (indel) mutations that are specifically found in the coding sequence of polypeptides. Here the number of nucleotides that are added or removed from the coding sequence are not multiples of three. They can arise from extremely simple mutations such as the addition or removal of a single nucleotide. Frameshift mutations do not include substitutions where a nucleotide replaces another. In substitution mutations, the polypeptide only changes by a single amino acid. Frameshift mutations also do not include indels in the non-coding or regulatory regions of the genome because these mutations do not have any direct effect on amino acid sequence, though protein regulation may change.

Effects of frameshift mutations

Frameshift mutations are among the most deleterious changes to the coding sequence of a protein. They are extremely likely to lead to large-scale changes to polypeptide length and chemical composition, resulting in a non-functional protein that often disrupts the biochemical processes of a cell. Frameshift mutations can lead to a premature end to translation of the mRNA as well as the formation of an extended polypeptide.

The amino acid sequences downstream of the frameshift mutation are also likely to be chemically distinct from the original sequence. For instance, if a frameshift mutation occurs in an integral transmembrane protein, it could vastly alter the stretch of hydrophobic residues that span the lipid bilayer making it impossible for the protein to be present in its subcellular location. When such errors occur, the cell often perceives the lack of functional protein and tries to compensate by upregulating the expression of the mutated gene. This can even overwhelm the translation machinery of the cell, result in a large number of misfolded proteins that could eventually lead to large-scale impairment of all functions of even cell death.

Diseases caused by frameshift mutations in genes include Crohn's disease, cystic fibrosis, and some forms of cancer. On the other hand, when some proteins become dysfunctional, they could have a protective effect, as seen in the resistance to HIV in people with a chemokine receptor gene (CCR5) containing a frameshift mutation. Since frameshift mutations are usually changes to the genetic material in every cell, it is rare to find a cure. Most interventions are palliative.

Genetic code

The core reason for the presence of frameshift mutations is the body's mechanism for translating genetic information into amino acid sequences through a triplet-based genetic code. This means that every set of three nucleotides on an mRNA represents either an amino acid or an instruction to cease translation.

Discovery of the genetic code: Mendel's initial experiments on the transmission of genetic traits pointed towards a discrete physical and chemical entity that carried genetic information. Based on the bulk biochemical analysis of cells, four major components were detected – carbohydrates, fats, proteins and nucleic acids. Any of these components could represent genetic material. Initial investigations into the chemical nature of the genome hypothesised that proteins, with 20 amino acids, were most likely to carry Mendel's factors or genes. However, later experiments indicated that nucleic acids were the carriers of genetic information. This presented an interesting difficulty. While nucleic acids had been analysed chemically as being polymers made of 4 different nucleotides, it wasn't clear how the information for the dazzling variety of forms and functions in the body could arise from just 4 nucleotides.

Triplet codon: A little later, the central dogma of molecular biology indicated that most organisms used RNA as the intermediate between DNA and proteins. This brought up the next question of how four bases could carry the information to encode 20 amino acids. If every nucleotide coded for a single amino acid, then only four amino acids could be reliably and reproducibly coded. If every two nucleotides encoded an amino acid, it would still lead to only 16 amino acids. Therefore, a minimum of three nucleotides was needed to code for 20 amino acids.

Lethal Mutation

Sometimes some mutations affect vital functions and the bacterial cell become nonviable. Hence those mutations that can kill the cell are called lethal mutation.

Suppressor Mutation

It is a reversal of a mutant phenotype by another mutation at a position on the DNA distinct from that of original mutation. True reversion or back mutation results in reversion of a mutant to original form, which occurs as a result of mutation occurring at the same spot once again.

Intragenic vs. intergenic suppression

Intragenic suppression: Intragenic suppression results from suppressor mutations that occur in the same gene as the original mutation. In a classic study, Francis Crick and others used intragenic suppression to study the fundamental nature of the genetic code. From this study it was shown that genes are expressed as non-overlapping triplets (codons). Researchers showed that mutations caused by either a single base insertion (+) or a single base deletion (–) could be 'suppressed' or restored by a second mutation of the opposite sign, as long as the two mutations occurred in the same vicinity of the gene. This led to the conclusion that genes needed to be read in a specific 'reading frame' and a single base insertion or deletion would shift the reading frame (frameshift mutation) in such a way that the remaining DNA would code for a different polypeptide than the one intended. Therefore, researchers concluded that the second mutation of opposite sign suppresses the original mutation by restoring the reading frame, as long as the portion between the two mutations is not critical for protein function.

In addition to the reading frame, Crick also used suppressor mutations to determine codon size. It was found that while one and two base insertions/deletions of the same sign resulted in a mutant phenotype, deleting or inserting three bases could give a wild type phenotype. From these results it was concluded that an inserted or deleted triplet does not disturb the reading frame and the genetic code is in fact a triplet.

Intergenic suppression: Intergenic (also known as extragenic) suppression relieves the effects of a mutation in one gene by a mutation somewhere else within the genome. The second mutation is not on the same gene as the original mutation. Intergenic suppression is useful for identifying and studying interactions between molecules, such as proteins. For example, a mutation which disrupts the complementary interaction between protein molecules may be compensated for by a second mutation elsewhere in the genome that restores or provides a suitable alternative interaction between those molecules. Several proteins of biochemical, signal transduction, and gene expression pathways have been identified using this approach. Examples of such pathways include receptor-ligand interactions as well as the interaction of components involved in DNA replication, transcription, and translation.

Suppressor mutations also occur in genes that code for virus structural proteins. To create a viable phage T4 virus, a balance of structural components is required. An amber mutant of phage T4 contains a mutation that changes a codon for an amino acid in a protein to the nonsense stop codon TAG (see stop codon and nonsense mutation). If, upon infection, an amber mutant defective in a gene encoding a needed structural component of phage T4 is weakly suppressed (in an *E. coli* host containing a specific altered tRNA – see nonsense suppressor), it will produce a reduced number of the needed structural component. As a consequence few if any viable phage are formed. However, it was found that viable phage could sometimes be produced in the host with the weak nonsense suppressor if a second amber mutation in a gene that encodes another structural protein is also present in the phage genome. It was found that the reason the second amber mutation could suppress the first one is that the two numerically reduced structural proteins would now be in balance. For instance, if the first amber mutation caused a reduction of tail fibres to one tenth the normal level, most phage particles produced would have insufficient tail fibres to be infective. However, if a second amber mutation is defective in a base plate component and causes one tenth the number of base plates to be made, this may restore the balance of tail fibres and base plates, and thus allow infective phage to be produced.

Conditional Lethal Mutation

Sometimes a mutation may affect an organism in such a way that the mutant can survive only in certain environmental condition. Example, a temperature sensitive mutant can survive at permissive temperature of 35°C but not at restrictive temperature of 39°C.

ISOLATION AND IDENTIFICATION OF MUTANTS

In general, changes at the amino acid level in a protein will have a consequential effect on the protein's activity, usually detrimental. Thus, an important metabolic pathway may be blocked by the lack of functional enzyme resulting in identifiable phenotypes. This phenotypes can be classified in to three main groups:

1. Mutants that are resistant to antibiotics, or to specific bacteriophages, toxic chemicals or any other agents that are usually lethal or inhibitory to the parent cell.

2. Auxotrophs, i.e. mutants that require some additional growth factor, such as an amino acid.

3. Mutants that are unable to use a particular growth substrate (usually a sugar).

Methods for mutant selection Replica Plating

In this procedure, the mutagenised culture is plated out to obtain single colonies on a nutrient medium on which mutants and parents will grow. After incubation, the colonies are replicated, using a sterile velvet pad, onto a minimal agar plate and then a similar plate to which the appropriate supplement (in this case, histidine, since we are looking specifically for histidine auxotrophs) has been added. Histidine requiring auxotrophs will be unable to grow on the first plate, but will grow on the second one. Thus, mutant colonies can be identified with localisation of colonies that have failed to grow in second plate in comparison with first one.

Penicillin enrichment

Some antibiotics (i.e. penicillin) acts only against growing bacteria. Cells that are stopped their growth for any reason, relatively not sensitive. Resuspending the bacteria in a minimal medium and adding penicillin will kill the parental cells, which are able to grow, while allowing the non-growing mutants to survive.

Ames test

The Ames test uses several strains of the bacterium *Salmonella typhimurium* (Fig. 15.1) that carry mutations in genes involved in histidine synthesis i.e. it is an auxotrophic mutant, so that they require histidine for growth. The method tests the capability of mutagen in creating mutations that can result in a reversion back to a non-auxotrophic state so that the cells can grow on a histidine-free medium. The bacteria are spread on an agar plate with a small amount of histidine. This small amount of histidine in the growth medium allows the bacteria to grow for an initial time and have the opportunity to mutate. When the histidine is depleted, only bacteria that have mutated to gain the ability to produce their own

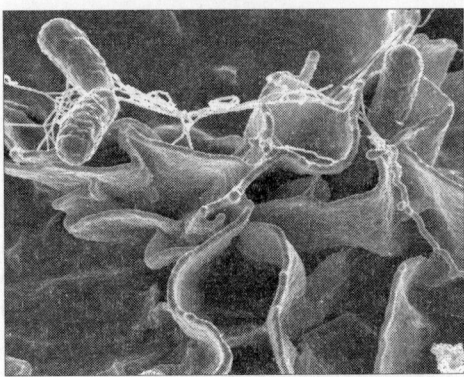

Fig. 15.1: *Salmonella typhimurium.*

histidine will survive. The plate is incubated for 48 hr. The mutagenicity of a substance is proportional to the number of colonies observed.

Use of chromogenic substrate

Mutants that are not able to utilise a particular carbon source (lactose, for example) can be isolated with use a chromogenic substrate that shows an easily detectable colour change when acted on by the enzyme concerned. In this case the enzyme is β-galactosidase, which catalyses the hydrolysis of lactose into its constituent sugars glucose and galactose. A commonly used chromogenic substrate for β-galactosidase is 5-bromo-4-chloro-3-indolyl-β-D-galactoside, more popularly known as X-gal. This is a synthetic analogue of the natural substrate, containing a dye linked to galactose. X-gal itself is colourless, the colour of the dye is only manifest when it is released by hydrolysis of the linkage by β-galactosidase. Lac+ colonies will be blue on a medium containing X-gal and colonies that do not produce β-galactosidase will be white.

Polymerase chain reaction (PCR) and Gel electrophoresis

In this method, target gen (mutant sequence in this case) can be increased exponentially. If the mutation has caused a significant change in the size of a specific gene (such as an insertion or a deletion) it will be detect by a change in the size of the PCR product, using gel electrophoresis.

Gene probes and Southern blotting

This method involves separating fragments of DNA by electrophoresis in an agarose gel and transferring them to a filter which can then be hybridised with the labelled probe. By using highly specific probes, detection of difference in the sequence is possible.

DNA sequencing

DNA sequencing template is amplified using PCR and oligonucleotide primers flanking the region of interest. The amplified fragment is directly cycle sequenced using fluorescent sequencing primers, Sanger dideoxy sequencing chemistry and an enzyme mixture of a mutant Taq DNA polymerase and thermostable pyrophosphatase. The sequence ladders produced are analysed on a real-time, automated four-colour sequencing system. The method produces sequence ladders from unpurified PCR fragments of sufficiently high quality such that heterozygotes can be reproducibly detected and identified by software that recognises signal-strength patterns indicative of mixed-base positions.

DNA microarray

Base-pairing or complementarity is the principle behind this emerging technology. The potential applications of microarray technology are gene expression profiling and identification of gene sequences (including sequences that bear mutations). In this method, a large number of DNA fragments are placed on a glass slide. The fragments are allowed to complement or bind with the labelled DNA (probes), which hybridise with the DNA on the glass slide. The amount of hybridisation is then analysed in each spot on the slide. The genes are given a colour where the hybridised ones are coloured red and the genes that are hybridised least are coloured green. It has been reported that microarray technology could be used in monitoring chromosome gains and losses, tumour classification, drug discovery and development.

Thus, mutations lead to variations in genes that are very important in evolution. A mutation is any heritable change in DNA sequence. Mutation can be beneficial or it can be detrimental. Mutations can be spontaneous due to cellular processes, or induced by a mutagen in the environment. Substitution of a nucleotide and deletion or addition of them is two mechanisms of mutation. Mutation in bacteria has some results that may, or may not, affect the phenotype of the organism. Several methods have been developed for the mutant detection, of these methods molecular methods due to the high sensitivity and specificity, and also more time saving than the classical methods is recommended.

Chapter 16

Genetically Modified Bacteriophages and their Ecology

INTRODUCTION

Phages or bacteriophages, viruses that infect and replicate inside bacteria, are the most abundant micro-organisms on earth. The realisation that antibiotic resistance poses a substantial risk to the world's health and global economy is revitalising phage therapy as a potential solution. The increasing ease by which phage genomes can be modified, owing to the influx of new technologies, has led to an expansion of their natural capabilities, and a reduced dependence on phage isolation from environmental sources. This chapter discusses the way synthetic biology has accelerated the construction of genetically modified phages and will describe the wide range of their applications. It will further provide insight into the societal and economic benefits that derive from the use of recombinant phages in various sectors, from health to biodetection, biocontrol and the food industry.

Current advances in synthetic biology have facilitated the rational design, modification and construction of recombinant phages – that contain genetically engineered DNA and/or have been through genetic recombination – enabling the extension of their innate phenotypes. The host specificity of phages is evolutionarily refined, with most phages targeting one species. This host recognition specificity is conferred by receptor binding domains (RBDs) that are found in either the tail-spike or tail fibre protein assemblies of the virions. Many researchers have altered the specificity of phages towards non-native hosts. In one such example, the host range of fd filamentous phage is altered by fusing a RBD from another filamentous phage (IKe), onto the infection-mediating protein of fd. Moving on to lytic phages, a genetically engineered T4 phage repository, was curated by randomising the T4 RBD using polymerases with less fidelity to PCR amplify non-conserved regions. The repository was found to propagate in *Yersinia ruckeri* and *Pseudomonas aeruginosa*, indicating that the host range of T4 had been re-directed from its native *Escherichia coli* host. Similarly, T3 (which naturally infects *E. coli*) and T7 phage (which infects *E. coli* and some species of *Yersinia*) was assembled in *Saccharomyces cerevisiae* with exogenous phage protein domains in order to alter its host range. As a proof of concept, it was demonstrated that modified T3 and T7 phage scaffolds could target pathogenic *Yersinia* and *Klebsiella bacteria* respectively. In addition, Klebsiella phage scaffolds were retargeted against *Escherichia coli* by swapping their phage tail components. Recombinant phages also function as vehicles for antimicrobials that are either incorporated into the phage or attached to its surface. For instance, they have been used to deliver light-activated antimicrobial agents (photosensitisers), which are seen as promising alternatives to antibiotics for treatment of common skin infections. Phages can also be engineered to suppress host SOS DNA repair system, enhancing the effectiveness of broad-spectrum antibiotics *in vitro*. Understandably, a natural concern about using engineered organisms is that the balance between natural phages in the environment may be affected. However, a recent study illustrated that phages endowed with gain of function mutations were out-competed by natural phages specific to the same host, suggesting that engineered phage genomes might not persist in the wild. Additionally, one strategy to a Wa commercialise phages is to re-engineer them to be non-replicative or non-lytic.

SYNTHETIC BIOLOGY TECHNOLOGIES FOR PHAGE ENGINEERING

Genome Engineering

A wide range of genome engineering methods have been applied to modify phage genomes and provide the desired characteristics for different applications. For simplicity, the methods have been divided into *in vitro* and *in vivo*.

In vitro methods: Restriction endonuclease-based methods have been used to construct recombinant genomes *in vitro*. For instance, the genome of T7 was redesigned to remove overlapping genetic elements among other modifications. The new version of the genome (T7.1) is divided into 73 'parts' belonging to six sections. The first two sections of T7.1 were synthesised and shown to be viable. An additional, *in vitro* method is reported for the genetic modification of lytic phages, called genome recombineering with electroporated DNA (BRED), where Smith and others used the P1vir phage as a proof of concept. BRED is based on the use of recombinases (obtained from bacterial heterologous over expression) to assemble phage genomes from purified phage genome and given synthetic DNA fragments. BRED has been recently used to genetically modify a P1vir phage. Specifically, a copy of the mobile element IS1 was removed from the genome of P1vir phage, with the use of BRED.

In vivo methods: *In vivo* methods have been used for bacteriophage engineering involving marker-based or marker-less selections of genetically modified bacteriophages. The most commonly used *in vivo* method is homologous recombination (HR), where the sequence to be inserted is cloned into a vector with flanking regions matching upstream and downstream of phage genome sequence. Phage that has undergone HR can then be selected from the phage population, with the methods described below.

Marker-based selection methods exploit genes promoting phage propagation. They could be genes encoded in the phage genome or host factors required for phage propagation. For the former, the gene has to be previously deleted from the genome, where the phage may require a strain expressing such gene to propagate. A first step would consist of the homologous recombination of the insert and the gene marker. Later, a marker-deficient strain could be used for selection. Alternatively, a host factor can be used. For instance, in order to identify a marker for T7 selection, *E. coli* BW25113 is screened for genes that promote T7 phage growth, and these can be used as selection markers when editing T7 phage genome. Two potential genes are identified: *cmk* and *trxA*. Deletion of the *trxA* gene appears to confer phage infection inhibition, whereas deletion of the *cmk* gene in the bacterial host shows a lower efficiency of plating of T7 bacteriophage in comparison to the control bacteria. The reduced efficiency of plating, but not a complete absence of plaques, indicates that despite the gene deletion, some degree of T7 infection is obtained. These false positives can be removed by serial dilutions. In this study the *E. coli* gene *cmk*, which encodes for CMP/dCMP kinase, was inserted instead of T7 gp5 by HR between wild-type T7 and a plasmid containing the cmk gene. The plated recombined phage was shown to be negative for growth on cells that were deficient in cmk, and which did not contain a plasmid expressing gp5. This expected phenotype was confirmed to be true at the genotypic level by sequencing.

False positives may occur in the marker-less selection method, CRISPR/Cas. Recently, CRISPR/Cas system, and specifically type I-E CRISPR/Cas system, was used to select for engineered T7 bacteriophage. The T7 phage genome was edited by homologous recombination and the recombinant phages were selected by targeting wild-type phages with the CRISPR/Cas system.

In another report, in addition to using CRISPR/Cas for the selection of engineered phage, CRISPR/Cas II-A system was used to *in vivo* modify phage 2972. Phage genome editing included gene exchange, point mutation and small or large deletions. For the gene exchange, orf33 in the phage 2972 was replaced with methyl transferase gene of the type II restriction/modification (R/M) system LlaDCHI from *L. lactis*. Since the results showed a successful gene swap and a fully functioning methyl transferase it was concluded that the CRISPR/Cas engineering system can be used for gene insertions into the phage's genome. CRISPR/Cas technology could be adapted to other phage genomes.

In another example, bacteriophage engineering is accomplished using an *in vivo* yeast platform as an alternative host for bacteriophage assembly. This platform is used to engineer phage with novel host ranges by swapping viral tail fibre scaffolds. Phage genomes are placed in *Saccharomyces cerevisiae*, allow gene modifications and result in generation of engineered phage. Each fragment of the phage genome is first amplified by PCR while retaining a homologous overhang. First and last fragments of the phage genome have a homology region with the yeast artificial chromosome (YAC). All amplified phage genome fragments as well as YAC are then transformed into yeast where gap repair facilitated joining of all the fragments and the YAC according to homology regions. After the purification of the vector the phage can then be initiated to form functional phages when transformed into bacteria. This yeast phage-engineering platform has a great potential because any genomic loci can be modified even by adding genes toxic to *E. coli*. One possible inconvenience is that the phage may have repeats at their ends (as it is the case for T7) and recombination may produce excision of the phage from the vector. This may be overcome by including a selective marker for yeast inside the phage genome.

Directed evolution methodologies: Directed evolution may be used to alter and optimise bacteriophage genomes providing a phenotypic or genotypic advantage in a given environment. It is possible to evolve bacteriophages via serial passaging, or continuous culture in a bioreactor. This platform was used to evolve lambda phage, which normally infects its host via LamB protein receptor, to infect via a novel OmpF receptor. In another remarkable study, a phage was optimised by serial passages in a living mouse providing a 13000 fold greater capacity of the phage to evade immune system and remain in the circulatory system. This was a result of a single mutation which led to amino acid substitution in the major lambda phage capsid protein E.

PACE (phage-assisted continuous evolution) combines continuous culture with increased mutagenesis to accelerate the evolution of M13 phagemids (non-replicative phages that require a strain carrying a helper system). PACE is used to evolve regulatory molecules rather than structural proteins in the virion. This is done by removing an essential gene (gpIII) from the phage and placing it, in an inactivated form, in the host strain. The gene responsible for the initiation of the evolution is introduced into the phage. The product of this gene must activate gpIII to produce infectious progeny. It is possible to use a similar methodology to evolve proteins from the phage such as those conferring host specificity or involved in replication. This method has been further expanded to evolve biomolecules with altered or highly specific new activities, using negative selection and modulation of selection stringency.

Phage display: Phage display is based on generating a library of synthetic or natural peptides and then fusing them onto a coat protein of a bacteriophage. Modified phages that bind strongly to the ligand displayed are enriched via sequential recovery from the surface and upon that they re-infect bacteria to propagate and increase in number. Filamentous phages M13 and fd are the most commonly used phages for phage display although T4, T7 and lambda phages have also been used. Traditionally phage display has been used for antibody production, proteomics, therapeutics, diagnostics (specially for cancer applications), infectious diseases and drug discovery. Phage display has also been used for epitope mapping, a method to identify the epitope of the antigen that interacts with an antibody. The identification of epitopes is important for the development of diagnostic tools, vaccines and new therapeutic targets. Additionally, phage display has proven useful in targeting membrane receptors via the identification of their agonists and antagonists, which present biological applications as drugs for various diseases. Phage display is also an excellent tool for the identification of protein–protein interactions. Its biggest advantage, compared to other methods established in the protein–protein interactions field, is that highly diverse peptide libraries can be constructed at low cost. These are some of the applications of phage display. The list is even broader and even more applications are expected to arise as the methodology evolves.

APPLICATIONS OF ENGINEERED PHAGES

Herein, we discuss how genetically modified phages (listed in Table 16.1) are used in different fields (presented in Fig. 16.1).

Table 16.1: Engineered bacteriophages and their applications.

Engineered bacteriophage	Applications
M13	Phage display, lethal delivery agent, engineered protein purification, nanomaterials, vaccinology
M13KE	Pathogen detection
T7	Phage display, gene therapy, biofilm control
Lambda (λ)	Phage display vaccinology, biocontrol
T4	Phage display, vaccinology
φA1122	Pathogen detection
A511	Pathogen detection
HK620	Pathogen detection
PBSPCA1	Agriculture
fd	Phage display, nanodevice fabrication and bottom-up manufacturing

Therapeutic Applications

Natural phages have multiple barriers that could prevent them from being developed into viable phage therapeutic products. Issues can arise both from their entry to mammalian cells and from circumventing the immune response of the host. Modified phages can be developed to avoid inactivation by the host defense system and persist in the body, thus enhancing their therapeutic potential. In this section, examples of recombinant phages as therapeutic agents for a variety of diseases are given. This includes phage therapy in mammalian hosts as well as phages as lethal delivery vehicles for prokaryotic hosts.

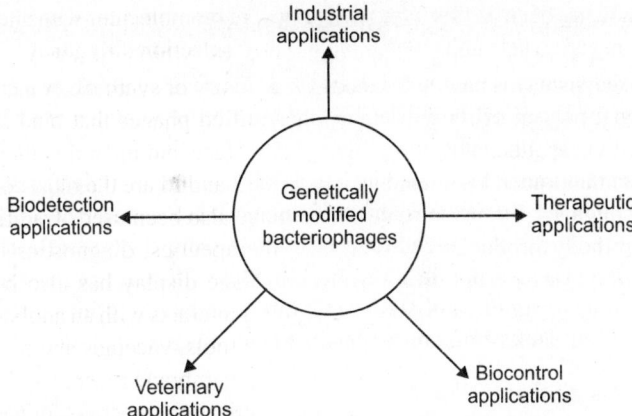

Fig. 16.1: A schematic representation of the synthetic bacteriophage applications.

The T7 bacteriophage was genetically modified for a potential therapy of hepatitis B. Globally HCC (hepatocellular carcinoma) is the fifth most common cancer in men, and the eighth most common in women, and it was estimated that during the year 2000, more than 500000 new cases arose. The first step of hepatitis B virus (HBV) infection is the interaction between a cell surface receptor and the HBV envelope protein (specifically the PreS1 region). T7 phage was modified to display polypeptides of varying length (up to fifty amino acids) of the PreS1 region. This was achieved by fusing the peptides of interest (PreSi region variants) to the C-terminus of the capsid protein gp10B fromT7. It was suggested that this system could be enhanced by displaying amino acids of the first half of the PreS1 fused proteins (which are heterologously expressed in insect cells).

The recombinant phages bind to the receptors on red blood cells and create a lattice structure of inter-connected virus and red blood cells. It is observed that two H5 influenza-specific monoclonal antibodies inhibit the binding of red blood cells to the recombinant phages. These modified phages mimic H5 influenza virus behavior by attaching to the red blood cells, this could potentially be exploited for the detection of influenza virus-specific antibodies in vaccine trials.

T4 phage is another example of engineered phage use in vaccinology. The outer capsid protein of T4 phage was fused to a protective antigen from *Bacillus anthracis*, to develop a vaccine for anthrax. The fusion protein was expressed in *E. coli*, purified, and *in vitro* added to the assembled phage. The PA-T4 particles presented immunogenicity inmice in the absence of an adjuvant. This study provides a promising system for construction of customised vaccines against anthrax.

Phages target bacteria more specifically than most antibiotics, and consequently have less effect on the human gut microbiome. However, lytic phages, whose concomitant cell lysis may result in the release of toxic substances (endotoxins) have encouraged the development of lysis-deficient phages. These lysis-deficient phages can be engineered by harnessing the phage machinery responsible for cell lysis. This consists of a membrane protein (normally deemed, holin) and endolysin or murein hydrolase. Holins form holes in the cell membrane, thus letting endolysin cross the membrane and degrade the peptidoglycan layer of the cell wall. An example of engineering a recombinant phage that is lysis-deficient involves *Staphylococcus aureus* phage P954 where its endolysin gene was inactivated by a loss of function insertion. Endolysin-deficient phages encoding lethal but non-lytic proteins are able to kill bacteria while reducing the endotoxin release. Engineered non-lytic phages have been shown to be efficient in treating mice infected with *P. aeruginosa*, *E. coli* or *S. aureus* which present higher survival rates, due to the lower levels of endotoxin release. Additionally, filamentous phages (which do not lyse the host) have been used for the specific delivery of lethal substances or genes to the site of infection. Among possible genes, those encoding for modified holin, lethal transcription regulator and addiction toxins (which induce programmed cell death) have been reported.

Modified phage particles can also be used as lethal delivery agents for efficient pathogen killing. A recent example is the engineering of the filamentous phage M13 to carry an integrin binding peptide and a fragment of the polymorphic membrane protein D from the sexually transmitted pathogen *Chlamydia trachomatis* (Ct), as a possible way to eliminate Ct infection. Based on this report, the engineered phage was able to significantly reduce Ct infection in both primary endocervical and HeLa cells, addressing the current lack of treatments against *Chlamydia trachomatis*.

Industrial Applications of Bacteriophage

High-gradient magnetic fishing (HGMF) partially purifies target products from heterogeneous bioprocess liquors. In HGMF, the target product is captured using magnetic adsorbent particles in combination with high-gradient magnetic separation equipment. HGMF binding capacity of microbeads was increased by placing an engineered M13 bacteriophage monolayer on a superparamagnetic (SPM) core of microbeads. This was achieved by genetic and chemical modification of the M13 coat proteins, pIII (minor coat) and pVIII (major coat) respectively. pIII protein was modified at its *N*-terminus to enable its binding onto nitrilotriacetic acid or silica coated SPMs, respectively. pVIII protein subunits of wild-type M13 were chemically cross-linked to a carboxyl-functionalised bead permitting side-on linkage of the phage to the SPMs. The phage-SPM particles, when used to fish the desired antibodies, led to 490% purified product from high protein solutions in one purification step.

fd filamentous phage has been engineered to increase the affinity of gold (Au) to its protein coat. This was achieved by substituting five amino acids on the *N*-terminal region of p8, the fd phage's major coat protein. These studies show how recombinant phages can be coated with a metal of interest, demonstrating the potential of recombinant phages as selfassembling templates for applications in bottom up manufacturing.

In addition, M13 filamentous bacteriophage has been used as a scaffold for the self-assembly of cobalt manganese oxide nanowires to make LiO_2 battery electrodes. Here, the phage coat protein gpVIII is modified to display peptides of negatively charged amino acids, and is able to interact with cationic metal precursors (such as cobalt and manganese) resulting in high production yield oxides. These oxides formed LiO_2 battery electrodes which were more porous and had a higher specific heat capacity in comparison to carbon electrodes.

Biodetection Applications of Bacteriophage

One area in which synthetic phages are proving useful is biodetection, where one of their main advantages is that they can be quickly amplified in the targeted live bacteria, compared to PCR or antibody-wash detection systems (which subsequently incur more false positives from the detection of dead bacteria). Early adoptions of biodetection with synthetic phages have focused on the insertion of reporter genes into naturally isolated phages. Most of these methods comprise of either inserting luciferase genes into the phage genome, or of fusing fluorescent proteins to the phage capsid, mimicking the engineering strategy employed in phage display. It should be emphasised that these systems are far from just academic enquires. Sample recently launched its DETECT/L kit on the back of luciferase-based recombinant phage technologies. The kit correctly identifies 50 Listeria species, as well as correctly excluding 30 non-listeria species that were subjected to testing. However, converting luciferase-based assays to more optimal multiplex assays (i.e. assays that detect more than one bacterial species in a given sample) may not be straight forward, which is an issue that could be circumvented by fluorescent-based reporter systems with compatible emission and excitation wavelengths.

The precision of phage host recognition has been explored for pathogen detection from environmental samples. Water quality control is one of the major concerns for public health as well as marine environment, and rapid methods need to be developed to allow accurate pathogen identification. One such method used a phage-based fluorescent biosensor 'phagosensor' prototype for enteric bacteria detection. In this system, the synthesis of the fluorescent protein only occurs after it is delivered to *E. coli* TD2158 by temperate bacteriophage HK620 carrying the fluorescent gene. The recombinant phages were incubated with the sample for one hour, followed by flow cytometry, which allowed sensitive detection of environmental *E. coli* TD2158 strain in diluted samples, and in mixed co-cultures. The established template was also successfully adapted to phage P22 to detect *Salmonella enterica Typhimurium*.

Colorimetry is another method for detecting pathogenic bacteria in water. In this instance, the target bacterial strain, ER2378, is trapped on a syringe filter followed by infection of a specific phage, M13KE.100 ER2378 is a lacZα-complementing strain of *E. coli* that expresses the ω-domain of the β-gal (ωGal) and the αGal peptide is cloned in an intergenetic region of the M13KE genome. Upon αGal peptide delivery to the bacterial strain, αGal is converted to the β-gal active form of αGal, which is detectable by colorimetric assay.

Another example of bacteriophage-based pathogen detection is the high-intensity fluorophage that can detect *Mycobacterium tuberculosis*. Phage A511 was modified to report cells of Listeria genus upon synthesis of a bacterial luciferase gene. The modified gene was placed downstream of the major capsid protein (cps) and was expressed upon phage infection of Listeria cells. Yersinia pestis is the etiological agent of the plague, which has seen a breakout of cases in America recently. To detect Yersinia pestis in blood samples, a recombinant reporter phage containing bacterial luxAB reporter genes was inserted in an early-transcribed noncoding region of the plague-diagnostic lytic phage fA1122 by homologous recombination.

Upon infection of Yersinia pestis with the recombinant fA1122, the bioluminescent phenotype was observed after 10 to 15 min. In a following study, the reporter phage was assessed as a diagnostic tool for Yersinia pestis in samples taken directly from the blood.

Even though it displayed 100% inclusivity for Yersinia pestis, some non-pestis *Yersinia* strains and *Enterobacteriaceae* also showed signal transduction. The reporter phage demonstrated rapid detection of antimicrobial susceptibility profiling upon antibiotic incubation of the blood samples. As a consequence these results suggest that the application of lytic reporter phages to detect bacterial pathogens in blood samples could reduce the time to diagnosis for patients afflicted with.

Phage-reporter systems were also developed for agricultural settings. *Pseudomonas cannabina* pv. *alisalensis* and *Pseudomonas syringae* pv. *maculicola* are both causative agents for diseases of *Brassicaceae* family. In a recent study, phage-based diagnostic was developed to identify the cause of bacterial blight. *P. cannabina* pv. *alisalensis* or PBSPCA1 phage was modified by integration of bacterial luxAB genes in the place of nonessential phoH gene using homologous recombination upon wild-type PBSPCA1 phage infection of *P. cannabina* pv. *alisalensis* BS91 containing luxAB expression cassette. A successful detection of Pseudomonas cannabina pv. alisalensis versus *Pseudomonas syringae* pv. *maculicola* resulted in more than 100-fold increase in bioluminescence within 4 hr of tissue harvesting.

Veterinary Applications of Bacteriophage

Genetically engineered phages have a wide range of applications in veterinary science and medicine. In the vast majority of cases, recombinant phages deliver antigens to be used for vaccination against animal diseases. Recombinant M13 bacteriophage has been used to vaccinate pigs against the tapeworm *Taenia solum*, which causes cysticercosis, a disease to which humans and pigs are susceptible. KETc1, KETc12 and GK1 peptides were fused to coat protein gpVIII and a recombinant antigen KETc7 was displayed on coat protein gpIII. The pooled phages were successful in reducing the number of cysts in the murine model (990 in mice receiving M13 vs. 338 immunised with the pool of recombinant phage). Preliminary work demonstrated sporadic effectiveness for a small sample of pigs, but further studies were needed to corroborate this evidence. Such a study was performed on a larger sample size, and significantly reduced the occurrence of cysticercosis in vaccinated pigs by 54.2%.

Phages lambda and T4, as mentioned earlier in this chapter, have been used to vaccinate against human diseases. In this section, we briefly mention their application as possible vaccines against pathogens that target animals. Recombinant lambda phage can be used as a potential vaccine against porcine Circovirus 246 a virus that causes post-weaning multisystemic wasting syndrome (PMWS), and has proved costly in the swine industry.

In another study, the T4 bacteriophage was used to develop a vaccine against infectious bursal disease virus (vvIBDV), a virus that causes infectious bursal disease (IBD) in chickens. Immunisation of chickens with the recombinant T4-VP2 phage resulted in no clinical death, however, some temporary bursal damages were observed.

Biocontrol Applications of Bacteriophage

Biocontrol is the regulation of pest/pathogen levels by biological means, a strategy that is being progressively favored by industry. One of the major problems in industrial processing is biofilm formation, and this is especially apparent in food industry. To this end, T7 bacteriophage was modified to express dispersin B (DspB), an enzyme produced by *Actinobacillus actinomycetemcomitans*. DspB acts via β-1,6-Nacetyl-D-glucosamine hydrolysis which disrupts biofilm formation and integrity. DspB was placed downstream of capsid gene 10B under the control of the strong T7 10 promoter. This allowed DspB to be expressed intracellularly so that its release would occur during cell lysis. The results showed that DspB expressing phage was significantly more effective at killing *E. coli* in comparison to wild-type T7 and wild-type T3 bacteriophages, and that this phage reduced the amount of biofilm by a factor of 2.6 in comparison to non-engineered T7 control phage.

In another study lambda phage was engineered to deliver CRISPR/Cas system to sensitise bacteria with antibiotic resistance genes. Once delivered to a pathogen, the CRISPR/Cas system was transferable between bacterial hosts so that bacteria with antibiotic genes would be outcompeted. In addition, pathogens with acquired CRISPR/Cas were no longer susceptible to engineered lytic phage infection. This system showed effective reduction in infections of antibiotic-resistant pathogens and thus offering a potential biocontrol system for hospital surface treatment.

NATURAL PHAGES

Natural phages may be a solution to a myriad of issues in agriculture, biocontrol, and medicine: in agriculture, they are applied against plant infections, in biocontrol, in the protection and control of crops and food products, and in medicine, a number of trials have explored their safety and efficacy. Phage therapy has reached a critical juncture in its development. Natural phages are, according to current legislature, unpatentable, as they are no longer considered novel, having first been introduced over a century ago. This prevents them from being commercially viable in industry, especially for big pharma corporations that have to undergo expensive clinical trials, and so is an impediment to the development of infrastructure that can deliver treatments to patients. The intellectual property of recombinant phages, on the other hand, can be secured, thus overcoming these issues. Yet recombinant phages do more than to provide opportunities for profit, they extend upon natural phages by creating additional functionalities (such as delivery of variety of cargos, e.g. depolymerase) as well as overcoming some of their limitations.

One such limitation is that natural phages can induce a mammalian immune response upon their entry, a response that could be avoided by modifying the phage's coat protein. Nonetheless, in some instances, an over excited immune response is desired, for example, when developing vaccines against viral particles. In the case of HBV, phage-displayed viral peptides can evoke immune response, and help identify the antibodies specific to these viral peptides.

Furthermore, by refactoring phage genomes, phages could have their sequences rejigged to avoid host restriction systems, by removing the palindromic sequences targeted by type II restriction enzymes, or by appending peptides that inhibit the CRISPR/Cas proteins. One can also envisage the swapping or addition of exogenous endo/exonucleases to cleave host genomes faster. Further work demonstrated that rational engineering of tail fibres can change host tropism of bacteriophages and pyocins (phage-like particles called bacteriocins, produced by some strains of Pseudomonas aeruginosa for use in intraspecies warfare). Employing this in combination with directed evolution, phage cocktails could be generated to target a given pathogen through separate, or a combination of, receptors, and adapted to circumvent the host-immune system. Importantly, new techniques are constantly being developed in the fields of genome engineering and gene synthesis, decreasing also the cost of gene synthesis. It is expected that also because of that, the engineering of recombinant bacteriophages will be further facilitated and will enable the corresponding broadening of their applications.

BACTERIOPHAGE ECOLOGY AND PLANTS

Plant biology cannot be fully appreciated absent microbial flora, and plant-associated bacteria are incompletely understood without an awareness of phage—the viruses of prokaryotes. Phage have been found in association with 'buds, leaves, root nodules (leguminous plants), roots, rotting fruit, seeds, stems and straw, crown gall tumours healthy or diseased alfalfa, barley, beans, broccoli, brussels sprouts, buckwheat, clover, cotton, cucumber, lucerne, mulberry, oats peas, peach trees, radish, rutabaga, ryegrass, rye, timothy, tobacco, tomatoes, and wheat'. In this section we will consider the myriad ways that phage can impact ecologically on plant-associated bacteria.

Phage Biology

Much is known of phage biology, particularly at the molecular level. This section focuses on the phage biology, starting with the phage life cycle, which consists of an extracellular search, attachment to susceptible bacteria, phage-genome uptake into bacteria, production (maturation) of phage progeny, and subsequent release of these progeny into the extracellular environment.

The phage itself, the virion particle, consists of a nucleic acid core that is made up, depending on the phage, of DNA or, less often, of RNA. Surrounding this nucleic-acid genome is a protein based capsid. The capsid plays three important roles in the phage life cycle: (i) protecting the phage genome during the extracellular search (e.g. from DNA-degrading enzymes), (ii) effecting phage adsorption, which is the attachment of the virion particle to a susceptible bacterium, and (iii) the subsequent delivery (uptake) of the phage genome into the cytoplasm of the now-infected bacterium. The extracellular search occurs via phage diffusion through an aqueous milieu. During this period the phage must avoid physical damage while waiting to encounter a susceptible bacterium. The likelihood that an individual phage will find a bacterium to adsorb is a function of time, the phage diffusion rate, and the local density of phage-susceptible bacteria, with more bacteria resulting in faster phage adsorption. A slightly different set of parameters governs the likelihood of phage attack on bacteria, with adsorption a function of time and the phage diffusion rate, but also of phage density, with more phage resulting in more bacteria infected.

Phage adsorption to bacteria furthermore is a function of phagebacteria chemical and physical interaction. Phage display proteins with high affinity to specific bacterial surface molecules-an association analogous to antigen recognition by immune systems. The host range of most phages, i.e. the species that they are capable of productively infecting, consequently is relatively narrow — typically limited to only a single bacterial genus, species, or, often, even to only a limited number of strains within a given species. Thus, while total phage densities can be enormous—as many as 100 million or more per gram of soil or ml of aquatic environment—the actual density of phages capable of infecting a particular bacterial strain usually is much smaller. Following uptake, the phage genome can rapidly subvert host-cell functions, directing bacterial metabolism during the phage latent period towards phage production. Depending on the phage, these virions either may accumulate within the bacterial cytoplasm (as is the case for so-called lytic phage) or, for filamentous phage, virions instead are released—over the course of an extended latent period—across an otherwise intact cell envelope.

Phage Ecology

Phage ecology is the study of the interaction of phage with their biotic and abiotic environments. Much of this section considers the ecological interaction between phage and bacteria within the context of plants and their surrounding soil, and in this section we introduce the basics of phage ecology. Following the traditions of ecology we can differentiate phage ecology into four general categories: (i) Phage organismal ecology is the study of the adaptations that phage employ to increases their likelihood of transmission between hosts such as virion desiccation resistance, ability during infection to repair ultraviolet (UV) light-mediated nucleic-acid damage, and so on. (ii) Phage population ecology is the study of phage life-history characteristics, particularly as they apply to phage growth and intraspecific (between-phage) competition. Understanding phage population growth within spatially structured environments, such as within the phyllosphere or rhizosphere, is particularly challenging. (iii) Phage community ecology focuses on the stability of phage-containing environments such as the propensity of phage to drive phage-sensitive bacteria to extinction. Phage community ecology is complicated by the continuous co-evolution of bacteria with their phage predators. In addition, phage play important roles in the horizontal transfer of DNA between bacteria. (iv) Phage ecosystem ecology considers the phage impact on energy flow and nutrient cycling within ecosystems. Phage, for example, can disrupt the soil bacteria responsible for nitrogen cycling.

Phage Temperance vs Virulence

Population and organismal ecologies are concerned with the adaptations that organisms employ to enhance their Darwinian fitness over the course of their life cycles. For phage, the life-cycle steps most under their control are the durability of the virion particle, the breadth of the host range, and the details of the infection strategy. In this section we take a population-ecology approach to contrasting two infection strategies: temperance versus virulence. Subsequently we consider the impact of plants on lysogeny.

For lytic phage, progeny release can occur only following the total destruction (lysis) of the host bacterial cell. One can differentiate lytic phage into two types, temperate phage and obligately lytic phage. Only temperate phage can display lysogeny, an infection that stalls shortly after the introduction of the phage genome into the host cell, which then (in most cases) integrates as a prophage into the bacterial chromosome. During lysogeny phages neither produce virions nor lyse bacteria. A temperate phage does not obligately enter into a lysogenic relationship with its host bacterium, in fact many temperate phage infections result in the immediate production of phage progeny, i.e. a lytic cycle rather than lysogeny. This decision is determined by characteristics of the infecting phage and the metabolic state of the host. When not induced, a phage in the lysogenic state replicates as a giant gene complex along with the host cell's genome.

Lysogeny typically results in bacterial resistance to infection by similar (i.e. homologous) phage. Mutant phage that are able to bypass this resistance are described as *vir* mutants (for *vir*ulence). One advantage that can be associated with such virulence is an ability to actively infect homologous lysogens (bacteria lysogenised by the same phage), though establishment of this Vir phenotype can require multiple phage mutations. Note, though, that a diversity of virulent phage exist that are not *vir* mutants but instead are unrelated to temperate phage. In addition to providing a safe home to the temperate-phage genome, and blocking the replication of non-virulent homologous phage, lysogeny has the potential to alter the phenotype of the host cell, a process known as phage (or lysogenic) conversion.

Ecology of Lysogeny

What advantages are bestowed upon a phage that displays a temperate lifestyle? We can describe obligately lytic phage as essentially *semelparous*, with the acquisition of a bacterial cell resulting in only a single reproductive episode. As such these phage are perhaps best understood as adapted to a so called *r* strategy of population growth, with a life-history emphasis on rapid population increase when resources are plentiful (resources for phage being susceptible bacteria). Aiding in this strategy is their (i) avoidance of physiological tradeoffs required for the display of lysogeny, (ii) a commitment of all progeny to lytic growth (rather than some fraction to lysogen formation), or (iii) an ability to infect lysogens. These advantages, however, come with requirements for long-term survival as free phage when bacteria are less numerous, and/or dissemination to new environments to find new bacterial hosts.

Temperate phage can also display the semelparous infection strategy of virulent phage (i.e. the lytic cycle). A fraction of infections, however, will instead result in lysogeny. Lysogeny represents an iteroparity of sorts, i.e. more than one reproductive episode per lifetime, at least so long as one is willing to accept a clonally related population of lysogens as a single individual and a sporadic induction of lytic cycles within this population as consecutive reproductive events. Such a life-history approach is the more *K*-like strategy whereby temperate prophage, by less-rapidly killing off their bacterial resource, may more readily sustain their population size at an environment's carrying capacity. Filamentous phage similarly display a more semelparous life-history strategy than virulent phage, with (i) a longer-term maintenance of the host infection, (ii) only a few phage progeny released over a given interval, and (iii) with multiple intervals (i.e. a long time) over which these phage progeny are released.

Though lysogeny often is framed as an adaptation to survival within relatively unstable environments, i.e. during 'hard times', one could similarly argue that lysogeny bestows a competitive advantage on phage that is useful when bacterial populations are relatively stable, i.e. not fluctuating in size. Lysogeny thusly can be an effective *K* strategy so long as lysogens are not being actively killed by lytic phage. Exposure to lytic phage may be less likely in well-structured environments that limit phage diffusion and in which lysogen microcolonies exist as relatively few cells, with low lysogen number minimising the potential for temperate-phage mutation to anti-lysogen virulence. Of course, arguing that well structured environments can favour lysogeny over virulence is nearly a restatement of the 'hard times' hypothesis whereby the 'long periods of dearth' required for this dominance is posited to be a consequence of environmental structure (e.g. insurmountable distances between bacterial microcolonies) rather than solely of temporal variation in resource availability.

Lysogeny in the Face of Plants

Gvozdyak has suggested that plants can induce bacterial lysogens (that is, cause them to initiate their lytic cycle), a strategy that plants could employ towards the elimination of bacterial pathogens. Perhaps similarly, Sato has shown that an extract of mulberry leaves could induce lysogens of *Pseudomonas syringae*. It may be that these induced prophage are 'abandoning ship' in response to the plant's release of antibacterial compounds, with the phage simply following an evolutionary algorithm based on the logic that it is better to take one's chances as a free phage than to continue to infect a dying bacterium. Also consistent with a shift away from lysogeny in the lysogeny-lytic cycle balance, Menzel and others have reported a negative impact of certain plant-growth regulators and herbicides on the initial establishment of lysogeny.

For many bacteria, plant association marks not a high likelihood of plant-induced bacterium death but, instead, a period of effective bacterial growth. Given heterogeneous bacterial populations it could be advantageous for temperate phage to lyse host bacteria when times are good since not only are healthy, uninfected bacteria potentially present, but those bacteria also could contain nonhomologous prophage capable of infecting and then lysing their own uninduced lysogens. That is, more effective bacterial growth could tip an environment from conditions that disfavour phage lytic growth and favour lysogen survival (i.e. environments in which it is better, from the phage perspective, to be a bacterium) to conditions that favour lytic growth and thereby disfavour a continued display of lysogeny.

Phage Rhizosphere

From the phage perspective much of what is of interest in understanding the phage-plant interaction has to do with the extracellular search, a province of phage organismal ecology. How exactly do phage manage to find new bacteria to infect before succumbing to the ravages of environmentally induced virion decay? Answering this question within the rhizosphere — the region consisting of plant roots and surrounding soil — involves examining the impact of soil structure and chemistry on the mobility and survival of free phage and their hosts.

In most crop environments, with a few notable exceptions, most of the time the soil is only partially hydrated. The lack of a continuous aqueous phase greatly complicates predictions regarding the diffusion of free phage, as for any soil colloid. This situation is complicated further by the propensity of free phage to become trapped within biofilms or reversibly adsorbed to particles, such as clays, that are commonly found in the soil. This non-specific and often reversible phage adsorbtion within soils is a function of sorbent and virion surface chemistry, virion size, and pH. Moreover, acidic soils can permanently inactivate free phage.

We can only speculate whether these phage-soil interactions help or hinder the phage in their search for a suitable host. Since sorption to solid substrates lowers the diffusion rates of free phage, it localises them to specific spatial regions, and thereby limits the maximum rate at which they can encounter a suitable host cell. On the other hand, adsorption to clays has been suggested to have a protective effect by holding phage within a hydrated environment. Both states are essentially in opposition only within undisturbed soil. If the soil itself is disseminated, becomes fully hydrated, or is otherwise well mixed, then associated phage, whether free or bound, may be disseminated. Soil-adsorbed phage thus could serve as a viable infectivity pool that is tapped only as bacteria grow, diffuse, or swim into the phage vicinity, or if the soil particle itself is transferred into or onto a bacterium-containing environment.

Phage can attack bacteria directly associated with plant roots. Given the close proximity of roots to soil it seems obvious that phage attack must occur via phage diffusion from either surrounding soil or from neighbouring roots. Rhizosphere bacteria, however, may gain an upper hand in what likely is a constant battle between the phage predator and bacteria prey by some combination of (i) relatively low viable counts of phage capable of infecting specific bacteria, (ii) relatively low rates of phage diffusion within soil, particularly under drier conditions or following phage adsorption to soil, (iii) relatively high rates of free-phage inactivation within soil, and (iv) physical (or spatial) refuges that provide bacteria with a degree of physical protection from phage. Indeed, one can envisage phage replication as equivalent to a nuclear chain reaction with anything damping the mobility or production of the phage 'neutron' serving to limit depletion of the bacterial 'fuel'. Significant bacterial depletion occurs only once bacteria first have achieved a critical 'mass' (i.e. sufficient density).

Phage researchers have significant experience handling phage within environments containing relatively low phage densities—and in which diffusion (and mixing) is limited — since these are the conditions under which phage growth typically occurs in solid media. Solid-media growth involves mixing a small number of phage with a large excess of bacteria, which is then poured into a thin layer over a regular plate of agar growth medium. The soft-agar in the top layer impedes phage and bacterial diffusion while the bottom agar layer maintains a relatively constant chemical and physical state for bacterial and phage growth. Within the soft agar layer, phage populations grow as plaques, which are expanding regions of phage induced bacterial lysis, each originating from a single phage infection. Plaques appear transparent or translucent against the background of the typically more-opaque bacterial lawn growing within the agar-based substrate. Of particular relevance to understanding host-phage ecology within the rhizosphere therefore is determination of the degree to which phage growth in soil systems approximates the better understood solid-phase phage growth in laboratory media. Though within agar plaque-development theory as well as techniques for plaque-growth quantification have been fairly well developed, to our knowledge similarly finescale investigation has not been attempted within a soil-based medium.

Individual soils likely vary spatially and temporally with regard to plaque-like growth-particularly as a function of soil composition, degree of hydration, density and physiological state of host bacteria, and rates of free-phage inactivation. Nevertheless, we predict that the basic principle of phage solid-phase population growth, i.e. a phage diffusion mediated expanding sphere of bacterial infection, could still apply. Thus, without active mixing of soil, e.g. via the action of invertebrates or other localised soil disruptions, we speculate that bacterial microcolonies within the rhizosphere may display periods of boom or bust with regard to phage attack, with increasing microcolony size, or mere time (i.e. chance), increasing the likelihood of phage-microcolony encounter. Infection of one bacterium within a localised bacterial clone could result in the destruction of part or all of a genetically homogeneous bacterial microcolony. Means by which such coordinated attack may be thwarted could include (i) variation in the physiological or anatomical state of the bacteria making up a clone, so that not all bacteria are equally susceptible to phage attack (including the formation of spores for those species that are able to, as well as hyphael aging for streptomycetes), (ii) display of motility such that bacteria progeny minimise co-location and thereby avoid serial infection (though with the caveat that active movement through soil might increase the likelihood that individual bacteria encounter phage), and (iii) sequestration away from the soil such as within root nodules colonised by rhizobia or perhaps following bacterial penetration into plants upon infection. Rarely encountering microcolonies could be antithetical to the prosperity or even survival of obligately lytic phage, but could provide numerous stable, otherwise phage-free niches for temperate-phage survival as bacterial lysogens.

Phage Phyllosphere

How phage interact with their bacterial hosts in the phyllosphere, the aerial plant structures, is even less understood than the phage ecology of the rhizosphere. The phyllosphere presents a less hospitable environment relative to the rhizosphere - given the exposure to UV, intense visible light, and desiccation that is likely on many above-soil plant surfaces. The harshness of the phyllosphere combined with its relative impermanence begs the question, particularly for obligately lytic phage: Where is the virion reservoir?

In the case of phages of the plant-pathogen *Erwinia amylovora*, some studies have noted that phage are less readily isolated from the aerial portions of trees, even during times of active infection by the host. By contrast, phage could almost always be isolated from the soil around infected trees. That would suggest that the phage reservoir is located in the soil, possibly with phage multiplying on stray bacteria that fall from the tree to the ground below. Other phage studies on the same host bacterium, however, have found abundant *E. amylovora* phages in the phyllosphere of infected trees (for review of similar observations in additional phage-plant pathogen systems). If the virion reservoir is the soil for at least some phage that attack plant epiphytes, then how do phage reach the phyllosphere of a tree, which may have foliage 3 or more feet off the ground? One possible explanation is that phage invade the phyllosphere upon plant germination and then remain a part of plant normal flora. Alternatively, phages could move from plant to plant within the phyllosphere with soil remaining a phyllosphere phage sink rather than source habitat.

The habitats of otherwise plant-associated phage can range beyond plants or plant-associated soil. Irrigation waters and agricultural drainage are known to contain phage capable of infecting plant-associated bacteria. *Erwinia* phage have been isolated from lakes as well as from sewage. The latter phage perhaps display broad host ranges, attacking enteric bacteria associated with humans as well as the bacteria associated with plants. Perhaps similarly, phage infecting phytopathogenic *Pseudomonas* have been isolated from sewage while *Agrobacterium*-infecting phage have been isolated from feces.

Erwinia phage have also been isolated from a corn flea beetle. This association between phage and insect is of interest since arthropods are known vectors for viruses that directly infect plants. However, the degree to which arthropods are responsible for phage transmission remains an open question. Indeed, phage movement within and between plants as well as between soil and plants presumably follows paths similar to those employed by bacteria, i.e. carriage by animals, dust, soil, seeds, and water, including splashing caused by hard rain, plus various human activities such as pruning. A case can be made that rain, by promoting epiphytic bacterial growth, can simultaneously supply phage with (i) healthy hosts, (ii) water in which to diffuse between bacteria, and (iii) a means of disseminating about individual plants as well as among populations of plants.

Phage and Agriculture

Though plants are surrounded by phage, the vast bulk of the phage impact on plants is mediated through plant-associated bacteria. Plant-associated symbiotic bacteria can range from helpful (mutuals) to harmful (pathogens), and the phage impact on bacteria also can range from mutualistic to parasitic. Despite these complications, the phage impact, either negative or positive on plants, tends to be limited (i) to phage-induced bacterial lysis, (ii) to selection for phage-resistance within bacterial communities, or (iii) to phage-associated modification of bacterial phenotypes (phage conversion). These we consider in order. There have been a number of reports of phage presence, in relatively small-scale experiments, that result in reduced plant growth or reduction in plant nitrogen content. Experimentally induced decline in the plant-protective bacterium, *Pseudomonas fluorescens*, has also been noted. However, it is uncertain how often wild phages negatively impact on plant growth under naturally occurring conditions. We speculate that extrapolation of observations from small to large scales is challenging due to ignorance of naturally occurring phage-bacteria dynamics and spatial heterogeneities that exist across large plots. Indeed, we are aware of only one report suggesting that phage may have obstructed plant growth on a large scale in a non-experimental agricultural setting, as mediated by reductions in soil rhizobia. Further exploration of this 'extrapolation' issue could be difficult assuming reluctance to conduct large-scale field tests of phage that are antagonistic to beneficial bacteria.

It is typically assumed that reduced plant growth correlated with phage presence is a consequence of phage antagonism against beneficial bacteria, e.g. phage-induced lysis. Lytic phage can also indirectly reduce the fitness of susceptible bacteria. This fitness reduction can be manifest either as a density decline of bacteria inhabiting specific niches, or by a decline only of susceptible bacteria, the latter suggesting a replacement of susceptible bacteria by similar but phage-resistant bacteria. The above-cited Demolon and Dunez study, for example, has been much discussed in the plantphage literature, with some authors concluding that the observed negative phage impact resulted from selection for a phage-resistant bacterial phenotype that was less effective at nitrogen fixation. This interpretation is consistent with more modern phage community-ecology theory, which posits that bacterial resistance to phage attack often comes at some metabolic cost to bacteria. Consequently, a bacterium that does not display phage resistance may be able to invade and even drive to extinction a phage-resistant population of otherwise-identical bacteria, at least so long as phage are not present.

From a plant's perspective, this change in bacterial prevalence upon phage attack is irrelevant unless phage-sensitive and phage resistant bacteria display differences in their ability to interact with plants. Such differences are often observed, though it is important to note that for many studies only a fraction of bacterial mutations to phage resistance result in significant change in plant-interaction phenotypes. Phage T4- and phage fEC2-resistant, mostly lypopolysaccharide (LPS)-defective mutants of the soft-rot Erwinias *E. carotovora* and *E. chrysanthemi*, for example, generally do not display a loss of virulence. Given a relative rarity of avirulence in phage-resistant mutants, an invasion of phage into a pathogen population and subsequent selection for phage-resistant variants may not impact negatively on the virulence of the surviving bacteria. Rather, the community impact may be seen as a decline of the pathogen population followed by recovery by similarly virulent but phage resistant bacteria.

Conversely, phage-resistant mutants of *Ralstonia solanacearum*, which display various defects in LPS synthesis, were predominantly avirulent in tobacco seedlings, as were approximately 50% of selected phage-resistant *Xanthomonas campestris* mutants.

Mutational phage resistance resulting from a loss of pili also has been shown to reduce *Rhizobium* nodulation in clover. Mutation to phage-resistance by *P. fluorescens* similarly can result in reduced protection of radishes from *Fusarium* wilt. The mechanism by which this loss occurs, however, appears to be not so much from a decline in *P. fluorescens* colonising ability as due to insufficient induction of cross-reactive systemic resistance by plants.

Like phage resistance, modification of bacterial phenotype can result from phage conversion, i.e. the expression of prophage genes over the course of lysogenic infection. Little is known of phage conversion positively affecting plant growth. There exists some evidence for the converse, however: lysogeny negatively impacting soyabean-*Bradyrhizobium japonicum* interaction. An example of phage conversion that could possibly be interpreted as positively affecting plant fitness, by poisoning a plant predator, occurs in the case of toxic annual ryegrass, *Lolium rigidum*. The developing seeds of this grass are susceptible to infection and gall formation by a nematode, *Anguina funesta*. If these nematodes are carrying certain strains of the bacterium *Clavibacter toxicus*, then the galls will contain corynetoxin. Related to tunicamycin-like antibiotics, corynetoxin inhibits protein glycosylation and can be fatal to grazing animals (i.e. sheep) that consume the infected grass.

Phage Therapy

Phage have been proposed as plant-pathogen control agents in a process known as phage therapy: the application of specific phages to specific ecosystems in order to reduce the population size of specific bacteria. That is, phage therapy is a form of biological control—the use of one organism to suppress another. Like other methods of biological control, one advantage of phage therapy is a reduction in the usage of chemical agents against pest species, which, in the case of phage, means a reduction in the usage of chemical antibiotics. Phages, such as the phage NCPPB 3778, are associated with the ability of *C. toxicus* to produce corynetoxin. It is not clear how the phage causes the production of the toxin, as the complicated glycolipid structure of corynetoxins would require an elaborate metabolic pathway to be expressed from the phage genome. However, associations between phage and bacterial virulence factors are quite common, being responsible for much of the virulence associated with such important human pathogens as *Corynebacterium diphtheria*, *Escherichia coli* O157:H7, and *Vibrio cholerae*. Note that the likelihood of phage conversion of non-toxogenic *C. toxicus* strains into toxigenic strains seems to be enhanced via the application various herbicides at the same time as phage exposure. Also of interest, phage Xf and Xf-2 infection of *X. campestris* results in an increase in this bacterium's virulence towards rice. Phage therapy was explored extensively by early phage workers as a means of controlling plant pathogens.

Circumstances in which phage therapy of plants or plant products has been attempted include against *Salmonella* associated with fresh cut fruit, to disinfest *Streptomyces scabies*-infected potato seed tuber, against bacterial leaf spot of mungbeans (particularly in combination with streptomycin), against *Xanthomonas pruni* associated bacterial spot of peaches, to control of *X. campestris* infections of peach trees as well as cabbage and pepper diseases, to control *Ralstonia solanacearum*, and to control soft rot and fire blight associated with *Erwinia*. Phage therapy has been used successfully against bacterial blotch of mushrooms caused by *Pseudomonas tolaasii*. In studies notable for the employment of phage host range mutants, phage therapy has also been employed against bacterial blight of geraniums and bacteria spot of tomatoes, both caused by pathovars of *X. campestris*. Phage can also be used to bias the survival of more-effective mutualistic bacteria. Basit and others, for example, have isolated phage that are ineffective against a preferred inoculum of *B. japonicum* but effective against naturally occurring competitors. By coating seeds with phage effective only against these potential competitors they can enhance nitrogen fixation. Though seemingly effective in certain situations, it is likely that phage therapy against bacterial plant pathogens will not prove to be a 'magic bullet' in all cases. Johnson proposed a general biological control model which suggests that the success of a particular treatment will be influenced by agent and target densities. An important component of this model is the possibility of the target residing in spatial refuges into which the biological control agent cannot penetrate. We would propose several additional factors that could contribute to the success or failure of a potential phage therapy system, such as the location or niche in which the target pathogen population resides (including the potential for refuges), the presence of adequate water as a medium for virion diffusion, rates of virion decay, the timing of phage application, phage *in situ* infection fecundity, and the relative fitness (and virulence) of phage-resistant bacterial mutants. Furthermore, due to the diversity of bacteria and their phages, extrapolation of phage therapy practices from one pathogen system to different systems will not always be practicable. Indeed, our nominal understanding of various aspects of the phage ecology of plants could hinder the development of phage therapy regimens that function reliably under diverse circumstances.

In summary, although there are still ethical, socio-economical, and experimental issues to resolve, the groundwork of phages appears promising, and will surely come to establish itself at the forefront of personalised therapeutics and diagnostics.

Bacteriophages in Chemotherapy and Medicines

INTRODUCTION

Phage therapy for eliminating multidrug resistant bacteria is gaining importance. The abundance of phages in the environment makes it a relatively simple task to isolate phages against any given pathogen which can be characterised using a series of known protocols. The timescale and costs for the development of a new phages for therapy will be a fraction of those for introducing a new antibiotic. Currently, many pathogenic bacteria have application of therapeutic phages in medicine acquired multiple drug resistance, which is a serious clinical problem. Phages, when properly selected, offer the most cost-effective alternative to antibiotics. These have proved to be efficient in bacterial elimination on single application and recently accepted for food treatment as well to counter food contamination during storage. Phages should be essentially free of contaminating bacterial toxin and also capable of evading the clearance by reticulendothelial system. Although some problems remain to be solved, many experts are of the opinion that phage therapy will find a niche in modern Western medicine in the future.

Phage lytic enzymes have a broad application in the treatment of bacterial diseases. Whenever there is a need to kill bacteria, phage enzymes may be freely utilised. They may be used not only to control pathogenic bacteria on human mucous membranes, but may find application in the food industry to control disease causing bacteria. Phage lytic enzymes have yet to be exploited. Because of the serious problems of resistant bacteria in hospitals, day care centers, and nursing homes, particularly *Staphylococci* and *Pneumococci*, such enzymes may be of immediate benefit in these environments.

For more than half a century, the doctors and clinicians have been relying primarily on antibiotics to treat infectious diseases caused by pathogenic bacteria. However, the emergence of bacterial resistance to antibiotics following widespread clinical, veterinary, and animal or agricultural usage has made antibiotics less and less effective. These days scientists are now facing the threat of superbugs, i.e. pathogenic bacteria resistant to most or all available antibiotics. During the last 30 years, no new classes of antibiotics have been found, even with the help of modern biotechnology such as genetic engineering. Pharmaceutical companies have mainly focused on the development of new products derived from the known classes of antibiotics which is a cause of major concern. Thus, exploring alternative approaches to develop antibacterial products is also a worthwhile task, and re-examining the potential of promising older methods might be of value. One of the possible replacements for antibiotics is the use of bacteriophages or simply phages as antimicrobial agents. Phage therapy involves the use of lytic phages for the treatment of bacterial infections, especially those caused by antibiotic resistant bacteria. In general, there are two major types of phages, lytic and lysogenic. Only the lytic phages (also known as virulent phages) are a good choice for developing therapeutic phage preparations. The bactericidal ability of phages has been used to treat human infections for years as a complement or alternative to antibiotic therapy. Bacteriophages, nature's tiniest viruses and it is estimated that there are about 1031 phages on earth making viruses the most abundant life form on earth. Bacteriophages not only help in the treatments of bacterial infections in animals and human beings but also used in birds, fishes, plants, food material and biofilm eradication.

BACTERIOPHAGES IN CHEMOTHERAPY

Therapeutic use of bacteriophages for the prevention and treatment of bacterial diseases, has been targeted since the discovery of phages in 1917 by Félix d'Hérelle. Following his discovery, he first attempted to use these against dysentery and since then, bacteriophages have been used to treat human infections as an alternative or a complement to antibiotic therapy. Particularly, from 1920s to 1950s, phage therapy has exploded and centres in the US, France and Georgia were established, however, there have been limitations to antibacterial phage therapy that hamper its application as an antibiotic alternative.

These have been summarised recently by Hermoso and others as follows: (i) phages generally have narrow host range and only strongly lytic phage against bacterial strain infecting the patient, should be given to the patient, (ii) phages may not always remain lytic under the physiological conditions and bacteria can become resistant to phages after infection, (iii) phage preparations should be free of bacteria and their toxic components to meet clinical safety requirements, but sterilisation of phage preparations could inactivate the phages, (iv) phages can be inactivated by a neutralising antibody, and there is some risk of promoting allergic reactions to them, (v) the pharmacokinetics of phage treatments are more complicated than those of chemical drugs because of their self-replicating nature, (vi) phages might endow bacteria with toxic or antibacterial resistance genes.

Due to the above-listed limitations of bacteriophage therapy, bacteriophages might have more value as tools in drug discovery such as for target discovery and validation, assay development and compound design, and some of these exploitations are discussed below.

Bacterial Virulence and Injection Mechanisms of Bacteriophages

Efficient host infection relies on bacterial virulence factors being localised outside the producing cell where they are identically placed to interact with host defences and subvert host cells for the pathogen's benefit. Pathogenic bacteria have thus developed powerful molecular strategies to deliver their virulence factors across the bacterial cell envelope as well as powerful mechanisms to adverse host cell plasma membrane. In Gram-negative bacteria, the cell envelopes have two hydrophobic inner and outer membranes with a hydrophilic space in between. The secreted hydrophobic molecules of proteins, enzymes or toxins have to travel through the hydrophobic environment of the membranes in an aqueous channel, or another type of conduit, that spans the cell envelope. These paths to the external medium are built by assembling macromolecular complexes, called secretion machines and they are distinguishable by the number and characteristics of the components such as types I, II and V secretion systems and they play important roles in the virulence of pathogens.

In type VI secretion systems (T6SS) of Gram-negative bacteria the lack of an outer membrane channel for the T6SS might suggest an alternative delivery strategy such as local puncturing of the cell envelope to avoid cell lysis whilst allowing transient assembly of the secretion machine. Filloux points out that the structural proteins of the T6SS are very similar to those that make up the injection machinery found in bacteriophages. Bacteriophages inject their DNA into bacterial cytosol and use the bacterium as a phage factory to replicate phage DNA. Bacterial cell envelope is perforated by bacteriophage puncturing device and its DNA is injected into bacterial cell via a tail tube. T6SS seems to use the same mechanism used by bacteriophages to inject their DNA into bacteria in which some components like the T6SS-specific exoproteins might have a similar tail-spike puncturing device of the T4 phage and might create a channel across the bacterial envelope which resembles the phage tail tube. T6SS translocation mechanism operate from the inside to the outside of the bacterial cell, and might be a mirror image of the phage translocation mechanism, which operates from outside to the inside of the bacterial cell Filloux. Therefore, a sound understanding of bacteriophage injection and bacterial secretion systems might bring new insights to the development of effective therapeutic agents.

Bacteriophage-guided Route to Biodiscovery

Bacteriophages have evolved multiple strategies to interfere with bacterial growth. As a result, improved understanding of the bacteriophage-host interactions can also bring a new perspective to drug discovery. Examples include successful use of phage encoded lytic enzymes to destroy bacterial targets and use of lysostaphin to achieve sterilisation in an endocarditis model. Furthermore, in a novel approach, Liu and others applied information deriving from phage genome to target discovery of gene products that inhibit pathogenic bacterium such as *Staphylococcus aureus*. They uncovered strategies used by bacteriophage to disable bacteria for design of a method, which uses key phage proteins to identify and validate vulnerable targets and exploit them in the identification of new antimicrobials.

Polysaccharide-specific phages were also suggested to treat encapsulated pathogenic bacteria since exolysaccharide production in bacteria involves biofilm formation and acts as a barrier to the penetration of therapeutic agents. Phages that can polymerise these substances and/or kill the bacteria may potentially be useful for control of bacteria forming biofilms on medical devices. Protein antibiotics, which are the gene products of some small phages that do not produce endolysins, have also been shown to inhibit cell wall synthesis. Genetic engineering of bacteriophages to carry toxic genes or proteins to produce cell death without lysis and hence avoiding the release of unwanted endotoxins has also been suggested. Furthermore, Hagens and others proposed a bacteriophage-based strategy to reduce effective doses of antibiotics during treatment for resensitisation of antibiotic resistant pathogen via the presence of phage *in vivo*. In addition, it has been reported that phage host-cell lysis proteins, encoded by holins and amidases and elaborated late in the infection cycle, maintain their potent antibacterial activity when administered from outside cell.

From Bacteriophage Genomics to Drug Discovery

Over evolutionary time, bacteriophages have developed unique proteins that arrest critical cellular processes to commit bacterial host metabolism to phage reproduction. Bacterial key metabolic processes can be shut off via inactivation of critical cellular proteins with these unique bacteriophage proteins, and host metabolism can be directed into the production of progeny phages. As an example, phages of *E. coli*, host physiology shuttoff is typically performed early during the phage lytic cycle by small phage-encoded proteins that target particularly vulnerable and accessible proteins involved in crucial host metabolic processes. Thus, Liu and others using a high-throughput bacteriophage genomics strategy, exploited the concept of phage-mediated inhibition of bacterial growth to systematically identify antimicrobial phage-encoded polypeptides. They found that four proteins of the *Staphylococcus aureus* DNA replication machinery were targeted by a total of seven unrelated phage polypeptides leading to a superior approach to currently available antibiotics which only target topoisomerases. In some cases, sequence-unrelated polypeptides from different phages were found to target the same proteins in *S. aureus*, and such susceptibility might have uses in antimicrobial drug discovery.

All these developments including increased understanding of the mechanism of injection, beginning with adsorption to the host and ending with complete delivery of genomic material are now paving the way towards recruitment of phages in the search for new antibiotics with previously unknown antibacterial mechanisms.

From Endolysins to Enzybiotics

Phages have different methods of progeny release from bacterial cells: filamentous phages are ejected from bacterial cell walls without destroying the host cell, whereas nonfilamentous phages induce lysis through lytic enzymes. Phage lytic enzymes are highly evolved murein hydrolases to quickly destroy the cell wall of the host bacterium to release the progeny. Lysis is a result of abrupt damage to the bacterial cell wall by means of specific proteins and as stated by Hermoso and others, it can be completed in two different ways: (i) inhibition of peptidoglycan synthesis by a single protein or (ii) enzymatic cleavage of peptidoglycan by lysins or holin-lysin system.

Tailed phages achieve correctly-timed lysis by the consequtive use of endolysins and holins. Holins are small hydrophobic proteins that are encoded by the phage and inserted into cytoplasmic membrane to form membrane lesions or holes for endolysin passage. Whereas endolysins are phage-coded enzymes that break down bacterial peptidoglycan at the terminal stage of the phage reproduction cycle. Target specificity in endolysin studies reveal differences such as bifunctional enzyme of *Streptococcus agalactiae* phage with glycosidase and endopeptidase activities or muramidase activity of *Lactobacillus helveticus* phage. However, most enzymes like amidases from phage that infect Gram-positive bacteria feature narrow lysis ranges, which can be genus-specific (*Streptomyces aureofaciens*) and even species-specific (*Clostridium perfringens*). Other examples include narrow specificity of endolysins only targeting *Clavibacter michiganensis* subspecies without affecting other bacteria in soil including closely related *Clavibacter* species.

Due to increasing antibiotic resistance, phage-derived lytic enzymes are now being exploited to control infections. In antibiotic resistant Gram-positive bacteria, it has been reported that even small quantities of purified recombinant lysin added externally lead to immediate lysis resulting in log-fold of death of the bacterial cells found on the mucosal surfaces and infected tissues. They have been suggested to make ideal anti infectives due to lysin specificity for the pathogen that does not disturb the normal flora, the low chance of bacterial resistance towards lysins, and their ability to kill colonising pathogens on mucosal surfaces illustrating a previously unavailable capacity. These enzymes are suggested to particularly be useful to control antibiotic resistant Gram-positive pathogens. In this group of bacteria, lysins can make direct contact with their cell wall carbohydrates and peptidoglycan externally making them suitable candidates in clinical applications.

Another example is *Mycobacterium*, phylogenetically related to Gram-positive bacteria but its cell envelope has a double-membrane structure similar to Gram-negative bacteria. Cell envelopes of mycobacteria contain peptidoglycan-arabinogalactan-mycolic acid complex. Mycobacteriophages must not only degrade the peptidoglycan layer but must also circumvent a mycolic acid-rich outer membrane covalently attached to the arabinogalactan-peptidoglycan complex. They utilise two lytic enzymes to produce lysis: (i) Lysin A that hydrolyses peptidoglycan, and (ii) Lysin B, a novel mycolylarabinogalactan esterase, that cleaves the mycolylarabinogalactan bond to release free mycolic acids and the study of phage ejection mechanisms in this group of bacteria might lead to the discovery of novel lytic systems and thus new antimicrobial agents.

Effective antimicrobial activity against Gram-positive bacterial pathogens including *Streptococcus pneumoniae* and *Bacillus anthracis* by exogenously applied phage-encoded endolysins has already been demonstrated. This approach has however, proved ineffective against Gram-negative bacteria since the outer membrane blocks access to the peptidoglycan targets. Due to their mycolic acid, rich outer membrane mycobacteria are likely to be similarly intractable to exogenously added endolysins. In order to overcome this resistance, a novel approach has been proposed by Payne and others to render mycobacterial pathogens such as *M. tuberculosis* susceptible to endolysin treatment through co-treatment with LysA and LysB proteins.

In-depth understanding of the host-phage interaction and the full lytic-system is required to design effective biocontrol strategies using bacteriophage lysins. In this search, another rich source for mycobacterial phages might be the activated sludge systems where fascinating suborder, family, genus and species-specific host-phage interactions occur. Recent genome sequencing of a *Tsukamurella* phage again isolated from an activated sludge system reveals a modular gene structure that shares some similarity with those of *Mycobacterium* phages. Accordingly, phylum level perspective and understanding of bacterial cell wall envelope architecture with particular emphasis on monoderm and diderm bacteria, and translation of this understanding to phage lytic activity will advance current knowledge and contribute towards design and application of new phage-derived therapeutics. *Actinobacteria*-specific proteins, mainly specific for the *Corynebacterium*, *Mycobacterium* and *Nocardia* subgroups, have also been reported and such specific proteins might have implications for the control of these pathogens. Mycetoma, a chronic granumatous infection persistent worldwide and endemic to tropical and subtropical regions, is another example and among bacteria *Actinomadura* species reportedly cause the disease. However, in spite of trials in many different laboratories, phages specific to *Actinomadura* species were not reported until early 1990s.

Phages isolated towards different species of *Actinomadura* from organic mulches used in avocado plantations revealed that they belonged to *Siphoviridae* (Fig. 17.1) group of phages.

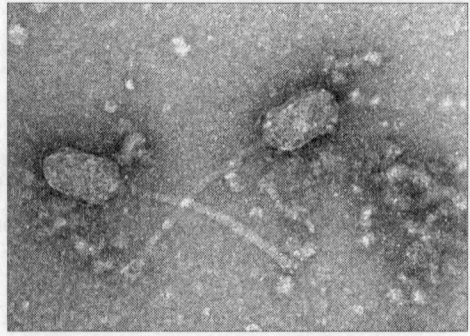

Fig. 17.1: *Siphoviridae.*

Further studies on the *Actinodamura* phage and host-cell-wall interactions might shed light on the development of effective treatment strategies deriving from phage lytic activity on the pathogenic host.

Furthermore, metagenomics sequencing studies of uncultured viral populations have provided new insights into bacteriophage ecology. The cloning of phage lytic enzymes from uncultured viral DNA, and observations into colony lysis following exposure to inducing agent, revealed the value of viral metagenomes as potential sources of recombinant proteins with biotechnological value. Functional screens of viral metagenomes will inevitably provide a large source of recombinant proteins which might subsequently be used to treat infections resulting from difficult to control pathogens.

BENEFITS OF PHAGE THERAPY OVER ANTIBIOTICS

Phages appear to be better therapeutic agents as they have several advantages over traditional antibiotics. Majority of them are summarised in the Table 17.1.

Table 17.1: Comparison of phages and antibiotics regarding their prophylactic and therapeutic use.

Bacteriophages	*Antibiotics*
Phages are highly effective in killing their targeted bacteria, i.e. their action is bactericidal	Some antibiotics are bacteriostatic, i.e. the inhibit the growth of bacteria, rather than killing them (e.g. chloramphenicol)
Production is simple and cheap	Production is complex and expensive
Phages are an 'intelligent' drug. They multiply at the site of the infection until there are no more bacteria. Then they are excreted.	They are metabolised and eliminated from the body and do not necessarily concentrate at the site of infection
The pharmacokinetics of bacteriophage therapy is such that the initial dose increases exponentially if the susceptible bacterial host is available. In such cases, there is no need to administer the phages repeatedly	Repeated doses of antibiotic is required to cure the bacterial disease
The high selectivity/specificity of bacteriophages permits the targeting of specific pathogens, without affecting desirable bacterial flora which means that phages are unlikely to affect the 'colonisation pressure' of the patients	Antibiotics demonstrate bactericidal or bacteriostatic effects not only on the cause of bacterial disease, but on all micro-organisms present in the body including the host normal microflora. Thus their non-selective action affects the patient's microbial balance, which may lead to various side effects
Because of phages specificity, their use is not likely to select for phage resistance in other (non-target) bacterial species	The broad spectrum activity of antibiotics may select for resistant mutants of many pathogenic bacterial species
Humans are exposed to phages throughout life, and well tolerate them. No serious side effects have been described	Multiple side effects, including intestinal disorders, allergies, and secondary infections (e.g. yeast infections) have been reported
Phage-resistant bacteria remain susceptible to other phages having a similar host range	Resistance to antibiotics is not limited to targeted bacteria
Phages are found throughout nature. This means that it is easy to find new phages when bacteria become resistant to them. Selecting a new phage (e.g. against phageresistant bacteria) is a rapid process and frequently can be accomplished in days	Developing a new antibiotic (against antibiotic resistant bacteria) is a time consuming process and may take several years to accomplish
Phages may be considered as good alternative for patients allergic to antibiotics	If patient is allergic to antibiotic, treatment is very difficult

There are also some disadvantages with the phage therapy approach. These include:

- The problem which requires attention is the rapid clearance of phage by the spleen, liver and other filtering organs of reticuloendothelial system . This can be taken care by doing serial passage in mice so as to obtain a phage mutant capable of evading the reticuloendothelial system and therefore capable of long circulation in the blood. The minor variations in their coat proteins enable some variants to be less easily recognised by the RES organs, allowing them in the circulation for longer periods than the 'average' wild-type phage.

- This therapy can not be used for intracellular bacteria as the host is not available for interaction.

- The shelf life of phages varies and needs to be tested and monitored.

- Phages are more difficult to administer than antibiotics. A physician needs special training in order to correctly prescribe and use phages.

- Theoretically development of neutralising antibodies against phages could be an obstacle to the use phage therapy in recurrent infections. This needs to be confirmed experimentally. However, in the immunocompromised host where the immune system is depressed such as chronic infections, the phage therapy may work in this situation.

SAFETY OF THE THERAPEUTIC PHAGE PREPARATION

During the long history of using phages as therapeutic agents through Eastern Europe and the former Soviet Union, there has been no report of serious complications associated with their use. Phages are extremely common in environment and regularly consumed in foods. In fact humans are exposed to phages from birth itself and therefore these constitute the normal microflora of the human body. They have been commonly found in human gastrointestinal tract, skin and mouth, where they are harboured in saliva and dental plaques. Phages are also abundant in environment including saltwater, freshwater, soil, plants and animals and they have been shown to be unintentional contents of some vaccines and sera commercially available in United States. Phages have high specificity for specific bacterial strains, a characteristic which requires careful targetting. Therefore, phage therapy can be used to lyse specific pathogens without disturbing normal bacterial flora and phages pose no risk to anything other than their specific bacterial host.

From a clinical standpoint, phage therapy appears to be very safe. Efficacy of natural phages against antibiotic-resistant *Streptococci, Escherichia, Pseudomonas, Proteus, Salmonella, Shigella, Serratia, Klebsiella, Enterobacter, Campylobacter, Yersinia, Acinetobacter* and *Brucella* are being evaluated by researchers. However, in the last few years, modified phages are being explored increasingly, due to the limitations of phage therapy using lytic phages. The safety concerns regarding spontaneously propagating live micro-organisms and the inconsistency of phage therapy results in the treatment of bacterial infections specifically induced scientists to explore more controllable phages. Phages can be modified to be an excellent therapeutic agent by directed mutation of the phage genome, recombination of phage genomes, artificial selection of phages *in vivo*, chimeric phages and other rational designs which confer new properties on the phages. These new modified phages have been shown to successfully overcome challenges to earlier phage therapy. As with antibiotic therapy and other methods of countering bacterial infections, endotoxins (lipopolysaccharide) are released by the gram negative bacteria as a component of outer membrane. This can cause symptoms of fever, or in extreme cases, toxic shock (Herxheimer reaction). To address the endotoxin release issue, recombinant phage derived from *P. aeruginosa* filamentous phage Pf3 was constructed by genetic modifications and the results showed that this filamentous phages could be used as effective anti-infection agent. This phage had the benefit of minimising the release of membrane associated endotoxins during phage therapy. In order not to compromise on the issue of the safe use of therapeutic phage preparation, rigorous characterisations of each phage to be used therapeutically should be done, in particular, especially looking for potentially harmful genes in their genome.

CLINICAL APPLICATION OF BACTERIOPHAGES

Whole Phage as Antimicrobial Agents

Phage therapy in humans

However, although d'Hérelle carried out the first human therapeutic phage trial, the first article documenting phage therapy was on research conducted in Belgium by Bruynoghe and Maisin in 1921. They reported that phages when injected in six patients targeted *Staphylococcus* near the base of cutaneous boils (furuncles and carbuncles), resulted in improvement within 48 hr and reduction in pain, swelling and fever. Merabishvili and workers used phage cocktail, consisting of exclusively lytic bacteriophages for the treatment of *Pseudomonas aeruginosa* and *Staphylococcus aureus* infections in burn wound patients in the Burn Centre of the Queen Astrid Military Hospital in Brussels, Belgium. The first controlled clinical trial of a therapeutic bacteriophage preparation (Biophage-PA) showed efficacy and safety in chronic otitis because of drug resistant *P. aeruginosa* in UCL Ear Institute and Royal National Throat, Nose and Ear Hospital, London, UK. Several clinical trials on phage therapy in humans were reported with the majority coming from researchers in Eastern Europe and the former Soviet Union. One of the most extensive studies evaluating the application of therapeutic phages for prophylaxis of infectious diseases was conducted in Tbilisi, Georgia, during 1963 and 1964 and involved phages against bacterial dysentery. The most detailed English language reports on phage therapy in humans were by Slopek and co workers who published a number of papers on the effectiveness of phages against infections caused by several bacterial pathogens, including multidrug-resistant mutants. Phages have been reported to be effective in treating various bacterial diseases such as cerebrospinal meningitis in a newborn, skin infections caused by *Pseudomonas, Staphylococcus, Klebsiella, Proteus, E. coli*, recurrent subphrenic and subhepatic abscesses, Staphylococcal lung infections Application of Therapeutic Phages in Medicine, *Pseudomonas aeruginosa* infections in cystic fibrosis patients, eye infections, neonatal sepsis, urinary tract infections, and cancer. Abdul-Hassan and others reported on the treatment of 30 cases of burn-wound associated antibiotic-resistant *Pseudomonas aeruginosa* sepsis. Bandages soaked with 1010 phages/ml were applied three times daily. Half of the cases were found to be improved. Markoishvili and others reported the use of PhagoBioDerm, the phage impregnated polymer, to treat infected venous stasis skin ulcers. To patients that had failed to respond to other treatment approaches, PhagoBioDerm was applied to ulcers both alone and, where appropriate, in combination with other treatment strategies. Complete healing of ulcers was observed in 70% of the patients.

Collin and others reported that a bacteriophage encoded enzyme, endosialidase E (endo E) selectively degrades the linear homopolymeric α-2, 8-linked *N*-acetylneuraminic acid capsule associated with the capacity of *E. coli* K1 strain to cause severe infection in the newborn infant. In one of the study, PhagoBioDerm (a wound-healing preparation consisting of a biodegradable polymer impregnated with ciprofloxacin and bacteriophages) was used in three Georgian lumberjacks from the village of Lia who were exposed to a strontium-90 source from two Soviet-era radiothermal generators they found near their village. In addition to systemic effects, two of them developed severe local radiation injuries which subsequently became infected with *Staphylococcus aureus*. Approximately 1 month after hospitalisation, treatment with phage bioderm was initiated. Purulent drainage stopped within 2–7 days. Clinical improvement was associated with rapid (7 days) elimination of the *S. aureus* resistant to many antibiotics (including ciprofloxacin), but susceptible to the bacteriophages contained in the PhagoBioDerm preparation. Leszczynski and co workers described the use of oral phage therapy for targeting Methicillin Resistant *Staphylococcus aureus* (MPSA) in a nurse who was a carrier. She had MRSA colonised in her gastrointestinal tract and also had a urinary tract infection. The result of phage therapy was complete elimination of culturable MRSA.

Animal trials

In Britain, Smith and Huggins carried out a series of excellent, well-controlled studies on the use of phages in systemic *E. coli* infections in mice and then in diarrheic disease in young calves and pigs. Bogovazova and othes studied the effectiveness of specific phage therapy in non inbred white mice, caused by intraperitoneal injection of *K. pneumoniae* K25053 into the animals. Soothill, examined the ability of bacteriophage to prevent the rejection of skin grafts of experimentally infected guinea pigs. His findings demonstrated that the phage-treated grafts were protected in six of seven cases, while untreated grafts failed uniformly, suggesting that phage might be useful for the prevention of *P. aeruginosa* infections in patients with burn wounds. Phage therapy has been successfully used to remove *E. coli* 0157:H7 from livestock. One of the most successful studies was carried out by Biswas and coworkers. These workers suggested that a single i.p. injection of 3×10^8 PFU of the phage strain, administered 45 minutes after the bacterial challenge (vancomycin-resistant *Enterococcus faecium* (VRE) was sufficient to rescue 100% of the animals. Even when treatment was delayed to the point where all animals were moribund, approximately 50% of them were rescued by a single injection of the phage. The protective effect of bacteriophage was assessed against experimental *S. aureus* infection in mice. Subsequent intraperitoneal administration of purified ØMR11 (MOI of 0.1) suppressed *S. aureus*–induced lethality. This lifesaving effect coincided with the rapid appearance of ØMR11 in the circulation, which remained at substantial levels until the bacteria were eradicated. Benedict & Flamiano, evaluated the use of bacteriophages as therapy for *Escherichia coli* induced bacteremia in mice. This experimental study showed clearly that a single dose of crude phage lysates administered by i.p. injection was enough to rescue bacteremic mice back to normal health after having been challenged with a lethal concentration of *E. coli*. Zogta and others studied the ability of bacterial viruses to rescue septicemic mice with multidrug resistant (MDR) Klebsiella pneumoniae isolated from neonatal septicemia. A single i.p. injection of 3×10^8 PFU of the phage strain administered 45 minutes after the bacterial challenge rescued 100% of the animals. Wills and colleagues also demonstrated the efficacy of bacteriophage therapy against *S. aureus* in a rabbit abscess model. 2×10^9 PFU of staphylococcal phage prevented abscess formation in rabbits when it was injected simultaneously with *S. aureus* (8×10^7 CFU) into the same subcutaneous site.

The sewerage-derived bacteriophage reduced the abscess area and the count of *S. aureus* in the abscess was lowered in a bacteriophage dose dependent way. Smith and others reported the treatment of a dog with chronic bilateral otitis external that had consistently grown *P. aeruginosa*. This infection had failed to be resolved after repeated courses of topical and systemic antibiotics. After inoculation with 400 PFU of bacteriophage into the auditory canal there was a marked improvement in the clinical signs, 27 hr after treatment. Wang and others examined the effectiveness of phages in the treatment of imipenem resistant *Pseudomonas aeruginosa* (IMPR-Pa) infection in an experimental mouse model. A single i.p. inoculation of the phage strain ØA392 (MOI > 0.01) at up to 60 min after the bacterial challenge was sufficient to rescue 100% of the animals. The workers demonstrated that the ability of the phage to rescue bacteremic animals was due to the functional capabilities of the phage and not to a non-specific immune effect. McVay and co-workers examined the efficacy of phage therapy in treating fatal *Pseudomonas aeruginosa* infections in mouse burn wound model. The results showed that a single dose of the *Pseudomonas aeruginosa* phage cocktail could significantly decrease the mortality of thermally injured, *Pseudomonas aeruginosa*-infected mice (from 6% survival without treatment to 22 to 87% survival with treatment) and that the route of administration was particularly important to the efficacy of the treatment, with the i.p. route providing the most significant (87%) protection. Watanabe and others examined the efficacy of bacteriophage by using a gut-derived sepsis model caused by *Pseudomonas aeruginosa* in mice. Oral administration of a newly isolated lytic phage strain (KPP10) significantly protected mice against mortality with survival rates, 66.7% for the phagetreated group as compared to 0% survival in saline treated control group. Mice treated with phage also had significantly lower numbers of viable *Pseudomonas aeruginosa* cells and lower level of inflammatory cytokines (tumor necrosis factor alpha TNF-a, interleukin-1b [IL-1a], and IL-6) in their blood and different organs such as liver and spleen. In recent years the phage therapy has received lot of attention due to an increase in the prevalence of antibiotic resistant strains in clinical settings. A numbers of recent experimental studies have proved the efficacy of phages in treating different infections. Chhibber and co workers had reported the therapeutic potential of phage SS in treating *Klebsiella pneumoniae* induced respiratory infection in mice. The use of lytic bacteriophages to rescue septicemic mice with multidrug-resistant (MDR) *Pseudomonas aeruginosa* infection was evaluated. A single i.p. injection of 109 PFU of the phage strain, administered 45 min after the bacterial challenge, was sufficient to rescue 100% of the animals. Malik and Chhibber investigated the protective effect of *K. pneumoniae*–specific bacteriophage KØ1 isolated from the environment in a mouse model of burn wound infection caused by *K. pneumoniae*. A substantial decrease in the bacterial load of blood, peritoneal lavage, and lung tissue was noted following treatment with the bacteriophage preparation. Recently in other studies, workers have successfully employed well characterised phages to treat burn wound infection induced by *Klebsiella pneumoniae* in mice. In this study, a single dose of phages, intraperitoneally (i.p.) at an MOI of 1.0, resulted in significant decrease in mortality, and this dose was found to be sufficient to completely cure *K. pneumoniae* infection in the burn wound model. Maximum decrease in bacterial counts in different organs was observed at 72 hr post infection. Kumari and co-workers evaluated the therapeutic potential of a well characterised phage Kpn5 in treating burn wound infection in mice as a single topical application of this phage was able to rescue mice from infection caused by *K. pneumoniae* B5055 in comparison to multiple applications of honey and Aloe vera gel. Recently, Kumari and co-workers evaluated the efficacy of silver nitrate and gentamicin in the treatment of burn wound infection and compared it with phage therapy using an isolated and well-characterised *Klebsiella* -specific phage, Kpn5. Phage Kpn5 mixed in hydrogel was applied topically at an MOI of 200 on the burn wound site. The efficacy of these antimicrobial agents was assessed on the basis of percentage survival of infected mice following treatment. The results showed that a single dose of phage Kpn5 resulted in a significant reduction in mortality (*P*<0.001) as compared to daily application of silver nitrate and gentamicin.

Phages in the eradication of biofilms

Biofilms are densely packed communities of micro-organisms growing on a range of biotic and abiotic surfaces and surround themselves with secreted extracellular polymer (EPS). Many bacterial species form biofilms and it is an important bacterial survival strategy. Biofilm formation is thought to begin when bacteria sense environmental conditions that trigger the transition to life on a surface. The structural and physiological complexity of biofilms has led to the idea that they are coordinated and cooperative groups, analogous to multicellular organisms. In humans biofilms are responsible for many pathologies, most of them associated with the use of medical devices. A major problem of biofilms is their inherent tolerance to host defences and antibiotic therapies. Therefore there is an urgent need to develop alternative ways to prevent and control biofilm-associated clinical infections. Bacteriophages have been suggested as effective antibiofilm agents. Use of indwelling catheters was often compromised as a result of biofilm formation. Curtin and Donlan investigated if hydrogel-coated catheters pretreated with coagulase negative bacteriophage would reduce *Staphylococcus epidermidis* biofilm formation. In one of the laboratory, efficacy of bacteriophage was assessed alone or in combination with amoxicillin, for the eradication of biofilm produced by *Klebsiella pneumoniae* B5055. Similarly Collin and others also evaluated the efficacy of lytic bacteriophage KPO1K2 alone or in combination with another antibiotic, ciprofloxacin for eradicating the biofilm of *Klebsiella pneumoniae in vitro*.

Despite the efficacy of antibiotics as well as bacteriophages in the treatment of bacterial infections, their role in treatment of biofilm associated infections is still under consideration especially in case of older biofilms. The ability of bacteriophage and their associated polysaccharide depolymerases was investigated to control enteric biofilm formation. The action of combined treatments of disinfectant and phage enzyme as a potentially effective biofilm control strategy was evaluated and the results showed that the combination of phage enzyme and disinfectant was found to be more effective than either of these when used alone. Since age of biofilm is a decisive factor in determining the outcome of antibiotic treatment, in one recent study, biofilm of *K. pneumoniae* was grown for extended periods and treated with ciprofloxacin and/or depolymerase producing lytic bacteriophage (KPO1K2). The reduction in bacterial numbers of older biofilm was greater after application of the two agents in combination as ciprofloxacin alone could not reduce bacterial biomass significantly in older biofilms.

Phage Products or Phage Lysins

With the increasing worldwide prevalence of antibiotic resistant bacteria, bacteriophage endolysins represent a very promising novel alternative class of antibacterial in the fight against infectious disease. Pathogenic bacteria are increasingly becoming resistant to antibiotics. For nearly a century, scientists have attempted to treat bacterial infections with whole phages. Vincent Fischetti was the first, however, to focus on the deadly weapons, the potent and specific enzymes called lysins produced by these viruses. These lysins create lethal holes in bacterial cell walls. Fischetti has identified lysins that can kill a wide range of Gram-positive pathogenic bacteria, and have proven their effectiveness in both preventing and treating infections in mice, an important step towards their potential application in human disease. As an alternative to 'classic' bacteriophage therapy, in which whole viable phage particles are used, one can also apply bacteriophageencoded lysis-inducing proteins, either as recombinant proteins or as lead structures for the development of novel antibiotics. Phage endolysins, or lysins, are enzymes that damage the cell walls' integrity by hydrolysing the four major bonds in its peptidoglycan component. A number of studies have shown the enormous potential of the use of phage endolysins, rather than the intact phage, as potential therapeutics. The great majority of human infections such as viral or bacterial start at mucous membrane site (upper and lower respiratory, intestinal, urogenital, and ocular) which are the reservoir for many pathogenic bacteria found in the environment (i.e. *pneumococci*, *staphylococci*, *streptococci*), many of which are reported to be resistant to antibiotics. Therefore, various animal models of mucosal colonisation were used to test the efficacy of phage lysins to kill organisms on these surfaces.

An oral colonisation model was developed for prevention and elimination of upper respiratory colonisation of mice by group A *streptococci* by using a purified C1 phage lysin C1. Phage lytic enzymes have recently been proposed for the reduction of nasopharyngeal carriage of *S. pneumoniae*. In both these cases, when the animals were colonised with their respective bacteria and treated with a small amount of lysin specific for the colonising organism, the animals were found to be free of application of therapeutic phages in medicine colonising bacteria two to five hours after lysin treatment. Group B *streptococci* are the leading cause of neonatal meningitis and sepsis all over the world. A vaginal model for group B streptococci was established to remove colonisation of the vagina and oropharynx of mice with a phage lysin (named PlyGBS). A single dose of PlyGBS significantly reduced bacterial colonisation in both the vagina and oropharynx. These results support the idea that such enzymes may be used in specific high-risk populations to control the reservoir of pathogenic bacteria and therefore control the disease. These phage enzymes are so efficient in killing pathogenic bacteria that they may be considered as valuable tools in controlling biowarfare bacteria.

To determine the feasibility of this approach, Schuch and co workers identified a lytic enzyme PlyG from the gamma phage that is specific for *Bacillus anthracis*. This approach may be used in post-exposure cases of anthrax, in which individuals can be treated intravenously with PlyG to control the bacilli entering the blood after germination because higher doses of phage lysin or multiple doses will result in nearly 100% protection. Recently, antimicrobial therapy of recombinant Cpl-1, a phage lysin specific for *Streptococcus pneumoniae* was reported to be effective in experimental pneumococcal meningitis using infant Wistar rats.

PHAGE APPLICATION IN FOOD INDUSTRY

Food contamination is a serious issue because it results in foodborne diseases. Food contamination can be microbial or environmental, with the former being more common. Meat and poultry can become contaminated during slaughter through cross-contamination from intestinal fecal matter. Similarly, fresh fruits and vegetables can be contaminated if they are washed using water contaminated with animal manure or human sewage. During food processing, contamination is also possible from infected food handlers. Food contamination usually causes abdominal discomfort and pain, and diarrhea, but symptoms vary depending on the type of infection. At the present time, the leading causes of death due to foodborne bacterial pathogens are *Listeria* and *Salmonella*, followed closely by other foodborne pathogens such as *Escherichia coli* (*E. coli* O157:H7, in particular) and *Campylobacter jejunii*. Bacteriophages may provide a natural, non-toxic, safe, and effective means for significantly reducing or eliminating contamination of foods with specific pathogenic bacteria, thereby eliminating the risk, or significantly reducing the magnitude and severity, of foodborne illness caused by the consumption of foods contaminated with those bacteria. The effectiveness of phage administration for the control of fish diseases and for food disinfection has also been documented. Nakai and co-workers and some other workers succeeded in saving the lives of cultured fish challenged by *Lactococcus garvieae* and *Pseudomonas plecoglossicida*, which are fish pathogens. The need for control of pathogens during the manufacture of food is reflected by the incidence of foodborne bacterial infections. The use of phage or phage products in food production has recently become an option for the food industry as a novel method for biocontrol of unwanted pathogens, enhancing the safety of especially fresh and ready-to-eat food products. Phages were also shown to be effective for the elimination of food poisoning pathogens such as *Listeria monocytogenes*, *Campylobacter jejuni* and *Salmonella* spp. from the surface of foods. The bacterial spot pathogen of tomato plants, *Xanthomonas campestris* pv. *vesicatoria* was successfully controlled with bacteriophage.

PHAGES AS ANTIBACTERIAL NANOMEDICINES

Now-a-days, apart from phage therapy, phages are also being used for phage display, DNA vaccine delivery, therapeutic gene delivery and bacterial typing Recently whole bacteriophage was constructed by fusing immunogenic peptides to modified coat proteins, which was found to be highly efficient DNA vaccine delivery vehicle (phage-display vaccination). Similarly the other approach has been incorporation of a eukaryotic promoterdriven vaccine gene within the phage genome (phage DNA vaccination). Bacteriophages (phages) have been used for about two decades as tools for the discovery of specific target-binding proteins and peptides, and for almost a decade as tools for vaccine development. Drug-carrying phage represents a versatile therapeutic nanoparticle which because of tailoring of its coat can be equipped with a targeting moiety, and its massive drug-carrying capacity may become an important general targeting drug-delivery platform. In comparison to particulate drug-carrying devices, such as liposomes or virus-like particles, the arrangement of drug that is conjugated in high density on the external surface of the targeted particle is unique. A dense coating of the phage with aminoglycosides and other drugs might produce advantages that have been regarded as challenges in the application of phages as therapeutic agent. Most important issue in this field is the immunogenicity of bacteriophages on *in vivo* administration. This problem can be tackled as it has been shown that drug-carrying phages are hardly recognised by commercial antiphage antibodies and generate significantly lower antiphage antibody titers when used to vaccinate mice (in comparison to 'naked' phages). Filamentous bacteriophages are the workhorse of antibody engineering and are gaining increasing importance in nanobiotechnology because of its nanometric dimentions.

Vaks and Benhar described a new application in the area of antibacterial nanomedicines where antibody targeted, chloramphenicol drug loaded filamentous phage (M13) was used for inhibiting the growth of *Staphylococcus aureus* bacteria. Systemic administration of chemotherapeutic agents, in addition to its anti-tumor benefits, results in indiscriminate drug distribution and severe toxicity. Therefore to solve this problem, Bar and coworkers used targeted anti-cancer therapy in the form of targeted drugcarrying phage nanoparticles. The bacteriophages are also being currently evaluated for their biosensor potential. In a recent study it has been proposed to develop a unique and innovative biosensor based on induced luminescence of captured Biowarfare bacterial agents and organic light emitting diode (OLED) technology. The system would use array of bacteriophage engineered to express fluorescent protein in infected Biowarfare agents. The specificity of the phage provides capture of only targets of interest, while the infection of the bacteria and natural replication of the expressed protein will provide the detection signal. Using novel OLED arrays, a phage array chip can be constructed similar to DNA chips for multianalyte detection.

SECTION VI

DNA Structure, DNA Replication and Genetic Techniques for DNA Analysis

Chapter 18

DNA Structure and Analysis

INTRODUCTION

DNA is the molecule that holds the instructions for all living things. DNA achieves this feat of storing, coding and transferring biological information though its unique structure. DNA analysis is any technique used to analyse genes and DNA.

DNA STRUCTURE

DNA (Deoxyribonucleic acid) is a molecule that carries most of the genetic instructions used in the development, functioning and reproduction of all known living organisms and many viruses. DNA is a nucleic acid, alongside proteins and carbohydrates, nucleic acids compose the three major macromolecules essential for all known forms of life. Most DNA molecules consist of two biopolymer strands coiled around each other to form a double helix. The two DNA strands are known as polynucleotides since they are composed of simpler units called nucleotides. Each nucleotide is composed of a nitrogen-containing nucleobase—either cytosine (C), guanine (G), adenine (A), or thymine (T)—as well as a monosaccharide sugar called deoxyribose and a phosphate group. The nucleotides are joined to one another in a chain by covalent bonds between the sugar of one nucleotide and the phosphate of the next, resulting in an alternating sugar-phosphate backbone. According to base pairing rules (A with T, and C with G), hydrogen bonds bind the nitrogenous bases of the two separate polynucleotide strands to make double-stranded DNA. The total amount of related DNA base pairs on Earth is estimated at 5.0×10^{37}, and weighs 50 billion tonnes. In comparison, the total mass of the biosphere has been estimated to be as much as 4 TtC (trillion tons of carbon).

DNA stores biological information. The DNA backbone is resistant to cleavage, and both strands of the double-stranded structure store the same biological information. Biological information is replicated as the two strands are separated. A significant portion of DNA (more than 98% for humans) is non-coding, meaning that these sections do not serve as patterns for protein sequences.

The two strands of DNA run in opposite directions to each other and are therefore anti-parallel. Attached to each sugar is one of four types of nucleobases (informally, bases). It is the sequence of these four nucleobases along the backbone that encodes biological information. Under the genetic code, RNA strands are translated to specify the sequence of amino acids within proteins. These RNA strands are initially created using DNA strands as a template in a process called transcription. Within cells, DNA is organised into long structures called chromosomes. During cell division these chromosomes are duplicated in the process of DNA replication, providing each cell its own complete set of chromosomes. Eukaryotic organisms (animals, plants, fungi, and protists) store most of their DNA inside the cell nucleus and some of their DNA in organelles, such as mitochondria or chloroplasts. In contrast, prokaryotes (bacteria and archaea) store their DNA only in the cytoplasm. Within the chromosomes, chromatin proteins such as histones compact and organise DNA. These compact structures guide the interactions between DNA and other proteins, helping control which parts of the DNA are transcribed.

Alternate DNA Structures

DNA exists in many possible conformations that include A-DNA, B-DNA, and Z-DNA forms, although, only B-DNA and Z-DNA have been directly observed in functional organisms (Fig. 18.1). The conformation that DNA adopts depends on the hydration level, DNA sequence, the amount and direction of supercoiling, chemical modifications of the bases, the type and concentration of metal ions, as well as the presence of polyamines in solution. The first published reports of A-DNA X-ray diffraction patterns—and also B-DNA—used analyses based on Patterson transforms that provided only a limited amount of structural information for oriented fibers of DNA. An alternate analysis was then proposed by Wilkins and others, in 1953, for the *in vivo* B-DNA X-ray diffraction/scattering patterns of highly hydrated DNA fibers in terms of squares of Bessel functions. In the same journal, James Watson and Francis Crick presented their molecular modelling analysis of the DNA X-ray diffraction patterns to suggest that the structure was a double-helix.

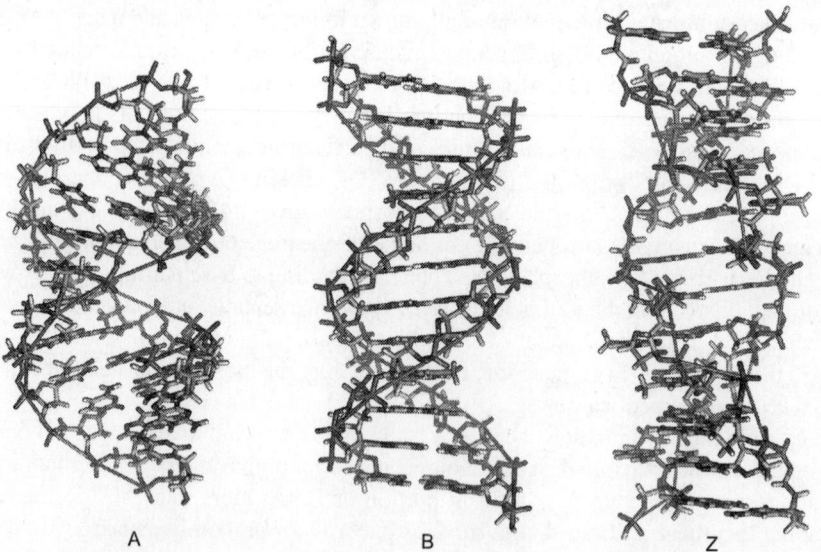

A   B   Z

Fig. 18.1: From left to right, the structures of A, B and Z DNA.

Although the 'B-DNA form' is most common under the conditions found in cells, it is not a well-defined conformation but a family of related DNA conformations that occur at the high hydration levels present in living cells. Their corresponding X-ray diffraction and scattering patterns are characteristic of molecular paracrystals with a significant degree of disorder.

Compared to B-DNA, the A-DNA form is a wider right-handed spiral, with a shallow, wide minor groove and a narrower, deeper major groove. The A form occurs under non-physiological conditions in partially dehydrated samples of DNA, while in the cell it may be produced in hybrid pairings of DNA and RNA strands, as well as in enzyme-DNA complexes. Segments of DNA where the bases have been chemically modified by methylation may undergo a larger change in conformation and adopt the Z form. Here, the strands turn about the helical axis in a left-handed spiral, the opposite of the more common B form. These unusual structures can be recognised by specific Z-DNA binding proteins and may be involved in the regulation of transcription.

Nucleic Acid Double Helices

By 1950, E. Chargaff had analysed the base ratios of DNAs from several animal and bacterial sources. Although the base ratios of different DNAs varied widely, certain regularities were apparent. Most fundamental was the molar equivalence of deoxyadenylate to deoxythymidylate and of deoxycytidylate to deoxyguanylate. The base ratios could be expressed simply as the per cent GC. That is, a DNA with 40% GC content has deoxyadenylate, deoxycytidylate and deoxythymidylate in the ratio of 30:20:20:30 to satisfy Chargaff's rule of molar equivalence. The structure of the DNA double helix is shown in Fig. 18.2. Another indication of the regular structure of DNA came from X-ray diffraction experiments, notably in studies by R. Franklin and M. Wilkins. When X-rays pass through ordered collections of DNA molecules and subsequently intercept a sheet of photographic film, the diffracted X-rays produce a regular pattern. Although the pattern is not a picture of the DNA molecule, it does show that the DNA molecule has a definite structure and can indicate whether a given model for the conformation of the polynucleotide chain in DNA is possibly valid or definitely not valid. The simplicity and certain other characteristics of the X-ray diffraction pattern of DNA fibers revealed to X-ray crystallographers that the DNA structure can be represented by a simple model that is helical.

In the early 1950s, concepts of the regular base composition and regular folding of the polynucleotide chain seemed to be in conflict with the presumed biological functions of DNA. DNA had been discovered as a major constituent of salmon sperm. O. T. Avery, C. M. MacLeod and M. McCarty had genetically changed (transformed) bacteria so that they elaborated a polysaccharide coat that they formerly were incapable of making. Avery and his colleagues showed in the 1940s that the 'transforming principle' was DNA from other strains of bacteria that normally produce the polysaccharide coat. Hershey and Chase had found that a bacteriophage (bacterial virus) injected its DNA, but not its protein coat, into the host bacterium to begin an infection.

Thus, the non-living DNA molecule seemed to be important to the genetics of animals, bacteria and viruses. It seemed reasonable to some that DNA would be found to be the molecule of which genes are made. How could genes for a polysaccharide coat and genes that direct the production of new bacteriphage particles be made from a molecule that seemed from X-ray crystallography and other physical and chemical studies to be so similar regardless of its biological source?

J. Watson and F. Crick reconciled the properties of uniform structure and diverse genetic function when they conceived their now well-known model for DNA structure, the most influential model of a biological molecule ever constructed. Figure 18.3 provides two representations of the model. Two polynucleotide chains are intertwined to form the familiar double-helix with the more polar, hydrophilic ('water-loving') deoxyribose and phosphate residues on the outside.

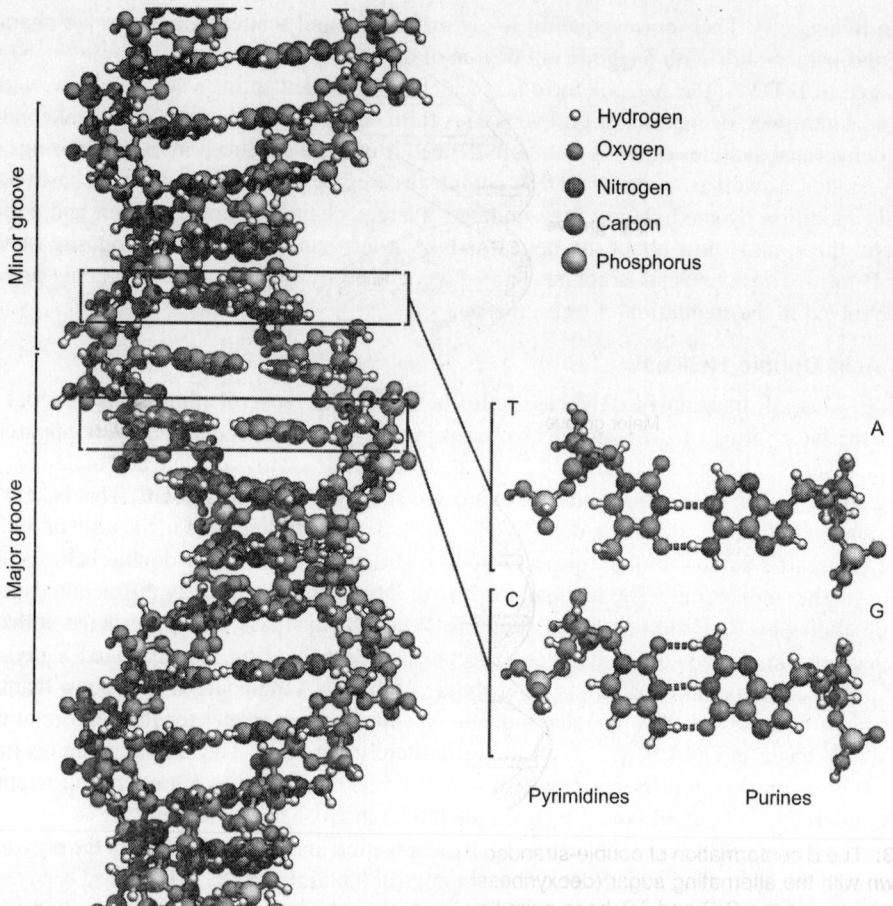

Hydrogen
Oxygen
Nitrogen
Carbon
Phosphorus

Minor groove

Major groove

T   A

C   G

Pyrimidines   Purines

Fig. 18.2: The structure of the DNA double helix. The atoms in the structure and element and the detailed structure of two base pairs are shown in the bottom right.

The less polar base pairs form the interior of the cylindrical molecule. In this model, the base pairs are roughly perpendicular to the long axis of the molecule and are stacked to give roughly the appearance of a spiral staircase. The bases of one base pair lie in the same plane. Thus, a base pair has approximately the same thickness as a base: 0.34 nm. One turn of the helix has ten base pairs, so the pitch (length of one full turn) of the helix is 3.4 nm. Note that the two strands of a helix are oriented in an antiparallel rather than parallel fashion. That is, the 5'-to-3' direction of the two chains is opposite. The base pairs are the conceptual, as well as the structural, core of the model. If we ignore for the moment steric restraints imposed by the polynucleotide chain, there are tens of ways that the nucleic acid bases could be juxtaposed or stacked in pairs. As indicated in Fig. 18.4, crucial features of the particular pairing proposed by Watson and Crick are:

1. The C-1' atoms of the deoxyribose residues are separated by the same distance in A:T and C:G base pairs.

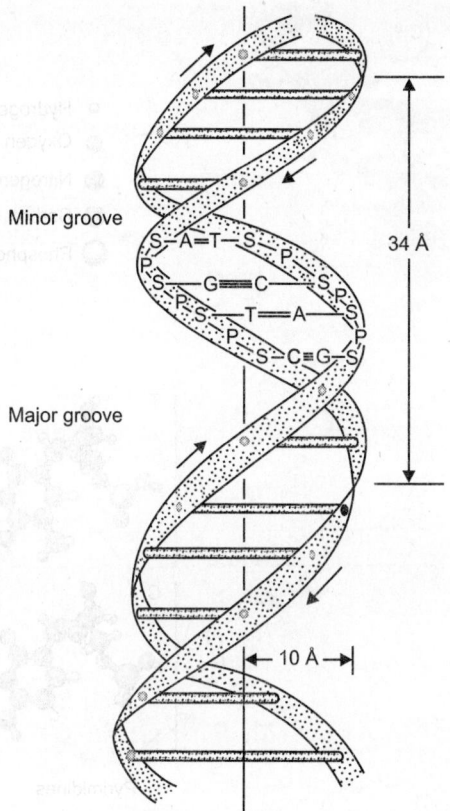

Fig. 18.3: The B conformation of double-stranded DNA. The course and opposite polarities of the two strands are shown with the alternating sugar (deoxyribose) and phosphate residues indicated by S—P—S—P—S. . . .. Also shown are the G:C and A:T base pairs that form the core of the molecule.

2. The angle formed between a line connecting the two C-1′ atoms of a base pair and an *N*-glycosidic bond is the same for all four nucleotide residues.

3. Strong, straight hydrogen bonds establish specific pairing between dA and dT residues and between dC and dG residues.

The proposed base pairs at once satisfied genetic and structural requirements, including Chargaff's rules. Similar dimensions of the two types of base pairs in two orientations allow a regular structure, but place no constraint on the sequence of nucleotide residues in one chain. Thus, any gene can be encoded in a sufficiently long strand of DNA and the locations of deoxyribose and phosphate residues will be the same. However, the nucleotide sequence in one strand dictates the nucleotide sequence in the other strand according to the Watson and Crick base pairing and the antiparallel structure.

This is illustrated by the following structure, written in a shorthand notation in which the strand with the 5′ to 3′ orientation is uppermost:

$$5' \ldots \text{pdGATCCGCG} \ldots 3'$$
$$3' \ldots \text{dCTAGGCGCp} \ldots 5'$$

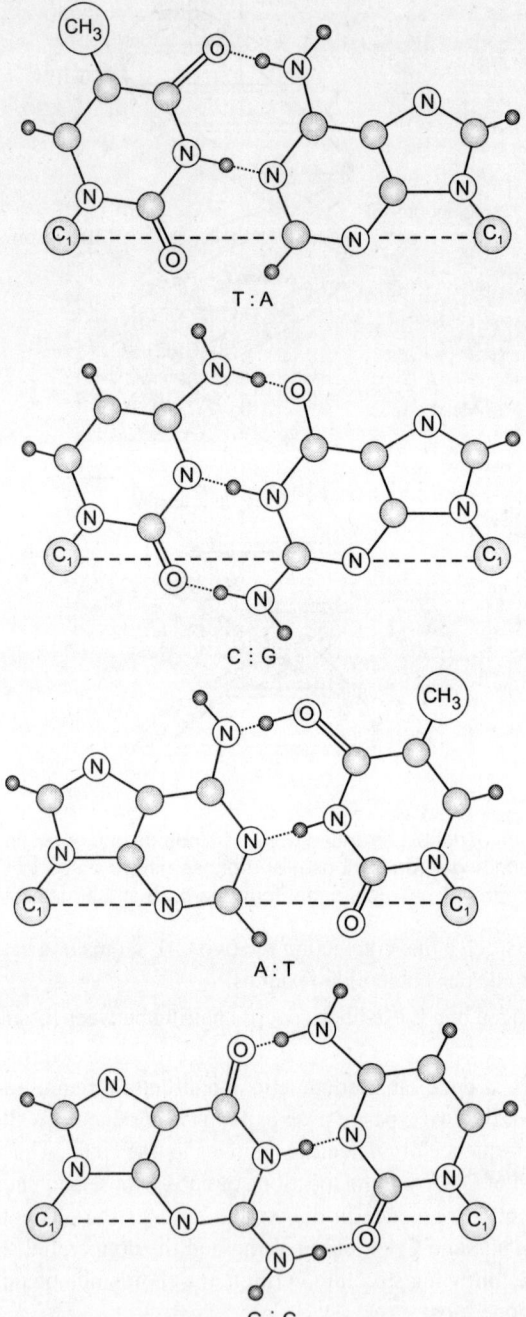

T : A

C : G

A : T

G : C

Fig. 18.4: The four possible Watson and Crick base pairs, representing the two possible orientations of a G : C and an A : T base pair within a double helix.

The structure described in Fig. 18.3 captures the essential features of ordinary DNA, that is, DNA with all four nucleotide residues well represented. It is designated the 'Watson-Crick B helix' to distinguish it from structures for DNA of unusual base composition or for DNA in water-poor environments. The correctness of the B structure was indicated not only by its agreement with Chargaff's rules and the genetic requirements for DNA function, but also because it correctly predicted the DNA X-ray scattering pattern, at least to a first approximation. It was stereochemically satisfactory, meaning that a space-filling molecular model could be built from correctly sized model atoms and the model was consistent with the known structures of mononucleotides. In the years since the publication of the B structure in 1953, modifications have been introduced to bring the structure into closer agreement with higher quality X-ray diffraction data.

DNA dissolved in buffered aqueous salt solutions behaves as if it is a Watson-Crick B helix except that it appears to have 10.5 rather than an even 10 base pairs per turn of the double helix. The diameter of the molecule, approximately 2 nm and the length per base pair, approximately 0.34 nm, are as predicted. These dimensions anticipate one of the most startling properties of DNA, the extraordinary length-to-diameter ratio. For example, the genome of the bacterium *Escherichia coli* is a single, circular DNA molecule of approximately 4.3 million base pairs (4300 kilobase pairs or 4300 kb). The chromosomes of higher organisms also appear to be composed of single DNA molecules. At 0.34 nm per base pair, the contour length of *E. coli* DNA is approximately 1.5 mm, giving a length-to-diameter ratio of 7,30,000. Because the DNA molecule is so long, the slightest disturbance of the solution can produce local regions that are flowing in different directions. This produces a stretching force on a long DNA molecule and may break it. Such 'shearing' forces normally break DNA molecules of the size of *E. coli* DNA into thousands of pieces and it is these pieces rather than the intact molecules that most often are studied in the laboratory.

Note that although the linear DNA double helix is composed of two intertwined, covalent, linear molecules, the convention is to refer to the two molecules together as the 'DNA molecule'. The two covalent units of this 'non-covalent' molecule obviously are held together by hydrogen bonds. The structure also is stabilised by the forces between the bases stacked one on another to form the 'spiral staircase' in the interior of the molecule. Destabilising the structure are the electrostatic repulsive forces between the negatively charged phosphodiester groups and thermal motion. The DNA molecule is not static but exhibits a random, dynamic and localised separation of bases and rapid reforming of the hydrogen-bonded base pairs. Raising the temperature increases thermal motion and shifts the equilibrium in favour of separation of bases, at a high enough temperature, the two strands of a linear DNA fragment unwind from each other and separate. This process is termed 'melting'. Extremes of pH also will melt DNA. DNA denaturation is a reversible process.

Some double-stranded DNAs are circular. The DNA will be circular whether one or both strands actually is a circular chain of nucleotide residues connected by phosphodiester bonds. If both strands are circular, the two strands are intertwined and cannot be separated so long as both strands are intact. Figure 18.5 shows diagrammatically how the two covalent, circular strands can be inseparable even though they are not covalently linked to each other. The Watson and Crick model predicts and the linear form of a double-stranded DNA defines, the number of turns that the B form DNA should have in its lowest energy form. The number of turns is approximately one per 10 base pairs. An important consequence of 'covalently closed' circular DNA is the possibility that the actual number of turns of the double helix, imposed by the two covalent circular strands, will be different than the number of turns in the corresponding linear DNA. An exact match of the number of turns of the helix and the number of turns anticipated by the Watson and Crick model for B-DNA will give a circular molecule without

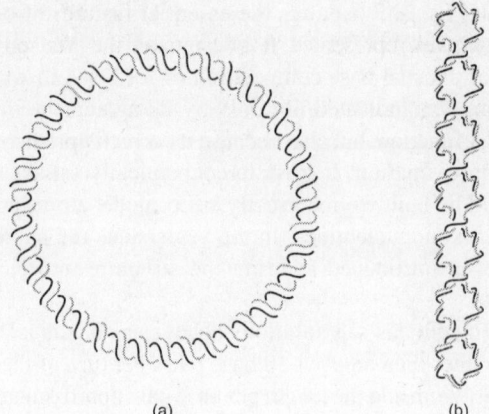

(a)   (b)

Fig. 18.5: Superhelical configuration of covalently closed circular DNA: (a) represents an imaginary circular DNA of only 500 base pairs, if we assume 10 base pairs per turn of the helix, the circular DNA will have 50 turns and (b) shows the superhelical form expected for a 500 base-pair circular DNA that has only 44 turns of the double helix rather than 50.

supercoils. In contrast, the supercoiled form of a circular, covalently-closed, double-stranded DNA molecule occurs when the actual number of turns in the helix is either greater or less than the number of turns that would occur if the molecule were linear. The conflict between: (i) the actual number of turns in the DNA strands and (ii) the number of turns that the low-energy form of B-DNA would assume if not constrained by the covalent circle results in supercoiling of the DNA. The spontaneous process of supercoiling allows the DNA to have the proper number of turns that the covalent structure of the covalently closed, circular DNA has prevented.

The phenomenon of supercoiling easily can be demonstrated with a rope. Lay the rope flat on a table and tape the ends together so as to form a covalent circle. The configuration of the rope then corresponds to Fig. 18.5a. Now, remove the tape. Hold one end of the rope and twist the other end of the rope one, two, three and so on complete rotations. Holding the rope in this tense form, tape the ends again. Notice that the rope assumes a configuration like that shown in Fig. 18.5b. Restriction endonucleases are among the most useful tools for analysing double-stranded DNA. We present information on these very important enzymes, which describe the origin and properties of restriction endo-nucleases and some of their applications in the study and manipulation of DNA sequences. Double-stranded DNA is not the only form of double-stranded nucleic acid. Double-stranded RNA is found in a few viruses and in small quantities in some fungi and plants. Double-stranded RNA is forced, because of steric constraints induced by the 2′ hydroxyl group, into a conformation that is called the A form. In the A form, the base pairs are tilted relative to the helix axis and certain other changes also distinguish this double helix from that of B-DNA. Artificially-formed DNA-RNA hybrids, with one strand of each type of polynucleotide, also assume the A conformation, as does double-stranded DNA in alcohol-water solutions.

CHARACTERISTICS AND PROPERTIES OF GENETIC MATERIAL

Characteristics of Genetic Material

The following are the properties and functions which should be fulfilled by a substance if it has to qualify as genetic material:

1. It should be present in every cell.
2. It must contain all the biologically useful information in a stable form.
3. It should be able to store information in the coded form for the control of biological functions of the cells, and also to express its information.
4. It should show diversity corresponding to the variety existing in the organisms.
5. It should be able to replicate precisely, and then faithfully pass over its true copies to the successive generation.
6. It should also be capable of variations, i.e. recombination and mutation. Further, such variations must be stable and inheritable.
7. The genetic material should be able to generate its own kind and also new kinds of molecules.
8. It should be capable of differential expression so that the various parts of an organism may acquire specific form, structure and functions in-spite of having the same genetic material.

Obviously, one would look for a macromolecule to satisfy the complex functions of genetic material present in the genes. Originally the proteins were thought to play the role of genetic material because they show enormous variety due to various combinations of their 20 constituent amino acids. However, they have no mechanism for replication (i.e. duplication), which is the most important feature of genetic material. Hence, they do not qualify to act as the genetic material.

However, it turned out on the basis of experimental evidences that Deoxyribonucleic Acid (DNA) is the genetic material. DNA shows a wide structural variety because the four types of nucleotide units it is composed of may be arranged in an endless manner in its molecules. It also fulfills all the requirements of the genetic material mentioned above.

Properties of DNA in Genetic Material

The following properties of DNA, present in all the cells of organisms, amply prove that it is genetic material:

1. It is present in all the cells of organisms. Each somatic cell of given species possesses double the amount of DNA than what is present in its gametes.
2. It shows a extremely wide variety due to unlimited sequences in which its monomers can exist.
3. It replicates precisely during interphase of the cell division, and its copies possessing genetic information are very faithfully transmitted to the daughter cells, representing successive generation, during mitosis.
4. Occasionally, it also produces mutations in the genes.
5. DNA stores genetic information as a 'triplet code' and expresses its genetic information by transcription of mRNA and synthesis of proteins. These proteins not only control the structure of the cells, but also control their metabolic activities by acting as enzymes.
6. Genes, composed of DNA, show differential gene activity that is responsible for the process of differentiation in the organism. In other words, different genes remain functional in different cell types so that the latter may acquire their specific structure and functions.
7. DNA, if damaged, can repair itself so as to preserve genetic information present in it.
8. DNA absorbs the same wavelengths of high-energy radiations that can cause maximum mutation (inheritable variation).

DNA AS A GENETIC MATERIAL

Transforming Principle

Frederick Griffith in 1928, carried out a series of experiments with *Streptococcus pneumoniae* (a bacterium that cause pneumonia). He observed that when these bacteria (*Streptococcus pneumonia*) are grown on a culture plate, some of them produce smooth, shiny colonies (S-type), whereas, the others produce rough colonies (R-type). This difference in character (smooth/rough) is due to a mucous (polysaccharide) coat present in the S-strain bacteria, which is not present in the R-strain.

In his experiments, Frederick Griffith first infected two separate groups of mice. The mice that were infected with the S-strain die from pneumonia.

Kindly Note:

'S' strains are the virulent strains causing pneumonia. The mice that were infected with the R-strain do not develop pneumonia and they live.

S-strain (virulent strain) → Inject into mice → Mice die

R-strain (non-virulent strain) → Inject into mice → Mice live

In the next set of experiments, Griffith killed the bacteria by heating them. The mice that were injected heat-killed S-strain bacteria did not die and lived, whereas the mice that were injected a mixture of heat-killed S-strain and live R-strain bacteria, died due to unexpected symptoms of pneumonia.

S-strain (heat killed) → Inject into mice → Mice live

S-strain (heat killed) + R-strain (live) → Inject into mice → Mice die

Griffith concluded that the live R-strain bacteria, were transformed by the heat-killed S-strain bacteria.

He proved that there was some 'transforming principle' that was transferred from the heat-killed S-strain, which helped the R-strain bacteria to synthesise a smooth polysaccharide coat and thus, become virulent. That was due to the transfer of the genetic material.

However, he was not able to define the biochemical nature of genetic material from his experiments.

Biochemical Characterisation of Transforming Principle

Oswald Avery, Colin MacLeod and Maclyn McCarty (1933–44) worked to determine the biochemical nature of 'transforming principle' in Griffith's experiment in an *in vitro* system.

From the heat-killed S-cells, they purified biochemicals (proteins, DNA, RNA, etc.) to observe, that which biochemicals could transform live R-cells into S-cells.

Therefore, they discovered that DNA alone from heat-killed S-type bacteria caused the transformation of non-virulent R-type bacteria into S-type virulent bacteria.

Protein-digesting enzymes (proteases) and RNA-digesting enzymes (RNases) did not cause this transformation. This proved that the 'transforming substance' was neither the protein no RNA.

DNA-digesting enzyme (DNase) caused inhibition of transformation, which suggests that the DNA caused the transformation. Thus, these scientists came to the conclusion that DNA is the hereditary material.

Hershey and chase experiment

The proof for DNA as a genetic material came from the experiment. Alfred Hershey and Martha Chase carried out some experiments with the viruses that infect bacteria. These viruses are called bacteriophages.

The genetic material of bacteriophage enters the bacterial cell after the bacteriophage gets attached to the bacteria. The bacterial cell treats the genetic material of the virus (bacteriophage) like its own genetic material and then produces more virus particles. Hershey and Chase experimented to find out whether it was protein or DNA from the virus that had entered into the bacteria.

For this, they took two separate media for growing these bacteriophages:

1. Out of two, one medium contained radioactive phosphorus and the other medium contained radioactive sulphur. Viruses (bacteriophage) were then grown on each medium.

   (a) The viruses grown in the presence of radioactive phosphorus (^{32}P) contained radioactive DNA (but not radioactive protein). This is because DNA contains phosphorus not protein.

   (b) In the same way, the viruses grown in the medium containing radioactive sulphur (^{35}S) now contained radioactive protein (not radioactive DNA). This is because DNA does not contain sulphur.

2. These radioactive viruses (bacteriophages) were then allowed to attach to bacteria (*E. coli*). As the process of infection with virus continued, the bacteria were agitated in a blender and the viral coats of the bacteria were removed.

3. When they were spinned in a centrifuge, the virus particles were separated from the bacteria.

4. They observed that the bacteria that were infected with virus containing radioactive DNA were radioactive, whereas the bacteria that were infected with radioactive proteins were not radioactive.

5. This indicates that only DNA not the protein coat entered the bacterial cell.

6. Thus, the genetic material that is passed from virus to bacteria is DNA.

Properties of Genetic Material

From the Hershey and Chase experiment, the fact was established that DNA acts as a genetic material. But later, studies revealed that in some viruses (e.g. Tobacco Mosaic Viruses, QB bacteriophage, etc.) RNA is the genetic material.

Following are the criteria that a molecule must fulfil to act as a genetic material:

- It should be able to replicate.
- It should be chemically and structurally stable.
- It should provide the scope for slow changes
- It should be able to express itself in the form of 'Mendelian characters'. According to these criteria, both DNA and RNA have the ability to direct their duplications (because of the rule of base pairing and complementarity). Both the nucleic acids (DNA and RNA) have the ability to direct their duplications, whereas the other molecules in the living system, fail to duplicate, e.g. protein.

DNA VIRUS

A DNA virus is a virus that has DNA as its genetic material and replicates using a DNA-dependent DNA polymerase. The nucleic acid is usually double-stranded DNA (dsDNA) but may also be single-stranded DNA (ssDNA). DNA viruses belong to either Group I or Group II of the Baltimore classification system for viruses. Single-stranded DNA is usually expanded to double-stranded in infected cells. Although Group VII viruses such as hepatitis B contain a DNA genome, they are not considered DNA viruses according to the Baltimore classification, but rather reverse transcribing viruses because they replicate through an RNA intermediate. Notable diseases like smallpox, herpes, and chickenpox are caused by such DNA viruses.

Group I: dsDNA Viruses

Genome organisation within this group varies considerably (Fig. 18.6). Some have circular genomes (Baculoviridae, Papovaviridae and Polydnaviridae) while others have linear genomes (Adenoviridae, Herpesviridae and some phages). Some families have circularly permuted linear genomes (phage T4 and some Iridoviridae). Others have linear genomes with covalently closed ends (Poxviridae and Phycodnaviridae).

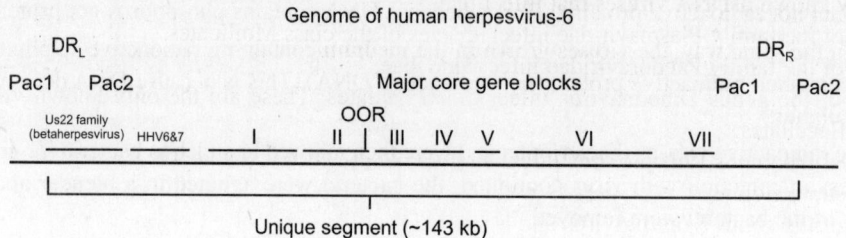

Fig. 18.6: Genome of human herpesvirus-6, a member of the Herpesviridae family.

A virus infecting archaea was first described in 1974. Several others have been described since: most have head-tail morphologies and linear double-stranded DNA genomes. Other morphologies have also been described: spindle shaped, rod shaped, filamentous, icosahedral and spherical. Additional morphological types may exist. Orders within this group are defined on the basis of morphology rather than DNA sequence similarity. It is thought that morphology is more conserved in this group than sequence similarity or gene order which is extremely variable. Three orders and 31 families are currently recognised. A fourth order–Megavirales–for the nucleocytoplasmic large DNA viruses has been proposed. Four genera are recognised that have not yet been assigned a family. The species Sulfolobus turreted icosahedral virus is so unlike any previously described virus that it will almost certainly be placed in a new family on the next revision of viral families.

Fifteen families are enveloped. These include all three families in the order Herpesvirales and the following families: Ascoviridae, Ampullaviridae, Asfarviridae, Baculoviridae, Fuselloviridae, Globuloviridae, Guttaviridae, Hytrosaviridae, Iridoviridae, Lipothrixviridae, Nimaviridae and Poxviridae.

Bacteriophages (viruses infecting bacteria) belonging to the families Tectiviridae and Corticoviridae have a lipid bilayer membrane inside the icosahedral protein capsid and the membrane surrounds the genome. The crenarchaeal virus Sulfolobus turreted icosahedral virus has a similar structure. The genomes in this group vary considerably from ~10 kilobases to over 2.5 megabases in length. The largest bacteriophage known is Klebsiella Phage vB_KleM-RaK2 which has a genome of 346 kilobases.

A recently proposed clade is the Megavirales which includes the nucleocytoplasmic large DNA viruses. This proposal has yet to be ratified by the ICTV.

Host range

Species of the order Caudovirales and of the families Corticoviridae and Tectiviridae infect bacteria.

Species of the order Ligamenvirales and the families Ampullaviridae, Bicaudaviridae, Clavaviridae, Fuselloviridae, Globuloviridae, Guttaviridae and Turriviridae infect hyperthermophilic archaea species of the Crenarchaeota.

Species of the order Herpesvirales and of the families Adenoviridae, Asfarviridae, Iridoviridae, Papillomaviridae, Polyomaviridae and Poxviridae infect vertebrates.

Species of the families Ascovirus, Baculovirus, Hytrosaviridae, Iridoviridae and Polydnaviruses and of the genus Nudivirus infect insects.

Species of the family Mimiviridae and the species Marseillevirus, Megavirus, Mavirus virophage and Sputnik virophage infect protozoa.

Species of the family Nimaviridae infect crustaceans.

Species of the family Phycodnaviridae and the species Organic Lake virophage infect algae. These are the only known dsDNA viruses that infect plants.

Species of the family Plasmaviridae infect species of the class Mollicutes.

Species of the family Pandoraviridae infect amoebae.

Species of the genus Dinodnavirus infect dinoflagellates. These are the only known viruses that infect dinoflagellates.

Species of the genus Rhizidiovirus infect stramenopiles. These are the only known dsDNA viruses that infect stramenopiles.

Species of the genus Salterprovirus and Sphaerolipoviridae infect species of the Euryarchaeota.

Taxonomy

- Order Caudovirales:
  - › Family Myoviridae–includes Enterobacteria phage T4
  - › Family Podoviridae–includes Enterobacteria phage T7
  - › Family Siphoviridae–includes Enterobacteria phage λ
- Order Herpesvirales:
  - › Family Alloherpesviridae
  - › Family Herpesviridae–includes human herpesviruses, Varicella Zoster virus
  - › Family Malacoherpesviridae
- Order Ligamenvirales:
  - › Family Lipothrixviridae
  - › Family Rudiviridae
- Unassigned families:
  - › Family Adenoviridae–includes viruses which cause human adenovirus infection
  - › Family Ampullaviridae
  - › Family Ascoviridae
  - › Family Asfarviridae–includes African swine fever virus
  - › Family Baculoviridae
  - › Family Bicaudaviridae
  - › Family Clavaviridae
  - › Family Corticoviridae
  - › Family Fuselloviridae
  - › Family Globuloviridae
  - › Family Guttaviridae
  - › Family Hytrosaviridae
  - › Family Iridoviridae

> Family Marseilleviridae
> Family Mimiviridae
> Family Nimaviridae
> Family Pandoraviridae
> Family Papillomaviridae
> Family Phycodnaviridae
> Family Plasmaviridae
> Family Polydnaviruses
> Family Polyomaviridae–includes Simian virus 40, JC virus, BK virus
> Family Poxviridae–includes Cowpox virus, smallpox
> Family Sphaerolipoviridae
> Family Tectiviridae
> Family Turriviridae
• Unassigned genera
> Dinodnavirus
  > Nudivirus
  > Salterprovirus
  > Rhizidiovirus
• Unassigned species
  > Abalone shriveling syndrome-associated virus
  > Bandicoot papillomatosis carcinomatosis virus
  > KIs-V
  > Haloarcula hispanica pleomorphic virus 1
  > Mavirus virophage
  > Megavirus
  > Organic Lake virophage
  > Pithovirus
  > Sputnik virophage
  > Sputnik virophage 2
  > Sulfolobus turreted icosahedral virus

Pleolipoviruses

A group known as the pleolipoviruses, although having a similar genome organisation, differ in having either single or double stranded DNA genomes. Within the double stranded forms have runs of single stranded DNA. This group does not fit into the current classification system and a new taxon is required.

These viruses are nonlytic and form virions characterised by a lipid vesicle enclosing the genome. They do not have nucleoproteins. The lipids in the viral membrane are unselectively acquired from host cell membranes. The virions contain two to three major structural proteins, which either are embedded in the membrane or form spikes distributed randomly on the external membrane surface.

This group includes the following viruses:
- Haloarcula hispanica pleomorphic virus 1
- Halogeometricum pleomorphic virus 1
- Halorubrum pleomorphic virus 1
- Halorubrum pleomorphic virus 2
- Halorubrum pleomorphic virus 3
- Halorubrum pleomorphic virus 6

Group II: ssDNA viruses

Although bacteriophages were first described in 1927, it was only in 1959 that Sinshemer working with phage Phi X 174 showed that they could possess single-stranded DNA genomes. Despite this discovery until relatively recently it was believed that the majority of DNA viruses belonged to the double-stranded clade. Recent work suggests that this may not be the case with single-stranded viruses forming the majority of viruses found in sea water, fresh water, sediment, terrestrial, extreme, metazoan-associated and marine microbial mats. Many of these 'environmental' viruses belong to the family Microviridae.

However, the vast majority has yet to be classified and assigned to genera and higher taxa. Because most of these viruses do not appear to be related or are only distantly related to known viruses additional taxa will be created for these.

Taxonomy

Families in this group have been assigned on the basis of the nature of the genome (circular or linear) and the host range. Ten families are currently recognised.
- Family Anelloviridae
- Family Bacillariodnaviridae
- Family Bidnaviridae
- Family Circoviridae
- Family Geminiviridae
- Family Inoviridae
- Family Microviridae
- Family Nanoviridae
- Family Parvoviridae
- Family Spiraviridae

Classification of circular single stranded viruses

A division of the circular single stranded viruses into four types has been proposed. This division seems likely reflects their phylogenetic relationships.

Type I genomes are characterised by a small circular DNA genome (approximately 2-kb), with the Rep protein and the major open reading frame (ORF) in opposite orientations. This type is characteristic of the circoviruses, geminiviruses and nanoviruses.

Type II genomes have the unique feature of two separate Rep ORFs.

Type III genomes contain two major ORFs in the same orientation. This arrangement is typical of the anelloviruses.

Type IV genomes have the largest genomes of nearly 4-kb, with up to eight ORFs. This type of genome is found in the Inoviridae and the Microviridae.

Given the variety of single stranded viruses that have been described this scheme– if it is accepted by the ICTV–will need to be extended.

Host range

The families Bidnaviridae and Parvoviridae have linear genomes while the other families have circular genomes. The Bidnaviridae have a two part genome and infect invertebrates. The Inoviridae and Microviridae infect bacteria, the Anelloviridae and Circoviridae infect animals (mammals and birds respectively), and the Geminiviridae and Nanoviridae infect plants. In both the Geminiviridae and Nanoviridae the genome is composed of more than a single chromosome. The Bacillariodnaviridae infect diatoms and have a unique genome: the major chromosome is circular (~6 kilobases in length): the minor chromosome is linear (~1 kilobase in length) and complementary to part of the major chromosome. Members of the Spiraviridae infect archaea.

Molecular biology

All viruses in this group require formation of a replicative form–a double stranded DNA intermediate– for genome replication. This is normally created from the viral DNA with the assistance of the host's own DNA polymerase.

Recently classified viruses

In the 9th edition of the viral taxonomy of the ICTV the Bombyx mori densovirus type 2 was placed in a new family–the Bidnaviridae on the basis of its genome structure and replication mechanism. This is currently the only member of this family but it seems likely that other species will be allocated to this family in the near future. A new genus–Bufavirus–was proposed on the basis of the isolation of two new viruses from human stool. These viruses have since been renamed Primate proto-parvovirus and been placed in the genus Protoparvovirus.

Unassigned species

A number of additional single stranded DNA viruses have been described but are as yet unclassified.

Animal viruses–vertebrates

Among these are the parvovirus like viruses. These have linear single stranded DNA genomes but unlike the parvoviruses the genome is bipartate. This group includes the Bombyx mori densovirus type 2, Hepatopancreatic parvo-like virus and Lymphoidal parvo-like virus. A new family Bidensoviridae has been proposed for this group but this proposal has not been ratified by the ICTV to date. Their closest relations appear to be the Brevidensoviruses (family Parvoviridae).

Another new genus–as yet unnamed–has been proposed. This genus includes the species bovine stool associated circular virus and chimpanzee stool associated circular virus. The closest relations to this genus appear to be the Nanoviridae but further work will be needed to confirm this. Another isolate that appears to be related to these viruses has been isolated from pig faeces in New Zealand. This isolate also appears to be related to the pig stool-associated single-stranded DNA virus. This virus has two large open reading frames one encoding the capsid gene and the other the Rep gene. These are bidirectionally transcribed and separated by intergenic regions. The name Gemycircularvirus has been proposed for this group of viruses. Another virus of this group has been reported again from pigs. Some of this group of viruses may infect fungi. An virus from this group has been isoalted from turkey faeces. Another ten viruses from this group have been isolated from pig faeces. Additional viruses from this group have been reported from dragonflies and damselflies.

Fur seal feces-associated circular DNA virus was isolate from the faeces of a fur seal (Arctocephalus forsteri) in New Zealand. The genome has 2 main open reading frames and is 2925 nucleotides in length. Another virus porcine stool associated virus 4 has been isolated that appears to be related to the fur seal virus. Two viruses have been isolated from human faeces—circo-like virus-Brazil hs1 and hs2—with genome lengths of 2526 and 2533 nucleotides respectively. These viruses have four open reading frames. These viruses appear to be related to three viruses previously isolated from wastewater, a bat and from a rodent. Another virus-Porcine stool-associated circular virus 5 has been reported. This appears to belong to a novel group.

Two viruses have been described from the nesting material yellow crowned parakeet (Cyanoramphus auriceps)–CynNCXV (2308 nt) and CynNCKV (2087 nt) Both viruses have two bidirectional open reading frames. Within these are the rolling-circle replication motifs I, II, III and the helicase motifs Walker A and Walker B. There is also a conserved nonanucleotide motif required for rolling-circle replication. CynNCKV has some similarity to the picobiliphyte nano-like virus (Picobiliphyte M5584-5) and CynNCXV has some similarity to the rodent stool associated virus (RodSCV M-45).

Psittacine beak and feather disease virus is a single stranded circular molecule of 1993 nucleotide bases encoding seven open reading frames—three in the virion strand and four in the complementary strand. The open reading frames have some homology to porcine circovirus, subterranean clover stunt virus and faba bean necrotic yellows virus. A virus with a circular genome–sea turtle tornovirus 1–has been isolated from a sea turtle with fibropapillomatosis. It is sufficiently unrelated to any other known virus that it may belong to a new family. The closest relations seem to be the Gyrovirinae. The proposed genus name for this virus is Tornovirus.

Animal viruses–invertebrates

A virus—Acheta domesticus volvovirus has been isolated from the house cricket (Acheta domesticus). The genome is circular, has four open reading frames and is 2517 nucleotides in length. It appears to be unrelated to previously described species. The genus name Volvovirus has been proposed for these species. The genomes in this genus are ~2.5 nucleotides in length and encode 4 open reading frames.

Two new viruses have been isolated from the copepods Acartia tonsa and Labidocera aestiva— Acartia tonsa copepod circo-like virus and Labidocera aestiva copepod circo-like virus respectively.

A virus has been isolated from the mud flat snail (Amphibola crenata). This virus has a single stranded circular genome of 2351 nucleotides that encoded 2 open reading frames that are oriented in opposite directions. The smaller open reading frame (874 nucleotides) encodes a protein with similarities to the Rep (replication) proteins of circoviruses and plasmids. The larger open reading frame (955 nucleotides) has no homology to any currently known protein. An unusual–and as yet unnamed – virus has been isolated from the flatwom Girardia tigrina. Because of its genome organisation, this virus appears to belong to an entirely new family. It is the first virus to be isolated from a flatworm. From the hepatopancreas of the shrimp (Farfantepenaeus duorarum) a circular single stranded DNA virus has been isolated. This virus does not appear to cause disease in the shrimp. A circo-like virus has been isolated from the shrimp (Penaeus monodon). The 1777-nucleotide genome is circular and single stranded. It has some similarity to the circoviruses and cycloviruses. Ten new circular viruses have been isolated from dragonfly larvae. The genomes range from 1628 to 2668 nucleotides in length.

Fungal

Most known fungal viruses have either double stranded DNA or RNA genomes. A single stranded DNA fungal virus–Sclerotinia sclerotiorum hypovirulence associated DNA virus 1–has been described. This virus appears to be related to the Geminiviridae but is distinct from them. A genus–Breviviridae–has been proposed for Sclerotinia sclerotiorum hypovirulence associated DNA virus 1 and a European badger fecal virus.

Plants

A virus–Cassava associated circular DNA virus–that has some similarity to Sclerotinia sclerotiorum hypovirulence associated DNA virus 1 has been isolated.

A circular single stranded DNA virus has been isolated from a grapevine. This species may be related to the family Geminiviridae but differs from this family in a number of important respects including genome size.

Grapevine red blotch associated virus and Grapevine cabernet franc associated virus are two single stranded DNA viruses associated with infections of grape vines.

A virus—Euphorbia caput medusae latent virus—is so divergent from the other members of the geminiviruses that a new genus has been proposed for it. The name of this new genus is proposed to be Capulavirus. Several viruses—baminivirus, nepavirus and niminivirus—related to geminvirus have also been reported.

Archaea

Although ~50 archaeal viruses are known, all but two have double stranded genomes. The first archaeal ssDNA virus to be isolated is the Halorubrum pleomorphic virus 1, which has a pleomorphic enveloped virion and a circular genome. The second single stranded DNA virus infecting Archaea is Aeropyrum coil-shaped virus (ACV). The genome is circular and with 24,893 nucleotides is currently the largest known ssDNA genome. The viron is nonenveloped, hollow, cylindrical and formed from a coiling fiber. The morphology and the genome appear to be unique. The new family Spiraviridae (from Latin spira, 'a coil') has been created by the ICTV to accommodate ACV.

Marine and other

Several hundred single stranded DNA viral genomes have been isolated from seawater. Their hosts have yet to be identified but are likely to be eukaryotic phytoplankton and zooplankton. They fall into at least 11 distinct groups that are unrelated to previously described viral families. A virus—Boiling Springs Lake virus—appears to have evolved by a recombination event between a DNA virus (circovirus) and an RNA virus (tombusvirus). The genome is circular and encodes two proteins—a Rep protein and a capsid protein. Further reports of viruses that appear to have evolved from recombination events between ssRNA and ssDNA viruses have been made. A new virus has been isolated from the diatom Chaetoceros setoensis. It has a single stranded DNA genome and does not appear to be a member of any previously described group.

Satellite viruses

Satellite viruses are small viruses with either RNA or DNA as their genomic material that require another virus to replicate. There are two types of DNA satellite viruses– the alphasatellites and the betasatellites–both of which are dependent on begomoviruses. At present satellite viruses are not classified into genera or higher taxa. Alphasatellites are small circular single strand DNA viruses that require a begomovirus for transmission. Betasatellites are small linear single stranded DNA viruses that require a begomovirus to replicate.

Phylogenetic relationships

Phylogenetic relationships between these families are difficult to determine. The genomes differ significantly in size and organisation. Most studies that have attempted to determine these relationships are based either on some of the more conserved proteins–DNA polymerase and others–or on common structural features. In general most of the proposed relationships are tentative and have not yet been used by the ICTV in their classification.

ds DNA viruses

Herpesviruses and caudoviruses: While determining the phylogenetic relations between the various known clades of viruses is difficult, on a number of grounds the herpesviruses and caudoviruses appear to be related. While the three families in the order Herpesvirales are clearly related on morpho-logical grounds, it has proven difficult to determine the dates of divergence between them because of the lack of gene conservation. On morphological grounds they appear to be related to the bacteriophages–specifically the Caudoviruses. The branching order among the herpesviruses suggests that Alloherpesviridae is the basal clade and that Herpesviridae and Malacoherpesviridae are sister clades. Given the phylogenetic distances between vertebrates and molluscs this suggests that herpesviruses were initially fish viruses and that they have evolved with their hosts to infect other vertebrates.

The vertebrate herpesviruses initially evolved ~400 million years ago and underwent subsequent evolution on the supercontinent Pangaea. The alphaherpesvirinae separated from the branch leading to the betaherpesvirinae and gammaherpesvirinae about 180 million years ago to 220 million years ago. The avian herpes viruses diverged from the branch leading to the mammalian species. The mammalian species divided into two branches–the Simplexvirus and Varicellovirus genera. This latter divergence appears to have occur around the time of the mammalian radiation.

Several dsDNA bacteriophages and the herpesviruses encode a powerful ATP driven DNA translocating machine that encapsidates a viral genome into a preformed capsid shell or prohead. The critical components of the packaging machine are the packaging enzyme (terminase) which acts as the motor and the portal protein that forms the unique DNA entrance vertex of prohead. The terminase complex consists of a recognition subunit (small terminase) and an endonuclease/translocase subunit (large terminase) and cuts viral genome concatemers. It forms a motor complex containing five large terminase subunits. The terminase-viral DNA complex docks on the portal vertex. The pentameric motor processively translocates DNA until the head shell is full with one viral genome. The motor cuts the DNA again and dissociates from the full head, allowing head-finishing proteins to assemble on the portal, sealing the portal, and constructing a platform for tail attachment. Only a single gene encoding the putative ATPase subunit of the terminase (UL15) is conserved among all herpesviruses. To a lesser extent this gene is also found also in T4-like bacteriophages suggesting a common ancestor for these two groups of viruses.

A common origin for the herpesviruses and the caudoviruses has been suggested on the basis of parallels in their capsid assembly pathways and similarities between their portal complexes, through which DNA enters the capsid. These two groups of viruses share a distinctive 12-fold arrangement of subunits in the portal complex.

Large DNA viruses

The family Ascoviridae appear to have evolved from the Iridoviridae. The family Polydnaviridae may have evolved from the Ascoviridae. Molecular evidence suggests that the Phycodnaviridae may have evolved from the family Iridoviridae. These four families (Ascoviridae, Iridoviridae, Phycodnaviridae and Polydnaviridae) may form a clade but more work is needed to confirm this.

Based on the genome organisation and DNA replication mechanism it seems that phylogenetic relationships may exist between the rudiviruses (Rudiviridae) and the large eukaryal DNA viruses: the African swine fever virus (*Asfarviridae*), *Chlorella viruses* (*Phycodnaviridae*) and poxviruses in birds is shown in Fig. 18.7 (*Poxviridae*).

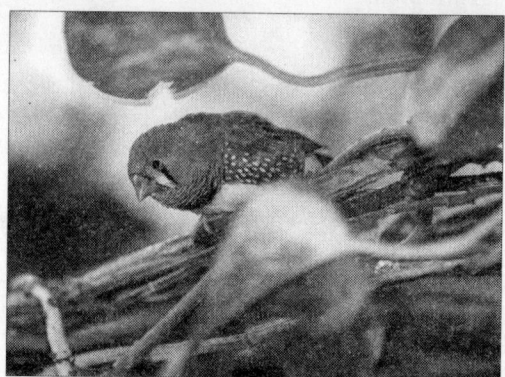

Fig. 18.7: Poxviruses in birds (*Poxviridae*).

Based on the analysis of the DNA polymerase the genus Dinodnavirus may be a member of the family *Asfarviridae*. Further work on this virus will required before a final assignment can be made.

The nucleocytoplasmic large DNA virus group (*Asfarviridae, Iridoviridae, Mar-seilleviridae, Mimiviridae, Phycodnaviridae* and *Poxviridae*) along with three other families–*Adenoviridde, Cortiviridae* (Fig. 18.8) and *Tectiviridae*–and the phage Sulfolobus turreted icosahedral virus and the satellite virus Sputnik all possess double β-barrel major capsid proteins suggesting a common origin.

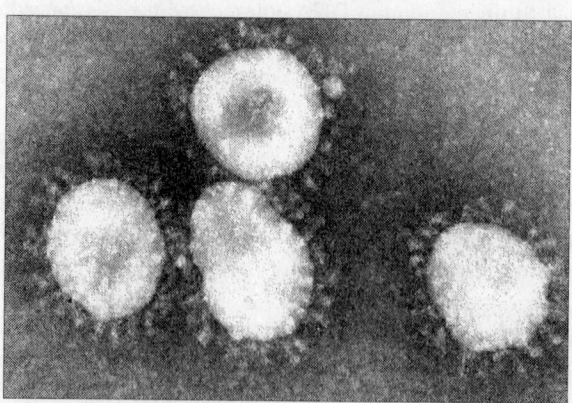

Fig. 18.8: Cortiviridae.

Some of the relations among the large viruses have been established. Mimiviruses are distantly related to Phycodnaviridae. Pandoraviruses share a common ancestor with Coccolithoviruses within the Phycodnaviridae family. Pithoviruses are related to Iridoviridae and Marseilleviridae.

Other viruses

Based on the analysis of the coat protein, Sulfolobus turreted icosahedral virus may share a common ancestry with the Tectiviridae.

- The families Adenoviridae and Tectiviridae appear to be related structurally.
- Baculoviruses evolved from the nudiviruses 310 million years ago.
- The Hytrosaviridae are related to the baculoviruses and to a lesser extent the nudiviruses suggesting they may have evolved from the baculoviruses.
- The Nimaviridae may be related to nudiviruses and baculoviruses.
- The Nudiviruses seem to be related to the polydnaviruses.
- A protein common to the families Bicaudaviridae, Lipotrixviridae and Rudiviridae and the unclassified virus Sulfolobus turreted icosahedral virus is known suggesting a common origin.

Examination of the pol genes that encode the DNA dependent DNA polymerase in various groups of viruses suggests a number of possible evolutionary relationships. All know viral DNA polymerases belong to the DNA pol families A and B. All possess a $3'$–$5'$-exonuclease domain with three sequence motifs Exo I, Exo II and Exo III. The families A and B are distinguishable with family A Pol sharing 9 distinct consensus sequences and only two of them are convincingly homologous to sequence motif B of family B. The putative sequence motifs A, B, and C of the polymerase domain are located near the C-terminus in family A Pol and more central in family B Pol.

Phylogenetic analysis of these genes places the adenoviruses (Adenoviridae), bacteriophages (Caudovirales) and the plant and fungal linear plasmids into a single clade. A second clade includes the alpha- and delta-like viral Pol from insect ascovirus (Ascoviridae), mammalian herpesviruses (Herpesviridae), fish lymphocystis disease virus (Iridoviridae) and chlorella virus (Phycoviridae). The pol genes of the African swine fever virus (Asfarviridae), baculoviruses (Baculoviridae), fish herpesvirus (Herpesviridae), T-even bacteriophages (Myoviridae) and poxviruses (Poxviridae) were not clearly resolved. A second study showed that poxvirus, baculovirus and the animal herpesviruses form separate and distinct clades. Their relationship to the Asfarviridae and the Myoviridae was not examined and remains unclear. The polymerases from the archaea are similar to family B DNA Pols. The T4-like viruses infect both bacteria and archaea and their pol gene resembles that of eukaryotes. The DNA polymerase of mitochondria resembles that of the T odd phages (Myoviridae). The virophage Mavirus may have evolved from a recombination between a transposon of the Polinton (Maverick) family and an unknown virus.

ss DNA viruses

The evolutionary history of this group is currently poorly understood. An ancient origin for the single stranded circular DNA viruses has been proposed. Capsid proteins of most icosahedral ssRNA and ssDNA viruses display the same structural fold, the eight-stranded beta-barrel, also known as the jelly-roll fold. On the other hand, the replication proteins of icosahedral ssDNA viruses belong to the superfamily of rolling-circle replication initiation proteins that are commonly found in prokaryotic plasmids. Based on these observations, it has been proposed that small DNA viruses have originated via recombination between RNA viruses and plasmids.

Circoviruses may have evolved from a nanovirus. Given the similarities between the rep proteins of the alphasatellites and the nanoviruses, it is likely that the alphasatellites evolved from the nanoviruses. Further work in this area is needed to clarify this. The geminiviruses may have evolved from phytoplasmal plasmids. Based on the three-dimensional structure of the Rep proteins the geminiviruses and parvoviruses may be related. The ancestor of the geminiviruses probably infected dicots.

The parvoviruses have frequently invaded the germ lines of diverse animal species including mammals, fishes, birds, tunicates, arthropods and flatworms. In particular they have been associated with the human genome for ~98 million years.

Members of the family Bidnaviridae have evolved from insect parvoviruses by replacing the typical replication-initiation endonuclease with a protein-primed family B DNA polymerase acquired from large DNA transposons of the Polinton/Maverick family. Some bidnavirus genes were also horizontally acquired from reoviruses (dsRNA genomes) and baculoviruses (dsDNA genomes).

Bacteriophage evolution

Since 1959 ~6300 prokaryote viruses have been described morphologically, including ~6200 bacterial and ~100 *archaeal* viruses. Archaeal viruses belong to 15 families and infect members of 16 *archaeal* genera. These are nearly exclusively hyperthermophiles or extreme halophiles. Tailed *archaeal* viruses are found only in the Euryarchaeota, whereas most filamentous and pleomorphic archaeal viruses occur in the Crenarchaeota. Bacterial viruses belong to 10 families and infect members of 179 bacterial genera: most these are members of the Firmicutes and γ-proteobacteria.

The vast majority (96.3%) are tailed with and only 230 (3.7%) are polyhedral, filamentous or pleomorphic. The family Siphoviridae is the largest family (>3600 descriptions: 57.3%). The tailed phages appear to be monophyletic and are the oldest known virus group. They arose repeatedly in different hosts and there are at least 11 separate lines of descent.

All of the known temperate phages employ one of only three different systems for their lysogenic cycle: lambda-like integration/excision, Mu-like transposition or the plasmid-like partitioning of phage N15. A putative course of evolution of these phages has been proposed by Ackermann.

Tailed phages originated in the early Precambrian, long before eukaryotes and their viruses. The ancestral tailed phage had an icosahedral head of about 60 nanometers in diameter and a long non contractile tail with sixfold symmetry. The capsid contained a single molecule of double stranded DNA of about 50 kilobases. The tail was probably provided with a fixation apparatus. The head and tail were held together by a connector. The viral particle contained no lipids, was heavier than its descendant viruses and had a high DNA content proportional to its capsid size (~50%). Most of the genome coded for structural proteins. Morphopoietic genes clustered at one end of the genome, with head genes preceding tail genes. Lytic enzymes were probably coded for. Part of the phage genome was nonessential and possibly bacterial. The virus infected its host from the outside and injected its DNA. Replication involved transcription in several waves and formation of DNA concatemers.

New phages were released by burst of the infected cell after lysis of host membranes by a peptidoglycan hydrolase. Capsids were assembled from a starting point, the connector and around a scaffold. They underwent an elaborate maturation process involving protein cleavage and capsid expansion. Heads and tails were assembled separately and joined later.

The DNA was cut to size and entered preformed capsids by a headful mechanism. Subsequently the phages evolved contractile or short tails and elongated heads. Some viruses become temperate by acquiring an integrase-excisionase complex, plasmid parts or transposons.

NCLDVs

The asfarviruses, iridoviruses, mimiviruses, phycodnaviruses and poxviruses have been shown to belong to a single group,–the large nuclear and cytoplasmic DNA viruses. These are also abbreviated 'NCLDV'. This clade can be divided into two groups:

- The iridoviruses-phycodnaviruses-mimiviruses group. The phycodnaviruses and mimiviruses are sister clades.
- The poxvirus-asfarviruses group.

It is probable that these viruses evolved before the separation of eukaryoyes into the extant crown groups. The ancestral genome was complex with at least 41 genes including: (i) the replication machinery, (ii) up to four RNA polymerase subunits, (iii) at least three transcription factors, (iv) capping and polyadenylation enzymes, (v) the DNA packaging apparatus (vi) and structural components of an icosahedral capsid and the viral membrane.

The evolution of this group of viruses appears to be complex with genes having been gained from multiple sources. It has been proposed that the ancestor of NCLDVs has evolved from large, virus-like DNA transposons of the Polinton/Maverick family. From Polinton/Maverick transposons NCLDVs might have inherited the key components required for virion morphogenesis, including the major and minor capsid proteins, maturation protease and genome packaging ATPase.

Another group of large viruses—the Pandoraviridae—has been described. Two species—Pandoravirus salinus and Pandoravirus dulcis—have been recognised. These were isolated from Chile and Australia respectively. These viruses are about one micrometer in diameter making them one of the largest viruses discovered so far. Their gene complement is larger than any other known virus to date. At present they appear to be unrelated to any other species of virus. An even larger genus, Pithovirus, has since been discovered, measuring about 1.5 μm in length.

Viruses of *Archaea*

A virus infecting archaea was first described in 1974. Several others have been described since then. Most have head-tail morphologies and linear double-stranded DNA genomes. Other morphologies have also been described including spindle shaped, rod shaped, filamentous, icosahedral, and spherical. Additional morphological types may exist.

Archaea can be infected by double-stranded DNA viruses that are unrelated to any other form of virus and have a variety of unusual shapes. These viruses have been studied in the most detail in thermophilics, particularly the orders Sulfolobales and Thermoproteales. Two groups of single-stranded DNA viruses that infect archaea have been recently isolated. One group is exemplified by the Halorubrum pleomorphic virus 1 (Pleolipoviridae) infecting halophilic archaea and the other one by the Aeropyrum coil-shaped virus.

Double-stranded DNA viruses infecting archaea

Bacteriophages (viruses infecting bacteria) belonging to the families Tectiviridae and Corticoviridae have a lipid bilayer membrane inside the icosahedral protein capsid and the membrane surrounds the genome. The crenarchaeal virus Sulfolobus turreted icosahedral virus has a similar structure.

Species of the order Ligamenvirales and the families Ampullaviridae, Bicaudaviridae, Clavaviridae, Fuselloviridae, Globuloviridae, and Guttaviridae infect hyperthermophilic archaea species of the Crenarchaeota.

Species of the genus Salterprovirus infect halophilic *archaea* species of the *Euryarchaeota*.

Single-stranded DNA viruses infecting archaea

Although around 50 archaeal viruses are known, all but two have double stranded genomes. The first archaeal ssDNA virus to be isolated is the Halorubrum pleomorphic virus 1, which has a pleomorphic enveloped virion and a circular genome. Defenses against these viruses may involve RNA interference from repetitive DNA sequences that are related to the genes of the viruses.

The second single stranded DNA virus infecting Archaea is Aeropyrum coil-shaped virus (ACV). The genome is circular and with 24,893 nucleotides is currently the largest known ssDNA genome. The viron is nonenveloped, hollow, cylindrical, and formed from a coiling fiber. The morphology and the genome appear to be unique. ACV has been suggested to represent a new viral family tentatively called 'Spiraviridae' (from Latin spira, 'a coil'). The Aeropyrum coil-shaped virus infects a hyperthermophilic (optimal growth at 90–95°C) host. Notably, the latter virus has the largest currently reported ssDNA genome. Figure 18.9 shows viruses infecting *archaea*.

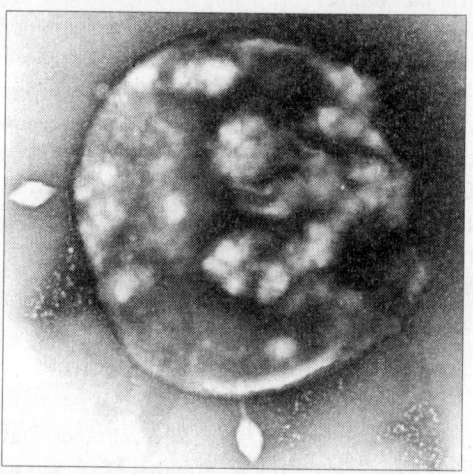

Fig. 18.9: Viruses infecting *archaea*.

Oncovirus

An oncovirus is a virus that can cause cancer. This term originated from studies of acutely transforming retroviruses in the 1950–60s, often called oncornaviruses to denote their RNA virus origin. It now refers to any virus with a DNA or RNA genome causing cancer and is synonymous with 'tumor virus' or 'cancer virus'. The vast majority of human and animal viruses do not cause cancer, probably because of long-standing coevolution between the virus and its host.

Worldwide, the WHO International Agency for Research on Cancer estimated that in 2002, 17.8% of human cancers were caused by infection, with 11.9% being caused by one of seven different viruses. The importance of this is that these cancers might be easily prevented through vaccination (e.g. papillomavirus vaccines), diagnosed with simple blood tests, and treated with less-toxic antiviral compounds.

Generally, tumor viruses cause little or no disease after infection in their hosts, or cause non-neoplastic diseases such as acute hepatitis for hepatitis B virus or mononucleosis for Epstein-Barr virus. A minority of persons (or animals) will go on to develop cancers after infection. This has complicated determining whether or not a given virus causes cancer. The well-known Koch's Postulates are 19th-century constructs developed by Robert Koch to establish the likelihood for Bacillus anthracis causing anthrax disease and are not applicable to viral diseases (Firstly, viruses cannot truly be isolated in pure culture-even stringent isolation techniques cannot exclude undetected contaminating viruses with similar density characteristics and viruses must be grown on cells. Secondly, asymptomatic virus infection and carriage is the norm for most tumor viruses, which violates Koch's third principle. Relman and Fredericks have elegantly described the difficulties in using Koch's postulates to virus-induced cancers. Finally, the host restriction for human viruses makes it unethical to experimentally transmit a suspected cancer virus.) Thus, other measures such as A.B. Hill's criteria are more relevant to cancer virology but also face some difficulties in determining causality.

Tumor viruses come in a variety of forms: viruses with a DNA genome, such as adenovirus, and viruses with an RNA genome, like the Hepatitis C virus (HCV) can cause cancers, as can retroviruses having both DNA and RNA genomes (Human T-lymphotropic virus and hepatitis B virus, which normally replicates as a mixed double and single-stranded DNA virus but also has a retroviral replication component). In many cases, tumor viruses do not cause cancer in their native hosts but only in dead-end species. For example, adenoviruses do not cause cancer in humans but are instead responsible for colds, conjunctivitis and other acute illnesses. They only become tumorigenic when infected into certain rodent species, such as Syrian hamsters. Some viruses are tumorigenic when they infect a cell and persist as circular episomes or plasmids, replicating separately from host cell DNA (Epstein-Barr virus and Kaposi's sarcoma-associated herpesvirus). Other viruses are only carcinogenic when they integrate into the host cell genome as part of a biological accident, such as polyomaviruses and papillomaviruses. Brain tumour virus is shown in Fig. 18.10.

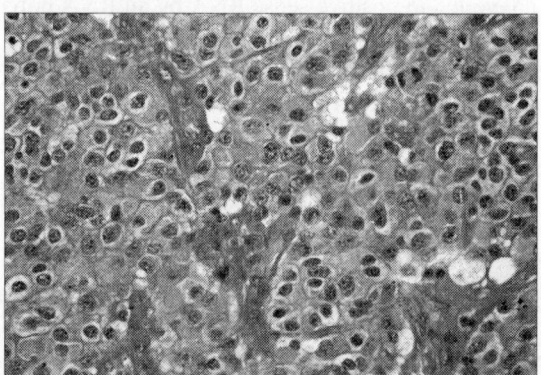

Fig. 18.10: Brain tumour virus.

A direct oncogenic viral mechanism involves either insertion of additional viral oncogenic genes into the host cell or to enhance already existing oncogenic genes (proto-oncogenes) in the genome. Indirect viral oncogenicity involves chronic nonspecific inflammation occurring over decades of infection, as is the case for HCV-induced liver cancer.

These two mechanisms differ in their biology and epidemiology: direct tumor viruses must have at least one virus copy in every tumor cell expressing at least one protein or RNA that is causing the cell to become cancerous. Because foreign virus antigens are expressed in these tumors, persons who are immunosuppressed such as AIDS or transplant patients are at higher risk for these types of cancers. Chronic indirect tumor viruses, on the other hand, can be lost (at least theoretically) from a mature tumor that has accumulated sufficient mutations and growth conditions (hyperplasia) from the chronic inflammation of viral infection. In this latter case, it is controversial but at least theoretically possible that an indirect tumor virus could undergo 'hit-and-run' and so the virus would be lost from the clinically diagnosed tumor. In practical terms, this is an uncommon occurrence if it does occur.

RNA Virus

An RNA virus is a virus that has RNA (ribonucleic acid) as its genetic material. This nucleic acid is usually single-stranded RNA (ssRNA), but may be double-stranded RNA (dsRNA). Notable human diseases caused by RNA viruses include Ebola hemorrhoragic fever, SARS, influenza, hepatitis C, West Nile fever, polio, and measles.

The ICTV classifies RNA viruses as those that belong to Group III, Group IV or Group V of the Baltimore classification system of classifying viruses, and does not consider viruses with DNA intermediates in their life cycle as RNA viruses. Viruses with RNA as their genetic material but that include DNA intermediates in their replication cycle are called retroviruses, and comprise Group VI of the Baltimore classification. Notable human retroviruses include HIV-1 and HIV-2, the cause of the disease AIDS. Another term for RNA viruses that explicitly excludes retroviruses is ribovirus.

Single-stranded RNA viruses and RNA Sense

RNA viruses can be further classified according to the sense or polarity of their RNA into negative-sense and positive-sense, or ambisense RNA viruses. Positive-sense viral RNA is similar to mRNA and thus can be immediately translated by the host cell. Negative-sense viral RNA is complementary to mRNA and thus must be converted to positive-sense RNA by an RNA polymerase before translation. As such, purified RNA of a positive-sense virus can directly cause infection though it may be less infectious than the whole virus particle. Purified RNA of a negative-sense virus is not infectious by itself as it needs to be transcribed into positive-sense RNA, each virion can be transcribed to several positive-sense RNAs. Ambisense RNA viruses resemble negative-sense RNA viruses, except they also translate genes from the positive strand.

Double-stranded RNA viruses

The double-stranded (ds)RNA viruses represent a diverse group of viruses that vary widely in host range (humans, animals, plants, fungi, and bacteria), genome segment number (one to twelve), and virion organisation (T-number, capsid layers, or turrets). Members of this group include the rotaviruses, renowned globally as the most common cause of gastroenteritis in young children, and picobirnaviruses, renowned worldwide as the most commonly occurring virus in fecal samples of both humans and animals with or without signs of diarrhea. Picobirnaviruses have also been recently reported in respiratory tract samples of pigs and bluetongue virus, an economically important pathogen of cattle and sheep. In recent years, remarkable progress has been made in determining, at atomic and subnanometeric levels, the structures of a number of key viral proteins and of the virion capsids of several dsRNA viruses, highlighting the significant parallels in the structure and replicative processes of many of these viruses.

Mutation rates

RNA viruses generally have very high mutation rates compared to DNA viruses, because viral RNA polymerases lack the proof-reading ability of DNA polymerases. This is one reason why it is difficult to make effective vaccines to prevent diseases caused by RNA viruses. Retroviruses also have a high mutation rate even though their DNA intermediate integrates into the host genome (and is thus subject to host DNA proofreading once integrated), because errors during reverse transcription are embedded into both strands of DNA before integration. Some genes of RNA virus are important to the viral replication cycles and mutations are not tolerated. For example, the region of the hepatitis C virus genome that encodes the core protein is highly conserved, because it contains an RNA structure involved in an internal ribosome entry site.

Replication

Animal RNA viruses are classified into three distinct groups depending on their genome and mode of replication (and the numerical groups based on the older Baltimore classification):

- Double-stranded RNA viruses (Group III) contain from one to a dozen different RNA molecules, each coding for one or more viral proteins.
- Positive-sense ssRNA viruses (Group IV) have their genome directly utilised as if it were mRNA, with host ribosomes translating it into a single protein that is modified by host and viral proteins to form the various proteins needed for replication. One of these includes RNA-dependent RNA polymerase (RNA replicase), which copies the viral RNA to form a double-stranded replicative form. In turn this directs the formation of new virions.
- Negative-sense ssRNA viruses (Group V) must have their genome copied by an RNA replicase to form positive-sense RNA. This means that the virus must bring along with it the RNA replicase enzyme. The positive-sense RNA molecule then acts as viral mRNA, which is translated into proteins by the host ribosomes. The resultant protein goes on to direct the synthesis of new virions, such as capsid proteins and RNA replicase, which is used to produce new negative-sense RNA molecules.

Retroviruses (Group VI) have a single-stranded RNA genome but, in general, are not considered RNA viruses because they use DNA intermediates to replicate. Reverse transcriptase, a viral enzyme that comes from the virus itself after it is uncoated, converts the viral RNA into a complementary strand of DNA, which is copied to produce a double-stranded molecule of viral DNA. After this DNA is integrated into the host genome using the viral enzyme integrase, expression of the encoded genes may lead to the formation of new virions.

Classification of RNA viruses

Classification of the RNA viruses has proven to be a difficult problem. This is in part due to the high mutation rates these genomes undergo. Classification is based principally on the type of genome (double-stranded, negative- or positive-single-strand) and gene number and organisation. Currently there are 5 orders and 47 families of RNA viruses recognised. There are also many unassigned species and genera. Related to but distinct from the RNA viruses are the viroids and the RNA satellite viruses. These are not currently classified as RNA viruses and are described on their own pages.

Positive strand RNA viruses

This is the single largest group of RNA viruses with 30 families. Attempts have been made to group these families in higher orders. These proposals were based on an analysis of the RNA polymerases and are still under consideration. To date, the suggestions proposed have not been broadly accepted because of doubts over the suitability of a single gene to determine the taxonomy of the clade. The proposed classification of positive-strand RNA viruses is based on the RNA-dependent RNA polymerase.

Three groups have been recognised:

1. Bymoviruses, comoviruses, nepoviruses, nodaviruses, picornaviruses, potyviruses, sobemoviruses and a subset of luteoviruses (beet western yellows virus and potato leafroll virus)—the picorna like group (Picornavirata).

2. Carmoviruses, dianthoviruses, flaviviruses, pestiviruses, tombusviruses, single-stranded RNA bacteriophages, hepatitis C virus and a subset of luteoviruses (barley yellow dwarf virus)—the flavi like group (Flavivirata).

3. Alphaviruses, carlaviruses, furoviruses, hordeiviruses, potexviruses, rubiviruses, tobraviruses, tricornaviruses, tymoviruses, apple chlorotic leaf spot virus, beet yellows virus and hepatitis E virus—the alpha like group (Rubivirata).

A division of the alpha-like (Sindbis-like) supergroup on the basis of a novel domain located near the N termini of the proteins involved in viral replication has been proposed. The two groups proposed are: the 'altovirus' group (alphaviruses, furoviruses, hepatitis E virus, hordeiviruses, tobamoviruses, tobraviruses, tricornaviruses and probably rubiviruses), and the 'typovirus' group (apple chlorotic leaf spot virus, carlaviruses, potexviruses and tymoviruses).

The alpha like supergroup can be further divided into three clades: the rubi-like, tobamo-like, and tymo-like viruses.

Additional work has identified five groups of positive-stranded RNA viruses containing four, three, three, three, and one orders, respectively. These fourteen orders contain 31 virus families (including 17 families of plant viruses) and 48 genera (including 30 genera of plant viruses). This analysis suggests that alphaviruses and flaviviruses can be separated into two families—the Togaviridae and Flaviridae, respectively—but suggests that other taxonomic assignments, such as the pestiviruses, hepatitis C virus, rubiviruses, hepatitis E virus, and arteriviruses, may be incorrect. The coronaviruses and toroviruses appear to be distinct families in distinct orders and not distinct genera of the same family as currently classified. The luteoviruses appear to be two families rather than one, and apple chlorotic leaf spot virus appears not to be a closterovirus but a new genus of the Potexviridae.

Evolution

The evolution of the picornaviruses based on an analysis of their RNA polymerases and helicases appears to date to the divergence of the eukaryotes. Their putative ancestors include the bacterial group II retroelements, the family of HtrA proteases and DNA bacteriophages.

Double-stranded RNA viruses

This analysis also suggests that the dsRNA viruses are not closely related to each other but instead belong to four additional classes—Birnaviridae, Cystoviridae, Partitiviridae, and Reoviridae—and one additional order (Totiviridae) of one of the classes of positive ssRNA viruses in the same subphylum as the positive-strand RNA viruses.

One study has suggested a that there are two large clades: One includes the Caliciviridae, Flaviviridae, and Picornaviridae families and a second that includes the Alphatetraviridae, Birnaviridae and Cystoviridae, Nodaviridae, and Permutotretra-viridae families.

Group III—dsRNA viruses

There are nine families and a number of unassigned genera and species recognised in this group.

- Family Birnaviridae

- Family Chrysoviridae
- Family Cystoviridae
- Family Endornaviridae
- Family Hypoviridae
- Family Megabirnaviridae
- Family Partitiviridae
- Family Picobirnaviridae
- Family Reoviridae—includes Rotavirus
- Family Totiviridae
- Unassigned species
  - › Botrytis porri RNA virus 1
  - › Circulifer tenellus virus 1
  - › Cucurbit yellows associated virus
  - › Sclerotinia sclerotiorum debilitation-associated virus
  - › Spissistilus festinus virus 1

Group IV—positive-sense ssRNA viruses

There are three orders and 33 families recognised in this group. In addition, there are a number of unclassified species and genera.

- Order Nidovirales
  - › Family Arteriviridae
  - › Family Coronaviridae—includes Coronavirus, SARS
  - › Family Mesoniviridae
  - › Family Roniviridae
- Order Picornavirales
  - › Family Dicistroviridae
  - › Family Iflaviridae
  - › Family Marnaviridae
  - › Family Picornaviridae—includes Poliovirus, Rhinovirus (a common cold virus), Hepatitis A virus
  - › Family Secoviridae includes subfamily Comovirinae
  - › Genus Bacillariornavirus
  - › Genus Labyrnavirus
- Order Tymovirales
  - › Family Alphaflexiviridae
  - › Family Betaflexiviridae
  - › Family Gammaflexiviridae
  - › Family Tymoviridae
- Unassigned

> Family Alphatetraviridae
> Family Alvernaviridae
> Family Astroviridae
> Family Barnaviridae
> Family Bromoviridae
> Family Caliciviridae—includes Norwalk virus
> Family Carmotetraviridae
> Family Closteroviridae
> Family Flaviviridae—includes Yellow fever virus, West Nile virus, Hepatitis C virus, Dengue fever virus
> Family Leviviridae
> Family Luteoviridae—includes Barley yellow dwarf virus
> Family Narnaviridae
> Family Nodaviridae
> Family Permutotetraviridae
> Family Potyviridae
> Family Togaviridae—includes Rubella virus, Ross River virus, Sindbis virus, Chikungunya virus
> Family Tombusviridae
> Family Virgaviridae
- Unassigned genera
  > Genus Benyvirus
  > Genus Blunervirus
  > Genus Cilevirus
  > Genus Hepevirus—includes Hepatitis E virus
  > Genus Higrevirus
  > Genus Idaeovirus
  > Genus Negevirus
  > Genus Ourmiavirus
  > Genus Polemovirus
  > Genus Sobemovirus
  > Genus Umbravirus
- Unassigned species
  > Acyrthosiphon pisum virus
  > Blueberry necrotic ring blotch virus
  > Botrytis virus F
  > Canine picodicistrovirus
  > Chronic bee paralysis associated satellite virus

> Extra small virus
> Heterocapsa circularisquama RNA virus
> Kelp fly virus
> Le Blanc virus
> Plasmopara halstedii virus
> Orsay virus
> Rosellinia necatrix fusarivirus 1
> Santeuil virus
> Solenopsis invicta virus 2
> Solenopsis invicta virus 3

Group V—negative-sense ssRNA viruses

There is one order and eight families recognised in this group. There are also a number of unassigned species and genera.

- Order Mononegavirales
  > Family Bornaviridae—Borna disease virus
  > Family Filoviridae—includes Ebola virus, Marburg virus
  > Family Paramyxoviridae—includes Measles virus, Mumps virus, Nipah virus, Hendra virus, RSV and NDV
  > Family Rhabdoviridae—includes Rabies virus
  > Family Nyamiviridae—includes Nyavirus
- Unassigned families:
  > Family Arenaviridae—includes Lassa virus
  > Family Bunyaviridae—includes Hantavirus, Crimean-Congo hemorrhagic fever
  > Family Ophioviridae
  > Family Orthomyxoviridae—includes Influenza viruses
- Unassigned genera:
  > Genus Deltavirus—includes Hepatitis D virus
  > Genus Dichorhavirus
  > Genus Emaravirus
  > Genus Nyavirus—includes Nyamanini and Midway viruses
  > Genus Tenuivirus
  > Genus Varicosavirus
- Unassigned species:
  > Taastrup virus
  > Sclerotinia sclerotiorum negative-stranded RNA virus 1

Notes: The majority of fungal viruses are double-stranded RNA viruses. A small number of positive-strand RNA viruses have been described. One report has suggested the possibility of a negative stranded virus.

MORPHOLOGY AND GENERAL PROPERTIES OF VIRUSES

Viruses occupy the twilight zone that separates the 'living' from the 'non-living'. They do not have a cellular organisation and contain only one type of nucleic acid, either DNA or RNA but never both.

The medical importance of viruses lies in their ability to cause a very large number of human diseases. Viral diseases range from minor ailments like common cold to terrifying diseases like rabies and AIDS. In this section, we shall be discussing the morphology and general properties of viruses.

Concept of Viruses in Relation to Other Organisms

Viruses occupy the twilight zone that separates the 'living' from the 'non-living'. They do not have a cellular organisation and contain only one type of nucleic acid, either DNA or RNA but never both. Viruses are obligate intracellular parasites. They lack the enzymes necessary for protein and nucleic acid synthesis. They are dependent for replication on the synthetic machinery of host cells. They multiply by a complex process and not by binary fission. They are unaffected by antibacterial antibiotics.

Morphology of Viruses

Size: The extracellular infectious virus particle is called virion. Viruses are much smaller than bacteria. They are too small to be seen under the light microscope. Some large viruses like the poxviruses can be seen under the light microscope when suitably stained.

The viruses range in size from 20 nm to 300 nm. Poxviruses are one of the largest viruses and parvoviruses are one of the smallest viruses. The earliest method of estimating the size of virus particles was by passing them through collodion membrane filters of graded porosity. The average pore diameter of the finest filter that permitted passage of the virion gave an estimate of its size. With the development of the ultracentrifuge, a second method became available. From the rate of sedimentation of the virus in the ultracentrifuge, the particle size could be calculated using Stoke's law. The third and the most direct method of measuring virus size is electron microscopy. By this method, both the shape and size of virions can be studied.

Structure, shape and symmetry: The virion consists essentially of a nucleic acid surrounded by a protein coat, the capsid. The capsid with the enclosed nucleic acid is called the nucleocapsid. The capsid protects the nucleic acid from harmful agents in the environment. It is composed of a large number of capsomers which form its morphological units. The chemical units of the capsid are polypeptide molecules which are arranged symmetrically. They form a shell around the nucleic acid.

Chemical properties: Viruses contain only one type of nucleic acid, either DNA or RNA. Viruses are unique because they carry genetic information on RNA. This property is not seen in any other organism in nature. Viruses also contain protein which makes up the capsid. Enveloped viruses contain lipids derived from the host cell membrane. Most viruses do not have enzymes for the synthesis of viral components or for energy production. Some viruses have enzymes, for example the influenza virus has neuraminidase.

Resistance: Viruses are destroyed by heat except a few. They are stable at low temperatures. For long term storage, they are kept at –70°C. A better method for prolonged storage is lyophilisation or freeze-drying. Viruses are inactivated by sunlight, UV rays and ionising radiation. They are, in general, more resistant than bacteria to chemical disinfectants. Phenolic disinfectants have a weak action on viruses.

Multiplication of Viruses

Multiplication of viruses is called viral replication. Viruses contain the genetic information for their replication but they lack the enzymes. They depend on host cell machinery for replication. The viral replication cycle can be divided into six phases – adsorption, penetration, uncoating, biosynthesis, maturation and release.

Adsorption: In this phase, the virus gets attached to the host cell. The host cell should have specific receptors on its surface. These receptors recognise viral surface components. This cell-virus interaction helps the virus to attach to the host cell surface.

Penetration: In this phase, the virus enters into the host cell. Bacteria have rigid cell wall. So, viruses which infect bacteria cannot penetrate into the bacterial cell. Only the nucleic acid of the virus enters the bacterial cell. Animal and human cells do not have cell walls. Therefore, whole virus enters the cell. Virus particle may be engulfed by a process called viropexis. In case of enveloped viruses, the viral envelope may fuse with the cell membrane of the host cell. Then the nucleocapsid is released into the cytoplasm.

Uncoating: This is the process in which the outer layers and capsid of the virus are removed. This mostly occurs by the action of lysosomal enzymes of the host cell. This can also occur by a viral uncoating enzyme. Finally, the viral nucleic acid is released into the cell.

Biosynthesis: In this phase, the viral nucleic acid and capsid are synthesised. The enzymes necessary in the various stages of viral synthesis, assembly and release are also synthesised. Certain 'regulator proteins' are synthesised.

They shut down the normal metabolism of the host cell. They direct the production of viral components. In general, most DNA viruses synthesise their nucleic acid in the host cell nucleus. Exceptions are the poxviruses. They are DNA viruses, but they synthesise all their components in the host cell cytoplasm. Most RNA viruses synthesise all their components in the cytoplasm. Orthomyxoviruses and some paramyxoviruses are exceptions. They synthesise some components in the host cell nucleus. Biosynthesis consists essentially of the following steps:

1. Transcription of messenger RNA (mRNA) from the viral nucleic acid.
2. Translation of mRNA into 'early proteins' or 'non-structural proteins'. They are enzymes responsible for the synthesis of viral components.
3. Replication of viral nucleic acid.
4. Synthesis of 'late proteins' or 'structural proteins'. They are the components of daughter virion capsids.

Maturation: This is the assembly of daughter virions following the synthesis of viral nucleic acid and proteins. It can take place in the host cell nucleus or cytoplasm. Herpesviruses and adenoviruses are assembled in the nucleus. Picornaviruses and poxviruses are assembled in the nucleus.

Release: Viruses which infect bacteria (bacteriophages) are released by lysis of the infected bacterium. Animal viruses are usually released without cell lysis. Myxoviruses are released by budding from the cell membrane. The host cell is unaffected. Daughter virions are released into the surrounding medium and may infect other cells. In some viruses (for, e.g. varicella), transmission occurs directly from cell to cell. In this case, there is very little free virus in the medium. The poliovirus causes cell damage and may be released by cell lysis.

From the stage of penetration till the appearance of mature daughter virions, the virus cannot be demonstrated inside the host cell. During this period, the virus seems to disappear. This is called the 'eclipse phase'. The time taken for a single cycle of replication is about 15–30 minutes for bacteriophages. It is about 15–30 hours for animal viruses. A single infected cell may release a large number of progeny virions.

Methods of Cultivation of Viruses

Viruses are obligate intracellular parasites. They donot grow on culture media used for bacteria. The methods used for cultivation of viruses are:

1. Animal inoculation: Monkeys were used for the isolation of the poliovirus by Landsteiner and Popper in 1909. Infant mice are used for the isolation of coxsackievirus and arboviruses (dengue, chikungunya). Mice may be inoculated by several routes–intracerebral, subcutaneous, intraperitoneal or subcutaneous. Other animals like guinea pigs, rabbits and ferrets are used in some situations.

2. Embryonated eggs: The embryonated hen's egg was first used for the cultivation of viruses by Goodpasture in 1931. This method was further developed by Burnet. Different parts of the egg are used for the cultivation of different viruses. Herpes simplex virus, when inoculated into the chorioallantoic membrane, produces visible lesions called pocks. Inoculation into the amniotic sac is done for the isolation of influenza virus. Yolk sac inoculation is done for the isolation of rabies virus.

3. Cell culture: Probably, the first application of tissue culture in virology was by Steinhardt and colleagues in 1913. They maintained the vaccinia virus in fragments of rabbit cornea. The turning point was the cultivation of poliovirus which was demonstrated by Enders, Weller and Robbins in 1949.

They showed that poliovirus, till then considered a strictly neurotropic virus, could be grown in tissue culture of non-neural origin.

The various types of tissue cultures are described as follows:

Organ culture: Small bits of organs can be maintained *in vitro* for days and weeks, preserving their original architecture and function. Organ culture is useful for viruses which are highly specialised parasites of certain organs. For example, tracheal ring organ culture is used for the isolation of coronavirus, a respiratory pathogen.

Explant culture: Fragments of minced tissue can be grown as 'explants' embedded in plasma clots. They may also be cultivated in suspension. Adenoid tissue explant cultures were used for the isolation of adenovirus.

Cell culture: This is routinely used for growing viruses. Tissues are dissociated into the component cells by the action of enzymes and mechanical shaking. The cells are washed, counted and suspended in a growth medium. The growth medium consists of essential amino acids, glucose, vitamins, salts and a buffer. Antibiotics are added to prevent bacterial contamination. The cell suspension is put into bottles, tubes and petridishes. The cells adhere to the glass or plastic surface, divide and form a confluent monolayer sheet within a week. Cell culture is further classified on the basis of origin, chromosomal characters and the number of generations through which they can be maintained. It is of three types– primary cell culture, diploid cell strain and continuous cell lines. Primary cell cultures are normal cells freshly taken from the body and cultured. They are capable of only limited growth in culture. They cannot be maintained in serial culture. Examples are monkey kidney, human embryonic kidney and chick embryo cell cultures. Diploid cell strains are cells of a single type that retain the original diploid chromosome number and karyotype during serial subcultivation for a limited number of times. After about fifty serial passages, they undergo 'senescence'.

Diploid strains developed from human fibroblasts are a good example. Continuous cell lines are cells of a single type, usually derived from cancer cells. They are capable of continuous serial cultivation indefinitely. Hela cell lines are derived from carcinoma of the cervix. Cell culture is used for the isolation of viruses and their cultivation for vaccine production.

Viruses in cell cultures can be detected by various methods like cytopathic effect, special staining techniques and detection of viral nucleic acid by molecular techniques like polymerase chain reaction (PCR). Cytopathic effect is the morphological change in the cultured cells which is produced by the virus growing in those cells. These changes can be seen by microscopic examination of the cell cultures.

The cytopathic effects (CPE) produced by different groups of viruses are characteristic and help in the presumptive identification of virus isolates. For example, measles virus produces syncytium formation, adenovirus produces large granular clumps resembling bunches of grapes, enteroviruses produce crenation of cells and degeneration of the entire cell sheet.

RETROVIRUS

Retroviridae is a family of enveloped viruses that replicate in a host cell through the process of reverse transcription. A retrovirus is a single-stranded RNA virus that stores its nucleic acid in the form of an mRNA genome (including the 5′ cap and 3′ PolyA tail) and, as an obligate parasite, targets a host cell. Once inside the host cell cytoplasm, the virus uses its own reverse transcriptase enzyme to produce DNA from its RNA genome, the reverse of the usual pattern, thus retro (backwards). This new DNA is then incorporated into the host cell genome by an integrase enzyme, at which point the retroviral DNA is referred to as a provirus. The host cell then treats the viral DNA as part of its own genome, translating and transcribing the viral genes along with the cell's own genes, producing the proteins required to assemble new copies of the virus. It is difficult to detect the virus until it has infected the host. At that point, the infection will persist indefinitely. In most viruses, DNA is transcribed into RNA, and then RNA is translated into protein.

However, retroviruses function differently–their RNA is reverse-transcribed into DNA, which is integrated into the host cell's genome (when it becomes a provirus), and then undergoes the usual transcription and translational processes to express the genes carried by the virus. So, the information contained in a retroviral gene is used to generate the corresponding protein via the sequence: RNA → DNA → RNA → polypeptide. This extends the fundamental process identified by Francis Crick, (one gene-one peptide), in which the sequence is: DNA → RNA → peptide, (proteins are made of one or more polypeptide chain, e.g. haemoglobin is a four chain peptide). Retroviruses are proving to be valuable research tools in molecular biology and have been used successfully in gene delivery systems.

Multiplication

When retroviruses have integrated their own genome into the germ line, their genome is passed on to a following generation. These endogenous retroviruses (ERVs), contrasted with exogenous ones, now make up 5–8% of the human genome. Most insertions have no known function and are often referred to as 'junk DNA'. However, many endogenous retroviruses play important roles in host biology, such as control of gene transcription, cell fusion during placental development in the course of the germination of an embryo, and resistance to exogenous retroviral infection. Endogenous retroviruses have also received special attention in the research of immunology-related pathologies, such as autoimmune diseases like multiple sclerosis, although endogenous retroviruses have not yet been proven to play any causal role in this class of disease.

While transcription was classically thought to occur only from DNA to RNA, reverse transcriptase transcribes RNA into DNA. The term 'retro' in retrovirus refers to this reversal (making DNA from RNA) of the central dogma of molecular biology. Reverse transcriptase activity outside of retroviruses has been found in almost all eukaryotes, enabling the generation and insertion of new copies of retrotransposons into the host genome. These inserts are transcribed by enzymes of the host into new RNA molecules that enter the cytosol. Next, some of these RNA molecules are translated into viral proteins. For example, the gag gene is translated into molecules of the capsid protein, the pol gene is translated into molecules of reverse transcriptase, and the env gene is translated into molecules of the envelope protein. It is important to note that a retrovirus must 'bring' its own reverse transcriptase in its capsid, otherwise it is unable to utilise the enzymes of the infected cell to carry out the task, due to the unusual nature of producing DNA from RNA.

Industrial drugs that are designed as protease and reverse transcriptase inhibitors are made such that they target specific sites and sequences within their respective enzymes. However these drugs can quickly become ineffective due to the fact that the gene sequences that code for the protease and the reverse transcriptase quickly mutate. These changes in bases cause specific codons and sites with the enzymes to change and thereby avoid drug targeting by losing the sites that the drug actually targets. Because reverse transcription lacks the usual proofreading of DNA replication, a retrovirus mutates very often. This enables the virus to grow resistant to antiviral pharmaceuticals quickly, and impedes the development of effective vaccines and inhibitors for the retrovirus. One drawback of retroviruses, such as the Moloney retrovirus, involves the requirement for cells to be actively dividing for transduction. As a result, cells such as neurons are very resistant to infection and transduction by retroviruses. There is concern that insertional mutagenesis due to integration into the host genome might lead to cancer or leukemia. This is unlike Lentivirus, a genus of Retroviridae, which are able to integrate their RNA into the genome of non-dividing host cells.

Cancer

Retroviruses that cause tumour growth include Rous sarcoma virus and Mouse mammary tumour virus. Cancer can be triggered by proto-oncogenes that were mistakenly incorporated into proviral DNA or by the disruption of cellular proto-oncogenes. Rous sarcoma virus contains the src gene that triggers tumour formation. Later it was found that a similar gene in cells is involved in cell signalling, which was most likely excised with the proviral DNA. Nontransforming viruses can randomly insert their DNA into proto-oncogenes, disrupting the expression of proteins that regulate the cell cycle. The promoter of the provirus DNA can also cause over expression of regulatory genes. Phylogeny of retroviruses is shown in Fig. 18.11.

METHODS FOR DETECTING PROTEIN–RNA INTERACTIONS

Proteins interact with RNA through electrostatic interactions, hydrogen bonding, hydrophobic interactions and base stacking in a manner similar to protein–DNA interactions. Protein–RNA interactions are also significantly influenced by the tertiary structure on the RNA molecules. Therefore, in assays to identify

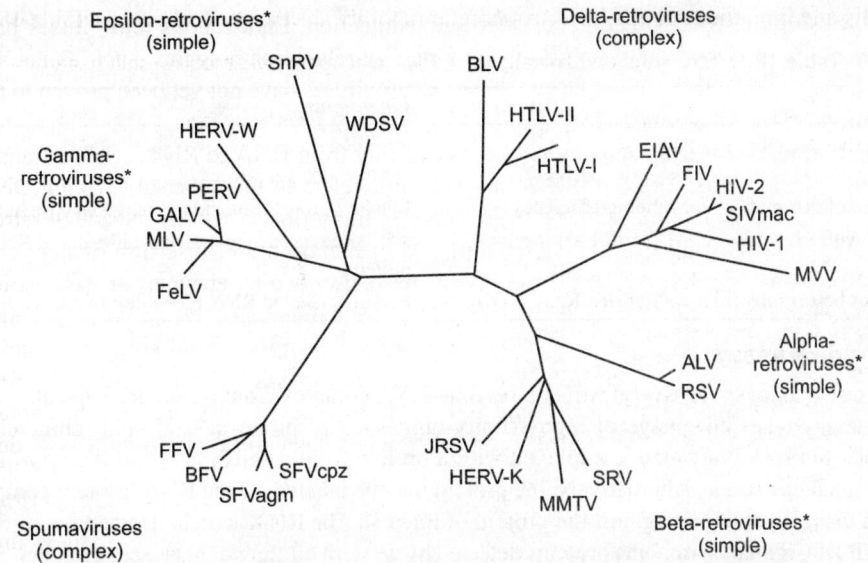

Fig. 18.11: Phylogeny of retroviruses.

protein–RNA interactions, both the RNA and protein(s) must be correctly folded to allow proper binding. RNA is very susceptible to degradation, so special care must be taken not to introduce RNases into the reaction. Protein–RNA interactions are required to both transport a messenger RNA molecule into the cytoplasm of a eukaryotic cell and for formation of the translation machinery.

The rate of translation and stability of RNA are also influenced by protein–RNA interactions as well as RNA–RNA interactions. The most common methods for studying protein–RNA interactions are discussed in this article.

RNA Electrophoretic Mobility Shift Assay (EMSA)

The RNA electrophoretic mobility shift assay (RNA EMSA) is an *in vitro* technique used to detect protein–RNA interactions through changes in migration speed during gel electrophoresis. First, a labeled RNA probe is incubated with a protein sample (typically from a cell lysate) to initiate binding and formation of the interaction complex. The binding reaction is then separated via non-denaturing polyacrylamide gel electrophoresis.

Like protein–DNA complexes, a protein–RNA complex migrates more slowly than a free RNA probe through a gel matrix. This causes a migration shift relative to the unbound RNA probe. Specificity is determined through a competition reaction, where excess unlabeled RNA is incubated in the binding reaction, resulting in a decrease in the shifted signal if the labeled and unlabeled RNA sequences compete for binding of the same protein.

Alternatively, the protein–RNA complex may be crosslinked and the reaction run on a denaturing gel. Specificity is determined through visualisation of a single shifted band. Traditionally, RNA probes are radioactively labeled for detection, although fluorescent and chemiluminescent detection is also possible. Non-radioactive RNA end-labelling techniques are limited, but more versatile biotin and fluorescent labelling methods are now available.

Strengths and limitations of RNA electrophoretic mobility shift assay is shown in Table 18.1.

Table 18.1: Strengths and limitations of RNA electrophoretic mobility shift assay.

Strengths	Limitations
Non-radioactive detection available	Homebrew experiments require significant reagent optimisation for success
Easy to screen RNA mutants for binding efficiency	Lengthy protocol including native electrophoresis step
Compatible with RNA labeled via runoff transcription	Antibodies needed to determine identity of RNA-binding protein
reactions, but best results from end-labeled RNA probes	Requires labeled RNA probe design and synthesis

RNA Pull-down Assays

RNA pull-down assays selectively extract a protein–RNA complex from a sample. Typically, the RNA pull-down assay takes advantage of high affinity tags, such as biotin or azido-phosphine chemistry. RNA probes can be biotinylated, complexed with a protein from a cell lysate, and then purified using agarose or magnetic beads. Alternatively, the protein may be labeled, or the RNA–protein complex may be isolated using an antibody against the protein of interest. The RNA is then detected by northern blot or through RT-PCR analysis and the proteins detected by western blotting or mass spectrometry. Strengths and limitations of RNA pull-down assays is shown in Table 18.2.

Table 18.2: Strengths and limitations of RNA pull-down assays.

Strengths	Limitations
Enrichment of low abundant targets	RNA secondary structure is important for function, so end-labelling is preferred
Isolation of intact complexes	Inefficient elution from the resin
Compatible with immunoblotting and mass spectrometry analysis	Nuclease-free conditions with the beads/resin

Oligonucleotide-targeted RNase H Protection Assays

The RNase protection assay (RPA) is a powerful method for detecting RNA and RNA fragments in cell extracts. Unlike northern blotting or RT-PCR analysis, RPA assays allow greater flexibility in the integrity of target RNA, requiring very short segments for hybridisation and detection. RPA assays can also be used to map protein–RNA interactions. In this adaptation of the RPA, RNase H is used to cleave a target RNA molecule at a specific site hybridised with a DNA probe. If a protein is bound to the RNA at the target sequence, it will block probe hybridisation, prevent cleavage by RNase H, and indicate a site of interaction between protein and RNA. RNase H requires only a four base pair hybrid with a DNA probe in order to cleave the RNA molecule of interest. Using many small probes allows the entire sequence of RNA to be mapped for sites of interaction. Oligonucleotide-targeted RNase H protection assays is shown in Table 18.3.

Table 18.3: Oligonucleotide-targeted RNase H protection assays.

Strengths	Limitations
Can be used for *in vitro* assays and crude cell extracts	Many probes required for detailed mapping
Allows detailed mapping of protein–RNA interactions	Difficult to optimise for rare RNA molecules
Can be used to for functional and mutational studies	Not compatible with high-throughput analysis

Fluorescent *In situ* Hybridisation Co-localisation

Fluorescent *in situ* hybridisation (FISH/ISH) co-localisation techniques require detection of both a RNA transcript and a protein of interest using RNA probes and antibodies. FISH/ISH detects the position and abundance of a RNA and protein in a cell or tissue sample. The readout is visual (usually imaged via microscopy), and a co-localised signal for both the RNA and protein of interest indicate possible complex formation. A labeled RNA probe must be generated for detection of a particular sequence of RNA, and the protein may be detected using antibody staining or fluorescent protein constructs. Fluorescent *in situ* hybridisation co-localisation is shown in Table 18.4.

Table 18.4: Fluorescent *in situ* hybridisation co-localisation.

Strengths	*Limitations*
Provides a snapshot of RNA–protein interactions as they occur *in vivo*	Tedious procedure, requiring denaturation, hybridisation and detection
Possible to multiplex with different substrates	Detection usually requires signal amplification
Delivers publication quality images	Cells/tissue must be preserved
	Quantitative software is necessary to determine co-localisation

Traditional FISH techniques using large oligonucleotide sequences labeled with one to five fluorophores are generally limited by high background and low sensitivity due to nonspecific binding and insufficient signal amplification. Invitrogen ViewRNA assays incorporate a proprietary probe set design and branched DNA (bDNA) signal amplification technology. A target-specific probe set of approximately 20 oligonucleotide pairs hybridises to the target RNA of interest. Signal amplification is achieved through specific hybridisation of adjacent oligonucleotide pairs to bDNA structures, which are formed by pre-amplifiers, amplifiers, and fluorochrome-conjugated label probes. This methodology results in greater specificity, lower background and higher signal-to-noise ratios.

NUCLEIC ACID ELECTROPHORESIS

Electrophoretic techniques have become the principle means for analysing and characterising recombinant DNA molecules. Both agarose (a linear polysach. of galactose and a 3,6-anhydrogalactose, cross-linked by hydrogen bonding) and polyacrilamide gels are used to separated DNA electrophoretically (following restriction digestion).

Principle of Gel Electrophoresis

Electrophoresis is the migration of charged particles or molecules in an electric field. This occurs when the substances are in aqueous solution. The speed of migration is dependent on the applied electric field strength and the charges of the molecules. Thus, differently charged molecules will form individual zones while they migrate. In order to keep diffusion of the zones to a minimum, electrophoresis is carried out in an anticonvective medium such as a viscous fluid or a gel matrix. Therefore, the speed of migration is also dependent on the size of the molecules. In this way fractionation of a mixture of substances is achieved with high resolution.

Principles of Electrophoresis

Molecules are resolved on the basis of size (mass or length), shape or conformation, magnitude of the net charge.

At neutral pH values, due to the ionised (negatively charged) phosphate groups of the phosphor-sugar backbone of DNA and RNA, they will migrate to the positive electrode called the anion in an electrical field. dsDNA have roughly the same net charge to mass ratio and will migrate to the anode at equal velocities. The viscosity (degree of cross-linking) of the medium affects the friction thus, molecular shape can be utilised to separated nucleic acids by size. The velocity is influenced by the size of the molecule and the pore. It is fairly independent of base composition or sequence.

- Agarose concentration: 3–0.1% (70–800,000bp).
- Polyacrilamide: 20–30% (6–1000bp)

Visualising DNA Molecules

Ethidium Bromide fluoresces when irradiated with UV light wavelength of 300nm. It can also intercalate between the stacked bases of RNA and DNA. The dye does not bind to agarose or polyacrilamide polymers. Illumination at 254 nm causes photo-nicking, dimerisation and rapid bleaching of the complex. Viewing at 302 nm is preferred, but does not give the same sensitivity as 254 nm for detection of faint bands.

- Eyes should be protected from UV light at all times.
- The intensity of the fluorescence is directly proportional to the size of the DNA fragments.
- The smallest amount of DNA detectable of any size class is less than 1 nanogram.
- EtBr, when bound to circular DNA, will convert the relaxed circle to a supercoiled molecule.
- DNA fragment migration is generally reduced by 10–15% by EtBr.
- The dye is added directly to the buffer to a concentration between 0.5 and 1.0 ug/ml.
- EtBr is a powerful mutagen and potential carcinogen. Always wear gloves manipulating gels. Do not dispose in sink.
- Photography: Digital image over a UV long-wave transilluminator is used to take pictures.

Tracking Dye Solution or Stop Mix

Serves three important functions:

1. Terminate enzymatic reactions.
2. A convenient means to load samples on the gel.
3. Monitor the progress of the electrophoresis.
   Usually contains:

- SDS or Urea to denature proteins.
- Ficoll or glycerol for viscosity.
- Ddye such as bromophenol blue.

Size Markers for Gels

- Bromophenol blue is used as a fairly accurate size marker for small DNA fragments.
- For accurate size estimation it is necessary to have a range of DNA fragments of known size.

Electrophoresis Conditions

- Run at room temperature (usually no cooling is needed).
- The same situation holds for gel length and gel concentration.

- If overheating occurs, the DNA bands can be distorted. Overheating depends upon gel dimensions and current.
- The optimal running current depends upon the degree of resolution, fragment size, and time. A balance has to be struck between sharpness and separation.

Electrophoretic Mobility

The electrophoretic mobility is dependent on external factors like electric field strength, viscosity, gel concentration and temperature, and intrinsic properties of the molecule like charge density, size and hydrophobicity. While proteins can be separated according to their net charges or their sizes, nucleic acid molecules are only distinguishable on size-based separations in which the properties of the separation medium have a large influence on the distribution of the zones.

Buffers

Electrophoretic separation is performed in buffers with a constant pH value and constant ionic strength. During electrophoresis, the buffer ions are carried through the gel just like the sample ions: negatively charged ions toward the anode, positively charged ones toward the cathode. To guarantee constant pH and buffer conditions, the supply of electrode buffers must be sufficient. For nucleic acids the mostly used buffer is composed of tris(hydroxymethyl)-aminoethane, borate and ethylenediaminetetraacetic acid (EDTA).

Joule Heat

Some of the electrical energy is transformed into Joule heat. Development of Joule heat is increased with high buffer concentrations. In order to prevent overheating effects, buffer strength and electric field strength must be limited, and – mostly for polyacrylamide gels – thermostating of the gels provides a homogeneous temperature distribution. When the conditions are not chosen correctly, a so-called 'smiling effect' will occur: the electrophoretic mobilities of ions are higher in the hot center of the gel plate than at the cooler lateral sides.

Gel Medium

The gel medium prevents diffusion and thermal convection of the zones, and serves as a molecular sieve. Two gel types are employed: agarose and polyacrylamide gels. Agarose gels are used as thick layers in flatbed chambers mainly for preparative purposes, whereas polyacrylamide gels are applied in thin layers in vertical or cooled flatbed systems, mainly for highresolution techniques like sequencing and genotyping.

Electroendosmosis

The stabilising medium, particularly agarose, can contain fixed carboxylic and sulfonic groups. In the presence of basic and neutral buffers, these groups will become deprotonated and thus negatively charged. In the electric field, the fixed negative charges are attracted by the anode. They cannot migrate, because they are a part of the matrix. A counterflow of hydrated protons toward the cathode will result in compensation, this effect is termed electroendosmosis. In gels, electroendosmosis is observed as a flow of water toward the cathode, which carries some of the solubilised substances along. The electrophoretic and electroosmotic migrations are subtractive, which results in blurred zones. Drying of the gel in the area of the anode can also occur.

Agarose Gel Electrophoresis

Properties of agarose gels

Agarose is a polysaccharide obtained from red seaweed. The pore size depends on the concentration of agarose (weight of agarose per volume). Agarose is dissolved in boiling water and forms a gel during cooling. During this process, double helices are built, which are joined laterally to form relatively thick filaments. This fact allows the preparation of gels with large pore sizes and high mechanical stability. Gels with a pore size from 150 nm at 1% (w/v) to 500 nm at 0.16% are used. This allows separation of nucleic acid fragment sizes in the range between 400 and 23000 base pairs (bp). Different agarose qualities are available. They are characterised by their gelling temperature (down to 35°C), melting point (down to 60°C) and the degree of electroendosmosis. The degree of electroendosmosis is dependent on the number of polar groups remaining from agaropectin.

Running Conditions and Properties

Electrophoresis setup

Agarose gels are run in simply designed flatbed chambers under a buffer layer to prevent drying due to electroendosmosis. The temperature is only controlled by the applied running conditions. The nucleic acids are separated under native conditions. Quick checks of multiple samples are performed in 96-well agarose gels in microtiter plate format without a buffer layer.

Migration of deoxyribonucleic acid fragments

Because of the sieving properties of agarose gels, the relative mobilities of deoxyribonucleic acid (DNA) and ribonucleic acid (RNA) molecules are dependent on the sizes of the molecules. At a defined pore size of the agarose gel, there is – within a certain molecule size range – a linear relationship between the logarithms of the fragment lengths and the relative migration distances.

Under the influence of the electric field, nucleic acid molecules are stretched and migrate through gel pores like a snake with a reptating movement. Above a certain molecule length of about 20 kilobase pairs (kbp), the electrophoretic mobilities of DNA molecules are similar, because these long chains keep to the same orientation. When the applied field strength exceeds a certain value, the DNA molecules are so strongly stretched that they become rigid rods. This results in poor separation.

Staining of the Bands

The bands are visualised with fluorescent dyes that are visible in UV light – ethidium bromide or SYBR Green. SYBR Green is less mutagenic and more sensitive than ethidium bromide. The best results and highest resolutions are obtained when the gels are stained after the run. When dyes are added to the gel or the sample during electrophoresis, the mobilities of the DNA fragments will be modified and the resolution will suffer.

Between 100 pg and 1 ng per band are detected. The dyes intercalate in the helix and stain proportionately to the length of the molecule. Therefore the sensitivity is dependent on the size of the DNA fragment, and is lower for single-stranded DNA and RNA. For a permanent record of the separation, instant photos are taken on a UV table or video documentation systems are employed. Agarose electrophoresis is the standard method for DNA restriction fragment analysis and purification of DNA and RNA fragments.

Blotting and Hybridisation

For restriction fragment length polymorphism (RFLP) analysis, the separated DNA fragments are transferred onto an immobilising membrane followed by hybridisation with radiolabeled probes. The molecules are transferred onto nitrocellulose or nylon membranes with capillary forces. The fragments are probed with radioactive DNA or RNA. The bound complementary nucleic acids are detected by autoradiography.

Recovery of DNA Fragments from Gels

Several different procedures are used for the isolation of nucleic acids from agarose gels: electroelution, absorption to DEAE paper, absorption to glass powder or resins, digestion of agarose with enzymes. For preparative electrophoresis, it is very important to use highly purified agarose that is free from polymerase and other enzyme inhibitors. Since the advent of polymerase chain reaction (PCR) technology, tiny amounts of DNA fragments can easily be amplified for further experiments.

Pulsed Field Gel Electrophoresis

DNA fragments longer than about 20 kb cannot be resolved in conventional agarose gel electrophoresis because long DNA molecules align themselves as rods and migrate with a mobility that is independent of their length. In pulsed field gel electrophoresis (PFGE), the molecules are subjected to two alternating electrical fields that are applied on the gel at an angle between 110° and 180°. The DNA fragments must change their orientation with changes in the electric field: their helical structure is first compressed and then stretched. The 'viscoelastic relaxation time' is dependent on the size of the molecule. In addition, large molecules need more time to change their direction than small ones. Because of the longer time needed for stretching and reorientation, larger molecules have less timeleft formigration in the electric field. InPFGE, the resulting electrophoreticmobilities depend on the pulse time: DNA molecules with fragment sizes up to about 10 megabases (Mb) can be resolved.

Pulse times of 1 s to 90 min are applied, depending on the length of the DNA molecules being analysed. Large molecules are better separated with long pulse times, small molecules need short pulse times. Separations can take several days.

In order to prevent chromosome-size molecules breaking by shear forces during pipetting, sample preparation including cell disruption is carried out inside little agarose blocks. These agarose blocks are inserted into preformed sample wells of the separation gel.

Pulsed field gel electrophoresis at different angles

The directions of the applied electric fields must differ at least by an angle of 110°. This is achieved by different arrangements: inhomogeneous fields created with point electrodes, hexagonal electrode sets, turning electrodes or turning gel tables. The resulting migration direction is diagonal.

Field inversion gel electrophoresis

Field inversion gel electrophoresis (FIGE) is performed in a standard agarose gel electrophoresis apparatus. The electric fields are just alternating in the direction of 180°. The resulting migration in one direction is achieved by applying a higher field strength or a longer pulse time in the separation direction. The advantage of this method is the simple design. The disadvantage is the long separation time, because the molecules migrate backwards for part of the time. A wide range of sizes ofDNAmolecules can be resolved in such gels.

Applications of pulsed field gel electrophoresis

The field of application of this technique includes chromosome mapping, isolation of intact chromosomal and chromosomal-sized DNA, large restriction fragment mapping and karyotyping. With PFGE, physical gene maps are created for the identification of genes responsible for hereditary diseases. Another important area of application is bacterial taxonomy.

Polyacrylamide Gel Electrophoresis

Properties of polyacrylamide gels

Polyacrylamide gels are prepared by chemical copolymerisation of acrylamide monomers with a cross-linking reagent, usually *N,N'*-methylenebisacrylamide. A clear transparent gel is obtained, which is chemically inert, mechanically stable and without electroendosmosis. Polymerisation of the acrylamide monomers and the cross-linker molecules occurs in the presence of free radicals. These are provided by ammonium persulphate as catalyst, tertiary amino groups, usually *N, N, N', N'*-tetramethylethylenediamine (TEMED), are required as accelerators.

The pore size is exactly controlled with the total acrylamide concentration (T) and the degree of crosslinking (C), which is determined by the amount of cross-linker relative to the total amount of acrylamide. The pore size decreases with increasing T value. With increasing cross-linking, the pore size follows a parabolic function: at high and low cross-linking, the pores are large and the minimum pore size is obtained at 4% cross-linking. Sequencing gels contain 5% cross-linking and gels for single-strand conformation polymorphism (SSCP) analysis 2% cross-linking.

Acrylamide monomers are toxic and should be handled with caution. Because oxygen is a scavenger of free radicals, polymerisation is performed in closed cassettes. Sample application wells for vertical gels are formed at the upper edge of the gel during polymerisation with the help of an inserted comb. Sample wells for flatbed gels are made by using self-adhesive tape glued onto one of the glass plates.

Running Conditions and Properties

For electrophoresis in vertical systems, the complete gel cassettes are placed into the buffer tanks, the gels are in direct contact with the electrode buffers. Gels for flatbed systems are polymerised on a film support and removed from the cassette before use.

Native conditions

In nondenaturing polyacrylamide gels, the mobility of DNA fragments is dependent on both size and sequence. A- and T-rich nucleic acids migrate faster, because they undergo fewer hydrophobic interactions with the gel matrix than C- and G-rich fragments. Therefore, nondenaturing polyacrylamide gels cannot be used for the determination of fragment length, but they are very sensitive to conformation differences of the secondary structure. Very sharp bands are obtained. Single-nucleotide polymorphisms and point mutations are detected with high sensitivity.

Denaturing conditions

In the presence of high molar formamide or urea, and at elevated temperature above 50°C, the DNA molecules are completely denatured and exist as single strands. In this case, the electrophoretic mobilities are strictly size dependent. When thin gel layers are used, the resolution reaches single-base difference within a range of around 1000–1200 bases, which makes DNA sequencing possible.

Detection of bands

Staining

Ethidium bromide and SYBR Green staining are rarely used for polyacrylamide gels, because the signals are weaker than in agarose gels. With silver staining, very high sensitivity independent of molecular size is reached, down to 15 pg per band. The staining method requires several steps, staining automates are available. The chemicals are less toxic than intercalating dyes, there is no radioactivity, no UV light and no photography is needed for inspection of the results. Silver-stained bands can be directly reamplified with PCR without any intermediate purification step.

Radioactive labelling

Labelling with radioactive phosphorus (^{32}P) during transcription or replication is employed for various applications because of its very high sensitivity of detection. After the run, the gels are dried and exposed on X-ray film. The major applications are sequencing, amplified fragment length polymorphism (AFLP), differential display reverse transcription (DDRT) and two-dimensional DNA typing.

Fluorescence labelling

Labelling of the DNA fragments with Cy5 and other fluorophors has replaced radiolabelling for many applications. It allows online detection of the migrating zones. The dyes are excited with a laser beam, and the emitted light – with a different wavelength – is measured with a diode detector.

DNA Sequencing Gels

For increasing the reading length, long gels in very thin layers are optimal. In order to achieve a straight front and straight band distribution over the entire gel width, the gels are mostly heated with thermoplates. Fluorescent labelling has generally replaced radiolabelling, which makes the long ultrathin layer gels and wedge gels unnecessary.

Denaturing Gradient Gel Electrophoresis

Denaturing gradient gel electrophoresis (DGGE) affords the detection of single-base exchanges in segments of DNA. Gels are prepared with a gradient from no additive to 7 mol L^{-1} urea and 40% formamide, and run at about 60°C. The differences in melting cause two fragments of DNA, which slow down at different levels of the gel. The obtained pattern displays single-base differences.

Temperature Gradient Gel Electrophoresis

Similar effects to DGGE can be achieved with temperature gradient gel electrophoresis (TGGE). In this technique, denaturing gels are run on a differentially thermostated plate with a cold side (15°C) at the cathode and a hot side (60°C) at the anode. The technique is mainly used for screening purposes.

GEL ELECTROPHORESIS OF NUCLEIC ACIDS

Factors Affecting Migration of Nucleic Acids

A number of factors can affect the migration of nucleic acids: the dimension of the gel pores, the voltage used, the ionic strength of the buffer, and the concentration intercalating dye such as ethidium bromide if used during electrophoresis.

Size of DNA

The gel sieves the DNA by the size of the DNA molecule whereby smaller molecules travel faster. Double stranded DNA moves at a rate that is approximately inversely proportional to the logarithm of the number of base pairs. This relationship however breaks down with very large DNA fragments and it is not possible to separate them using standard agarose gel electrophoresis. The limit of resolution depends on gel composition and field strength. and the mobility of larger circular DNA may be more strongly affected than linear DNA by the pore size of the gel. Separation of very large DNA fragments requires pulse field gel electrophoresis (PFGE). In field inversion gel electrophoresis (FIGE, a kind of PFGE), it is possible to have 'band inversion' where large molecules may move faster than small molecules.

Conformation of DNA

The conformation of the DNA molecule can significantly affect the movement of the DNA, for example, supercoiled DNA usually moves faster than relaxed DNA because it is tightly coiled and hence more compact. In a normal plasmid DNA preparation, multiple forms of DNA may be present, and gel from the electrophoresis of the plasmids would normally show a main band which would be the negatively supercoiled form, while other forms of DNA may appear as minor fainter bands. These minor bands may be nicked DNA (open circular form) and the relaxed closed circular form which normally run slower than supercoiled DNA, and the single-stranded form (which can sometimes appear depending on the preparation methods) may move ahead of the supercoiled DNA. The rate at which the various forms move however can change using different electrophoresis conditions, for example linear DNA may run faster or slower than supercoiled DNA depending on conditions, and the mobility of larger circular DNA may be more strongly affected than linear DNA by the pore size of the gel. Unless supercoiled DNA markers are used, the size of a circular DNA like plasmid therefore may be more accurately gauged after it has been linearised by restriction digest. DNA damage due to increased cross-linking will also reduce electrophoretic DNA migration in a dose-dependent way.

Concentration of ethidium bromide

Circular DNA are more strongly affected by ethidium bromide concentration than linear DNA if ethidium bromide is present in the gel during electrophoresis. All naturally occurring DNA circles are underwound, but ethidium bromide which intercalates into circular DNA can change the charge, length, as well as the superhelicity of the DNA molecule, therefore its presence during electrophoresis can affect its movement in gel. Increasing ethidium bromide intercalated into the DNA can change it from a negatively supercoiled molecule into a fully relaxed form, then to positively coiled superhelix at maximum intercalation. Agarose gel electrophoresis can be used to resolve circular DNA with different supercoiling topology.

Gel concentration

The concentration of the gel determines the pore size of the gel which affect the migration of DNA. The resolution of the DNA changes with the percentage concentration of the gel. Increasing the agarose concentration of a gel reduces the migration speed and improves separation of smaller DNA molecules, while lowering gel concentration permits large DNA molecules to be separated. For a standard agarose gel electrophoresis, a 0.7% gives good separation or resolution of large 5–10kb DNA fragments, while 2% gel gives good resolution for small 0.2–1kb fragments. Up to 3% can be used for separating very tiny fragments but a vertical polyacrylamide gel would be more appropriate for resolving small fragments. High concentrations gel however requires longer run times (sometimes days) and high percentage gels are often brittle and may not set evenly. High percentage agarose gels should be run with PFGE or FIGE. Low percentage gels (0.1–0.2%) are fragile and may break. 1% gels are common for many applications.

Applied field

At low voltages, the rate of migration of the DNA is proportional to the voltage applied, i.e. the higher the voltage, the faster the DNA moves. However, in increasing electric field strength, the mobility of high-molecular-weight DNA fragments increases differentially, and the effective range of separation decreases and resolution therefore is lower at high voltage. For optimal resolution of DNA greater than 2kb in size in standard gel electrophoresis, 5 to 8 V/cm is recommended. Voltage is also limited by the fact that it heats the gel and may cause the gel to melt if a gel is run at high voltage for a prolonged period, particularly for low-melting point agarose gel. The mobility of DNA however may change in an unsteady field. In a field that is periodically reversed, the mobility of DNA of a particular size may drop significantly at a particular cycling frequency. This phenomenon can result in band inversion whereby larger DNA fragments move faster than smaller ones in PFGE.

Mechanism of Migration and Separation

The negative charge of its phosphate backbone moves the DNA towards the positively charged anode during electrophoresis. However, the migration of DNA molecules in solution, in the absence of a gel matrix, is independent of molecular weight during electrophoresis, i.e. there is no separation by size without a gel matrix. Hydrodynamic interaction between different parts of the DNA are cut off by streaming counterions moving in the opposite direction, so no mechanism exists to generate a dependence of velocity on length on a scale larger than screening length of about 10 nm. This makes it different from other processes such as sedimentation or diffusion where long-ranged hydrodynamic interaction are important.

The gel matrix is therefore responsible for the separation of DNA by size during electrophoresis, however the precise mechanism responsible the separation is not entirely clear. A number of models exists for the mechanism of separation of biomolecules in gel matrix, a widely accepted one is the Ogston model which treats the polymer matrix as a sieve consisting of randomly distributed network of inter-connected pores. A globular protein or a random coil DNA moves through the connected pores large enough to accommodate its passage, and the movement of larger molecules is more likely to be impeded and slowed down by collisions with the gel matrix, and the molecules of different sizes can therefore be separated in this process of sieving.

The Ogston model however breaks down for large molecules whereby the pores are significantly smaller than size of the molecule. For DNA molecules of size greater than 1 kb, a reptation model (or its variants) is most commonly used. This model assumes that the DNA can crawl in a 'snake-like' fashion (hence 'reptation') through the pores as an elongated molecule. At higher electric field strength, this turned into a biased reptation model, whereby the leading end of the molecule become strongly biased in the forward direction, and this leading edge pulls the rest of the molecule along. In the fully biased mode, the mobility reached a saturation point and DNA beyond a certain size cannot be separated. Perfect parallel alignment of the chain with the field however is not observed in practice as that would mean the same mobility for long and short molecules. Further refinement of the biased reptation model takes into account of the internal fluctuations of the chain.

The biased reptation model has also been used to explain the mobility of DNA in PFGE. The orientation of the DNA is progressively built up by reptation after the onset of a field, and the time it reached the steady state velocity is dependent on the size of the molecule. When the field is changed, larger molecules take longer to reorientate, it is therefore possible to discriminate between the long chains that cannot reach its steady state velocity from the short ones that travel most of the time in steady velocity. Other models, however, also exist.

Real-time fluorescence microscopy of stained molecules showed more subtle dynamics during electrophoresis, with the DNA showing considerable elasticity as it alternately stretching in the direction of the applied field and then contracting into a ball, or becoming hooked into a U-shape when it gets caught on the polymer fibres. This observation may be termed the 'caterpillar' model. Other model proposes that the DNA gets entangled with the polymer matrix, and the larger the molecule, the more likely it is to become entangled and its movement impeded.

Visualisation

The most common dye used to make DNA or RNA bands visible for agarose gel electrophoresis is ethidium bromide, usually abbreviated as EtBr. It fluoresces under UV light when intercalated into the major groove of DNA (or RNA). By running DNA through an EtBr-treated gel and visualising it with UV light, any band containing more than ~20 ng DNA becomes distinctly visible. EtBr is a known mutagen, and safer alternatives are available, such as GelRed, produced by Biotium, which binds to the minor groove.

SYBR Green I is another dsDNA stain, produced by Invitrogen. It is more expensive, but 25 times more sensitive, and possibly safer than EtBr, though there is no data addressing its mutagenicity or toxicity in humans.

SYBR Safe is a variant of SYBR Green that has been shown to have low enough levels of mutagenicity and toxicity to be deemed nonhazardous waste under US Federal regulations. It has similar sensitivity levels to EtBr, but, like SYBR Green, is significantly more expensive. In countries where safe disposal of hazardous waste is mandatory, the costs of EtBr disposal can easily outstrip the initial price difference, however.

Since EtBr stained DNA is not visible in natural light, scientists mix DNA with negatively charged loading buffers before adding the mixture to the gel. Loading buffers are useful because they are visible in natural light (as opposed to UV light for EtBr stained DNA), and they co-sediment with DNA (meaning they move at the same speed as DNA of a certain length). Xylene cyanol and Bromophenol blue are common dyes found in loading buffers, they run about the same speed as DNA fragments that are 5000 bp and 300 bp in length respectively, but the precise position varies with percentage of the gel. Other less frequently used progress markers are Cresol Red and Orange G which run at about 125 bp and 50 bp, respectively.

Visualisation can also be achieved by transferring DNA after SDS-PAGE to a nitrocellulose membrane followed by exposure to a hybridisation probe. This process is termed Southern blotting.

For fluorescent dyes, after electrophoresis the gel is illuminated with an ultraviolet lamp (usually by placing it on a light box, while using protective gear to limit exposure to ultraviolet radiation). The illuminator apparatus mostly also contains imaging apparatus that takes an image of the gel, after illumination with UV radiation. The ethidium bromide fluoresces reddish-orange in the presence of DNA, since it has intercalated with the DNA. The DNA band can also be cut out of the gel, and can then be dissolved to retrieve the purified DNA. The gel can then be photographed usually with a digital or polaroid camera. Although the stained nucleic acid fluoresces reddish-orange, images are usually shown in black and white. UV damage to the DNA sample can reduce the efficiency of subsequent manipulation of the sample, such as ligation and cloning. Shorter wavelength UV radiations (302 or 312 nm) cause greater damage, for example exposure for as little as 45 seconds can significantly reduce transformation efficiency. Therefore if the DNA is to be use for downstream procedures, exposure to a shorter wavelength UV radiations should be limited, instead higher-wavelength UV radiation (365 nm) which cause less damage should be used. Higher wavelength radiations however produces weaker fluorescence, therefore if it is necessary to capture the gel image, a shorter wavelength UV light can be used a short time. Addition of Cytidine or guanosine to the electrophoresis buffer at 1 mM concentration may protect the DNA from damage. Alternatively, a blue light excitation source with a blue-excitable stain such as SYBR Green or GelGreen may be used.

Chapter 19

DNA Replication

INTRODUCTION

Replication is the process by which a double-stranded DNA molecule is copied to produce two identical DNA molecules. DNA replication is one of the most basic processes that occurs within a cell. Each time a cell divides, the two resulting daughter cells must contain exactly the same genetic information, or DNA, as the parent cell. To accomplish this, each strand of existing DNA acts as a template for replication.

ORIGIN OF REPLICATION

The origin of replication (also called the replication origin) is a particular sequence in a genome at which replication is initiated. This can either involve the replication of DNA in living organisms such as prokaryotes and eukaryotes, or that of DNA or RNA in viruses, such as double-stranded RNA viruses. DNA replication may proceed from this point bidirectionally or unidirectionally. The specific structure of the origin of replication varies some what from species to species, but all share some common characteristics such as high AT content (repeats of adenine and thymine are easier to separate because their base stacking interactions are not as strong as those of guanine and cytosine). The origin of replication binds the pre-replication complex, a protein complex that recognises, unwinds, and begins to copy DNA.

TYPES OF REPLICATION

Prokaryotic

The genome of *E. coli* consists of a single circular DNA molecule of approximately 4.6×10^6 nucleotide pairs. DNA replication typically begins at a single origin of replication. In *E. coli,* the origin of replication ―oriC―consists of three A–T rich 13-mer repeats and four 9-mer repeats. Ten to 20 monomers of the replication initiator protein DnaA bind to the 9-mer repeats, and the DNA coils around this protein complex forming a protein core. This coiling stimulates the AT rich region in the 13-mer sequence to unwind, allowing the helicase loader DnaC to load the replicative helicase DnaB to each of the two unwound DNA strands. The helicase DnaB forms the basis of the primosome, a complex of enzymes to which DNA polymerase III is recruited before replication can occur.

Many bacteria, including *E. coli*, contain plasmids that each contain an origin of replication, usually named oriV for vegetative replication. They in general still work by binding DnaA. These are separate from the origins of replication that are used by the bacteria to copy their genome and are regulated differently. For example, the *E. coli* plasmid pBR322 uses a protein called Rop/Rom (derived from pMB1, a relative of ColE1) to regulate the number of plasmids that are within each bacterial cell. This limits the number of plasmids per cell – the copy number – to 30–40. The pUC series of plasmids, including pUC19, is more commonly used. Compared to pBR322, it uses ori with a single point mutation and has the regulatory Rop/Rom gene removed. With those changes, the bacteria can produce up to 500 copies pUC19 per cell. This allows genetic engineers to produce large quantities of DNA for research purposes. Other origins of plasmid replication include pSC101 (derived from Salmonella, around 5 copies per cell), 15A origin (derived from p15A, 10–20 copies per cell) and Bacterial artificial chromosomes (1 copy per cell). During conjugation, the rolling circle mode of replication starts at the oriT ('T' for transfer) sequence of the FAT plasmid.

Eukaryotic

In eukaryotes, the budding yeast *Saccharomyces cerevisiae* were first identified by their ability to support the replication of mini-chromosomes or plasmids, giving rise to the name Autonomously replicating sequences or ARS elements. Each budding yeast origin consists of a short (~11 bp) essential DNA sequence (called the ARS consensus sequence or ACS) that recruits replication proteins.

In other eukaryotes, including humans, the base pair sequences at the replication origins vary. Despite this sequence variation, all the origins form a base for assembly of a group of proteins known collectively as the pre-replication complex (pre-RC):

- First, the origin DNA is bound by the origin recognition complex (ORC) which, with help from two further protein factors (Cdc6 and Cdt1), load the mini chromosome maintenance (or MCM) protein complex.
- Once assembled, this complex of proteins indicates that the replication origin is ready for activation. Once the replication origin is activated, the cell's DNA will be replicated.

In metazoans, pre-RC formation is inhibited by the protein geminin, which binds to and inactivates Cdt1. Regulation of replication prevents the DNA from being replicated more than once each cell cycle.

In humans an origin of replication has been originally identified near the Lamin B2 gene on chromosome 19 and the ORC binding to it has extensively been studied.

There are also significant differences between prokaryotic and eukaryotic:

- Most bacteria have a single circular molecule of DNA, and typically only a single origin of replication per circular chromosome.
- Most *archaea* have a single circular molecule of DNA, and several origins of replication along this circular chromosome.
- Eukaryotes often have multiple origins of replication on each linear chromosome that initiate at different times (replication timing), with up to 100,000 present in a single human cell. Having many origins of replication helps to speed the duplication of their (usually) much larger store of genetic material. The segment of DNA that is copied starting from each unique replication origin is called a replicon. The replicons range from 40 kb length, in yeast and Drosophila, to 300 kb in plants.
- Mitochondrial DNA in many organisms has two ori sequences. In humans, they are called oriH and oriL for the heavy and light strand of the DNA, each being the origin of replication for single-

stranded replication. The two Chloroplast DNA ori sequences in Nicotiana tabacum, the tobacco plant, has been characterised as oriA and oriB.

Origins of replication are typically assigned names containing 'ori'. When it comes to plasmids, origins of replication are classified in two ways:

- Narrow or broad host range.
- High- or low-copy number.

DNA REPLICATION

Every time a cell divides, its DNA must be duplicated so that each daughter cell receives an identical copy of instructions. The size of a DNA molecule alone makes replication an amazing undertaking. For example, human cells contain 3 billion base pairs of DNA divided into chromosomes ranging in size from about 50–250 million base pairs. If they were completely stretched out, these DNA molecules would range in length from about 1.7–8.5 cm. Many enzymes and proteins are required to physically manipulate these large polymers and to catalyse the synthesis of new DNA. These enzymes and the process of DNA replication are regulated by the cell so that replication is complete and genomes are duplicated only once every cell division.

DNA replication begins at a specific time in the cell cycle and at specific sites, origins of replication, in the genome. The DNA duplex is unwound at these replication origins to allow the enzymes that synthesise DNA access to the individual DNA strands (Fig. 19.1). Each strand of parental DNA serves as a template for a DNA polymerase to make a new strand of DNA. Single nucleotide monomers that form Watson-Crick pairs with template bases are incorporated into a new DNA polymer by DNA polymerases. As the new DNA grows, the parental duplex is progressively unwound forming replication forks that move away from the origin. DNA replication is semi-conservative, ultimately forming two DNA double helices that contain one strand of parental DNA and one strand of new DNA. In bacteria, replication forks move at a rate of about 500 nucleotides per second while in eukaryotes they move

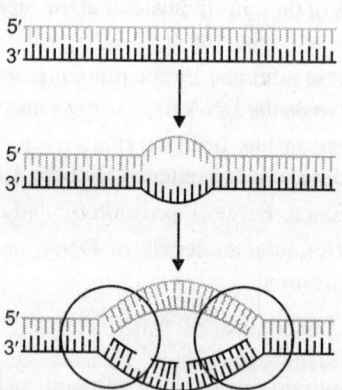

Fig. 19.1: Unwinding DNA at the origin of replication and the formation of replication forks. DNA replication begins at specific sites known as origins of replication. Origin binding proteins recognise, these sites and initiate unwinding of the DNA duplex so that replication proteins can access the individual strands of DNA. Initially a small bubble is formed that is opened further by the activity of a DNA helicase. Replication complexes assemble on both sides of the bubble and these replication forks (circled) move away from the origin in both directions so that replication is bidirectional. At, each fork, two new copies of DNA are synthesised using the parental strands as a templates.

somewhat slower. Because genomes of eukaryotes are in general larger than bacteria and replication fork movement is slower, replication in eukaryotes is initiated at several origins instead of a single origin so that DNA duplication can be accomplished in a reasonable amount of time.

Much of what we know about DNA replication is based on studies in bacteria and viruses. However, more recent investigations of eukaryotic systems are revealing that many of the features of the bacterial replication machinery are also common to eukaryotes. Because replication in bacteria has been studied in greater detail to date, the *Escherichia coli* replication machinery will be presented for illustrative purposes and compared to eukaryotic systems.

Initiation of DNA Replication

Origins of DNA replication contain two general DNA sequence elements, an element that is relatively easy to unwind, and an element that is recognised by initiation proteins. The genome of *E. coli* exists as a single circular DNA molecule of about 4.5 million base pairs and contains a single 245 base pair (bp) origin of replication, ori*C*. Within ori*C* are three 13-bp AT-rich regions of DNA that are relatively easy to unwind and four 9-bp regions that are recognised by the *E. coli* initiator protein, DnaA. A complex containing several DnaA molecules binds to ori*C* in the region containing the 9-bp repeats and bends the DNA. This bending helps to unwind the DNA helix at the 13-bp AT-rich sequences. Many of the steps in DNA replication and repair, such as the unwinding of the origin, require energy to manipulate the structures of macromolecules and disrupt noncovalent interactions such as hydrogen bonding. The enzymes catalysing these changes utilise the chemical energy stored in the phosphate bonds of adenosine-5'-triphosphate (ATP) to do the mechanical work. The DnaA protein utilises the energy gained from ATP hydrolysis to power the unwinding of DNA at the origin. An origin recognition complex also exists in eukaryotes but its mechanism of action has not yet been completely defined.

Once the DNA duplex is opened, a DNA helicase can be loaded onto the single-stranded DNA to continue the unwinding process. DNA helicases are enzymes that utilise the energy from hydrolysis of ribonucleoside 5-triphosphates, most commonly ATP, to break hydrogen bonding interactions between complementary DNA strands and unwind nucleic acid duplexes. In *E. coli*, six molecules of the DnaB protein form a ring-shaped hexamer that encircles single-stranded DNA and functions as a helicase. This hexameric helicase structure is common to other organisms including eukaryotes where the MCM (Mini-Chromosome Maintenance) proteins are believed to perform the function of replicative DNA helicase. In *E. coli*, the DnaB hexamer is assembled around DNA by the ATP-dependent activity of DnaC.

Before DNA synthesis can begin, RNA primers must be made. DNA polymerases are unable to synthesise DNA *de novo* and can only extend RNA (or DNA) primers that are already paired with the template to be copied. Primases synthesise these primers using ribonucleoside 5'-triphosphates as building blocks to form a short strand of RNA complementary to the DNA template. The *E. coli* primase interacts with the DnaB helicase and begins synthesis of RNA primers shortly after DnaB has begun to unwind DNA. In eukaryotes, a hybrid RNA-DNA primer is synthesised by an enzyme complex containing both primase and DNA polymerase α. Once primers are formed, they can be extended by a DNA polymerase.

Enzymes at the Replication Fork

Assembly of a replisome is complete when the replicative DNA polymerase and its accessory proteins join the helicase and primase at the replication fork (Fig. 19.2). The replisome will then continue to synthesise new DNA, unwinding the parental duplex as it goes. The actual synthesis of new DNA is catalysed by a DNA polymerase contained within the replisome. Cells contain many different DNA

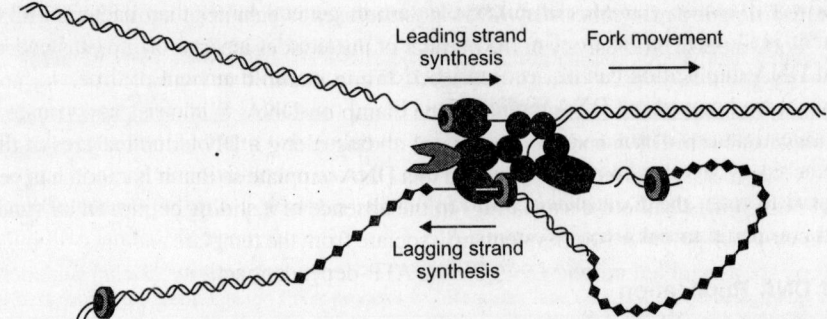

Fig. 19.2: Proteins at the *E. coli* replication fork. The dimeric polymerase complex is capable coordinated DNA synthesis on the leading and lagging strands. The leading strand polymerase synthesises new DNA in the direction of fork movement and the lagging strand polymerase synthesises DNA in the opposite direction.

polymerases that have different functions in DNA replication and repair. There are 5 known DNA polymerases in *E. coli* and at least a dozen in humans. In *E. coli*, DNA polymerase III catalyses the bulk of DNA synthesis during replication and DNA polymerase δ does so in eukaryotes.

All DNA polymerases use 2′-deoxyribonucleoside-5′-triphosphates (dNTPs) as monomeric building blocks for making DNA. They catalyse the attack of the 3′ hydroxyl group of the nucleotide at the primer end on the α-phosphoryl group of an incoming dNTP displacing pyrophosphate (Fig. 19.3, upper panel). Thus, DNA polymerases extend DNA polymers in the 5′ to 3′ direction by incorporation of 2′-deoxyribonucleoside monophosphates. Watson-Crick base pairing interactions between the incoming dNTP and the next unpaired template base direct incorporation of correct nucleotides. Frequencies of adding incorrect nucleotides can be as low as one in a million, but even with this low error frequency mistakes will be made. To further reduce error frequencies, the DNA polymerases that function in replication contain a 3′ to 5′ exonuclease activity that allows them to proof read nucleotides that have been incorporated. This exonuclease activity catalyses the hydrolysis of phosphodiester bonds to remove the last nucleotide added to the 3′ primer end (Fig. 19.3, lower panel). Thus, a nucleotide that has been added incorrectly can be removed.

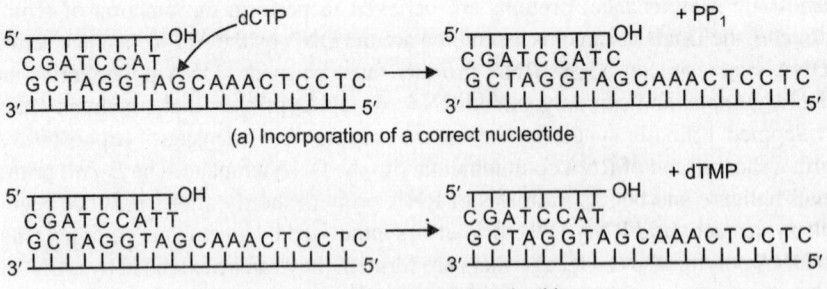

Fig. 19.3: Reactions catalysed by DNA polymerases. (a) 2′-Deoxyribonucleoside 5′-triphosphates are used as substrates by DNA polymerases to extend a primer in template-directed reactions. The net reaction is incorporation of 2′-deoxyribonucleoside monophosphates onto the 3′ hydroxyl of a primer with loss of pyrophosphate. (b) DNA polymerases can proof read newly incorporated nucleotides and excise incorrect nucleotides. The excision reaction removes the last nucleoside monophosphate that was incorporated.

The overall efficiency of synthesis by DNA polymerases is enhanced by accessory proteins which increase DNA polymerase processivity or the number of nucleotides incorporated per DNA binding event. These accessory proteins consist of a ring-shaped sliding clamp that binds both DNA and the DNA polymerase and a clamp loader that assembles the clamp on DNA. Sliding clamps, made of identical protein subunits, encircle DNA and are capable of sliding along a DNA duplex. By binding a sliding clamp, a DNA polymerase is effectively tethered to a DNA template so that it is capable of incorporating thousands of nucleotides without dissociating. In the absence of a sliding clamp, DNA synthesis is less efficient because DNA polymerases frequently dissociate from the template and must rebind to continue. Sliding clamps are assembled around DNA by the ATP-dependent activity of clamp loaders.

Leading and Lagging Strand Synthesis

In *E. coli*, a complex containing a dimeric DNA polymerase and accessory proteins interacts with the helicase and primase to form a replisome. This interaction stimulates the activity of the helicase and increases the rate of fork movement. The replisome, which contains two copies of DNA polymerase III, is capable of simultaneously copying both strands of parental DNA at the replication fork. But the two DNA polymerases must work in opposite directions to do this because DNA strands in a duplex are antiparallel and DNA polymerases can only synthesise DNA in the 5′ to 3′ direction. To accomplish this, one DNA polymerase working on the leading strand, synthesises DNA in a single continuous piece moving in the direction of the replication fork. The other DNA polymerase working on the opposite or lagging strand, synthesises DNA in shorter fragment named *Okazaki* fragments after Reiji Okazaki whose work led to their discovery. In *E. coli*, Okazaki fragments are 1000–2000 nt in length and in eukaryotes they are 100–200 nt. As the fork progresses, a loop of single-stranded DNA is created on the lagging strand and an RNA primer is synthesised by an enzyme called primase to begin each Okazaki fragment. The lagging strand polymerase extends these primers in the direction opposite to fork movement until it encounters a completed Okazaki fragment. Then, the polymerase dissociates and rebinds a new primer closer to the fork and extends it. Thus, the lagging strand polymerase must repeatedly dissociate from completed Okazaki fragments and rebind to new primers to continue DNA synthesis in a discontinuous manner. Overall, DNA synthesis is semi-discontinuous because it is made in one continuous strand on the leading strand and in discontinuous fragments on the lagging strand.

To complete DNA replication, RNA primers must be replaced by DNA and Okazaki fragments must be joined together to form a continuous strand. In *E. coli*, removal of RNA primers and synthesis of DNA can be accomplished by a single enzyme, DNA polymerase I. The 5′ to 3′ exonuclease activity of DNA polymerase I degrades RNA primers while the 5′ to 3′ polymerase activity simultaneously synthesises DNA to replace the RNA. In eukaryotes, separate enzymes are responsible for degrading the RNA and replacing it with DNA. Finally, DNA fragments on the lagging strand are joined by a DNA ligase to form one continuous polymer. DNA ligase catalyses the formation of a phosphodiester bond between the 3′ hydroxyl group at the end of one Okazaki fragment and the 5′ phosphate at the beginning of the next. Any nick in one strand of a DNA duplex that has a 3′ hydroxyl on one side and 5′ phosphate on the other can be sealed by the activity of a DNA ligase.

FIDELITY OF DNA REPLICATION AND MISMATCH REPAIR

DNA replication can be accomplished with as few as one mistake in a billion nucleotides incorporated. This amazing accuracy or fidelity of synthesis is achieved for the most part by the DNA polymerase but is enhanced by a group of mismatch repair enzymes that function to detect and correct replication errors. One main feature of a DNA polymerase that contributes to its fidelity is the geometry of the active site, which is optimised for binding Watson-Crick base pairs where the overall shape of both A·T and G·C pairs are the same. Mismatches such as G·T deviate from this ideal geometry so that incorrect nucleotides are incorporated much less efficiently. Frequencies of adding an incorrect nucleotide range from 1 in 1000 to 1 in 10,00,000 nucleotides depending on the nucleotide added. In the rare instant when a mistake is made, DNA polymerases have the ability to remove the incorrect nucleotide using the 3′ to 5′ exonuclease activity contained in the enzymes. This proof reading capability is further enhanced by a reduced efficiency of adding the next correct nucleotide onto a primer that ends with an incorrect nucleotide. Thus, when a mistake is made, the rate of adding more nucleotides is greatly reduced which allows the exonuclease time to remove the incorrect nucleotide. Once an incorrect nucleotide is removed, rapid incorporation of correct nucleotides by the DNA polymerase activity resumes. This proof reading activity increases the accuracy of DNA synthesis by a factor of about 10–100.

Mismatches that escape proof reading by the DNA polymerase can be corrected by the postreplicative mismatch repair process (Fig. 19.4). The net result is the removal of a segment of DNA containing the incorrect nucleotide and resynthesis of DNA to replace the segment that was excised. The key enzymes responsible for mismatch repair in *E. coli* are MutS, MutL, MutH and MutU. Mismatches are detected in double-stranded DNA by MutS which then interacts with the MutL protein. Together MutS and MutL signal where the mismatch is located to MutH and MutU. MutH is an endonuclease that is stimulated by MutL to cut the DNA strand containing the incorrect nucleotide. MutU is a DNA helicase that unwinds the duplex displacing the strand containing the incorrect nucleotide which is then degraded by an exonuclease. New DNA is synthesised to replace the segment that was removed. Homologs to MutS and MutL exist in eukaryotic cells and the overall repair process is similar.

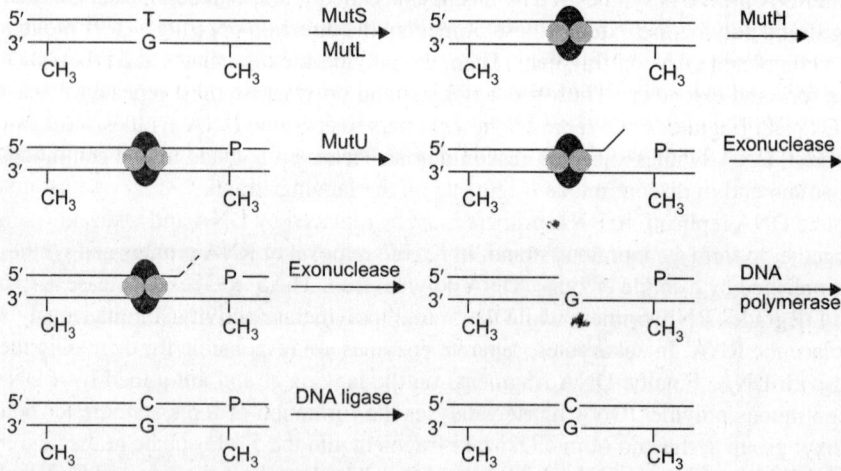

Fig. 19.4: Methyl-directed mismatch repair in *E. coli*. MutS protein recognises and binds mismatches such as G·T in DNA and is joined by the MutL protein. MutL within the MutS-MutL-mismatched DNA complex stimulates the endonuclease activity of MutH to cleave the unmethylated DNA strand at the GATC sequence closest to the protein-mismatched DNA complex. The cut DNA strand is unwound by the activity of MutU helicase and then degraded by an exonuclease until the mismatch is removed. The missing segment of DNA is replaced by a DNA polymerase and the DNA strands are joined together by the activity of a DNA ligase. The letter P indicates a 5′ phosphate group.

How do the mismatch repair enzymes recognise which nucleotide of the mismatch is incorrect? In *E. coli*, the methylation status of the DNA allows the mismatch repair enzymes to distinguish between the newly synthesised DNA strand and the parental strand. Adenine is methylated in the *E. coli* genome when it appears in the sequence 5′GATC. This methylation of the genome occurs shortly after replication, so for a short time, the daughter strand is unmethylated while the parent strand is methylated. These 5′GATC sequences are also recognised by MutH which cuts the unmethylated daughter strand. These cut sites can be up to 1000–2000 nt away from the mismatch so a fairly large segment of DNA may be removed and replaced. While the overall process of mismatched repair is similar in eukaryotes, it is not yet clear how the eukaryotic enzymes distinguish between the newly synthesised strand and the parental strand.

SEMICONSERVATIVE REPLICATION

Semiconservative replication describes the mechanism of DNA replication in all known cells. It derives its name from the fact that it produces two copies of the original DNA molecule, each of which contains one of original strand, and one newly-synthesised strand. The structure of DNA (as deciphered by Watson and Crick in 1953) suggested that each strand of the double helix would serve as a template for synthesis of a new strand. However, it was not known how newly synthesised strands combined with template strands to form two double helical DNA molecules. The semiconservative model of replication seemed most reasonable since it would allow each daughter strand to remain associated with its template strand. The semiconservative model was anticipated by Nikolai Koltsov, is supported by the Meselson-Stahl experiment as well as subsequent experiments that enabled autoradiographic visualisation of the distribution of old and new strands within replicated chromosomes. Experimental evidence confirmed that two lines were observed, therefore offering compelling evidence for the semi-conservative theory. Figure 19.5 shows a summary of the three postulated methods of DNA synthesis.

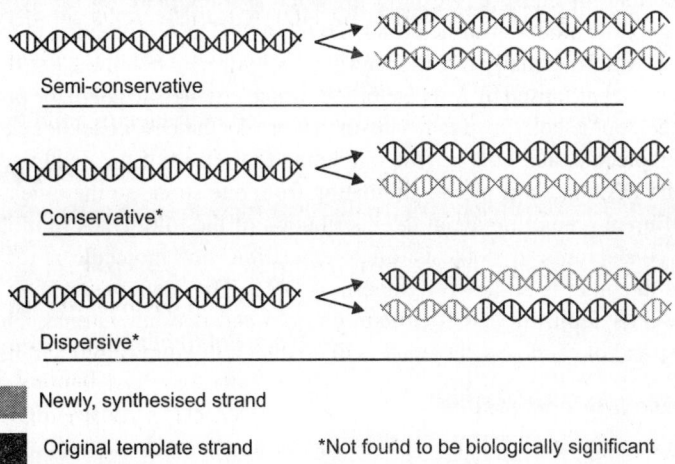

Fig. 19.5: A summary of the three postulated methods of DNA synthesis.

Proposed Models of Replication

Semiconservative replication derives its name from the fact that this mechanism of transcription was one of three models originally proposed for DNA replication:

1. Semiconservative replication would produce two copies that each contained one of the original strands and one new strand.
2. Conservative replication would leave the two original template DNA strands together in a double helix and would produce a copy composed of two new strands containing all of the new DNA base pairs.
3. Dispersive replication would produce two copies of the DNA, both containing distinct regions of DNA composed of either both original strands or both new strands.

Meselson–Stahl Experiment

The Meselson–Stahl experiment is an experiment by Matthew Meselson and Franklin Stahl in 1958 which supported Watson and Crick's hypothesis that DNA replication was semiconservative. In semiconservative replication, when the double stranded DNA helix is replicated, each of the two new double-stranded DNA helices consisted of one strand from the original helix and one newly synthesised. It has been called 'the most beautiful experiment in biology.' Meselson and Stahl decided the best way to tag the parent DNA would be to change one of the atoms in the parent DNA molecule. Since nitrogen is found in the nitrogenous bases of each nucleotide, they decided to use an isotope of nitrogen to distinguish between parent and newly copied DNA. The isotope of nitrogen had an extra neutron in the nucleus, which made it heavier.

Hypothesis

Three hypotheses had been previously proposed for the method of replication of DNA. In the semi-conservative hypothesis, proposed by Watson and Crick, the two strands of a DNA molecule separate during replication. Each strand then acts as a template for synthesis of a new strand. The conservative hypothesis proposed that the entire DNA molecule acted as a template for the synthesis of an entirely new one. According to this model, histone proteins bind to the DNA, revolving the strand and exposing the nucleotide bases (which normally line the interior) for hydrogen bonding. The dispersive hypothesis is exemplified by a model proposed by Max Delbrück, which attempts to solve the problem of unwinding the two strands of the double helix by a mechanism that breaks the DNA backbone every 10 nucleotides or so, untwists the molecule, and attaches the old strand to the end of the newly synthesised one. This would synthesise the DNA in short pieces alternating from one strand to the other. Each of these three models makes a different prediction about the distribution of the 'old' DNA in molecules formed after replication. In the conservative hypothesis, after replication, one molecule is the entirely conserved 'old' molecule, and the other is all newly synthesised DNA. The semiconservative hypothesis predicts that each molecule after replication will contain one old and one new strand. The dispersive model predicts that each strand of each new molecule will contain a mixture of old and new DNA.

Experimental procedure and results

Nitrogen is a major constituent of DNA. ^{14}N is by far the most abundant isotope of nitrogen, but DNA with the heavier (but non-radioactive) ^{15}N isotope is also functional. E. coli was grown for several generations in a medium containing NH_4Cl with ^{15}N. When DNA is extracted from these cells and centrifuged on a salt (CsCl) density gradient, the DNA separates out at the point at which its density equals that of the salt solution. The DNA of the cells grown in ^{15}N medium had a higher density than cells grown in normal ^{14}N medium. After that, E. coli cells with only ^{15}N in their DNA were transferred to a ^{14}N medium and were allowed to divide, the progress of cell division was monitored by microscopic cell counts and by colony assay. DNA was extracted periodically and was compared to pure ^{14}N DNA and ^{15}N DNA. After one replication, the DNA was found to have intermediate density. Since conservative replication would result in equal amounts of DNA of the higher and lower densities (but no DNA of an intermediate density), conservative replication was excluded. However, this result was consistent with both semiconservative and dispersive replication. Semiconservative replication would result in double-stranded DNA with one strand of 15N DNA, and one of ^{14}N DNA, while dispersive replication would result in double-stranded DNA with both strands having mixtures of ^{15}N and ^{14}N DNA, either of which would have appeared as DNA of an intermediate density.

Smith and others continued to sample cells as replication continued. DNA from cells after two replications had been completed was found to consist of equal amounts of DNA with two different densities, one corresponding to the intermediate density of DNA of cells grown for only one division in ^{14}N medium, the other corresponding to DNA from cells grown exclusively in ^{14}N medium. This was inconsistent with dispersive replication, which would have resulted in a single density, lower than the intermediate density of the one-generation cells, but still higher than cells grown only in ^{14}N DNA medium, as the original ^{15}N DNA would have been split evenly among all DNA strands. The result was consistent with the semiconservative replication hypothesis.

Rate and Accuracy

The rate of semiconservative DNA replication in a living cell was first measured as the rate of phage T4 DNA strand elongation in phage-infected *E. coli*. During the period of exponential DNA increase at 37°C, the rate of strand elongation was 749 nucleotides per second. The mutation rate per base pair per round of replication during phage T4 DNA synthesis is 2.4×10^{-8}. Thus semiconservative DNA replication is both rapid and accurate.

ENZYMES INVOLVED IN DNA REPLICATION OF PROKARYOTES

The following points highlight the seven important enzymes involved in the process of DNA replication of prokaryotes. The enzymes are: (i) DNA polymerase, (ii) primase, (iii) polynucleotide ligase, (iv) endonucleases, (v) pilot proteins, (vi) helicase, and (vii) single-strand binding (SSB) protein.

Enzyme # 1 DNA Polymerase

DNA polymerase is the chief enzyme of DNA replication. DNA polymerase activity was discovered by Kornberg in 1956, this activity was due to DNA polymerase I. *E. coli* has four more enzymes, DNA polymerase II, III, IV and V, DNA polymerase III (Pol III) is concerned with DNA replication, while the remaining four enzymes are involved in DNA repair.

All DNA polymerases require the following:

1. A template DNA strand.
2. A short primer (either RNA or DNA).
3. A free 3′-OH in the primer.

They add one nucleotide at a time to the free 3′-OH of the primer, and extend the primer chain in $5' \rightarrow 3'$ direction.

DNA polymerase I

DNA polymerase I enzyme provides the major part of activity in *E. coli*. It is chiefly a DNA repair enzyme, and is used for *in vitro* DNA replication.

This enzyme has the following three activities:

1. The 5′ → 3′ polymerase activity is responsible for primer extension or DNA synthesis.
2. The 5′ → 3′ exonuclease activity is involved in excision of DNA strands during DNA repair, it removes ~ 10 bases at a time. An exonuclease digests nucleic acids (here DNA) from one end, and it does not cut DNA internally.
3. The 3′ → 5′exonuclease activity is responsible for proof-reading.

In this case, only one nucleotide is removed at a time. The polymerase action does commit errors in DNA synthesis. DNA polymerase is known to scrutinise the new bases added to the growing chain and to delete or remove the wrong bases, this is called proof-reading. Proof-reading activity reduces errors in replication by over 100 – fold.

DNA polymerase I is encoded by gene polA, has a single polypeptide, and can initiate replication *in vitro* at a nick in a DNA duplex. It can be cleaved by proteolytic treatments into a large and a small fragments. This large fragment, called Klenow fragment, lacks 5′ → 3′ exonuclease activity and is used for *in vitro* DNA replication.

DNA polymerase II

DNA polymerase II enzyme functions in DNA-repair. It has 5′ → 3′ polymerase and 3′ → 5′ exonuclease activities, and uses as template only such DNA duplexes that have short gaps.

DNA polymerase III

DNA polymerase III enzyme is responsible for DNA replication *in vivo*. It has 5′ → 3′ polymerase and 3′ → 5′ exonuclease activities. It catalyses DNA synthesis at very high rates, e.g. 15,000 bases/min at 37°C. It is composed of several subunits. A DNA polymerase molecule has the following 4 functional sites involved in polymerase activity.

Schematic representation of crystal structure of DNA polymerase belonging to *E. coli* pol I family

- Template site binds the strand serving as template during replication.
- Primer site binds to the primer used for DNA replication.
- Primer terminus site binds only to such primers that have free 3′-OH.
- The nucleotide triphosphate site binds to the deoxynucleotide 5′-triphosphate that is complementary to the corresponding nucleotide of the template. It also catalyses the formation of phosphodiester bond between the 5′ phosphate of this nucleotide and the 3′-OH of the terminal primer nucleotide.

[In addition, the polymerase molecule has a 3′ → 5′ exonuclease site and a 5′ → 3′ exo-nuclease site (in case of DNA polymerase I only)].

In case of eukaryotes, at least nine different DNA polymerases are found. DNA polymerase δ replicates the leading strand, while DNA polymerase δ synthesises the lagging strand. DNA polymerase a catalyses priming of both the strands. DNA polymerases ξ, η, τ, and κ are all nuclear DNA repair enzymes. DNA polymerase y is found in mitochondria and catalyses replication of mtDNA.

Enzyme # 2 Primase

This enzyme activity catalyses the synthesis of RNA primers to initiate DNA replication. In *E. coli*, DnaG functions as primase. But in eukaryotes, DNA polymerase a provides this function. There are, however, several other ways in which primers are produced, e.g. the 3′-OH generated by a nick in the template DNA molecule.

Enzyme # 3 Polynucleotide Ligase

DNA ligase or polynucleotide ligase catalyses the formation of phosphodiester linkage between two immediate neighbour nucleotides of a DNA strand. Thus it seals the nicks remaining in a DNA strand either following DNA replication or DNA repair. However, this enzyme cannot fill the gaps in DNA strands.

Enzyme # 4 Endonucleases

An endonuclease produces an internal cut (single- or double-stranded) in a DNA molecule. But a restriction endonuclease produces cuts only at those sites that have a specific base sequence. During DNA replication, an endonuclease may induce a nick to initiate DNA replication, or it may induce nicks to generate a swivel for DNA unwinding. Restriction endonucleases are required for DNA repair.

Enzyme # 5 Pilot Proteins

Pilot proteins are produced by most viruses. The type of pilot proteins associated with viral genome determines whether the viral DNA will undergo replication or it would support transcription.

Enzyme # 6 Helicase

Helicase effects strand separation at the forks and uses one ATP molecule for each base that is separated. In *E. coli*, DNA functions as helicase, this protein is a hexamer and it moves with the replication fork.

Enzyme # 7 Single-Strand Binding (SSB) Protein

SSB protein binds to single-stranded DNA, and prevents it from forming duplex DNA or secondary structures. SSB binds as a monomer, but it binds cooperatively in that binding of one SSB molecule facilitates binding of more SSB monomers to the same DNA strand. *E. coli* SSB is a tetramer.

EUKARYOTIC DNA REPLICATION

Eukaryotic DNA replication is a conserved mechanism that restricts DNA replication to once per cell cycle. Eukaryotic DNA replication of chromosomal DNA is central for the duplication of a cell and is necessary for the maintenance of the eukaryotic genome.

DNA replication is the action of DNA polymerases synthesising a DNA strand complementary to the original template strand. To synthesise DNA, the double-stranded DNA is unwound by DNA helicases ahead of polymerases, forming a replication fork containing two single-stranded templates. Replication processes permit the copying of a single DNA double helix into two DNA helices, which are divided into the daughter cells at mitosis. The major enzymatic functions carried out at the replication fork are well conserved from prokaryotes to eukaryotes, but the replication machinery in eukaryotic DNA replication is a much larger complex, coordinating many proteins at the site of replication, forming the replisome. The replisome is responsible for copying the entirety of genomic DNA in each proliferative cell. This process allows for the high-fidelity passage of hereditary/genetic information from parental cell to daughter cell and is thus essential to all organisms. Much of the cell cycle is built around ensuring that DNA replication occurs without errors.

In G1 phase of the cell cycle, many of the DNA replication regulatory processes are initiated. In eukaryotes, the vast majority of DNA synthesis occurs during S phase of the cell cycle, and the entire genome must be unwound and duplicated to form two daughter copies. During G2, any damaged DNA or replication errors are corrected. Finally, one copy of the genomes is segregated to each daughter cell at mitosis or M phase. These daughter copies each contain one strand from the parental duplex DNA and one nascent antiparallel strand. This mechanism is conserved from prokaryotes to eukaryotes and is known as semiconservative DNA replication. The process of semiconservative replication for the site of DNA replication is a fork-like DNA structure, the replication fork, where the DNA helix is open, or unwound, exposing unpaired DNA nucleotides for recognition and base pairing for the incorporation of free nucleotides into double-stranded DNA.

Initiation

Initiation of eukaryotic DNA replication is the first stage of DNA synthesis where the DNA double helix is unwound and an initial priming event by DNA polymerase a occurs on the leading strand. The priming event on the lagging strand establishes a replication fork. Priming of the DNA helix consists of synthesis of an RNA primer to allow DNA synthesis by DNA polymerase a. Priming occurs once at the origin on the leading strand and at the start of each Okazaki fragment on the lagging strand.

DNA replication is initiated from specific sequences called origins of replication, and eukaryotic cells have multiple replication origins. To initiate DNA replication, multiple replicative proteins assemble on and dissociate from these replicative origins. The individual factors described below work together to direct the formation of the pre-replication complex (pre-RC), a key intermediate in the replication initiation process. Association of the origin recognition complex (ORC) with a replication origin recruits the cell division cycle 6 protein (Cdc6) to form a platform for the loading of the minichromosome maintenance (Mcm 2-7) complex proteins, facilitated by the chromatin licensing and DNA replication factor 1 protein (Cdt1). The ORC, Cdc6, and Cdt1 together are required for the stable association of the Mcm2-7 complex with replicative origins during G1 phase of the cell cycle.

Pre-replicative complex

Eukaryotic origins of replication control the formation of a number of protein complexes that lead to the assembly of two bidirectional DNA replication forks. These events are initiated by the formation of the pre-replication complex (pre-RC) at the origins of replication. This process takes place in the G1 stage of the cell cycle. The pre-RC formation involves the ordered assembly of many replication factors including the origin recognition complex (ORC), Cdc6 protein, Cdt1 protein, and minichromosome maintenance proteins (Mcm2-7). Once the pre-RC is formed, activation of the complex is triggered by two kinases, cyclin-dependent kinase 2 (CDK) and Dbf4-dependent kinase (DDK) that help transition the pre-RC to the initiation complex prior to the initiation of DNA replication. This transition involves the ordered assembly of additional replication factors to unwind the DNA and accumulate the multiple eukaryotic DNA polymerases around the unwound DNA.

Origin recognition complex

The first step in the assembly of the pre-replication complex (pre-RC) is the binding of the origin recognition complex (ORC) to the replication origin. In late mitosis, Cdc6 protein joins the bound ORC followed by the binding of the Cdt1-Mcm2-7 complex. ORC, Cdc6, and Cdt1 are all required to load the six protein minichromosome maintenance (Mcm 2–7) complex onto the DNA. The ORC is a six-subunit, Orc1p-6, protein complex that selects the replicative origin sites on DNA for initiation of replication and ORC binding to chromatin is regulated through the cell cycle. Generally, the function and size of the ORC subunits are conserved throughout many eukaryotic genomes with the difference being their diverged DNA binding sites.

The most widely studied origin recognition complex is that of *Saccharomyces cerevisiae* or yeast which is known to bind to the autonomously replicating sequence (ARS). The *S. cerevisiae* ORC interacts specifically with both the A and B1 elements of yeast origins of replication, spanning a region of 30 base pairs. The binding to these sequences requires ATP.

The atomic structure of the *S. cerevisiae* ORC bound to ARS DNA has been determined. Orc1, Orc2, Orc3, Orc4, and Orc5 encircle the A element by means of two types of interactions, base non-specific and base-specific, that bend the DNA at the A element. All five subunits contact the sugar phosphate backbone at multiple points of the A element to form a tight grip without base specificity. Orc1 and Orc2 contact the minor groove of the A element while a winged helix domain of Orc4 contacts the methyl groups of the invariant Ts in the major groove of the A element via an insertion helix (IH). The absence of this IH in metazoans partly explains the lack of sequence specificity in human ORC. The ARS DNA is also bent at the B1 element through interactions with Orc2, Orc5 and Orc6. The bending of origin DNA by ORC appears to be evolutionarily conserved suggesting that it may be required for the Mcm2-7 complex loading mechanism.

When the ORC binds to DNA at replication origins, it serves as a scaffold for the assembly of other key initiation factors of the pre-replicative complex. This pre-replicative complex assembly during the G1 stage of the cell cycle is required prior to the activation of DNA replication during the S phase. The removal of at least part of the complex (Orc1) from the chromosome at metaphase is part of the regulation of mammalian ORC to ensure that the pre-replicative complex formation prior to the completion of metaphase is eliminated. Central to the question of how bidirectional replication forks are established at replication origins is the mechanism by which ORC recruits two head-to-head Mcm2-7 complexes to every replication origin.

Cdc6 protein

Binding of the cell division cycle 6 (Cdc6) protein to the origin recognition complex (ORC) is an essential step in the assembly of the pre-replication complex (pre-RC) at the origins of replication. Cdc6 binds to the ORC on DNA in an ATP-dependent manner, which induces a change in the pattern of origin binding that requires Orc1 ATPase. Cdc6 requires ORC in order to associate with chromatin and is in turn required for the minichromosome maintenance proteins (Mcm2-7) to bind to the chromatin. The ORC-Cdc6 complex forms a ring-shaped structure and is analogous to other ATP-dependent protein machines. The levels and activity of Cdc6 regulate the frequency with which the origins of replication are utilised during the cell cycle.

Cdt1 protein

The chromatin licensing and DNA replication factor 1 (Cdt1) protein is required for the licensing of chromatin for DNA replication. In *S. cerevisiae*, Cdt1 facilitates the loading of the Mcm2-7 complex one at a time onto the chromosome by stabilising the left-handed open-ring structure of the Mcm2-7 single hexamer. Cdt1 has been shown to associate with the C terminus of Cdc6 to cooperatively promote the association of Mcm proteins to the chromatin. The cryo-EM structure of the OCCM (ORC-Cdc6-Cdt1-MCM) complex shows that the Cdt1-CTD interacts with the Mcm6-WHD. In metazoans, Cdt1 activity during the cell cycle is tightly regulated by its association with the protein geminin, which both inhibits Cdt1 activity during S phase in order to prevent re-replication of DNA and prevents it from ubiquitination and subsequent proteolysis.

Minichromosome maintenance protein complex

The minichromosome maintenance (Mcm) proteins were named after a genetic screen for DNA replication initiation mutants in *S. cerevisiae* that affect plasmid stability in an ARS-specific manner. Mcm2, Mcm3, Mcm4, Mcm5, Mcm6 and Mcm7 form a hexameric complex that has an open-ring structure with a gap between Mcm2 and Mcm5. The assembly of the Mcm proteins onto chromatin requires the coordinated function of the origin recognition complex (ORC), Cdc6, and Cdt1. Once the Mcm proteins have been loaded onto the chromatin, ORC and Cdc6 can be removed from the chromatin without preventing subsequent DNA replication. This observation suggests that the primary role of the pre-replication complex is to correctly load the Mcm proteins.

The Mcm proteins on chromatin form a head-to-head double hexamer with the two rings slightly tilted, twisted and off-centred to create a kink in the central channel where the bound DNA is captured at the interface of the two rings. Each hexameric Mcm2-7 ring serves as the scaffold for the assembly of the replisome and then as the core of the catalytic CMG (Cdc45-MCM-GINS) helicase, which is a main component of the replisome. Each Mcm protein is highly related to all others, but unique sequences distinguishing each of the subunit types are conserved across eukaryotes. All eukaryotes have exactly six Mcm protein analogs that each fall into one of the existing classes (Mcm2-7), indicating that each Mcm protein has a unique and important function.

Minichromosome maintenance proteins are required for DNA helicase activity. Inactivation of any of the six Mcm proteins during S phase prevents further progression of the replication fork suggesting that the helicase cannot be recycled and must be assembled at replication origins. Along with the minichromosome maintenance protein complex helicase activity, the complex also has associated ATPase activity. A mutation in any one of the six Mcm proteins reduces the conserved ATP binding sites, which indicates that ATP hydrolysis is a coordinated event involving all six subunits of the Mcm complex. Studies have shown that within the Mcm protein complex are specific catalytic pairs of Mcm proteins that function together to coordinate ATP hydrolysis. For example, Mcm3 but not Mcm6 can activate Mcm6 activity. These studies, confirmed by cryo-EM structures of the Mcm2-7 complexes, suggest that the Mcm complex is a hexamer with Mcm3 next to Mcm7, Mcm2 next to Mcm6, and Mcm4 next to Mcm5. Both members of the catalytic pair contribute to the conformation that allows ATP binding and hydrolysis and the mixture of active and inactive subunits create a coordinated ATPase activity that allows the Mcm protein complex to complete ATP binding and hydrolysis as a whole.

The nuclear localisation of the minichromosome maintenance proteins is regulated in budding yeast cells. The Mcm proteins are present in the nucleus in G1 stage and S phase of the cell cycle, but are exported to the cytoplasm during the G2 stage and M phase. A complete and intact six subunit Mcm complex is required to enter into the cell nucleus. In *S. cerevisiae*, nuclear export is promoted by cyclin-dependent kinase (CDK) activity. Mcm proteins that are associated with chromatin are protected from CDK export machinery due to the lack of accessibiiity to CDK.

Initiation complex

During the G1 stage of the cell cycle, the replication initiation factors, origin recognition complex (ORC), Cdc6, Cdt1, and minichromosome maintenance (Mcm) protein complex, bind sequentially to DNA to form the pre-replication complex (pre-RC). At the transition of the G1 stage to the S phase of the cell cycle, S phase–specific cyclin-dependent protein kinase (CDK) and Cdc7/Dbf4 kinase (DDK) transform the pre-RC into an active replication fork. During this transformation, the pre-RC is disassembled with the loss of Cdc6, creating the initiation complex. In addition to the binding of the Mcm proteins, cell division cycle 45 (Cdc45) protein is also essential for initiating DNA replication. Studies have shown that Mcm is critical for the loading of Cdc45 onto chromatin and this complex containing both Mcm and Cdc45 is formed at the onset of the S phase of the cell cycle. Cdc45 targets the Mcm protein complex, which has been loaded onto the chromatin, as a component of the pre-RC at the origin of replication during the G1 stage of the cell cycle.

Cdc45 protein

Cell division cycle 45 (Cdc45) protein is a critical component for the conversion of the pre-replicative complex to the initiation complex. The Cdc45 protein assembles at replication origins before initiation and is required for replication to begin in *Saccharomyces cerevisiae*, and has an essential role during elongation. Thus, Cdc45 has central roles in both initiation and elongation phases of chromosomal DNA replication.

Cdc45 associates with chromatin after the beginning of initiation in late G1 stage and during the S phase of the cell cycle. Cdc45 physically associates with Mcm5 and displays genetic interactions with five of the six members of the Mcm gene family and the ORC2 gene. The loading of Cdc45 onto chromatin is critical for loading other various replication proteins, including DNA polymerase a, DNA polymerase e, replication protein A (RPA) and proliferating cell nuclear antigen (PCNA) onto chromatin. Within a Xenopus nucleus-free system, it has been demonstrated that Cdc45 is required for the unwinding of plasmid DNA. The Xenopus nucleus-free system also demonstrates that DNA unwinding and tight RPA binding to chromatin occurs only in the presence of Cdc45.

Binding of Cdc45 to chromatin depends on Clb-Cdc28 kinase activity as well as functional Cdc6 and Mcm2, which suggests that Cdc45 associates with the pre-RC after activation of S-phase cyclin-dependent kinases (CDKs). As indicated by the timing and the CDK dependence, binding of Cdc45 to chromatin is crucial for commitment to initiation of DNA replication. During S phase, Cdc45 physically interacts with Mcm proteins on chromatin, however, dissociation of Cdc45 from chromatin is slower than that of Mcm's, which indicates that the proteins are released by different mechanisms.

GINS

The six minichromosome maintenance proteins and Cdc45 are essential during initiation and elongation for the movement of replication forks and for unwinding of the DNA. GINS are essential for the interaction of Mcm and Cdc45 at the origins of replication during initiation and then at DNA replication forks as the replisome progresses. The GINS complex is composed of four small proteins Sld5 (Cdc105), Psf1 (Cdc101), Psf2 (Cdc102) and Psf3 (Cdc103), GINS represents 'go, ichi, ni, san' which means '5, 1, 2, 3' in Japanese.

Mcm10

Mcm10 is essential for chromosome replication and interacts with the minichromosome maintenance 2–7 helicase that is loaded in an inactive form at origins of DNA replication. Mcm10 chaperones the catalytic DNA polymerase a and helps stabilise the polymerase.

DDK and CDK kinases

At the onset of S phase, the pre-replicative complex must be activated by two S phase-specific kinases in order to form an initiation complex at an origin of replication. One kinase is the Cdc7-Dbf4 kinase called Dbf4-dependent kinase (DDK) and the other is cyclin-dependent kinase (CDK). Chromatin binding assays of Cdc45 in yeast and Xenopus have shown that a downstream event of CDK action is loading of Cdc45 onto chromatin. Cdc6 has been speculated to be a target of CDK action, because of the association between Cdc6 and CDK, and the CDK-dependent phosphorylation of Cdc6. The CDK-dependent phosphorylation of Cdc6 has been considered to be required for entry into the S phase. Both the catalytic subunits of DDK and Cdc7, and the activator protein, Dbf4, are conserved in eukaryotes and are required for the onset of S phase of the cell cycle. Both DDK and Cdc7 are required for the loading of Cdc45 onto chromatin origins of replication. The target for binding of the DDK kinase is the Mcm complex, possibly Mcm2. DDK targets the Mcm complex, and its phosphorylation leads to the possible activation of Mcm helicase activity.

Dpb11, Sld3, and Sld2 proteins

Sld3, Sld2, and Dpb11 interact with many replication proteins. Sld3 and Cdc45 form a complex that associated with the pre-RC at the early origins of replication even in the $G1_1$ phase and with the later origins of replication in the S phase in a mutually Mcm-dependent manner. Dpb11 and Sld2 interact with Polymerase ε and cross-linking experiments have indicated that Dpb11 and Polymerase ε coprecipitate in the S phase and associate with replication origins. Sld3 and Sld2 are phosphorylated by CDK, which enables the two replicative proteins to bind to Dpb11. Dpb11 had two pairs of BRCA1 C-Terminus (BRCT) domains which are known as a phosphopeptide-binding domains. The N-terminal pair of the BRCT domains binds to phosphorylated Sld3, and the C-terminal pair binds to phosphorylated Sld2. Both of these interactions are essential for CDK-dependent activation of DNA budding in yeast.

Dpb11 also interacts with GINS and participates in the initiation and elongation steps of chromosomal DNA replication. GINS are one of the replication proteins found at the replication forks and forms a complex with Cdc45 and Mcm. These phosphorylation-dependent interactions between Dpb11, Sld2, and Sld3 are essential for CDK-dependent activation of DNA replication, and by using cross-linking reagents within some experiments, a fragile complex was identified called the pre-loading complex (pre-LC). This complex contains Pol ε, GINS, Sld2, and Dpb11. The pre-LC is found to form before any association with the origins in a CDK-dependent and DDK-dependent manner and CDK activity regulates the initiation of DNA replication through the formation of the pre-LC.

Elongation

The formation of the pre-replicative complex (pre-RC) marks the potential sites for the initiation of DNA replication. Consistent with the minichromosome maintenance complex encircling double stranded DNA, formation of the pre-RC does not lead to the immediate unwinding of origin DNA or the recruitment of DNA polymerases. Instead, the pre-RC that is formed during the G1 of the cell cycle is only activated to unwind the DNA and initiate replication after the cells pass from the G1 to the S phase of the cell cycle.

Once the initiation complex is formed and the cells pass into the S phase, the complex then becomes a replisome. The eukaryotic replisome complex is responsible for coordinating DNA replication. Replication on the leading and lagging strands is performed by DNA polymerase ε and DNA polymerase δ. Many replisome factors including Claspin, And1, replication factor C clamp loader and the fork protection complex are responsible for regulating polymerase functions and coordinating DNA synthesis with the unwinding of the template strand by Cdc45-Mcm-GINS complex. As the DNA is unwound the twist number decreases. To compensate for this the writhe number increases, introducing positive supercoils in the DNA. These supercoils would cause DNA replication to halt if they were not removed. Topoisomerases are responsible for removing these supercoils ahead of the replication fork.

The replisome is responsible for copying the entire genomic DNA in each proliferative cell. The base pairing and chain formation reactions, which form the daughter helix, are catalysed by DNA polymerases. These enzymes move along single-stranded DNA and allow for the extension of the nascent DNA strand by 'reading' the template strand and allowing for incorporation of the proper purine nucleobases, adenine and guanine, and pyrimidine nucleobases, thymine and cytosine. Activated free deoxyribonucleotides exist in the cell as deoxyribonucleotide triphosphates (dNTPs). These free nucleotides are added to an exposed 3'-hydroxyl group on the last incorporated nucleotide. In this reaction, a pyrophosphate is released from the free dNTP, generating energy for the polymerisation reaction and exposing the 5' monophosphate, which is then covalently bonded to the 3' oxygen. Additionally, incorrectly inserted nucleotides can be removed and replaced by the correct nucleotides in an energetically favorable reaction. This property is vital to proper proof reading and repair of errors that occur during DNA replication.

Replication fork

The replication fork is the junction between the newly separated template strands, known as the leading and lagging strands, and the double stranded DNA. Since duplex DNA is antiparallel, DNA replication occurs in opposite directions between the two new strands at the replication fork, but all DNA polymerases synthesise DNA in the 5' to 3' direction with respect to the newly synthesised strand. Further coordination is required during DNA replication. Two replicative polymerases synthesise DNA in opposite orientations. Polymerase ε synthesises DNA on the 'leading' DNA strand continuously as it is pointing in the same direction as DNA unwinding by the replisome. In contrast, polymerase δ synthesises DNA on the 'lagging' strand, which is the opposite DNA template strand, in a fragmented or discontinuous manner. The discontinuous stretches of DNA replication products on the lagging strand are known as Okazaki fragments (Fig. 19.6) and are about 100 to 200 bases in length at eukaryotic replication forks. The lagging strand usually contains longer stretches of single-stranded DNA that is coated with single-stranded binding proteins, which help stabilise the single-stranded templates by preventing a secondary structure formation. In eukaryotes, these single-stranded binding proteins are a heterotrimeric complex known as replication protein A (RPA).

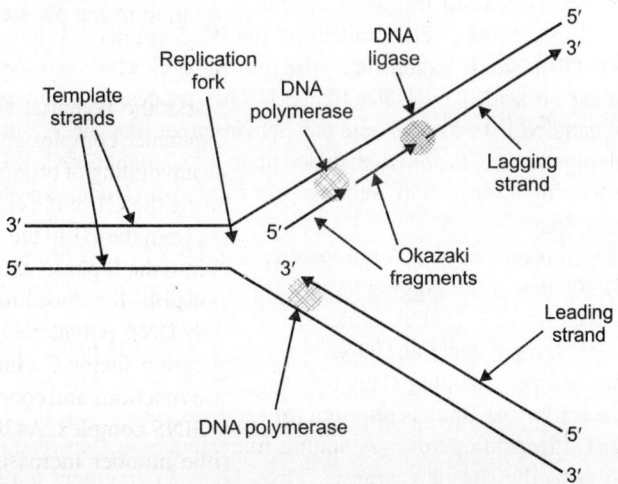

Fig. 19.6: Depiction of DNA replication at replication fork.

Each Okazaki fragment is preceded by an RNA primer, which is displaced by the procession of the next Okazaki fragment during synthesis. RNase H recognises the DNA:RNA hybrids that are created by the use of RNA primers and is responsible for removing these from the replicated strand, leaving behind a primer:template junction. DNA polymerase a, recognises these sites and elongates the breaks left by primer removal. In eukaryotic cells, a small amount of the DNA segment immediately upstream of the RNA primer is also displaced, creating a flap structure. This flap is then cleaved by endonucleases. At the replication fork, the gap in DNA after removal of the flap is sealed by DNA ligase I, which repairs the nicks that are left between the 3'-OH and 5'phosphate of the newly synthesised strand. Owing to the relatively short nature of the eukaryotic Okazaki fragment, DNA replication synthesis occurring discontinuously on the lagging strand is less efficient and more time consuming than leading-strand synthesis. DNA synthesis is complete once all RNA primers are removed and nicks are repaired.

Leading strand

During DNA replication, the replisome will unwind the parental duplex DNA into a two single-stranded DNA template replication fork in a 5' to 3' direction. The leading strand is the template strand that is being replicated in the same direction as the movement of the replication fork. This allows the newly synthesised strand complementary to the original strand to be synthesised 5' to 3' in the same direction as the movement of the replication fork. Once an RNA primer has been added by a primase to the 3' end of the leading strand, DNA synthesis will continue in a 3' to 5' direction with respect to the leading strand uninterrupted. DNA Polymerase ε will continuously add nucleotides to the template strand therefore making leading strand synthesis require only one primer and has uninterrupted DNA polymerase activity.

Lagging strand

DNA replication on the lagging strand is discontinuous. In lagging strand synthesis, the movement of DNA polymerase in the opposite direction of the replication fork requires the use of multiple RNA primers. DNA polymerase will synthesise short fragments of DNA called Okazaki fragments which are added to the 3' end of the primer. These fragments can be anywhere between 100–400 nucleotides long in eukaryotes. At the end of Okazaki fragment synthesis, DNA polymerase d runs into the previous Okazaki fragment and displaces its 5' end containing the RNA primer and a small segment of DNA. This generates an RNA-DNA single strand flap, which must be cleaved, and the nick between the two Okazaki fragments must be sealed by DNA ligase I. This process is known as Okazaki fragment maturation and can be handled in two ways: one mechanism processes short flaps, while the other deals with long flaps. DNA polymerase δ is able to displace up to 2 to 3 nucleotides of DNA or RNA ahead of its polymerisation, generating a short 'flap' substrate for Fen1, which can remove nucleotides from the flap, one nucleotide at a time.

By repeating cycles of this process, DNA polymerase d and Fen1 can coordinate the removal of RNA primers and leave a DNA nick at the lagging strand. It has been proposed that this iterative process is preferable to the cell because it is tightly regulated and does not generate large flaps that need to be excised. In the event of deregulated Fen1/DNA polymerase d activity, the cell uses an alternative mechanism to generate and process long flaps by using Dna2, which has both helicase and nuclease activities. The nuclease activity of Dna2 is required for removing these long flaps, leaving a shorter flap to be processed by Fen1. Electron microscopy studies indicate that nucleosome loading on the lagging strand occurs very close to the site of synthesis. Thus, Okazaki fragment maturation is an efficient process that occurs immediately after the nascent DNA is synthesised.

Replicative DNA polymerases

After the replicative helicase has unwound the parental DNA duplex, exposing two single-stranded DNA templates, replicative polymerases are needed to generate two copies of the parental genome. DNA polymerase function is highly specialised and accomplish replication on specific templates and in narrow localisations. At the eukaryotic replication fork, there are three distinct replicative polymerase complexes that contribute to DNA replication: Polymerase α, Polymerase δ, and Polymerase ε. These three polymerases are essential for viability of the cell.

Because DNA polymerases require a primer on which to begin DNA synthesis, polymerase α (Pol α) acts as a replicative primase. Pol α is associated with an RNA primase and this complex accomplishes the priming task by synthesising a primer that contains a short 10 nucleotide stretch of RNA followed by 10 to 20 DNA bases. Importantly, this priming action occurs at replication initiation at origins to begin leading-strand synthesis and also at the 5′ end of each Okazaki fragment on the lagging strand.

However, Pol α is not able to continue DNA replication and must be replaced with another polymerase to continue DNA synthesis. Polymerase switching requires clamp loaders and it has been proven that normal DNA replication requires the coordinated actions of all three DNA polymerases: Pol α for priming synthesis, Pol ε for leading-strand replication, and the Pol δ, which is constantly loaded, for generating Okazaki fragments during lagging-strand synthesis.

- Polymerase α (Pol α): Forms a complex with a small catalytic subunit (PriS) and a large noncatalytic (PriL) subunit. First, synthesis of an RNA primer allows DNA synthesis by DNA polymerase alpha. Occurs once at the origin on the leading strand and at the start of each Okazaki fragment on the lagging strand. Pri subunits act as a primase, synthesising an RNA primer. DNA Pol α elongates the newly formed primer with DNA nucleotides. After around 20 nucleotides, elongation is taken over by Pol ε on the leading strand and Pol δ on the lagging strand.

- Polymerase δ (Pol δ): Highly processive and has proof reading, 3′->5′ exonuclease activity. In vivo, it is the main polymerase involved in both lagging strand and leading strand synthesis.

- Polymerase ε (Pol ε): Highly processive and has proof reading, 3′->5′ exonuclease activity. Highly related to pol δ, *in vivo* it functions mainly in error checking of pol δ.

Cdc45–Mcm–GINS helicase complex

The DNA helicases and polymerases must remain in close contact at the replication fork. If unwinding occurs too far in advance of synthesis, large tracts of single-stranded DNA are exposed. This can activate DNA damage signalling or induce DNA repair processes. To thwart these problems, the eukaryotic replisome contains specialised proteins that are designed to regulate the helicase activity ahead of the replication fork. These proteins also provide docking sites for physical interaction between helicases and polymerases, thereby ensuring that duplex unwinding is coupled with DNA synthesis.

For DNA polymerases to function, the double-stranded DNA helix has to be unwound to expose two single-stranded DNA templates for replication. DNA helicases are responsible for unwinding the double-stranded DNA during chromosome replication. Helicases in eukaryotic cells are remarkably complex. The catalytic core of the helicase is composed of six minichromosome maintenance (Mcm2-7) proteins, forming a hexameric ring. Away from DNA, the Mcm2-7 proteins form a single heterohexamer and are loaded in an inactive form at origins of DNA replication as a head-to-head double hexamers around double-stranded DNA. The Mcm proteins are recruited to replication origins then redistributed throughout the genomic DNA during S phase, indicative of their localisation to the replication fork.

Loading of Mcm proteins can only occur during the G1 of the cell cycle, and the loaded complex is then activated during S phase by recruitment of the Cdc45 protein and the GINS complex to form the active Cdc45–Mcm–GINS (CMG) helicase at DNA replication forks. Mcm activity is required throughout the S phase for DNA replication. A variety of regulatory factors assemble around the CMG helicase to produce the 'Replisome Progression Complex' which associates with DNA polymerases to form the eukaryotic replisome, the structure of which is still quite poorly defined in comparison with its bacterial counterpart. The isolated CMG helicase and Replisome Progression Complex contain a single Mcm protein ring complex suggesting that the loaded double hexamer of the Mcm proteins at origins might be broken into two single hexameric rings as part of the initiation process, with each Mcm protein complex ring forming the core of a CMG helicase at the two replication forks established from each origin. The full CMG complex is required for DNA unwinding, and the complex of CDC45-Mcm-GINS is the functional DNA helicase in eukaryotic cells.

Ctf4 and And1 proteins

The CMG complex interacts with the replisome through the interaction with Ctf4 and And1 proteins. Ctf4/And1 proteins interact with both the CMG complex and DNA polymerase α. Ctf4 is a polymerase a accessory factor, which is required for the recruitment of polymerase a to replication origins.

Mrc1 and Claspin proteins

Mrc1/Claspin proteins couple leading-strand synthesis with the CMG complex helicase activity. Mrc1 interacts with polymerase ε as well as Mcm proteins. The importance of this direct link between the helicase and the leading-strand polymerase is underscored by results in cultured human cells, where Mrc1/Claspin is required for efficient replication fork progression. These results suggest that efficient DNA replication also requires the coupling of helicases and leading-strand synthesis.

Proliferating cell nuclear antigen

DNA polymerases require additional factors to support DNA replication. DNA polymerases have a semiclosed 'hand' structure, which allows the polymerase to load onto the DNA and begin translocating. This structure permits DNA polymerase to hold the single-stranded DNA template, incorporate dNTPs at the active site, and release the newly formed double-stranded DNA. However, the structure of DNA polymerases does not allow a continuous stable interaction with the template DNA.

To strengthen the interaction between the polymerase and the template DNA, DNA sliding clamps associate with the polymerase to promote the processivity of the replicative polymerase. In eukaryotes, the sliding clamp is a homotrimer ring structure known as the proliferating cell nuclear antigen (PCNA). The PCNA ring has polarity with surfaces that interact with DNA polymerases and tethers them securely to the DNA template. PCNA-dependent stabilisation of DNA polymerases has a significant effect on DNA replication because PCNAs are able to enhance the polymerase processivity up to 1000-fold. PCNA is an essential cofactor and has the distinction of being one of the most common interaction platforms in the replisome to accommodate multiple processes at the replication fork, and so PCNA is also viewed as a regulatory cofactor for DNA polymerases.

Replication factor C

PCNA fully encircles the DNA template strand and must be loaded onto DNA at the replication fork. At the leading strand, loading of the PCNA is an infrequent process, because DNA replication on the leading strand is continuous until replication is terminated. However, at the lagging strand, DNA polymerase d needs to be continually loaded at the start of each Okazaki fragment. This constant initiation of Okazaki fragment synthesis requires repeated PCNA loading for efficient DNA replication.

PCNA loading is accomplished by the replication factor C (RFC) complex. The RFC complex is composed of five ATPases: Rfc1, Rfc2, Rfc3, Rfc4 and Rfc5. RFC recognises primer-template junctions and loads PCNA at these sites. The PCNA homotrimer is opened by RFC by ATP hydrolysis and is then loaded onto DNA in the proper orientation to facilitate its association with the polymerase. Clamp loaders can also unload PCNA from DNA, a mechanism needed when replication must be terminated.

Stalled replication fork

DNA replication at the replication fork can be halted by a shortage of deoxynucleotide triphosphates (dNTPs) or by DNA damage, resulting in replication stress. This halting of replication is described as a stalled replication fork. A fork protection complex of proteins stabilises the replication fork until DNA damage or other replication problems can be fixed. Prolonged replication fork stalling can lead to further DNA damage. Stalling signals are deactivated if the problems causing the replication fork are resolved.

Termination of Eukaryotic DNA Replication

Termination of eukaryotic DNA replication requires different processes depending on whether the chromosomes are circular or linear. Unlike linear molecules, circular chromosomes are able to replicate the entire molecule. However, the two DNA molecules will remain linked together. This issue is handled by decatenation of the two DNA molecules by a type II topoisomerase. Type II topoisomerases are also used to separate linear strands as they are intricately folded into a nucleosome within the cell.

As previously mentioned, linear chromosomes face another issue that is not seen in circular DNA replication. Due to the fact that an RNA primer is required for initiation of DNA synthesis, the lagging strand is at a disadvantage in replicating the entire chromosome. While the leading strand can use a single RNA primer to extend the 5′ terminus of the replicating DNA strand, multiple RNA primers are responsible for lagging strand synthesis, creating Okazaki fragments. This leads to an issue due to the fact that DNA polymerase is only able to add to the 3′ end of the DNA strand. The 3′-5′ action of DNA polymerase along the parent strand leaves a short single-stranded DNA (ssDNA) region at the 3′ end of the parent strand when the Okazaki fragments have been repaired. Since replication occurs in opposite directions at opposite ends of parent chromosomes, each strand is a lagging strand at one end. Over time this would result in progressive shortening of both daughter chromosomes. This is known as the end replication problem.

The end replication problem is handled in eukaryotic cells by telomere regions and telomerase. Telomeres extend the 3′ end of the parental chromosome beyond the 5′ end of the daughter strand. This single-stranded DNA structure can act as an origin of replication that recruits telomerase. Telomerase is a specialised DNA polymerase that consists of multiple protein subunits and an RNA component. The RNA component of telomerase anneals to the single stranded 3′ end of the template DNA and contains 1.5 copies of the telomeric sequence. Telomerase contains a protein subunit that is a reverse transcriptase called telomerase reverse transcriptase or TERT. TERT synthesises DNA until the end of the template telomerase RNA and then disengages. This process can be repeated as many times as needed with the extension of the 3′ end of the parental DNA molecule. This 3′ addition provides a template for extension of the 5′ end of the daughter strand by lagging strand DNA synthesis. Regulation of telomerase activity is handled by telomere-binding proteins.

Replication fork barriers

Eukaryotic DNA replication is bidirectional, within a replicative origin, replisome complexes are created at each end of the replication origin and replisomes move away from each other from the initial starting point. In prokaryotes, bidirectional replication initiates at one replicative origin on the circular chromosome and terminates at a site opposed from the initial start of the origin. These termination regions have DNA sequences known as Ter sites. These Ter sites are bound by the Tus protein. The Ter-Tus complex is able to stop helicase activity, terminating replication.

In eukaryotic cells, termination of replication usually occurs through the collision of the two replicative forks between two active replication origins. The location of the collision varies on the timing of origin firing. In this way, if a replication fork becomes stalled or collapses at a certain site, replication of the site can be rescued when a replisome traveling in the opposite direction completes copying the region. There are programmed replication fork barriers (RFBs) bound by RFB proteins in various locations, throughout the genome, which are able to terminate or pause replication forks, stopping progression of the replisome.

Cell Cycle Regulation

DNA replication is a tightly orchestrated process that is controlled within the context of the cell cycle. Progress through the cell cycle and in turn DNA replication is tightly regulated by the formation and activation of pre-replicative complexes (pre-RCs) which is achieved through the activation and inactivation of cyclin-dependent kinases (Cdks, CDKs). Specifically it is the interactions of cyclins and cyclin dependent kinases that are responsible for the transition from G1 into S-phase.

During the G1 phase of the cell cycle there are low levels of CDK activity. This low level of CDK activity allows for the formation of new pre-RC complexes but is not sufficient for DNA replication to be initiated by the newly formed pre-RCs. During the remaining phases of the cell cycle there are elevated levels of CDK activity. This high level of CDK activity is responsible for initiating DNA replication as well as inhibiting new pre-RC complex formation. Once DNA replication has been initiated the pre-RC complex is broken down. Due to the fact that CDK levels remain high during the S phase, G2, and M phases of the cell cycle no new pre-RC complexes can be formed. This all helps to ensure that no initiation can occur until the cell division is complete.

In addition to cyclin dependent kinases a new round of replication is thought to be prevented through the downregulation of Cdt1. This is achieved via degradation of Cdt1 as well as through the inhibitory actions of a protein known as geminin. Geminin binds tightly to Cdt1 and is thought to be the major inhibitor of re-replication. Geminin first appears in S-phase and is degraded at the metaphase-anaphase transition, possibly through ubiquination by anaphase promoting complex (APC). Various cell cycle checkpoints are present throughout the course of the cell cycle that determine whether a cell will progress through division entirely. Importantly in replication the G1, or restriction, checkpoint makes the determination of whether or not initiation of replication will begin or whether the cell will be placed in a resting stage known as G0. Cells in the G0 stage of the cell cycle are prevented from initiating a round of replication because the minichromosome maintenance proteins are not expressed. Transition into the S-phase indicates replication has begun. Cell cycle for eukaryotic cells is shown in Fig. 19.7.

Replication checkpoint proteins

In order to preserve genetic information during cell division, DNA replication must be completed with high fidelity. In order to achieve this task, eukaryotic cells have proteins in place during certain points in the replication process that are able to detect any errors during DNA replication and are able to preserve

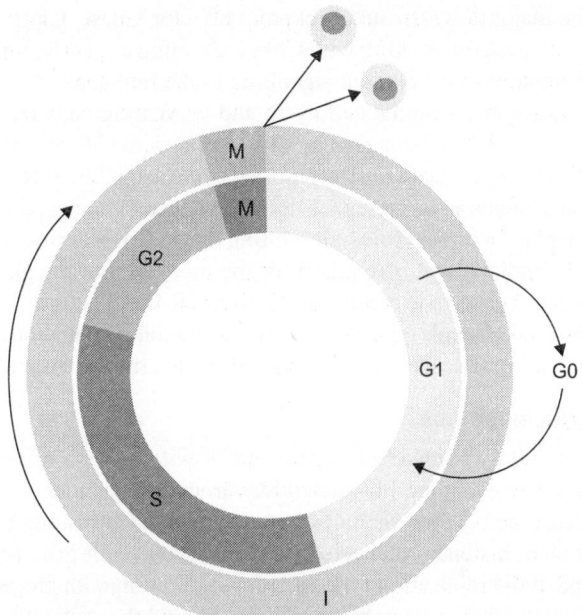

Fig. 19.7: Cell cycle for eukaryotic cells.

genomic integrity. These checkpoint proteins are able to stop the cell cycle from entering mitosis in order to allow time for DNA repair. Checkpoint proteins are also involved in some DNA repair pathways, while they stabilise the structure of the replication fork to prevent further damage. These checkpoint proteins are essential to avoid passing down mutations or other chromosomal aberrations to offspring.

Eukaryotic checkpoint proteins are well conserved and involve two phosphatidylinositol 3-kinase-related kinases (PIKKs), ATR and ATM. Both ATR and ATM share a target phosphorylation sequence, the SQ/TQ motif, but their individual roles in cells differ. ATR is involved in arresting the cell cycle in response to DNA double-stranded breaks. ATR has an obligate checkpoint partner, ATR-interacting-protein (ATRIP), and together these two proteins are responsive to stretches of single-stranded DNA that are coated by replication protein A (RPA). The formation of single-stranded DNA occurs frequently, more often during replication stress. ATR-ATRIP is able to arrest the cell cycle to preserve genome integrity. ATR is found on chromatin during S phase, similar to RPA and claspin.

The generation of single-stranded DNA tracts is important in initiating the checkpoint pathways downstream of replication damage. Once single-stranded DNA becomes sufficiently long, single-stranded DNA coated with RPA are able to recruit ATR-ATRIP. In order to become fully active, the ATR kinase rely on sensor proteins that sense whether the checkpoint proteins are localised to a valid site of DNA replication stress. The RAD9-HUS1-Rad1 (9-1-1) heterotrimeric clamp and its clamp loader RFCRad17 are able to recognise gapped or nicked DNA. The RFCRad17 clamp loader loads 9-1-1 onto the damaged DNA. The presence of 9-1-1 on DNA is enough to facilitate the interaction between ATR-ATRIP and a group of proteins termed checkpoint mediators, such as TOPBP1 and Mrc1/claspin. TOPBP1 interacts with and recruits the phosphorylated Rad9 component of 9-1-1 and binds ATR-ATRIP, which phosphorylates Chk1. Mrc1/Claspin is also required for the complete activation of ATR-ATRIP that phosphorylates Chk1, the major downstream checkpoint effector kinase. Claspin is a component of the replisome and contains a domain for docking with Chk1, revealing a specific function of Claspin during DNA replication: the promotion of checkpoint signalling at the replisome.

Chk1 signalling is vital for arresting the cell cycle and preventing cells from entering mitosis with incomplete DNA replication or DNA damage. The Chk1-dependent Cdk inhibition is important for the function of the ATR-Chk1 checkpoint and to arrest the cell cycle and allow sufficient time for completion of DNA repair mechanisms, which in turn prevents the inheritance of damaged DNA. In addition, Chk1-dependent Cdk inhibition plays a critical role in inhibiting origin firing during S phase. This mechanism prevents continued DNA synthesis and is required for the protection of the genome in the presence of replication stress and potential genotoxic conditions. Thus, ATR-Chk1 activity further prevents potential replication problems at the level of single replication origins by inhibiting initiation of replication throughout the genome, until the signalling cascade maintaining cell-cycle arrest is turned off.

Replication through Nucleosomes

Eukaryotic DNA must be tightly compacted in order to fit within the confined space of the nucleus. Chromosomes are packaged by wrapping 147 nucleotides around an octamer of histone proteins, forming a nucleosome. The nucleosome octamer includes two copies of each histone H2A, H2B, H3, and H4. Due to the tight association of histone proteins to DNA, eukaryotic cells have proteins that are designed to remodel histones ahead of the replication fork, in order to allow smooth progression of the replisome. There are also proteins involved in reassembling histones behind the replication fork to reestablish the nucleosome conformation. There are several histone chaperones that are known to be involved in nucleosome assembly after replication. The FACT complex has been found to interact with DNA polymerase α-primase complex, and the subunits of the FACT complex interacted genetically with replication factors. The FACT complex is a heterodimer that does not hydrolyse ATP, but is able to facilitate 'loosening' of histones in nucleosomes, but how the FACT complex is able to relieve the tight association of histones for DNA removal remains unanswered.

Another histone chaperone that associates with the replisome is Asf1, which interacts with the Mcm complex dependent on histone dimers H3-H4. Asf1 is able to pass newly synthesised H3-H4 dimer to deposition factors behind the replication fork and this activity makes the H3-H4 histone dimers available at the site of histone deposition just after replication. Asf1 (and its partner Rtt109) has also been implicated in inhibiting gene expression from replicated genes during S-phase.

The heterotrimeric chaperone chromatin assembly factor 1 (CAF-1) is a chromatin formation protein that is involved in depositing histones onto both newly replicated DNA strands to form chromatin. CAF-1 contains a PCNA-binding motif, called a PIP-box, that allows CAF-1 to associate with the replisome through PCNA and is able to deposit histone H3-H4 dimers onto newly synthesised DNA. The Rtt106 chaperone is also involved in this process, and associated with CAF-1 and H3-H4 dimers during chromatin formation. These processes load newly synthesised histones onto DNA.

After the deposition of histones H3-H4, nucleosomes form by the association of histone H2A-H2B. This process is thought to occur through the FACT complex, since it already associated with the replisome and is able to bind free H2A-H2B, or there is the possibility of another H2A-H2B chaperone, Nap1. Electron microscopy studies show that this occurs very quickly, as nucleosomes can be observed forming just a few hundred base pairs after the replication fork. Therefore, the entire process of forming new nucleosomes takes place just after replication due to the coupling of histone chaperones to the replisome.

Comparisons between Prokaryotic and Eukaryotic DNA Replication

When compared to prokaryotic DNA replication, the completion of eukaryotic DNA replication is more complex and involves multiple origins of replication and replicative proteins to accomplish. Prokaryotic DNA is arranged in a circular shape, and has only one replication origin when replication starts. By contrast, eukaryotic DNA is linear. When replicated, there are as many as one thousand origins of replication.

Eukaryotic DNA is bidirectional. Here the meaning of the word bidirectional is different. Eukaryotic linear DNA has many origins (called O) and termini (called T). 'T' is present to the right of 'O'. One 'O' and one 'T' together form one replicon. After the formation of pre-initiation complex, when one replicon starts elongation, initiation starts in second replicon. Now, if the first replicon moves in clockwise direction, the second replicon moves in anticlockwise direction, until 'T' of first replicon is reached. At 'T', both the replicons merge to complete the process of replication. Meanwhile, the seco nond replicon is moving in forward direction also, to meet with the third replicon. This clockwise and counter-clockwise movement of two replicons is termed as bidirectional replication.

Eukaryotic DNA replication requires precise coordination of all DNA polymerases and associated proteins to replicate the entire genome each time a cell divides. This process is achieved through a series of steps of protein assemblies at origins of replication, mainly focusing the regulation of DNA replication on the association of the MCM helicase with the DNA. These origins of replication direct the number of protein complexes that will form to initiate replication. In prokaryotic DNA replication regulation focuses on the binding of the DnaA initiator protein to the DNA, with initiation of replication occurring multiple times during one cell cycle. Both prokaryotic and eukaryotic DNA use ATP binding and hydrolysis to direct helicase loading and in both cases the helicase is loaded in the inactive form. However, eukaryotic helicases are double hexamers that are loaded onto double stranded DNA whereas prokaryotic helicases are single hexamers loaded onto single stranded DNA.

Segregation of chromosomes is another difference between prokaryotic and eukaryotic cells. Rapidly dividing cells, such as bacteria, will often begin to segregate chromosomes that are still in the process of replication. In eukaryotic cells chromosome segregation into the daughter cells is not initiated until replication is complete in all chromosomes. Despite these differences, however, the underlying process of replication is similar for both prokaryotic and eukaryotic DNA is shown in Table 19.1.

Table 19.1: Difference between prokaryotic and eukaryotic DNA replication.

Prokaryotic DNA replication	Eukaryotic DNA replication
Occurs inside the cytoplasm	Occurs inside the nucleus
Only one origin of replication per molecule of DNA	Have many origins of replication in each chromosome
Origin of replication is about 100–200 or more nucleotides in length	Each origin of replication is formed of about 150 nucleotides
Replication occurs at one point in each chromosome	Replication occurs at several points simultaneously in each chromosome
Only have one origin of replication	Has multiple origins of replication
Initiation is carried out by protein DnaA and DnaB	Initiation is carried out by the origin recognition complex
Topoisomerase is needed	Topoisomerase is needed
Replication is very rapid	Replication is very slow

PROKARYOTIC DNA REPLICATION

Prokaryotic DNA replication is the process by which a prokaryote duplicates its DNA into another copy that is passed on to daughter cells. Although it is often studied in the model organism *E. coli*, other bacteria show many similarities. Replication is bi-directional and originates at a single origin of replication (OriC). It consists of three steps: Initiation, elongation, and termination.

Initiation

All cells must finish DNA replication before they can proceed for cell division. Media conditions that support fast growth in bacteria also couples with shorter inter-initiation time in them, i.e. the doubling time in fast growing cells is less as compared to the slow growth. In other words, it is possible that in fast growth conditions the grandmother cells starts replicating its DNA for grand daughter cell. For the same reason, the initiation of DNA replication is highly regulated. Bacterial origins regulate orisome assembly, a nuclei-protein complex assembled on the origin responsible for unwinding the origin and loading all the replication machinery. In *E. coli*, the direction for orisome assembly are built into a short stretch of nucleotide sequence called as origin of replication (oriC) which contains multiple binding sites for the initiator protein DnaA (a highly homologous protein amongst bacterial kingdom). DnaA has four domains with each domain responsible for a specific task. There are 11 DnaA binding sites/boxes on the *E. coli* origin of replication out of which three boxes R1, R2 and R4 (which have a highly conserved 9 bp consensus sequence 5'-TTATC/ACACA) are high affinity DnaA boxes. They bind to DnaA-ADP and DnaA-ATP with equal affinities and are bound by DnaA throughout most of the cell cycle and forms a scaffold on which rest of the orisome assembles. The rest eight DnaA boxes are low affinity sites that preferentially bind to DnaA-ATP. During initiation, DnaA bound to high affinity DnaA box R4 donates additional DnaA to the adjacent low affinity site and progressively fill all the low affinity DnaA boxes. Filling of the sites changes origin conformation from its native state. It is hypothesised that DNA stretching by DnaA bound to the origin promotes strand separation which allows more DnaA to bind to the unwound region. The DnaC helicase loader then interacts with the DnaA bound to the single-stranded DNA to recruit the DnaB helicase, which will continue to unwind the DNA as the DnaG primase lays down an RNA primer and DNA Polymerase III holoenzyme begins elongation.

Regulation

Chromosome replication in bacteria is regulated at the initiation stage. DnaA-ATP is hydrolysed into the inactive DnaA-ADP by RIDA (Regulatory Inactivation of DnaA), and converted back to the active DnaA-ATP form by DARS (DnaA Reactivating Sequence, which is itself regulated by Fis and IHF). However, the main source of DnaA-ATP is synthesis of new molecules. Meanwhile, several other proteins interact directly with the oriC sequence to regulate initiation, usually by inhibition. In *E. coli* these proteins include DiaA, SeqA, IciA, HU, and ArcA-P, but they vary across other bacterial species. A few other mechanisms in *E. coli* that variously regulate initiation are DDAH (datA-Dependent DnaA Hydrolysis, which is also regulated by IHF), inhibition of the dnaA gene (by the SeqA protein), and reactivation of DnaA by the lipid membrane.

Elongation

Once priming is complete, DNA polymerase III holoenzyme is loaded into the DNA and replication begins. The catalytic mechanism of DNA polymerase III involves the use of two metal ions in the active site, and a region in the active site that can discriminate between deoxyribonucleotides and ribonucleotides.

The metal ions are general divalent cations that help the 3′ OH initiate a nucleophilic attack onto the alpha phosphate of the deoxyribonucleotide and orient and stabilise the negatively charged triphosphate on the deoxyribonucleotide. Nucleophilic attack by the 3′ OH on the alpha phosphate releases pyrophosphate, which is then subsequently hydrolysed (by inorganic phosphatase) into two phosphates. This hydrolysis drives DNA synthesis to completion.

Furthermore, DNA polymerase III must be able to distinguish between correctly paired bases and incorrectly paired bases. This is accomplished by distinguishing Watson-Crick base pairs through the use of an active site pocket that is complementary in shape to the structure of correctly paired nucleotides. This pocket has a tyrosine residue that is able to form van der Waals interactions with the correctly paired nucleotide. In addition, dsDNA (double stranded DNA) in the active site has a wider major groove and shallower minor groove that permits the formation of hydrogen bonds with the third nitrogen of purine bases and the second oxygen of pyrimidine bases. Finally, the active site makes extensive hydrogen bonds with the DNA backbone. These interactions result in the DNA polymerase III closing around a correctly paired base. If a base is inserted and incorrectly paired, these interactions could not occur due to disruptions in hydrogen bonding and van der Waals interactions.

DNA is read in the 3′→5′ direction, therefore, nucleotides are synthesised (or attached to the template strand) in the 5′→3′ direction. However, one of the parent strands of DNA is 5′→3′ while the other is 5′→3′. To solve this, replication occurs in opposite directions. Heading towards the replication fork, the leading strand is synthesised in a continuous fashion, only requiring one primer. On the other hand, the lagging strand, heading away from the replication fork, is synthesised in a series of short fragments known as Okazaki fragments, consequently requiring many primers. The RNA primers of Okazaki fragments are subsequently degraded by RNase H and DNA Polymerase I (exonuclease), and the gaps (or nicks) are filled with deoxyribonucleotides and sealed by the enzyme ligase.

Rate of replication

The rate of DNA replication in a living cell was first measured as the rate of phage T4 DNA elongation in phage-infected *E. coli*. During the period of exponential DNA increase at 37°C, the rate was 749 nucleotides per second. The mutation rate per base pair per replication during phage T4 DNA synthesis is 1.7 per 108.

Termination of DNA Replication

Termination of DNA replication in *E. coli* is completed through the use of termination sequences and the 'Tus' protein. These sequences allow the two replication forks to pass through in only one direction, but not the other. DNA replication initially produces two catenated or linked circular DNA duplexes, each comprising one parental strand and one newly synthesised strand (by nature of semiconservative replication). This catenation can be visualised as two interlinked rings which cannot be separated. Topoisomerase 2 in *E. coli* unlinks or decatenates the two circular DNA duplexes by breaking the phosphodiester bonds present in two successive nucleotides of either parent DNA or newly formed DNA and thereafter the ligating activity ligates that breaked DNA strand and so the two DNA gets formed.

LINEAR CHROMOSOME

A linear chromosome is a type of chromosome, found in most eukaryotic cells, in which the DNA is arranged in multiple linear molecules of DNA. In contrast, most prokaryotic cells contain circular chromosomes, where the DNA is arranged in one large circular molecule. However, linear chromosomes are not limited to eukaryotic organisms, some prokaryotic organisms do have linear chromosomes as well, such as *Borrelia burgdorferi*. It is possible to take a prokaryotic cell with a circular chromosome, linearise the chromosome, and still have a viable organism. Linear chromosomes have a few advantages and disadvantages to circular chromosomes. One reason that many organisms have evolved to having linear chromosomes is the size of their genome. Linear chromosomes make it easier for transcription and replication of large genomes. If an organism had a very large genome arranged in a circular chromosome, it would have the potential problems when unwinding due to torsional strain. As mentioned before, linear chromosomes are not perfect and have their disadvantages, the biggest being the terminal ends of the chromosomes, or telomeres.

Generally, telomeres tend to be unstable and lead to mutations or tumors. Additionally, due to the methods of DNA replication the ends of the telomeres will not completely be replicated and will be lost, which is known as the 'end replication problem'. Most eukaryotic cells are able to prevent crucial DNA from being lost by the use of telomerase, an enzyme that synthesises telomeric DNA, which allows the telomeric DNA to be cut short instead of cutting crucial DNA. Lastly, even though an organism may have evolved to having linear chromosomes, it is still possible for said organism to revert to having a circular chromosome. When this happens, the organism will essentially delete part of or all of its telomere ends of their linear chromosomes and recombine the strands into the circular shape.

Chapter 20

Genetics Techniques for DNA Analysis

INTRODUCTION

Before the 1980s, finding the genotype of an individual usually involved various laboratory assays for a gene product—the protein or enzyme. The cases of the ABO and Rhesus blood groups are classic examples of how one infers genotypes from the reaction of gene products with certain chemicals. In the mid 1980s, genetic technology took a great leap forward with the ability to genotype the DNA itself. The geneticist could now examine the DNA directly without going through the laborious process of developing assays to detect individual differences in proteins and enzymes. Direct DNA analysis had the further advantage of being able to identify alleles in sections of DNA that did not code for polypeptide chains. As a result of these new advances, the number of genetic loci that could be detected increased exponentially and soon led to the identification of the genes for disorders that had remained a mystery for the better part of this century.

BASIC TOOLS AND TECHNIQUES

Basic Tools: Cloning

In popular imagination, the term 'cloning' is associated with Brave New World, science fiction, and a famous sheep called Dolly. To the molecular geneticist, however, the term 'cloning' simply means the copying of a desired section of DNA. Historically, cloning began by isolating a small (i.e. several thousand base pairs) section of human DNA and then, after an elaborate series of steps, incorporating this segment into the DNA of another organism. The 'other' organism is called a vector, and of course, not any type of vector will do. To make many copies of the human DNA segment, one desires a vector that can reproduce rapidly. Hence, the most common vectors are the smallest organisms with dramatic reproductive potential— plasmids, virus, bacteria, and yeast. There are several major reasons for cloning human DNA. One purpose is to obtain large amounts of a human DNA sequence that can then be used as a probe in other types of molecular genetic techniques. A second reason is to construct DNA libraries, a topic discussed later in this chapter. Finally, cloning is also used for therapeutic genetic engineering. Here, the hope is that the vector with a cloned copy of the 'good' gene missing in a patient might be incorporated into the patient's cells and produce the missing protein or enzyme.

Basic Tools: Electrophoresis

Electrophoresis is a technique that separates small biological molecules by their molecular weight. It may be applied to molecules as large as proteins and enzymes as well as to small snippets of DNA and RNA. One begins the procedure by constructing a 'gel' a highly viscous material the actual chemistry of which need not concern us. Purified copies of the biological specimen are then injected into a 'starting lane' at one end of the gel. Finally, a weak electric current is passed through the gel for a specified amount of time. Gravity and the electric current cause the biological molecules to migrate to the opposite end of the gel. The extent to which any molecule moves depends upon its electrical charge, molecular weight, the viscosity of the gel, the strength of the current, and the amount of time that the current is applied. With constant charge, viscosity, current, and time, smaller molecules will migrate further through the gel than larger molecules (Fig. 20.1).

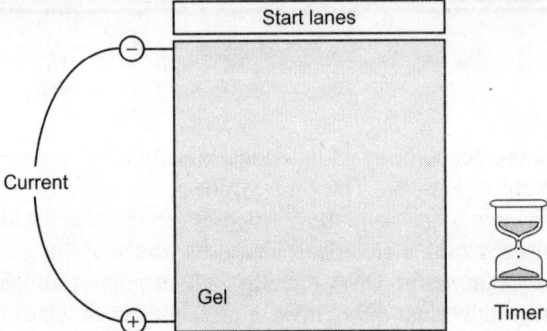

Fig. 20.1: Gel electrophoresis. Biological material (DNA, proteins, etc.) is placed in the start lane and an electrical current is turned on for a specified amount of time. Molecules will migrate to the opposite end of the gel according to their molecular weights. Smaller molecules will move further than larger ones.

Basic Tools: Probes

A probe is a segment of single stranded DNA or RNA with a known nucleotide sequence. The probe is either synthesised or cloned in a laboratory in very large amounts and is then placed into physical contact with human DNA that has been treated to become single-stranded. Because of complementary base pairing, the probe will bind to the DNA segment that contains the specific nucleotide sequence that complements the probe's sequence. An example is given in Fig. 20.2.

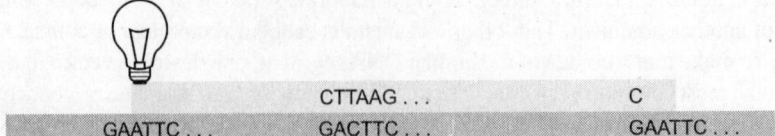

Fig. 20.2: An example of a probe. Probes are manufactured segments of single-stranded DNA that carry a 'lightbulb,' usually a florescent tag, and bind to its complementary single-stranded DNA sequence.

Basic Tools: Light Bulbs

Purified DNA and RNA resemble viscous water. If many small sections of single stranded DNA are subjected to gel electrophoresis, the sections will migrate to the opposite side of the gel according to their size, but they will be invisible. If probes are added, they will bind to the appropriate complementary snippets of the single-stranded DNA, forming a double strand. But the probes, being composed of nucleotides, will also be invisible. To locate the probe after it binds to the DNA, it is necessary to engineer the probe so that it carries the biological equivalent of a light bulb. Two major types of light bulbs are used in molecular genetics. The first type is constructed by labelling the probe with radioactive isotopes. The second type of probe uses special fluorescent dyes that allow the probe to be visualised and photographed under specialised lighting conditions. For many types of DNA analyses, radioactive probes are still the method of choice, but fluorescent technology is quickly replacing it.

Basic Tools: Restriction Enzyme

A restriction enzyme is an enzyme that recognises a specific nucleotide sequence and cuts DNA at the sequence. For example, the restriction enzyme EcoRI (for *E. Coli* Restriction enzyme number I) recognises the sequence GAATTC and slices the DNA right after the G. Restriction enzymes are used in a wide variety of techniques. One major advantage is that they can cut DNA (or 'digest' DNA, as the microbiologists prefer to call it) into fragments of manageable lengths. Without digestion using restriction enzymes, human DNA segments would simply be too long to allow them to be cloned or subject to many kinds of electrophoresis. Restriction enzymes also play an important role in detecting human polymorphisms.

Basic Tools: Polymerase Chain Reaction (PCR)

The polymerase chain reaction or PCR is a technique used to 'amplify' DNA, i.e. make a sufficient number of copies of a DNA segment to permit it to be used for other types of techniques. Many people are familiar with the forensic application of PCR. When only a tiny drop of blood, semen, or other biological specimen is available at a crime scene, PCR is used to make a sufficient amount of DNA to permit genotyping. PCR methodology makes use of many of the concepts outlined above, so it will be explained in some detail (Fig. 20.3). The procedure begins with purifying DNA from a biological specimen and then heating it almost to the boiling point of water. The heat separates the double-stranded DNA

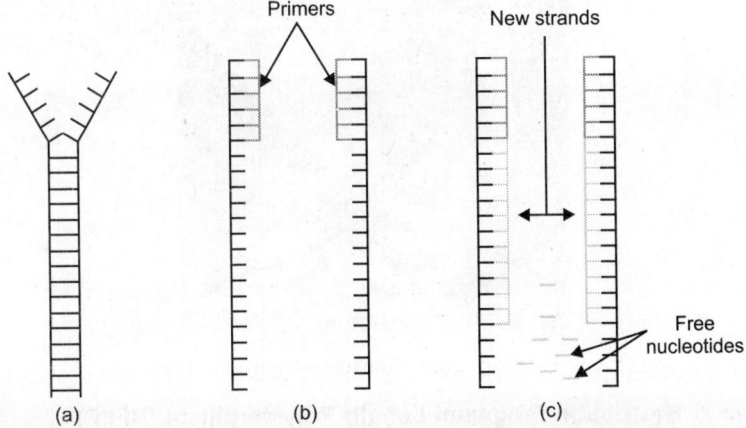

Fig. 20.3: PCR: The polymerase chain reaction. (a) With heating DNA becomes single-stranded, (b) a primer section of DNA is added, it will bind with its complementary base pairs on the original DNA, (c) free nucleotides and enzymes are added that will synthesise a new chain starting at the end of the primer.

into two single-strands. Once the DNA has become single-stranded, large amounts of specialised probe are added to the mixture along with an enzyme and a large number of free nucleotides. The probe binds to the DNA and then the enzyme synthesises a complementary strand to the DNA beginning with the end of the probe and continuing to the end of the DNA segment. If we began with a single copy of DNA, then the end of this process will result in two copies of the DNA molecule. By repeating the process of heating, bathing the DNA with probes, and adding the enzyme and nucleotides, we would now have four molecules of the desired DNA segment. Continuous repetition results in a geometric progression of DNA copies—8, then 16, then 32—until a sufficient amount of DNA is available for genotyping. Today, PRC is machine automated and is often done in conjunction with a robot that automatically sequences the amplified DNA. The advantage here is that PCR avoids the complicated laboratory procedures necessary to harvest enough DNA required for other types of genotyping. Automation also reduces the time and cost of genotyping. The biggest disadvantage of PCR is that the technique is so sensitive that it is susceptible to contamination from other DNA. Hence, careful laboratory protocol must be followed.

TYPES OF DNA POLYMORPHISMS

Polymorphisms 1: Blood groups

In the early days of human genetics, the majority of polymorphisms were those associated with proteins in blood. When your blood is typed, you are informed that you are blood group O+ or AB– or A+, etc. The letter in this blood group gives your phenotype at the ABO locus, and the plus (+) or minus (–) sign denotes your phenotype at the Rhesus locus. A number of other loci such as Kell, Duffy, MN, and Kidd can also be phenotyped from blood. These polymorphisms are still used today to assess suitability of donors and recipients for blood transfusions (ABO locus) and to assess Rhesus incompatibility between a mother and her fetus. However, blood group polymorphisms have given way to other, more sophisticated techniques in modern human genetic research. Rhesus monkey is shown in Fig. 20.4

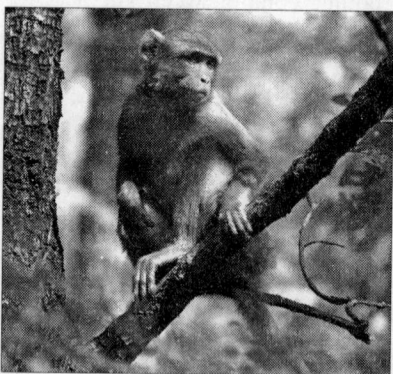

Fig. 20.4: Rhesus monkey.

Polymorphisms 2: Restriction Fragment Length Polymorphism (RFLP)

At this point, it is helpful to describe a genotyping technique that will use all the tools outlined above even though it is not the preferred method for todays research. The restriction fragment length polymorphism or RFLP was the technology that began the dramatic explosion in genetic technology by allowing the field to locate genes for Mendelian disorders like Huntington's disease (Fig. 20.5) and cystic fibrosis. The procedure is illustrated in Fig. 20.6. First a probe must be constructed that will bind with a known sequence of DNA. The sequence is the gene that we want to examine. The probe for this example was previously given in Fig. 20.2.

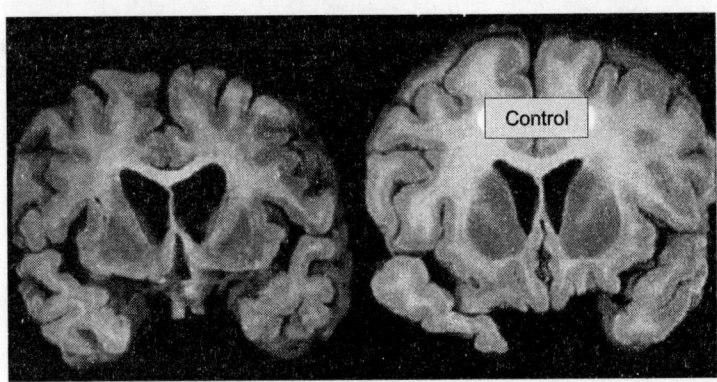

Fig. 20.5: Huntington's disease.

The DNA of an individual—I will use myself as the example—is then purified and the bonds connecting the two strands of the DNA molecule are cut, making the DNA single stranded. I happen to be a heterozygote at the locus at which the probe will bind. The difference in the alleles is subtle, but it appears in the middle nucleotide sequence for alleles 1 and 2 in Fig. 20.6. Allele 1 contains the sequence GACTTC while allele 2 contains the sequence GAATTC. The third nucleotide in this series differs. But this sequence is an important one because it is the one that is recognised by the EcoRI restriction enzyme. Suppose now that we take my DNA and place it into a solution with this restriction enzyme. Panels (b) and (c) show this for respectively my alleles. Allele 2 contains the necessary sequence for the restriction enzyme to cut the gene in the middle (in addition, of course, to cutting it at the beginning and end of the gene). This allele will now have two fragments. The first will begin with the sequence AATTC and will end with the G close to the middle. The second will begin with the AATTC near the middle and will end with the terminal G. For allele 1, on the other hand, the EcoRI enzyme recognises the initial sequence GAATTC and cuts the DNA between the G and the A. EcoRI will also recognise the last (rightmost) nucleotide sequence and cut the DNA after the G. EcoRI does not recognise the middle sequence, so it will not cut it there. Hence, allele 1 will contain one very long DNA fragment.

Now let us subject these fragments to electrophoresis. Allele 1, being quite long, will not move much from the start lane. The two fragments from allele 2, however, are considerably shorter than the single one for allele 1. These two fragments will move much further along the gel, the smaller of the two migrating more than the larger. We now have to 'light up' the invisible DNA strands by bathing everything in the probe. The single stranded probe will bind to all three of my DNA fragments—the long one from allele 1 and two shorter ones from allele 2. When the probe 'lights up,' all three strands will be revealed—see the panel (d) of Fig. 20.6. The laboratory now knows my genotype at this locus.

Polymorphisms 3: Tandem Repeat Polymorphisms

Although RFLPs were the first of the modern molecular methods used to detect polymorphisms, they have given ground to other, more discerning techniques. One generic class of polymorphisms has their

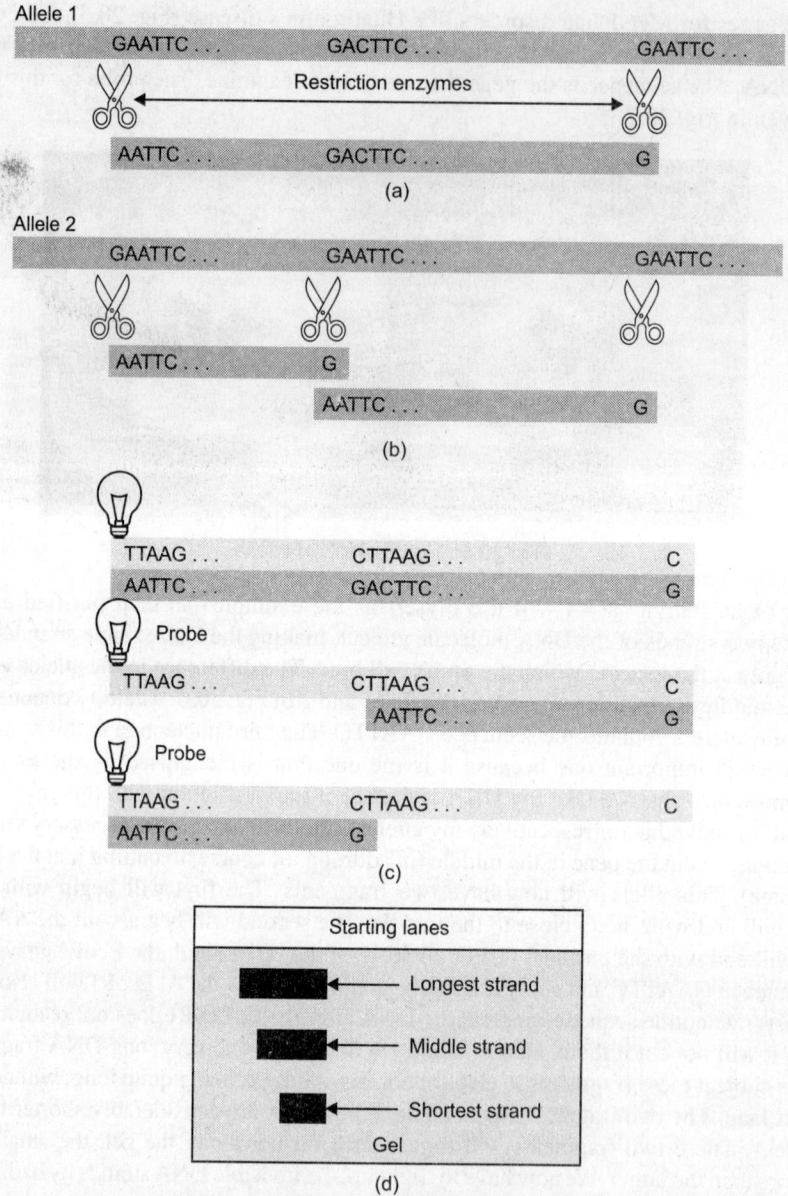

Fig. 20.6: The restriction fragment length polymorphism (RFLP). Panel (a): Allele 1 has two restriction sites; incubating this allele in the restriction enzyme will result in one long fragment. Panel (b): Allele 2 has three restriction sites; incubating this allele with the restriction enzyme results in two fragments. Panel (c): After the restriction enzyme cuts the DNA, the DNA is subjected to electrophoresis that separates the fragments according to size. A probe is then added to bind to the gene of interest. The binding of the probe after electrophoresis is illustrated in this panel. Panel (d): The gel is then viewed under special lighting or photographic film is placed on it. The result will be the characteristic bands illustrated in this panel.

origin in DNA nucleotide sequences that are repeated a certain number of times, one right after the other. These 'tandem repeats' are highly polymorphic in the sense that a large number of alleles may be found at any given locus. For example, one allele at a locus may have the sequence CAG repeated four times, another may have it repeated eight times, while yet a third may have it repeated 20 times.

Unfortunately, even though the concept of the tandem repeat is quite simple, the terminology for referring to these polymorphisms is quite confusing to the uninitiated. For simplicity's sake, we will lump all these fine distinctions together into the single category of tandem repeat polymorphisms.

Figure 20.7 illustrates this type of polymorphism. The repetitive nucleotide sequence is GAAC, which is contained eight times in allele 1 but only four times in allele 2. The probe in this case contains the repetitive complement CTTG.

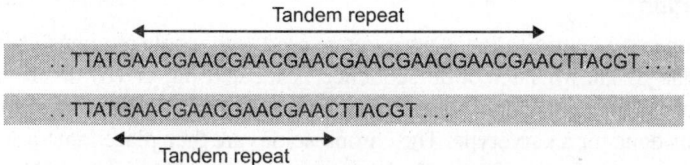

Fig. 20.7: Example of a tandem repeat polymorphism. The polymorphism consists in the number of times that a nucleotide sequence is repeated, GAAC in this case.

There are several different ways to genotype for tandem repeats. When the number of nucleotides in a sequence is fairly large (e.g. a series of 25 nucleotides is repeated over and over), then separating alleles by electrophoresis is often done. When the number is small (e.g. repeats of two to four nucleotides), then PCR is commonly used. Here, a special probe for the gene of interest is constructed for the area before the repeated sequence. PCR is then done to amplify the DNA that is then placed into a special sequencing machine that counts the number of repeats.

Polymorphisms 4: Single Nucleotide Polymorphisms (SNP)

A single nucleotide polymorphism or SNP is a sequence of DNA on which humans vary by one and only one nucleotide. Because humans by one nucleotide per every several hundred nucleotides, there are likely to be hundreds of thousands of SNPs scattered throughout the human genome.

The major advantage of SNPs, however, lies in the fact that they can be detected in a highly automated way using DNA chips. This avoids the laborious process of using gel electrophoresis and thus many more people and many more loci can be genotyped within a given amount of time. Genotyping begins with PCR to amplify the region containing a SNP. The resulting DNA is then heated to make it single stranded and placed onto a special chip that contains single-stranded DNA and microcircuitry. Specialised computer software can then 'read' the specific polymorphism. The potential of SNPs is so great that the Human Genome Project has established a special group, the SNP Consortium, to develop the technology and to locate SNPs.

Polymorphisms 5: Gene Sequencing

Nothing surpasses finding the ordering of the nucleotide sequence for a gene, a technique known as *sequencing*, for the detection of polymorphisms. Although this is the ultimate knowledge for the geneticist and will in time overshadow all other types of polymorphism detection, it is too time consuming and expensive to be used anywhere but in the more advanced research centers.

Here, we eschew explanation of sequencing procedures for one major reason. The Human Genome Project is devoting large amounts of its resources to automating the process of sequencing, so it is difficult to predict the methods of choice by the time these words hit print. Suffice it to say that within the next few decades, the computerised laboratory robots now available to the well-funded genetics laboratory will encounter the dramatic price discounts witnessed by the electronic calculator and later, the personal computer. Every hospital—as well as many laboratories researching individual differences in human behaviour—will eventually have a 'DNAnalyser' sitting in the corner of a room spurting out sequence information about genotypes.

Other Molecular Techniques

In situ hybridisation

In situ (Latin for 'on site') hybridisation is a technique used with whole chromosomes to: (i) find which chromosome a gene of known nucleotide sequence is located on, or (ii) determine if a section of chromosome has been deleted or duplicated. The technique begins by preparing chromosomes much in the same way that is done for a karyotype. The chromosomes are then placed into a solution with a large amount of either radioactively labelled or fluorescent probe. Combinations of chemicals and heat are used to split the double-stranded DNA in the chromosomes into single stranded DNA, permitting the probe to bind with the DNA. Excess probe is washed away and the chromosomes are then stained. If a section of a chromosome 'lights up' then we know that it has the nucleotide sequence complementary to that of the probe.

Mutational screening

Once a probe for a section of a protein-coding gene is identified, the curious geneticist can hardly resist the temptation to see if patients with a particular disorder have an irregularity at the locus. A classic example would be schizophrenia and the genes for dopamine receptors. For a long time, it was known that many drugs that diminish the florid hallucinations and delusions of the schizophrenic had important influences on dopamine receptors. Hence, when the gene for a dopamine receptor was first cloned, it was a natural matter to question if schizophrenics differed from nonschizophrenics in this gene.

Except for direct sequencing, many of the techniques outlined above are not suitable for screening the genotypes of patients. For example, RFLPs will only detect DNA differences at a restriction site, and the chances are quite remote that the aberration in the schizophrenic dopamine receptor allele happens to be at just this site. Several other techniques, collectively known as mutational screening, are preferred in this circumstance.

The two most widely developed mutational screens use souped up versions of electrophoresis to find small and subtle differences in DNA. One technique uses a gel that aries in temperature from the top to the bottom of the gel. As the DNA moves through the gel, the increased temperature will cause it to denature into its single strands and the resolution of the procedure permits detection of small sequence differences between a patient and a control. Once such a difference is detected, then the patient's DNA is sequenced to find the exact nucleotide variations.

The second technique is conceptually identical with the exception that the gel does not have a temperature gradient. It relies on the fact that small differences in the nucleotide sequence between two strands of DNA can be resolved in different bands on a specialised gel. Again, the patient's DNA is sequenced after a difference is found.

Finding the Gene for a Trait

Having surveyed the various tools and techniques of modern DNA genotyping, we now present the logic of going about the labour-intensive task of actually finding a gene for a trait. The first task is to make certain that the trait has some genetic influence on it. In the case of simple Mendelian disorders, the rarity of the disorder and the risk to different classes of relatives are usually sufficient to implicate a single gene. More complicated methods must be used for complex phenotypes.

The first challenge is to identify the chromosome on which the gene is located. Without knowing either the gene or its product, it is necessary to use a statistical procedure called linkage analysis to achieve this goal. Linkage begins with a host of genetic loci called markers or marker loci. A marker locus is a polymorphic locus with a known location on a chromosome. Linkage does not try to locate the precise position of the disease gene. Rather, it tries to identify which marker loci are close to the disease gene. In this way, a rough area of a particular chromosome will be targeted for further analysis. With current linkage maps, a disease gene can be located to anywhere within 1Mb (million base pairs) to 2Mb of its exact location. The major advantage of new technology is that it has greatly expanded the number of polymorphic loci that can be used as markers in a linkage study.

Before the human genome was fully sequenced, positive linkage findings were followed up by a procedure called positional cloning or gene walking to identify the location of the disease gene. Because the actual DNA sequence is now known, contemporary researchers power up their computers and download the nucleotide sequence for the region with the positive linkage. They then try to locate genes within this region by looking for promoter regions, initiation codons, stop codons, etc.

SECTION VII

Genetic Code and Transcription, RNA Editing and RNA Polymerase

Chapter 21

Genetic Code

INTRODUCTION

The genetic code is the set of rules by which a gene is translated into a functional protein. Each gene consists of a specific sequence of nucleotides encoded in a DNA (or sometimes RNA) strand, a correspondence between nucleotides, the basic building blocks of genetic material, and amino acids, the basic building blocks of proteins, must be established for genes to be successfully translated into functional proteins. Sets of three nucleotides, known as codons, each correspond to a specific amino acid or to a signal, three codons are known as 'stop codons' and, instead of specifying a new amino acid, alert the translation machinery that the end of the gene has been reached. There are 64 possible codons (four possible nucleotides at each of three positions, hence 4^3 possible codons) and only 20 standard amino acids, hence the code is redundant and multiple codons can specify the same amino acid. The correspondence between codons and amino acids is nearly universal among all known living organisms (Fig. 21.1).

CRACKING THE GENETIC CODE

After the structure of DNA was deciphered by James Watson, Francis Crick, Maurice Wilkins and Rosalind Franklin, serious efforts to understand the nature of the encoding of proteins began. George Gamow postulated that a three-letter code must be employed to encode the 20 standard amino acids used by living cells to encode proteins (because 3 is the smallest integer n such that 4^n is at least 20). The fact that codons consist of three DNA bases was first demonstrated in the Crick and Brenner experiment. They used a cell-free system to translate a polyuracil RNA sequence (e.g. UUUUU...) and discovered that the polypeptide that they had synthesised consisted of only the amino acid phenylalanine. They thereby deduced from this polyphenylalanine that the codon UUU specified the amino acid phenylalanine. Extending this work, Nirenberg and Philip Leder revealed the triplet nature of the genetic code and allowed the codons of the standard genetic code to be deciphered. In these experiments various combinations of mRNA were passed through a filter which contained ribosomes, the components of cells that translate RNA into protein. Unique triplets promoted the binding of specific tRNAs to the ribosome. Leder and Nirenberg were able to determine the sequences of 54 out of 64 codons in their experiments.

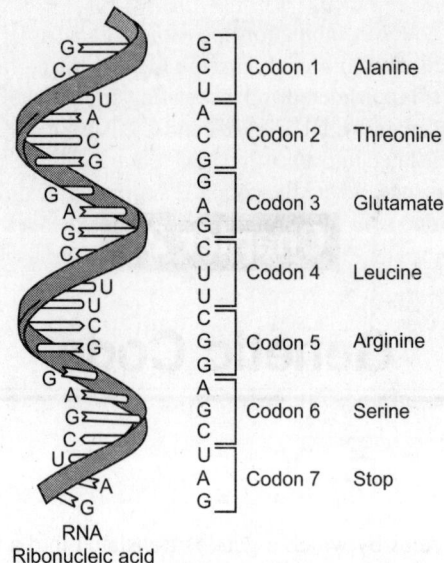

RNA
Ribonucleic acid

Fig. 21.1: Schematic diagram of a single-stranded RNA molecule illustrating the position of three-base codons.

Transfer of Information via the Genetic Code

The genome of an organism is inscribed in DNA, or in the case of some viruses, RNA. The portion of the genome that codes for a protein or an RNA is referred to as a gene. Those genes that code for proteins are composed of trinucleotide units called codons, each coding for a single amino acid. Each nucleotide subunit consists of a phosphate, deoxyribose sugar and one of the four nitrogenous nucleotide bases. The purine bases adenine (A) and guanine (G) are larger and consist of two aromatic rings. The pyrimidine bases cytosine (C) and thymine (T) are smaller and consist of only one aromatic ring. In the double-helix configuration, two strands of DNA are joined to each other by hydrogen bonds in an arrangement known as base pairing. These bonds almost always form between an adenine base on one strand and a thymine on the other strand and between a cytosine base on one strand and a guanine base on the other. This means that the number of A and T residues will be the same in a given double helix, as will the number of G and C residues. In RNA, thymine (T) is replaced by uracil (U), and the deoxyribose is substituted by ribose.

Each protein-coding gene is transcribed into a template molecule of the related polymer RNA, known as messenger RNA or mRNA. This, in turn, is translated on the ribosome into an amino acid chain or polypeptide. The process of translation requires transfer RNAs specific for individual amino acids with the amino acids covalently attached to them, guanosine triphosphate as an energy source, and a number of translation factors.

tRNAs have anticodons complementary to the codons in mRNA and can be 'charged' covalently with amino acids at their 3′ terminal CCA ends. Individual tRNAs are charged with specific amino acids by enzymes known as aminoacyl tRNA synthetases, which have high specificity for both their cognate amino acids and tRNAs. The high specificity of these enzymes is a major reason why the fidelity of protein translation is maintained.

There are $4^3 = 64$ different codon combinations possible with a triplet codon of three nucleotides, all 64 codons are assigned for either amino acids or stop signals during translation. If, for example, an RNA sequence, UUUAAACCC is considered and the reading-frame starts with the first U (by convention, 5′ to 3′), there are three codons, namely, UUU, AAA and CCC, each of which specifies one amino acid. This RNA sequence will be translated into an amino acid sequence, three amino acids long. A comparison may be made with computer science, where the codon is similar to a word, which is the standard 'chunk' for handling data (like one amino acid of a protein), and a nucleotide is similar to a bit, in that it is the smallest unit.

Salient Features

Sequence reading frame

A codon is defined by the initial nucleotide from which translation starts. For example, the string GGGAAACCC, if read from the first position, contains the codons GGG, AAA and CCC, and, if read from the second position, it contains the codons GGA and AAC, if read starting from the third position, GAA and ACC. Every sequence can thus be read in three reading frames, each of which will produce a different amino acid sequence (in the given example, Gly-Lys-Pro, Gly-Asn, or Glu-Thr, respectively). With double-stranded DNA there are six possible reading frames, three in the forward orientation on one strand and three reverse on the opposite strand.

The actual frame in which a protein sequence is translated is defined by a start codon, usually the first AUG codon in the mRNA sequence. Mutations that disrupt the reading frame by insertions or deletions of a non-multiple of 3 nucleotide bases are known as frameshift mutations. These mutations may impair the function of the resulting protein, if it is formed, and are thus rare in *in vivo* protein coding sequences. Such misformed proteins are often targeted for proteolytic degradation. In addition, a frame shift mutation is very likely to cause a stop codon to be read, which truncates the creation of the protein. One reason for the rareness of frame-shifted mutations being inherited is that, if the protein being translated is essential for growth under the selective pressures the organism faces, absence of a functional protein may cause death before the organism is viable.

Start/stop codons

Translation starts with a chain initiation codon (start codon). Unlike stop codons, the codon alone is not sufficient to begin the process. Nearby sequences (such as the Shine-Dalgarno sequence in *E. coli*) and initiation factors are also required to start translation. The most common start codon is AUG which is read as methionine or, in bacteria, as formylmethionine.

Alternative start codons (depending on the organism), include 'GUG' or 'UUG', which normally code for valine or leucine, respectively. However, when used as a start codon, these alternative start codons are translated as methionine or formylmethionine.

The three stop codons have been given names: UAG is amber, UGA is opal (sometimes also called umber), and UAA is ochre. 'Amber' was named by discoverers Richard Epstein and Charles Steinberg after their friend Harris Bernstein, whose last name means 'amber' in German. The other two stop codons were named 'ochre' and 'opal' in order to keep the 'colour names' theme. Stop codons are also called termination or nonsense codons and they signal release of the nascent polypeptide from the ribosome due to binding of release factors in the absence of cognate tRNAs with anticodons complementary to these stop signals.

Effect of mutations

Frameshift mutations altering the sequence reading frame, and nonsense mutations causing a stop codon are examples of point mutations. In addition, there may be missense mutations that cause exchange of one amino acid for another. Clinically important missense mutations generally change the properties of the coded amino acid residue between being basic, acidic polar or nonpolar, while nonsense mutations result in a stop codon.

Degeneracy of the genetic code

The genetic code has redundancy but no ambiguity. For example, although codons GAA and GAG both specify glutamic acid (redundancy), neither of them specifies any other amino acid (no ambiguity). The codons encoding one amino acid may differ in any of their three positions. For example the amino acid glutamic acid is specified by GAA and GAG codons (difference in the third position), the amino acid leucine is specified by UUA, UUG, CUU, CUC, CUA, CUG codons (difference in the first or third position), while the amino acid serine is specified by UCA, UCG, UCC, UCU, AGU, AGC (difference in the first, second or third position).

A position of a codon is said to be a four-fold degenerate site if any nucleotide at this position specifies the same amino acid. For example, the third position of the glycine codons (GGA, GGG, GGC, GGU) is a fourfold degenerate site, because all nucleotide substitutions at this site are synonymous, i.e. they do not change the amino acid. Only the third positions of some codons may be fourfold degenerate. A position of a codon is said to be a twofold degenerate site if only two of four possible nucleotides at this position specify the same amino acid. For example, the third position of the glutamic acid codons (GAA, GAG) is a twofold degenerate site. In twofold degenerate sites, the equivalent nucleotides are always either two purines (A/G) or two pyrimidines (C/U), so only transversional substitutions (purine to pyrimidine or pyrimidine to purine) in two-fold degenerate sites are nonsynonymous. A position of a codon is said to be a non-degenerate site if any mutation at this position results in amino acid substitution. There is only one threefold degenerate site where changing three of the four nucleotides may have no effect on the amino acid (depending on what it is changed to), while changing the fourth possible nucleotide always results in an amino acid substitution. This is the third position of an isoleucine codon: AUU, AUC or AUA all encode isoleucine, but AUG encodes methionine. In computation this position is often treated as a twofold degenerate site.

There are three amino acids encoded by six different codons: serine, leucine, arginine. Only two amino acids are specified by a single codon, one of these is the amino-acid methionine, specified by the codon AUG, which also specifies the start of translation, the other is tryptophan, specified by the codon UGG. The degeneracy of the genetic code is what accounts for the existence of synonymous mutations.

Degeneracy results because a triplet code designates 20 amino acids and a stop codon. Because there are four bases, triplet codons are required to produce at least 21 different codes. For example, if there were two bases per codon, then only 16 amino acids could be coded for ($4^2 = 16$). Because at least 21 codes are required, then 4^3 gives 64 possible codons, meaning that some degeneracy must exist.

These properties of the genetic code make it more fault-tolerant for point mutations. For example, in theory, four-fold degenerate codons can tolerate any point mutation at the third position, although codon usage bias restricts this in practice in many organisms, twofold degenerate codons can tolerate one out of the three possible point mutations at the third position. Since transition mutations (purine to purine or pyrimidine to pyrimidine mutations) are more likely than transversion (purine to pyrimidine or vice-versa) mutations, the equivalence of purines or that of pyrimidines at two-fold degenerate sites adds a further fault-tolerance. A practical consequence of redundancy is that some errors in the genetic code only cause a silent mutation or an error that would not affect the protein because the hydrophilicity or hydrophobicity is maintained by equivalent substitution of amino acids, for example, a codon of NUN (where N = any nucleotide) tends to code for hydrophobic amino acids. NCN yields amino acid residues that are small in size and moderate in hydropathy, NAN encodes average size hydrophilic residues. These tendencies may result from that the aminoacyl tRNA synthetases related the such codons share a common ancestry (Fig. 21.2).

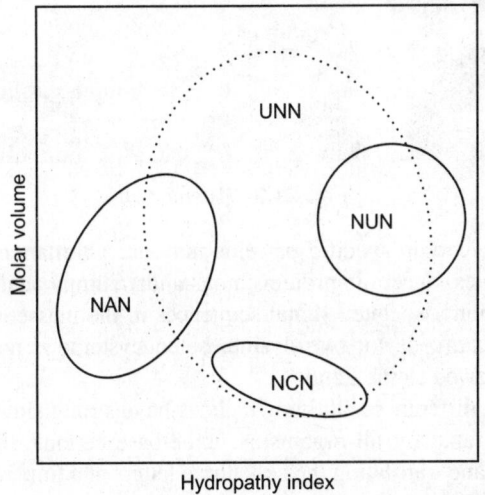

Fig. 21.2: Grouping of codons by amino acid residue molar volume and hydropathy.

Even so, single point mutations can still cause dysfunctional proteins. For example, a mutated haemoglobin gene causes sickle-cell disease. In the mutant haemoglobin a hydrophilic glutamate (Glu) is substituted by the hydrophobic valine (Val), that is, GAA or GAG becomes GUA or GUG. The substitution of glutamate by valine reduces the solubility of β-globin which causes haemoglobin to form linear polymers linked by the hydrophobic interaction between the valine groups causing sickle-cell deformation of erythrocytes. Sickle-cell disease is generally not caused by a *de novo* mutation. Rather it is selected for in malarial regions (in a way similar to thalassemia), as heterozygous people have some resistance to the malarial *Plasmodium* (Fig. 21.3) parasite (heterozygote advantage).

These variable codes for amino acids are allowed because of modified bases in the first base of the anticodon of the tRNA, and the base-pair formed is called a wobble base pair. The modified bases include inosine and the Non-Watson-Crick U-G basepair.

Variations to the Standard Genetic Code

While slight variations on the standard code had been predicted earlier, none were discovered until 1979, when researchers studying human mitochondrial genes discovered they used an alternative code. Many slight variants have been discovered since, including various alternative mitochondrial codes, as well as small variants such as Mycoplasma translating the codon UGA as tryptophan and Candida species translating CUG as a serine rather than a leucine. In bacteria and *archaea*, GUG and UUG are common start codons.

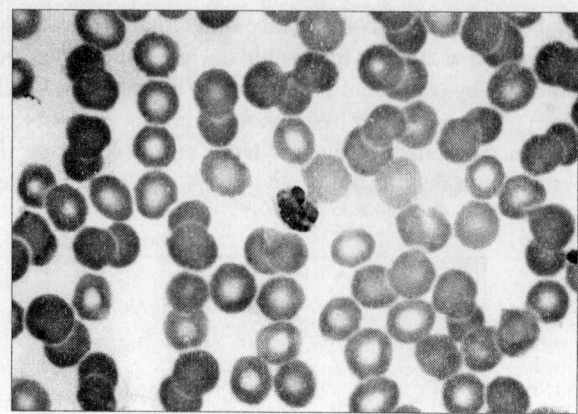

Fig. 21.3: *Plasmodium.*

However, in rare cases, certain specific proteins may use alternative initiation (start) codons not normally used by that species. In certain proteins, nonstandard amino acids are substituted for standard stop codons, depending upon associated signal sequences in the messenger RNA: UGA can code for selenocysteine and UAG can code for pyrrolysine. Selenocysteine is now viewed as the 21st amino acid, and pyrrolysine is viewed as the 22nd.

Not with standing these differences, all known codes have strong similarities to each other, and the coding mechanism is the same for all organisms: three-base codons, tRNA, ribosomes, reading the code in the same direction and translating the code three letters at a time into sequences of amino acids.

DECODING THE CODONS AND ROLE OF TRANSFER RNAs

Nucleic acids and proteins are like two languages written with different types of letters. This is the reason why protein synthesis is referred to as translation. Translation requires that information encoded in the nucleotide sequence of an mRNA be decoded and use to direct the sequential assembly of amino acids into a polypeptide chain. Decoding the information in an mRNA is accomplished by transfer RNAs, which act as adaptors. On one hand, each tRNA is linked to a specific amino acid (as an aa-tRNA), while on the other hand, that same tRNa is able to recognise a particular codon in the mRNA. The interaction between successive codons in the mRNA and specific aa-tRNAs leads to the synthesis of a polypeptide with an ordered sequence of amino acids. To understand how this occurs, we must first consider the structure of tRNAs.

Structure of tRNA

The major role of tRNA is to translate mRNA sequence into amino acid sequence. A tRNA molecule consists of 70–80 nucleotides. The tertiary structure of tRNA are shown in Fig. 21.4. Some nucleotides in tRNA have been modified, such as dihydrouridine (D), pseudouridine (Ψ), and inosine (I). In dihydrouridine, a hydrogen atom is added to each C5 and C6 of uracil. In pseudouridine, the ribose is attached to C5, instead of the normal N1. Inosine plays an important role in codon recognition. In addition to these modifications, a few nucleosides are methylated.

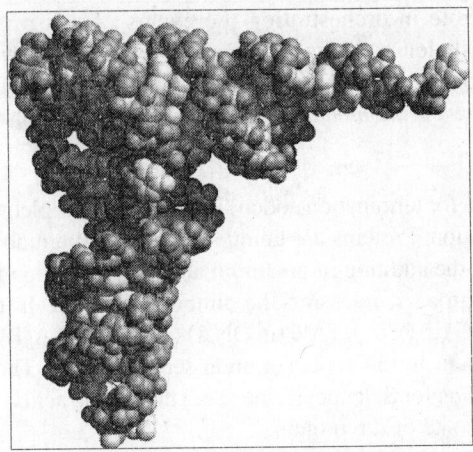

Fig. 21.4: The tertiary structure of tRNA.

TRANSLATING GENETIC INFORMATION

Protein synthesis, or translation, may be the most complex synthetic activity in a cell. The assembly of a protein requires all the various tRNAs with their attached amino acids, ribosomes, a messenger RNA, numerous proteins having different functions, cations, and GTP. The complexity is not surprising considering that protein synthesis requires in incorporation of 20 different amino acids in the precise sequence dictated by a coded message written in a language that uses different characters. In the following discussion, we will draw most heavily on translation mechanisms as they operate in bacterial cells, which is simpler and better understood. The process is remarkably similar in eukaryotic cells.

The synthesis of a polypeptide chain can be divided into three rather distinct activities: initiation of the chain, elongation of the chain, and termination of the chain. These activities are discussed below.

Initiation

Once it attaches to an mRNA, a ribosome always moves along the mRNA from one codon to the next, that is, in consecutive blocks of three nucleotides. This ensure that the proper triplets are read, the ribosome attaches to the mRNA at a precise site, termed the initiation codon, which is specified as AUG. Binding to this codon automatically puts the ribosome in the proper reading frame so that it correctly reads the entire message from that point on.

Elongation Factor

Elongation factors are a set of proteins that facilitate the events of translational elongation, the steps in protein synthesis from the formation of the first peptide bond to the formation of the last one.

Elongation is the most rapid step in translation:

1. In prokaryotes it proceeds at a rate of 15 to 20 amino acids added per second (about 60 nucleotides per second).
2. In eukaryotes the rate is about two amino acids per second.

Elongation factors play a role in orchestrating the events of this process, and in ensuring the 99.99 per cent accuracy of translation at this speed. *Corynebacterium diphtheriae* produces a toxin that alters protein function in the host by inactivating elongation factor (EF-2). This causes pharyngitis and 'pseudomembrane' in the throat. *Pseudomonas aeruginosa's* exotoxin A also inhibits EF-2.

Termination Codon

In the genetic code, a stop codon (or termination codon) is a nucleotide triplet within messenger RNA that signals a termination of translation. Proteins are unique sequences of amino acids, and most codons in messenger RNA correspond to the addition of an amino acid to a growing protein chain—stop codons signal the termination of this process, releasing the amino acid chain. In the standard genetic code, there are three stop codons: UAG (in RNA)/TAG (in DNA) (amber), UAA/TAA (ochre), and UGA/TGA (opal or umber), several variations to this most common set are known. The UGA codon has recently been identified as the codon coding for Selenocysteine (Sec) this amino acid is found in 25 selenoproteins where it is located in the active site of the protein.

Transcription of this codon is enabled by proximity of the SECIS element (SElenoCysteine Incorporation Sequence). Nonsense mutations are changes in DNA sequence which introduce a premature stop codon, causing any resulting protein to be abnormally shortened. This often causes a loss of function in the protein as critical parts of the amino acid chain are no longer created. Because of this terminology, stop codons have also been referred to as nonsense codons.

Amber, ochre, and opal nomenclature

Stop codons were historically given many different names as they each corresponded to a distinct class of mutants that all behaved in a similar manner. These mutants were first isolated within bacteriophages (T4 and lambda), viruses that infect the bacteria *Escherichia coli*. Mutations in viral genes weakened their infectious ability, sometimes creating viruses that were only able to infect and grow within certain varieties of *E coli*. Amber mutations were the first set of nonsense mutations to be discovered, isolated by graduate student Harris Bernstein in experiments designed to resolve a debate between Richard Epstein and Charles Steinberg. Bernstein (whose last name means 'amber' in German) had been offered the reward of having any discovered mutants named after himself.

Viruses with amber mutations are characterised by their ability to only infect certain strains of bacteria, known as amber suppressors. These bacteria carry their own mutation which allow a recovery of function in the mutant viruses. For example, a mutation in the tRNA which recognises the amber stop codon allows translation to 'read through' the codon and produce full length protein, thereby recovering the normal form of the protein and 'suppressing' the amber mutation. Thus, amber mutants are an entire class of virus mutants which can grow in bacteria that contain amber suppressor mutations.

The ochre mutation was the second stop codon mutation to be discovered. Given a colour name to match the name of amber mutants, ochre mutant viruses had a similar property in that they recovered infectious ability within certain suppressor strains of bacteria. The set of ochre suppressors was distinct from amber suppressors, so ochre mutants were inferred to correspond to a different nucleotide triplet. Through a series of mutation experiments comparing these mutants with each other and other known amino acid codons, Sydney Brenner concluded that the amber and ochre mutations corresponded to the nucleotide triplets UAG and UAA. The third and last stop codon in the standard genetic code was discovered soon after, corresponding to the nucleotide triplet UGA. Nonsense mutations that created this premature stop codon were later called opal mutations or umber mutations.

Transcription

The process of genetic transcription produces a single-stranded RNA molecule known as messenger RNA, whose nucleotide sequence is complementary to the DNA from which it was transcribed. The DNA strand whose sequence matches that of the RNA is known as the coding strand and the strand from which the RNA was synthesised is the template strand. Transcription is performed by an enzyme called an RNA polymerase, which reads the template strand in the 3' to 5' direction and synthesises the RNA from 5' to 3'. To initiate transcription, the polymerase first recognises and binds a promoter region of the gene. Thus a major mechanism of gene regulation is the blocking or sequestering of the promoter region, either by tight binding by repressor molecules that physically block the polymerase or by organising the DNA so that the promoter region is not accessible.

In prokaryotes, transcription occurs in the cytoplasm, for very long transcripts, translation may begin at the 5' end of the RNA while the 3' end is still being transcribed. In eukaryotes, transcription necessarily occurs in the nucleus, where the cell's DNA is sequestered, the RNA molecule produced by the polymerase is known as the primary transcript and must undergo post-transcriptional modifications before being exported to the cytoplasm for translation. The splicing of introns present within the transcribed region is a modification unique to eukaryotes, alternative splicing mechanisms can result in mature transcripts from the same gene having different sequences and thus coding for different proteins. This is a major form of regulation in eukaryotic cells.

Translation

Translation is the process by which a mature mRNA molecule is used as a template for synthesising a new protein. Translation is carried out by ribosomes, large complexes of RNA and protein responsible for carrying out the chemical reactions to add new amino acids to a growing polypeptide chain by the formation of peptide bonds. The genetic code is read three nucleotides at a time, in units called codons, via interactions with specialised RNA molecules called transfer RNA (tRNA). Each tRNA has three unpaired bases known as the anticodon that are complementary to the codon it reads, the tRNA is also covalently attached to the amino acid specified by the complementary codon. When the tRNA binds to its complementary codon in an mRNA strand, the ribosome ligates its amino acid cargo to the new polypeptide chain, which is synthesised from amino terminus to carboxyl terminus. During and after its synthesis, the new protein must fold to its active three-dimensional structure before it can carry out its cellular function.

CHARACTERISTICS OF THE GENETIC CODE

The genetic code consists of 64 triplets of nucleotides. These triplets are called codons. With three exceptions, each codon encodes for one of the 20 amino acids used in the synthesis of proteins. That produces some redundancy in the code: most of the amino acids being encoded by more than one codon. The genetic code is the set of rules by which information encoded in genetic material (DNA or RNA sequences) is translated into proteins (amino acid sequences) by living cells. The genetic code, once thought to be identical in all forms of life, has been found to diverge slightly in certain organisms and in the mitochondria of some eukaryotes. Nevertheless, these differences are rare, and the genetic code is identical in almost all species, with the same codons specifying the same amino acids.

1. Triplet nature: A triplet code could make a genetic code for 64 different combinations ($4 \times 4 \times 4$) genetic code and provide plenty of information in the DNA molecule to specify the placement of

all 20 amino acids. When experiments were performed to crack the genetic code it was found to be a code that was triplet. These three letter codes of nucleotides (AUG, AAA, etc.) are called codons.

2. Degeneracy: The code is degenerate which means that the same amino acid is coded by more than one base triplet. For example, the three amino acids arginine, alanine and leucine each have six synonymous codons.

3. Non-overlapping: The genetic code is non-overlapping, i.e. the adjacent codons do not overlap. A non-overlapping code means that the same letter is not used for two different codons. In other words, no single base can take part in the formation of more than one codon.

4. Commaless: There is no signal to indicate the end of one codon and the beginning of the next. The genetic code is commaless (or comma-free).

5. Non-ambiguity: A particular codon will always code for the same amino acid. While the same amino acid can be coded by more than one codon (the code is degenerate), the same codon shall not code for two or more different amino acids (non-ambiguous).

6. Universality: Although the code is based on work conducted on the bacterium *Escherichia coli* but it is valid for other organisms. This important characteristic of the genetic code is called its universality. It means that the same sequences of 3 bases encode the same amino acids in all life forms from simple microorganisms to complex, multi celled organisms such as human beings.

7. Polarity: The genetic code has polarity, that is, the code is always read in a fixed direction, i.e. in the 5′→3′ direction.

8. Chain initiation codons: The triplets AUG and GUG play double roles in *E. coli*. When they occur in between the two ends of a cistron (intermediate position), they code for the amino acids methionine and valine, respectively in an intermediate position in the protein molecule.

9. Chain termination codons: The 3 triplets UAA, UAG, UGA do not code for any amino acid. They were originally described as non-sense codons, as against the remaining 61 codons, which are termed as sense codons

NIRENBERG AND MATTHAEI EXPERIMENT

The Nirenberg and Matthaei experiment was a scientific experiment performed on May 15, 1961, by Marshall W. Nirenberg and his post doctoral fellow, J. Heinrich Matthaei. The experiment deciphered the first of the 64 triplet codons in the genetic code by using nucleic acid homopolymers to translate specific amino acids.

In the experiment, an extract from bacterial cells that could make protein even when no intact living cells were present was prepared. Adding an artificial form of RNA consisting entirely of uracil-containing nucleotides, the polyuridylic acid (or poly-U), to this extract caused it to make a protein composed entirely of the amino acid phenylalanine. This experiment cracked the first codon of the genetic code and showed that RNA controlled the production of specific types of protein.

Discoveries by Frederick Griffith and improved on by Oswald Avery discovered that the substance responsible for producing inheritable change in the disease-causing bacteria (*Streptococcus pneumoniae*) was neither a protein nor a lipid, rather deoxyribonucleic acid (DNA). In 1944, he and his colleagues Colin MacLeod and Maclyn McCarty suggested that DNA was responsible for transferring genetic information. Later, Erwin Chargaff (1950) discovered that the makeup of DNA differs from one species to another. These experiments helped pave the way for the discovery of the structure of DNA. In 1953, with the help of Maurice Wilkins and Rosalind Franklin's X-ray crystallography, James Watson and

Francis Crick proposed DNA is structured as a double helix. In the 1960s, one main DNA mystery scientists needed to figure out was the number of bases found in each code word, or codon, during transcription. Scientists knew there was a total of four bases (guanine, cytosine, adenine, and thymine). They also knew that were 20 known amino acids. George Gamow suggested that the genetic code was made of three nucleotides per amino acid. He reasoned that because there are 20 amino acids and only four bases, the coding units could not be single (4 combinations) or pairs (only 16 combinations). Rather, he thought triplets (64 possible combinations) were the coding unit of the genetic code. However, he proposed that the triplets were overlapping and non-degenerate (later explained by Crick in his Wobble concept).

Seymour Benzer in the late 1950s had developed an assay using phage mutations which provided the first detailed linearly structured map of a genetic region. Crick felt he could use mutagenesis and genetic recombination phage to further delineate the nature of the genetic code. In the Crick, Brenner and others experiment, using these phages, the triplet nature of the genetic code was confirmed. They used frameshift mutations and a process called reversions, to add and delete various numbers of nucleotides. When a nucleotide triplet was added or deleted to the DNA sequence the encoded protein was minimally affected. Thus, they concluded that the genetic code is a triplet code because it did not cause a frameshift in the reading frame. They correctly concluded that the code is degenerate (triplets are not overlapping) and that each nucleotide sequence is read from a specific starting point.

Marshall Nirenberg and Johann Matthaei both longed to understand how information gets transmitted from DNA to protein. At this time there was a race to crack the code of the DNA language. At the same time, Severo Ochoa was busy working on the coding problem with the help of Leon Heppel, a skillful biochemist capable of making artificial RNAs of defined compositions. Ochoa had a big staff, and Nirenberg was worried he would not be able to keep up. Many NIH scientists helped Nirenberg in deciphering the mRNA codons for amino acids. Nirenberg and his post doctoral fellow Matthaei started their experiments in a lab in Germany and completed them in a National Institutes of Health (NIH) laboratory campus in Maryland.

Experimental Work

In order to decipher this biological mystery, Nirenberg and Matthaei needed a cell-free system that would build amino acids into proteins. Following the work of Alfred Tissieres and after a few failed attempts, they created a stable system by rupturing *E. coli* bacteria cells and releasing the contents of the cytoplasm. This allowed them to synthesise protein, but only when the correct kind of RNA was added, allowing Nirenberg and Matthaei to control the experiment. They created synthetic RNA molecules outside the bacterium and introduced this RNA to the *E. coli* system. The experiment used 20 test tubes, each filled with a different amino acid. For each individual experiment, 19 amino acids were 'cold', and one was radioactively tagged with ^{14}C so they could detect the tagged amino acid later. They varied the 'hot' amino acid in each round of the experiment, seeking to determine which amino acid would be incorporated into a protein following the addition of a particular type of synthetic RNA. In their experiments in late May 1961 they had narrowed down the amino acids encoded by Poly-U to Phenylalanine or Tyrosine. At 3 am on May 27 Matthaei used phenylalanine for the 'hot' test tube. After an hour, the control tubes showed a background level of 70 counts, whereas the hot tube showed 38,000 counts per milligram of protein. The experiment showed that a chain of the repeated uracil bases produced a protein chain made of one repeating amino acid, phenylalanine. Therefore, polyU coded for polyphenylalanine, consistent with UUU coding for phenylalanine. At the time the number of bases per codon could not be determined.

The two kept their breakthrough a secret from the larger scientific community until they could complete further experiments with other strands of synthetic RNA (such as Poly-A) and prepare papers for publication. Using the three-letter poly-U experiment as a model, the research team discovered that AAA (three adenines) was the code word or 'codon' for the amino acid lysine, and CCC (three cytosines) was the code word for proline. They also discovered that by replacing one or two units of a triplet with other nucleotides, they could direct the production of other amino acids. They found, for example, that a synthetic RNA GUU codes for a valine to be added to a developing amino acid chain.

Reception and Legacy

In August 1961, at the International Congress of Biochemistry in Moscow, Nirenberg presented his paper. The experimentation with synthetic RNA in a cell-free system was a key technical innovation. In 1961, when they announced their methods for decoding the relationship of mRNA to amino acids, there was still a lot of experimentation required before the entire code was deciphered. The scientists had to determine which bases made up each codon, then determine the sequence of bases in the codons. This proved to be a tremendous amount of work.

In 1964 and 1965, Nirenberg's postdoctoral researcher, Philip Leder, developed a filtration machine that allowed the NIH research team determine the order of the nucleotides in the codons. This development sped up the process of assigning code words to amino acids. By 1966, Nirenberg announced that he had deciphered the sixty-four RNA codons for all twenty amino acids.

For his ground-breaking work on the genetic code, Nirenberg was awarded the 1968 Nobel Prize in Physiology or Medicine. He shared the award with Har Gobind Khorana and Robert W. Holley. Working independently, Khorana had mastered the synthesis of nucleic acids, and Holley had discovered the exact chemical structure of transfer-RNA. The New York Times reported on Nirenberg's discovery by explaining that 'the science of biology has reached a new frontier,' leading to 'a revolution far greater in its potential significance than the atomic or hydrogen bomb.' Most of the scientific community saw these experiments as highly important and beneficial. However, there were some who were concerned with the new area of Molecular Genetics. For example, Arne Wilhelm Kaurin Tiselius, the 1948 Nobel Laureate in Chemistry, asserted that knowledge of the genetic code could 'lead to methods of tampering with life, of creating new diseases, of controlling minds, of influencing heredity, even perhaps in certain desired directions.'

IMPORTANT PROPERTIES OF GENETIC CODE

Genetic Code refers to the relationship between the sequence of nitrogenous bases (UCAG) in mRNA and the sequence of amino acids in a polypeptide chain. In other words, the relationship between the 4 letters language of nucleotides and twenty letters language of amino acids is known as genetic code.

DNA (or RNA) carries all the genetic information and it is expressed in the form of proteins. Proteins are made of 20 different amino acids. The information about the number and sequence of these amino acids forming protein is present in DNA, and during transcription is passed over to mRNA. The form in which it is transferred was not understood for long.

Sugar (pentose) and phosphate of DNA could not perform this job of passing on the genetic message to mRNA because sugar is only of one type and so also the phosphate. This leaves only four nucleotides to form the message for 20 amino acids, but 4 nucleotides are too few for twenty amino acids. This difficult problem was solved with the discovery that a codon (hereditary unit of a gene) containing coded information for one amino acid consists three nucleotides (i.e. a triplet code). Thus for twenty amino acids, 64 (4 × 4 × 4 or 43 = 64) possible permutation are available. This break through resulted into 64 codons dictionary — the Genetic Code.

According to Bark the genetic code is a code for amino acids, specifically it is concerned with as to what codons specify what amino acids. Genetic code is the outcome of experiments performed by M. Nirenberg, S. Ochoa, H. Khorana, F. Crick and Mathaei. Professor M. Nirenberg was awarded Nobel Prize in 1961 for this outstanding work.

The dictionary of genetic code employs the letters in RNA (U, C, A, G, i.e. A = Adenine, U = Uracil, C = Cytosine, G = Guanine). The codon for the amino acids, which are the same in all known life forms, have been determined experimentally. They are given in Fig. 21.5.

In Fig. 21.5 note that more than one codon can signal a particular amino acid to be incorporated into a protein. In addition, some codons serve special functions.

Second letter

	U	C	A	G	
U	UUU ⎤ Phe UUC ⎦ UUA ⎤ Leu UUG ⎦	UCU ⎤ UCC ⎥ Per UCA ⎥ UCG ⎦	UAU ⎤ Tyr UAC ⎦ UAA Stop UAG Stop	UGU ⎤ CyS UGC ⎦ UGA Stop UGG Stop	U C A G
C	CUU ⎤ CUC ⎥ Leu CUA ⎥ CUG ⎦	CCU ⎤ CCC ⎥ Pro CCA ⎥ CCG ⎦	CAU ⎤ His CAC ⎦ CAA ⎤ Gln CAG ⎦	CGU ⎤ CGC ⎥ Arg CGA ⎥ CGG ⎦	U C A G
A	AUU ⎤ AUC ⎥ Ile AUA ⎦ AUG Met	ACU ⎤ ACC ⎥ Thr ACA ⎥ ACG ⎦	AAU ⎤ Asn AAC ⎦ AAA ⎤ Lys AAG ⎦	AGU ⎤ Ser AGC ⎦ AGA ⎤ Arg AGG ⎦	U C A G
G	GUU ⎤ GUC ⎥ Val GUA ⎥ GUG ⎦	GCU ⎤ GCC ⎥ Ala GCA ⎥ GCG ⎦	GAU ⎤ Asp GAC ⎦ GAA ⎤ Glu GAG ⎦	GGU ⎤ GGC ⎥ Gly GGA ⎥ GGG ⎦	U C A G

(First letter — left axis; Third letter — right axis)

Fig. 21.5: The triplet codons code for specific amino acids.

For example, the codon AUG serves two functions:

1. As an initiator codon signalling for the start of synthesis of a peptide, and

2. For the incorporation of methionine into the growing chain of a peptide. Other special-purpose codons are UAA (Ochre), UAG (Amber), and UGA (Umber), all of which signal STOP.

When the ribosomal synthesis site encounters one of these stop codons, the peptide chain is released and assumes its secondary and tertiary structures. Since UAA (Ochre), UAG (Amber) and UGA (Umber) do not specify any amino acid they are also called nonsense codons.

BACTERIOPHAGE MS2

The bacteriophage MS2 is an icosahedral, positive-sense single-stranded RNA virus that infects the bacterium *Escherichia coli* and other members of the *Enterobacteriaceae* (Fig. 21.6). MS2 is a member of a family of closely related bacterial viruses that includes bacteriophage f2, bacteriophage Qβ, R17, and GA.

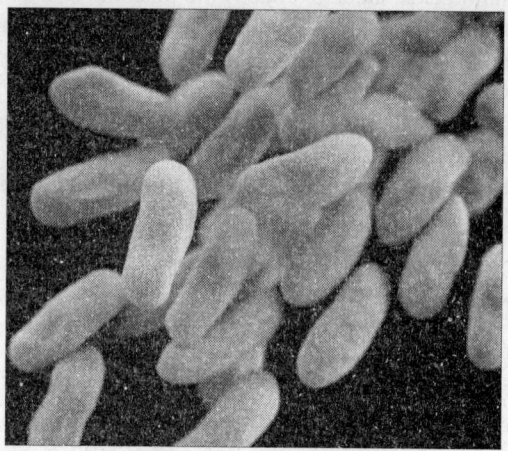

Fig. 21.6: *Enterobacteriaceae.*

Virology

Genome and gene products

The MS2 genome is one of the smallest known, consisting of 3569 nucleotides of single-stranded RNA. It encodes just four proteins: The maturation protein (A-protein), the lysis protein, the coat protein, and the replicase protein. The gene encoding lysis protein (lys) overlaps both the 3′-end of the upstream gene (cp) and the 5′-end of the downstream gene (rep), and was one of the first known examples of overlapping genes (Fig. 21.7). The positive-stranded RNA genome serves as messenger RNA, and is translated upon viral uncoating within the host cell. Although the four proteins are encoded by the same messenger/ viral RNA, they are not all expressed at the same levels, expression of these proteins is regulated by a complex interplay between translation and RNA secondary structure.

Gene	Gene length	Gene product	Amino acids
cp (MS2g2)	510 nt	Coat protein	130
lys (MS2g3)	295 nt	Lysis protein	75
rep (MS2g4)	2055 nt	RNA replicase, beta subunit	545
mat (MS2g1)	1487 nt	Maturation protein	393

Capsid structure

An MS2 virion (viral particle) is about 27 nm in diameter, as determined by electron microscopy. It consists of one copy of the maturation protein and 180 copies of the coat protein (organised as 90 dimers) arranged into an icosahedral shell with triangulation number T = 3, protecting the genomic RNA inside. The virion has an isoelectric point (pI) of 3.9.

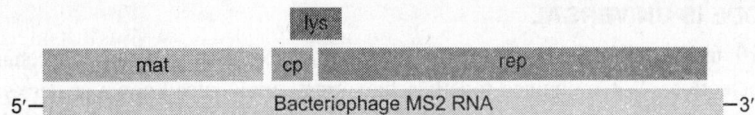

Fig. 21.7: Location of protein-coding genes within bacteriophage MS2 RNA. Note that the lys gene overlaps segments of both the cp and rep genes.

The structure of the coat protein is a five-stranded β-sheet with two α-helices and a hairpin. When the capsid is assembled, the helices and hairpin face the exterior of the particle, while the β-sheet faces the interior.

Life cycle

MS2 infects enteric bacteria carrying the fertility (F) factor, a plasmid that allows cells to serve as DNA donors in bacterial conjugation. Genes on the F plasmid lead to the production of an F pilus, which serves as the viral receptor. MS2 attaches to the side of the pilus via its single maturation protein. The precise mechanism by which phage RNA enters the bacterium is unknown.

Once the viral RNA has entered the cell, it begins to function as a messenger RNA for the production of phage proteins. The gene for the most abundant protein, the coat protein, can be immediately translated. The translation start of the replicase gene is normally hidden within RNA secondary structure, but can be transiently opened as ribosomes pass through the coat protein gene. Replicase translation is also shut down once large amounts of coat protein have been made, coat protein dimers bind and stabilise the RNA 'operator hairpin', blocking the replicase start. The start of the maturation protein gene is accessible in RNA being replicated but hidden within RNA secondary structure in the completed MS2 RNA, this ensures translation of only a very few copies of maturation protein per RNA. Finally, the lysis protein gene can only be initiated by ribosomes that have completed translation of the coat protein gene and 'slip back' to the start of the lysis protein gene, at about a 5% frequency.

Replication of the plus-strand MS2 genome requires synthesis of the complementary minus strand RNA, which can then be used as a template for synthesis of a new plus strand RNA. MS2 replication has been much less well studied than replication of the highly related bacteriophage Qβ, partly because the MS2 replicase has been difficult to isolate, but is likely to be similar.

The formation of the virion is thought to be initiated by binding of maturation protein to the MS2 RNA, in fact, the complex of maturation protein and RNA is infectious. The assembly of the icosahedral shell or capsid from coat proteins can occur in the absence of RNA, however, capsid assembly is nucleated by coat protein dimer binding to the operator hairpin, and assembly occurs at much lower concentrations of coat protein when MS2 RNA is present. Bacterial lysis and release of newly formed virions occurs when sufficient lysis protein has accumulated. Lysis protein forms pores in the cytoplasmic membrane, which leads to loss of membrane potential and breakdown of the cell wall.

Applications of MS2

Since 1998, the MS2 operator hairpin and coat protein have found utility in the detection of RNA in living cells. MS2 and other viral capsids are also currently under investigation as agents in drug delivery, tumour imaging, and light harvesting applications. MS2, due to its structural similarities to noroviruses, its similar optimum proliferation conditions, and non-pathogenicity to humans, has been used as substitute for noroviruses in studies of disease transmission.

GENETIC CODE IS UNIVERSAL

All life on Earth uses nucleic acids to transmit information. Nucleic acids are long chains of individual units called nucleotides. When chained together, they create molecules known as deoxyribonucleic acid, DNA, or ribonucleic acid, RNA. Those molecules carry information through generations of a species and through the cells of an organism. The information is contained in the specific sequence of nucleotides, and the genetic code is the way in which an organism uses the order of nucleotides to direct its development. It's the same among plants, animals, bacteria and fungi - that's why it's called 'universal.'

DNA AND RNA

The four nucleotides that make up DNA are adenosine monophosphate, guanosine monophosphate, cytosine monophosphate and deoxythymidine monophosphate. In a DNA molecule, these are usually referred to by the initials A, G, C and T. RNA has no deoxythymidine monophosphate, instead it has uridine monophosphate, which goes by the initial U. For most organisms, DNA is the hereditary molecule. That is, it's responsible for transmitting traits from one generation to the next. Those traits are visible because of the actions of proteins in an organism. For example, hair, skin and eye colour are produced by the action of proteins. So DNA must somehow direct the action of proteins.

DNA and Proteins

Organisms transfer traits from generation to generation through DNA, but those traits are the visible manifestation of microscopic proteins. So DNA must somehow carry information that is used to build proteins. It does this through a two-step process: First DNA is transcribed into RNA, then RNA is translated into protein. Transcription uses a strand of DNA as a model for a strand of RNA. Where DNA has a G, RNA will have a C, and where DNA has a C, RNA will have a G. Where DNA has a T, RNA will have an A, and where DNA has an A, RNA will have a U. In some sense, that's the code used to convert a DNA molecule to an RNA molecule.

Transcription and Codons

Where DNA and RNA are built from more-or-less the same components, RNA and proteins are quite different. Proteins are built from sequences of amino acids, each of a much different structure than the nucleotides in the RNA. There is not a one-for-one correspondence between a G, for example, and a specific amino acid. There is not even a correspondence between an amino acid and two nucleotides, a UC, for example. There is, however, a match between three-letter sequences of RNA and amino acids. For example, CGU in an RNA molecule will direct the assembly of an arginine amino acid onto a protein. Other three-letter sequences, called codons, encode for the other 19 common amino acids.

Universal Code

There is no reason that the genetic code needed to be the way it is. It could just as easily have happened that CCU would encode for arginine instead of proline. But it turns out that the genetic code - the three-letter codons—direct the assembly of exactly the same amino acids in nearly every organism on Earth. Bacteria, plants and you all use exactly the same genetic code. Although there are a few minor differences in a very small percentage of organisms, those are exceptions that prove the rule. That's why biologists say the genetic code is universal.

OVERLAPPING GENES

An overlapping gene is a gene whose expressible nucleotide sequence partially overlaps with the expressible nucleotide sequence of another gene. In this way, a nucleotide sequence may make a contribution to the function of one or more gene products. Overprinting refers to a type of overlap in which all or part of the sequence of one gene is read in an alternate reading frame from another gene at the same locus.

Overprinting has been hypothesised as a mechanism for de novo emergence of new genes from existing sequences, either older genes or previously non-coding regions of the genome. Overprinted genes are particularly common features of the genomic organisation of viruses, likely to greatly increase the number of potential expressible genes from a small set of viral genetic information.

Classification of Genes

Genes may overlap in a variety of ways and can be classified by their positions relative to each other.

- Unidirectional or tandem overlap: The 3′ end of one gene overlaps with the 5′ end of another gene on the same strand. This arrangement can be symbolised with the notation $\rightarrow \rightarrow$ where arrows indicate the reading frame from start to end.
- Convergent or end-on overlap: The 3′ ends of the two genes overlap on opposite strands. This can be written as $\rightarrow \leftarrow$.
- Divergent or tail-on overlap: The 5′ ends of the two genes overlap on opposite strands. This can be written as $\leftarrow \rightarrow$.

Overlapping genes can also be classified by phases, which describe their relative reading frames:

- In-phase overlap occurs when the shared sequences use the same reading frame. This is also known as 'phase 0'. Unidirectional genes with phase 0 overlap are not considered distinct genes, but rather as alternative start sites of the same gene.
- Out-of-phase overlaps occurs when the shared sequences use different reading frames. This can occur in 'phase 1' or 'phase 2', depending on whether the reading frames are offset by 1 or 2 nucleotides. Because a codon is three nucleotides long, an offset of three nucleotides is an in-phase, phase 0 frame.

Evolution of Genes

Overlapping genes are particularly common in rapidly evolving genomes, such as those of viruses, bacteria, and mitochondria. They may originate in three ways:

1. By extension of an existing open reading frame (ORF) downstream into a contiguous gene due to the loss of a stop codon.
2. By extension of an existing ORF upstream into a contiguous gene due to loss of an initiation codon.
3. By generation of a novel ORF within an existing one due to a point mutation.

The use of the same nucleotide sequence to encode multiple genes may provide evolutionary advantage due to reduction in genome size and due to the opportunity for transcriptional and translational co-regulation of the overlapping genes. Gene overlaps introduce novel evolutionary constraints on the sequences of the overlap regions.

Origins of new genes

A cladogram indicating the likely evolutionary trajectory of the gene-dense pX region in human T-lymphotropic virus 1 (HTLV1), a deltaretrovirus associated with blood cancers. This region contains numerous overlapping genes, several of which likely originated de novo through overprinting. In 1977, Pierre-Paul Grassé proposed that one of the genes in the pair could have originated de novo by mutations to introduce novel ORFs in alternate reading frames, he described the mechanism as overprinting. It was later substantiated by Susumu Ohno, who identified a candidate gene that may have arisen by this mechanism. Some *de novo* genes originating in this way may not remain overlapping, but subfunctionalise following gene duplication, contributing to the prevalence of orphan genes. Which member of an overlapping gene pair is younger can be identified bioinformatically either by a more restricted phylogenetic distribution, or by less optimised codon usage. Younger members of the pair tend to have higher intrinsic structural disorder than older members, but the older members are also more disordered than other proteins, presumably as a way of alleviating the increased evolutionary constraints posed by overlap. Overlaps are more likely to originate in proteins that already have high disorder.

Taxonomic Distribution

Overlapping genes occur in all domains of life, though with varying frequencies. They are especially common in viral genomes.

Viruses

The RNA silencing suppressor p19 from tomato bushy stunt virus, a protein encoded by an overprinted gene. The protein specifically binds siRNAs produced as part of the plants RNA silencing defense against viruses.

The existence of overlapping genes was first identified in viruses, the first DNA genome ever sequenced, of the bacteriophage FX174, contained several examples. Overlapping genes are particularly common in viral genomes. Some studies attribute this observation to selective pressure toward small genome sizes mediated by the physical constraints of packaging the genome in a viral capsid, particularly one of icosahedral geometry. However, other studies dispute this conclusion and argue that the distribution of overlaps in viral genomes is more likely to reflect overprinting as the evolutionary origin of overlapping viral genes. Overprinting is a common source of *de novo* genes in viruses.

Studies of overprinted viral genes suggest that their protein products tend to be accessory proteins which are not essential to viral proliferation, but contribute to pathogenicity. Overprinted proteins often have unusual amino acid distributions and high levels of intrinsic disorder. In some cases overprinted proteins do have well-defined, but novel, three-dimensional structures, one example is the RNA silencing suppressor p19 found in Tombusviruses, which has both a novel protein fold and a novel binding mode in recognising siRNAs.

Prokaryotes

Estimates of gene overlap in bacterial genomes typically find that around one third of bacterial genes are overlapped, though usually only by a few base pairs. Most studies of overlap in bacterial genomes find evidence that overlap serves a function in gene regulation, permitting the overlapped genes to be transcriptionally and translationally co-regulated. In prokaryotic genomes, unidirectional overlaps are most common, possibly due to the tendency of adjacent prokaryotic genes to share orientation. Among unidirectional overlaps, long overlaps are more commonly read with a one-nucleotide offset in reading frame (i.e. phase 1) and short overlaps are more commonly read in phase 2. Long overlaps of greater than 60 base pairs are more common for convergent genes, however, putative long overlaps have very high rates of misannotation. Robustly validated examples of long overlaps in bacterial genomes are rare, in the well-studied model organism *Escherichia coli*, only four gene pairs are well validated as having long, overprinted overlaps.

Eukaryotes

Compared to prokaryotic genomes, eukaryotic genomes are often poorly annotated and thus identifying genuine overlaps is relatively challenging. However, examples of validated gene overlaps have been documented in a variety of eukaryotic organisms, including mammals such as mice and humans. Eukaryotes differ from prokaryotes in distribution of overlap types: while unidirectional (i.e. same-strand) overlaps are most common in prokaryotes, opposite or antiparallel-strand overlaps are more common in eukaryotes. Among the opposite-strand overlaps, convergent orientation is most common. Most studies of eukaryotic gene overlap have found that overlapping genes are extensively subject to genomic reorganisation even in closely related species, and thus the presence of an overlap is not always well-conserved. Overlap with older or less taxonomically restricted genes is also a common feature of genes likely to have originated de novo in a given eukaryotic lineage.

Chapter 22

Transcription, RNA Editing and RNA Polymerase

INTRODUCTION

The processes of transcription, RNA processing (in eukaryotes), and translation constitute the pathway that leads to the conversion of genetic information in the linear sequence of bases in genomic DNA into the linear amino acid sequences of functional proteins. Thus, DNA undergoes transcription to synthesise a primary RNA transcript, which in eukaryotes undergoes RNA processing to produce a mature messenger RNA (mRNA), then mRNAs are translated into functional polypeptides. Each of these cellular processes will be described below.

The process of transcription involves the sequential and enzyme-catalysed polymerisation of ribonucleotide triphosphates into a single-stranded linear RNA molecule that is complementary to, and encoded by, one strand of a DNA template. This process in eukaryotes occurs in the nucleus. The growth of the nascent RNA chain proceeds from the 5′ end to the 3′ end of the chain, elongating by adding nucleotides to the –OH group at the 3′ end of the RNA. As depicted in Fig. 22.1, polymerisation occurs by formation of a phosphodiester bond between the –OH group of the ribose moiety at the 3′ end of the elongating RNA and the 5′ phosphate of the ribonucleotide triphosphate (rNTP) precursor to be added to the growing RNA chain. Thus, unidirectional growth of the RNA chain occurs in the 5′ to 3′ direction. The phosphodiester bond is synthesised by a condensation reaction involving the 3′ –OH group of the sugar and the α phosphate group of the rNTP, with release of pyrophosphate (PPi). As shown in Fig. 22.1, the nucleotide sequence of the elongating RNA chain is specified by the nucleotide sequence of one strand of the duplex DNA template.

Following the rules of Watson-Crick base pairing, adenine, cytosine, guanine and thymine in the template DNA sequence direct the addition of uracil, guanine, cytosine, and adenine, respectively, to the RNA sequence. In most cases, only one strand of a given region of double-stranded DNA is transcribed into RNA, though a small but increasing number of eukaryotic genes show transcription from both strands over all or a portion of the gene. In several cases, a gene encodes a functional sense transcript as well as a so-called anti-sense transcript (often of unknown function) that extends over the

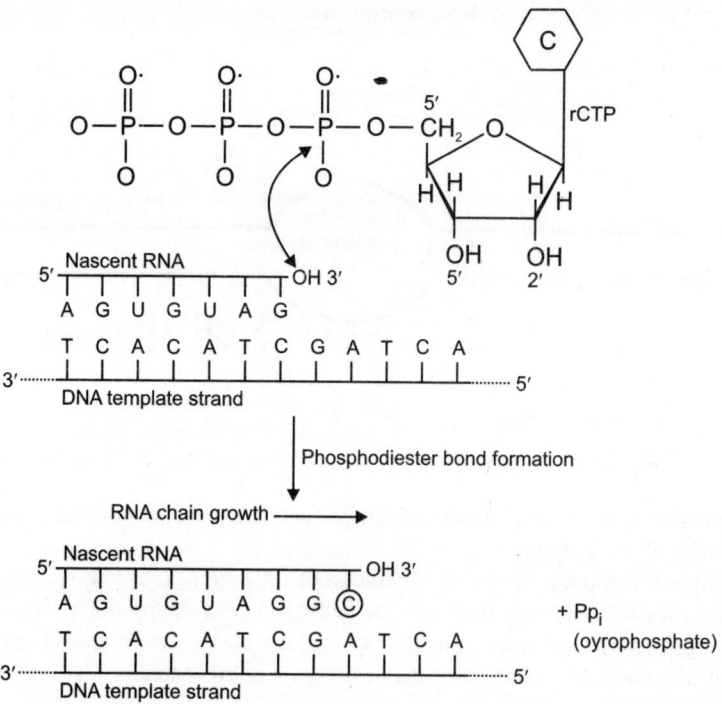

Fig. 22.1: DNA-dependent synthesis of RNA. In this example, a cytidine triphosphate (rCTP) precursor is added to the 3′ end of an elongating RNA chain by forming a phosphodiester bond between the 5′ phosphate of the rCTP precursor and the 3′ OH of the previously added nucleotide. The nucleotide sequence of the nascent RNA is specified by the complementary nucleotide sequence of the DNA template strand according to Watson-Crick base pairing. The circled C residue indicates the position of the newly added nucleotide.

entire region encoding the sense transcript. Some of these anti-sense transcripts have been postulated to regulate the expression of the sense transcript.

The synthesis of RNA from a DNA template is catalysed by the enzyme RNA polymerase. Most, if not all, RNA synthesis in prokaryotes is directed by a single RNA polymerase, while RNA synthesis in eukaryotes is catalysed by three different RNA polymerases, pol I, pol II and pol III, each of which transcribes a different class of genes. The high-resolution structure of both bacterial RNA polymerase and eukaryotic RNA polymerase II has recently been determined by X-ray crystallography. The amino acid homology of certain subunits in the prokaryotic and eukaryotic polymerases and their many shared structural features are notable though not unexpected due to their similar functions.

The macromolecular complex formed during the process of transcription consists of RNA polymerase, the DNA template and the nascent RNA (Fig. 22.2). The double stranded DNA template is melted to form a transcription bubble (of approximately 12 base pairs) within the bubble the elongating nascent RNA forms an approximately 9 bp RNA:DNA duplex with the template strand of the DNA at its 3′ end. As the polymerase moves downstream along the DNA template, the double-stranded DNA helix is unwound at the front of the bubble and rewound behind the bubble. Growth of the nascent RNA occurs by the addition of nucleotides at the 3′ end of the nascent RNA within the bubble, with nucleotide

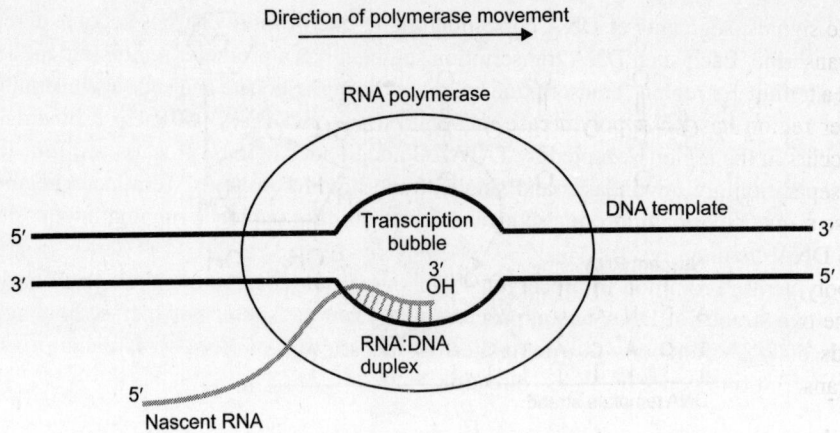

Fig. 22.2: Schematic of the transcription elongation complex.

triphosphate precursors presumably translocated to the active site of the enzyme via a pore and channel within the structure of the polymerase.

Regulation of transcription, particularly regulation of transcription initiation, is a major mechanism that regulates macromolecular biosynthesis in the cell. However, the processes by which transcription is initiated and regulated in prokaryotes and eukaryotes are notably different. Therefore, a description of each of these processes in prokaryotes and eukaryotes is presented.

TRANSCRIPTION OR SYNTHESIS OF RNA OVER DNA TEMPLATE

Transcription or Synthesis of RNA over DNA Template

In eucaryotes, transcription occurs at G1 and G2 phase of cell cycle inside the nucleus and the transcription products move out into cytoplasm for translation. In prokaryotes, transcription occurs in contact with the cytoplasm as their DNA lies in the cytoplasm.

Transcription requires a DNA dependent enzyme RNA polymerase. Transcribing segment of DNA has promoter and terminator regions. Besides a promoter, eukaryotes may also require an enhancer.

A termination factor called Rho (ρ) factor present in DNA is required for termination of transcription. A number of other factors are also required for unwinding of DNA duplex, stabilisation of unwound DNA strand, base pairing, separation and processing of transcribed RNA.

Activation of ribonucleotides

Ribonucle-otides differ from deoxyribonucleotides in having ribose sugar instead of deoxyribose sugar. Thymi-dine monophosphate is replaced by uridine monophosphate. The four types of ribonucleotides are adenosine monophosphate (AMP), guanosine monophosphate (GMP), uridine monosphosphate (UMP) and cytidine monophosphate (CMP).

They occur freely in the nucleoplasm. Prior to transcription the nucleotides are activated through phosphorylation. Enzyme phosphorylase is required alongwith energy. The activated or phos- phorylated ribonucleotides are adenosine triphosphate (ATP), guanosine triphosphate (GTP), uridine triphosphate (UTP) and cytidine triphosphate (CTP).

DNA template

On specific signals, segments of DNA corresponding to one or more cistrons become derepressed and ready to transcribe. Each such DNA transcription segment has a promoter region initiation site, coding region and a terminator region. Transcription begins at the initiation site and ends at the terminator region. A promoter region has RNA polymerase recognition site and RNA polymerase binding site. Chain opening occurs in the region occupied by TATAAG nucleotides in most procaryotes. Enzymes required for chain separation are unwindases and single strand binding proteins. Terminator region has either poly A base sequence or pallindromic sequence (identical base sequence running in opposite directions in the two DNA chains).

RNA polymerase (common in procaryotes and specific in eucaryotes) binds itself to the promoter region. The two strands of DNA uncoil progressively from the site of polymerase binding. One of the two strands of DNA functions as a template for transcription of RNA. It is called master or sense strand. Transcription occurs in $5' \rightarrow 3'$ direction.

Base pairing

Ribonucleoside triphosphates present in the surrounding medium come to lie opposite the nitrogen bases of the DNA template (sense strand). They form complementary pairs, U opposite A, A opposite T, C opposite G, and G opposite C. With the help of pyrophos-phatase, the two extra phosphates present on the ribonucleoside triphosphates (ribonucleotide diphosphates) separate.

Energy is released in the process:

$$\text{Ribonculeoside triphosphate} \xrightarrow{\text{Pyrophosphatase}} \text{Ribonucleotide} + \text{PPi} + \text{Energy}$$

Chain formation

With the help of RNA polymerase the adjacent ribonucleotides held over DNA template join to form RNA chain in prokaryotes. Transcription factors are already distinct from RNA polymerase in eukaryotes. As the RNA chain formation initiates, the sigma (σ) factor of the RNA polymerase separates. RNA polymerase (core enzyme) moves along the DNA template causing elongation of RNA chain at the rate of some 30 nucleotides per second. RNA synthesis stops as soon as polymerase reaches the terminator region. Rho factor (ρ) is required for this. Terminator region has a stop signal. It also possesses 4–8 A-nucleotides.

Separation of RNA

Termination or rho factor has ATP-ase activity. It helps in the release of completed RNA chain. The released RNA is called primary transcript. It is processed to form functional RNAs. In many prokaryotes, the structural genes of related functions are generally grouped together in operons. An operon is transcribed as a single unit. Such a transcription unit is polycistronic mRNA. In eukaryotes, the transcription unit is a monocistronic mRNA.

Duplex formation

After the release of primary transcript, the two strands of DNA establish linkages amongst complementary base pairs. Gyrases, unwindases and SSB proteins are released. Consequently the double helical form of DNA is resumed.

Post-transcription processing

Primary transcript is often larger than the functional RNAs. It is called heterogeneous or hnRNA especially in case of mRNA. Post-transcription processing is required to convert primary transcript into functional RNAs. It is of four types:

1. Cleavage: Larger RNA precursors are cleaved to form smaller RNAs. Primary transcript of rRNA is 45S in eucaryotes. It is cleaved to form the following:

$$45S \rightarrow 41S \nearrow \begin{array}{l} 32S \rightarrow 28S + 5.8S \\ \\ 20S \rightarrow 18S \end{array}$$

   Primary transcript is cleaved by ribonuclease-P (an RNA enzyme). A primary transcript may form 5–7 tRNA precursors.

2. Splicing: Eucaryotic transcripts possess extra segments (introns or intervening sequences). The functional coding sequences are called exons. Splicing is removal of introns and fusion of exons to form functional RNAs. Each intron starts with dinucleotide GU and ends with dinucleotide AG (GU-AG rule). They are recognised by components of splicing apparatus of Sn- RNPs (pronounced as snurps) or small nuclear ribonucleoproteins (viz. Ul, U2, U4, U5, and U6).

   A complex called spliceosome is formed between 5′ end (GU) and 3′ end (AG) of intron. Energy is obtained from ATP. It removes the intron. The adjacent exons are brought together. The ends are sealed by RNA ligase.

   Introns are not recent development. They appeared when RNA-centric genetic machinery was in place. Therefore, split genes and split transcrips are ancient features of the genetic system. Splicing continues to be RNA mediated catalytic function. Many more such RNA dependent processes are coming to light.

3. Terminal additions (Capping and Tailing): Additional nucleotides are added to the ends of RNAs for specific functions, e.g. CCA segment in tRNA, cap nucleotides at 5′ end of mRNA or poly-A segments (200–300 residues) at 3′ end of mRNA. Cap is formed by modification of GTP into 7-methyl guanosine or 7mG.

4. Nucleotide Modifications: They are most common in tRNA—methylation (e.g. methyl cytosine, methyl guanosine), deamination (e.g. inosine from adenine), dihydrouracil, pseudouracil, etc. In parkaryotes mRNA does not require any elaborate processing to become active. Further, transcription and translation occur in the same region. It results in beginning of translation even before mRNA is fully formed. *In vitro* synthesis of RNA was first performed by Ochoa.

TRANSCRIPTION IN PROKARYOTES

Transcription of prokaryotic genes is accomplished by a single RNA polymerase. The prototype of the prokaryotic RNA polymerase is the polymerase of *Escherichia coli*. It is composed of four different polypeptide subunits, α, β, β′ and σ. The RNA polymerase core enzyme, which functions in transcription elongation, is composed of two α subunits and one each of the β and β′ subunits. The RNA polymerase holoenzyme, which initiates transcription, is organised as the core enzyme plus one copy of the σ subunit.

   To initiate transcription, RNA polymerase holoenzyme first binds to DNA sequences immediately upstream of a gene. This region upstream of the gene, termed the promoter, contains DNA sequences specifically recognised and bound by the RNA polymerase holoenzyme. The σ subunit confers upon the holoenzyme the ability to recognise and bind to the promoter in a DNA sequence-specific manner, and to initiate transcription at a site specifically from the template strand of the DNA. Different σ subunits, such as σ^{54} and σ^{70}, recognise and bind different subsets of prokaryotic promoter sequences. For example, σ^{70}-containing holoenzyme recognises and contacts (via the σ subunit) specific promoter sequences surrounding positions -10 and -35 (upstream of the transcription initiation site).

Initial binding of the polymerase to the promoter leads to formation of a closed binary complex where the polymerase-bound DNA duplex remains double-stranded. This closed complex is then converted to a more stable open complex where melting of the DNA duplex occurs and the two strands of the promoter DNA undergo separation. The DNA duplex is melted over ~12 bp, from the -10 region to just downstream of the transcription initiation site (i.e. the deoxynucleotide in the DNA, encoding the first ribonucleotide in the RNA transcript). Both the closed and open promoter complexes are composed of multiple intermediate forms, with formation of an open complex accompanied by a major conformation change in the RNA polymerase. Conversion to an open promoter complex is followed by entry of ribonucleotide triphosphates (rNTPs) and binding of the initial (rNTP) to form a ternary complex. For σ^{70} promoters, conversion and stability of the open promoter complex does not require rNTP hydrolysis, though for some promoters (e.g. certain σ^{54} promoters) this conversion from a closed to open complex requires interaction with activator proteins bound to the DNA upstream of the promoter as well as hydrolysis of ATP. After forming the open ternary complex, active transcription begins with the synthesis of a series of abortive transcripts. These are short transcripts <10 nucleotides in length that are repetitively synthesised and released without release of the polymerase from the promoter. Once a nascent transcript reaches a length of 8–10 nucleotides, σ factor is released from the holoenzyme and RNA polymerase escapes and clears the promoter to begin committed elongation of the transcript. The transcription elongation complex (TEC) is a stable association of the core polymerase with the DNA template and nascent RNA. Elongation proceeds by movement of the TEC down the linear DNA template, with sequential and continuous addition of nucleotides to the 3' end of the nascent transcript. The exact ribonucleotide added to the elongating RNA chain is specified by the next base in the DNA template sequence according to Watson-Crick base pairing (i.e. A:U, C:G, G:C, T:A for DNA:RNA base pairs). Misincorporation of a nucleotide in the nascent RNA or pausing of the polymerase along the DNA template during elongation, leads the polymerase to backtrack along a short stretch of the DNA, cleavage of the newly synthesised portion of the nascent RNA at the 3' end and continuation of elongation from the newly truncated nascent RNA (including resynthesis of the cleaved portion of the RNA).

Termination of transcription in prokaryotes occurs at specific sites downstream of the coding region of genes and is accomplished by either of two possible mechanisms. One, termed *rho-dependent termination*, is mediated by the action of the rho termination protein and requires the hydrolysis of ATP. The second mechanism is rho-independent termination and occurs via formation of specific hairpin structures in the nascent RNA that destabilises the ternary complex immediately downstream of the hairpin and leads to dissociation of the ternary complex and transcription termination. Rho-independent termination can also occur via terminators formed by an RNA:DNA hybrid between the nascent RNA and the DNA template just upstream of the elongation complex.

Following termination of transcription and release of the RNA polymerase from the DNA template and the RNA transcript, the free core polymerase is able to rebind another σ factor and reinitiate another round of transcription. Regulation of transcription in prokaryotes occurs by a wealth of different mechanisms that often involve activator and repressor proteins.

Initiation and Regulation of Transcription in Eukaryotes

The three eukaryotic RNA polymerases all synthesise RNA transcripts encoded by a DNA template, but transcribe different subsets of genes. RNA pol I synthesises the precursor of ribosomal RNAs (rRNAs) which is eventually processed into the mature 5.8S, 18S and 28S rRNAs. The bulk of RNA synthesis in a cell is carried out by pol I. RNA pol II primarily transcribes the mRNA encoding genes and therefore is responsible for transcription of the largest and most diverse subset of genes in the cell. RNA pol III catalyses synthesis of an assortment of small RNAs including tRNAs and 5S rRNA. Unlike the prokaryotic RNA polymerase, highly purified eukaryotic RNA polymerases do not recognise promoter sequences by themselves or initiate transcription by binding directly to specific DNA sequences in eukaryotic promoters. Rather eukaryotic polymerases are recruited to promoter regions via protein-protein interactions by both proteins that bind to specific DNA sequences in promoter and other regulatory regions as well as additional proteins that interact with these DNA-binding proteins.

RNA EDITING

RNA editing is a molecular process through which some cells can make discrete changes to specific nucleotide sequences within an RNA molecule after it has been generated by RNA polymerase. RNA editing may include the insertion, deletion, and base substitution of nucleotides within the RNA molecule. RNA editing is relatively rare, with common forms of RNA processing (e.g. splicing, 5'-capping, and 3'-polyadenylation) are not usually considered as editing. RNA editing has been observed in some tRNA, rRNA, mRNA, or miRNA molecules of eukaryotes and their viruses, archaea, and prokaryotes. RNA editing occurs in the cell nucleus and cytosol, as well as within mitochondria and plastids. In vertebrates, editing is rare and usually consists of a small number of changes to the sequence of affected molecules. In other organisms, extensive editing (pan-editing) can occur, in some cases the majority of nucleotides in an mRNA sequence may result from editing. RNA-editing processes show great molecular diversity, and some appear to be evolutionarily recent acquisitions that arose independently. The diversity of RNA editing phenomena includes nucleobase modifications such as cytidine (C) to uridine (U) and adenosine (A) to inosine (I) deaminations, as well as non-templated nucleotide additions and insertions. RNA editing in mRNAs effectively alters the amino acid sequence of the encoded protein so that it differs from that predicted by the genomic DNA sequence.

Editing by Insertion or Deletion

RNA editing through the addition and deletion of uracil has been found in kinetoplasts from the mitochondria of Trypanosoma brucei Because this may involve a large fraction of the sites in a gene, it is sometimes called 'pan-editing' to distinguish it from topical editing of one or a few sites.

Pan-editing starts with the base-pairing of the unedited primary transcript with a guide RNA (gRNA), which contains complementary sequences to the regions around the insertion/deletion points. The newly formed double-stranded region is then enveloped by an editosome, a large multi-protein complex that catalyses the editing. The editosome opens the transcript at the first mismatched nucleotide and starts inserting uridines. The inserted uridines will base-pair with the guide RNA, and insertion will continue as long as A or G is present in the guide RNA and will stop when a C or U is encountered. The inserted nucleotides cause a frameshift, and result in a translated protein that differs from its gene.

The mechanism of the editosome involves an endonucleolytic cut at the mismatch point between the guide RNA and the unedited transcript. The next step is catalysed by one of the enzymes in the complex, a terminal U-transferase, which adds Us from UTP at the 3' end of the mRNA. The opened ends are held in place by other proteins in the complex. Another enzyme, a U-specific exoribonuclease, removes the unpaired Us. After editing has made mRNA complementary to gRNA, an RNA ligase rejoins the ends of the edited mRNA transcript. As a consequence, the editosome can edit only in a 3′ to 5′ direction along the primary RNA transcript. The complex can act on only a single guide RNA at a time. Therefore, a RNA transcript requiring extensive editing will need more than one guide RNA and editosome complex is shown in Fig. 22.3.

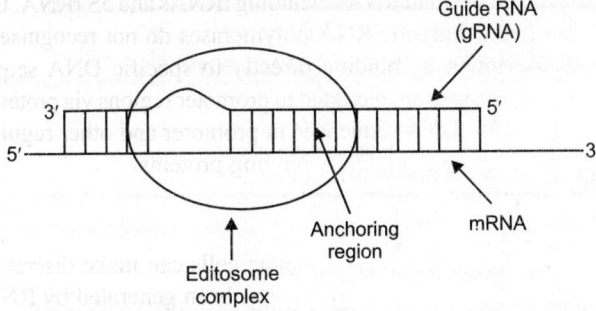

Fig. 22.3: Editosome complex.

Editing by Deamination

C-to-U editing

The editing involves cytidine deaminase that deaminates a cytidine base into a uridine base. An example of C-to-U editing is with the apolipoprotein B gene in humans. Apo B100 is expressed in the liver and apo B48 is expressed in the intestines. In the intestines, the mRNA has a CAA sequence edited to be UAA, a stop codon, thus producing the shorter B48 form. C-to-U editing often occurs in the mitochondrial RNA of flowering plants. Different plants have different degrees of C-to-U editing, for example, eight (8) editing events occur in mitochondria of the moss Funaria hygrometrica, whereas over 1700 editing events occur in the lycophytes Isoetes engelmanii. C-to-U editing is performed by members of the pentatricopeptide repeat (PPR) protein family. Angiosperms have large PPR families, acting as *trans*-factors for *cis*-elements lacking a consensus sequence, Arabidopsis has around 450 members in its PPR family. There have been a number of discoveries of PPR proteins in both plastids and mitochondria.

A-to-I editing

Adenosine-to-inosine (A-to-I) modifications contribute to nearly 90% of all editing events in RNA. The deamination of adenosine is catalysed by the double-stranded RNA-specific adenosine deaminase (ADAR), which typically acts on pre-mRNAs. The deamination of adenosine to inosine disrupts and destabilises the dsRNA base pairing, therefore rendering that particular dsRNA less able to produce siRNA, which interferes with the RNAi pathway. Effect of uracil insertion in pre-mRNA transcripts is shown in Fig.22.4.

The wobble base pairing causes deaminated RNA to have a unique but different structure, which may be related to the inhibition of the initiation step of RNA translation. Studies have shown that I-RNA (RNA with many repeats of the I-U base pair) recruits methylases that are involved in the formation of heterochromatin and that this chemical modification heavily interferes with miRNA target sites. There is active research into the importance of A-to-I modifications and their purpose in the novel concept of epitranscriptomics, in which modifications are made to RNA that alter their function. A long established

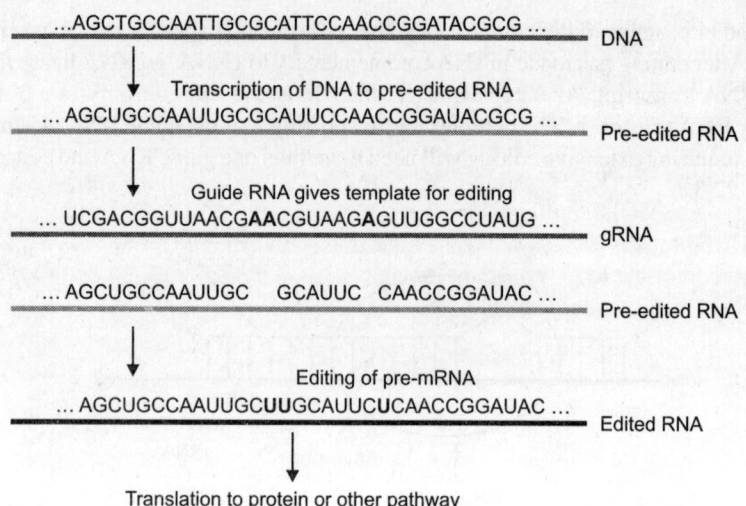

Fig. 22.4: Effect of uracil insertion in pre-mRNA transcripts.

consequence of A-to-I in mRNA is the interpretation of I as a G, therefore leading to functional A-to-G substitution, e.g. in the interpretation of the genetic code by ribosomes. Newer studies however, have weakened this correlation by showing that I's can also be decoded by the ribosome (although in a lesser extent) as A's and U's. Furthermore it was shown that I's lead to the stalling of ribosomes on the I-rich mRNA. The development of high-throughput sequencing in recent years has allowed for the development of extensive databases for different modifications and edits of RNA. RADAR (Rigorously Annotated Database of A-to-I RNA editing) was developed in 2013 to catalog the vast variety of A-to-I sites and tissue-specific levels present in humans, mice, and flies. The addition of novel sites and overall edits to the database are ongoing. The level of editing for specific editing sites, e.g. in the filamin A transcript, is tissue-specific. The efficiency of mRNA-splicing is a major factor controlling the level of A-to-I RNA editing.

Alternative mRNA editing

Alternative U-to-C mRNA editing was first reported in WT1 (Wilms Tumour-1) transcripts, and non-classic G-A mRNA changes were first observed in HNRNPK (heterogeneous nuclear ribonucleoprotein K) transcripts in both malignant and normal colourectal samples. The latter changes were also later seen alongside non-classic U-to-C alterations in brain cell TPH2 (tryptophan hydroxylase 2) transcripts. Although the reverse amination might be the simplest explanation for U-to-C changes, transamination and transglycosylation mechanisms have been proposed for plant U-to-C editing events in mitochondrial transcripts. A recent study reported novel G-to-A mRNA changes in WT1 transcripts at two hotspots, proposing the APOBEC3A (apolipoprotein B mRNA editing enzyme, catalytic polypeptide 3A) as the enzyme implicated in this class of alternative mRNA editing. It was also shown that alternative mRNA changes were associated with canonical WT1 splicing variants, indicating their functional significance.

RNA Editing in Plant Mitochondria and Plastids

It has been shown in previous studies that the only types of RNA editing seen in the plants mitochondria and plastids are conversion of C-to-U and U-to-C (very rare). RNA-editing sites are found mainly in the coding regions of mRNA, introns, and other non-translated regions. In fact, RNA editing can restore the functionality of tRNA molecules. The editing sites are found primarily upstream of mitochondrial or plastid RNAs. While the specific positions for C to U RNA editing (Fig. 22.5) events have been fairly well studied in both the mitochondrion and plastid, the identity and organisation of all proteins comprising the editosome have yet to be established. Members of the expansive PPR protein family have been shown to function as *trans*-acting factors for RNA sequence recognition. Specific members of the MORF (Multiple organellar RNA editing factor) family are also required for proper editing at several sites. As some of these MORF proteins have been shown to interact with members of the PPR family, it is possible MORF proteins are components of the editosome complex. An enzyme responsible for the *trans*- or deamination of the RNA transcript remains elusive, though it has been proposed that the PPR proteins may serve this function as well.

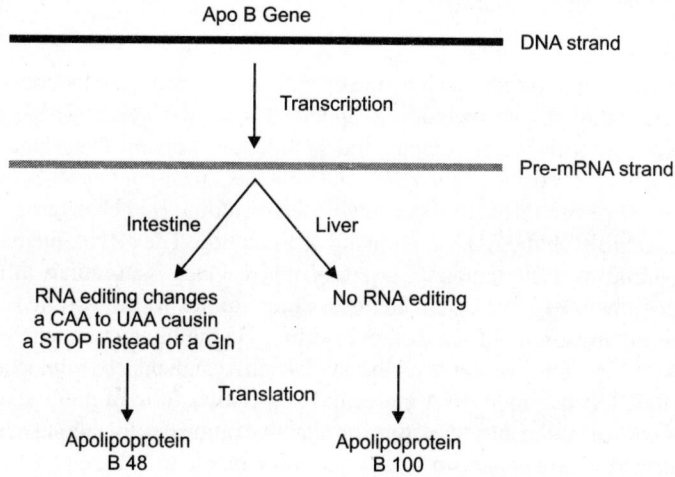

Fig. 22.5: Effect of C-to-U RNA editing on the human ApoB gene.

RNA editing is essential for the normal functioning of the plants translation and respiration activity. Editing can restore the essential base-pairing sequences of tRNAs, restoring functionality. It has also been linked to the production of RNA-edited proteins that are incorporated into the polypeptide complexes of the respiration pathway. Therefore, it is highly probable that polypeptides synthesised from unedited RNAs would not function properly and hinder the activity of both mitochondria and plastids. C-to-U RNA editing can create start and stop codons, but it cannot destroy existing start and stop codons. A cryptic start codon is created when the codon ACG is edited to be AUG. Figure 22.6 shows summary of the various functions of RNA editing.

RNA Editing in Viruses

RNA editing in viruses (i.e. measles, mumps, or parainfluenza) is used for stability and generation of protein variants. Viral RNAs are transcribed by a virus-encoded RNA-dependent RNA polymerase, which is prone to pausing and 'stuttering' at certain nucleotide combinations. In addition, up to several hundred non-templated A's are added by the polymerase at the 3' end of nascent mRNA. These As help stabilise the mRNA. Furthermore, the pausing and stuttering of the RNA polymerase allows the incorporation of one or two Gs or As upstream of the translational codon. The addition of the non-templated nucleotides shifts the reading frame, which generates a different protein.

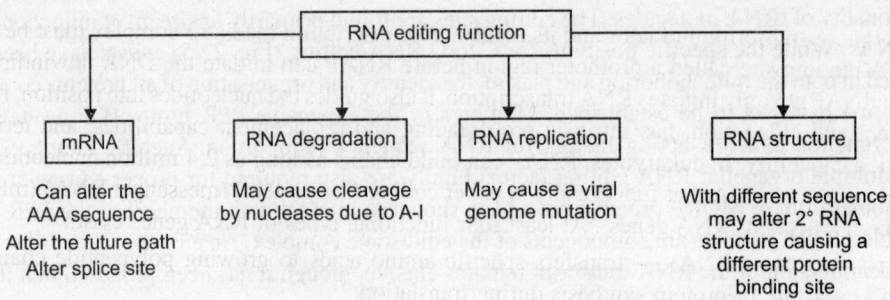

Fig. 22.6: Summary of the various functions of RNA editing.

Origin and Evolution of RNA Editing

The RNA-editing system seen in the animal may have evolved from mononucleotide deaminases, which have led to larger gene families that include the apobec-1 and adar genes. These genes share close identity with the bacterial deaminases involved in nucleotide metabolism. The adenosine deaminase of *E. coli* cannot deaminate a nucleoside in the RNA, the enzyme's reaction pocket is too small to for the RNA strand to bind to. However, this active site is widened by amino acid changes in the corresponding human analog genes, APOBEC1 and ADAR, allowing deamination. The gRNA-mediated pan-editing in trypanosome mitochondria, involving templated insertion of U residues, is an entirely different biochemical reaction. The enzymes involved have been shown in other studies to be recruited and adapted from different sources. But the specificity of nucleotide insertion via the interaction between the gRNA and mRNA is similar to the tRNA editing processes in the animal and Acanthamoeba mithochondria. Eukaryotic ribose methylation of rRNAs by guide RNA molecules is a similar form of modification.

Thus, RNA editing evolved more than once. Several adaptive rationales for editing have been suggested. Editing is often described as a mechanism of correction or repair to compensate for defects in gene sequences. However, in the case of gRNA-mediated editing, this explanation does not seem possible because if a defect happens first, there is no way to generate an error-free gRNA-encoding region, which presumably arises by duplication of the original gene region. This thinking leads to an evolutionary proposal called 'constructive neutral evolution' in which the order of steps is reversed, with the gratuitous capacity for editing preceding the 'defect'.

RNA Editing may be involved in RNA Degradation

A study looked at the involvement of RNA editing in RNA degradation. The researchers specifically looked at the interaction between ADAR and UPF1, an enzyme involved in the nonsense-mediated mRNA decay pathway (NMD). They found that ADAR and UPF1 are found within the suprasliceosome and they form a complex that leads to the down-regulation of specific genes. The exact mechanism or the exact pathways that these two are involved in are unknown at this time. The only fact that this research has shown is that they form a complex and down-regulate specific genes.

RNA POLYMERASE

RNA polymerase (ribonucleic acid polymerase), both abbreviated RNAP or RNApol, official name DNA-directed RNA polymerase, is an enzyme that synthesises RNA from a DNA template. RNAP locally opens the double-stranded DNA (usually about four turns of the double helix) so that one strand of the exposed nucleotides can be used as a template for the synthesis of RNA, a process called transcription. A transcription factor and its associated transcription mediator complex must be attached to a DNA binding site called a promoter region before RNAP can initiate the DNA unwinding at that position. RNAP not only initiates RNA transcription, it also guides the nucleotides into position, facilitates attachment and elongation, has intrinsic proofreading and replacement capabilities, and termination recognition capability. In eukaryotes, RNAP can build chains as long as 2.4 million nucleotides.

RNAP produces RNA that functionally is either coding (for protein) (messenger RNA) (mRNA), or non-coding: so-called 'RNA genes'. At least four functional types of RNA genes exist:

1. Rransfer RNA (tRNA) — transfers specific amino acids to growing polypeptide chains at the ribosomal site of protein synthesis during translation.

2. Ribosomal RNA (rRNA) — incorporates into ribosomes.

3. Micro RNA (miRNA) — regulates gene activity.

4. Catalytic RNA (ribozyme) — functions as an enzymatically active RNA molecule.

RNA polymerase is essential to life, and is found in all living organisms and many viruses. Depending on the organism, a RNA polymerase can be a protein complex (multi-subunit RNAP) or only consist of one subunit (single-subunit SNAP, ssSNAP), each representing an independent lineage. The former is found in bacteria, archaea, and eukaryotes alike, sharing a similar core structure and mechanism. The latter is found in phages as well as eukaryotic chloroplasts and mitochondria, and is related to modern DNA polymerases. Eukaryotic and archaeal RNAPs have more subunits than bacterial ones do, and are controlled differently.

Bacteria and archaea only have one RNA polymerase. Eukaryotes have multiple types of nuclear RNAP, each responsible for synthesis of a distinct subset of RNA. RNA polymerase I synthesises a pre-rRNA 45S (35S in yeast), which matures and will form the major RNA sections of the ribosome. RNA polymerase II synthesises precursors of mRNAs and most snRNA and microRNAs. RNA polymerase III synthesises tRNAs, rRNA 5S and other small RNAs found in the nucleus and cytosol. RNA polymerase IV and V found in plants are less-understood, they make siRNA. In addition to the ssSNAPs, chloroplasts also encode and use a bacteria-like RNAP.

Structure

The 2006 Nobel Prize in Chemistry was awarded to Roger D. Kornberg for creating detailed molecular images of RNA polymerase during various stages of the transcription process. In most prokaryotes, a single RNA polymerase species transcribes all types of RNA. RNA polymerase 'core' from *E. coli* consists of five subunits: two alpha (α) subunits of 36 kDa, a beta (β) subunit of 150 kDa, a beta prime subunit (β') of 155 kDa, and a small omega (ω) subunit. A sigma (σ) factor binds to the core, forming the holoenzyme. After transcription starts, the factor can unbind and let the core enzyme proceed with its work. The core RNA polymerase complex forms a 'crab claw' or 'clamp-jaw' structure with an internal channel running along the full length. Eukaryotic and archaeal RNA polymerases have a similar core structure and work in a similar manner, although they have many extra subunits. All RNAPs contain metal cofactors, in particular zinc and magnesium cations which aid in the transcription process.

Function

Control of the process of gene transcription affects patterns of gene expression and, thereby, allows a cell to adapt to a changing environment, perform specialised roles within an organism, and maintain basic metabolic processes necessary for survival. Therefore, it is hardly surprising that the activity of RNAP is long, complex, and highly regulated. In *Escherichia coli* bacteria, more than 100 transcription factors have been identified, which modify the activity of RNAP. RNAP can initiate transcription at specific DNA sequences known as promoters. It then produces an RNA chain, which is complementary to the template DNA strand. The process of adding nucleotides to the RNA strand is known as elongation, in eukaryotes, RNAP can build chains as long as 2.4 million nucleotides (the full length of the dystrophin gene). RNAP will preferentially release its RNA transcript at specific DNA sequences encoded at the end of genes, which are known as terminators.

Products of RNAP include:

- Messenger RNA (mRNA)—template for the synthesis of proteins by ribosomes.
- Non-coding RNA or 'RNA genes'—a broad class of genes that encode RNA that is not translated into protein. The most prominent examples of RNA genes are transfer RNA (tRNA) and ribosomal RNA (rRNA), both of which are involved in the process of translation. However, since the late 1990s, many new RNA genes have been found, and thus RNA genes may play a much more significant role than previously thought.

   o   Transfer RNA (tRNA)—transfers specific amino acids to growing polypeptide chains at the ribosomal site of protein synthesis during translation.

   o   Ribosomal RNA (rRNA)—a component of ribosomes.

   o   Micro RNA—regulates gene activity.

   o   Catalytic RNA (Ribozyme)—enzymatically active RNA molecules.

RNAP accomplishes de novo synthesis. It is able to do this because specific interactions with the initiating nucleotide hold RNAP rigidly in place, facilitating chemical attack on the incoming nucleotide. Such specific interactions explain why RNAP prefers to start transcripts with ATP (followed by GTP, UTP, and then CTP). In contrast to DNA polymerase, RNAP includes helicase activity, therefore no separate enzyme is needed to unwind DNA.

Action

Initiation

RNA polymerase binding in bacteria involves the sigma factor recognising the core promoter region containing the -35 and -10 elements (located before the beginning of sequence to be transcribed) and also, at some promoters, the a subunit C-terminal domain recognising promoter upstream elements. There are multiple interchangeable sigma factors, each of which recognises a distinct set of promoters. For example, in E. coli, s70 is expressed under normal conditions and recognises promoters for genes required under normal conditions ('housekeeping genes'), while s32 recognises promoters for genes required at high temperatures ('heat-shock genes'). In archaea and eukaryotes, the functions of the bacterial general transcription factor sigma are performed by multiple general transcription factors that work together. The RNA polymerase-promoter closed complex is usually referred to as the 'transcription preinitiation complex.'

After binding to the DNA, the RNA polymerase switches from a closed complex to an open complex. This change involves the separation of the DNA strands to form an unwound section of DNA of approximately 13 bp, referred to as the 'transcription bubble'. Supercoiling plays an important part in polymerase activity because of the unwinding and rewinding of DNA. Because regions of DNA in front of RNAP are unwound, there are compensatory positive supercoils. Regions behind RNAP are rewound and negative supercoils are present.

Promoter escape

RNA polymerase then starts to synthesise the initial DNA-RNA heteroduplex, with ribonucleotides base-paired to the template DNA strand according to Watson-Crick base-pairing interactions. As noted above, RNA polymerase makes contacts with the promoter region. However these stabilising contacts inhibit the enzymes ability to access DNA further downstream and thus the synthesis of the full-length product. In order to continue RNA synthesis, RNA polymerase must escape the promoter. It must maintain promoter contacts while unwinding more downstream DNA for synthesis, 'scrunching' more downstream DNA into the initiation complex. During the promoter escape transition, RNA polymerase is considered a 'stressed intermediate.' Thermodynamically the stress accumulates from the DNA-unwinding and DNA-compaction activities. Once the DNA-RNA heteroduplex is long enough (~10 bp), RNA polymerase releases its upstream contacts and effectively achieves the promoter escape transition into the elongation phase. The heteroduplex at the active center stabilises the elongation complex.

However, promoter escape is not the only outcome. RNA polymerase can also relieve the stress by releasing its downstream contacts, arresting transcription. The paused transcribing complex has two options: (i) release the nascent transcript and begin anew at the promoter or (ii) reestablish a new 3'OH on the nascent transcript at the active site via RNA polymerases catalytic activity and recommence DNA scrunching to achieve promoter escape. Abortive initiation, the unproductive cycling of RNA polymerase before the promoter escape transition, results in short RNA fragments of around 9 bp in a process known as abortive transcription. The extent of abortive initiation depends on the presence of transcription factors and the strength of the promoter contacts.

Elongation

The 17-bp transcriptional complex has an 8-bp DNA-RNA hybrid, that is, 8 base-pairs involve the RNA transcript bound to the DNA template strand. As transcription progresses, ribonucleotides are added to the 3' end of the RNA transcript and the RNAP complex moves along the DNA. The characteristic elongation rates in prokaryotes and eukaryotes are about 10–100 nts/sec. Aspartyl (asp) residues in the RNAP will hold on to Mg^{2+} ions, which will, in turn, coordinate the phosphates of the ribonucleotides. The first Mg^{2+} will hold on to the α-phosphate of the NTP to be added. This allows the nucleophilic attack of the 3'OH from the RNA transcript, adding another NTP to the chain. The second Mg^{2+} will hold on to the pyrophosphate of the NTP. The overall reaction equation is:

$$(NMP)n + NTP \rightarrow (NMP)n+1 + PPi$$

Fidelity

Unlike the proof reading mechanisms of DNA polymerase those of RNAP have only recently been investigated. Proof reading begins with separation of the mis-incorporated nucleotide from the DNA template. This pauses transcription. The polymerase then backtracks by one position and cleaves the dinucleotide that contains the mismatched nucleotide. In the RNA polymerase this occurs at the same active site used for polymerisation and is therefore markedly different from the DNA polymerase where proofreading occurs at a distinct nuclease active site. The overall error rate is around 10^{-4} to 10^{-6}.

Termination

In bacteria, termination of RNA transcription can be rho-independent or rho-dependent. The former relies on the rho factor, which destablises the DNA-RNA heteroduplex and causes RNA release. The latter, also known as intrinsic termination, relies on a palindromic region of DNA. Transcribing the region causes the formation of a 'hairpin' structure from the RNA transcription looping and binding upon itself. This hairpin structure is often rich in G-C base-pairs, making it more stable than the DNA-RNA hybrid itself. As a result, the 8 bp DNA-RNA hybrid in the transcription complex shifts to a 4 bp hybrid. These last 4 base pairs are weak A-U base pairs, and the entire RNA transcript will fall off the DNA. Transcription termination in eukaryotes is less well understood than in bacteria, but involves cleavage of the new transcript followed by template-independent addition of adenines at its new 3′ end, in a process called polyadenylation. Figure 22.7 shows RNA Polymerase II Transcription: the process of transcript elongation facilitated by disassembly of nucleosomes.

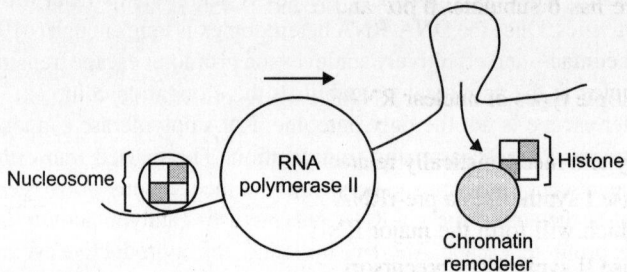

Fig. 22.7: RNA Polymerase II Transcription: the process of transcript elongation facilitated by disassembly of nucleosomes.

Other Organisms

Given that DNA and RNA polymerases both carry out template-dependent nucleotide polymerisation, it might be expected that the two types of enzymes would be structurally related. However, X-ray crystallographic studies of both types of enzymes reveal that, other than containing a critical Mg^{2+} ion at the catalytic site, they are virtually unrelated to each other, indeed template-dependent nucleotide polymerising enzymes seem to have arisen independently twice during the early evolution of cells. One lineage led to the modern DNA Polymerases and reverse transcriptases, as well as to a few single-subunit RNA polymerases (ssRNAP) from phages and organelles. The other multi-subunit RNAP lineage formed all of the modern cellular RNA polymerases.

Bacteria

In bacteria, the same enzyme catalyses the synthesis of mRNA and non-coding RNA (ncRNA). RNAP is a large molecule. The core enzyme has five subunits (~400 kDa):

- β′: The β′ subunit is the largest subunit, and is encoded by the rpoC gene. The β′ subunit contains part of the active center responsible for RNA synthesis and contains some of the determinants for non-sequence-specific interactions with DNA and nascent RNA. It is split into two subunits in Cyanobacteria and chloroplasts.

- β: The β subunit is the second-largest subunit, and is encoded by the rpoB gene. The β subunit contains the rest of the active center responsible for RNA synthesis and contains the rest of the determinants for non-sequence-specific interactions with DNA and nascent RNA.

- α: Theβα subunit is the third-largest subunit and is present in two copies per molecule of RNAP, aI and aII (one and two). Each a subunit contains two domains: αNTD (N-Terminal domain) and αCTD (C-terminal domain). αNTD contains determinants for assembly of RNAP. αCTD

(C-terminal domain) contains determinants for interaction with promoter DNA, making non-sequence-non-specific interactions at most promoters and sequence-specific interactions at upstream-element-containing promoters, and contains determinants for interactions with regulatory factors.

- ω: The ω subunit is the smallest subunit. The ω subunit facilitates assembly of RNAP and stabilises assembled RNAP.

In order to bind promoters, RNAP core associates with the transcription initiation factor sigma (σ) to form RNA polymerase holoenzyme. Sigma reduces the affinity of RNAP for nonspecific DNA while increasing specificity for promoters, allowing transcription to initiate at correct sites. The complete holoenzyme therefore has 6 subunits: $\beta'\beta\alpha^I$ and $\alpha^{II}\omega\sigma$ (~450 kDa).

Eukaryotes

Eukaryotes have multiple types of nuclear RNAP, each responsible for synthesis of a distinct subset of RNA.

All are structurally and mechanistically related to each other and to bacterial RNAP:

- RNA polymerase I synthesises a pre-rRNA 45S (35S in yeast), which matures into 28S, 18S and 5.8S rRNAs which will form the major RNA sections of the ribosome.
- RNA polymerase II synthesises precursors of mRNAs and most snRNA and microRNAs. This is the most studied type, and, due to the high level of control required over transcription, a range of transcription factors are required for its binding to promoters.
- RNA polymerase III synthesises tRNAs, rRNA 5S and other small RNAs found in the nucleus and cytosol.
- RNA polymerase IV synthesises siRNA in plants.
- RNA polymerase V synthesises RNAs involved in siRNA-directed heterochromatin formation in plants.

Eukaryotic chloroplasts contain an RNAP very highly similar to bacterial RNAP ('plastid-encoded polymerase, PEP'). They use sigma factors encoded in the nuclear genome. Chloroplast also contain a second, structurally and mechanistically unrelated, single-subunit RNAP ('nucleus-encoded polymerase, NEP'). Eukaryotic mitochondria use POLRMT (human), a nucleus-encoded single-subunit RNAP. Such phage-like polymerases are referred to as RpoT in plants.

Archaea

Archaea have a single type of RNAP, responsible for the synthesis of all RNA. Archaeal RNAP is structurally and mechanistically similar to bacterial RNAP and eukaryotic nuclear RNAP I-V, and is especially closely structurally and mechanistically related to eukaryotic nuclear RNAP II. The history of the discovery of the archaeal RNA polymerase is quite recent. The first analysis of the RNAP of an archaeon was performed in 1971, when the RNAP from the extreme halophile Halobacterium cutirubrum was isolated and purified. Crystal structures of RNAPs from Sulfolobus solfataricus and Sulfolobus shibatae set the total number of identified archaeal subunits at thirteen.

Archaea has the subunit corresponding to Eukaryotic Rpb1 split into two. There is no homolog to eukaryotic Rpb9 (POLR2I) in the *S. shibatae* complex, although TFS (TFIIS homolog) has been proposed as one based on similarity. There is an additional subunit dubbed Rpo13, together with Rpo5 it occupies a space filled by an insertion found in bacterial β' subunits (1377–1420 in Taq). An earlier, lower-resolution study on *S. solfataricus* structure did not find Rpo13 and only assigned the space to

Rpo5/Rpb5. Rpo3 is notable in that it's an iron–sulfur protein. RNAP I/III subunit AC40 found in some eukaryotes share similar sequences, but does not bind iron. This domain, in either case, serves a structural function.

Archaeal RNAP subunit previously used an 'RpoX' nomenclature where each subunit is assigned a letter in a way unrelated to any other systems. In 2009, a new nomenclature based on Eukaryotic Pol II subunit 'Rpb' numbering was proposed.

Viruses

T7 RNA polymerase producing a mRNA from a DNA template. The protein is shown as a purple ribbon. Image derived from PDB 1MSW Orthopoxviruses and some other Nucleocytoplasmic large DNA viruses synthesise RNA using a virally encoded multi-subunit RNAP. They are most similar to Eukaryotic RNAPs, with some subunits minified or removed. Most other viruses that synthesise RNA use unrelated mechanics. Many viruses use a single-subunit DNA-dependent RNAP (ssRNAP) that is structurally and mechanistically related to the single-subunit RNAP of eukaryotic chloroplasts and mitochondria and, more distantly, to DNA polymerases and reverse transcriptases. Perhaps the most widely studied such single-subunit RNAP is bacteriophage T7 RNA polymerase. ssRNAPs cannot proofread. Other viruses use a RNA-dependent RNAP (an RNAP that employs RNA as a template instead of DNA). This occurs in negative strand RNA viruses and dsRNA viruses, both of which exist for a portion of their life cycle as double-stranded RNA. However, some positive strand RNA viruses, such as poliovirus, also contain RNA-dependent RNAP.

History

RNAP was discovered independently by Charles Loe, Audrey Stevens, and Jerard Hurwitz in 1960. By this time, one half of the 1959 Nobel Prize in Medicine had been awarded to Severo Ochoa for the discovery of what was believed to be RNAP, but instead turned out to be polynucleotide phosphorylase.

Purification

RNA polymerase can be isolated in the following ways:

- By a phosphocellulose column.
- By glycerol gradient centrifugation.
- By a DNA column.
- By an ion chromatography column.

And also combinations of the above techniques.

TRANSMISSION ELECTRON MICROSCOPY DNA SEQUENCING

Transmission electron microscopy (TEM) DNA sequencing is a single-molecule sequencing technology that uses transmission electron microscopy techniques. The method was conceived and developed in the 1960s and 70s, but lost favour when the extent of damage to the sample was recognised. In order for DNA to be clearly visualised under an electron microscope, it must be labelled with heavy atoms. In addition, specialised imaging techniques and aberration corrected optics are beneficial for obtaining the resolution required to image the labelled DNA molecule. In theory, transmission electron microscopy DNA sequencing could provide extremely long read lengths, but the issue of electron beam damage may still remain and the technology has not yet been commercially developed.

Principle of Electron Microscope

The electron microscope has the capacity to obtain a resolution of up to 100 pm, whereby microscopic biomolecules and structures such as viruses, ribosomes, proteins, lipids, small molecules and even single atoms can be observed. Although DNA is visible when observed with the electron microscope, the resolution of the image obtained is not high enough to allow for deciphering the sequence of the individual bases, i.e. DNA sequencing. However, upon differential labelling of the DNA bases with heavy atoms or metals, it is possible to both visualise and distinguish between the individual bases. Therefore, electron microscopy in conjunction with differential heavy atom DNA labeling could be used to directly image the DNA in order to determine its sequence.

Workflow

Step 1 – DNA denaturation

As in a standard polymerase chain reaction (PCR), the double stranded DNA molecules to be sequenced must be denatured before the second strand can be synthesised with labelled nucleotides.

Step 2 – Heavy atom labelling

The elements that make up biological molecules (C, H, N, O, P, S) are too light (low atomic number, Z) to be clearly visualised as individual atoms by transmission electron microscopy. To circumvent this problem, the DNA bases can be labelled with heavier atoms (higher Z). Each nucleotide is tagged with a characteristic heavy label, so that they can be distinguished in the transmission electron micrograph.

- ZS Genetics proposes using three heavy labels: bromine (Z=35), iodine (Z=53), and trichloro-methane (total Z=63). These would appear as differential dark and light spots on the micrograph, and the fourth DNA base would remain unlabelled.
- Halcyon molecular, in collaboration with the Toste group, proposes that purine and pyrimidine bases can be functionalised with platinum diamine or osmium tetraoxide bipyridine, respectively. Heavy metal atoms such as osmium (Z=76), iridium (Z=77), gold (Z=79), or uranium (Z=92) can then form metal-metal bonds with these functional groups to label the individual bases.

Step 3 – DNA alignment on substrate

The DNA molecules must be stretched out on a thin, solid substrate so that order of the labelled bases will be clearly visible on the electron micrograph. Molecular combing is a technique that utilises the force of a receding air-water interface to extend DNA molecules, leaving them irreversibly bound to a silane layer once dry. This is one means by which alignment of the DNA on a solid substrate may be achieved.

Step 4 – TEM imaging

Transmission electron microscopy (TEM) produces high magnification, high resolution images by passing a beam of electrons through a very thin sample. Whereas atomic resolution has been demonstrated with conventional TEM, further improvement in spatial resolution requires correcting the spherical and chromatic aberrations of the microscope lenses. This has only been possible in scanning transmission electron microscopy where the image is obtained by scanning the object with a finely focused electron beam, in a way similar to a cathode ray tube. However, the achieved improvement in resolution comes together with irradiation of the studied object by much higher beam intensities, the concomitant sample damage and the associated imaging artefacts.

Different imaging techniques are applied depending on whether the sample contains heavy or light atoms:

- Annular dark-field imaging measures the scattering of electrons as they deflect off the nuclei of the atoms in the transmission electron microscopy sample. This is best suited to samples containing heavy atoms, as they cause more scattering of electrons. The technique has been used to image atoms as light as boron, nitrogen, and carbon, however, the signal is very weak for such light atoms. If annular dark-field microscopy is put to use for transmission electron microscopy DNA sequencing, it will certainly be necessary to label the DNA bases with heavy atoms so that a strong signal can be detected.

- Annular bright-field imaging detects electrons transmitted directly through the sample, and measures the wave interference produced by their interactions with the atomic nuclei. This technique can detect light atoms with greater sensitivity than annular dark-field imaging methods. In fact, oxygen, nitrogen, lithium, and hydrogen in crystalline solids have been imaged using annular bright-field electron microscopy. Thus, it is theoretically possible to obtain direct images of the atoms in the DNA chain, however, the structure of DNA is much less geometric than crystalline solids, so direct imaging without prior labeling may not be achievable.

Step 5 – Data analysis

Dark and bright spots on the electron micrograph, corresponding to the differentially labelled DNA bases, are analysed by computer software.

Applications of Transmission Electron Microscopy

Transmission electron microscopy DNA sequencing is not yet commercially available, but the long read lengths that this technology may one day provide will make it useful in a variety of contexts.

De novo genome assembly

When sequencing a genome, it must be broken down into pieces that are short enough to be sequenced in a single read. These reads must then be put back together like a jigsaw puzzle by aligning the regions that overlap between reads, this process is called *de novo* genome assembly. The longer the read length that a sequencing platform provides, the longer the overlapping regions, and the easier it is to assemble the genome. From a computational perspective, microfluidic Sanger sequencing is still the most effective way to sequence and assemble genomes for which no reference genome sequence exists. The relatively long read lengths provide substantial overlap between individual sequencing reads, which allows for greater statistical confidence in the assembly. In addition, long Sanger reads are able to span most regions of repetitive DNA sequence which otherwise confound sequence assembly by causing false alignments. However, *de novo* genome assembly by Sanger sequencing is extremely expensive and time consuming. Second generation sequencing technologies, while less expensive, are generally unfit for *de novo* genome assembly due to short read lengths. In general, third generation sequencing technologies, including transmission electron microscopy DNA sequencing, aim to improve read length while maintaining low sequencing cost. Thus, as third generation sequencing technologies improve, rapid and inexpensive *de novo* genome assembly will become a reality.

Full haplotypes

A haplotype is a series of linked alleles that are inherited together on a single chromosome. DNA sequencing can be used to genotype all of the single nucleotide polymorphisms (SNPs) that constitute a haplotype. However, short DNA sequencing reads often cannot be phased, that is, heterozygous variants cannot be confidently assigned to the correct haplotype. In fact, haplotyping with short read DNA sequencing data requires very high coverage (average >50x coverage of each DNA base) to accurately identify SNPs, as well as additional sequence data from the parents so that Mendelian transmission can be used to estimate the haplotypes. Sequencing technologies that generate long reads, including transmission electron microscopy DNA sequencing, can capture entire haploblocks in a single read. That is, haplotypes are not broken up among multiple reads, and the genetically linked alleles remain together in the sequencing data. Therefore, long reads make haplotyping easier and more accurate, which is beneficial to the field of population genetics.

Copy number variants

Genes are normally present in two copies in the diploid human genome, genes that deviate from this standard copy number are referred to as copy number variants (CNVs). Copy number variation can be benign (these are usually common variants, called copy number polymorphisms) or pathogenic. CNVs are detected by fluorescence in situ hybridisation (FISH) or comparative genomic hybridisation (CGH). To detect the specific breakpoints at which a deletion occurs, or to detect genomic lesions introduced by a duplication or amplification event, CGH can be performed using a tiling array (array CGH), or the variant region can be sequenced. Long sequencing reads are especially useful for analysing duplications or amplifications, as it is possible to analyse the orientation of the amplified segments if they are captured in a single sequencing read.

Cancer

Cancer genomics, or oncogenomics, is an emerging field in which high-throughput, second generation DNA sequencing technology is being applied to sequence entire cancer genomes. Analysing this short read sequencing data encompasses all of the problems associated with *de novo* genome assembly using short read data. Furthermore, cancer genomes are often aneuploid.

These aberrations, which are essentially large scale copy number variants, can be analysed by second-generation sequencing technologies using read frequency to estimate the copy number. Longer reads would, however, provide a more accurate picture of copy number, orientation of amplified regions, and SNPs present in cancer genomes.

Microbiome sequencing

The microbiome refers the total collection of microbes present in a micro environment and their respective genomes. For example, an estimated 100 trillion microbial cells colonise the human body at any given time. The human microbiome is of particular interest, as these commensal bacteria are important for human health and immunity. Most of the Earth bacterial genomes have not yet been sequenced, undertaking a microbiome sequencing project would require extensive *de novo* genome assembly, a prospect which is daunting with short read DNA sequencing technologies. Longer reads would greatly facilitate the assembly of new microbial genomes.

Advantages and Disadvantages of TEM

Compared to other second- and third-generation DNA sequencing technologies, transmission electron microscopy DNA sequencing has a number of potential key strengths and weaknesses, which will ultimately determine its usefulness and prominence as a future DNA sequencing technology.

Advantages of TEM

- Longer read lengths: ZS Genetics has estimated potential read lengths of transmission electron microscopy DNA sequencing to be 10000 to 20000 base pairs with a rate of 1.7 billion base pairs per day. Such long read lengths would allow easier *de novo* genome assembly and direct detection of haplotypes, among other applications.
- Lower cost.
- No dephasing: Dephasing of the DNA strands due to loss in synchronicity during synthesis is a major problem of second-generation sequencing technologies. For transmission electron microscopy DNA sequencing and several other third-generation sequencing technologies, sychronisation of the reads is unnecessary as only one molecule is being read at a time.
- Shorter turnaround time: The capacity to read native fragments of DNA renders complex template preparation an unnecessary step in the general workflow of whole genome sequencing. Consequently, shorter turnaround times are possible.

Disadvantages of TEM

- High capital cost: A transmission electron microscope with sufficient resolution required for transmission electron microscopy DNA sequencing costs approximately US$1,000,000, therefore pursuing DNA sequencing by this method requires a substantial investment.
- Technically challenging: Selective heavy atom labeling and attaching and straightening the labeled DNA to a substrate are a serious technical challenge. Further, the DNA sample should be stable to the high vacuum of electron microscope and irradiation by a focused beam of high-energy electrons.
- Potential PCR bias and artefacts: Although PCR is only being utilised in transmission electron microscopy DNA sequencing as a means to label the DNA strand with heavy atoms or metals, there could be the possibility of introducing bias in template representation or errors during the single amplification.

Comparison to other sequencing technologies

Many non-Sanger second- and third-generation DNA sequencing technologies have been or are currently being developed with the common aim of increasing throughput and decreasing cost such that personalised genetic medicine can be fully realised. Both the US$10 million Archon X Prize for Genomics supported by the X Prize Foundation (Santa Monica, CA, USA) and the US$70 million in grant awards supported by the National Human Genome Research Institute of the National Institutes of Health (NIH-NHGRI) are fueling the rapid burst of research activity in the development of new DNA sequencing technologies. Since different approaches, techniques, and strategies are what define each DNA sequencing technology, each has its own strengths and weaknesses.

References

Allen, M.G., *Introduction to Genetics*, CRC Press, USA.

Bergeron, R.S, *Principles of Genetics,* Harper & Row, New York.

Brazma, K.D., *Population Genetics*, Elsevier Applied Science, London.

Bryan, M.E., *Molecular Genetics*. Cambridge University Press, Cambridge, England.

Close, K.W., *Genetics and Molecular Biology*, Prentice Hall, New York.

Coffee, L. *Human Genetic Diseases*, Academic Press, USA.

Craig, T.H., *The Wonder of Genetics*, Tata-Mcgraw-Hill, New York.

De Jong, K.A., *Basic Concepts of Genetics*, Elsevier, New York.

Dorian, L., *Quantitative Genetics*, Harper & Row, New York.

Duncan, M.E., *Human Molecular Genetics*, Cambridge University Press, New Delhi.

Freund, R.D., *Forensic Genetics*, Marcel Dekker, Inc., New York.

Godfrey, D.I., *Genetics of Bacteria*, Tata-Mcgraw-Hill, New York.

Gold, K.W., *Molecular Genetics*, Oxford University Press, New Delhi.

Gregor Mendle, Mendle's Principles of Heredity, Cambridge University Press, London.

Hampel, T.F., *Conservation Genetics*, Academic Press, Inc., London.

Harper, L.J., *Molecular Genetics*. Harvard University Press, Cambridge.

Henikoff, S., *Genetics Disorder*, Wiley, New York.

Ian, R.L., *Fundamentals or Genetics*, Marcel Dekker, Inc., New York.

James, C.W., *Genetic Analysis,* McGraw-Hill, New York

Jenni, P.R., *Principles of Genetics*, Plenum, New York.

Johnson, V.K., *Behavioural Genetics,* Elsevier, Philadelphia.

Kimbrell, D.A., *Genetics and Genomes*, CRC Press, USA.

Leinster Murray, *Human Heredity*, Pergamon Press, Oxford, London.

Lewis, L.J., *Human Genetics*, Academic Press, Inc., London.

Maalouf Amin, *Viral Genetics,* Academic Press, New York.

MacLeod, I.R., *Population Genetics*. Macmillan, New York.

Marrett Damian, *Principles of Cancer Genetics*, Springer, USA.

Mount, D.W., *Genetics of Genomics*, University of Hertfordshire Press, UK.

Munn, R.F., *Bacteria and Genetics*, Elsevier, New York.

Painter, D.E., *Reproductive Genetics*, Lippincott Williams & Wilkins, Philadelphia.

Pevzner, P.A., *Population Genetics*, John Wiley and Sons, Inc, New Jersey.

Ricci, F.G., *Molecular Genetics*, Saunders Elsevier, Philadelphia.

Richard M. Twyman, *Genetics of Bacteria*, John Wiley and Sons, Inc, New Jersey.

Schrowebel, J., *Genomes*, Pergamon Press, Oxford, London.

Smith, T.F., Anthony J. Murgo, *Fundamentals of Genetics,* CRC Press, USA.

Snell, I.D., *Genetic Engineering,* Saunders Elsevier, Philadelphia.

Waterman, M.S., *Genetics and Molecular Biology*, CRC Press, USA.

Wilbur, W.J., *Genetics*, McGraw Hill, New York.

Willam Bateston, Problems of Genetics, Cambridge University Press, London.

Index

Genetics

Volume II

Highlights

- Gene Mutation, DNA Repair, Transposable Elements and Ames Test
- Regulation of Gene Expression, Transcription Attenuation, RNA Splicing and RNA Silencing
- Cell Cycle Regulation, Genetics of Cancer, Cancer and the Environment
- Recombinant DNA, Methods of Creating DNA Molecules, Genomic Library and DNA Sequencing
- Genomics, Proteomics and Genome Annotation
- Genome Mapping
- Evolutionary and Conservation Genetics
- Ethical Issues and Intellectual Property Rights of Genetic Engineering

Contents at a Glance

Genetics

Volume II

MM Morris

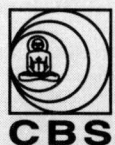

CBS

CBS Publishers & Distributors Pvt Ltd

New Delhi • Bengaluru • Chennai • Kochi • Kolkata • Mumbai
Bhopal • Bhubaneswar • Hyderabad • Jharkhand • Nagpur • Patna • Pune
Uttarakhand • Dhaka (Bangladesh) • Kathmandu (Nepal)

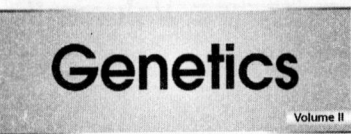

Genetics
Volume II

ISBN: 978-93-89688-55-9

Copyright © Author and Publisher

First Edition: 2020

Published by Satish Kumar Jain and produced by Varun Jain for

CBS Publishers & Distributors Pvt Ltd

4819/XI Prahlad Street, 24 Ansari Road, Daryaganj, New Delhi 110 002, India.
Ph: 23289259, 23266861, 23266867 Website: www.cbspd.com
Fax: 011-23243014   e-mail: delhi@cbspd.com; cbspubs@airtelmail.in.
Corporate Office: 204 FIE, Industrial Area, Patparganj, Delhi 110 092

Ph: 4934 4934   Fax: 4934 4935   e-mail: publishing@cbspd.com; publicity@cbspd.com

Branches

- **Bengaluru:** Seema House 2975, 17th Cross, K.R. Road,
  Banasankari 2nd Stage, Bengaluru 560 070, Karnataka
  Ph: +91-80-26771678/79   Fax: +91-80-26771680   e-mail: bangalore@cbspd.com
- **Chennai:** 7, Subbaraya Street, Shenoy Nagar, Chennai 600 030, Tamil Nadu
  Ph: +91-44-26680620, 26681266   Fax: +91-44-42032115   e-mail: chennai@cbspd.com
- **Kochi:** 68/1534, 35, 36, Power House Road, Opp. KSEB, Kochi 682018, Kerala
  Ph: +91-484-4059061-65   Fax: +91-484-4059065   e-mail: kochi@cbspd.com
- **Kolkata:** 6/B, Ground Floor, Rameswar Shaw Road, Kolkata-700 014, West Bengal
  Ph: +91-33-22891126, 22891127, 22891128   e-mail: kolkata@cbspd.com
- **Mumbai:** 83-C, Dr E Moses Road, Worli, Mumbai-400018, Maharashtra
  Ph: +91-22-24902340/41   Fax: +91-22-24902342   e-mail: mumbai@cbspd.com

Representatives

• **Bhopal** 0-8319310552	• **Bhubaneswar** 0-9911037372	• **Hyderabad** 0-9885175004	• **Jharkhand** 0-9811541605
• **Nagpur** 0-9421945513	• **Patna** 0-9334159340	• **Pune** 0-9623451994	• **Uttarakhand** 0-9716462459
• **Dhaka (Bangladesh)** 01912-003485	• **Kathmandu (Nepal)** 977-9818742655		

Printed at Mudrak, Noida, UP, India

Preface

Genetics is the study of genes. Genetics is about how and why physical characteristics such as eye colour are passed on from one generation to another about how diseases and conditions can run in families the study of patterns in genetic information, such as the patterns used in DNA fingerprinting and profiling and genetics is about how variation occurs in and between animals, plants or humans. Genetics affects us all in many ways. Genetics can help us to understand why people look the way they do and why some people are more prone to certain diseases than others. Genetics can help healthcare professionals to identify certain conditions in babies before they are born using techniques such as prenatal testing. Genetic technologies are also being used to help develop targeted medicines for certain diseases. In addition to its use in healthcare, genetics has a range of other applications.

To understand genetics, it is important to know something about cells, chromosomes and DNA. All living things are made up of cells. The cell is the basic building block of life. A human body contains millions and millions of cells. An average adult has an estimated ten to one hundred thousand million cells. Each cell is so small that you can only see it using a microscope. Genetics allows us to understand how thalassaemia is passed on in families. Blood tests and genetic investigations can help us to determine whether an individual has the disease or is a carrier. Our improved understanding of the causes of the condition may even raise the possibility of future gene-based therapies that may offer a cure.

This reference textbook on *Genetics* is divided in two volumes. Second volume is divided into 10 sections and comprises 1 to 25 chapters.

Section I discusses translation, neurospora, haemoglobin and protein–structure and domains. Chapter 1 is devoted to translation, neurospora and haemoglobin. Translation refers to the process of creating proteins from an mRNA template. Chapter 2 deals with proteins–structure and domains. Proteins are an important class of biological macromolecules present in all biological organisms, made up of such elements as carbon, hydrogen, nitrogen, oxygen, and sulphur. All proteins are polymers of amino acids.

Section II discusses gene mutation, DNA repair, transposable elements and Ames test. Chapter 3 focuses on gene mutations, DNA repair and transposable elements. Chapter 4 explains Ames test. The Ames test is a widely employed method that uses bacteria to test whether a given chemical can cause mutations in the DNA of the test organism. More formally, it is a biological assay to assess the mutagenic potential of chemical compounds.

Section III discusses regulation of gene expression, transcription attenuation, RNA splicing and RNA silencing. Chapter 5 concentrates on regulation of gene expression. Gene expression is the process by which information from a gene is used in the synthesis of a functional gene product. These products are often proteins, but in non-protein coding genes such as rRNA genes or tRNA genes, the product is a functional RNA. Chapter 6 is devoted to transcription attenuation. Attenuation (in genetics) is a proposed mechanism of control in some bacterial operons which results in premature termination of transcription and is based on the fact that, in bacteria, transcription and translation proceed simultaneously. Chapter 7 deals with RNA splicing and RNA silencing. In molecular biology, splicing is a modification of an RNA after transcription, in which introns are removed and exons are joined. This is needed for the typical eukaryotic messenger RNA before it can be used to produce a correct protein through translation.

Section IV discusses cell cycle regulation, genetics of cancer, cancer and the environment. Chapter 8 concentrates on cell cycle and cancer. The cell cycle, the process by which cells progress and divide, lies at the heart of cancer. In normal cells, the cell cycle is controlled by a complex series of signalling pathways by which a cell grows, replicates its DNA and divides. Chapter 9 focuses on genetics of cancer. Cancer is a genetic disease—that is, cancer is caused by certain changes to genes that control the way our cells function, especially how they grow and divide. Chapter 10 explains cancer and the environment. Cancer is a generic term for a large group of diseases that can affect any part of the body. Exposure to a wide variety of natural and man-made substances in the environment accounts for at least two-thirds of all the cases of cancer in the United States. These environmental factors include lifestyle choices like cigarette smoking, excessive alcohol consumption, poor diet, lack of exercise, excessive sunlight exposure, and sexual behaviour that increases exposure to certain viruses.

Section V discusses recombinant DNA, methods of creating DNA molecules, genomic library and DNA sequencing. Chapter 11 is devoted to recombinant DNA and gene cloning. Recombinant DNA, which is often shortened to rDNA, is an artificially made DNA strand that is formed by the combination of two or more gene sequences. This new combination may or may not occur naturally, but is engineered specifically for a purpose to be used in one of the many applications of recombinant DNA. Chapter 12 deals with method of creating recombinant DNA molecules. Chapter 13 focuses on genomic library and DNA sequencing. A genomic library is an organism specific collection of DNA covering the entire genome of an organism. It contains all DNA sequences such as expressed genes, non-expressed genes, exons and introns, promoter and terminator regions and intervening DNA sequences.

Section VI discusses genomics, proteomics, genome annotation, bacterial and eukaryotic genomes, comparative and minimal genomics and genome mapping. Chapter 14 concentrates on genomics, proteomics and genome annotation. Chapter 15 explains bacterial and eukaryotic genomes. Bacterial genomes are generally smaller and less variant in size between species when compared with genomes of animals and single cell eukaryotes. Chapter 16 is devoted to comparative and minimal genomics. Comparative genomics is a field of biological research in which the genomic features of different organisms are compared. The genomic features may include the DNA sequence, genes, gene order, regulatory sequences, and other genomic structural landmarks. Chapter 17 deals with genome mapping. Gene mapping, also called genome mapping, is the creation of a genetic map assigning DNA fragments to chromosomes. When a genome is first investigated, this map is nonexistent.

Section VII discusses developmental genetics and genetic control of development. Chapter 18 focuses on developmental genetics. Developmental genetics is the study of the way in which genes control the growth and development of an organism throughout its life-cycle. A newly fertilised egg cell or zygote contains a unique collection of genes that will control its development from a single cell into an embryo through patterns of differential gene expression in the process of embryogenesis. Chapter 19 concentrates on genetic control of development.

Section VIII discusses quantitative and population genetics. Chapter 20 is devoted to quantitative genetics. Quantitative genetics is a branch of population genetics that deals with phenotypes that vary continuously—as opposed to discretely identifiable phenotypes and gene-products. Chapter 21 deals with population genetics. Population genetics is the study of the distributions and changes of allele frequency in a population, as the population is subject to the four main evolutionary processes: natural selection, genetic drift, mutation and gene flow.

Section IX discusses evolutionary and conservation genetics. Chapter 22 explains evolutionary genetics. Evolution is the cornerstone of modern biology. It unites all the fields of biology under one theoretical umbrella. Evolution is a change in the gene pool of a population over time. A gene is a hereditary unit that can be passed on unaltered for many generations. Chapter 23 focuses on conservation genetics. Conservation genetics is concerned with population genetic variation, population viability, and the future evolution of species. Conservation genetics, ecology, and habitat management together provide the technical underpinnings of conservation biology, a crisis oriented science of biodiversity management.

Section X discusses ethical issues and intellectual property rights of genetic engineering. Chapter 24 is devoted to ethical issues of genetics. Ethical issues raised by genetics at the start of the twenty-first century reveals a wide spectrum of possibilities, potential benefits, and ethical issues, as well as numerous efforts to devise policy structures that will ensure that newly acquired genetic knowledge is used ethically. Chapter 25 deals with genetic inventions and intellectual property rights. This chapter provides a brief factual overview of the patenting of genetic inventions. It relates the basic principles of intellectual property protection, summarises the key issues in patent protection, and describes how patent protection for genetic inventions currently works. It also provides a brief review of the types of reform proposals being debated which would influence the patenting and licensing of genetic inventions.

Diagrams, figures, tables and index supplement the text. All topics have been covered in a cogent and lucid style to help the reader grasp the information quickly and easily.

It may not be wrong to hold that the present reference textbook of *Genetics* is a complete treatise on this subject. It is essential reading for BTech (environmental biotechnology/microbiology/food microbiology/biomedical and biochemical engineering) and students pursuing BSc/MSc course in biotechnology and microbiology. Besides students, this book will prove useful to industrialists, consultants and researchers in the respective fields.

The reference textbook also caters to the requirement of the syllabus prescribed by various universities for undergraduate and postgraduate courses in the above subjects. It has been prepared with meticulous care, aiming at making the book error-free. Constructive suggestions are always welcome from users of this book.

MM Morris

Contents

Section III
REGULATION OF GENE EXPRESSION, TRANSCRIPTION ATTENUTION, RNA SPLICING AND RNA SILENCING

Section VI
GENOMICS, PROTEOMICS, GENOME ANNOTATION, BACTERIAL AND EUKARYOTIC GENOMES, COMPARATIVE AND MINIMAL GENOMICS AND GENOME MAPPING

Section IX
EVOLUTIONARY AND CONSERVATION GENETICS

Section X
ETHICAL ISSUES AND INTELLECTUAL PROPERTY RIGHTS OF GENETIC ENGINEERING

SECTION I

Translation, Neurospora, Haemoglobin and
Protein–Structure and Domains

Chapter 1

Translation, Neurospora and Haemoglobin

INTRODUCTION

Translation refers to the process of creating proteins from an mRNA template. The sequence of nucleotides on the RNA is translated into the amino acid sequence of proteins and this reaction is carried out by ribosomes. Ribosomes and tRNA dock on a mature mRNA transcript and recruit multiple enzymes in an energy intensive process that uses ATP as well as GTP. The control of the cell cycle and cell proliferation also involves regulation of protein synthesis, and malignant transformation of cells involves loss of certain translational regulatory controls. In fact, several translation initiation factors are over-expressed in certain cancers and play key roles in tumour development and progression. The process of protein synthesis and important examples of its regulation are now understood at the molecular level. We will discuss the mechanism and regulation of protein synthesis, elucidating this complex area of gene regulation with specific examples. Many viruses compete with their infected host cell and often dominate the protein synthetic machinery to maintain viral production and thwart innate (intracellular) anti-viral responses. For many viruses, the inhibition of host cell protein synthesis is an important component of their ability to propagate and destroy the infected cell. The infected cell, in turn, responds by enacting antiviral activities that include the production of potent biological molecules such as α-interferon that function, in part, to inhibit protein synthesis. Finally, a large proportion of antibiotics currently in use or under development inhibit protein synthesis in bacteria but not animal cells by exploiting differences in the structure of prokaryotic and eularyotic ribosomes.

PROTEIN BIOSYNTHESIS

Protein synthesis is the process whereby biological cells generate new proteins, it is balanced by the loss of cellular proteins via degradation or export. Translation, the assembly of amino acids by ribosomes, is an essential part of the biosynthetic pathway, along with generation of messenger RNA (mRNA), aminoacylation of transfer RNA (tRNA), co-translational transport, and post-translational modification. Protein biosynthesis is strictly regulated at multiple steps. They are principally during transcription (phenomena of RNA synthesis from DNA template) and translation (phenomena of amino acid assembly from RNA).

3

The cistron DNA is transcribed into the first of a series of RNA intermediates. The last version is used as a template in synthesis of a polypeptide chain. Protein will often be synthesised directly from genes by translating mRNA. However, when a protein must be available on short notice or in large quantities, a protein precursor is produced. A proprotein is an inactive protein containing one or more inhibitory peptides that can be activated when the inhibitory sequence is removed by proteolysis during posttranslational modification. A preprotein is a form that contains a signal sequence (an N-terminal signal peptide) that specifies its insertion into or through membranes, i.e. targets them for secretion. The signal peptide is cleaved off in the endoplasmic reticulum. Preproproteins have both sequences (inhibitory and signal) still present.

In protein synthesis, a succession of tRNA molecules charged with appropriate amino acids are brought together with an mRNA molecule and matched up by base-pairing through the anti-codons of the tRNA with successive codons of the mRNA. The amino acids are then linked together to extend the growing protein chain, and the tRNAs, no longer carrying amino acids, are released. This whole complex of processes is carried out by the ribosome, formed of two main chains of RNA, called ribosomal RNA (rRNA), and more than 50 different proteins. The ribosome latches onto the end of an mRNA molecule and moves along it, capturing loaded tRNA molecules and joining together their amino acids to form a new protein chain. Protein biosynthesis, although very similar, is different for prokaryotes and eukaryotes.

TRANSLATION

Translation, the second part of the central dogma of molecular biology, describes how the genetic code is used to make amino acid chains. This chapter, explore the mechanics involved in polypeptide synthesis and describes the three major steps of translation and tRNA, mRNA, and ribosomes.

Translation is the second step in the central dogma that describes how the genetic code is converted into amino acids. It is well known about how the mRNA codes are recognised by tRNA and how the amino acids are linked together by peptide bonds. A chain of amino acids is also called a polypeptide. Polypeptides are assembled inside the ribosomes, which are tiny organelles on the rough ER of a cell.

Now that we are learning more about the mechanics of translation, we are going to have to start putting the pieces together. We already understand the role of the ribosome and the amino acids in the process of translation, but how does polypeptide assembly actually occur? There are three important steps to the process of translation. There's a beginning step, called initiation, a middle step, called elongation, and a final step, called termination. These three words may sound familiar to you. The same terms are used in transcription to describe the steps involved in making the mRNA strand. But, here in translation, we are making a polypeptide strand. In either case, we are making a long molecule out of a chain of smaller subunits. So, whether we are referring to transcription or translation, the three terms accurately describe the mechanics of the process.

Initiation

We'll start with initiation. During initiation, the mRNA, the tRNA, and the first amino acid all come together within the ribosome. The mRNA strand remains continuous, but the true initiation point is the start codon, AUG. Remember that the start codon is the set of three nucleotides that begins the coded sequence of a gene. Remember also that the start codon specifies the amino acid methionine.

So, methionine is the name of the amino acid that is brought into the ribosome first. And how did methionine get itself to the ribosome? By attaching to the tRNA that contains the right anticodon. The anticodon for AUG is UAC. We know that because of the rules of complementary base pairing. The tRNA with the anticodon UAC will automatically match to the codon AUG, bringing the methionine along for the ride. So, there you have it-mRNA is attached to tRNA, and tRNA is attached to methionine. That's initiation.

Elongation

The next step makes up the bulk of translation. It's called elongation, and it's the addition of amino acids by the formation of peptide bonds. Elongation is just what it sounds like: a chain of amino acids grows longer and longer as more amino acids are added on. This will eventually create the polypeptide. Now that we've begun with the start codon, the mRNA shifts a little through the ribosome so that the next codon is up for grabs. Let's say the next codon is UAU. So, now we need a tRNA that has the matching anticodon, AUA. Oh, look! Here's a tRNA with the right anticodon, and it's brought along a tyrosine. Tyrosine is the amino acid that is specified by the codon UAU. The tRNA attaches to the mRNA in the ribosome and lines up tyrosine right next to the waiting methionine. A peptide bond forms between the two amino acids. Then the first tRNA leaves everyone else behind and floats off to find more work to do. Poor methionine! Now it's just drifting around like a lonely kite in the wind! That tRNA left methionine hanging by only one anchor: its peptide bond with tyrosine. The tyrosine is still attached to its own tRNA, which, in turn, is clinging to the mRNA inside the ribosome. Already we can see the beginnings of a polypeptide elongating outward.

Should we walk through that process one more time? Let's keep everything just as we have it here and move on to add our third amino acid. mRNA shifts over again, and now the third codon is ready for a match. What's that codon? CAC. Here comes a tRNA with the matching anticodon, GUG. It's also brought us a histidine, since CAC codes for histidine. The tRNA's anticodon matches up with the mRNA's codon, putting the histidine in perfect position for making a peptide bond with tyrosine.

So now we have methionine, tyrosine, and histidine all connected. We won't be needing tyrosine's tRNA anymore, so that tRNA detaches and floats away, just like the first one did in the beginning. Now we have an even longer kite, methionine and tyrosine are drifting around with only their peptide bonds to hold them down to the ribosome. But the histidine is still connected to its own tRNA, and it'll stay that way until it has the next amino acid to latch onto. You can see how this chain of amino acids would grow longer as each new codon is translated. The addition process and peptide bond formation continues over and over again until the chain is about one hundred amino acids long.

FROM GENES TO PROTEINS

Transcription and Translation

RNA plays a central role in the production of proteins according to the DNA's instructions. RNA transcribes the message from DNA and then the RNA message is translated into a protein. Just as with DNA synthesis the RNA strand is synthesised using DNA as a template. The RNA is then used to determine the linear sequence of amino acids in the protein.

DNA, RNA and Protein

RNA differs from DNA in two ways

The sugar in RNA is ribose not deoxyribose and RNA does not have thymine instead this pyrimidine is replaced by uracil. DNA and RNA are both nucleic acids and are each made up of four nucleotides that differ in their nitrogenous bases (A, (T or U) G, C). Each RNA or DNA molecule is hundreds of thousands of nucleotides long and each gene has a specific linear sequence of the four possible bases. Transcription–the synthesis of RNA using DNA as a template. A gene's unique nucleotide sequence is transcribed from DNA to a complementary nucleotide sequence in the messenger RNA (mRNA). mRNA carries the instructions to the protein assembly machinery the rough endoplasmic reticulum.

Translation–Synthesis of a polypeptide occurs under the direction of mRNA. During translation the linear sequence of bases in the mRNA is translated into the linear sequence of amino acids in a polypeptide. Translation occurs on ribosomes which are made up of ribosomal RNA (rRNA) and protein. Ribosomes facilitate the orderly linking of amino acids into polypeptide chains.

Triplet code

There are four bases and 20 amino acids to code for. Therefore you cannot use a 1 to 1 or even 2 to 1 mapping of bases to amino acids. Two base pair mapping could code for only 42, i.e. 16 different amino acids. Three base pair mapping could code for 43 different amino acids, i.e. 64 different ones. The smallest code that will do the job is a triplet code. The genetic code is based on triplets. The triplet 'words' are called codons.

Codon is a three base sequence in mRNA that specifies which amino acids will be added to a growing polypeptide chain or that signals termination. It is the basic unit of the gentic code. The mRNA is complementary to the template strand of DNA with U substituted for T. During translation the linear sequence of codons in the mRNA is translated into the linear sequence of amino acids in a polypeptide.

1960's how do we translate the genetic code? Marshall Nirenberg at NIH. He made poly U (by putting uracil in with the appropriate chemicals) and then put it into the protein making apparatus and got out a chain of phenylalanine. Therefore, UUU = phenylalanine. By the mid 1960's the code had been deciphered. 61 of 64 codons code for amino acids. Three are 'stop' codons (UAA, UAG, UGA) and AUG codes for both methionine and is the 'start' codon. The genetic code is redundant, but not ambiguous. Redundancy means more than one codon codes for a particular amino acid. For example, AGU and AGC both code for serine. No ambiguity means that no codon codes for more than one amino acid.

TRANSCRIPTION–PRODUCING AN RNA MESSAGE FROM DNA

Three stages binding and initiation, elongation, and termination takes place in the nucleus.

Binding and Initiation

Transcription begins when RNA polymerases bind to the DNA, separate it into two strands and add nucleotides to the 3' end of the growing RNA molecule. A specific initiation sequence identifies the location to begin transcription and a second sequence, the termination sequence terminates the copying. This 'transcription unit' is a single gene in eukaryotes (in prokaryotes it may be several functionally related proteins). It consists of the gene and the initiation and termination signals. Initiation and termination sequences are not the same as the start and stop codons.

RNA polymerases bind to regions of the DNA known as promoters. The Promoter consists of the initiation site where transcription begins and some dozens of nucleotides upstream from the Initiation site. Certain regions of the promoter must be present for the RNA polymerases to bind. For example, RNA polymerase II keys on a region called the TATA box. The RNA polymerase cannot bind to the DNA directly unless a transcription factor (a protein has bound to the region) first. The RNA polymerase aparently recognises the complex of the transcription factor and the initiation site together. Once RNA polymerase has bound to the initiation site elongation of the RNA strand can begin.

Elongation

RNA Polymerase II moves along the DNA and performs two main functions: (i) it untwists the DNA one turn about 10 bases at a time and (ii) adds nucleotides to the 3′ end of the growing RNA. As the RNA polymerase moves along the growing mRNA molecule trails along behind. Transcription goes about 60 nucleotides per second. More than one RNA polymerase can act on the same gene and as a result cells can make large amounts of mRNA (and proteins) very rapidly.

Termination

Transcription proceeds until the RNA polymerase reaches a termination site on the DNA (the most common stop sequence is AATAAA). At this point, no more RNA nucleotides are added and the mRNA is released. Post-transcriptional modification of RNA. In prokaryotes mRNA is complete and is not further modified after it is transcribed. Translation may begin even before the mRNA has been fully transcribed. In eukaryotes, however, some modifications to the mRNA occur.

First there are tail modifications a poly-AAA tail up to 200 bases long, that may be needed to get it out of the nucleus is attached at the 3′ end and a guanosine tri-phosphate cap is added to the 5′ end. The two ends may protect the molecule from degradation. In addition the 5′ cap and the first non-coding section of RNA the leader act as an 'attach here' sign for ribosomes. Messenger RNA moves out of the nucleus into the cytoplasm.

TRANSLATION-BUILDING A POLYPEPTIDE

Structure of Transfer RNA – tRNA

Like all RNA's, tRNA's are made in the nucleus and then travel to the cytoplasm where they function. A tRNA can be used repeatedly. tRNA's are odd t-shaped structures. tRNA's cannot bind to amino acids by themselves. An enzyme (Aminoacyl tRNA synthetase) is responsible and the reaction takes energy. Each tRNA molecule consists of an L-shaped stretch of RNA about 80 nucleotides long with at one end an attachment site for an amino acid and at the other end an anticodon binding site.

tRNA's shuttle amino acids for attachment on to growing polypeptides

Ribosomes are where polypeptide assembly takes place. There are two types free ribosomes and attached ribosomes. Free ribosomes are loose in the cytosol. Bound ribsomes are attached to the endoplasmic reticulum. Free ribosomes make proteins intended for use in the cytosol, bound ribosomes make proteins for inclusion in organelles such as lysosomes or for export from the cell. Ribosomes made up of two subunits a large and a small. They are made up of ribosomal RNA (rRNA) and protein. Constructed in the nucleoli and migrate from there through pores in the nuclear mebrane into the cytoplasm.

Ribosome has three binding sites. One to attach to mRNA and two sites for attaching tRNA's. The P-site holds the tRNA attached to the growing polypeptide chain and the other the A-site holds the tRNA attached to the next amino acid to be added to the chain. Translation takes place in the cytoplasm. During translation proteins are synthesised based on the message encoded in the mRNA. Three steps–initiation, elongation, termination.

Initiation

Without wading through the details, the small ribosomal subunit attaches to the mRNA at the initiation codon site and the first tRNA attaches. Then the big ribosomal subunit attaches with the tRNA in the P-site

Elongation

Transfer RNA (tRNA) translates the mRNA into the amino acid sequence. tRNA attaches by its anticodon to the codon of mRNA sitting in the A-site. The two amino acids are joined together. The first tRNA is detached, the ribosome moves and the tRNA moves into the P-site and the process is repeated. tRNA gathers amino acids from the cytoplasm and transfers them to the ribosome. One end of the tRNA attaches to a specific amino acid. The other end attaches to an mRNA codon by base pairing with its anticodon. Anticodon is a nucleotide triplet in tRNA that pairs with a complementary codon in the mRNA. tRNa's decde the message codon by codon and as the tRNS'a deposit the amino acids in the correct order, ribosomal enzymes link them into a chain.

Termination

Elongation continues until a stop codon is encountered. UAA, UAG, UGA. A protein called a release factor binds in the A-site to the termination codon and the ribosomes adds a water molecule to ttheend of the now complete polypeptide chain.

Post-translational modification of polypeptides

Once the new protein has been produced it may have to be further modified to be functional. A variety of things may happen.

Addition of molecules such as sugars, lipids or phosphate groups.

Some amino acids may be removed from the leading end.

A single chain may be cleaved into two pieces, e.g. Insulin converted from one chain to two to be active. Multiple polypeptides may be joined together to make a functional protein. For example haemoglobin made up of 4 polypeptide chains.

Information flows in only one direction

DNA leads to the production of proteins. Modifications to proteins or other bodily structures have no effect on the DNA.

Result of transcription and translation

DNA	RNA	Protein
DNA sequence	ATA -- CGC -- GTC -- GCC	
RNA sequence	UAU -- GCG --CAG – CGG	Transcription
Amino Acid Sequence	Tyrosine – Alanine -- Glycine -- Arginine	Translation

Mutations – mutations are changes in the genetic makeup of a cell. Point mutations are mutations that are chemical changes in one nucleotide in one gene. If a point mutation occurs in a gamete, it may be passed on the future generations.

Types of Point Mutations

Substitutions

A substitution occurs when a nucleotide and its partner from the complemntary strand are replaced by another base pair. Some are silent mutations because the new amino acid coded for is the same as the previous one. For example if CCG à CCA the RNA coded for would go from GGC à GGU but the amino acid coded for would still be Glycine.

Other Mutations

Missense mutations - a substitution leads to a different amino acid being inserted in the protein. For example sickle cell anemia.

PROKARYOTIC TRANSLATION

Prokaryotic translation is the process by which messenger RNA is translated into proteins in prokaryotes.

Initiation

Initiation of translation in prokaryotes involves the assembly of the components of the translation system, which are: the two ribosomal subunits (50S and 30S subunits), the mature mRNA to be translated, the tRNA charged with N-formylmethionine (the first amino acid in the nascent peptide), guanosine triphosphate (GTP) as a source of energy, the prokaryotic elongation factor EF-P and the three prokaryotic initiation factors IF1, IF2, and IF3, which help the assembly of the initiation complex. Variations in the mechanism can be anticipated.

The ribosome has three active sites: the A-site, the P-site, and the E-site. The A-site is the point of entry for the aminoacyl tRNA (except for the first aminoacyl tRNA, which enters at the P-site). The P-site is where the peptidyl tRNA is formed in the ribosome. And the E-site which is the exit site of the now uncharged tRNA after it gives its amino acid to the growing peptide chain.

The selection of an initiation site (usually an AUG codon) depends on the interaction between the 30S subunit and the mRNA template. The 30S subunit binds to the mRNA template at a purine-rich region (the Shine-Dalgarno sequence) upstream of the AUG initiation codon. The Shine-Dalgarno sequence is complementary to a pyrimidine rich region on the 16S rRNA component of the 30S subunit. During the formation of the initiation complex, these complementary nucleotide sequences pair to form a double stranded RNA structure that binds the mRNA to the ribosome in such a way that the initiation codon is placed at the P-site.

Elongation

Elongation of the polypeptide chain involves addition of amino acids to the carboxyl end of the growing chain. The growing protein exits the ribosome through the polypeptide exit tunnel in the large subunit.

Elongation starts when the fMet-tRNA enters the P-site, causing a conformational change which opens the A-site for the new aminoacyl-tRNA to bind. This binding is facilitated by elongation factor-Tu (EF-Tu), a small GTPase. For fast and accurate recognition of the appropriate tRNA, the ribosome utilises large conformational changes (conformational proofreading). Now the P-site contains the beginning of the peptide chain of the protein to be encoded and the A-site has the next amino acid to be added to the peptide chain. The growing polypeptide connected to the tRNA in the P-site is detached from the tRNA in the P-site and a peptide bond is formed between the last amino acids of the polypeptide and the amino acid still attached to the tRNA in the A-site. This process, known as peptide bond formation, is catalysed by a ribozyme (the 23S ribosomal RNA in the 50S ribosomal subunit). Now, the A-site has the newly formed peptide, while the P-site has an uncharged tRNA (tRNA with no amino acids). The newly formed peptide in the A-site tRNA is known as dipeptide and the whole assembly is called dipeptidyl-tRNA. The tRNA in the P-site minus the amino acid is known to be deacylated. In the final stage of elongation, called translocation, the deacylated tRNA (in the P-site) and the dipeptidyl-tRNA (in the A-site) along with its corresponding codons move to the E and P-sites, respectively, and a new codon moves into the A-site. This process is catalysed by elongation factor G (EF-G). The deacylated tRNA at the E-site is released from the ribosome during the next A-site occupation by an aminoacyl-tRNA again facilitated by EF-Tu. The ribosome continues to translate the remaining codons on the mRNA as more aminoacyl-tRNA bind to the A-site, until the ribosome reaches a stop codon on mRNA(UAA, UGA, or UAG).

The translation machinery works relatively slowly compared to the enzyme systems that catalyse DNA replication. Proteins in prokaryotes are synthesised at a rate of only 18 amino acid residues per second, whereas bacterial replisomes synthesise DNA at a rate of 1000 nucleotides per second. This difference in rate reflects, in part, the difference between polymerising four types of nucleotides to make nucleic acids and polymerising 20 types of amino acids to make proteins. Testing and rejecting incorrect aminoacyl-tRNA molecules takes time and slows protein synthesis. In bacteria, translation initiation occurs as soon as the 5′ end of an mRNA is synthesised, and translation and transcription are coupled. This is not possible in eukaryotes because transcription and translation are carried out in separate compartments of the cell (the nucleus and cytoplasm).

Termination

Termination occurs when one of the three termination codons moves into the A-site. These codons are not recognised by any tRNAs. Instead, they are recognised by proteins called release factors, namely RF1 (recognising the UAA and UAG stop codons) or RF2 (recognising the UAA and UGA stop codons). These factors trigger the hydrolysis of the ester bond in peptidyl-tRNA and the release of the newly synthesised protein from the ribosome. A third release factor RF-3 catalyses the release of RF-1 and RF-2 at the end of the termination process.

Recycling

The post-termination complex formed by the end of the termination step consists of mRNA with the termination codon at the A-site, an uncharged tRNA in the P-site, and the intact 70S ribosome. Ribosome recycling step is responsible for the disassembly of the post-termination ribosomal complex. Once the nascent protein is released in termination, Ribosome Recycling Factor and Elongation Factor G (EF-G) function to release mRNA and tRNAs from ribosomes and dissociate the 70S ribosome into the 30S and 50S subunits. IF3 then replaces the deacylated tRNA releasing the mRNA. All translational components are now free for additional rounds of translation.

Polysomes

Translation is carried out by more than one ribosome simultaneously. Because of the relatively large size of ribosomes, they can only attach to sites on mRNA 35 nucleotides apart. The complex of one mRNA and a number of ribosomes is called a polysome or polyribosome.

Regulation of Translation

When bacterial cells run out of nutrients, they enter stationary phase and downregulate protein synthesis. Several processes mediate this transition. For instance, in *E. coli*, 70S ribosomes form 90S dimers upon binding with a small 6.5 kDa protein, ribosome modulation factor RMF. These intermediate ribosome dimers can subsequently bind a hibernation promotion factor (the 10.8 kDa protein, HPF) molecule to form a mature 100S ribosomal particle, in which the dimerisation interface is made by the two 30S subunits of the two participating ribosomes. The ribosome dimers (Fig. 1.1) represent a hibernation state and are translationally inactive. A third protein that can bind to ribosomes when *E. coli* cells enter the stationary

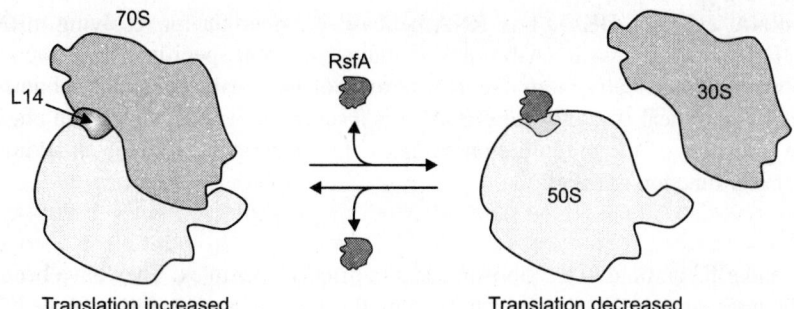

Fig. 1.1: Mechanism of ribosomal subunit dissociation by RsfS (= RsfA).

phase is YfiA (previously known as RaiA). HPF and YfiA are structurally similar, and both proteins can bind to the catalytic A- and P-sites of the ribosome. RMF blocks ribosome binding to mRNA by preventing interaction of the messenger with 16S rRNA. When bound to the ribosomes the C-terminal tail of *E. coli* YfiA interferes with the binding of RMF, thus preventing dimerisation and resulting in the formation of translationally inactive monomeric 70S ribosomes.

In addition to ribosome dimerisation, the joining of the two ribosomal subunits can be blocked by RsfS (formerly called RsfA or YbeB). RsfS binds to L14, a protein of the large ribosomal subunit, and thereby blocks joining of the small subunit to form a functional 70S ribosome, slowing down or blocking translation entirely. RsfS proteins are found in almost all eubacteria (but not archaea) and homologs are present in mitochondria and chloroplasts (where they are called C7orf30 and iojap, respectively). However, it is not known yet how the expression or activity of RsfS is regulated.

Effect of Antibiotics

Several antibiotics exert their action by targeting the translation process in bacteria. They exploit the differences between prokaryotic and eukaryotic translation mechanisms to selectively inhibit protein synthesis in bacteria without affecting the host.

EUKARYOTIC INITIATION FACTOR

Eukaryotic initiation factors (eIF) are proteins involved in the initiation phase of eukaryotic translation. They function in forming a complex with the 40S ribosomal subunit and Met-tRNAi called the 43S preinitation complex (PIC), recognising the 5′ cap structure of mRNA and recruiting the 43S PIC to mRNA, promoting ribosomal scanning of mRNA and regulating recognition of the AUG initiation codon, and joining of the 60S ribosomal subunit to create the 80S ribosome. There exist many more eukaryotic initiation factors than prokaryotic initiation factors due to greater biological complexity of eukaryotic cells. The protein RLI is known to have an essential, probably catalytic role in the formation of initiation complexes as well.

eIF4 (eIF4F)

The eIF4 initiation factors include eIF4A, eIF4B, eIF4E, and eIF4G. eIF4F is often used to refer to the complex of eIF4A, eIF4E, and eIF4G. eIF4G is a scaffolding protein that interacts with eIF3, as well as the other members of the eIF4F complex. eIF4E recognises and binds to the 5′ cap structure of mRNA, while eIF4G binds to Poly(A)-binding protein, which binds the poly(A) tail, circularising and activating the bound mRNA. eIF4A–a DEAD box RNA helicase–is important for resolving mRNA secondary structures. eIF4B contains two RNA-binding domains–one non-specifically interacts with mRNA, whereas the second specifically binds the 18S portion of the small ribosomal subunit. It acts as an anchor, as well as a critical co-factor for eIF4A. It is a substrate of S6K, and, when phosphorylated, it promotes the formation of the pre-initiation complex. In vertebrates, eIF4H is an additional initiation factor with similar function to eIF4B.

eIF1 & eIF3

eIF1, eIF1A, and eIF3 all bind to the ribosome subunit-mRNA complex. They have been implicated in preventing the large ribosomal subunit from binding the small subunit before it is ready to commence elongation. In mammals, eIF3 is the largest scaffolding initiation factor, made up of 13 subunits (a-m). It is roughly ~750 kDa and it controls the assembly of 40S ribosomal subunit on mRNA that have a 5' cap or an IRES (Internal Ribosomal Entry Site). eIF3 uses the eIF4F complex or IRES from viruses to position the mRNA strand near the exit site of the 40S ribosome subunit, thus promoting the assembly of the pre-initiation complex.

In many cancers, eIF3 is overexpressed. Under serum-deprived conditions (inactive state), eIF3 is bound to S6K1. On stimulation by either mitogens, growth factors, or drugs, mTOR/Raptor complex gets activated and, in turn, binds and phosphorylates S6K1 on T389 (linker region), causing a conformational change that causes the kinase S6K1 to dissociate from eIF3. The T389 phosphorylated S6k1 is then further phosphorylated by PDK1 on T229. This second phosphorylation fully activates the S6K1 kinase, which can then phosphorylate eIF4B, S6, and other protein targets.

Mammalian 17-kDa eukaryotic initiation factor, eIF1A (formerly designated eIF-4C), is essential for transfer of the initiator Met-tRNAf (as Met-tRNAf·eIF2·GTP ternary complex) to 40 S ribosomal subunits in the absence of mRNA to form the 40 S preinitiation complex (40 S·Met-tRNAf·eIF2·GTP). Furthermore, eIF1A acts catalytically in this reaction to mediate highly efficient transfer of the Met-tRNAf·eIF2·GTP ternary complex to 40 S ribosomal subunits.

The 40 S complex formed is free of eIF1A which indicates that its role in 40 S preinitiation complex formation is not to stabilise the binding of Met-tRNAf to 40 S ribosomes. Additionally, the eIF1A-mediated 40 S initiation complex formed in the presence of AUG codon efficiently joins 60 S ribosomal subunits in an eIF5-dependent reaction to form a functional 80 S initiation complex. Though found in some reports, eIF1A probably plays no role either in the subunit joining reaction or in the generation of ribosomal subunits from 80 S ribosomes. The major function of eIF1A is to mediate the transfer of Met-tRNAf to 40 S ribosomal subunits to form the 40 S preinitiation complex.

eIF2

eIF2 is a GTP-binding protein responsible for bringing the initiator tRNA to the P-site of the pre-initiation complex. It has specificity for the methionine-charged initiator tRNA, which is distinct from other methionine-charged tRNAs specific for elongation of the polypeptide chain. Once it has placed the initiator tRNA on the AUG start codon in the P-site, it hydrolyses GTP into GDP, and dissociates. This hydrolysis, also signals for the dissociation of eIF3, eIF1, and eIF1A, and allows the large subunit to bind. This signals the beginning of elongation.

eIF2 has three subunits, eIF2-α, β, and γ. The former is of particular importance for cells that may need to turn off protein synthesis globally. When phosphorylated, it sequesters eIF2B (not to be confused with beta), a GEF. Without this GEF, GDP cannot be exchanged for GTP, and translation is repressed.

eIF2a-induced translation repression occurs in reticulocytes when starved for iron. In addition, protein kinase R (PKR) phosphorylates eIF2a when dsRNA is detected in many multicellular organisms, leading to cell death.

eIF5 & eIF5B

eIF5A is a GTPase-activating protein, which helps the large ribosomal subunit associate with the small subunit. It is required for GTP-hydrolysis by eIF2 and contains the unusual amino acid hypusine.

eIF5B is a GTPase, and is involved in assembly of the full ribosome (which requires GTP hydrolysis).

eIF6: eIF6 performs the same inhibition of ribosome assembly as eIF3, but binds with the large subunit.

EF-Tu

EF-Tu (elongation factor thermo unstable) is one of the prokaryotic elongation (Fig. 1.2) factors. Elongation factors are part of the mechanism that synthesises new proteins by translation at the ribosome. Individual amino acid links are added to the protein chain by transfer RNA (tRNA). Messenger RNA (mRNA) carries a codon that codes for each amino acid. tRNA carries the amino acid and an anticodon for that amino acid. The ribosome creates a protein chain by following the mRNA code and selecting the next tRNA and its amino acid.

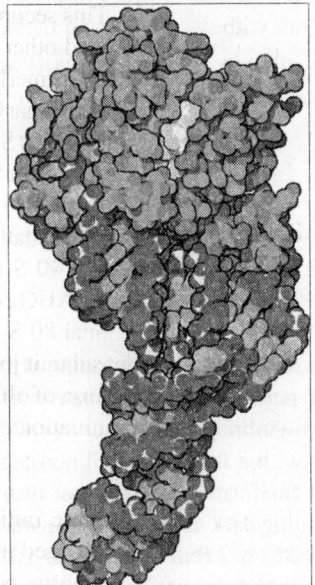

Fig. 1.2: EF-Tu (elongation factor thermo unstable) prokaryotic elongation.

The prokaryotic factor EF-Tu helps the aminoacyl-tRNA move onto a free site on the ribosome. In the cytoplasm, EF-Tu binds an aminoacylated, or charged, tRNA molecule. This complex enters the ribosome. There are 3 tRNA attachment sites on the ribosome: aminoacyl (A), peptidyl (P) and exit (E). The tRNA complex first binds to the A-site, then moves to the P-site, and is released at the E-site.

The tRNA anticodon domain associates with the mRNA codon domain in the ribosomal A-site. If the codon-anticodon pairing is correct, EF-Tu hydrolyses guanosine triphosphate (GTP) into guanosine diphosphate (GDP) and inorganic phosphate. This creates a conformational change in EF-Tu that causes EF-Tu to dissociate from the tRNA of the ternary complex (and therefore leave the ribosome). The aminoacyl-tRNA then fully enters the A-site, where its amino acid is brought near the P-site's polypeptide and the ribosome catalyses the covalent transfer of the polypeptide onto the amino acid. The tRNA on the P-site (without peptide) moves to the E-site and is then released.

EF-Tu contributes to translational accuracy in three ways. It delays GTP hydrolysis if the tRNA in the ribosome's A-site does not match the mRNA codon, thus preferentially increasing the likelihood for the incorrect tRNA to leave the ribosome. It also adds a second delay (regardless of tRNA matching) after freeing itself from tRNA, before the aminoacyl-tRNA fully enters the A-site. This delay period is a second opportunity for incorrectly paired tRNA (and their bound amino acids) to move out of the A-site before the incorrect amino acid is irreversibly added to the polypeptidic chain. A third mechanism is the less well understood function of EF-Tu to crudely check aminoacyl-tRNA associations and reject complexes where the amino acid is not bound to the correct tRNA coding for it.

Eukaryotic Elongation Factors

'EF2' redirects here. For the tornado intensity rating, see Enhanced Fujita Scale.

Eukaryotic elongation factors are very similar to those in prokaryotes.

Elongation in eukaryotes is carried out with two elongation factors: eEF-1 and eEF-2.

- The first is eEF-1, and has two subunits, α and $\beta\gamma$. α acts as counterpart to prokaryotic EF-Tu, mediating the entry of the aminoacyl tRNA into a free site of the ribosome. $\beta\gamma$ acts as counterpart to prokaryotic EF-Ts, serving as the guanine nucleotide exchange factor for a, catalysing the release of GDP from α.

- The second elongation factor is eEF-2, the counterpart to prokaryotic EF-G, catalysing the translocation of the tRNA and mRNA down the ribosome at the end of each round of polypeptide elongation.

NEUROSPORA

Neurospora species are molds with broadly spreading colonies, with abundant production of ascomata. Ascomata are superficial or immersed, perithecial and ostiolate or cleistothecial and non-ostiolate, hairy or glabrous, dark coloured. Peridium membranaceous, asci cylindrical, clavate or subspherical, with a persistent or evanescent wall, usually with a thickened and non-amyloid annular structure at the apex, usually 8-spored. Ascospores broadly fusiform, ellipsoidal, or nearly spherical, unicellular, hyaline to yellowish brown or olive-brown, becoming dark and opaque at maturity, ascospore wall with longitudinal ribs or pitted, occasionally nearly smooth, 1–2 (but rarely up to 12) germ pores disposed at the ends of the ascospores, gelatinous sheaths or appendages are absent. Anamorphs are known in only a relatively small number of species, which belong to the fungi imperfecti genus Chrysonilia. The type species of the genus is *Neurospora sitophila* Shear.

Systematics

The former genera Gelasinospora and Neurospora are closely related and not resolved as monophyletic groups, thus the former genus is nowadays included in Neurospora.

As model organisms

Neurospora is widely used in genetics as a model organism (especially *N. crassa*) because it is quickly reproducing, is easy to culture, and can survive on minimal media (inorganic salts, glucose, water and biotin in agar).

The first studies of sexual reproduction in Neurospora were made by BO Dodge. Neurospora was later used by George Wells Beadle and Edward Lawrie Tatum in X-ray mutation experiments in order to discover mutants that would differ in nutritional requirements. The results of their experiments led them to the one gene-one enzyme hypothesis, in which they postulated that every enzyme was encoded with its own gene.

Research with Neurospora is reported semi-annually at the Neurospora Meeting at Asilomar, California, coordinated by the Fungal Genetics Stock Center. Mutant and wild-type strains of Neurospora are available from the FGSC. The FGSC also publishes the Fungal Genetics Reports.

Important people in Neurospora research:

- Bernard Ogilvie Dodge (1872–1960)
- George Beadle (Nobel Prize in Physiology or Medicine, 1958)
- Edward Tatum (Nobel Prize in Physiology or Medicine, 1958)
- Esther Lederberg
- Norman Giles
- David Perkins
- Robert Metzenberg
- Norman Horowitz
- Herschel Mitchell
- Mary B. Mitchell
- Martha Merrow

Sexual Reproduction

In the heterothallic species Neurospora crassa, interaction of haploid strains of opposite mating type is necessary for the occurrence of sexual reproduction and the production of ascospores by meiosis. Ascospores then restore haploid individuals of either mating type. The life cycle phase is thus predominantly haploid, however, upon mating, the nuclei do not immediately fuse: karyogamy is delayed until the very onset of meiosis. The resulting mycelium is called a heterokaryon, and is neither diploid, nor haploid. The genus Neurospora also includes homothallic species in which a single haploid individual carries both mating type loci and can undergo self-fertilisation leading to meiosis and sexual reproduction. Neurospora africana is an example of such a species. Additionally, some 'Neurospora' species are said pseudohomothallic. They carry both mating types, but in separate nuclei in the same individual. Two haploid nuclei originating from the same meiosis are packaged into one ascospore. The individual is thus permanently heterokaryotic. Examples of this mating system include 'Neurospora tetrasperma' and 'Neurospora tetraspora'. Because heterothallic species necessarily undergo some degree of out-crossing they may benefit from a higher efficiency of selection because of higher effective recombination rates. In contrast, pseudohomothallic and homothallic species do not outcross (or rarely) and do not experience these benefits: in homothallics a reduced efficiency of negative selection has been shown. However, both hetero- and pseudohomothallic species benefit from the masking of deleterious recessive alleles in the heterokaryotic phase. In addition, all species derive the benefits of meiosis that include the removal of stress-induced DNA damages by homologous recombinational repair, and the formation of stress-resistant ascospores.

HAEMOGLOBIN

We've all experienced the sensation of having to stop to catch our breath until our lungs can absorb enough oxygen to transport through the bloodstream to our waiting muscles. Imagine what life would be like if we had to rely only on our lungs and the water in our blood to transport oxygen through our bodies. Various haemolgoin levels are shown in Fig. 1.3. O_2 is a nonpolar molecule, and therefore does not dissolve well in the aqueous environment of the blood. The evolution of large, multicellular animals depended on a mechanism that could enhance oxygen delivery to the tissues. Haemoglobin increases O_2 solubility in blood by about a hundredfold. This means that without haemoglobin, in order to provide sufficient oxygen to the tissues, blood would have to make a complete circuit through the body in less than a second, instead of the minute that it actually takes. That would take a mighty powerful heart! In this chapter, we will take a detailed look at haemoglobin and its chemical cousin, myoglobin, to see how they work together to deliver O_2 to our waiting muscles.

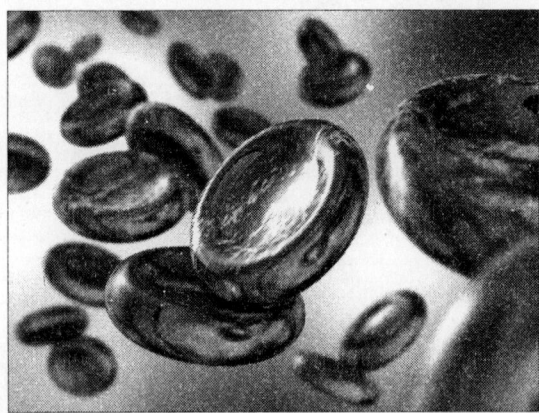

Fig. 1.3: Haemolgoin levels.

Structures and Functions of Haemoglobin vs Myoglobin

Whereas haemoglobin is the oxygen-carrying protein of blood, myoglobin is the oxygen-carrying protein of the muscle. Myoglobin is particularly abundant in the muscles of diving mammals, like seals and whales, allowing them to continue to use oxygen even when they are underwater for extended periods of time. The structures of haemoglobin and myoglobin have some notable similarities, which are related to their oxygen-binding functions. None of the amino acids are well suited to bind oxygen, so both of these proteins have an additional iron-containing group (heme) as part of their structure. Fe^{2+} is commonly used in biological systems to reversibly bind O_2. A notable difference between the two proteins, which relates to their specific roles in the body, is that haemoglobin contains four polypeptide chains but myoglobin has only one. Each chain with its attached heme group is called a 'subunit.' Myoglobin with polypeptide chain is shown in Fig. 1.4.

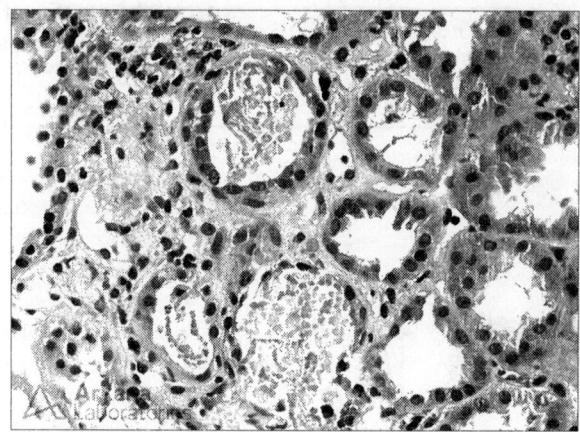

Fig. 1.4: Myoglobin with polypeptide chain.

O$_2$ Binding of Haemoglobin vs Myoglobin

Let's follow the path of oxygen from the lungs to the peripheral tissues. Oxygen diffuses from the alveoli of the lungs- little sacs at the end of the finely divided air passageways in the lung- into the capillaries of the bloodstream and then into the red blood cells, where it binds to haemoglobin. The concentration of oxygen is relatively high in the alveoli, about 100 mm Hg1.

Taking a look at Fig. 1.5, we see that haemoglobin is virtually 100% saturated in the lungs, meaning that essentially all four heme groups have an O$_2$ molecule bound to them. As haemoglobin circulates in the bloodstream to the working muscles, the pressure of oxygen decreases to about 25 mm Hg. At these lower levels of oxygen, haemoglobin is only about 50% saturated. Where did this oxygen go? It was released into the muscles, where myoglobin is found. Returning to Fig. 1.5, we can see that at 25 mm Hg, myoglobin is almost fully saturated, meaning that it will bind the oxygen released by the haemoglobin. The amount of oxygen in the mitochondria, where fuels are burned to release energy, is even lower (1 or 2 mm Hg), allowing myoglobin to release most of its oxygen where it is most needed in the cell. Thus, haemoglobin picks up oxygen in the lungs, circulates through the bloodstream to the muscles (and other tissues), and drops off oxygen there. Myoglobin picks up the oxygen and delivers it to the mitochondria, where it is used to oxidise fuel molecules.

The shape of hemoglobins oxygen binding curve is sigmoidal ('S'-shaped), with the steep part of the curve occurring at about the oxygen pressure found within the tissues, allowing haemoglobin to deliver a significant amount of oxygen over a fairly narrow range of pressures. That is, it binds oxygen at the relatively high partial pressures in the lungs and releases oxygen at the lower partial pressures in the peripheral tissues.

On the other hand, the shape of myoglobins oxygen binding curve is hyperbolic, meaning that it holds onto oxygen much tighter. Only when the amount of oxygen is extremely low, as in the mitochondria of working muscle, does myoglobin release its oxygen. Therefore, the distinct binding curves of these two proteins reflect their functions: haemoglobin, which is well suited for oxygen binding in the lungs, transport in the bloodstream, and delivery to the tissues, and myoglobin, which is well suited for oxygen storage in the muscles and delivery to mitochondria when needed.

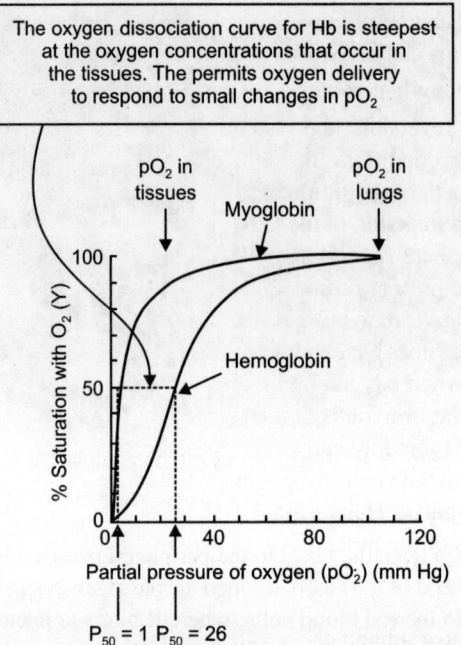

The oxygen dissociation curve for Hb is steepest at the oxygen concentrations that occur in the tissues. The permits oxygen delivery to respond to small changes in pO_2

Fig. 1.5: At higher concentrations of O_2, both haemoglobin and myoglobin have more oxygen bound.

Haemoglobin Structure Influences O_2 Delivery

The secret to hemoglobins success as an oxygen delivery molecule is the fact that it has four subunits that 'talk' to each other. Evidence for this is provided by hemoglobins 'cooperativity' in oxygen binding. In other words, the binding of one O_2 molecule affects the binding of others, as we can see by the following:

- In order to achieve 25% saturation (an average of 1 O_2 molecule per haemoglobin), the amount of O_2 needs to be about 18 mm Hg.
- In order to achieve 50% saturation (an average of 2 O_2 molecules per haemoglobin), the amount of O_2 needs to be about 26 mm Hg.

Therefore, it is easier to bind the second molecule of O_2 than the first. (Otherwise, it would require 2×18 mm Hg, or 36 mm Hg, to bind the second.) In order to understand how this is possible, we need to take a detailed look at the structure of haemoglobin.

Max Perutz, the scientist who originally determined the structure of the haemoglobin molecule, using a technique called X-ray diffraction, noted during his experiments that haemoglobin can be found in two different forms, or shapes. These different shapes depended on whether oxygen was present or absent, so he called the forms oxyhaemoglobin and deoxy-haemoglobin, respectively. Further experiments revealed that deoxy-haemoglobin has a relatively low attraction for oxygen, but when one molecule of oxygen binds to a heme group, the structure changes to the oxygenated form, which has a greater attraction for oxygen. Therefore, the second molecule of O_2 binds more easily, and the third and fourth even more easily.

The oxygen affinity of oxyhaemoglobin is many times greater than that of deoxy-haemoglobin. The relationship between these forms can be written as follows:

$$\text{Deoxy-haemoglobin} + O_2 \leftrightarrow \text{Oxyhaemoglobin}$$

Because oxygen binding is reversible, the two forms of haemoglobin are said to be in equilibrium with one another. Under certain conditions, the deoxy form is favoured, and under other conditions the oxy form is favoured. Changing the conditions can shift the equilibrium in either direction. For example, adding more O_2 would shift the reaction to the right, producing more oxyhaemoglobin.

In contrast to haemoglobin, there is only one form of myoglobin. That is, the structure of myoglobin is the same whether oxygen is present or not. The origin of the two different forms of haemoglobin, which account for its cooperative oxygen binding, is the fact that haemoglobin has four subunits. Myoglobin, with its single chain, does not exhibit cooperative oxygen binding. Lets look at what happens to the haemoglobin molecule when oxygen binds.

In the deoxygenated state, the iron ion is domed out of the heme plane because of its attraction to a histidine side chain (His F8). O_2 binding causes the iron ion to move such that it becomes planar with the rest of the heme group, which then pulls the histidine with it, causing a relatively large-scale structural change in the protein. His F8 is part of Helix F, which is attached to the rest of the haemoglobin molecule, and when it moves, other parts of the protein also move with it. The result is a switch to the oxy form, with its enhanced ability to bind oxygen. Binding of subsequent molecules of O_2 to the other subunits is therefore easier.

In summary, when O_2 binds to a subunit of deoxyhemoglobin, it causes subtle changes in the structure of the protein, altering the way that the four subunits fit together. This in turn affects the structure of each subunit, making it easier for a subsequent molecule of oxygen to bind to the next subunit. Thus, with the binding of the first oxygen molecule to one subunit, the remaining subunits become more receptive to oxygen.

Factors that Effects Hemoglobins Equilibrium

Other substances can also alter the binding of oxygen to haemoglobin. (In general, such molecules are called 'allosteric effectors' in biochemistry.) Hydrogen ions (protons), CO_2, and the molecule 2,3-bis-phosphoglycerate (BPG) all promote the release of oxygen by shifting the equilibrium towards the deoxygenated form of haemoglobin. Since these effectors bind to distinct sites, their effects are cumulative. All these molecules play a key role in metabolism of the exercising athlete.

Bohr Effect

Hydrogen ions (such as produced by lactic acid) and CO_2 are found in high concentrations around actively metabolising tissues. In the capillaries, binding of these allosteric effectors prompts the release of oxygen from haemoglobin, which can then be taken up by the high affinity myoglobin in the tissues and delivered to the mitochondria. The specific reaction of hydrogen ions and carbon dioxide with haemoglobin causing the release of O_2 is called the Bohr effect.

The reactions of the Bohr effect are reversible. When deoxygenated haemoglobin returns to the lungs, the concentrations of H^+ and CO_2 are low. This causes these compounds to be released from haemoglobin. The carbon dioxide is expelled out of the body through expired air. Therefore, haemoglobin not only carries oxygen to the cells, but it also carries waste products from the cells to the lungs for elimination from the body.

BPG and Altitude Adjustment

In addition to hydrogen ions and carbon dioxide, a key allosteric effector of haemoglobin is BPG, a small molecule made in red blood cells. BPG affects oxygen-binding affinity by binding in a small central cavity of deoxygenated haemoglobin. This shifts the equilibrium towards deoxy-hemoglobin, promoting oxygen release to actively respiring tissues. At high altitude, when oxygen in the atmosphere is scarce because the air is 'thinner,' production of BPG is greatly increased, helping haemoglobin to release more of its bound oxygen. It takes about 24 hr for BPG levels to rise, and over longer periods of time, the levels continue to increase as part of the acclimation effect. BPG production is one reason that athletes train at high altitudes to increase their aerobic capacity. Interestingly, BPG does not bind to fetal haemoglobin. This results in tighter binding of oxygen relative to maternal haemoglobin, giving the developing fetus better access to oxygen from the mother's bloodstream.

Summary of Allosteric Effectors

In summary, several molecules influence oxygen binding to haemoglobin, binding to the deoxy form and therefore shifting the equilibrium to the left, promoting oxygen release to the tissues when needed:

$$\text{Deoxyy Hb-(BPG)-(CO}_2\text{)-H}^+ + O_2 \leftrightarrow \text{oxy Hb} + CO_2 + \text{BPG} + H^+$$

Adapting to Altitude

High altitude environments pose a number of unique physiological challenges to animal life. In addition to the characteristically cold temperatures, high altitude environments also have lower partial pressures of oxygen (relative to low altitude environments at similar latitudes). Since there is less oxygen in each breath, there is an accompanying reduction in the O_2 saturation of arterial blood. In order to compensate, physiological adjustments are required to ensure an adequate supply of O_2 to the cells of aerobically metabolising tissues. Although the genetic basis of low oxygen (hypoxia) tolerance has yet to be fully elucidated in any species, evidence from a number of animals suggests that modifications of haemoglobin function often plays a key role in adaptation to high-altitude hypoxia.

One strategy for adapting hypoxic conditions is through altered O_2 affinity of haemoglobin. In several high-altitude species, various haemoglobin mutations result in increased O_2 affinity by stabilisation of the oxy haemoglobin form.

For example, the bar-headed goose (*Anser indicus*) spends its breeding season on high alpine lakes on the Tibetan Plateau but winters in wetland habitats in India. This requires an annual round-trip migratory flight over the crest of the Himalaya Mountains at altitudes of nearly 10000 meters. The bar-headed goose is well suited for this lifestyle because of its hemoglobins exceptionally high O_2 affinity relative to most other birds. A few key differences in the amino acid sequence of haemoglobin account for the increased oxygen binding of the bar-headed goose.

Adaptation to hypoxic conditions has also allowed many population groups, from Andeans to Tibetans, to thrive at high altitude. When people from lower elevations move above about 4000 meters, where oxygen levels are about 40% lower than at sea level, they typically tire easily, develop headaches, produce babies with lower birth weights, and have a higher infant mortality rate. Tibetans have none of these problems, despite relatively low oxygen saturation in their blood and haemoglobin levels. In order to gain insight into such physiological adaptations, scientists recently completed a genetic comparison of Tibetans and Han Chinese (lowland relatives of the Tibetans). Their findings revealed that Tibetans split off from the Han less than 3000 years ago and since then have rapidly evolved a unique ability to thrive at high altitudes and low oxygen levels. One mutation in particular spread from fewer than 10% of the Han Chinese to nearly 90% of all Tibetans. This mutation is near a gene called EPAS1, a socalled 'super athlete gene' identified several years ago and named because some variants of the gene are associated with improved athletic performance. This gene codes for a protein involved in regulating haemoglobin in the blood as a response to oxygen levels. Individuals with two copies of the mutation function well in high altitude despite a relatively low haemoglobin concentration in their blood. The mutation seems to provide an inborn mechanism for dealing with the low oxygen levels.

Anemia

Some individuals have inadequate levels of haemoglobin, a condition known as anemia. Anemia can occur when the body is unable to produce enough red blood cells, destroys too many red blood cells, or experiences significant blood loss. The most common cause of anemia is iron deficiency due to insufficient dietary intake or absorption to meet the body's needs.

Anemia is especially common in athletes for several reasons. First, hard training stimulates an increase in haemoglobin and red blood cell production, increasing the demand for iron, particularly in endurance athletes training at high intensity. Second, 'footstrike' damage to red blood cells in the feet from running on hard surfaces, especially with poor quality shoes, contributes to iron loss. Finally, iron is lost in sweat. The term 'sports anemia' is commonly used to describe iron depletion and consequent reductions in haemoglobin to anemic levels in athletes who dramatically increase their training intensity.

Avoidance of red meat can also contribute to anemia. The iron in animal products is largely in the form of heme, which is better absorbed than the iron found in plant products. However, there are lots of non-meat sources of iron, including legumes (like beans), soyabean products (like tofu), dark green leafy vegetables (like spinach), and dried fruits (like raisins). Iron absorption can be enhanced by eating foods rich in vitamin C (like orange juice) with the iron-containing food. On the other hand, iron absorption can be inhibited by tannic acid found in tea and coffee and phosphoric acid found in soda.

Blood loss also contributes to anemia. For example, a significant amount of iron can be lost in feces. This problem is particularly severe for runners, with up to 85% of runners testing positive for blood in their stools following a strenuous run. Blood loss because of menstruation increases the risk of anemia in women. This problem is exacerbated by the fact that women tend to eat less than men on average. In fact, 75% of women aged 18 to 44 do not eat enough iron-rich foods.

When haemoglobin levels are low, the tissues and organs do not receive enough oxygen. Symptoms of irondeficiency anemia include muscle burning from increased lactic acid production, shortness of breath during exercise, nausea, frequent illness and a pale, washed-out appearance. Anemia also causes fatigue, weakness, and an inability to concentrate, making it difficult to exercise or even perform day-to-day activities, so remember to eat your spinach!

GENETICS OF HAEMOGLOBIN

Haemoglobin consists of protein subunits (the 'globin' molecules), and these proteins, in turn, are folded chains of a large number of different amino acids called polypeptides. The amino acid sequence of any polypeptide created by a cell is in turn determined by the stretches of DNA called genes. In all proteins, it is the amino acid sequence that determines the protein's chemical properties and function.

There is more than one haemoglobin gene: in humans, haemoglobin A (the main form of haemoglobin present) is coded for by the genes, HBA1, HBA2, and HBB. The amino acid sequences of the globin proteins in hemoglobins usually differ between species. These differences grow with evolutionary distance between species. For example, the most common haemoglobin sequences in humans and chimpanzees are nearly identical, differing by only one amino acid in both the alpha and the beta globin protein chains. These differences grow larger between less closely related species.

Even within a species, different variants of haemoglobin always exist, although one sequence is usually a 'most common' one in each species. Mutations in the genes for the haemoglobin protein in a species result in haemoglobin variants. Many of these mutant forms of haemoglobin cause no disease. Some of these mutant forms of haemoglobin, however, cause a group of hereditary diseases termed the hemoglobinopathies. The best known hemoglobinopathy is sickle-cell disease, which was the first human disease whose mechanism was understood at the molecular level. A (mostly) separate set of diseases called thalassemias involves underproduction of normal and sometimes abnormal hemoglobins, through problems and mutations in globin gene regulation. All these diseases produce anemia.

Protein alignment of human haemoglobin proteins, alpha, beta, and delta subunits respectively. The alignments were created using Uniprot's alignment tool available online.

Variations in haemoglobin amino acid sequences, as with other proteins, may be adaptive. For example, haemoglobin has been found to adapt in different ways to high altitudes. Organisms living at high elevations experience lower partial pressures of oxygen compared to those at sea level. This presents a challenge to the organisms that inhabit such environments because haemoglobin, which normally binds oxygen at high partial pressures of oxygen, must be able to bind oxygen when it is present at a lower pressure. Different organisms have adapted to such a challenge. For example, recent studies have suggested genetic variants in deer mice that help explain how deer mice that live in the mountains are able to survive in the thin air that accompanies high altitudes.

A researcher from the University of Nebraska-Lincoln found mutations in four different genes that can account for differences between deer mice that live in lowland prairies versus the mountains. After examining wild mice captured from both highlands and lowlands, it was found that: the genes of the two breeds are 'virtually identical—except for those that govern the oxygen-carrying capacity of their haemoglobin'. 'The genetic difference enables highland mice to make more efficient use of their oxygen', since less is available at higher altitudes, such as those in the mountains.

Mammoth haemoglobin featured mutations that allowed for oxygen delivery at lower temperatures, thus enabling mammoths to migrate to higher latitudes during the Pleistocene. This was also found in hummingbirds that inhabit the Andes. Hummingbirds already expend a lot of energy and thus have high oxygen demands and yet Andean hummingbirds have been found to thrive in high altitudes. Non-synonymous mutations in the hemoglobin gene of multiple species living at high elevations (*Oreotrochilus*, *A. castelnaudii*, *C. violifer*, *P. gigas*, and *A. viridicuada*) have caused the protein to have less of an affinity for inositol hexaphosphate (IHP), a molecule found in birds that has a similar role as 2,3-BPG in humans, this results in the ability to bind oxygen in lower partial pressures.

Birds unique circulatory lungs also promote efficient use of oxygen at low partial pressures of O_2. These two adaptations reinforce each other and account for birds remarkable high-altitude performance.

Hemoglobin adaptation extends to humans, as well. Studies have found that a small number of native Tibetan women have a genotype which codes for hemoglobin to be more highly saturated with oxygen. Natural selection seems to be the main force working on this gene because the mortality rate of offspring is significantly lower for women with higher hemoglobin-oxygen affinity when compared to the mortality rate of offspring from women with low hemoglobin-oxygen affinity. While the exact genotype and mechanism by which this occurs is not yet clear, selection is acting on these women's ability to bind oxygen in low partial pressures, which overall allows them to better sustain crucial metabolic processes.

Synthesis

Hemoglobin (Hb) is synthesised in a complex series of steps. The heme part is synthesised in a series of steps in the mitochondria and the cytosol of immature red blood cells, while the globin protein parts are synthesised by ribosomes in the cytosol. Production of Hb continues in the cell throughout its early development from the proerythroblast to the reticulocyte in the bone marrow. At this point, the nucleus is lost in mammalian red blood cells, but not in birds and many other species. Even after the loss of the nucleus in mammals, residual ribosomal RNA allows further synthesis of Hb until the reticulocyte loses its RNA soon after entering the vasculature (this hemoglobin-synthetic RNA in fact gives the reticulocyte its reticulated appearance and name).

POST-TRANSLATIONAL MODIFICATION

Post-translational modification (PTM) refers to the covalent and generally enzymatic modification of proteins following protein biosynthesis. Proteins are synthesised by ribosomes translating mRNA into polypeptide chains, which may then undergo PTM to form the mature protein product. PTMs are important components in cell signalling, as for example when prohormones are converted to hormones.

Post-translational modifications can occur on the amino acid side chains or at the protein's C- or N- termini. They can extend the chemical repertoire of the 20 standard amino acids by modifying an existing functional group or introducing a new one such as phosphate. Phosphorylation is a very common mechanism for regulating the activity of enzymes and is the most common post-translational modification. Many eukaryotic proteins also have carbohydrate molecules attached to them in a process called glycosylation, which can promote protein folding and improve stability as well as serving regulatory functions. Attachment of lipid molecules, known as lipidation, often targets a protein or part of a protein attached to the cell membrane.

Other forms of post-translational modification consist of cleaving peptide bonds, as in processing a propeptide to a mature form or removing the initiator methionine residue. The formation of disulphide bonds from cysteine residues may also be referred to as a post-translational modification. For instance, the peptide hormone insulin is cut twice after disulphide bonds are formed, and a propeptide is removed from the middle of the chain, the resulting protein consists of two polypeptide chains connected by disulphide bonds.

Some types of post-translational modification are consequences of oxidative stress. Carbonylation is one example that targets the modified protein for degradation and can result in the formation of protein aggregates. Specific amino acid modifications can be used as biomarkers indicating oxidative damage.

Sites that often undergo post-translational modification are those that have a functional group that can serve as a nucleophile in the reaction: the hydroxyl groups of serine, threonine, and tyrosine, the amine forms of lysine, arginine, and histidine, the thiolate anion of cysteine, the carboxylates of aspartate and glutamate, and the N- and C-termini.

In addition, although the amide of asparagine is a weak nucleophile, it can serve as an attachment point for glycans. Rarer modifications can occur at oxidised methionines and at some methylenes in side chains.

Post-translational modification of proteins can be experimentally detected by a variety of techniques, including mass spectrometry, Eastern blotting, and Western blotting. Additional methods are provided in the external links sections.

PTMs Involving Addition of Functional Groups

Addition by an enzyme in vivo

Hydrophobic groups for membrane localisation:
* Myristoylation (a type of acylation), attachment of myristate, a C14 saturated acid.
* Palmitoylation (a type of acylation), attachment of palmitate, a C16 saturated acid.
* Isoprenylation or prenylation, the addition of an isoprenoid group (e.g. farnesol and geranylgeraniol)
  o Farnesylation
  o Geranilgeranilatyon
* Glipyatyon, glycosylphosphatidylinositol (GPI) anchor formation via an amide bond to C-terminal tail.

Cofactors for enhanced enzymatic activity:
* Lipoylation (a type of acylation), attachment of a lipoate (C8) functional group.
* Flavin moiety (FMN or FAD) may be covalently attached.
* Heme C attachment via thioether bonds with cysteines.
* hosphopantetheinylation, the addition of a 4'-phosphopantetheinyl moiety from coenzyme A, as in fatty acid, polyketide, non-ribosomal peptide and leucine biosynthesis.
* Retinylidene Schiff base formation.

Modifications of translation factors:
* Diphthamide formation (on a histidine found in eEF2).
* Ethanolamine phosphoglycerol attachment (on glutamate found in eEF1a).
* Hypusine formation (on conserved lysine of eIF5A (eukaryotic) and aIF5A (archaeal).
* Beta-Lysine addition on a conserved lysine of the elongation factor P (EFP) in most bacteria. EFP is an homolog to eIF5A (eukaryotic) and aIF5A (archaeal).

Smaller chemical groups

* Acylation, e.g. O-acylation (esters), N-acylation (amides), S-acylation (thioesters).
  o Acetylation, the addition of an acetyl group, either at the N-terminus of the protein or at lysine residues. See also histone acetylation. The reverse is called deacetylation.
  o Formylation
* Alkylation, the addition of an alkyl group, e.g. methyl, ethyl.
  o Methylation the addition of a methyl group, usually at lysine or arginine residues. The reverse is called demethylation.
* Amidation at C-terminus. Formed by oxidative dissociation of a C-terminal Gly residue.
* Amide bond formation.
  o Amino acid addition:
    Arginylation, a tRNA-mediation addition.
    Polyglutamylation, covalent linkage of glutamic acid residues to the N-terminus of tubulin and some other proteins.

Polyglycylation, covalent linkage of one to more than 40 glycine residues to the tubulin C-terminal tail.

- Butyrylation
- Gamma-carboxylation dependent on Vitamin K.
- Glycosylation, the addition of a glycosyl group to either arginine, asparagine, cysteine, hydroxylysine, serine, threonine, tyrosine, or tryptophan resulting in a glycoprotein. Distinct from glycation, which is regarded as a nonenzymatic attachment of sugars.
  - o Polysialylation, addition of polysialic acid, PSA, to NCAM.
- Malonylation
- Hydroxylation: Addition of an oxygen atom to the side-chain of a Pro or Lys residue.
- Iodination: Addition of an iodine atom to the aromatic ring of a tyrosine residue (e.g. in thyroglobulin).
- Nucleotide addition such as ADP-ribosylation.
- Phosphate ester (O-linked) or phosphoramidate (N-linked) formation:
  - o Phosphorylation, the addition of a phosphate group, usually to serine, threonine, and tyrosine (O-linked), or histidine (N-linked).
  - o Adenylylation, the addition of an adenylyl moiety, usually to tyrosine (O-linked), or histidine and lysine (N-linked).
  - o Uridylylation, the addition of an uridylyl-group (i.e. uridine monophosphate, UMP), usually to tyrosine.
- Propionylation
- Pyroglutamate formation.
- S-glutathionylation
- S-nitrosylation
- S-sulphenylation (aka S-sulphenylation), reversible covalent addition of one oxygen atom to the thiol group of a cysteine residue.
- S-sulphinylation, normally irreversible covalent addition of two oxygen atoms to the thiol group of a cysteine residue.
- S-sulphonylation, normally irreversible covalent addition of three oxygen atoms to the thiol group of a cysteine residue, resulting in the formation of a cysteic acid residue.
- Succinylation addition of a succinyl group to lysine.
- Sulphation, the addition of a sulphate group to a tyrosine.

Non-enzymatic additions in vivo

- Glycation, the addition of a sugar molecule to a protein without the controlling action of an enzyme.
- Carbamylation the addition of Isocyanic acid to a protein's N-terminus or the side-chain of Lys.
- Carbonylation the addition of carbon monoxide to other organic/inorganic compounds.
- Spontaneous isopeptide bond formation, as found in many surface proteins of Gram-positive bacteria.

Non-enzymatic additions in vitro

- Biotinylation: Covalent attachment of a biotin moiety using a biotinylation reagent, typically for the purpose of labeling a protein.
- Carbamylation: The addition of Isocyanic acid to a protein's N-terminus or the side-chain of Lys or Cys residues, typically resulting from exposure to urea solutions.
- Oxidation: Addition of one or more Oxygen atoms to a susceptible side-chain, principally of Met, Trp, His or Cys residues. Formation of disulphide bonds between Cys residues.
- Pegylation: Covalent attachment of polyethylene glycol (PEG) using a pegylation reagent, typically to the N-terminus or the side-chains of Lys residues. Pegylation is used to improve the efficacy of protein pharmaceuticals.

Other Proteins or Peptides

- ISGylation, the covalent linkage to the ISG15 protein (Interferon-Stimulated Gene 15).
- SUMOylation, the covalent linkage to the SUMO protein (Small Ubiquitin-related MOdifier).
- Ubiquitination, the covalent linkage to the protein ubiquitin.
- Neddylation, the covalent linkage to Nedd.
- Pupylation, the covalent linkage to the Prokaryotic ubiquitin-like protein.

Chemical Modification of Amino Acids

- Citrullination, or deimination, the conversion of arginine to citrulline.
- Deamidation, the conversion of glutamine to glutamic acid or asparagine to aspartic acid.
- Eliminylation, the conversion to an alkene by beta-elimination of phosphothreonine and phosphoserine, or dehydration of threonine and serine.

Structural Changes

- Disulphide bridges, the covalent linkage of two cysteine amino acids.
- Proteolytic cleavage, cleavage of a protein at a peptide bond.
- Isoaspartate formation, via the cyclisation of asparagine or aspartic acid amino-acid residues racemisation.
    - o Of serine by protein-serine epimerase.
    - o Of alanine in dermorphin, a frog opioid peptide.
    - o Of methionine in deltorphin, also a frog opioid peptide.
- Protein splicing, self-catalytic removal of inteins analogous to mRNA processing.

Chapter 2

Proteins - Structure and Domains

INTRODUCTION

Proteins are an important class of biological macromolecules present in all biological organisms, made up of such elements as carbon, hydrogen, nitrogen, oxygen, and sulphur. All proteins are polymers of amino acids. According to their physical size, proteins are nanoparticles (definition: 1–100 nm). The polymers, also known as polypeptides, consist of a sequence of 20 different L-α-amino acids, also referred to as residues. For chains under 40 residues the term peptide is frequently used instead of protein. To be able to perform their biological function, proteins fold into one or more specific spatial conformations, driven by a number of noncovalent interactions such as hydrogen bonding, ionic interactions, van der Waals forces and hydrophobic packing. To understand the functions of proteins at a molecular level, it is often necessary to determine their three-dimensional structure.

FUNCTIONS OF PROTEINS

Most of the functions of proteins fall into the categories of binding, catalysis, conduction or transport, contraction, nutrition and/or structure. Often, a protein will have more than one of these functions and the categories are in any case not mutually exclusive. Consider some examples of binding. A protein that binds to a specific portion of a nucleic acid molecule may be able to control the expression of the genetic information encoded in nearby regions of that molecule. A cell surface protein receptor that binds insulin molecules may be able, in effect, to let the cell 'sense' the concentration of insulin in its environment, providing a link between the hormone and the hormone's action. Serum antifreeze proteins that are crucial to the survival of certain cold water fishes appear to act by binding to the surface of ice crystals.

The tremendous variety of chemical reactions within the cell must all be carried out within the narrow ranges of temperature, pH and so on, under which the cell is active. The cell does not have the option of using extremes of temperature or pH to facilitate a reaction. Instead, catalysts of specific reactions are used. Virtually all of the important catalysts of the cell are proteins: the enzymes. Enzymes, of course, bind the molecules on which they act, but they also transform them, breaking and making covalent and non-covalent bonds. Without enzymes, clearly there would be no metabolism. Some proteins facilitate the movement of compounds through cell membranes. The movement may be passive, a conduction of the substance through the membrane from a concentrated to a less concentrated solution. However, often the transport is active. In an energy-requiring process, a substance moves against a gradient of its concentration. Conduction and transport involve binding and contribute to such processes as nutrient uptake and nerve conduction. Contraction is, of course, a property of muscles. Muscles are principally protein and it is the sliding motion of muscle proteins, one relative to the other, that is responsible for contraction of muscles. Some proteins contribute to motion and coordination directly through their contraction. The storage proteins of seeds supply much of the necessary nitrogen and energy to support growth of the plant until it can be supported by photosynthesis. Prolamins, the most abundant class of cereal storage proteins, make up a significant fraction of the protein consumed by man and domestic animals. Collagen, a fibrous protein of skin and bone, is just one example of the many structural proteins. Thus, proteins influence almost every facet of the cell's activity.

PROTEINS AS POLYMERS OF AMINO ACIDS

The abundance of proteins and their relatively high content of nitrogen, roughly 15 to 18 per cent by weight, brought them to the attention of pioneering biochemists. Nitrogen is an essential constituent of proteins because proteins are polymers of amino acids. Because the amino group is on the carbon atom adjacent to the carboxyl group, the amino acids having this general formula are known as α-amino acids. It is also apparent that if R in this structure is not equal to H, the α-carbon atom is asymmetric. The α-amino acids are chiral or 'optically active' compounds. It is well-known that all the naturally occurring amino acids found in proteins have the same configuration.

With respect to the reference compound for carbohydrates, D-glyceraldehyde, the amino acids that occur in proteins have the opposite or L-configuration. This relationship is shown in Structure 2.1 where, in the ball-and-stick model and the Fischer projection, the amino group of L-serine is on the left when the carboxyl group is written at the top of the formula. An early accomplishment in biochemistry was the conversion of L-serine into L-glyceraldehyde by a series of chemical reactions that did not modify the configuration of the α-carbon atom. In this way, the absolute configuration of L-serine was established. Other amino acids are compared, for absolute configuration about the α-carbon atom, to L-serine as the reference compound. (When reference is made to the absolute configuration of L-serine rather than to the actual optical rotation of the amino acid, the notation L_s is often used.) Note that the amino group is below the α-carbon atom in the structure of an L-amino acid when the carboxyl group is written to the right in the projection formula. As with the carbohydrates, it is important to stress that the use of L and D conventions refers only to the relative configuration of these compounds and does not provide any information regarding the direction in which these optically active compounds rotate polarised light. Note that the amino acids are represented in different ionic forms in Structures 2.1. The zwitterionic form of the amino acid, as represented in Structure 2.1, most closely represents the state of ionisation of the amino acids in solutions of neutral pH.

The fundamental structural unit of proteins is the α-amino acid is easily demonstrated by hydrolysing purified proteins by either chemical or enzymatic procedures. For example, a protein may be hydrolysed completely or nearly completely to its constituent amino acids in a period of 18 to 24 hr by the action of $6N$ HCl at 110°C in a sealed tube. Under these conditions, 17 of the 20 common protein amino acids are released in good yield. Isolating 17 distinct amino acids from a hydrolysate by crystallisation and other classical techniques of organic chemistry was a considerable accomplishment of pioneering biochemists. An amino acid analysis, which gives the relative amounts of the amino acids that survive the hydrolysis procedure, is an important step in the preliminary characterisation of a newly purified protein.

Ball-and-stick model

COO⁻ (structure)

CHO (structure)

Fischer projection formula

$$H_3\overset{+}{N}—\overset{|}{\underset{|}{C}}—H$$
COO⁻ / CH₂OH

$$H—\overset{|}{\underset{|}{C}}—OH$$
CHO / CH₂OH

L-Serine   D-Glyceraldehyde

Structure 2.1

Early investigators realised, from certain physical properties of proteins, that they must be high molecular weight substances. High molecular weight substances already were well known in the chemistry laboratory. The tars that accumulate in some reactions and the colloidal substances formed by an electric arc between two metal electrodes under water are examples. Such high molecular weight substances are said to be 'polydisperse' because they are, in fact, mixtures of compounds of related chemical structure but highly variable size. Tars and colloidal substances, as well as haemoglobin and certain other oxygen-transporting proteins, all were examined by applying strong centrifugal fields to their solutions or suspensions. The relatively large size of the molecules in tars and proteins or the aggregates in colloidal substances caused them to move much more rapidly than low molecular solutes, such as salts, in the centrifugal field. However, purified proteins, such as haemoglobin, behaved very differently from tars and colloids. Only the proteins migrated in the centrifugal field in such a way as to give a sharp, discrete boundary. This was observed because proteins are high molecular weight compounds, meaning that they have a definite atomic composition. Each constituent of a tar or colloid will have its characteristic rate of sedimentation in the centrifugal field. However, since the constituents are of different sizes, no sharp, discrete boundary could be observed for these substances.

The atomic composition of haemoglobin, stripped of its oxygen-bearing heme groups, is:

$$C_{2796}H_{4592}O_{832}N_{812}S_8$$

This atomic composition is typical of protein molecules, which usually are 30 to 33 per cent C, roughly 50 per cent H, 9 to 11 per cent O and 7 to 9 per cent N, with small amounts of S.

PRIMARY STRUCTURE OF PROTEINS

The covalent structure of a protein is essentially linear. Amino acids are connected together to form a chain, the connection being a peptide bond. The peptide bond is simply an amide bond between the carbonyl carbon of one amino acid and the amino nitrogen of another.

$$—\overset{O}{\overset{||}{C}}—\overset{|}{\underset{|}{N}}—$$
H

Conceptually, the formation of the peptide bond may be considered to result from the removal of two protons and one oxygen atom (i.e., one molecule of water) from a pair of amino acids. In the reaction shown below, the oxygen atom may be considered to have been removed from the carboxylate group of amino acid 1 and two protons from the alkyl ammonium group of amino acid 2. The polypeptide character of a protein is shown in Fig. 2.1.

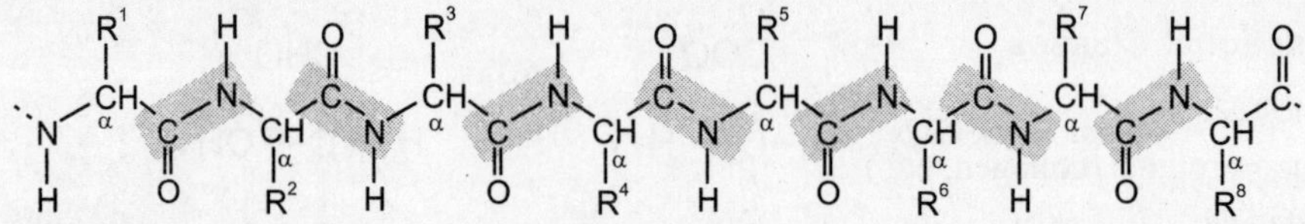

Fig. 2.1: A generalised structure of a polypeptide chain showing the linkage of adjacent amino acid residues through peptide bonds.

Obviously, there is no theoretical limit to the molecular weight attainable with such a chain structure and proteins vary in molecular weight from a few thousands to a few millions.

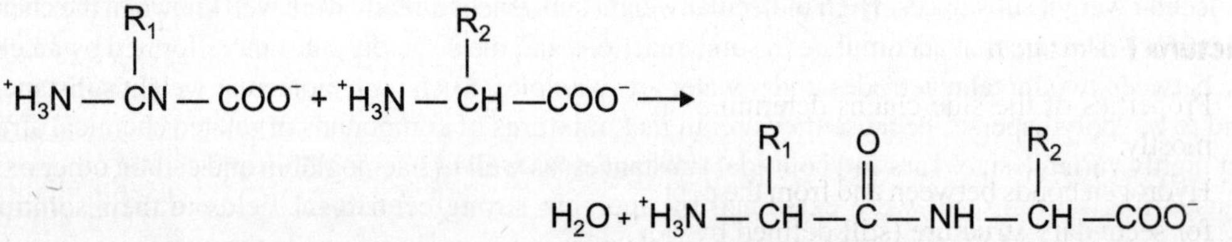

$$^+H_3N - CN - COO^- + {}^+H_3N - CH - COO^- \longrightarrow$$
$$\overset{R_1}{\underset{}{}} \qquad \qquad \overset{R_2}{\underset{}{}}$$

$$H_2O + {}^+H_3N - CH - C - NH - CH - COO^-$$
$$\overset{R_1}{\underset{}{}} \quad \overset{O}{\underset{}{}} \qquad \overset{R_2}{\underset{}{}}$$

When an amino acid has been incorporated into a polypeptide chain, it is referred to as an 'amino acid residue' rather than simply an amino acid. The reason for this is that water has been 'split out' in the process of forming the peptide bond, so that what remains does not correspond to the full structure of an amino acid. Twenty different amino acid residues account for the vast majority of protein structures. With the exception of the imino acid proline (whose structure follows), these all are α-amino acids, which means that they differ only in the R groups. The average weight of a protein amino acid residue is approximately 110, which means that proteins have from a few tens to about ten thousand amino acid residues. The primary structure of a protein is simply the order of amino acid residues in the polypeptide chain. In the remainder of this section, we present the structures of the 20 common protein amino acids and of a few less common protein amino acids.

These could be classified according to the chemical nature (aliphatic, aromatic, heterocyclic) of their R groups into appropriate sub-classes. More meaningful, however, is a classification-based on the polarity of the R group or residue because it emphasises the possible functional roles that the different amino acids can play in proteins and their possible contributions to the folding of the polypeptide chain. In this classification, the 20 amino acids commonly found in proteins may be described as:

1. Non-polar or hydrophobic.
2. Polar but uncharged.
3. Polar because of a negative charge at the physiological pH of 7.
4. Polar because of a positive charge at physiological pH.

Hydrophobic means 'water hating'. It is a term used to describe aliphatic and aromatic hydrocarbon compounds or portions of molecules or other chemical groups, that share the property of having only very limited solubility in water.

CELLULAR FUNCTIONS OF PROTEINS

- Produced by living cells, translated from the encoding gene.
- May function inside the cell (in its various compartments, e.g. nucleus -DNA binding proteins- or cytosol or on the cell membrane or be secreted out (e.g. microbial enzymes such as cellulases, etc. animals growth factors, antibodies, lysozyme, proteases, etc. (food processing in the stomach, gut).

Protein Functional Classes

- Enzymes
- Structural proteins (collagen, etc.)
- Ion channels
- Transporters (haemoglobin, through membrane transport)
- Immune system proteins (binding)
- Other binding proteins (growth factors, DNA binding proteins, chaperones)
- Often functionalities are specific to specific domains.

Structure Formation

- Properties of the side chains determine the higher order structure of proteins, and functionality, mostly.
- Hydrogen bonds between and from the peptide 'backbone' amide and carbonyl groups are important for secondary structure (still defined by side chains).
- Peptide bond is planar (important!).
- Proteins can be (i) fibrious/filamentous (collagen, silk, muscles myosin and actin), (ii) soluble (e.g. enzymes, growth factors, insulin, etc.) or in the cell lipid membrane, (iii) 'membrane proteins' (hydrophobic/lipid soluble) (ion channels and pumps, control of cell homeostatis, transporters and receptors (G-protein coupled receptors, signalling).
- Typically cell surface receptors have a intramembrane domain + extracellular ligand binding domain + intracellular region for signalling inside the cell.

Secondary Structure

- Fold/structure of the protein stabilised in secondary structure, α-helices or β-strands.
- Sequencial arrangement (topology) and spacial organisation of these elements defines the FOLD of the protein.
- Amino acids have different propensies for forming particular secondary structure (e.g. Ala and non-β branced residues in α-helices.

Proteins Folds

- Some protein folds are unique, but the 'fold-space' must be limited.
- Many proteins have several domains.
- Most proteins fold into already-known structures:
  - o Even when there is no sequence homology (<10–20%).
  - o Structure preserved much longer than sequence.

- Some common folds:
  - o β/α barrel
  - o 7-TM receptor
  - o 4-helix bundle
  - o β-sanwich domains (immunoglobulin-like), etc.

β/α barrel

- 40% of unique proteins
- Usually enzymes

7-TM fold

- Example is Bovine rhodopsin
- >500 such folds in humans
- 7 transmembrane helices
- Signal transduction
  - o Signals very varied

Protein Folding

- The protein folding problem
  - o Complex, vs e.g. DNA/RNA structure
  - o Can't predict the structure ab initio
  - o But there are cases of success for small proteins
- What stabilises the folded (native) state
- Driving forces
- Mechanisms

Folded/Native State

- Free energy minimum, typical functional proteins have a single defined native state.
- Hydrophobic and aromatic residues inside.
- Charged/polar residues on the outside OR hydrogen bonded (solvation by the protein).

PROTEIN DOMAIN

A protein domain is a conserved part of a given protein sequence and tertiary structure that can evolve, function, and exist independently of the rest of the protein chain. Each domain forms a compact three-dimensional structure and often can be independently stable and folded. Many proteins consist of several structural domains. One domain may appear in a variety of different proteins. Molecular evolution uses domains as building blocks and these may be recombined in different arrangements to create proteins with different functions. In general, domains vary in length from between about 50 amino acids up to 250 amino acids in length. The shortest domains, such as zinc fingers, are stabilised by metal ions or disulphide bridges. Domains often form functional units, such as the calcium-binding EF hand domain of calmodulin. Because they are independently stable, domains can be 'swapped' by genetic engineering between one protein and another to make chimeric proteins. The concept of the domain was first proposed in 1973 by Wetlaufer after X-ray crystallographic studies of hen lysozyme and papain and by limited proteolysis studies of immunoglobulins. Wetlaufer defined domains as stable units of protein structure that could fold autonomously. In the past domains have been described as units of:

- Compact structure.
- Function and evolution.
- Folding.

Each definition is valid and will often overlap, i.e. a compact structural domain that is found amongst diverse proteins is likely to fold independently within its structural environment. Nature often brings several domains together to form multidomain and multifunctional proteins with a vast number of possibilities. In a multidomain protein, each domain may fulfill its own function independently, or in a concerted manner with its neighbours. Domains can either serve as modules for building up large assemblies such as virus particles or muscle fibres, or can provide specific catalytic or binding sites as found in enzymes or regulatory proteins. Pyruvate kinase, a protein with three domains are shown in Fig. 2.2.

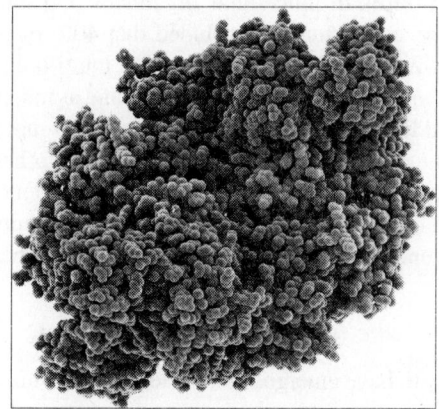

Fig. 2.2: Pyruvate kinase, a protein with three domains.

Domains as Evolutionary Modules

Nature is a tinkerer and not an inventor, new sequences are adapted from pre-existing sequences rather than invented. Domains are the common material used by nature to generate new sequences, they can be thought of as genetically mobile units, referred to as 'modules'. Often, the C and *N* termini of domains are close together in space, allowing them to easily be 'slotted into' parent structures during the process of evolution. Many domain families are found in all three forms of life, Archaea, Bacteria and Eukarya. Protein modules are a subset of protein domains which are found across a range of different proteins with a particularly versatile structure. Examples can be found among extracellular proteins associated with clotting, fibrinolysis, complement, the extracellular matrix, cell surface adhesion molecules and cytokine receptors. Four concrete examples of widespread protein modules are the following domains: SH2, immunoglobulin, fibronectin type 3 and the kringle.

Molecular evolution gives rise to families of related proteins with similar sequence and structure. However, sequence similarities can be extremely low between proteins that share the same structure.

Protein structures may be similar because proteins have diverged from a common ancestor. Alternatively, some folds may be more favoured than others as they represent stable arrangements of secondary structures and some proteins may converge towards these folds over the course of evolution. There are currently about 110000 experimentally determined protein 3D structures deposited within the Protein Data Bank (PDB). However, this set contains many identical or very similar structures. All proteins should be classified to structural families to understand their evolutionary relationships. Structural comparisons are best achieved at the domain level. For this reason many algorithms have been developed to automatically assign domains in proteins with known 3D structure, see 'Domain definition from structural co-ordinates'.

The CATH domain database classifies domains into approximately 800 fold families, ten of these folds are highly populated and are referred to as 'super-folds'. Super-folds are defined as folds for which there are at least three structures without significant sequence similarity. The most populated is the α/β-barrel super-fold, as described previously.

Multidomain Proteins

The majority of proteins, two-thirds in unicellular organisms and more than 80% in metazoa, are multidomain proteins. However, other studies concluded that 40% of prokaryotic proteins consist of multiple domains while eukaryotes have approximately 65% multi-domain proteins.

Many domains in eukaryotic multidomain proteins can be found as independent proteins in prokaryotes, suggesting that domains in multidomain proteins have once existed as independent proteins. For example, vertebrates have a multi-enzyme polypeptide containing the GAR synthetase, AIR synthetase and GAR transformylase domains (GARs-AIRs-GARt, GAR: glycinamide ribonucleotide synthetase/transferase, AIR: aminoimidazole ribonucleotide synthetase). In insects, the polypeptide appears as GARs-(AIRs)2-GARt, in yeast GARs-AIRs is encoded separately from GARt, and in bacteria each domain is encoded separately.

Origin

Multidomain proteins are likely to have emerged from selective pressure during evolution to create new functions. Various proteins have diverged from common ancestors by different combinations and associations of domains. Modular units frequently move about, within and between biological systems through mechanisms of genetic shuffling:

- Transposition of mobile elements including horizontal transfers (between species).
- Gross rearrangements such as inversions, translocations, deletions and duplications.
- Homologous recombination.
- Slippage of DNA polymerase during replication.

Types of Organisation

The simplest multidomain organisation seen in proteins is that of a single domain repeated in tandem. The domains may interact with each other (domain-domain interaction) or remain isolated, like beads on string. The giant 30000 residue muscle protein titin comprises about 120 fibronectin-III-type and Ig-type domains. In the serine proteases, a gene duplication event has led to the formation of a two β-barrel domain enzyme. The repeats have diverged so widely that there is no obvious sequence similarity between them. The active site is located at a cleft between the two β-barrel domains, in which functionally important residues are contributed from each domain. Genetically engineered mutants of the chymotrypsin serine protease were shown to have some proteinase activity even though their active site residues were abolished and it has therefore been postulated that the duplication event enhanced the enzymes activity.

Modules frequently display different connectivity relationships, as illustrated by the kinesins and ABC transporters. The kinesin motor domain can be at either end of a polypeptide chain that includes a coiled-coil region and a cargo domain. ABC transporters are built with up to four domains consisting of two unrelated modules, ATP-binding cassette and an integral membrane module, arranged in various combinations.

Not only do domains recombine, but there are many examples of a domain having been inserted into another. Sequence or structural similarities to other domains demonstrate that homologues of inserted and parent domains can exist independently. An example is that of the 'fingers' inserted into the 'palm' domain within the polymerases of the Pol I family. Since a domain can be inserted into another, there should always be at least one continuous domain in a multidomain protein. This is the main difference between definitions of structural domains and evolutionary/functional domains. An evolutionary domain will be limited to one or two connections between domains, whereas structural domains can have unlimited connections, within a given criterion of the existence of a common core. Several structural domains could be assigned to an evolutionary domain.

A superdomain consists of two or more conserved domains of nominally independent origin, but subsequently inherited as a single structural/functional unit. This combined superdomain can occur in diverse proteins that are not related by gene duplication alone. An example of a superdomain is the protein tyrosine phosphatase–C2 domain pair in PTEN, tensin, auxilin and the membrane protein TPTE2. This superdomain is found in proteins in animals, plants and fungi. A key feature of the PTP-C2 superdomain is amino acid residue conservation in the domain interface.

Domains are Autonomous Folding Units

Folding

Protein folding: The unsolved problem: Since the seminal work of Anfinsen in the early 1960s, the goal to completely understand the mechanism by which a polypeptide rapidly folds into its stable native conformation remains elusive. Many experimental folding studies have contributed much to our understanding, but the principles that govern protein folding are still based on those discovered in the very first studies of folding. Anfinsen showed that the native state of a protein is thermodynamically stable, the conformation being at a global minimum of its free energy.

Folding is a directed search of conformational space allowing the protein to fold on a biologically feasible time scale. The Levinthal paradox states that if an averaged sized protein would sample all possible conformations before finding the one with the lowest energy, the whole process would take billions of years. Proteins typically fold within 0.1 and 1000 seconds. Therefore, the protein folding process must be directed some way through a specific folding pathway. The forces that direct this search are likely to be a combination of local and global influences whose effects are felt at various stages of the reaction.

Advances in experimental and theoretical studies have shown that folding can be viewed in terms of energy landscapes, where folding kinetics is considered as a progressive organisation of an ensemble of partially folded structures through which a protein passes on its way to the folded structure. This has been described in terms of a folding funnel, in which an unfolded protein has a large number of conformational states available and there are fewer states available to the folded protein. A funnel implies that for protein folding there is a decrease in energy and loss of entropy with increasing tertiary structure formation. The local roughness of the funnel reflects kinetic traps, corresponding to the accumulation of misfolded intermediates. A folding chain progresses toward lower intra-chain free-energies by increasing its compactness. The chains conformational options become increasingly narrowed ultimately toward one native structure.

Advantage of domains in protein folding

The organisation of large proteins by structural domains represents an advantage for protein folding, with each domain being able to individually fold, accelerating the folding process and reducing a potentially large combination of residue interactions. Furthermore, given the observed random distribution of hydrophobic residues in proteins, domain formation appears to be the optimal solution for a large protein to bury its hydrophobic residues while keeping the hydrophilic residues at the surface.

However, the role of inter-domain interactions in protein folding and in energetics of stabilisation of the native structure, probably differs for each protein. In T4 lysozyme, the influence of one domain on the other is so strong that the entire molecule is resistant to proteolytic cleavage. In this case, folding is a sequential process where the C-terminal domain is required to fold independently in an early step, and the other domain requires the presence of the folded C-terminal domain for folding and stabilisation.

It has been found that the folding of an isolated domain can take place at the same rate or sometimes faster than that of the integrated domain, suggesting that unfavourable interactions with the rest of the protein can occur during folding. Several arguments suggest that the slowest step in the folding of large proteins is the pairing of the folded domains. This is either because the domains are not folded entirely correctly or because the small adjustments required for their interaction are energetically unfavourable, such as the removal of water from the domain interface.

Domains and Protein Flexibility

Protein domain dynamics play a key role in a multitude of molecular recognition and signalling processes. Protein domains, connected by intrinsically disordered flexible linker domains, induce long-range allostery via protein domain dynamics. The resultant dynamic modes cannot be generally predicted from static structures of either the entire protein or individual domains. They can however be inferred by comparing different structures of a protein (as in Database of Molecular Motions). They can also be suggested by sampling in extensive molecular dynamics trajectories and principal component analysis, or they can be directly observed using spectra measured by neutron spin echo spectroscopy.

Domain definition from structural co-ordinates

The importance of domains as structural building blocks and elements of evolution has brought about many automated methods for their identification and classification in proteins of known structure. Automatic procedures for reliable domain assignment is essential for the generation of the domain databases, especially as the number of known protein structures is increasing. Although the boundaries of a domain can be determined by visual inspection, construction of an automated method is not straightforward. Problems occur when faced with domains that are discontinuous or highly associated. The fact that there is no standard definition of what a domain really is has meant that domain assignments have varied enormously, with each researcher using a unique set of criteria.

A structural domain is a compact, globular sub-structure with more interactions within it than with the rest of the protein. Therefore, a structural domain can be determined by two visual characteristics: its compactness and its extent of isolation. Measures of local compactness in proteins have been used in many of the early methods of domain assignment and in several of the more recent methods.

Methods

One of the first algorithms used a Cα-Cα distance map together with a hierarchical clustering routine that considered proteins as several small segments, 10 residues in length. The initial segments were clustered one after another based on inter-segment distances, segments with the shortest distances were clustered and considered as single segments thereafter. The stepwise clustering finally included the full protein. Go also exploited the fact that inter-domain distances are normally larger than intra-domain distances, all possible Cα-Cα distances were represented as diagonal plots in which there were distinct patterns for helices, extended strands and combinations of secondary structures.

The method by Sowdhamini and Blundell clusters secondary structures in a protein based on their Cα-Cα distances and identifies domains from the pattern in their dendrograms. As the procedure does not consider the protein as a continuous chain of amino acids there are no problems in treating discontinuous domains. Specific nodes in these dendrograms are identified as tertiary structural clusters of the protein, these include both super-secondary structures and domains. The DOMAK algorithm is used to create the 3Dee domain database. It calculates a 'split value' from the number of each type of contact when the protein is divided arbitrarily into two parts. This split value is large when the two parts of the structure are distinct.

The method of Wodak and Janin was based on the calculated interface areas between two chain segments repeatedly cleaved at various residue positions. Interface areas were calculated by comparing surface areas of the cleaved segments with that of the native structure. Potential domain boundaries can be identified at a site where the interface area was at a minimum. Other methods have used measures of solvent accessibility to calculate compactness.

The PUU algorithm incorporates a harmonic model used to approximate inter-domain dynamics. The underlying physical concept is that many rigid interactions will occur within each domain and loose interactions will occur between domains. This algorithm is used to define domains in the FSSP domain database.

Swindells developed a method, DETECTIVE, for identification of domains in protein structures based on the idea that domains have a hydrophobic interior. Deficiencies were found to occur when hydrophobic cores from different domains continue through the interface region.

RigidFinder is a novel method for identification of protein rigid blocks (domains and loops) from two different conformations. Rigid blocks are defined as blocks where all inter residue distances are conserved across conformations.

A general method to identify dynamical domains, that is protein regions that behave approximately as rigid units in the course of structural fluctuations, has been introduced by Potestio and other and, among other applications was also used to compare the consistency of the dynamics-based domain subdivisions with standard structure-based ones. The method, termed PiSQRD, is publicly available in the form of a webserver. The latter allows users to optimally subdivide single-chain or multimeric proteins into quasi-rigid domains based on the collective modes of fluctuation of the system. By default the latter are calculated through an elastic network model, alternatively pre-calculated essential dynamical spaces can be uploaded by the user.

Example domains

- Armadillo repeats: Named after the β-catenin-like Armadillo protein of the fruit fly *Drosophila*.
- Basic Leucine zipper domain (bZIP domain): Is found in many DNA-binding eukaryotic proteins. One part of the domain contains a region that mediates sequence-specific DNA-binding properties

and the Leucine zipper that is required for the dimerisation of two DNA-binding regions. The DNA-binding region comprises a number of basic aminoacids such as arginine and lysine.

- Cadherin repeats: Cadherins function as Ca^{2+}-dependent cell–cell adhesion proteins. Cadherin domains are extracellular regions which mediate cell-to-cell homophilic binding between cadherins on the surface of adjacent cells.

- Death effector domain (DED): Allows protein–protein binding by homotypic interactions (DED-DED). Caspase proteases trigger apoptosis via proteolytic cascades. Pro-Caspase-8 and pro-caspase-9 bind to specific adaptor molecules via DED domains and this leads to autoactivation of caspases.

- EF hand: A helix-turn-helix structural motif found in each structural domain of the signalling protein calmodulin and in the muscle protein troponin-C.

- Immunoglobulin-like domains: Are found in proteins of the immunoglobulin superfamily (IgSF). They contain about 70–110 amino acids and are classified into different categories (IgV, IgC1, IgC2 and IgI) according to their size and function. They possess a characteristic fold in which two beta sheets form a 'sandwich' that is stabilised by interactions between conserved cysteines and other charged amino acids. They are important for protein–protein interactions in processes of cell adhesion, cell activation, and molecular recognition. These domains are commonly found in molecules with roles in the immune system.

- Phosphotyrosine-binding domain (PTB): PTB domains usually bind to phosphorylated tyrosine residues. They are often found in signal transduction proteins. PTB-domain binding specificity is determined by residues to the amino-terminal side of the phosphotyrosine. Examples: the PTB domains of both SHC and IRS-1 bind to a NPXpY sequence. PTB-containing proteins such as SHC and IRS-1 are important for insulin responses of human cells.

- Pleckstrin homology domain (PH): PH domains bind phosphoinositides with high affinity. Specificity for PtdIns(3)P, PtdIns(4)P, PtdIns(3,4)P2, PtdIns(4,5)P2, and PtdIns(3,4,5)P3 have all been observed. Given the fact that phosphoinositides are sequestered to various cell membranes (due to their long lipophilic tail) the PH domains usually causes recruitment of the protein in question to a membrane where the protein can exert a certain function in cell signalling, cytoskeletal reorganisation or membrane trafficking.

- Src homology 2 domain (SH2): SH2 domains are often found in signal transduction proteins. SH2 domains confer binding to phosphorylated tyrosine (pTyr). Named after the phosphotyrosine binding domain of the src viral oncogene, which is itself a tyrosine kinase.

- Zinc finger DNA binding domain (ZnF_GATA): ZnF_GATA domain-containing proteins are typically transcription factors that usually bind to the DNA sequence [AT]GATA[AG] of promoters.

Domains of Unknown Function

A large fraction of domains are of unknown function. A domain of unknown function (DUF) is a protein domain that has no characterised function. These families have been collected together in the Pfam database using the prefix DUF followed by a number, with examples being DUF2992 and DUF1220. There are now over 3000 DUF families within the Pfam database representing over 20% of known families.

PROTEIN–PROTEIN INTERACTION

Protein–protein interactions (PPIs) refer to intentional physical contacts established between two or more proteins as a result of biochemical events and/or electrostatic forces. In fact, proteins are vital macromolecules, at both cellular and systemic levels, but they rarely act alone. Diverse essential molecular processes within a cell are carried out by molecular machines that are built from a large number of protein components organised by their PPIs.

Indeed, these interactions are at the core of the entire interactomics system of any living cell and so, unsurprisingly, aberrant PPIs are on the basis of multiple diseases, such as Creutzfeld-Jacob, Alzheimer's disease, and cancer. PPIs have been studied from different perspectives: biochemistry, quantum chemistry, molecular dynamics, signal transduction, among others. All this information enables the creation of large protein interaction networks–similar to metabolic or genetic/epigenetic networks–that empower the current knowledge on biochemical cascades and disease pathogenesis, as well as provide putative new therapeutic targets.

Examples of Protein-protein Interactions

Signal transduction

The activity of the cell is regulated by extracellular signals. Signals propagation to inside and/or along the interior of cells depends on PPIs between the various signalling molecules. This process, called signal transduction, plays a fundamental role in many biological processes and in many diseases (e.g. Parkinson's disease and cancer).

Transport across membranes

A protein may be carrying another protein (for example, from cytoplasm to nucleus or vice versa in the case of the nuclear pore importins).

Cell metabolism

In many biosynthetic processes enzymes interact with each other to produce small compounds or other macromolecules.

Muscle contraction

Physiology of muscle contraction involves several interactions. Myosin filaments act as molecular motors and by binding to actin enables filament sliding. Furthermore, members of the skeletal muscle lipid droplet-associated proteins family associate with other proteins, as activator of adipose triglyceride lipase and its coactivator comparative gene identification-58, to regulate lipolysis in skeletal muscle.

Types of Protein-protein Interactions

Protein complex assembly can result in the formation of homo-oligomeric or hetero-oligomeric complexes. In addition to the conventional complexes, as enzyme-inhibitor and antibody-antigen, interactions can also be established between domain-domain and domain-peptide. Moreover, interactions can be classified into stable or transient, and also according to the nature of the chemical bonds established between proteins.

Homo-oligomers vs hetero-oligomers

Homo-oligomers are macromolecular complexes constituted by only one type of protein subunit. Protein subunits assembly is guided by the establishment of non-covalent interactions in the quaternary structure of the protein. Disruption of homo-oligomers in order to return to the initial individual monomers often requires denaturation of the complex. Several enzymes, carrier proteins, scaffolding proteins, and transcriptional regulatory factors carry out their functions as homo-oligomers. Distinct protein subunits interact in hetero-oligomers, which are essential to control several cellular functions. The importance of the communication between heterologous proteins is even more evident during cell signalling events and such interactions are only possible due to structural domains within the proteins.

Stable interactions vs transient interactions

Stable interactions involve proteins that interact for a long time, taking part of permanent complexes as subunits, in order to carry out structural or functional roles. These are usually the case of homo-oligomers (e.g. cytochrome c), and some hetero-oligomeric proteins, as the subunits of ATPase. On the other hand, a protein may interact briefly and in a reversible manner with other proteins in only certain cellular contexts–cell type, cell cycle stage, external factors, presence of other binding proteins, etc.–as it happens with most of the proteins involved in biochemical cascades. These are called transient interactions. For example, some G protein-coupled receptors only transiently bind to Gi/o proteins when they are activated by extracellular ligands, while some Gq-coupled receptors, such as muscarinic receptor M3, pre-couple with Gq-proteins prior to the receptor-ligand binding.

Covalent vs non-covalent

Covalent interactions are those with the strongest association and are formed by disulphide bonds or electron sharing. Although being rare, these interactions are determinant in some post-translational modifications, as ubiquitination and SUMOylation. Non-covalent bonds are usually established during transient interactions by the combination of weaker bonds, such as hydrogen bonds, ionic interactions, Van der Waals forces, or hydrophobic bonds.

Techniques to Study the Molecular Structure of Protein Complexes

The molecular structures of many protein complexes have been unlocked by the technique of X-ray crystallography. The first structure to be solved by this method was that of sperm whale myoglobin by Sir John Cowdery Kendrew. In this technique the angles and intensities of a beam of X-rays diffracted by crystalline atoms are detected in a film, thus producing a three-dimensional picture of the density of electrons within the crystal.

Later, nuclear magnetic resonance also started to be applied with the aim of unravelling the molecular structure of protein complexes. One of the first examples was the structure of calmodulin-binding domains bound to calmodulin. This technique is based on the study of magnetic properties of atomic nuclei, thus determining physical and chemical properties of the correspondent atoms or the molecules. Nuclear magnetic resonance is advantageous for characterising weak PPIs.

Properties of Protein-protein Interface

The study of the molecular structure can give fine details about the interface that enables the interaction between proteins. When characterising PPI interfaces it is important to take into account the type of complex. Parameters evaluated include size (measured in absolute dimensions Å2 or in solvent-accessible surface area (SASA)), shape, complementarity between surfaces, residue interface propensities, hydrophobicity, segmentation and secondary structure, and conformational changes on complex formation. The great majority of PPI interfaces reflects the composition of protein surfaces, rather than the protein cores, inspite of being frequently enriched in hydrophobic residues, particularly in aromatic residues. PPI interfaces are dynamic and frequently planar, although they can be globular and protruding as well.

Based on three structures –insulin dimer, trypsin-pancreatic trypsin inhibitor complex, and oxyhaemoglobin –Cyrus Chothia and Joel Janin found that between 1,130 and 1,720 Å of surface area was removed from contact with water indicating that hydrophobicity is a major factor of stabilisation of PPIs. Later studies refined the buried surface area of the majority of interactions to $1,600 \pm 350$ Å2.

However, much larger interaction interfaces were also observed and were associated with significant changes in conformation of one of the interaction partners. PPIs interfaces exhibit both shape and electrostatic complementarity. It has been shown that PPI interfaces assemble to mitigate the protein-water interfacial tension (epistructural tension) of individual binding partners. The epistructural tension is mostly caused by a type of protein structural defect known as dehydron.

Factors that Regulate Protein-protein Interactions

- Protein concentration, which in turn are affected by expression levels and degradation rates.
- Protein affinity for proteins or other binding ligands.
- Ligands concentrations (substrates, ions, etc.).
- Presence of other proteins, nucleic acids, and ions.
- Electric fields around proteins.
- Occurrence of covalent modifications.

Structural Domains Involved in Protein-protein Interactions

Proteins hold structural domains that allow their interaction with and bind to specific sequences on other proteins.

Src homology 2 (SH2) domain

SH2 domains are structurally composed by three-stranded twisted beta sheet sandwiched flanked by two alpha-helices. The existence of a deep binding pocket with high affinity for phosphotyrosine, but not for phosphoserine or phosphothreonine, is essential for the recognition of tyrosine phosphorylated proteins, mainly autophosphorylated growth factor receptors. Growth factor receptor binding proteins and phospholipase Cg are examples of proteins that have SH2 domains.

Src homology 3 (SH3) domain

Structurally, SH3 domains are constituted by a beta barrel formed by two orthogonal beta sheets and three anti-parallel beta strands. These domains recognise proline enriched sequences, as polyproline type II helical structure (PXXP motifs) in cell signalling proteins like protein tyrosine kinases and the growth factor receptor bound protein 2 (Grb2).

Phosphotyrosine-binding (PTB) domain

PTB domains interact with sequences that contain a phosphotyrosine group. These domains can be found in the insulin receptor substrate.

LIM domain

LIM domains were initially identified in three homeodomain transcription factors (lin11, is11, and mec3). In addition to this homeodomain proteins and other proteins involved in development, LIM domains have also been identified in non-homeodomain proteins with relevant roles in cellular differentiation, association with cytoskeleton and senescence. These domains contain a tandem cysteine-rich Zn^{2+}-finger motif and embrace the consensus sequence CX2CX16–23HX2CX2CX2CX16–21CX2C/H/D. LIM domains bind to PDZ domains, bHLH transcription factors, and other LIM domains.

Sterile alpha motif (SAM) domain

SAM domains are composed by five helices forming a compact package with a conserved hydrophobic core. These domains, which can be found in the Eph receptor and the stromal interaction molecule (STIM) for example, bind to non-SAM domain-containing proteins and they also appear to have the ability to bind RNA.

PDZ domain

PDZ domains were first identified in three guanylate kinases: PSD-95, DlgA and ZO-1. These domains recognise carboxy-terminal tri-peptide motifs (S/TXV), other PDZ domains or LIM domains and bind them through a short peptide sequence that has a C-terminal hydrophobic residue. Some of the proteins identified as having PDZ domains are scaffolding proteins or seem to be involved in ion receptor assembling and receptor-enzyme complexes formation.

FERM domain

FERM domains contain basic residues capable of binding PtdIns(4,5)P2. Talin and focal adhesion kinase (FAK) are two of the proteins that present FERM domains.

Calponin homology (CH) domain

CH domains are mainly present in cytoskeletal proteins as parvin.

Pleckstrin homology domain

Pleckstrin homology domains bind to phosphoinositides and acid domains in signalling proteins.

WW domain

WW domains bind to proline enriched sequences.

WSxWS motif

Found in cytokine receptors.

Methods to Investigate Protein–protein Interactions

There are a multitude of methods to detect them. Each of the approaches has its own strengths and weaknesses, especially with regard to the sensitivity and specificity of the method. The most conventional and widely used high-throughput methods are yeast two-hybrid screening and affinity purification coupled to mass spectrometry.

Yeast two-hybrid screening

This system was firstly described in 1989 by Fields and Song using *Saccharomyces cerevisiae* as biological model. Yeast two hybrid allows the identification of pairwise PPIs (binary method) *in vivo*, indicating non-specific tendencies towards sticky interactions.

Yeast cells are transfected with two plasmids: the bait (protein of interest fused with the DNA-binding domain of a yeast transcription factor, like Gal4), and the prey (a library of cDNA fragments linked to the activation domain of the transcription factor. Transcription of reporter genes does not occur unless bait and prey interact with each other and form a functional transcription factor. Thus, the interaction between proteins can be inferred by the presence of the products resultant of the reporter gene expression.

Despite its usefulness, the yeast two-hybrid system has limitations: specificity is relatively low, uses yeast as main host system, which can be a problem when studying other biological models, the number of PPIs identified is usually low because some transient PPIs are lost during purification steps, and, understates membrane proteins, for example. Limitations have been overcoming by the emergence of yeast two-hybrid variants, such as the membrane yeast two-hybrid (MYTH) and the split-ubiquitin system, which are not limited to interactions that occur in the nucleus, and, the bacterial two-hybrid system, performed in bacteria.

Affinity purification coupled to mass spectrometry

Affinity purification coupled to mass spectrometry mostly detects stable interactions and thus better indicates functional *in vivo* PPIs. This method starts by purification of the tagged protein, which is expressed in the cell usually at *in vivo* concentrations, and its interacting proteins (affinity purification). One of the most advantageous and widely used method to purify proteins with very low contaminating background is the tandem affinity purification, developed by Bertrand Seraphin and Mathias Mann and respective colleagues. PPIs can then be quantitatively and qualitatively analysed by mass spectrometry using different methods: chemical incorporation, biological or metabolic incorporation (SILAC), and label-free methods.

Other potential methods

Diverse techniques to identify PPIs have been emerging along with technology progression. These include co-immunoprecipitation, protein microarrays, analytical ultracentrifugation, light scattering, fluorescence spectroscopy, luminescence-based mammalian interactome mapping (LUMIER), resonance-energy transfer systems, mammalian protein-protein interaction trap, electro-switchable biosurfaces, surface plasmon resonance, protein-fragment complementation assay, and calorimetry.

Text-mining methods

Recently text-mining methods were implemented to extract automatically protein-protein interactions from the literature. These methods generally detect binary relations between interacting proteins from individual sentences using machine learning and rule/pattern based information extraction and machine learning approaches.

Protein-protein Interaction Databases

Large scale identification of PPIs generated hundreds of thousands interactions, which were collected together in specialised biological databases that are continuously updated in order to provide complete interactomes. The first of these databases was the Database of Interacting Proteins (DIP). Since that time, the number of public databases has been increasing. Databases can be subdivided into primary databases, meta-databases, and prediction databases.

- Primary databases collect information about published PPIs proven to exist via small-scale or large-scale experimental methods. Examples: DIP, Biomolecular Interaction Network Database (BIND), Biological General Repository for Interaction Datasets (BioGRID), Human Protein

Reference Database (HPRD), IntAct Molecular Interaction Database, Molecular Interactions Database (MINT), MIPS Protein Interaction Resource on Yeast (MIPS-MPact), and MIPS Mammalian Protein-Protein Interaction Database (MIPS-MPPI).

- Meta-databases normally result from the integration of primary databases information, but can also collect some original data. Examples: Agile Protein Interaction DataAnalyser (APID), The Microbial Protein Interaction Database (MPID8), and Protein Interaction Network Analysis (PINA) platform.

- Prediction databases include many PPIs that are predicted using several techniques. Examples: Michigan Molecular Interactions (MiMI), Human Protein-Protein Interaction Prediction Database (PIPs), Online Predicted Human Interaction Database (OPHID), Known and Predicted Protein-Protein Interactions (STRING), and Unified Human Interactome (UniHI).

Protein-protein Interaction Networks

Information found in PPIs databases supports the construction of interaction networks. Although the PPI network of a given query protein can be represented in textbooks, diagrams of whole cell PPIs are frankly complex and difficult to generate.

One example of a manually produced molecular interaction map is the Kurt Kohn's 1999 map of cell cycle control. Drawing on Kohn's map, Schwikowski and others in 2008 published a paper on PPIs in yeast, linking together 1548 interacting proteins determined by two-hybrid screening. They used a layered graph drawing method to find an initial placement of the nodes and then improved the layout using a force-based algorithm.

Bioinformatic tools have been developed to simplify the difficult task of visualise molecular interaction networks and complement them with other types of data. For instance, Cytoscape is an open-source software widely used and lots of plugins are currently available. Pajek software is advantageous for the visualisation and analysis of very large networks. The awareness of the major roles of PPIs in numerous physiological and pathological processes has been driving the challenge of unravel many interactomes. Examples of published interactomes are the thyroid specific DREAM interactome and the PP1α interactome in human brain.

Protein-protein Interaction as Therapeutic Targets

Modulation of PPI is challenging and is receiving increasing attention by the scientific community. Several properties of PPI such as allosteric sites and hotspots, have been incorporated into drug-design strategies. The relevance of PPI as putative therapeutic targets for the development of new treatments is particularly evident in cancer, with several ongoing clinical trials within this area. The consensus among these promising targets is, nonetheless, denoted in the already available drugs on the market to treat a multitude of diseases. Examples are Titrobifan, inhibitor of the glycoprotein IIb/IIIa, used as a cardiovascular drug, and Maraviroc, inhibitor of the CCR5-gp120 interaction, used as anti-HIV drug.

PROTEIN–PROTEIN INTERACTION PREDICTION

Protein–protein interaction prediction is a field combining bioinformatics and structural biology in an attempt to identify and catalog physical interactions between pairs or groups of proteins. Understanding protein–protein interactions is important for the investigation of intracellular signalling pathways, modelling of protein complex structures and for gaining insights into various biochemical processes.

Experimentally, physical interactions between pairs of proteins can be inferred from a variety of experimental techniques, including yeast two-hybrid systems, protein-fragment complementation assays (PCA), affinity purification/mass spectrometry, protein microarrays, fluorescence resonance energy transfer (FRET), and Microscale Thermophoresis (MST). Efforts to experimentally determine the interactome of numerous species are ongoing, and a number of computational methods for interaction prediction have been developed in recent years.

Methods

Proteins that interact are more likely to co-evolve, therefore, it is possible to make inferences about interactions between pairs of proteins based on their phylogenetic distances. It has also been observed in some cases that pairs of interacting proteins have fused orthologues in other organisms. In addition, a number of bound protein complexes have been structurally solved and can be used to identify the residues that mediate the interaction so that similar motifs can be located in other organisms.

Phylogenetic profiling

Phylogenetic profiling finds pairs of protein families with similar patterns of presence or absence across large numbers of species. This method is based on the hypothesis that potentially interacting proteins should co-evolve and should have orthologs in closely related species. That is, proteins that form complexes or are part of a pathway should be present simultaneously in order for them to function. A phylogenetic profile is constructed for each protein under investigation. The profile is basically a record of whether the protein is present in certain genomes. If two proteins are found to be present and absent in the same genomes, those proteins are deemed likely to be functionally related. A similar method can be applied to protein domains, where profiles are constructed for domains to determine if there are domain interactions. Some drawbacks with the phylogenetic profile methods are that they are computationally expensive to perform, they rely on homology detection between distant organisms, and they only identify if the proteins being investigated are functionally related (part of complex or in same pathway) and not if they have direct interactions.

Prediction of co-evolved protein pairs based on similar phylogenetic trees

It was observed that the phylogenetic trees of ligands and receptors were often more similar than due to random chance. This is likely because they faced similar selection pressures and co-evolved. This method uses the phylogenetic trees of protein pairs to determine if interactions exist. To do this, homologs of the proteins of interest are found (using a sequence search tool such as BLAST) and multiple-sequence alignments are done (with alignment tools such as Clustal) to build distance matrices for each of the proteins of interest. The distance matrices should then be used to build phylogenetic trees. However, comparisons between phylogenetic trees are difficult, and current methods circumvent this by simply comparing distance matrices. The distance matrices of the proteins are used to calculate a correlation coefficient, in which a larger value corresponds to co-evolution. The benefit of comparing distance matrices instead of phylogenetic trees is that the results do not depend on the method of tree building that was used. The downside is that difference matrices are not perfect representations of phylogenetic trees, and inaccuracies may result from using such a shortcut. Another factor worthy of note is that there are background similarities between the phylogenetic trees of any protein, even ones that do not interact. If left unaccounted for, this could lead to a high false-positive rate. For this reason, certain methods construct a background tree using 16S rRNA sequences which they use as the canonical tree of life.

The distance matrix constructed from this tree of life is then subtracted from the distance matrices of the proteins of interest. However, because RNA distance matrices and DNA distance matrices have different scale, presumably because RNA and DNA have different mutation rates, the RNA matrix needs to be rescaled before it can be subtracted from the DNA matrices. By using molecular clock proteins, the scaling coefficient for protein distance/RNA distance can be calculated. This coefficient is used to rescale the RNA matrix.

Rosetta stone method: A Rosetta stone protein is a protein chain composed of two fused proteins. It is observed that proteins or domains that interact with one another tend to have homologs in other genomes that are fused into a Rosetta stone protein. It is thought that the fusion helps optimise the co-expression of these proteins. The most obvious drawback of this method is that there are many protein interactions that cannot be discovered this way, it relies on the presence of Rosetta stone proteins. Also, like phylogenetic profile methods, the Rosetta stone method does not necessarily find interacting proteins, as there can be other reasons for the fusion of two proteins.

Classification methods

Classification methods use data to train a programme (classifier) to distinguish positive examples of interacting protein/domain pairs with negative examples of non-interacting pairs. Popular classifiers used are Random Forest Decision (RFD) and Support Vector Machines. RFD produces results based on the domain composition of interacting and non-interacting protein pairs. When given a protein pair to classify, RFD first creates a representation of the protein pair in a vector. The vector contains all the domain types used to train RFD, and for each domain type the vector also contains a value of 0, 1, or 2. If the protein pair does not contain a certain domain, then the value for that domain is 0. If one of the proteins of the pair contains the domain, then the value is 1. If both proteins contain the domain, then the value is 2. Using training data, RFD constructs a decision forest, consisting of many decision trees. Each decision tree evaluates several domains, and based on the presence or absence of interactions in these domains, makes a decision as to if the protein pair interacts.

The vector representation of the protein pair is evaluated by each tree to determine if they are an interacting pair or a non-interacting pair. The forest tallies up all the input from the trees to come up with a final decision. The strength of this method is that it does not assume that domains interact independent of each other. This makes it so that multiple domains in proteins can be used in the prediction. This is a big step up from previous methods which could only predict based on a single domain pair. The limitation of this method is that it relies on the training dataset to produce results. Thus, usage of different training datasets could influence the results.

Inference of interactions from homologous structures: This group of methods makes use of known protein complex structures to predict and structurally model interactions between query protein sequences. The prediction process generally starts by employing a sequence based method (e.g. interolog) to search for protein complex structures that are homologous to the query sequences. These known complex structures are then used as templates to structurally model the interaction between query sequences. This method has the advantage of not only inferring protein interactions but also suggests models of how proteins interact structurally, which can provide some insights into the atomic level mechanism of that interaction. On the other hand, the ability for these methods to make a prediction is constrained by a limited number of known protein complex structures.

Association methods

Association methods look for characteristic sequences or motifs that can help distinguish between interacting and non-interacting pairs. A classifier is trained by looking for sequence-signature pairs where one protein contains one sequence-signature, and its interacting partner contains another sequence-signature. They look specifically for sequence-signatures that are found together more often than by chance. This uses a log-odds score which is computed as $\log_2(Pij/PiPj)$, where Pij is the observed frequency of domains i and j occurring in one protein pair, Pi and Pj are the background frequencies of domains i and j in the data. Predicted domain interactions are those with positive log-odds scores and also having several occurrences within the database. The downside with this method is that it looks at each pair of interacting domains separately, and it assumes that they interact independently of each other.

Identification of structural patterns

This method builds a library of known protein–protein interfaces from the PDB, where the interfaces are defined as pairs of polypeptide fragments that are below a threshold slightly larger than the van der Waals radius of the atoms involved. The sequences in the library are then clustered based on structural alignment and redundant sequences are eliminated. The residues that have a high (generally >50%) level of frequency for a given position are considered hotspots. This library is then used to identify potential interactions between pairs of targets, providing that they have a known structure (i.e. present in the PDB).

Bayesian network modelling: Bayesian methods integrate data from a wide variety of sources, including both experimental results and prior computational predictions, and use these features to assess the likelihood that a particular potential protein interaction is a true positive result. These methods are useful because experimental procedures, particularly the yeast two-hybrid experiments, are extremely noisy and produce many false positives, while the previously mentioned computational methods can only provide circumstantial evidence that a particular pair of proteins might interact.

Domain-pair exclusion analysis: The domain-pair exclusion analysis detects specific domain interactions that are hard to detect using Bayesian methods. Bayesian methods are good at detecting nonspecific promiscuous interactions and not very good at detecting rare specific interactions. The domain-pair exclusion analysis method calculates an E-score which measures if two domains interact. It is calculated as log(probability that the two proteins interact given that the domains interact/probability that the two proteins interact given that the domains don't interact). The probabilities required in the formula are calculated using an Expectation Maximisation procedure, which is a method for estimating parameters in statistical models. High E-scores indicate that the two domains are likely to interact, while low scores indicate that other domains form the protein pair are more likely to be responsible for the interaction. The drawback with this method is that it does not take into account false positives and false negatives in the experimental data.

Supervised learning problem: The problem of PPI prediction can be framed as a supervised learning problem. In this paradigm the known protein interactions supervise the estimation of a function that can predict whether an interaction exists or not between two proteins given data about the proteins (e.g. expression levels of each gene in different experimental conditions, location information, phylogenetic profile, etc.).

Relationship to Docking Methods

The field of protein–protein interaction prediction is closely related to the field of protein–protein docking, which attempts to use geometric and steric considerations to fit two proteins of known structure into a bound complex. This is a useful mode of inquiry in cases where both proteins in the pair have known structures and are known (or at least strongly suspected) to interact, but since so many proteins do not have experimentally determined structures, sequence-based interaction prediction methods are especially useful in conjunction with experimental studies of an organism's interactome.

PROTEIN–PROTEIN INTERACTION SCREENING

The screening of protein–protein interactions refers to the identification of protein interactions with high-throughput screening methods such as computer- and/or robot-assisted plate reading, flow cytometry analysing. The interactions between proteins are central to virtually every process in a living cell. Information about these interactions improves understanding of diseases and can provide the basis for new therapeutic approaches.

Methods to Screen Protein–protein Interactions

Though there are many methods to detect protein–protein interactions, the majority of these methods— such as Co-immunoprecipitation, Fluorescence resonance energy transfer (FRET) and dual polarisation interferometry—are not screening approaches.

Ex vivo or in vivo methods

Methods that screen protein–protein interactions in the living cells.

- Bimolecular fluorescence complementation (BiFC) is a new technique for observing the interactions of proteins. Combining it with other new techniques DERB can enable the screening of protein–protein interactions and their modulators.
- The yeast two-hybrid screen investigates the interaction between artificial fusion proteins inside the nucleus of yeast. This approach can identify the binding partners of a protein without bias. However, the method has a notoriously high false-positive rate, which makes it necessary to verify the identified interactions by co-immunoprecipitation.

In vitro methods

- The Tandem affinity purification (TAP) method allows the high-throughput identification of proteins interactions. In contrast with the Y2H approach, the accuracy of the method can be compared to those of small-scale experiments and the interactions are detected within the correct cellular environment as by co-immunoprecipitation. However, the TAP tag method requires two successive steps of protein purification, and thus cannot readily detect transient protein–protein interactions. Recent genome-wide TAP experiments were performed by Krogan and Gavin providing updated protein interaction data for yeast organisms.
- Chemical cross-linking is often used to 'fix' protein interactions in place before trying to isolate/ identify interacting proteins. Common cross-linkers for this application include the non-cleavable [NHS-ester] cross-linker, [bis-sulpho-succinimidyl suberate] (BS3), a cleavable version of BS3, [dithiobis (sulpho-succinimidyl propionate)](DTSSP), and the [imidoester] crosslinker [dimethyl dithiobispropionimidate] (DTBP) that is popular for fixing interactions in ChIP assays.

SECTION II

Gene Mutation, DNA Repair, Transposable Elements and Ames Test

Chapter 3

Gene Mutations, DNA Repair and Transposable Elements

INTRODUCTION

Recall that the flow of information within a cell involves the transcription of DNA to mRNA and the translation of mRNA to protein. Recall also, that the flow of information between generations involves DNA replication and distribution to two daughter cells. Therefore, we would expect a change in DNA to be replicated and passed on to future generations and to affect protein structure and function if the change occurred in a gene that coded for that protein. These changes are called mutations.

Point mutations are the most common type of mutation. A single point mutation, also called a base substitution, occurs when a single nucleotide is replaced with a different nucleotide. A point mutation results in a base pair substitution after replication and possibly a mutant protein after transcription and translation. Various types of mutations are discussed in volume I in Chapter 15.

CREATIONARY CLASSIFICATION OF MUTATIONS

Mutations are normally classified according to their proximal effect on an organism's fitness, whether beneficial, deleterious, or neutral. While this is a very useful first-pass categorisation of mutations, the realisation that mutations are not always haphazard, but in fact may be part of a regulated design, means that creationists should be looking for a deeper classification of mutations based on whether or not they conform to their organism's design. Design-consistent mutations are those which occur within the pattern expected by the genome's architecture, and design-inconsistent mutations are those which occur outside of the genome's architecture. Features such as metabolic consistency, mutational mechanism, mutation rate, reversibility, and preservation of genome semantics can be used by biologists to assess whether or not a mutation is design-consistent or design-inconsistent.

Modern biochemistry has shown that the cell is a much more fascinating piece of machinery than ever would have been expected a century earlier. It has moved in our understanding from being a blob of protoplasm to an intricate wonder of nanotechnology. Likewise, our understanding of the genome and its intricacies has increased by leaps and bounds over the last few decades. While it was previously thought that only protein-coding genes would be relevant, it is now known that the regulation of protein-coding genes is just as important, if not more so. While it was previously thought to be intellectually irresponsible to consider a biological function for transposable elements, we are now understanding their ubiquity and importance in shaping the genome.

Our understanding of the process of mutation is undergoing a similar revolution. Historically, creationists and evolutionists have been in agreement that mutations which occur in organisms are haphazard—that is, there is no designed purpose for them. However, this understanding is beginning to change. It is becoming increasingly apparent that the cell itself can induce mutational processes in the right genes to produce beneficial changes at appropriate times. The most well-studied of these systems is the somatic hypermutation (SMH) system in the vertebrate immune system. In order to increase the binding potential of immunoglobulins to antigens, the cells direct mutations to a specific region of a specific gene in order to produce immunoglobulins that have a higher affinity to the antigens.

This mutational process skips the region of the gene which attaches to the B-cell entirely, and focuses only on the region of the gene which binds to the antigen. It is not deterministic—that is, the specific changes which are made seem to be stochastic—but the changes are focused to the right gene in the right situation, bypassing well over 99.99% of the genome and focusing on the correct few hundred base pairs which would matter.

More and more examples of focused mutations have been explored. Some transposable elements are triggered in direct response to specific cell stressors. For instance, Hall showed that *E. coli* can use insertion sequences to activate the gene required to metabolise beta-glucoside sugars. Simple sequence repeats (SSRs) have shown to mutate primarily in copy-number, acting as a genomic tuning knob or state switch. King, Trifonov, and Kashi enumerate several, including an AC repeat in a promoter which causes variation in body weight in Angus beef cattle, and an AC repeat in tilapia fish with similar effects. Bayless and Moxon report that a 4-nucleotide repeat (CAAC) can cause the lic2A gene of H. influenzae to switch between three states—off, low expression, and high expression—as it alters the reading frame on which the ATG start codon is found.

Semi-palindromic DNA often points to potentially beneficial areas where mutations might take place. For instance, one study of the genetic adaptation of *E. coli* to low glucose concentrations found identical modifications of the mgl operator sequence (mglO) in multiple populations. These were later found to be in loops that were near stem-loop structures in DNA, formed by semipalindromic sequences. Caporale has synthesised this new research into what she terms an 'implicit genome'. That is, a genome has an implicit range of mutations which are likely to occur, and these mutations are part of evolutionary strategies for organisms to survive changing environments. While Caporale and others attribute the creation of implicit genomes to indirect selection, this idea also seems to play well into a creationary understanding of the way that genomes should work. In fact, understanding cells to have internal mechanisms for large-scale genetic adaptation has been steadily growing in creation thinking over the last decade.

Need for a Second-Order Classification of Mutations

In the current literature of both creationists and evolutionists, mutations are often classified according to their effect on an organism's survival within a specific environment. A mutation is considered beneficial if it helps the organism survive, 'deleterious' if it hinders the organism, and 'neutral' or 'nearly-neutral' if there is little observed effect. This convention of using beneficial/neutral/deleterious for categorisation is useful because it can often be measured directly and quantitatively. Unfortunately, many people take these categorisations to signify more than can be inferred from them. For example, those who view all mutations as haphazard often view beneficial mutations as evidence of evolution. Likewise, those who view mutations as being possibly internally generated by a guided process within an organism may view the fact that a mutation is beneficial as being prima facie evidence that a mutation was internally generated, and likewise view the fact that a mutation is deleterious to be prima facie evidence that a mutation was haphazard.

Upon closer examination, however, knowing whether a mutation is 'beneficial', 'deleterious', or 'neutral' does not by itself tell us whether or not a given mutation occurred according to design or not. For instance, in order to survive large-scale environmental changes, populations of organisms may keep a supply of organisms with alternative biochemical configurations through a mutational process. Compared to the overall population of organisms, these mutations would actually be phenotypically deleterious, even though they are part of the overall biological design for hedging against possible environmental changes.

Likewise, a phenotypically beneficial mutation is not necessarily part of an overall design. Behe has termed this sort of event 'trench warfare'—the mutation may give a phenotypic advantage within a competitive environment, but at the cost of debilitating some important function of the organism. An easy example of this would be sickle-cell anemia—while it may be beneficial in some circumstances because it prevents malaria, the way it debilitates the person who has it overall leads to the conclusion that this was not a designed feature. Many other such locally beneficial mutations which have an overall deleterious effect on the complexity of a cell's biochemistry have been documented. Therefore, while the scale of beneficial/neutral/deleterious works well for a first-order classification of mutations, creation biologists should be looking deeper into a second-order classification based on its consistency with the design of the organism. This classification separates mutations into one of two possibilities—'design-consistent' mutations, and 'design-inconsistent' mutations. A 'design consistent' mutation is one which appears to have occurred within the genome's implicit range, and a 'design-inconsistent' mutation is one which appears to be haphazard (that is, philosophically random as described by Bartlett).

Guidelines for Determining Second Order Classification

The problem with a second-order classification system is that since we do not have total knowledge of the original plan, it makes it difficult to determine whether a mutation was consistent with that design or not. However, creationists can apply theological concepts to achieve a basic understanding of the plan, which can then illuminate our investigations, even in absence of full prior knowledge of the full plan. The notion of a Genesis 'created kind' (called baramins in creation biology) is a key theological notion which will aid our investigation. Because God created the animals according to their kinds (Genesis 1:11, 1:21, 1:24, 1:25), it can be presumed that the biological plan is a sort of dynamic stasis, where basic patterns are preserved, yet variance is allowed to aid in both survival of the baramin and the fulfillment of the baramin's role. The extent of the intended dynamic and static elements of the baramin are not known a priori. The criteria presented here should help creation biologists take the basic theological concepts provided by scripture, and combine these with the data of biology to achieve a fuller understanding of the pattern of life that God created. The following are several parameters which can be considered which will help make the second-order classification of mutations based on the assumed dynamic stasis of the original kinds.

Metabolic consistency

One of the major ways of determining whether or not a mutation is design-consistent is to look at the internal operation of the organism, examining the consistency of function of organisms with and without the mutation. Design-consistent mutations should maintain internal consistency whether or not they are beneficial within the current environment. It is hard to separate problems which occur from internal metabolic problems as opposed to those caused from the outside. However, a decent test of metabolic consistency in single-celled organisms would be whether or not a mutation caused metabolic problems for an organism which was growing in a nutrient-rich environment free of competition, predation, and toxic compounds. Similar stress-free environments could be constructed for testing the metabolic consistency of mutations in multicellular organisms.

Sickle-cell anemia, for instance, while it is beneficial as far as preventing malaria, causes large-scale functional problems for the organism even in the best environments. Therefore, the mutation causing sickle cell anemia is metabolically inconsistent, even though it may provide benefit in certain circumstances. Anderson pointed out that most drug resistant mutations of bacteria involve a fitness cost in most normal environments. However, for some of the mutations cited, the fitness cost was not severe, and therefore, by this criteria, would be considered metabolically consistent. In *Mycobacterium tuberculosis* (Fig. 3.1), for example, some mutations which confer rifampin resistance also do well in normal cultures. In the three mutations isolated by Billington, McHugh, and Gillespie, one mutation type had no relative fitness decreases, and another one had only moderate relative fitness decreases, thus indicating that they are metabolically consistent. One of the mutations had a drastic reduction in relative fitness, indicating that this mutation was probably not metabolically consistent.

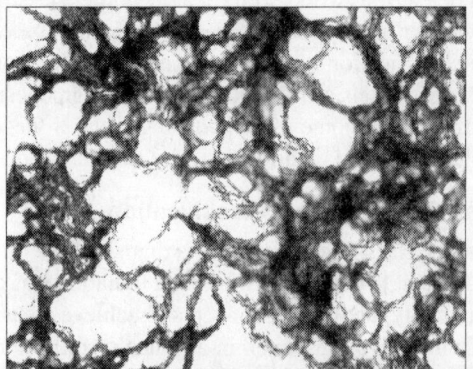

Fig. 3.1: *Mycobacterium tuberculosis.*

Mutational mechanism

A mutation which is in response to a specific stress or group of stresses, or is timed to occur with a particular stage of life for an organism, or for which there is an enzyme whose core function is to produce such a mutation, is likely to be design-consistent. Williams uses mutational mechanism as the primary differentiator between design-consistent mutations, which he terms as 'recombination', and design-inconsistent mutations, which he terms as simply 'mutations'. Other creationists have followed this approach as well. This criteria by itself is not sufficient, especially considering that the physical cause of many mutations is unknown. In addition, some design-consistent mutational events may be the result of DNA sequence alone, and may occur without specialised enzyme assistance. In addition, some mutational mechanisms may become mistargeted due to either a problem in the mutational mechanism or the sites which are targeted. An obvious example of a mutational mechanism would be the V(D)J recombination system used in the production of immunoglobulins. This system recombines three types of gene fragments (variable, diversity, and joining) into a nearly-limitless array of immunoglobulins. This system uses a combination of a pair of enzymes (RAG1 and RAG2) and a recombination signal sequence (RSS), to cut and splice gene fragments at the appropriate locations. However, this targeting mechanism can also lead to cancers when cryptic RSS sequences (sequences similar to the RSS used by V(D)J reactions, but in other parts of the genome) become accessible to the recombination enzymes.

As already mentioned that *E. coli* can use insertion sequences to activate the gene required to metabolise betaglucoside sugars. Because this mutation only occurs under the conditions where the mutation is needed, it can be inferred that this is the result of a cellular mechanism.

Mutation rate

A mutation which occurs at a significantly higher rate than the average mutation rate for the organism is likely to be design-consistent. This points to the mutation being part of the phenotype of the organism, rather than the mutation occurring arbitrarily. Even though we are living in a post-fall world, we assume that most of our biological systems function properly according to their design on a daily basis. Thus, a high mutation rate, especially across an entire population, is suggestive that a mutation is design-consistent. As with other considerations, this one must be used with care. Problematic mutations can cause a site to become mutationally active when it should not be. One test suggested by Bartlett in differentiating between a design-consistent and a design-inconsistent hotspot would be to compare the average fitness effects of mutations at that hotspot with the average fitness effects of induced arbitrary mutations. If the mutations in the hotspot tend to be metabolically consistent, and their relative fitness is greater than the relative fitness of organisms with arbitrary mutations, then this is evidence of a mutational hotspot being design-consistent. In the human genome, this appears to hold as a general pattern. Chuang and Li have noted that mutational hotspots tend to occur in genomic regions involved in extracellular communication, while mutational coldspots tend to occur in cellular housekeeping functions. Thus, the mutations seem to be targeted at areas which would provide adaptation to new environments, and silenced at areas which would more likely cause metabolic inconsistencies.

Reversibility

If a mutation is easily reversible (that is, the frequency of reversion is significantly greater than what would be expected from the overall mutation rate), this is good evidence that the mutation is design-consistent. If one of the purposes of mutations is to provide a hedge against environmental changes, then it would be reasonable to think that if the hedge is successful, the organism needs to be able to make a future hedge of going back to the original configuration. Therefore, reversibility is a key indicator of designconsistent mutations. SSRs are quite interesting subjects because, in general, they are both highly mutable as well as being easily reversible. Historically, they have been viewed as evolutionary by-products, or junk DNA. However, current research is continually finding new ways in which SSRs allow for the genome to adapt to changing circumstances.

Preservation of genomic semantics

Every day we are learning more and more about the semantics of the genome. The genome's semantics can be considered its internal logic—how different sequences serve to regulate and format the genome's function and adaptation. In computer programming, a programmes semantics is the set of rules, conventions, and axioms which are assumed to hold true as the programme progresses. Many mutations that lead to sickness are those which cause certain regions of the genome to operate in a semantically different way than before. For instance, some mutations have transformed a non-SSR sequence into an SSR. This causes the cell to modify the SSR's copy number where it would not have before. One example of this is in a heritable form of colorectal cancer. In this cancer, a T to A mutation creates a novel SSR. In later generations, the expansion of this SSR leads to colorectal cancer. Other types of signals may also be created improperly due to mutation, which could cause other systems to act on the wrong site (see for instance the previous discussion about V(D)J recombination).

Therefore, in many cases, the altering of the semantics of the genome often points to a design inconsistent mutation. However, this criteria should be used with care. DNA might contain a large quantity of meta-information. Meta-information is 'information about information'. If, for instance, the cell has sufficient meta-information about the roles of different DNA sequences (as opposed to simply the sequences themselves), there is no reason to think that it could not add or remove semantic elements as needed, using the meta-information as a guide. Dipterans, for example, have a class of transposable elements known as *mini-me* elements (microsatellite initiating mobile elements), which are retro-transposons that contain primers for SSRs. The functions of these are not well-characterised, but their abundance within Diptera (comprising, for instance, 1.2% of the *Drosophila melanogaster* genome), indicates that they are probably a part of the organism's design. Since scientific knowledge of genome semantics is still in its infancy, other factors such as metabolic consistency and precision should be considered in determining whether or not a violation of genomic semantics has taken place, or if the mutation is simply a part of a higher-level or undiscovered semantic within the cell.

Other considerations

These heuristic guidelines are certainly not complete, nor do any of them stand on their own. Nonetheless, when used in combination, they can open up a new way for creationists to look at mutational processes within cells. Hopefully as this categorisation is applied, additional considerations will be supplied to this list. Also note that the weighting of the various criteria are dependent on our understanding of God's general plan for organisms. If the goal is a dynamic stasis, then reversibility should be a heavily weighted factor. If the goal is for life to proceed according to a specific direction, then mutation rate should be weighted higher.

While the first-level classifications of mutations as beneficial, neutral, or deleterious is certainly useful, the perspective of creation biology can add additional depth by looking at whether or not a mutation is consistent with the cell's overall architecture, or if the mutation goes against that architecture. Only distinguishing between mutations on the basis of immediate fitness gains or losses can blind biologists to the architecture in which those mutations are made. By differentiating between design-consistent and design-inconsistent mutations, creation biologists can better understand the overall architecture of each baramin, and ultimately understand both God's purposes for these organisms as well as how humans can best cooperate with their designs in ecological and biotechnical endeavors.

EXPERIMENTAL METHODOLOGY

A basic outline of how an experimenter could test each of these criteria is given below. Because experimental mutational studies are generally easier on single-celled organisms which can be grown in a laboratory setting, these methodologies are tailored to that environment. Thus, the further work can expand upon these methodologies and demonstrate the most effective ways of experimentally determining whether mutations are design-consistent or design-inconsistent.

Metabolic Consistency

Metabolic consistency to determine metabolic consistency, plate both the wild-type and the mutant-type on several different media, and examine the relative fitness of the mutant-type on each. Compare the best fitness scores of both the wild-type and mutant-type. If the relative fitness of the mutant-type on its best media is significantly lower than the fitness of the wild-type on its best media, then the mutation is probably metabolically inconsistent. Further experimental work comparing relative fitness values of mutations in the context of the other criteria is required for determining what the relative fitness value ranges should be for a mutation to be considered metabolically consistent.

Mutational Mechanism

Mutational mechanism—this criteria is easy to rule in (by knowing a mutational mechanism capable of producing the mutation) but hard to rule out. If no known mutational mechanism causes the mutation, but a specific environmental inducer causes a specific or semi-specific mutational response, then it is reasonable to infer a mutational mechanism even without knowing what it is.

Mutation Rate

Mutation Rate—the rate of mutation should be compared to other sites within this organism's genome. If the production of this mutation is significantly higher than the average site for the organism, then a high mutation rate is established.

Reversibility

Reversibility—the reversion rate for a given mutation should be compared to the mutation rate for the mutant's original production. It is best if the specific gene sequences can be obtained for the wild-type, the mutant, and the reversion, in order to determine if the reversion is a true genetic reversion, or if a different mutation supplied the missing functionality. If the original mutation was a spontaneous mutation by the fluctuation test or the Lederberg test, then it is reasonable to think that the reversions should be spontaneous, too. If the original mutation is adaptive, however, then the reversion mutation might require a specific environmental signal to occur, and it might take some effort for the experimenter to determine what this signal is.

Preservation of Genomic Semantics

Preservation of Genomic Semantics—the interplay of the mutant sequence and the surrounding genetic context should be examined. Known genetic sequence motifs should be identified, as well as the mutation's impact on those motifs. If the mutation corrupts an existing motif, then it is likely that the mutation is violating genomic semantics. However, if a set of mutations are consistently altering motifs in narrow ways, then it is possible that the mutations are following an as-yet-unknown semantic rule within the cell.

DNA REPAIR MECHANISMS

Cells cannot function if DNA damage corrupts the integrity and accessibility of essential information in the genome (but cells remain superficially functional when so-called 'nonessential' genes are missing or damaged). Depending on the type of damage inflicted on the DNA's double helical structure, a variety of repair strategies have evolved to restore lost information. If possible, cells use the unmodified complementary strand of the DNA or the sister chromatid as a template to recover the original information.

Without access to a template, cells use an error-prone recovery mechanism known as translesion synthesis as a last resort (Fig. 3.2). Damage to DNA alters the spatial configuration of the helix and such alterations can be detected by the cell. Once damage is localised, specific DNA repair molecules bind at or near the site of damage, inducing other molecules to bind and form a complex that enables the actual repair to take place. The types of molecules involved and the mechanism of repair that is mobilised depend on the type of damage that has occurred and the phase of the cell cycle that the cell is in.

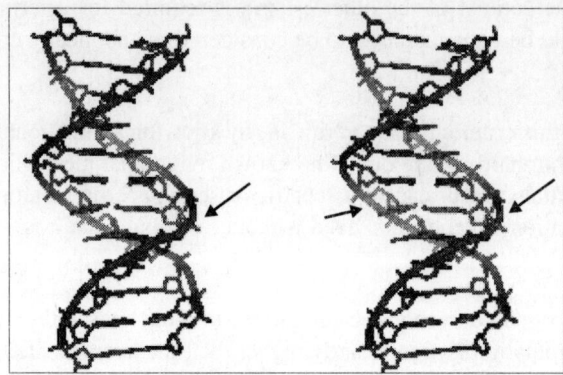

Fig. 3.2: Single strand and double strand DNA damage.

Direct Reversal

Cells are known to eliminate three types of damage to their DNA by chemically reversing it. These mechanisms do not require a template, since the types of damage they counteract can only occur in one of the four bases. Such direct reversal mechanisms are specific to the type of damage incurred and do not involve breakage of the phosphodiester backbone. The formation of thymine dimers (a common type of cyclobutyl dimer) upon irradiation with UV light results in an abnormal covalent bond between adjacent thymidine bases. The photoreactivation process directly reverses this damage by the action of the enzyme photolyase, whose activation is obligately dependent on energy absorbed from blue/UV light (300–500 nm wavelength) to promote catalysis. Another type of damage, methylation of guanine bases, is directly reversed by the protein methyl guanine methyl transferase (MGMT), the bacterial equivalent of which is called ogt. This is an expensive process because each MGMT molecule can only be used once, that is, the reaction is stoichiometric rather than catalytic. A generalised response to methylating agents in bacteria is known as the adaptive response and confers a level of resistance to alkylating agents upon sustained exposure by upregulation of alkylation repair enzymes. The third type of DNA damage reversed by cells is certain methylation of the bases cytosine and adenine.

Single Strand Damage

When only one of the two strands of a double helix has a defect, the other strand can be used as a template to guide the correction of the damaged strand. In order to repair damage to one of the two paired molecules of DNA, there exist a number of excision repair mechanisms that remove the damaged nucleotide and replace it with an undamaged nucleotide complementary to that found in the undamaged DNA strand.

1. Base excision repair (BER), which repairs damage to a single base caused by oxidation, alkylation, hydrolysis or deamination. The damaged base is removed by a DNA glycosylase. The 'missing

tooth' is then recognised by an enzyme called AP endonuclease, which cuts the phosphodiester bond. The missing part is then resynthesised by a DNA polymerase, and a DNA ligase performs the final nick-sealing step.

2. Nucleotide excision repair (NER), which recognises bulky, helix-distorting lesions such as pyrimidine dimers and 6,4-photoproducts. A specialised form of NER known as transcription-coupled repair deploys NER enzymes to genes that are being actively transcribed.

3. Mismatch repair (MMR), which corrects errors of DNA replication and recombination that result in mispaired (but undamaged) nucleotides.

Double-strand breaks

A double-strand break (DSBs) occurs in one of the paired DNAs followed by enzymatic trimming back of nucleotides on the new single-strand ends.

A free 3'-end invades the unbroken helix and displaces a loop of single strand DNA. A DNA polymerase elongates the free 3'-end of the invading strand, further displacing the looped out strand, which then pairs with an exposed single-strand on the opposing helix. The displaced strand serves as a template for enzymatic extension from the 3'-end of the paired single strand, which eventually crosses the junction and switches templates. As 3'- and 5'-ends meet, strands join to form two Holliday junctions.

There are two ways to resolve each Holliday junction by single cleavage and rejoining, so there are four ways to resolve the double Holliday structure by two cleavages and rejoinings. Two of these combinations of cleavage and rejoining generate non-crossover recombinants. The other two combinations of cleavage and rejoining generate crossover recombinants. All recombinants include heteroduplex segments. Double-strand breaks, in which both strands in the double helix are severed, are particularly hazardous to the cell because they can lead to genome rearrangements. Three mechanisms exist to repair DSBs: non-homologous end joining (NHEJ), microhomology-mediated end joining (MMEJ) and homologous recombination.

Homologous recombination requires the presence of an identical or nearly identical sequence to be used as a template for repair of the break. The enzymatic machinery responsible for this repair process is nearly identical to the machinery responsible for chromosomal crossover during meiosis. This pathway allows a damaged chromosome to be repaired using a sister chromatid (available in G2 after DNA replication) or a homologous chromosome as a template. DSBs caused by the replication machinery attempting to synthesise across a single-strand break or unrepaired lesion cause collapse of the replication fork and are typically repaired by recombination.

Topoisomerases introduce both single- and double-strand breaks in the course of changing the DNA's state of supercoiling, which is especially common in regions near an open replication fork. Such breaks are not considered DNA damage because they are a natural intermediate in the topoisomerase biochemical mechanism and are immediately repaired by the enzymes that created them.

Translesion synthesis

Translesion synthesis is a DNA damage tolerance process that allows the DNA replication machinery to replicate past DNA lesions such as thymine dimers or AP sites. It involves switching out regular DNA polymerases for specialised translesion polymerases (e.g. DNA polymerase V), often with larger active sites that can facilitate the insertion of bases opposite damaged nucleotides. The polymerase switching is thought to be mediated by, among other factors, the post-translational modification of the replication processivity factor PCNA. Translesion synthesis polymerases often have low fidelity (high propensity to insert wrong bases) relative to regular polymerases. However, many are extremely efficient at inserting correct bases opposite specific types of damage. For example, Pol η mediates error-free by-pass of lesions induced by UV irradiation, whereas Pol ζ introduces mutations at these sites. From a cellular perspective, risking the introduction of point mutations during translesion synthesis may be preferable to resorting to more drastic mechanisms of DNA repair, which may cause gross chromosomal aberrations or cell death.

GLOBAL RESPONSE TO DNA DAMAGE

Cells exposed to ionising radiation, ultraviolet light or chemicals are prone to acquire multiple sites of bulky DNA lesions and double-strand breaks. Moreover, DNA damaging agents can damage other biomolecules such as proteins, carbohydrates, lipids and RNA. The accumulation of damage, specifically double strand breaks or adducts stalling the replication forks, are among known stimulation signals for a global response to DNA damage. The global response to damage is an act directed toward the cells' own preservation and triggers multiple pathways of macromolecular repair, lesion by-pass, tolerance or apoptosis. The common features of global response are induction of multiple genes, cell cycle arrest, and inhibition of cell division.

DNA Damage Checkpoints

After DNA damage, cell cycle checkpoints are activated. Checkpoint activation pauses the cell cycle and gives the cell time to repair the damage before continuing to divide. DNA damage checkpoints occur at the G1/S and G2/M boundaries. An intra-S checkpoint also exists. Checkpoint activation is controlled by two master kinases, ATM and ATR. ATM responds to DNA double-strand breaks and disruptions in chromatin structure, whereas ATR primarily responds to stalled replication forks. These kinases phosphorylate downstream targets in a signal transduction cascade, eventually leading to cell cycle arrest.

Prokaryotic SOS Response

The SOS response is the term used to describe changes in gene expression in *Escherichia coli* and other bacteria in response to extensive DNA damage. The prokaryotic SOS system is regulated by two key proteins: LexA and RecA. The LexA homodimer is a transcriptional repressor that binds to operator sequences commonly referred to as SOS boxes. In *Escherichia coli* it is known that LexA regulates transcription of approximately 48 genes including the lexA and recA genes. The SOS response is known to be widespread in the bacteria domain, but it is mostly absent in some bacterial phyla, like the Spirochetes. The most common cellular signals activating the SOS response are regions of single-stranded DNA (ssDNA), arising from stalled replication forks or double-strand breaks, which are processed by DNA helicase to separate the two DNA strands. In the initiation step, RecA protein binds to ssDNA in an ATP hydrolysis driven reaction creating RecA–ssDNA filaments. RecA–ssDNA filaments activate LexA autoprotease activity which ultimately leads to cleavage of LexA dimer and subsequent LexA degradation. The loss of LexA repressor induces transcription of the SOS genes and allows for further signal induction, inhibition of cell division and an increase in levels of proteins responsible for damage processing. In *Escherichia coli*, SOS boxes are 20-nucleotide long sequences near promoters with palindromic structure and a high degree of sequence conservation. In other classes and phyla, the sequence of SOS boxes varies considerably, with different length and composition, but it is always highly conserved and one of the strongest short signals in the genome. The high information content of SOS boxes permits differential binding of LexA to different promoters and allows for timing of the SOS response. Logically, the lesion repair genes are induced at the beginning of SOS response. The error prone translesion polymerases, for example: UmuCD'2 (also called DNA polymerase V), are induced later on as a last resort. Once the DNA damage is repaired or by-passed using polymerases or through recombination, the amount of single-stranded DNA in cells is decreased, lowering the amounts of RecA filaments decreases cleavage activity of LexA homodimer which subsequently binds to the SOS boxes near promoters and restores normal gene expression.

Eukaryotic Transcriptional Responses to DNA Damage

Eukaryotic cells exposed to DNA damaging agents also activate important defensive pathways by inducing multiple proteins involved in DNA repair, cell cycle checkpoint control, protein trafficking and degradation. Such genome wide transcriptional response is very complex and tightly regulated, thus allowing coordinated global response to damage. Exposure of yeast *Saccharomyces cerevisiae* to DNA damaging agents results in overlapping but distinct transcriptional profiles.

Similarities to environmental shock response indicates that a general global stress response pathway exist at the level of transcriptional activation. In contrast, different human cell types respond to damage differently indicating an absence of a common global response. The probable explanation for this difference between yeast and human cells may be in the heterogeneity of mammalian cells. In an animal different types of cells are distributed amongst different organs which have evolved different sensitivities to DNA damage.

In general global response to DNA damage involves expression of multiple genes responsible for postreplication repair, homologous recombination, nucleotide excision repair, DNA damage checkpoint, global transcriptional activation, genes controlling mRNA decay and many others. A large amount of damage to a cell leaves it with an important decision: undergo apoptosis and die, or survive at the cost of living with a modified genome. An increase in tolerance to damage can lead to an increased rate of survival which will allow a greater accumulation of mutations. Yeast Rev1 and human polymerase η are members of Y family translesion DNA polymerases present during global response to DNA damage and are responsible for enhanced mutagenesis during a global response to DNA damage in eukaryotes.

DNA REPAIR AND AGEING

Pathological Effects of Poor DNA Repair

Experimental animals with genetic deficiencies in DNA repair often show decreased lifespan and increased cancer incidence. For example, mice deficient in the dominant NHEJ pathway and in telomere maintenance mechanisms get lymphoma and infections more often, and consequently have shorter lifespans than wild-type mice.

Similarly, mice deficient in a key repair and transcription protein that unwinds DNA helices have premature onset of ageing-related diseases and consequent shortening of lifespan. However, not every DNA repair deficiency creates exactly the predicted effects, mice deficient in the NER pathway exhibited shortened lifespan without correspondingly higher rates of mutation.

If the rate of DNA damage exceeds the capacity of the cell to repair it, the accumulation of errors can overwhelm the cell and result in early senescence, apoptosis or cancer. Inherited diseases associated with faulty DNA repair functioning result in premature ageing, increased sensitivity to carcinogens, and correspondingly increased cancer risk. On the other hand, organisms with enhanced DNA repair systems, such as *Deinococcus radiodurans*, the most radiation-resistant known organism, exhibit remarkable resistance to the double-strand break-inducing effects of radioactivity, likely due to enhanced efficiency of DNA repair and especially NHEJ.

Longevity and Caloric Restriction

A number of individual genes have been identified as influencing variations in lifespan within a population of organisms. The effects of these genes is strongly dependent on the environment, particularly on the organism's diet. Caloric restriction reproducibly results in extended lifespan in a variety of organisms, likely via nutrient sensing pathways and decreased metabolic rate. The molecular mechanisms by which such restriction results in lengthened lifespan are as yet unclear, however, the behaviour of many genes known to be involved in DNA repair is altered under conditions of caloric restriction (Fig. 3.3).

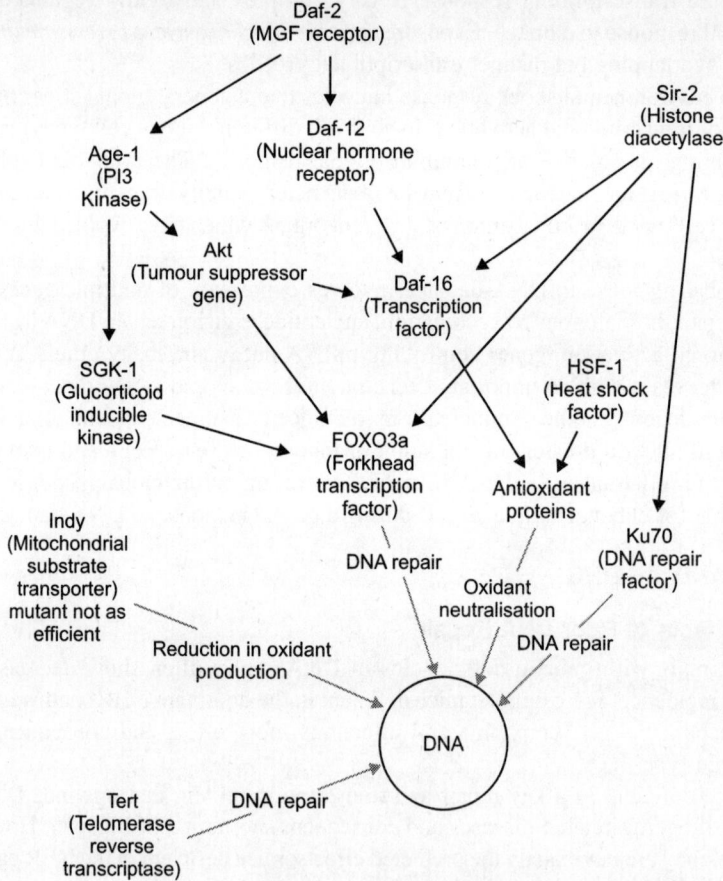

Fig. 3.3: Most lifespan influencing genes affect the rate of DNA damage.

For example, increasing the gene dosage of the gene Sir-2, which regulates DNA packaging in the nematode worm *Caenorhabditis elegans*, can significantly extend lifespan. The mammalian homologue of Sir-2 is known to induce downstream DNA repair factors involved in NHEJ, an activity that is especially promoted under conditions of caloric restriction. Caloric restriction has been closely linked to the rate of base excision repair in the nuclear DNA of rodents, although similar effects have not been observed in mitochondrial DNA.

Interestingly, the *C. elegans* gene AgE-1, an upstream effector of DNA repair pathways, confers dramatically extended life span under free-feeding conditions but leads to a decrease in reproductive fitness under conditions of caloric restriction. This observation supports the pleiotropy theory of the biological origins of ageing, which suggests that genes conferring a large survival advantage early in life will be selected for even if they carry a corresponding disadvantage late in life.

MEDICINE AND DNA REPAIR MODULATION

Hereditary DNA Repair Disorders

Defects in the NER mechanism are responsible for several genetic disorders, including:

1. Xeroderma pigmentosum: Hypersensitivity to sunlight/UV, resulting in increased skin cancer incidence and premature ageing.
2. Cockayne syndrome: Hypersensitivity to UV and chemical agents.
3. Trichothiodystrophy: Sensitive skin, brittle hair and nails.

Mental retardation often accompanies the latter two disorders, suggesting increased vulnerability of developmental neurons.

Other DNA repair disorders include:

1. Werner's syndrome: Premature ageing and retarded growth.
2. Bloom's syndrome: Sunlight hypersensitivity, high incidence of malignancies (especially leukemias).
3. Ataxia telangiectasia: Sensitivity to ionising radiation and some chemical agents.

All of the above diseases are often called 'segmental progerias' (accelerated ageing diseases) because their victims appear elderly and suffer from ageing-related diseases at an abnormally young age, while not manifesting all the symptoms of old age. Other diseases associated with reduced DNA repair function include Fanconi's anemia, hereditary breast cancer and hereditary colon cancer.

DNA Repair and Cancer

Inherited mutations that affect DNA repair genes are strongly associated with high cancer risks in humans. Hereditary nonpolyposis colorectal cancer (HNPCC) is strongly associated with specific mutations in the DNA mismatch repair pathway. BRCA1 and BRCA2, two famous mutations conferring a hugely increased risk of breast cancer on carriers, are both associated with a large number of DNA repair pathways, especially NHEJ and homologous recombination.

Cancer therapy procedures such as chemotherapy and radiotherapy work by overwhelming the capacity of the cell to repair DNA damage, resulting in cell death. Cells that are most rapidly dividing—most typically cancer cells—are preferentially affected. The side effect is that other noncancerous but rapidly dividing cells such as stem cells in the bone marrow are also affected. Modern cancer treatments attempt to localise the DNA damage to cells and tissues only associated with cancer, either by physical means (concentrating the therapeutic agent in the region of the tumour) or by biochemical means (exploiting a feature unique to cancer cells in the body).

DNA REPAIR AND EVOLUTION

The basic processes of DNA repair are highly conserved among both prokaryotes and eukaryotes and even among bacteriophage (viruses that infect bacteria), however, more complex organisms with more complex genomes have correspondingly more complex repair mechanisms. The ability of a large number of protein structural motifs to catalyse relevant chemical reactions has played a significant role in the elaboration of repair mechanisms during evolution. For an extremely detailed review of hypotheses relating to the evolution of DNA repair. Nucleic acids became the sole and universal means of encoding genetic information, requiring DNA repair mechanisms that in their basic form have been inherited by all extant life forms from their common ancestor. The emergence of earth's oxygen-rich atmosphere (known as the 'oxygen catastrophe') due to photosynthetic organisms, as well as the presence of potentially damaging free radicals in the cell due to oxidative phosphorylation, necessitated the evolution of DNA repair mechanisms that act specifically to counter the types of damage induced by oxidative stress.

Rate of Evolutionary Change

On some occasions, DNA damage is not repaired or is repaired by an error-prone mechanism which results in a change from the original sequence. When this occurs, mutations may propagate into the genomes of the cell's progeny. Should such an event occur in a germ line cell that will eventually produce a gamete, the mutation has the potential to be passed on to the organism's offspring. The rate of evolution in a particular species (or, more narrowly, in a particular gene) is a function of the rate of mutation. Consequently, the rate and accuracy of DNA repair mechanisms have an influence over the process of evolutionary change.

TRANSPOSABLE GENETIC ELEMENTS

Transposable genetic elements are segments of DNA that have the capacity to move from one location to another (i.e. jumping genes).

Properties of Transposable Genetic Elements

1. Random movement: Transposable genetic elements can move from any DNA molecule to any DNA other molecule or even to another location on the same molecule. The movement is not totally random, there are preferred sites in a DNA molecule at which the transposable genetic element will insert.

2. Not capable of self replication: The transposable genetic elements do not exist autonomously and thus, to be replicated they must be a part of some other replicon.

3. Transposition mediated by site-specific recombination: Transposition requires little or no homology between the current location and the new site. The trans-position event is mediated by an enzyme transposase that is coded by the transposable genetic element. Recombination that does not require homology between the recombining molecules is called illegitimate or nonhomologous recombination.

4. Transposition can be accompanied by duplication: In many instances transposition of the transposable genetic element results in removal of the element from the original site and insertion at a new site. However, in some cases the transposition event is accompanied by the duplication of the transposable genetic element. One copy remains at the original site and the other is transposed to the new site.

Types of Transposable Genetic Elements

1. Insertion sequences (IS): Insertion sequences are transposable genetic elements that carry no known genes except those that are required for transposition. Insertion sequences are small stretches of DNA that have at their ends repeated sequences, which are involved in transposition. In between the terminal repeated sequences there are genes involved in transposition and sequences that can control the expression of the genes but no other nonessential genes are present.

2. Importance of IS:
   (a) Mutation: The introduction of an insertion sequence into a bacterial gene will result in the inactivation of the gene.
   (b) The sites at which plasmids insert into the bacterial chromosome are at or near insertion sequence in the chromosome.
   (c) Phase Variation: In *Salmonella* there are two genes, which code for two antigenically different flagellar antigens. The expression of these genes is regulated by an insertion sequences.

3. Transposons: Transposons are transposable genetic elements that carry one or more other genes in addition to those, which are essential for transposition. The structure of a transposon is similar to that of an insertion sequence. The extra genes are located between the terminal repeated sequences.

Importance of transposons: Many antibiotic resistance genes are located on transposons. Since transposons can jump from one DNA molecule to another, these antibiotic resistance transposons are a major factor in the development of plasmids, which can confer multiple drug resistance on a bacterium harbouring such a plasmid. These multiple drug resistance plasmids have become a major medical problem.

GENETIC MECHANISM OF DRUG RESISTANCE

Antibiotic resistance in bacteria may either be intrinsic or acquired. Intrinsic resistance means that the bacteria were resistant to the antibiotic even before the antibiotic was introduced. Acquired resistance means that a bacterium that was previously sensitive to an antibiotic has now turned resistant. It is the acquired resistance that is of great importance because it would result in treatment failure as well as potential dissemination of resistance to other bacteria.

The physiological mechanisms of antibiotic resistance include:

1. Inactivation of the antibiotic by enzymes produced by the bacteria.
2. Alteration of target proteins such that the antibiotic doesn't bind or binds with decreased affinity.
3. Alteration of the membrane which decreases the permeability of the antibiotic.
4. Active efflux of the antibiotic.
5. Development of alternate metabolic pathway to bypass the action of antibiotic.

TEN THINGS WE SHOULD KNOW ABOUT TRANSPOSABLE ELEMENTS

1. Transposable elements come in many different forms and shapes: Transposable elements (TEs) are DNA sequences that have the ability to change their position within a genome. As a result of their deep evolutionary origins and continuous diversification, TEs come in a bewildering variety of forms and shapes. TEs can be divided into two major classes based on their mechanism of

transposition, and each class can be subdivided into subclasses based on the mechanism of chromosomal integration. Class 1 elements, also known as retrotransposons, mobilise through a 'copy-and-paste' mechanism whereby a RNA intermediate is reverse-transcribed into a cDNA copy that is integrated elsewhere in the genome. For long terminal repeat (LTR) retrotransposons, integration occurs by means of a cleavage and strand-transfer reaction catalysed by an integrase much like retroviruses. For non-LTR retrotransposons, which include both long and short interspersed nuclear elements (LINEs and SINEs), chromosomal integration is coupled to the reverse transcription through a process referred to as target-primed reverse transcription. Class 2 elements, also known as DNA transposons, are mobilised via a DNA intermediate, either directly through a 'cut-and-paste' mechanism or, in the case of Helitrons, a 'peel-and-paste' replicative mechanism involving a circular DNA intermediate. Each TE subclass is further divided into subgroups (or superfamilies) that are typically found across a wide range of organisms, but share a common genetic organisation and a monophyletic origin. For example, Ty3/gypsy and Ty1/copia elements are two major superfamilies of LTR retrotransposons that occur in virtually all major groups of eukaryotes. Similarly, Tc1/mariner, hAT (hobo-Ac-Tam3), and MULEs (Mutator-like elements) are three superfamilies of DNA transposons that are widespread across the eukaryotic tree. At the most detailed level of TE classification, elements are grouped into families or subfamilies, which can be defined as a closely related group of elements that can be traced as descendants of a single ancestral unit. This ancestral copy can be inferred as a consensus sequence, which is representative of the entire (sub)family. Thus, in principle, every TE sequence in a genome can be affiliated to a (sub)family, superfamily, subclass, and class. However, much like the taxonomy of species, the classification of TEs is in constant flux, perpetually subject to revision due to the discovery of completely novel TE types, the introduction of new levels of granularity in the classification, and ongoing development of methods and criteria to detect and classify TEs.

2. TEs are not randomly distributed in the genome: The genome may be viewed as an ecosystem inhabited by diverse communities of TEs, which seek to propagate and multiply through sophisticated interactions with each other and with other components of the cell. These interactions encompass processes familiar to ecologists, such as parasitism, cooperation, and competition. Thus, it is perhaps not surprising that TEs are rarely, if ever, randomly distributed in the genome. TEs exhibit various levels of preference for insertion within certain features or compartments of the genome. These are often guided by opposite selective forces, a balancing act of facilitating future propagation while mitigating deleterious effects on host cell function. At the most extreme end of the site-selection spectrum, many elements have evolved mechanisms to target specific loci where their insertions are less detrimental to the host but favorable for their propagation. For instance, several retrotransposons in species as diverse as slime mold and budding and fission yeast have evolved independently, but convergently, the capacity to target the upstream regions of genes transcribed by RNA polymerase III, where they do not appear to affect host gene expression but retain the ability to be transcribed themselves.

Natural selection and genetic drift are also powerful forces shaping the distribution and accumulation of TEs. Insertions that are strongly deleterious are rapidly removed from the population. Insertions that have little or no effects on genome function and host fitness may reach fixation according to the efficiency of selection and drift at purging these insertions from the population, which vary greatly among species. Selective forces can explain why some elements are more likely to be retained in certain genomic locations than others. For instance, *de novo* insertions of the human

LINE 1 (L1) retrotransposon readily occur within (and disrupt) gene exons, but very few if any L1 elements have been fixed within the coding region of human genes. Similarly, no LTR retrotransposon is known to exhibit insertion preference with regard to which DNA strand is transcribed, and yet these elements are strongly depleted in the sense orientation within human introns—most likely due to their propensity to interfere with gene splicing and polyadenylation when inserted in sense orientation. Perhaps because of some of these shared properties, the evolutionary trajectories of TE accumulation in mammals were found to be conserved across species in spite of clade specific differences in TE content. Thus, the success and diversity of TEs in a genome are shaped both by properties intrinsic to the elements as well as evolutionary forces acting at the level of the host species. A solid comprehension of how these forces act together is paramount to understanding the impact of TEs on organismal biology.

3. TEs are an extensive source of mutations and genetic polymorphisms: TEs occupy a substantial portion of the genome of a species, including a large fraction of the DNA unique to that species. In maize, where Barbara McClintock did her seminal work, an astonishing 60 to 70% of the genome is comprised of LTR retrotransposons, many of which are unique to this species or its close wild relatives, but the less prevalent DNA transposons are currently the most active and mutagenic. Similarly, the vast majority of TE insertions in *Drosophila melanogaster* are absent at the orthologous site in its closest relative *D. simulans* (and *vice versa*), and most are not fixed in the population. Many TE families are still actively transposing and the process is highly mutagenic, more than half of all known phenotypic mutants of D. melanogaster isolated in the laboratory are caused by spontaneous insertions of a wide variety of TEs. Transposition events are also common and mutagenic in laboratory mice, where ongoing activity of several families of LTR elements are responsible for 10–15% of all inherited mutant phenotypes. This contribution of TEs to genetic diversity may be underestimated, as TEs can be more active when organisms are under stress, such as in their natural environment.

Because TE insertions rarely provide an immediate fitness advantage to their host, those reaching fixation in the population do so largely by genetic drift and are subsequently eroded by point mutations that accumulate neutrally. Over time, these mutations result in TEs that can no longer encode transposition enzymes and produce new integration events. For instance, our (haploid) genome contains ~500000 L1 copies, but more than 99.9% of these L1 copies are fixed and no longer mobile due to various forms of mutations and truncations. It is estimated that each person carries a set of ~100 active L1 elements, and most of these are young insertions still segregating within the human population. Thus, as for any other organism, the 'reference' human genome sequence does not represent a comprehensive inventory of TEs in humans. Thousands of 'non-reference', unfixed TE insertions have been catalogued through whole genome sequencing and other targeted approaches. On average, any two human haploid genomes differ by approximately a thousand TE insertions, primarily from the L1 or Alu families. The number of TE insertion polymorphisms in a species with much higher TE activity such as maize dwarfs the number in humans.

If TEs bring no immediate benefit to their host and are largely decaying neutrally once inserted, how do they persist in evolution? One key to this conundrum is the ability of TEs not only to propagate vertically but also horizontally between individuals and species. There is now a large body of evidence supporting the idea that horizontal transposon transfer is a common phenomenon that affects virtually every major type of TE and all branches of the tree of life. While the cellular mechanisms underlying horizontal transposon transfer remain murky, it is increasingly apparent that the intrinsic mobility of TEs and ecological interactions between their host species, including those with pathogens and parasites, facilitate the transmission of elements between widely diverged taxa.

4. TEs are associated with genome rearrangements and unique chromosome features: Transposition represents a potent mechanism of genome expansion that over time is counteracted by the removal of DNA via deletion. The balance between the two processes is a major driver in the evolution of genome size in eukaryotes. Several studies have demonstrated the impact and range of this shuffling and cycling of genomic content on the evolution of plant and animal genomes. Because the insertion and removal of TEs is often imprecise, these processes can indirectly affect surrounding host sequences. Some of these events occur at high enough frequency to result in vast amounts of duplication and reshuffling of host sequences, including genes and regulatory sequences. For example, a single group of DNA transposons (MULEs) has been responsible for the capture and reshuffling of ~1000 gene fragments in the rice genome. Such studies have led to the conclusion that the rate at which TEs transpose, which is in part under host control, is an important driver of genome evolution.

   In addition to rearrangements induced as a byproduct of transposition, TEs can promote genomic structural variation long after they have lost the capacity to mobilise. In particular, recombination events can occur between the highly homologous regions dispersed by related TEs at distant genomic positions and result in large-scale deletions, duplications, and inversions. TEs also provide regions of microhomology that predispose to template switching during repair of replication errors leading to another source of structural variants. These non-transposition-based mechanisms for TE-induced or TE-enabled structural variation have contributed substantially to genome evolution. These processes can also make the identification of actively transposing elements more difficult in population studies that infer the existence of active elements through the detection of non-reference insertions.

   TEs also contribute to specialised chromosome features. An intriguing example is in *Drosophila*, where LINE-like retrotransposons form and maintain the telomeres in replacement of the telomerase enzyme which has been lost during dipteran evolution. This domestication event could be viewed as a replay of what might have happened much earlier in eukaryotic evolution to solve the 'end problem' created by the linearisation of chromosomes. Indeed, the reverse transcriptase component of telomerase is thought to have originated from an ancient lineage of retroelements. TE sequences and domesticated transposase genes also play structural roles at centromeres.

5. There is an intrinsic balance between TE expression and repression: To persist in evolution, TEs must strike a delicate balance between expression and repression. Expression should be sufficient to promote amplification, but not so vigorous as to lead to a fitness disadvantage for the host that would offset the benefit to the TE of increased copy numbers. This balancing act may explain why TE-encoded enzymes are naturally suboptimal for transposition and why some TEs have evolved self-regulatory mechanisms controlling their own copy numbers. A variety of host factors are also employed to control TE expression, which includes a variety of small RNA, chromatin, and DNA modification pathways, as well as sequence-specific repressors such as the recently profiled KRAB zinc-finger proteins. However, many of these silencing mechanisms must be at least partially released to permit developmental regulation of host gene expression programmes, particularly during early embryonic development. For example, genome-wide loss of DNA methylation is necessary to reset imprinted genes in primordial germ cells. This affords TEs an opportunity, as

reduced DNA methylation often promotes TE expression. Robust expression of a TE in the germ lineage (but not necessarily in the gametes themselves) is often its own downfall. In one example of a clever trick employed by the host, TE repression is relieved in a companion cell derived from the same meiotic product as flowering plant sperm. However, this companion cell does not contribute genetic material to the next generation. Thus, although TEs transpose in a meiotic product, the events are not inherited. Instead, TE activity in the companion cell may further dampen TE activity in sperm via the import of TE-derived small RNAs.

Another important consequence of the intrinsic expression/repression balance is that the effects of TEs on a host can vary considerably among tissue types and stages of an organism's life cycle. From the TE's perspective, an ideal scenario is to be expressed and active in the germline, but not in the soma, where expression would gain the TE no advantage, only disadvantage. This is indeed observed among many species, with ciliates representing an extreme example of this division—TEs are actively deleted from the somatic macronucleus but retained in the micronucleus, or germline. Another example is the P-elements in *Drosophila*, which are differentially spliced in the germline versus soma. Many organisms, including plants, do not differentiate germ lineage cells early in development, rather, they are specified from somatic cells shortly before meiosis commences. Thus, TEs that transpose in somatic cells in plants have the potential to be inherited, which suggests that the interest of TEs and host are in conflict across many more cells and tissues than in animals with a segregated germline.

6. TEs are insertional mutagens in both germline and soma: Like other species, humans contend with a contingent of currently active TEs where the intrinsic balance between expression and repression is still at play. For us, this includes L1 and other mobile elements that depend on L1-encoded proteins for retrotransposition. These elements are responsible for new germline insertions that can cause genetic disease. More than 120 independent TE insertions have been associated with human disease. The rate of *de novo* germline transposition in humans is approximately one in 21 births for Alu and one in 95 births for L1.

Historically, little attention has been given to transposition in somatic cells and its consequences, because somatic transposition may be viewed as an evolutionary dead-end for the TE with no long-term consequences for the host species. Yet, there is abundant evidence that TEs are active in somatic cells in many organisms. In humans, L1 expression and transposition have been detected in a variety of somatic contexts, including early embryos and certain stem cells. There is also a great deal of interest in mobile element expression and activity in the mammalian brain, where L1 transposition has been proposed to diversify neuronal cell populations. One challenge for assessing somatic activity has rested with the development of reliable single cell insertion site mapping strategies.

Somatic activity has also been observed in human cancers, where tumors can acquire hundreds of new L1 insertions. Just like for human polymorphisms, somatic activity in human cancers is caused by small numbers of so-called 'hot' L1 loci. The activities of these master copies varies depending on the individual, tumor type, and timeframe in the clonal evolution of the tumor. Some of these *de novo* L1 insertions disrupt critical tumor suppressors and oncogenes and thus drive cancer formation, although the vast majority appear to be 'passenger' mutations. Host cells have evolved several mechanisms to keep TEs in check. However, as the force of natural selection begins to diminish with age and completely drops in post-reproductive life, TEs may become more active.

7. TEs can be damaging in ways that do not involve transposition: TEs are best known for their mobility, in other words their ability to transpose to new locations. While the breakage and insertion of DNA associated with transposition represents an obvious source of cell damage, this is not the only or perhaps even the most common mechanism by which TEs can be harmful to their host. Reactivated transposons harm the host in multiple ways. First, de-repression of transposon loci, including their own transcription, may interfere with transcription or processing of host mRNAs through a myriad of mechanisms. Genome-wide transcriptional de-repression of TEs has been documented during replicative senescence of human cells and several mouse tissues, including liver, muscle, and brain. De-repression of LTR and L1 promoters can also cause oncogene activation in cancer. Second, TE-encoded proteins such as the endonuclease activity of L1 ORF2p can induce DNA breaks and genomic instability. Third, accumulation of RNA transcripts and extrachromosomal DNA copies derived from TEs may trigger an innate immune response leading to autoimmune diseases and sterile inflammation. Activation of interferon response is now a well-documented property of transcripts derived from endogenous retroviruses and may give immunotherapies a boost in identifying and attacking cancer cells. The relative contribution of all the above mechanisms in organismal pathologies remains to be determined.

Following transcription (and sometimes splicing) of TEs, the next step in the process involves translation of the encoded proteins and, for retroelements, reverse transcription of the TEs into cDNA substrates suitable for transposition. Once engaged by a TE-encoded reverse transcriptase protein, the resulting cytosolic DNAs and RNA:DNA hybrids can alert inflammatory pathways. An example of this is seen in patients with Aicardi–Goutières syndrome, where accumulation of TE-derived cytosolic DNA is due to mutations in pathways that normally block TE processing or degrade TE-derived DNA. Although not all TEs encode functional proteins, some do, including a few endogenous retroviruses capable of producing Gag, Pol, or envelope (Env) proteins. Over expression of these Env proteins can be cytotoxic, and has been linked to at least two neuro-degenerative diseases, multiple sclerosis and amytrophic lateral sclerosis. Small accessory proteins produced by the youngest human endogenous retrovirus (HERV) group, HERV-K (HML-2), may play a role in some cancers but the evidence remains circumstantial.

8. A number of key coding and non-coding RNAs are derived from TEs: Although usually detrimental, there is growing evidence that TE insertions can provide raw material for the emergence of protein-coding genes and non-coding RNAs, which can take on important and, in some cases essential, cellular function. The process of TE gene 'domestication' or exaptation over evolutionary time contributes to both deeply conserved functions and more recent, species-specific traits. Most often, the ancestral or a somewhat modified role of a TE-encoded gene is harnessed by the host and conserved, while the rest of the TE sequence, and hence its ability to autonomously transpose, has been lost. Spectacular examples of deeply conserved TE-derived genes are Rag1 and Rag2, that catalyse V(D)J somatic recombination in the vertebrate immune system. Both genes, and probably the DNA signals they recognise, were derived from an ancestral DNA transposon around 500 million years ago. Indeed, DNA transposases have been co-opted multiple times to form new cellular genes.

The gag and env genes of LTR retrotransposons or endogenous retroviruses (ERVs) have also been domesticated numerous times to perform functions in placental development, contribute to host defense against exogenous retroviruses, act in brain development, and play other diverse roles. One of the most intriguing examples of TE domestication is the repeated, independent capture of ERV env genes, termed syncytins, which appear to function in placentation by facilitating cell–cell fusion and syncytiotrophoblast formation. Notably, one or more such syncytin genes have been found in virtually every placental mammalian lineage where they have been sought, strongly suggesting that ERVs have played essential roles in the evolution and extreme phenotypic variability of the mammalian placenta. Another example of a viral-like activity re-purposed for host cell function is provided by the neuronal Arc gene, which arose from the gag gene from a LTR retrotransposon domesticated in the common ancestor of tetrapod vertebrates. Genetic and biochemical studies of murine Arc show that it is involved in memory and synaptic plasticity and has preserved most of the ancestral activities of Gag, including the packaging and intercellular trafficking of its own RNA. Remarkably, flies appear to have independently evolved a similar system of trans-synaptic RNA delivery involving a gag-like protein derived from a similar yet distinct lineage of LTR retrotransposons. Thus, the biochemical activities of TE-derived proteins have been repeatedly co-opted during evolution to foster the emergence of convergent cellular innovations in different organisms.

TEs can donate their own genes to the host, but they can also add exons and rearrange and duplicate existing host genes. In humans, intronic Alu elements are particularly prone to be captured as alternative exons through cryptic splice sites residing within their sequences. L1 and SVA (SINE/VNTR/Alu) elements also contribute to exon shuffling through transduction events of adjacent host sequences during their mobilisation. The reverse transcriptase activity of retroelements is also responsible for the trans-duplication of cellular mRNAs to create 'processed' retrogenes in a wide range of organisms. The L1 enzymatic machinery is thought to be involved in the generation of tens of thousands of retrogene copies in mammalian genomes, many of which remain transcribed and some of which have acquired new cellular functions. This is a process still actively shaping our genomes, it has been estimated that 1 in every 6000 humans carries a novel retrogene insertion. TEs also make substantial contributions to non-protein coding functions of the cell. They are major components of thousands of long non-coding RNAs in human and mouse genomes, often transcriptionally driven by retroviral LTRs. Some of these TE-driven lncRNAs appear to play important roles in the maintenance of stem cell pluripotency and other developmental processes. Many studies have demonstrated that TE sequences embedded within lncRNAs and mRNAs can directly modulate RNA stability, processing, or localisation with important regulatory consequences. Furthermore, TE-derived microRNAs and other small RNAs processed from TEs can also adopt regulatory roles serving host cell functions. The myriad of mechanisms by which TEs contribute to coding and non-coding RNAs illustrate the multi-faceted interactions between these elements and their host.

9. TEs contribute *cis*-regulatory DNA elements and modify transcriptional networks: *Cis*-regulatory networks coordinate the transcription of multiple genes that function in concert to orchestrate entire pathways and complex biological processes. In line with Barbara McClintock's insightful predictions, there is now mounting evidence that TEs have been a rich source of material for the modulation of eukaryotic gene expression. Indeed, TEs can disperse vast amounts of promoters and enhancers, transcription factor binding sites, insulator sequences, and repressive elements. The varying coat colours of agouti mice provides a striking example of a host gene controlling coat colour whose expression can be altered by the methylation levels of a TE upstream of its promoter. In the oil palm, the methylation level of a TE that sits within a gene important for flowering ultimately controls whether or not the plants bear oil-rich fruit.

As TE families typically populate a genome as a multitude of related copies, it has long been postulated that they have the potential to donate the same *cis*-regulatory module to 'wire' batteries of genes dispersed throughout the genome. An increasing number of studies support this model and suggest that TEs have provided the building blocks for the assembly and remodeling of *cis*-regulatory networks during evolution, including pathways underlying processes as diverse as pregnancy, stem cell pluripotency, neocortex development, innate immunity in mammals, or the response to abiotic stress in maize. Indeed, TE sequences harbor all the necessary features of a 'classical' gene regulatory network. They are bound by diverse sets of transcription factors integrate multiple inputs (activation/repression), respond to signals in both *cis* and trans, and are capable of co-ordinately regulating gene expression. In this context, TEs are highly suitable agents to modify biological processes by creating novel *cis*-regulatory circuits and fine-tuning pre-existing networks.

10. Analysing TEs requires specialised tools: TEs have been historically neglected and remain frequently ignored in genomic studies in part because of their repetitive nature, which poses a number of analytical challenges and often requires the use of specialised tools. As genomes can harbor thousands of copies of very similar TE sequences, uniqueness or, alternatively, repetitiveness of substrings within these regions need to be taken into consideration during both experimental design and analysis. As an example, short DNA oligos targeting a specific TE instance in the genome for PCR, short hairpin RNA, or CRISPR-Cas9 have to be carefully designed and validated to ensure that they are truly specific and target unique regions of the genome. In some scenarios, it can be acceptable or even desirable to target many elements simultaneously or an entire TE family. Similarly, uniqueness and repetitiveness are important concepts to consider when aligning reads from next generation sequencing and analysing TEs. Various strategies exist to assign reads that could originate from multiple genomic locations: (i) mapping reads to consensus sequences of TE subfamilies, (ii) mapping to the genome and keeping only uniquely-mapping reads, (iii) assigning multiple mapping reads at random between possible candidates, (iv) redistributing them according to various algorithms, such as maximum likelihood. The choice is ultimately guided by the technique (such as ChIP-seq and RNA-seq) and the purpose of the analysis—is information about individual TE instances needed, or is a high-level tally of results for each subfamily sufficient? Notably, these issues of uniqueness will differ substantially depending on the species studied and the presence or absence of recently, or currently, active TE families. For example, mapping reads to TEs in the human genome will be less challenging than in the mouse genome given the more recent and mobile TE landscape of the latter species. Finally, as sequencing technology and bioinformatics pipelines improve, notably with the increasing length of sequencing reads, many of the hurdles faced by earlier studies will be progressively removed.

Outlook

As potent insertional mutagens, TEs can have both positive and negative effects on host fitness, but it is likely that the majority of TE copies in any given species—and especially those such as humans with small effective population size—have reached fixation through genetic drift alone and are now largely neutral to their host. When can we say that TEs have been co-opted for cellular function? The publication of the initial ENCODE paper, which asserted 'function for 80% of the genome', was the subject of much debate and controversy. Technically speaking, ENCODE assigned only 'biochemical' activity to this large fraction of the genome. Yet critics objected to the grand proclamations in the popular press (The Washington Post Headline: 'Junk DNA concept debunked by new analysis of the human genome') and to the ENCODE consortium's failure to prevent this misinterpretation. To these critics, ignoring evolutionary definitions of function was a major misstep.

This debate can be easily extended to include TEs. TEs make up the vast majority of what is often referred to as 'junk DNA'. Today, the term is mostly used (and abused) by the media, but it has in fact deep roots in evolutionary biology. Regardless of the semantics, what evidence is needed to assign a TE with a function? Many TEs encode a wide range of biochemical activities that normally benefit their own propagation. For example, TEs often contain promoter or enhancer elements that highjack cellular RNA polymerases for transcription and autonomous elements encode proteins with various biochemical and enzymatic activities, all of which are necessary for the transposon to replicate. Do these activities make them functional?

The vast differences in TEs between species make standard approaches to establish their regulatory roles particularly challenging. For example, intriguing studies on the impact of HERVs, in particular HERV-H, in stem cells and pluripotency must be interpreted using novel paradigms that do not invoke deep evolutionary conservation to imply function, as these particular ERVs are absent outside of great apes. Evolutionary constraint can be measured at shorter time scales, including the population level, but this remains a statistically challenging task especially for non-coding sequences. Natural loss-of-function alleles may exist in the human population and their effect on fitness can be studied if their impact is apparent, but these are quite rare and do not allow systematic studies. It is possible to engineer genetic knockouts of a particular human TE locus to test its regulatory role but those are restricted to in-vitro systems, especially when the orthologous TE does not exist in the model species. In this context, studying the impact of TEs in model species with powerful genome engineering tools and vast collections of mutants and other genetic resources, such as plants, fungi, and insects, will also continue to be extremely valuable.

Finally, a growing consensus is urging more rigor when assigning cellular function to TEs, particularly for the fitness benefit of the host. Indeed, a TE displaying biochemical activity (such as those bound by transcription factors or lying within open chromatin regions) cannot be equated to a TE that shows evidence of purifying selection at the sequence level or, when genetically altered, result in a deleterious or dysfunctional phenotype. Recent advances in editing and manipulating the genome and the epigenome en masse yet with precision, including repetitive elements, offer the promise for a systematic assessment of the functional significance of TEs.

Chapter 4

Ames Test

INTRODUCTION

The Ames test is a widely employed method that uses bacteria to test whether a given chemical can cause mutations in the DNA of the test organism. More formally, it is a biological assay to assess the mutagenic potential of chemical compounds. A positive test indicates that the chemical is mutagenic and therefore may act as a carcinogen, because cancer is often linked to mutation. The test serves as a quick and convenient assay to estimate the carcinogenic potential of a compound because standard carcinogen assays on mice and rats are time-consuming (taking two to three years to complete) and expensive. However, false-positives and false-negatives are known.

GENERAL PROCEDURE

The Ames test uses several strains of the bacterium *Salmonella typhimurium* that carry mutations in genes involved in histidine synthesis. These strains are auxotrophic mutants, i.e. they require histidine for growth, but cannot produce it. The method tests the capability of the tested substance in creating mutations that result in a return to a 'prototrophic' state, so that the cells can grow on a histidine-free medium. The tester strains are specially constructed to detect either frameshift (e.g. strains TA-1537 and TA-1538) or point (e.g. strain TA-1531) mutations in the genes required to synthesise histidine, so that mutagens acting via different mechanisms may be identified.

Some compounds are quite specific, causing reversions in just one or two strains. The tester strains also carry mutations in the genes responsible for lipopolysaccharide synthesis, making the cell wall of the bacteria more permeable, and in the excision repair system to make the test more sensitive. Ames test procedure is shown in Fig. 4.1.

Larger organisms like mammals have metabolic processes that could potentially turn a chemical considered not mutagenic into one that is or one that is considered mutagenic into one that is not. Therefore, to more effectively test a chemical compounds mutagenicity in relation to larger organisms, rat liver enzymes can be added in an attempt to replicate the metabolic processes effect on the compound being tested in the Ames Test. Rat liver extract is optionally added to simulate the effect of metabolism, as some compounds, like benzo[a]pyrene, are not mutagenic themselves but their metabolic products are.

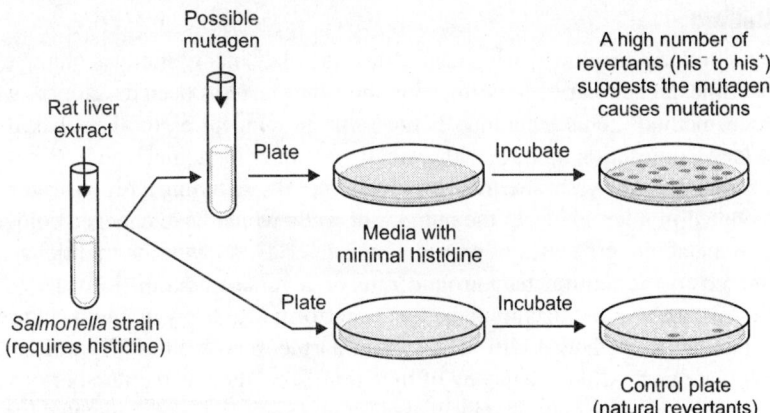

Fig. 4.1: Ames test procedure.

The bacteria are spread on an agar plate with small amount of histidine. This small amount of histidine in the growth medium allows the bacteria to grow for an initial time and have the opportunity to mutate. When the histidine is depleted only bacteria that have mutated to gain the ability to produce its own histidine will survive. The plate is incubated for 48 hours. The mutagenicity of a substance is proportional to the number of colonies observed.

Ames Test and Carcinogens

Mutagens identified via Ames test are also possible carcinogens, and early studies by Ames showed that 90% of known carcinogens may be identified via this test. Later studies however showed identification of 50–70% of known carcinogens. The test was used to identify a number of compounds previously used in commercial products as potential carcinogens. Examples include tris(2,3-dibromopropyl) phosphate, which was used as a flame retardant in plastic and textiles such as children's sleepwear, and furylfuramide which was used as an antibacterial additive in food in Japan in 1960s and 1970s. Furylfuramide in fact had previously passed animal test, but more vigorous tests after its identification in the Ames test showed it to be carcinogenic. Their positive tests resulted in those chemicals being withdrawn from use in consumer products.

One interesting result from the Ames test is that the dose response curve using varying concentrations of chemical is almost always linear, indicating that there is no threshold concentration for mutagenesis. It therefore suggests that, as with radiations, there may be no safe threshold for chemical mutagens or carcinogens. However some proposed that organisms can tolerate low level of mutagens due to protective mechanisms such as DNA repair, and threshold may exist for certain chemical mutagens. Bruce Ames himself argued against linear dose-response extrapolation from the high dose used in carcinogenesis tests in animal systems to the lower dose of chemicals normally encountered in human exposure, as the results may be false positives due to mitogenic response caused by the artificially high dose of chemicals used in such tests. He also cautioned against the 'hysteria over tiny traces of chemicals that may or may not cause cancer', that 'completely drives out the major risks you should be aware of'.

The Ames test is often used as one of the initial screens for potential drugs to weed out possible carcinogens, and it is one of the eight tests required under the Pesticide Act (USA) and one of six tests required under the Toxic Substances Control Act (USA).

Fluctuation Method

The Ames test was initially developed using agar plates (the plate incorporation technique), as described above. Since that time, an alternative to performing the Ames test has been developed, which is known as the 'fluctuation method'. This technique is the same in concept as the agar-based method, with bacteria being added to a reaction mixture with a small amount of histidine, which allows the bacteria to grow and mutate, returning to synthesise their own histidine. By including a pH indicator, the frequency of mutation is counted in microplates as the number of wells which have changed colour (caused by a drop in pH due to metabolic processes of reproducing bacteria). As with the traditional Ames test, the sample is compared to the natural background rate of reverse mutation in order to establish the genotoxicity of a substance. The fluctuation method is performed entirely in liquid culture and is scored by counting the number of wells that turn yellow from purple in 96-well or 384-well microplates.

In the 96-well plate method the frequency of mutation is counted as the number of wells out of 96 which have changed colour. The plates are incubated for up to five days, with mutated (yellow) colonies being counted each day and compared to the background rate of reverse mutation using established tables of significance to determine the significant differences between the background rate of mutation and that for the tested samples.

In the more scaled-down 384-well plate microfluctuation method the frequency of mutation is counted as the number of wells out of 48 which have changed colour after 2 days of incubation. A test sample is assayed across 6 dose levels with concurrent zero-dose (background) and positive controls which all fit into one 384-well plate. The assay is performed in triplicates to provide statistical robustness. It uses the recommended OECD Guideline 471 tester strains (histidine auxotrophs and tryptophan auxotrophs).

The fluctuation method is comparable to the traditional pour plate method in terms of sensitivity and accuracy, however, it does have a number of advantages: it needs less test sample, it has a simple colorimetric endpoint, counting the number of positive wells out of possible 96 or 48 wells is much less time consuming than counting individual colonies on an agar plate. Several commercial kits are available. Most kits have consumable components in a ready-to-use state, including lyophilised bacteria, and tests can be performed using multichannel pipettes. The fluctuation method also allows for testing higher volumes of aqueous samples (up to 75% v/v), increasing the sensitivity and extending its application to low-level environmental mutagens.

Limitations

Salmonella typhimurium is a prokaryote, therefore it is not a perfect model for humans. Rat liver S9 fraction is used to mimic the mammalian metabolic conditions so that the mutagenic potential of metabolites formed by a parent molecule in the hepatic system can be assessed; however, there are differences in metabolism between human and rat that can affect the mutagenicity of chemicals being tested. The test may therefore be improved by the use of human liver S9 fraction; its use was previously limited by its availability, but it is now available commercially and therefore may be more feasible. An adapted in vitro model has been made for eukaryotic cells, for example yeast.

Mutagens identified in the Ames test need not necessarily be carcinogenic, and further tests are required for any potential carcinogen identified in the test. Drugs that contain the nitrate moiety sometimes come back positive for Ames when they are indeed safe. The nitrate compounds may generate nitric oxide, an important signal molecule that can give a false positive. Nitroglycerin is an example that gives a positive Ames yet is still used in treatment today. Nitrates in food however may be reduced by bacterial action to nitrites which are known to generate carcinogens by reacting with amines and amides.

Long toxicology and outcome studies are needed with such compounds to disprove a positive Ames test. Detail description of Ames test is discussed below.

AMES TEST

The Ames test was developed in the 1970s by Bruce Ames, Professor of Biochemistry at UC-Berkeley, as a fast and sensitive assay of the ability of a chemical compound or mixture to induce mutations in DNA. Because the assay does not use a live animal model, it is inexpensive, easy, and fast. Bruce Ames published his work in a series of papers, including 'Identifying Environmental Chemicals Causing Mutations and Cancer' in the journal Science. Dr. Ames work was critical in linking mutations in DNA to carcinogenesis. His work identified many mutagens including pesticides such as DDT, the food additive AF-2 (no longer used), the flame retardant 'tris-BP', and mutagenic compounds in commercial hair dyes.

ASSAY

Since DNA is chemically the same in all organisms, any living organism can be used to test for mutagens. Thus, bacteria can be used as a first step in identifying potential human carcinogens without waiting for long-lived mammals to develop cancer. In this assay, mutant strains of the bacteria *Salmonella tymphimurium* (*S. typhimurium*) will be used. These haploid bacteria already contain particular mutations in the gene encoding an enzyme used to synthesise the amino acid histidine; their genotype is given as his$^-$. Since the bacteria require histidine to make many of their proteins, these mutant bacteria will die unless the media in which they are grown contains histidine.

It is known that secondary mutations occur at a low spontaneous rate, these mutants are called revertants because they have reverted to the his$^+$ genotype and phenotype and can now grow just fine in media lacking histidine. The assay then involves plating his$^-$ *S. typhimurium* onto media with trace amounts histidine and adding chemicals to be tested for mutagenicity. The number of colonies growing on the plate indicates the number of revertants. In a true testing situation, a variety of concentrations of each chemical would be tested to generate a dose-response curve.

A CAVEAT

The rate of mutagenicity in various organisms can still differ however, due to the rate of chemical absorption by cells and differential metabolism of compounds, in the mammalian liver for example. In the original Ames test, a liver extract is added to the plates as well, simulating how mammalian liver enzymes can modify compounds. In some cases, the liver de-toxifies compounds, but some compounds are actually rendered more toxic after modification. Note that compounds that test positive in the Ames test would be subjected to further testing in mammalian model systems such as in mice or rats before being labelled as a human carcinogen.

Experiment for Ames Test

The experiment is in two parts: the exposure of *S. typhimurium* strains to potential mutagens (The Ames Test itself) and measurement of the number of bacteria in the cultures used to allow you to quantitatively assess the mutagenicity of the chemicals tested.

BACTERIAL STRAINS

We will use two his$^-$ *S. typhimurium* strains in screen for mutagens. TA1535 contains a T to C missense mutation in the *hisG* gene, leading to a leucine to proline amino acid substitution. TA1538 has a deletion of 1 base pair (C) in the *hisD* gene, which causes α–1 frameshift mutation. This changes two amino acids and brings a stop codon into the reading frame133 amino acids prematurely. Because there are different his⁻ mutations in these strains, reversion to the his⁺ phenotype will require different molecular lesions (mutations). Since different mutagens can exert their effect on DNA through different mechanisms, using strains containing different mutations allows us to identify mutagens that have differing effects on DNA. Using our knowledge of gene structure and translation, we should try to predict what kinds of mutations could lead to reversion in each case. We should know that there are additional mutations in the bacterial strains used in the Ames test. Both of the strains have a defect in the lipopolysaccharide cell wall causing them to be more vulnerable to exogenous mutagens. Additionally, both strains have defective DNA excision-repair mechanisms. These mechanisms would normally correct mutations arising during DNA replication or from exogenous mutagens.

A WORD ABOUT SAFETY

During the procedure we will be handling strains of *S. typhimurium* and known or suspected mutagens. *S. typhimurium* is a pathogenic organism responsible for certain types of food poisoning, so be sure to follow proper microbiological technique. The mutagens chosen in this lab are not very harmful to humans and they are provided in low concentrations. Nonetheless, this is a good time to practice lab safety. Wear gloves when working with the bacteria or mutagens and keep these materials localised in one place on our bench. Known mutagens will only be applied to our plates in one place in the lab. Dispose of all gloves/plates/pipette tips in the biohazard containers (not the normal trash). Wash your hands before and after this weeks lab.

PART I: DETERMINING THE NUMBER OF BACTERIA IN OVERNIGHT CULTURES

To quantitatively determine the mutagenicity of a compound, one must not only determine the number of mutant bacteria produced, but also the total number of cells exposed to the mutagen to begin with. This is particularly important if one wishes to compare experiments done on different days or with different bacterial cultures. For example, say a new drug undergoing clinical trials causes allergic reactions in 20 patients. Before we make an assessment of the potential allergic properties of this drug, we need to know how many patients were exposed to the drug: were there 200 or 20000 patients exposed?

We will do our Ames test with a bacterial culture that was grown overnight. That is, the population of bacteria had been doubling by binary fission for about 10 hours. How many living cells are in that culture, say, per mL? How can we figure this out? We could use a spectrophotometer to determine the cell number per mL, as each cell scatters light when it is in solution. However, overnight cultures are saturated, that is, they are at or near the carrying capacity of the nutrient broth in which they are growing, so some cells are dying but will still scatter light. It would be better to directly measure the number of living cells per mL. Each living cell is capable of dividing to produce 2 cells and so on – on a solid surface these aggregate cells will form a colony. We will thus measure colony-forming units (CFUs) in a culture. Overnight cultures of bacteria like *S. typhimurium* exhibit variation in CFU concentration, typically containing 2×10^8–2×10^9 CFUs/mL. The human eye obviously cannot distinguish such a large number of individual colonies, so we will determine the number of CFUs in a given culture by spreading serial dilutions of the overnight cultures on nutrient-rich agar plates and counting the resulting colonies after about 20 hr of growth at 37°C.

The steps involved in calculating CFU concentration are not difficult, but they do require exacting precision when using the pipetters. Think about how a small error at one of the first few dilutions could affect all the subsequent dilutions. How much would a pipetting error of 0.1 mL be magnified after six or seven serial dilutions? With this in mind, take your time and be sure to conduct this experiment with care. Our data will reflect our pipetting skills and plating consistency.

We will want to count 100 or fewer colonies on we plates. We will be plating 100 µl of our dilutions – remember that 1000 µl = 1 mL or, 100 µl = 0.1 mL. If we expect your overnight culture to contain $2 \times 10^8 - 2 \times 10^9$ CFUs/mL, how many 1 in 10 or 1:1 serial dilutions should we do? Plan to plate 2 dilutions, one of which is 50% less concentrated than the other. Recall that a 1 in 10 dilution means adding 1 volume of a liquid to 9 volumes of a liquid (as in 1 mL culture + 9 mLs water or 100 µl culture + 900 µl water). Serial dilutions means diluting a stock solution, then diluting the dilution that you just made even further, then diluting that dilution. Determine how many serial dilutions you need to make and what the dilution factor is. Lastly, determine how you can make one last dilution that is only half the concentration of the previous dilution. Plan to plate the contents of the last 2 dilutions. Before actually creating the dilutions, check your protocol with the instructor or lab assistant to be sure you have an appropriate plan.

When we count the number of colonies on your plate, you can simply multiply the colony number by the dilution factor to determine how many CFUs were in the 100 µl that you plated. Then multiply by 10 to determine the CFUs/mL of the overnight culture. Will a 10^6 concentration be dilute enough for your experiment?

Creating and Plating Serial Dilutions

1. Determine the number of serial dilutions that you will perform, and what the final dilution factor of each of your dilutions will be. Write all of these concentrations on labelling tape and apply to the microcentrifuge tubes (include the strain name and your initials). Make sure you label all the intermediate dilutions, as it is easy to lose track of which one you are on.

2. Apply Bacdown to your work area and allow it to dry.

3. Gently vortex your overnight solution to mix up the sediment at the bottom of the test tube (approximately 5–10 seconds).

4. Pipet approximately 900 µl of your overnight culture into your first empty microcentrifuge tube. Vortex thoroughly for approximately 5 seconds.

5. Pipet 900 µl of the sterile water into every microcentrifuge tube except the ones containing the original overnight culture solution and the final dilution.

6. Pipet 100 µl of your full strength overnight solution into your first serial dilution microcentrifuge tube (should contain 900 µl of sterile water). Vortex thoroughly.

7. Repeat this process for all of your serial dilutions.

8. Label your Petri dishes with the strain name, concentration, group initials, and date. Write in small letters around the edges of the bottom of the dish. The lids may get mixed up, but the Petri dish will always stay with the agar!

9. Pipet 100 µl of one of your serial dilutions onto the center of the L medium agar plate. Perform this step carefully, as the liquid tends to bead up and roll around the dish. The desired result is one large drop in the center of the dish. Don't puncture the surface of the agar- this is a surface application.

10. Flame sterilise the hockey stick spreader, briefly touch it to the agar away from the bacteria, and then spread the bacteria over the surface of the agar.

11. Repeat steps 9–10 for one other serial dilution. Think about why having data from two different dilutions is important.

12. Allow the plates to sit for about 10 minutes, invert and put together with tape, then incubate for 24 hr at 37°C.

13. Count the resulting colonies and record your observations.

14. Using the estimated concentrations of your serial dilutions, determine the CFU/mL content of your original solution and express the standard error as a ± value.

Find the average of both the dilutions (you will have to adjust for the differences in concentration). Note that you only plated 0.1 mL of the dilutions, not a full mL.

PART II: AMES TEST

Experimental design: The material is given to prepare an experiment in which a total of 10 plates may be used. Each plate will eventually contain 1 strain of bacteria exposed to one concentration of one chemical, for example. The person should be design a carefully controlled experiment using both TA1535 and TA1538. Determine what will work best as positive and negative controls. Two chemicals with known mutagenicity are available.

Sodium azide (NaN_3) is a white solid that is highly soluble in water. Because it easily kills bacteria in high enough concentration, it is used as a preservative in some chemical solutions; its degradation via electric shock is used to inflate car airbags. 4-nitro-o-phenylenediame (4NOP) is an orange-red powder previously used in hair dyes. In the late 1970 s the National Cancer Institute (NCI) noticed that there was an abnormally high incidence of bladder cancer among workers in the dye industry, so they requested a bioassay of 4NOP to determine its mutagenic potential. 4NOP produced positive results in the Ames test and it is considered a potential mutagen.

While choosing your mutagens, you should think about the nature of the organism you are testing. Although the strains of *S. typhimurium* used in the Ames test are his⁻, most bacteria are not. The incubation conditions used in this experiment are idea for many micro-organisms, and many types of fungi and bacteria will readily grow on both top agar and Vogel-Bonner medium.

We should be meticulous in your sterile procedure to ensure that no outside contaminants enter our Petri dishes. Furthermore, we should do our best to ensure that there are not micro-organisms in the mutagens we are testing.

For example, that nasty week-old casserole in your mini-fridge will probably produce many bacterial colonies if we test it as a potential mutagen. This does not necessarily mean your casserole is mutagenic. If we choose a potential mutagen that may have micro-organisms in it (e.g. river water), talk to your instructor or lab assistant as soon as possible to see if it is autoclavable. If we suspect your potential mutagen may already have bacteria that can survive on a nutrient-deficient medium, think about how you could test this. Finally, remember that *S. typhimurium* is affected by anti-microbial substances.

Determine what mutagens you will be testing, and discuss your concentrations and application procedure with your professor.

Ensure that your plates are labelled to reflect the mutagens you will test and their concentrations.

The potential mutagens are put into solution at the concentration as suggested by lab assistant. Typically most mutagens will be suspended in 1 mL of water and placed in an microcentrifuge tubes.

Exposing *S. Typhimurium* to Different Mutagens

While allowing the top agar to harden completely, you may prepare your potential mutagens for use. Several potential mutagens will be supplied for you and you will have brought some of your own as well. Solid substances can be blended with sterile water as aqueous substances will diffuse in the agar and contact the maximum number of bacteria. Waxy materials might be easily melted in the microwave and then applied to filters. We find that placing mutagen solutions on sterile filter paper disks produces consistent results. If your mutagen is difficult to put into solution, direct application is a viable option.

The following steps are for application of a mutagen in solution:

- Flame sterilise your forceps after dipping them in 95% ethanol and allow the forceps to cool for a few seconds.
- Using the lid of the glass *Petri dish* as a protective cover, remove one sterile filter paper disk with your forceps.
- Ensure that the cover for your microcentrifuge tube is secured and lightly flick the tube to evenly distribute your mutagen in the solution.

  This is especially important with 4NOP because it is highly insoluble in water. Repeat this step every time you use a mutagen.
- Pipette 10 μL of the test solution directly onto the center of the filter paper.
- Using the lid of the *Petri dish* as a protective cover, place the filter paper (mutagen-side down) onto the top agar.
- Repeat this process for each plate.
- Tape your plates together, label them with the date and your group initials, invert the plates (to prevent condensation) and incubate for approximately 48 hr at 37°C.

Counting the Revertant Colonies on Your Plates

1. Remove nutrient-rich plates (CFU concentration experiment) after 18–24 hr of incubation.
2. Make notes on colony characteristics such as size, shape, and colour.
3. Count each colony on your plates. Make sure to be consistent in your definition of a colony. All colonies come from one revertant bacterium, so all colonies should be counted the same, regardless of size. If there are an excessive number of revertant colonies on a plate (over 400), you may want to count only ¼ of the plate and then multiply your final result by four. This is known as the quadrant counting method, and it is less accurate than counting all the colonies on a given plate.
4. Remove nutrient-deficient plates (Ames test) after about 48 hr.
5. Repeat steps 2+3 for these plates.
6. Calculate reversion frequency as # of revertant colonies per mL/total # of CFUs per mL of appropriate overnight culture.
7. Select one plate which contains revertant colonies you wish to test for molecular lesions. Label one of the provided large test tubes (this should contain approximately 5mL of L. medium) with the same information that is on your selected plate. Place your plate in the 4°C refrigerator and replace the test tube in the appropriate area.

Thus, prepare one colony from your selected plate in an overnight culture solution before the next laboratory period.

Materials Needed in Lab

Materials for each group (groups of 2):

- 10 mL overnight L medium broth culture of each of the following strains: TA1538, TA1535.
- 12- L medium plates (L. medium+1.5% bacto agar)- 12 plates per lab group
- 10 Vogel-Bonner medium E plates
- 11 tubes of 3 mL bio-his top agar, liquified (autoclaved) in hot water bath (57°C)
- 1 test tube rack (for large test tubes)
- 1 test tube containing 5ml of sterile L. medium
- 1 p1000
- 1 p200
- 1 p20
- 1 pipetman rack
- 1 box p200 tips
- 1 box p1000 tips (can probably share between groups- only need 20 or so)
- 1 pipette tip bucket
- 1 Bunsen burner
- 1 bottle Bacdown
- 1 Miracloth
- 1 jar 95% ethanol
- 1 Plating hockey stick
- 1 vortex mixer
- 1 bottle sterile ddH$_2$O
- Labelling Tape

Materials for Lab

- 1 mL of sodium azide @ 0.05 mg/mL
- 1 mL of 4-nitro-o-phenylenediamine @ 0.5 mg/mL
- 3 large hot water baths (set to 57°C)
- 1 Box each size glove
- 1 biohazard trash bag
- 3 bottles of sterile H$_2$O
- 3 sterile forceps
- 2–3 Petri dishes of sterilised filter paper disks
- 1 jar 95% ethanol
- 3 blenders
- 5 microfuge racks

- 1 beaker sterile microfuge tubes
- 1 square bottle sterile H_2O
- 1 area of Benchkote for very hazardous chemicals
- 2 beakers of sterile 1.5 ml microcentrifuge tubes
- Forceps and alcohol and matches near mutagens (or move near gas jet)

REVERSION: PHENOTYPE TO DNA

Since in the lab we exposed his⁻ mutant strains of *S. typhimurium* to suspected mutagens. Some of his⁻ bacteria reverted to a his⁺ phenotype but how this happened? As we remember, different mutagens affect DNA in different ways. However, even though a specific mutagen will typically cause one type of mutation, this is not necessarily the only mutation that particular mutagen can induce. Furthermore, we know that TA1535 and TA1538 have contain different mutations, so perhaps different secondary mutations can lead to the his⁺ phenotype. This section discusses how we prepared DNA to identify the molecular changes that confer the revertant phenotype.

Isolation of Genomic DNA from *S. Typhimurium*

Before we can amplify the most probable areas of mutation, we must isolate the genomic DNA from your revertants. An overnight culture of the revertant bacteria you selected will be provided and it is your job to extract genomic DNA from these bacteria. We will use DNeasy' his mini-prep spin columns to isolate genomic DNA away from cell membranes, proteins, and RNA. This kit can be used to isolate DNA from a variety of sources, including blood, tissue samples, plants, and bacteria. To obtain genomic DNA, you will first lyse the bacteria with a buffered Proteinase K solution and a high temperature incubation. Then we will pipet the lysed bacteria onto the spin column membrane and centrifuge the sample. The bacterial genomic DNA will adhere to the membrane, but all contaminants (proteins, salts, divalent cations, etc.) will flow through the membrane and be discarded. The spin column membrane should be watch several times to ensure the purity of your DNA, and then we will dry the membrane. Finally, we will elute the DNA into a microcentrifuge tube to use as a template for PCR.

Please be careful with while pipetting and check off each step of the protocol as you complete it.

Protocol for Bacterial Genomic DNA Extraction (Qiagen mini-prep spin column):

1. Vortex your overnight culture solution for approximately 15 seconds.
2. Using the P1000, transfer approximately 2×10^8 cells (1.5 mls) from your solution into a small labelled microcentrifuge tube. Use your calculations from the CFU concentration experiment to determine how many µL this will be. This is a separate overnight solution, but the number should be relatively close.
3. Centrifuge the solution for 10 minutes at 7500 rpm. Check to ensure that a small pellet has formed after this step. If no pellet forms, repeat centrifugation.
4. Remove the supernatant with a P1000 and discard. Be careful not to disturb the pellet.
5. Resuspend the pellet in 180 µL of Buffer ATL. You may need to perform multiple up and down pipettings to ensure uniform suspension.
6. Add 20 µL of proteinase K solution and mix by vortexing for at least 10 seconds.
7. Incubate bacteria for approximately one hour at 56°C in a hot water bath. Vortex twice during the incubation period to ensure complete lysis of the cells.

8. After incubation is complete, pulse vortex your sample for 15 seconds.

9. Add 400 µL of Buffer AL/ethanol solution and vortex immediately for approximately 15 seconds. You should have a homogenous solution at this point. Vortex the sample again if there is an excessive amount of precipitate.

10. Pipette this mixture into the Qiagen DNeasy™ spin column (the column should come pre-packaged in a 2 mL collection tube). Centrifuge for 1 minute at 8000 rpm.

11. Discard the flow-through in the appropriate waste disposal area and place the spin column in a new collection tube.

12. Pipette 500 µL of Buffer AW1 into the spin column and spin for 1 min. at 8000 rpm.

13. Discard the flow-through and place the spin column in a new collection tube.

14. Pipet 500 µL of Buffer AW2 into the spin column and centrifuge for 3 minutes at 14000 rpm. This will dry the spin column membrane, so be sure that the column is empty after this step. Do not allow the flow-through to touch the spin column.

15. Discard the flow-through and place the spin column back in the collection tube and respin for 1 minute. Discard the flow-through and the collection tube. Place the spin column into a clean (labeled) 1.5 ml eppendorf tube. This tube will contain your DNA prep, so be clearly label it. Additionally, place an uppercase P on the side of the tube to indicate that it is a DNA Prep.

16. Pipette 200 µL of Buffer AE into the spin column (directly onto the membrane). Allow the spin column to sit at room temperature for approximately one minute.

17. Centrifuge the spin column at 8000 rpm to elute.

18. Place your DNA prep on ice and turn it in to your lab assistant.

Amplifying the *hisG* or *hisD* Gene via PCR

We should now have an isolated preperation of genomic DNA from our revertant colony. However, this DNA is from the entire genome of your bacteria, and we are only interested in determining what causes the his+ phenotype, most likely due to changes in the coding regions of the His operon. Since we know where the mutations are that render TA1535 and TA1538 his⁻, and since the bacteria will have to somehow overcome these mutations, we will be amplifying these specific regions of the *hisG* and *hisD* genes.

We will use a polymerase chain reaction (PCR) to amplify portions of the *hisG* (mutant in TA1535) and *hisD* (mutant in TA1538) genes surrounding the original mutations which confer the his⁻ phenotype. The final amplified regions will be approximately 500 base pairs long.

The two primer sets have different optimum annealing temperatures and will require separate thermocycling. The primer sets are:

hisG primer set (optimum annealing temperature of 38°C):

> *hisG* 919 PS: CGCTTACGCATAGCT
>
> *hisG* 1440 PA: AGCTTCAAGCGTCGC

hisD primer set (optimum annealing temperature of 44°C):

> *hisD* 2611 PS: CCGTCTGAAGTACTG
>
> *hisD* 3114 PA: TCAATGGTTGATGCC

Protocol for PCR Amplification

Important note: To ensure that you obtain good results from your PCR, you do not want contaminants getting into your sterile 0.2 mL PCR tube, be sure to use fresh pipette tips every time you transfer a new solution. Keep reagents on ice at all times.

1. Obtain a 0.2 mL thin-walled PCR tube and label the top with your group initials.
2. Determine which primer set you will use and obtain the appropriate set of primers.
3. Pipette 10.5 μL of nuclease-free water into your reaction tube.
4. Pipet 0.5 μL of each desired primer into the PCR tube (6.25 pmole each primer). You should have two primers in your reaction, so there will be 1 μL added to your total reaction volume in this step.
5. Add 1 μL of your bacterial genomic DNA prep to the PCR tube. Try to pipette the DNA directly into the reaction mixture.
6. Add 12.5 μL of the Promega Master Mix to the reaction tube. This contains the Taq polymerase, $MgCl_2$, reaction buffer, and dNTP mixture.
7. Gently vortex the tube to mix all the components and briefly centrifuge to collect the reagents at the bottom of the PCR tube.
8. Place the PCR tube in a thermocycler. Your PCR products will be removed after the reaction is complete and stored at −20°C until they are needed.

Technical Information about PCR

1. PCR master mix contains the following ingredients:
   - 3mM $MgCl_2$
   - 400uM dNTP's (each dATP, dGTP, dCTP, dTTP)
   - 50units/mL
2. The thermocycler programme is:
   - 92°C-5 minutes (denatures DNA)
   - 30 cycles of:
     94°C-2 minutes (separation)
     38°C/44°C (*hisD* primers/*hisD* primers)- 30 seconds (annealing)
     72°C- 2 minutes (extension)
   - 72°C- 20 minutes (elongation)
   - 4°C- hold temperature

Purifying PCR Products for Sequencing

We will employ Sanger DNA sequencing to look for mutations associated with reversion to the his⁺ phenotype. Recall that Sanger sequencing is basically DNA replication from a single primer hybridised to one of the two strands of template DNA. Because the PCR reaction includes many extra copies of two different primers, the amplified DNA fragment must be purified away from the primers. We will use another spin column to purify the DNA fragment (PCR product) away from the primers, dNTPs, and TAQ polymerase. Once you have purified your DNA fragment, you will add a portion of it, along with just one of the PCR primers, to a clean tube. We will send these samples to a DNA sequencing facility and you will get a data file of the finished sequence. Be sure to obtain a sample number from your instructor so that your sample can be identified when the sequences are returned. We will then use software and a sequence file you can find on Moodle to compare the original TA1535 or TA1538 sequence to the sequence of your revertant.

Protocol for Purifying PCR Products

1. Add 125 µL of Buffer PBI (should have a yellow colour) to your PCR product and pipette to mix. Check to make sure that the mixture is still yellow. If the mixture has a violet hue you will need to adjust the pH with 3M sodium acetate (pH 5.0) until the colour is yellow. Obtaining the appropriate pH is essential for efficient purification of your PCR products.

2. Apply this mixture to the spin column and centrifuge for one minute at 14000 rpm to bind the DNA.

3. Discard the flow-through and place the spin column back in the same collection tube. Add 650 µL of Buffer PE to the column and centrifuge for 60 seconds at 14000 rpm.

4. Discard the flow-through and place the column back in the same collection tube.

5. Centrifuge for an additional minute at 14000 rpm to completely dry the column.

6. Discard the flow-through and place the column in a clean labeled 1.5 mL microcentrifuge tube. This tube contains your final purified PCR product, so be sure it is clearly labeled.

7. Add 50 µL of Buffer EB and centrifuge for one minute at 14000 rpm.

Verifying Results

Typically one would run a gel of the final purified PCR products to determine DNA concentration and confirm the success of PCR amplification.

Preparing your Sample to Send off for Sequencing

1. Obtain a sterile 0.5 mL PCR tube, close it, and label it with a unique number obtained from your instructor. Fill in the small form that details which strain you began with and the mutagen used to create your revertant. Record your number so you can identify your sequence.

2. Add 8.7 µL of nuclease free water to your microcentrifuge tube.

3. Add 0.3 µL of one sense primer (12.5 pm/L) to your microcentrifuge tube. You only need to use one primer, so you should use either His G 919 PS, or His D 2611 PS, same as one primer from the primer set you used for PCR.

4. Add 3.0 µL of your purified PCR product to your microcentrifuge tube.

5. Close the lid tightly, invert to ensure that it is sealed, and give your tube to your instructor or lab assistant.

6. Enter your purified PCR product into the PCR product library.

Materials Needed in the Lab, Ames Test parts 2 and 3

Material for each group

- 1 p1000
- 1 p200

- 1 p20
- 1 pipetman rack
- 1 pipette tip bucket
- 1 box p200 tips
- 1 labelling marker
- 1 ice bucket
- 1 microcentrifuge tube block

Materials for lab

- 2 thermocyclers
- 2 tubes of Promega Master Mix (clear)
- 6 tubes of nuclease free water (for PCR)
- 50uL each of HisG919, HisG1440, HisD2611, and HisD3114 primers
- 4 microcentrifuges (more if they are available)
- 4 small hot water baths (for microcentrifuge tubes)
- 2 square bottles sterile H_2O
- 1 box each size glove
- 1 jar labeled Salmonella Waste (to be autoclaved)
- 1 biohazard trash bag
- 2 boxes p1000 tips
- 2 boxes p2 tips
- 2 beakers of sterile 1.5ml microcentrifuge tubes
- 1 beaker sterile PCR tubes (thin pink ones)
- 2 Qiagen DNeasy Blood+Tissue DNA prep kits (50 tubes per kit)
- 2 10ml containers of 1:1 Buffer AL (Qiagen product)/100% ethanol
- 2 Qiagen Qiaquick PCR purification kits (50 tubes/kit)
- 1 roll of parafilm
- 1 beaker sterile 1.5 ml microcentrifuge tube
- Two primers from last lab-HisG919, HisD2611 (@ 12.5pm/μL)
- 1 ice bucket (for the primers)
- 4 tubes of nuclease free water

AMES TEST: DATA ANALYSIS

Part I: Reversion Frequencies

Compute both CFU/per ml and the reversion frequencies for controls and each potential mutagen tested. Be sure these are reported in visual and prose form in your manuscript.

Part II: Sequence Analysis

Download FASTA DNA sequence files that are available on Moodle. These are stored in .txt format, so use whatever text editor programme you have to open and manipulate these.

At step one, use the pull-down menu to select 'DNA' rather than 'protein.' You do not need to change any of the parameters, simply copy in each sequence, hitting return between each one that you enter. Do include the line at the top that identifies the sequence; it will look like: >HisD blah blah...Then press the 'submit' button. The output will be the best alignment possible. Be sure you can tell which sequence is which by the first label in the name (the first line that begins with > is the label). It is this line that makes the text file a FASTA file. Wherever the sequences are all identical, there will be an asterisk under the sequence alignment. Look for the differences between mutant and wild type first.

To 'conceptually translate' a DNA sequence into amino acid sequence, there are many programmes available.

Input your sequence via copy/paste (leave off that first labelling line this time), then hit translate. All 6 reading frames will be displayed. One should be an open reading frame that starts on the first ATG start codon. Using your alignment, you should be able to find the location of the mutation. You may then copy and save these protein sequences into a text file and do an alignment in ClustalW, this time using 'Protein' rather than 'DNA.' Be sure to indicate how the DNA sequence and the protein sequence correlates with the histindine phenotype for each bacterial strain you analyse. You must analyse the wild type sequence, the original his⁻ mutant sequence, and at least two different revertant sequences for each of the TA1538 and TA1535 strains.

SECTION III

Regulation of Gene Expression, Transcription Attenuation, RNA Splicing and RNA Silencing

SECTION III

Chapter 5

Regulation of Gene Expression

INTRODUCTION

Gene expression is the process by which information from a gene is used in the synthesis of a functional gene product. These products are often proteins, but in non-protein coding genes such as rRNA genes or tRNA genes, the product is a functional RNA. The process of gene expression is used by all known life—eukaryotes (including multicellular organisms), prokaryotes (bacteria and *archaea*) and viruses — to generate the macromolecular machinery for life.

Several steps in the gene expression process may be modulated, including the transcription, RNA splicing, translation, and post-translational modification of a protein. Gene regulation gives the cell control over structure and function, and is the basis for cellular differentiation, morphogenesis and the versatility and adaptability of any organism. Gene regulation may also serve as a substrate for evolutionary change, since control of the timing, location, and amount of gene expression can have a profound effect on the functions (actions) of the gene in a cell or in a multicellular organism. In genetics gene expression is the most fundamental level at which genotype gives rise to the phenotype.

The genetic code is 'interpreted' by gene expression, and the properties of the expression products give rise to the organism's phenotype (Fig. 5.1).

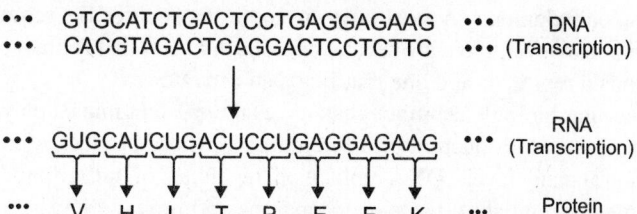

Fig. 5.1: Genes are expressed by being transcribed into RNA and this transcript may then be translated into protein.

Regulation of gene expression ordinarily occurs at the transcriptional, post-transcriptional, translational or post-translational levels. Transcriptional regulation includes all mechanisms that control the information transfer from DNA to RNA by RNA polymerase. Post-transcriptional regulation involves all modifications of the primary RNA transcript before it is translated into proteins. Translational regulation involves those factors that determine the rate of translation of mature mRNA molecules. Post-translational regulation involves mechanisms that control the processing of the primary translation product into the mature protein product. The environmental and metabolic state of the cell has a direct and significant effect on the control of gene expression. Usually, small extracellular or intracellular metabolites trigger the complex mechanisms that result either in stimulation or inhibition of gene expression. The regulation of the expression of genes is absolutely essential for the growth, development, differentiation and the very existence of an organism.

In prokaryotes such as *Escherichia coli* (*E. coli*), regulation of gene expression occurs primarily at the level of transcription and in general, is mediated by the binding of *trans*-acting proteins to *cis*-acting regulatory elements on their single DNA molecule (chromosome). Prokaryotes are not as structurally complex as eukaryotes, and were once thought not to have any internal structures enclosed by lipid membranes. The controls that act on gene expression (i.e. the ability of a gene to produce a biologically active protein) are much more complex in eukaryotes than in prokaryotes. A major difference is the presence in eukaryotes of a nuclear membrane, which prevents the simultaneous transcription and translation that occurs in prokaryotes. Whereas, in prokaryotes, control of transcriptional initiation is the major point of regulation, in eukaryotes the regulation of gene expression is controlled nearly equivalently from many different points. In bacteria, genes are clustered into operons: gene clusters that encode the proteins necessary to perform coordinated function, such as biosynthesis of a given amino acid. RNA that is transcribed from prokaryotic operons is polycistronic a term implying that multiple proteins are encoded in a single transcript.

In bacteria, control of the rate of transcriptional initiation is the predominant site for control of gene expression. As with the majority of prokaryotic genes, initiation is controlled by two DNA sequence elements that are approximately 35 bases and 10 bases, respectively, upstream of the site of transcriptional initiation and as such are identified as the –35 and –10 positions. These two sequence elements are termed promoter sequences, because they promote recognition of transcriptional start sites by RNA polymerase. The activity of RNA polymerase at a given promoter is in turn regulated by interaction with accessory proteins, which affect its ability to recognise start sites. These regulatory proteins can act both positively (activators) and negatively (repressors). The accessibility of promoter regions of prokaryotic DNA is in many cases regulated by the interaction of proteins with sequences termed operators. The operator region is adjacent to the promoter elements in most operons and in most cases the sequences of the operator bind a repressor protein. However, there are several operons in *E. coli* that contain overlapping sequence elements, one that binds a repressor and one that binds an activator.

Application of molecular biology techniques can have an important impact on yield and productivity of recombinant bioprocesses. Introduction of a foreign gene whose product is not utilised by the host can perturb cell function at many levels: DNA replication, regulation of transcription, ribosome functions, RNA turnover, activities of regulatory proteins, chaperone and protease levels, membrane energetics, postranslational processing, and energy and intermediary metabolism. Thus, r-protein production processes must be carefully designed to reduce negative effects of host-vector interactions. Recombinant bioprocesses are determined in many ways by the selection of the host and vector. For instance, a prokaryotic host requires totally different production and purification schemes than a mammalian expression system. Several issues must be considered upon vector and host selection, such as intrinsic r-product characteristics (size, postranslational modifications), product performance (stability, activity, authenticity) and even financial considerations (final use, quantity required, cost/added value, time for development, market). Additionally, many production parameters (cultivation mode, medium composition, environmental conditions, and others) have an important relationship with gene expression, plasmid copy number, plasmid stability, etc. Such information is necessary for properly selecting an expression system for industrial r-protein production. Thus, the process of gene expression simply refers to the events that transfer the information content of the gene into the production of a functional product, usually a protein. Although there are genes whose functional product is an RNA, including the genes encoding the ribosomal RNAs as well as the transfer RNAs and certain other small RNAs, the vast majority of genes within the cell are protein-encoding genes.

GENE REGULATION

The phenotype of a cell as well as the organism as a whole, is the consequence of the regulated expression of a group of genes. Every cell in the organism contains the exact same complement of genes, nevertheless, there are unique proteins produced in the brain that are not produced in the liver, proteins are expressed at a particular time in the cell cycle, proteins are produced in response to hormones, etc. Clearly, an understanding of the molecular basis for the control gene expression is critical to an overall understanding of the basis for cell phenotype.

Regulation of Gene Expression is Responsible for Tissue Differences and Many other Cellular Phenotypes

Since the expression of a gene is ultimately the production of the protein product of the gene, control must be defined as any process that alters the production of the protein. Control of gene expression can be most easily visualised by the pattern of proteins produced in one circumstance versus another. For instance, as schematically depicted in the Fig. 5.2, a two-dimensional gel analysis of proteins (a method that can separate thousands of individual proteins in a sample) in the brain versus in the liver reveals a number of proteins that are common (black spots) but a number of others that are unique to each tissue type.

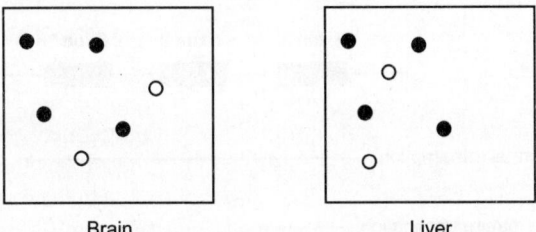

Brain   Liver

Fig. 5.2: Two-dimensional gel analysis of proteins.

Thus, even though both tissues possess the exact same complement of genetic information, the expression of this information differs - gene control clearly does exist. The question is - what is the basis for this control? What are the underlying mechanisms? Gene control in prokaryotes and simple unicellular eukaryotes is largely a response to environmental signals - nutrients, etc. In higher eukaryotes (metazoans), the major form of gene control relates to cellular differentiation. Thus, in most cases it is long term and permanent. An example can be seen in the comparison of proteins synthesised in the brain versus in the liver, as analysed by two dimensional gel electrophoresis. Although the majority of proteins that are synthesised are the same in each tissue, one can find examples of species that are unique to one or the other.

Complexity of Eukaryotic Gene Expression Provides Multiple Opportunities for Gene Control

As discussed previously, the events associated with the expression of any given gene in a eukaryotic cell is a very complex process, involving multiple processing events as well as transport from the nuclear to the cytoplasm in order to achieve the final production of afunctional mRNA. Thus, alterations in any of the steps in mRNA biogenesis could alter the final concentration of functional mRNA. Moreover, control of gene expression could also result from an alteration in the translation efficiency of the mRNA or alterations in the stability of the protein product.

Transcription Control

The initial step in gene expression is transcription of the gene and it is now clear from a variety of studies that the control of transcription is a critical regulatory step in the control of gene expression. In considering transcription control, and particularly when carrying out measurements of transcription, one usually defines the transcriptional unit which is that segment of the chromosome (DNA) that specificies the start and the end of transcription. This includes all of the signals necessary for proper transcription.

Transcription regulation could take the form of either initiation control or termination control . Clearly, the control of initiation will determine whether the primary transcript, and thus the funtional mRNA, will be produced and thus represents the most basic form of gene control. Termination can also be a factor if it occurs prior to the completion of the transcript (premature termination). This has in fact been demonstrated to be an important control in the expression of several oncogenes such as the c-myc gene (Fig. 5.3). A similar example of control of transcription elongation can be found in the control of HIV transcription. In the absence of viral regulatory proteins, HIV transcripts initiate properly but fail to efficiently elongate. One of the early viral proteins produced, known as *Tat*, functions to promote elongation and thus increase the efficiency of viral transcript production. Interestingly, the mechanism for the action of *Tat* is unique in that the protein recognises sequences in the 5′ end of the initiated RNA transcript rather than DNA promoter sequences.

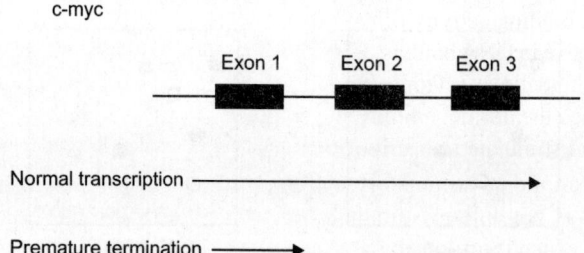

Fig. 5.3: Control in the expression of several oncogenes such as the c-myc gene.

How does one measure transcription, and thus determine transcription control? It is important in this regard to distinguish steady state RNA levels from synthesis which requires that the events of transcription must be separated from subsequent processing steps. Analysis of the RNA in a cellular extract provides a measure of the steady state level - thus, a combination of both transcription and subsequent events. Transcription must be measured by pulse-labeling, usually with a radioactive precursor to RNA, for short time such that no processing has taken place. In short, one is measuring the synthesis of the RNA not the accumulation of the RNA. In actual practice, this is accomplished by incubating cells with radioactive RNA precursors and then measuring the amount of radioactivity incorporated into the RNA, usually by hybridisation to a DNA probe. Once a gene has been isolated and the promoter/enhancer has been identified, it is also possible to study transcription control, particularly the identification of regulatory sequences, through the use of a reporter gene. The promoter to be studied is fused to a gene that can be easily assayed (a reporter) and then assayed by introduction into appropriate cells, or into animals, scoring for the expression of the reporter. For instance, if a suspected promoter element is placed upstream of a β-galactosidase gene (the reporter), activity of the promoter, and thus transcriptional activity, can be assessed by measuring the production of β-galactosidase activity as shown below:

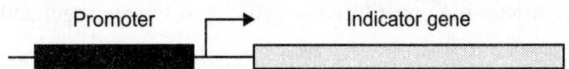

In this way, transcription is being separated from RNA processing contributions by only analysing the role of DNA sequences that contribute to transcription control. Given the fact that transcription is the key first step in gene expression, and the fact that the binding of *trans*-acting factors to promoter elements is critical for transcription, gene expression can be regulated by controlling the activity of these *trans*-acting factors.

Mechanisms regulating transcription factor activity

1. Control of synthesis of the transcription factor: This is primarily the basis for tissue specific control, i.e. a key regulatory factor or factors is only found in the cell type that the target gene is expressed. For example, the albumin gene is transcribed in the liver but not the brain because the necessary transcription factors are not found in the brain. Another example is the myc transcription factor that functions to regulate the transcription of genes important for cell proliferation. The myc protein is not found in quiescent cells because the myc gene is inactive. Upon stimulation of cell growth, the myc promoter is activated and transcription of the gene is induced. As already discussed, the control of termination of transcription of the myc gene is also a factor in the regulation of myc gene expression.

2. Control of the DNA binding activity of the factor: In this case, the protein (transcription factor) is present but it is not active in DNA binding. For example, the steroid hormone receptors are transcription factors. These are intracellular (cytoplasmic) proteins that bind specifically to the hormone when it enters the cell. Once the hormone binds, the receptor is then activated and can enter the nucleus, bind to the gene, and stimulate transcription.

3. Control of the transcriptional stimulatory activity of the factor: In this instance, the protein can bind to DNA but it is not able to stimulate transcription. For instance, the activity of the E2F transcription factor, which is responsible for the control of transcription of various genes important for DNA replication and cell growth, is regulated by interaction with the retinoblastoma (Rb) tumour suppressor protein. When Rb binds to E2F, the resulting complex can still bind to DNA but it is inactive in stimulating transcription. In fact, the complex can function in just the opposite fashion by serving as a repressor of transcription. The interaction of Rb with E2F is regulated by phosphorylation. That is, unphosphorylated Rb can bind to and regulate E2F but when Rb is phosphorylated by cell cycle regulated protein kinases, it loses the capacity to bind to E2F.

Practical importance of defining transcription control elements

In considering strategies for gene therapy, one must be able to express the protein of interest (for instance, the cystic fibrosis gene product) in the right cell type, at the right time, and in the proper amounts. Thus, an understanding of the mechanisms controlling the expression of the gene to be used is essential in designing the gene therapy vector.

To understand the basis for alterations in transcription control that occur in disease conditions such as cancer, it is critical to know the normal mechanisms of function of the gene. Such alterations can take two general forms:

1. Mutation of *trans*-acting factors: This could involve an inactivation of a factor as the result of a specific mutation or deletion or it could involve the creation of a factor with altered properties. For instance, it might become constitutively active (no longer regulated) or it might acquire an altered specificity.

2. Alteration of *cis*-acting elements of a promoter/enhancer: This could involve mutation of the element resulting in a loss of binding of the transcription factor or it could involve chromosomal alterations that create new elements resulting in a change in the transcription of the gene.

Alterations of transcription regulation in disease

By developing an understanding of normal gene structure, as well as the components of transcription regulation, it has been possible to define the molecular basis for alterations in gene control events that underlie certain disease states. Several such examples are given here. Retrovirus mediated promoter insertion resulting in activation of the c-myc gene As discussed above, transcription of the myc gene, which encodes a transcription factor that controls cell cycle progression, is normally tightly controlled by cell growth regulation.

This normal control can be disrupted as the result of an insertion of a retrovirus (ALV) into the promoter region of the c-myc gene. As a result of this insertion, the myc gene is now controlled by the retrovirus promoter which does not respond to the cell growth regulatory signals. Although this is a rare event, it does raise the potential danger of the use of retrovirus vectors in gene therapy protocols, that is, the inadvertant activation of an oncogene as a result of the retrovirus insertion.

This was a critically important discovery that led directly to the discovery of myc gene rearrangements in human tumours as shown below:

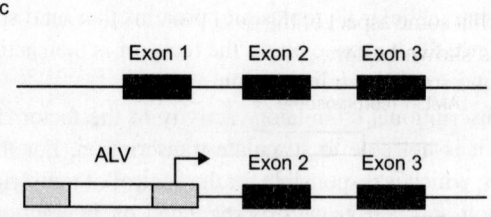

Rearrangement of the c-myc gene in B cell lymphomas

The expression of the c-myc gene is also deregulated in many tumours as the result of chromosome rearrangements, once again resulting from a change in the transcriptional regulatory sequences. For instance, many B cell lymphomas contain a translocation involving chromosome 8 and chromosome 14 that places the c-myc gene in the chromosomal environment of the immunoglobulin heavy chain gene enhancer. In this case, the normal regulation of the myc gene is disrupted with control now being directed by the immunoglobulin enhancer.

This then confers a high level of transcription that is B cell-specific and non-cell cycle regulated as shown below:

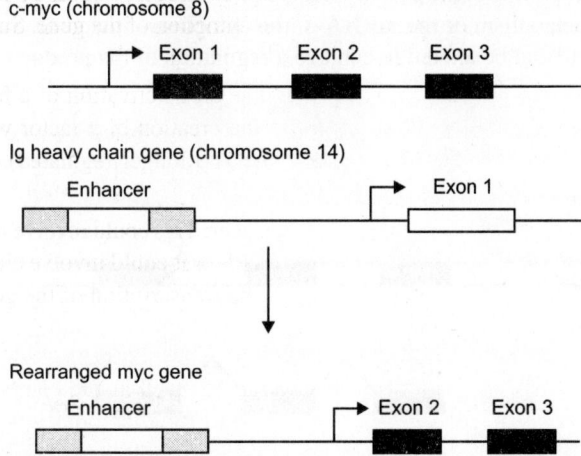

Creation of a chimeric transcription factor in AML by chromosome rearrangments

Whereas the changes detailed above regarding the myc gene result in alterations in regulation of expression of the gene, but still producing the normal protein, another form of transcriptional deregulation can be seen in a chromosomal rearrangement that alters the structure of the encoded protein. The most common chromosomal rearrangment seen in acute myelogenous leukemia is a translocation that fuses a portion of chromosome 8 with a portion of chromosome 21, a so called 8:21 translocation.

The breakpoints involve a gene on chromosome 21 known as AML-1 which encodes a transcription factor and a gene on chromosome 8 known as ETO of unknown function. As a result of the translocation, a new gene is created that encodes a chimeric protein containing sequence from AML-1, including the DNA binding domain, and sequence from ETO. Although the nature of the effect on AML-1 function is unknown, one presumes that some aspect of the specificity or the regulatory properties of the transcription factor has been altered as shown below:

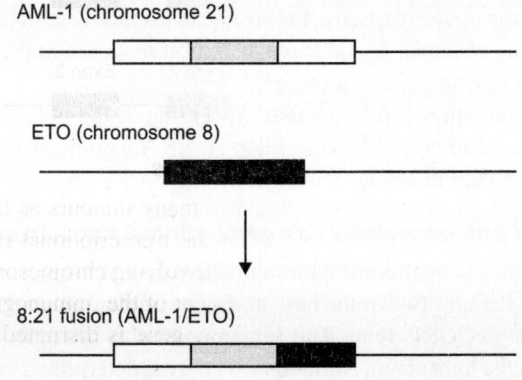

Post-Transcriptional Gene Control

Each one of the steps of mRNA biogenesis following transcription has been demonstrated to participate in gene regulation. Thus, splicing of the primary transcript, 3′ end cleavage and polyadenylation, transport to the cytoplasm, and metabolism of the mRNA in the cytoplasm, including translation efficiency and stability of the mRNA, all can be altered to achieve a regulation of the production of the product of the gene as shown below:

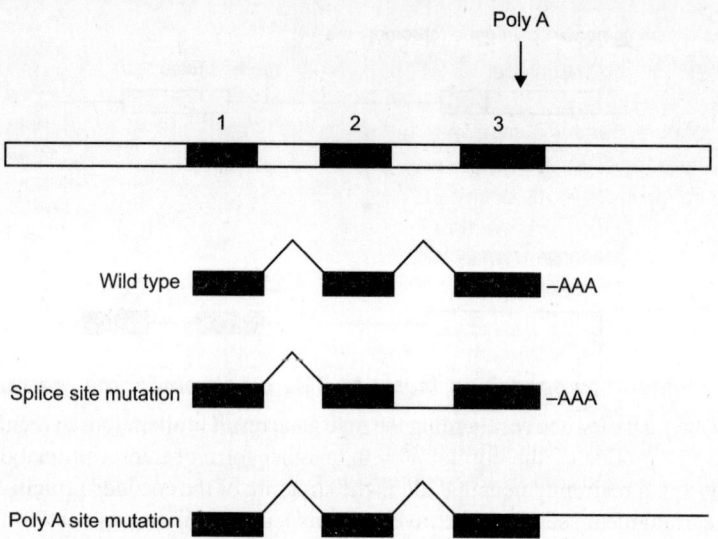

A variety of transcription units have now been shown to possess the potential to produce more than one mRNA as a result of alternative processing. This can include both alternative splicing as well as polyadenylation. A selective use of exons in a primary transcript can thus define a distinct protein product. If this selection is regulated, changing under one circumstance or another, then such changes are defined as events regulating the expression of the gene.

It is also clear that mutation of either critical splice site sequences or poly A site sequences can impair gene expression. Although such mutations would not alter the coding sequences directly, they can result in alterations that do affect the coding capacity. For instance, a splice site mutation that altered the splice donor following exon 2 in the example, would leave the intron sequence in the mRNA which would lead to a frameshift and likely a non-functional protein.

Likewise, a poly A site mutation would prevent processing at the poly A site resulting in an RNA with an extended 3′ terminus and no poly A tail. Such an RNA would not be efficiently transported to the cytoplasm and would be very unstable.

Alternative splicing and polyadenylation as gene control mechanisms

There are a variety of examples of gene control through alternative RNA processing events, both splicing as well as polyadenylation. Perhaps two of the best studies examples include the immunoglobulin heavy chain gene and the calcitonin/CGRP gene. The immunoglobulin heavy is composed of two protein molecules, a heavy chain and a light chain. Antibody diversity is determined by variation in the sequence in both the heavy chain and the light chain as a consequence of gene rearrangement as well as mutation.

In addition, the production of the heavy chain is regulated during B cell differentiation. In a mature B cell, the heavy chain, together with the light chain, is inserted into the B cell membrane and serves as an antigen receptor. When antigen binds, the B cell is stimulated to mature to a plasma cell where the immunoglobulin molecule is now secreted as a antibody. This switch in immunoglobulin expression is the result of alternative splicing as well as polyadenylation of the primary transcript of the gene as indicated below. This brings a different set of exon sequences into the 3' position of the transcript. The Cμ4 exon encodes the secreted form of the protein whereas the M1 and M2 exons encode the membrane bound form of the protein.

Another example can be found in the calcitonin gene which encodes a calcium regulating hormone that is produced in the thyroid. This locus also encodes a distinct separate product known as CGRP (calcitonin gene related peptide), a neuropeptide produced in the brain. Thus, alternative RNA splicing and polyadenylation, that occurs in a tissue specific manner (brain versus thyroid), results in the production of two distinct gene products with distinct function. Finally, one very striking example of the role of alternative RNA processing in the control of gene expression can be seen in the large variety of products that can be generated from the alpha-tropomyosin locus in a tissue-specific fashion.

Other forms of post-transcription gene control

Control of RNA transport: Although there are no clear examples whereby the nuclear/cytoplasmic transport of a cellular mRNA is regulated, there are at least two instances in viral infections in which RNA transport is affected.

First, adenovirus infection results in the inhibition of transport of most cellular mRNAs - a specific viral gene product is required for this to occur and at the same time, this protein facilitates the transport of viral RNA.

Second, as indicated previously, studies of Bryan Cullen and colleagues here at Duke have shown that the product of the HIV rev gene is required for the efficient transport of unspliced viral RNA from the nucleus to the cytoplasm.

Control of mRNA stability: The stability of mRNAs varies over a large range. Some RNAs are quite stable with half lives approaching the cell division time. Other RNAs turn over very rapidly (half lives of a few minutes). As a general rule, RNAs that are expressed in a transient fashion often are short lived. Many RNAs that encode cytokines as well as early responses to mitogens are unstable, dependent on specific sequences in the 3' untranslated region of the RNA. The unstable nature of the mRNA as a result of recognition of this sequence is associated with shortening of the poly A tail.

Translation control: General control - alterations of translation factors can alter the translation efficiency of mRNAs. For instance, phosphorylation of eIF2 inhibits is action. Translation efficiency is also determined by *cis*-acting sequences in the mRNA - particularly the sequences that surround the AUG initiation codon.

OPERON

An operon is a functioning unit of genomic material containing a cluster of genes under the control of a single regulatory signal or promoter. The genes are transcribed together into a mRNA strand and either translated together in the cytoplasm or undergo *trans*-splicing to create monocistronic mRNAs that are translated separately, i.e. several strands of mRNA that each encode a single gene product. The result of this is that the genes contained in the operon are either expressed together or not at all. Originally operons were thought to exist solely in prokaryotes but since the discovery of the first operons in eukaryotes in the early 1990s, more evidence has arisen to suggest they are more common than previously assumed. Several genes must be both co-transcribed and co-regulated to define an operon.

Operons occur primarily in prokaryotes but also in some eukaryotes, including nematodes, *Drosophila melanogaster* flies, and *C. elegans*. rRNA genes often exist in operons that have been found in a range of eukaryotes including chordates. An operon is made up of several structural genes arranged under a common promoter and regulated by a common operator. It is defined as a set of adjacent structural genes, plus the adjacent regulatory signals that affect transcription of the structural genes. The regulators of a given operon, including repressors, corepressors, and activators, are not necessarily coded for by that operon. The location and condition of the regulators, promoter, operator and structural DNA sequences can determine the effects of common mutations.

Operons are related to regulons and stimulons. Whereas operons contain a set of genes regulated by the same operator, regulons contain a set of genes under regulation by a single regulatory protein, and stimulons contain a set of genes under regulation by a single cell stimulus.

Operon as a Unit of Transcription

An operon contains one or more structural genes which are transcribed into one polycistronic mRNA: a single mRNA molecule that codes for more than one protein. Upstream of the structural genes lies a promoter sequence which provides a site for RNA polymerase to bind and initiate transcription. Close to the promoter lies a section of DNA called an operator. The operon may also contain regulatory genes such as a repressor gene which codes for a regulatory protein that binds to the operator and inhibits transcription. Regulatory genes need not be part of the operon itself, but may be located elsewhere in the genome. The repressor molecule will reach the operator to block the transcription of the structural genes.

lac Operon

The *lac* operon is an operon required for the transport and metabolism of lactose in *Escherichia coli* and some other enteric bacteria. It consists of three adjacent structural genes, a promoter, a terminator, and an operator. The *lac* operon is regulated by several factors including the availability of glucose and of lactose. Gene regulation of the *lac* operon was the first complex genetic regulatory mechanism to be elucidated and is one of the foremost examples of prokaryotic gene regulation (Fig. 5.4).

lac operon

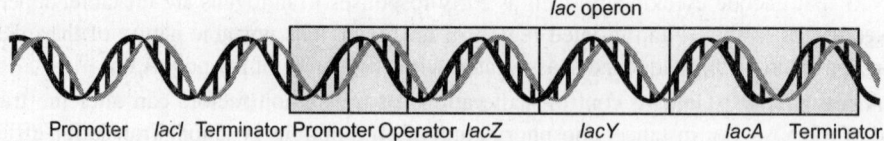

Promoter *lacI* Terminator Promoter Operator *lacZ*   *lacY*   *lacA* Terminator

Fig. 5.4: Prokaryotic gene regulation.

In its natural environment, the *lac* operon is a complex mechanism to digest lactose efficiently. The cell can use lactose as an energy source by producing the enzyme β-galactosidase to digest that lactose into glucose. However, it would be inefficient to produce enzymes when there is no lactose available, or if there is a more readily-available energy source available such as glucose. The *lac* operon uses a two-part control mechanism to ensure that the cell expends energy producing β-galactosidase, β-galactoside permease and thiogalactoside transacetylase (also known as galactoside O-acetyltransferase) only when necessary. It achieves this with the *lac* repressor, which halts production in the absence of lactose, and the catabolite activator protein (CAP), which assists in production in the absence of glucose. This dual control mechanism causes the sequential utilisation of glucose and lactose in two distinct growth phases, known as diauxie. Similar diauxic growth patterns have been observed in bacterial growth on mixtures of other sugars as well, such as mixtures of glucose and xylose or of glucose and arabinose, etc. The genetic control mechanisms underlying such diauxic growth patterns are known as *xyl* operon and *ara* operon, etc.

trp Operon

The *trp* operon (Fig. 5.5) encodes the genes for the synthesis of tryptophan. This cluster of genes, like the *lac* operon, is regulated by a repressor that binds to the operator sequences. The activity of the *trp* repressor for binding the operator region is enhanced when it binds tryptophan, in this capacity, tryptophan is known as a corepressor. Since the activity of the *trp* repressor is enhanced in the presence of tryptophan, the rate of expression of the *trp* operon is graded in response to the level of tryptophan in the cell.

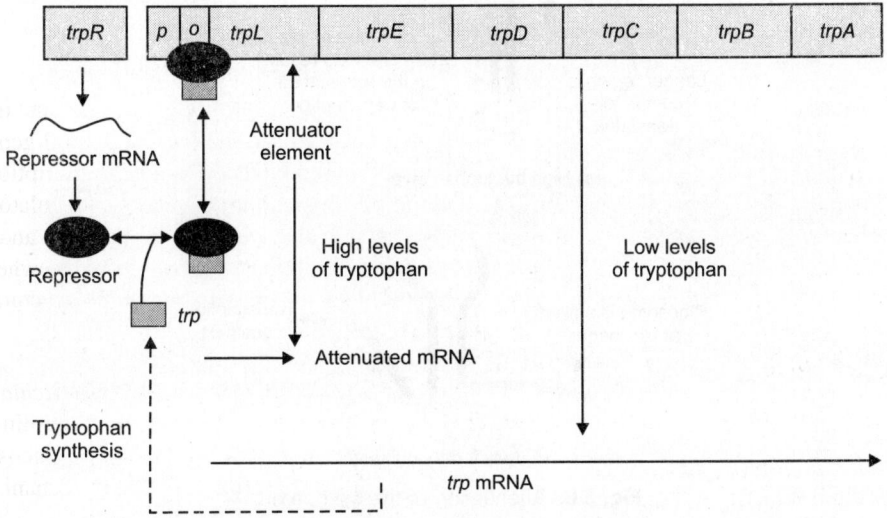

Fig. 5.5: Structure of the *trp* operon.

Expression of the *trp* operon is also regulated by attenuation. The attenuator region, which is composed of sequences found within the transcribed RNA, is involved in controlling transcription from the operon after RNA polymerase has initiated synthesis. The attenuator of sequences of the RNA are found near the 5′ end of the RNA termed the leader region of the RNA. The leader sequences are located prior to the start of the coding region for the first gene of the operon (the *trpE* gene). The attenuator region contains codons for a small leader polypeptide, that contains tandem tryptophan codons. This region of the RNA is also capable of forming several different stable stem-loop structures.

Depending on the level of tryptophan in the cell and hence the level of charged *trp*-tRNAs, the position of ribosomes on the leader polypeptide and the rate at which they are translating allows different stem-loops to form. If tryptophan is abundant, the ribosome prevents stem-loop 1–2 from forming and thereby favours stem-loop 3–4. The latter is found near a region rich in uracil and acts as the transcriptional terminator loop. Consequently, RNA polymerase is dislodged from the template.

The operons coding for genes necessary for the synthesis of a number of other amino acids are also regulated by this attenuation mechanism. It should be clear, however, that this type of transcriptional regulation is not feasible for eukaryotic cells. Regulation of the *trp* operon in *E. coli*. The *trp* operon is controlled by both a repressor protein binding to the operator region as well as by translation-induced transcriptional attenuation. The *trp* repressor binds the operator region of the *trp* operon only when bound to tryptophan. This makes tryptophan a co-repressor of the operon. The *trpL* gene encodes a non-functional leader peptide which contains several adjacent trp codons. The structural genes of the operon responsible for tryptophan biosynthesis are *trpE, D, C, B* and *A*. When trptophan level are high some binds to the repressor which then binds to the operator region and inhibits transcription. The mechanism of attenuation of the *trp* operon is shown in Fig. 5.6.

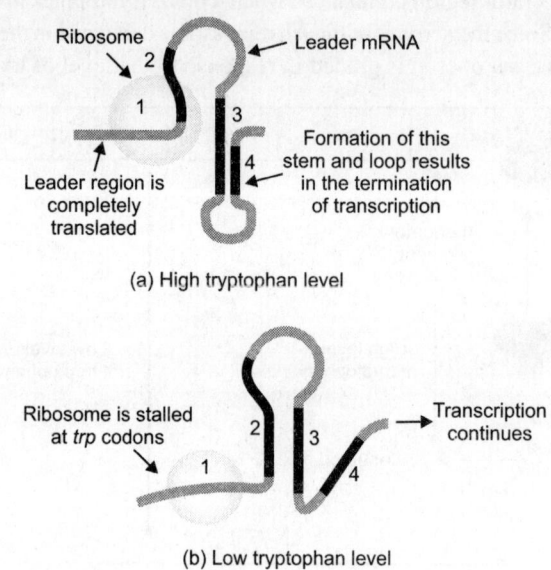

(a) High tryptophan level

(b) Low tryptophan level

Fig. 5.6: Attenuation of the *trp* operon.

Attenuation of the *trp* operon. The attenuation region of the *trp* operon contains sequences that allow the resulting mRNA to form several different stem-loop structures. These regions are identified as 1 through 4. The stem-loops that are significant as to whether transcription is attenuated or not are formed between regions 2 and 3 or between regions 3 and 4. When tryptophan levels are high there is plenty of charged *trp*-tRNAs available and ribosomes translating the leader peptide encoded by the *trpL* gene do not stall at the repeated *trp* codons in the leader peptide. Under these conditions the ribosomes rapidly cover regions 1 and 2 of the mRNA which allows the stem-loop composed of regions 3 and 4 to form. The stem-loop formed by regions 3–4 results in a transcriptional termination structure and transcription of the *trp* operon ceases, that is attenuated. Conversely, when tryptophan levels are low the level of charged *trp*-tRNAs will also be low.

This leads to a stalling of the ribosomes within the leader peptide when they encounter the *trp* codon repeats. The ribosome stalls over region 1 of the mRNA which allows step-loop 2–3 to form and prevents the transcriptional termination stem-loop 3–4 from forming. The inability of this structure to form allows the entire operon to be transcribed and the tryptophan biosynthetic enzymes to be produced.

Repression

This is a negative repressive feedback mechanism. The repressor for the *trp* operon is produced upstream by the *trpR* gene, which is continually expressed at a low level. It creates monomers, which associate into tetramers. These tetramers are inactive and 'floating' around within the cell. When tryptophan is present, these tetramers bind to the tryptophan repressor tetramers causing a change in conformation, which allows the repressor to bind the operator. This prevents RNA polymerase from binding to and transcribing the operon, so tryptophan is not produced from its precursor. When tryptophan is not present, the repressor is in its native conformation and cannot bind the operator region, so transcription is not inhibited by the repressor.

lac Operon of E. Coli

- The *lac* operon of *E. coli* contains genes involved in lactose metabolism. It's expressed only when lactose is present and glucose is absent.
- Two regulators turn the operon 'on' and 'off' in response to lactose and glucose levels: the *lac* repressor and catabolite activator protein (CAP).
- The *lac* repressor acts as a lactose sensor. It normally blocks transcription of the operon, but stops acting as a repressor when lactose is present. The *lac* repressor senses lactose indirectly, through its isomer allolactose.
- Catabolite activator protein (CAP) acts as a glucose sensor. It activates transcription of the operon, but only when glucose levels are low. CAP senses glucose indirectly, through the 'hunger signal' molecule cAMP.

Lactose can be an excellent meal for *E. coli* bacteria. With that for context, what exactly is the *lac* operon? The *lac* operon is an operon, or group of genes with a single promoter (transcribed as a single mRNA). The genes in the operon encode proteins that allow the bacteria to use lactose as an energy source.

lac Operon Turn In

E. coli bacteria can break down lactose, but it's not their favorite fuel. If glucose is around, they would much rather use that. Glucose requires fewer steps and less energy to break down than lactose. However, if lactose is the only sugar available, the *E. coli* will go right ahead and use it as an energy source.

To use lactose, the bacteria must express the *lac* operon genes, which encode key enzymes for lactose uptake and metabolism. To be as efficient as possible, *E. coli* should express the *lac* operon only when two conditions are met:

- Lactose is available.
- Glucose is not available.

How are levels of lactose and glucose detected, and how how do changes in levels affect *lac* operon transcription? Two regulatory proteins are involved:

- One, the *lac* repressor, acts as a lactose sensor.
- The other, catabolite activator protein (CAP), acts as a glucose sensor.

These proteins bind to the DNA of the *lac* operon and regulate its transcription based on lactose and glucose levels.

Structure of the *lac* Operon

The *lac* operon contains three genes: *lacZ*, *lacY*, and *lacA*. These genes are transcribed as a single mRNA, under control of one promoter (Fig. 5.7).

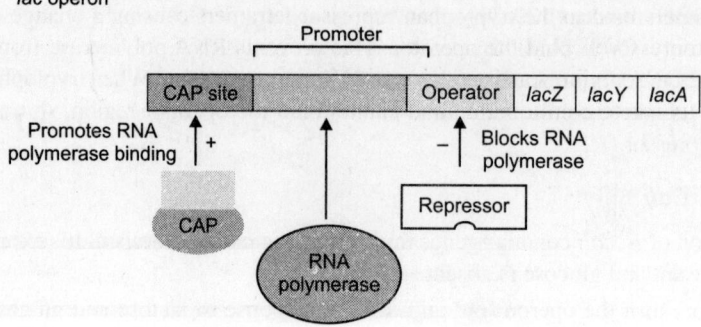

Fig. 5.7: Structure of the *lac* operon.

Genes in the *lac* operon specify proteins that help the cell utilise lactose. *lacZ* encodes an enzyme that splits lactose into monosaccharides (single-unit sugars) that can be fed into glycolysis. Similarly, lacY encodes a membrane-embedded transporter that helps bring lactose into the cell.

In addition to the three genes, the *lac* operon also contains a number of regulatory DNA sequences. These are regions of DNA to which particular regulatory proteins can bind, controlling transcription of the operon.

- The promoter is the binding site for RNA polymerase, the enzyme that performs transcription.
- The operator is a negative regulatory site bound by the *lac* repressor protein. The operator overlaps with the promoter, and when the *lac* repressor is bound, RNA polymerase cannot bind to the promoter and start transcription.
- The CAP binding site is a positive regulatory site that is bound by catabolite activator protein (CAP). When CAP is bound to this site, it promotes transcription by helping RNA polymerase bind to the promoter.

lac Repressor

The *lac* repressor is a protein that represses (inhibits) transcription of the *lac* operon. It does this by binding to the operator, which partially overlaps with the promoter. When bound, the *lac* repressor gets in RNA polymerase's way and keeps it from transcribing the operon.

When lactose is not available, the *lac* repressor binds tightly to the operator, preventing transcription by RNA polymerase. However, when lactose is present, the *lac* repressor loses its ability to bind DNA. It floats off the operator, clearing the way for RNA polymerase to transcribe the operon.

This change in the *lac* repressor is caused by the small molecule allolactose, an isomer (rearranged version) of lactose. When lactose is available, some molecules will be converted to allolactose inside the cell. Allolactose binds to the *lac* repressor and makes it change shape so it can no longer bind DNA.

Allolactose is an example of an inducer, a small molecule that triggers expression of a gene or operon. The *lac* operon is considered an inducible operon because it is usually turned off (repressed), but can be turned on in the presence of the inducer allolactose.

Catabolite Activator Protein

Catabolite activator protein (Fig. 5.8) (CAP, also known as cAMP receptor protein, CRP) is a *trans-acting* transcriptional activator that exists as a homodimer in solution. Each subunit of CAP is composed of a ligand-binding domain at the *N*-terminus (CAPN, residues 1-138) and a DNA-binding domain at the C-terminus (DBD, residues 139-209). Two cAMP (cyclic AMP) molecules bind dimeric CAP with negative cooperativity. Cyclic AMP functions as an allosteric effector by increasing CAP's affinity for DNA. CAP binds a DNA region upstream from the DNA binding site of RNA polymerase. CAP activates transcription through protein-protein interactions with the α-subunit of RNA polymerase.

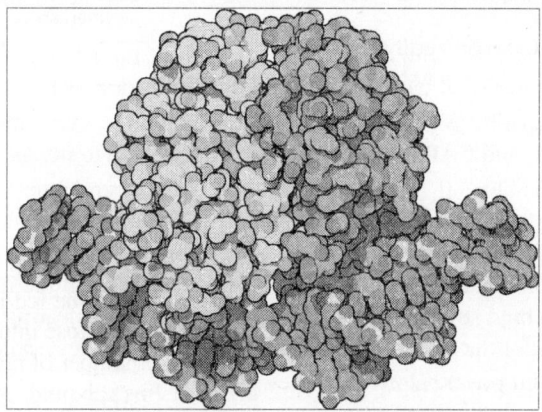

Fig. 5.8: Catabolite activator protein.

This protein-protein interaction is responsible for (i) catalysing the formation of the RNAP-promoter closed complex, and (ii) isomerisation of the RNAP-promoter complex to the open confirmation. CAP's interaction with RNA polymerase causes bending of the DNA near the transcription start site, thus effectively catalysing the transcription initiation process. CAP's name is derived from its ability to affect transcription of genes involved in many catabolic pathways. For example, when the amount of glucose transported into the cell is low, a cascade of events results in the increase of cytosolic cAMP levels. This increase in cAMP levels is sensed by CAP, which goes on to activate the transcription of many other catabolic genes. CAP has a characteristic helix-turn-helix motif structure that allows it to bind to successive major grooves on DNA. The two helices are reinforcing, each causing a 43° turn in the structure, with an overall 94° turn in the DNA. This interaction opens up the DNA molecule, allowing RNA polymerase to bind and transcribe the genes involved in lactose catabolism. cAMP-CAP is required for transcription activation of the *lac* operon. This requirement reflects the greater simplicity with which glucose may be metabolised in comparison to lactose. The cell 'prefers' glucose, and, if it is available, the *lac* operon is not activated, even when lactose is present. This is an effective way of integrating the two different signals. This phenomenon is known as catabolite repression. CAP plays an important role in catabolite repression, a well-known example of a modulon and also plays a role in the Mal regulon.

When lactose is present, the *lac* repressor loses its DNA-binding ability. This clears the way for RNA polymerase to bind to the promoter and transcribe the *lac* operon. That sounds like the end of the story, right?

Well not quite. As it turns out, RNA polymerase alone does not bind very well to the *lac* operon promoter. It might make a few transcripts, but it won't do much more unless it gets extra help from catabolite activator protein (CAP). CAP binds to a region of DNA just before the *lac* operon promoter and helps RNA polymerase attach to the promoter, driving high levels of transcription.

CAP is not always active (able to bind DNA). Instead, it's regulated by a small molecule called cyclic AMP (cAMP). cAMP is a 'hunger signal' made by *E. coli* when glucose levels are low. cAMP binds to CAP, changing its shape and making it able to bind DNA and promote transcription. Without cAMP, CAP cannot bind DNA and is inactive. CAP is only active when glucose levels are low (cAMP levels are high). Thus, the *lac* operon can only be transcribed at high levels when glucose is absent. This strategy ensures that bacteria only turn on the *lac* operon and start using lactose after they have used up all of the preferred energy source (glucose).

So, when does the *lac* Operon really Turn On?

The *lac* operon will be expressed at high levels if two conditions are met:

- Glucose must be unavailable: When glucose is unavailable, cAMP binds to CAP, making CAP able to bind DNA. Bound CAP helps RNA polymerase attach to the *lac* operon promoter.
- Lactose must be available: If lactose is available, the *lac* repressor will be released from the operator (by binding of allolactose). This allows RNA polymerase to move forward on the DNA and transcribe the operon.

These two events in combination – the binding of the activator and the release of the repressor – allow RNA polymerase to bind strongly to the promoter and give it a clear path for transcription. They lead to strong transcription of the *lac* operon and production of enzymes needed for lactose utilisation.

These can be summarised given below:

- Glucose present, lactose absent: No transcription of the *lac* operon occurs. That is because the *lac* repressor remains bound to the operator and prevents transcription by RNA polymerase. Also, cAMP levels are low because glucose levels are high, so CAP is inactive and cannot bind DNA.
- Glucose present, lactose present: Low-level transcription of the *lac* operon occurs. The *lac* repressor is released from the operator because the inducer (allolactose) is present. cAMP levels, however, are low because glucose is present. Thus, CAP remains inactive and cannot bind to DNA, so transcription only occurs at a low, leaky level.
- Glucose absent, lactose absent: No transcription of the *lac* operon occurs. cAMP levels are high because glucose levels are low, so CAP is active and will be bound to the DNA. However, the *lac* repressor will also be bound to the operator (due to the absence of allolactose), acting as a roadblock to RNA polymerase and preventing transcription.
- Glucose absent, lactose present: Strong transcription of the *lac* operon occurs. The *lac* repressor is released from the operator because the inducer (allolactose) is present. cAMP levels are high because glucose is absent, so CAP is active and bound to the DNA. CAP helps RNA polymerase bind to the promoter, permitting high levels of transcription.

Summary of *lac* Operon Responses

Glucose	Lactose	CAP binds	Repressor binds	Level of transcription
+	−	−	+	No transcription
+	+	−	−	Low-level transcription
−	−	+	+	No transcription
−	+	+	−	Strong transcription

Chapter 6

Transcription Attenuation

INTRODUCTION

Attenuation (in genetics) is a proposed mechanism of control in some bacterial operons which results in premature termination of transcription and is based on the fact that, in bacteria, transcription and translation proceed simultaneously. Attenuation involves a provisional stop signal (attenuator), located in the DNA segment that corresponds to the leader sequence of mRNA. During attenuation, the ribosome becomes stalled (delayed) in the attenuator region in the mRNA leader. Depending on the metabolic conditions, the attenuator either stops transcription at that point or allows read-through to the structural gene part of the mRNA and synthesis of the appropriate protein.

Attenuation is a regulatory feature found throughout *Archaea* and Bacteria causing premature termination of transcription. Attenuators are 5′-*cis* acting regulatory regions which fold into one of two alternative RNA structures which determine the success of transcription. The folding is modulated by a sensing mechanism producing either a Rho-independent terminator, resulting in interrupted transcription and a non-functional RNA product, or an anti-terminator structure, resulting in a functional RNA transcript.

There are now many equivalent examples where the translation, not transcription, is terminated by sequestering the Shine-Dalgarno sequence (ribosomal binding site) in a hairpin-loop structure. While not meeting the previous definition of (transcriptional) attenuation, these are now considered to be variants of the same phenomena and are included in this chapter.

Attenuation is an ancient regulatory system, prevalent in many bacterial species providing fast and sensitive regulation of gene operons and is commonly used to repress genes in the presence of their own product (or a downstream metabolite).

CLASSIFICATION OF ATTENUATORS

Attenuators may be classified according to the type of molecule which induces the change in RNA structure. It is likely that transcription attenuation mechanisms developed early, perhaps prior to the *archaea*/bacteria separation and have since evolved to use a number of different sensing molecules (the tryptophan biosynthetic operon has been found to use three different mechanisms in different organisms.)

Small-molecule-mediated Attenuation (Riboswitches)

Riboswitch sequences (in the mRNA leader transcript) bind molecules such as amino acids, nucleotides, sugars, vitamins, metal ions and other small ligands which cause a conformational change in the mRNA. Most of these attenuators are inhibitory and are employed by genes for biosynthetic enzymes or transporters whose expression is inversely related to the concentration of their corresponding metabolites.

Example: Cobalamine biosynthesis, Cyclic AMP-GMP switch , lysin biosynthesis, glycine biosynthesis, fluoride switch, etc.

T-boxes

These elements are bound by specific uncharged tRNAs and modulate the expression of corresponding aminoacyl-tRNA synthetase operons. High levels of uncharged tRNA promote the anti-terminator sequence leading to increased concentrations of charged tRNA. These are considered by some to be a separate family of riboswitches but are significantly more complex than the previous class of attenuators.

Protein-mediated attenuation

Protein-RNA interactions may prevent or stabilise the formation of an anti-terminator structure.

Ribosome-mediated attenuation

In this situation RNA polymerase is dependent on (lagging) ribosome activity, if the ribosome pauses due to insufficient charged tRNA then the anti-terminator structure is favoured. The canonical attenuator example of the *trp* operon uses this mechanism in *E. coli*.

RNA thermometers

Temperature dependent loop formations introduce temperature-dependence in the expression of downstream operons. All such elements act in a translation-dependent manner by controlling the accessibility of the Shine-Dalgarno sequence, for example the expression of pathogenicity islands of some bacteria upon entry to a host. Recent data predict the existence of temperature-dependent alternative secondary structures (including Rho-independent terminators) upstream of cold shock proteins in *E. coli*.

Discovery of Operon

Attenuation was first observed by Charles Yanofsky in the *trp* operon of *E. coli*. The first observation was linked to two separate scientific facts. Mutations which knocked out the *trp* R (repressor) gene still showed some regulation of the *trp* operon (these mutants were not fully induced/repressed by tryptophan). The total range of *trp* operon regulation is about 700 X (on/off). When the *trp* repressor was knocked out, one still got about 10 X regulation by the absence or presence of *trp*. When the sequence of the beginning of the *trp* operon was determined an unusual open reading frame (ORF) was seen immediately preceding the ORFs for the known structural genes for the tryptophan biosynthetic enzymes. The general structural information shown below was observed from the sequence of the *trp* operon.

First, Yanofsky observed that the ORF contained two tandem *Trp* codons and the protein had a *Trp* percent composition which was about 10X normal.

Second, the mRNA in this region contained regions of dyad symmetry which would allow it to form two mutually exclusive secondary structures. One of the structures looked exactly like a rho-independent transcription termination signal. The other secondary structure, if formed, would prevent the formation of this secondary structure and thus the terminator. This other structure is called the 'preemptor'.

trp Operon

An example is the *trp* gene in bacteria. When there is a high level of tryptophan in the region, it is inefficient for the bacterium to synthesise more. When the RNA polymerase binds and transcribes the *trp* gene, the ribosome will start translating. (This differs from eukaryotic cells, where RNA must exit the nucleus before translation starts.) The attenuator sequence, which is located between the mRNA leader sequence (5′ UTR) and *trp* operon gene sequence, contains four domains, where domain 3 can pair with domain 2 or domain 4.

The attenuator sequence at domain 1 contains instruction for peptide synthesis that requires tryptophans. A high level of tryptophan will permit ribosomes to translate the attenuator sequence domains 1 and 2, allowing domains 3 and 4 to form a hairpin structure, which results in termination of transcription of the *trp* operon. Since the protein coding genes are not transcribed due to rho independent termination, no tryptophan is synthesised.

In contrast, a low level of tryptophan means that the ribosome will stall at domain 1, causing the domains 2 and 3 to form a different hairpin structure that does not signal termination of transcription. Therefore, the rest of the operon will be transcribed and translated, so that tryptophan can be produced. Thus, domain 4 is an attenuator. Without domain 4, translation can continue regardless of the level of tryptophan. The attenuator sequence has its codons translated into a leader peptide, but is not part of the *trp* operon gene sequence. The attenuator allows more time for the attenuator sequence domains to form loop structures, but does not produce a protein that is used in later tryptophan synthesis.

Attenuation is a second mechanism of negative feedback in the *trp* operon. While the *Trp*R repressor decreases transcription by a factor of 70, attenuation can further decrease it by a factor of 10, thus allowing accumulated repression of about 700-fold. Attenuation is made possible by the fact that in prokaryotes (which have no nucleus), the ribosomes begin translating the mRNA while RNA polymerase is still transcribing the DNA sequence. This allows the process of translation to directly affect transcription of the operon.

At the beginning of the transcribed genes of the *trp* operon is a sequence of 140 nucleotides termed the leader transcript (*trp*L). This transcript includes four short sequences designated 1–4. Sequence 1 is partially complementary to sequence 2, which is partially complementary to sequence 3, which is partially complementary to sequence 4. Thus, three distinct secondary structures (hairpins) can form: 1–2, 2–3 or 3–4. The hybridisation of strands 1–2 to form the 1–2 structure prevents the formation of the 2–3 structure, while the formation of 2–3 prevents the formation of 3–4. The 3–4 structure is a transcription termination sequence, once it forms RNA polymerase will disassociate from the DNA and transcription of the structural genes of the operon will not occur.

Part of the leader transcript codes for a short polypeptide of 14 amino acids, termed the leader peptide. This peptide contains two adjacent tryptophan residues, which is unusual, since tryptophan is a fairly uncommon amino acid (about one in a hundred residues in a typical *E. coli* protein is tryptophan). If the ribosome attempts to translate this peptide while tryptophan levels in the cell are low, it will stall at either of the two *trp* codons. While it is stalled, the ribosome physically shields sequence 1 of the transcript, thus preventing it from forming the 1–2 secondary structure. Sequence 2 is then free to hybridise with sequence 3 to form the 2–3 structure, which then prevents the formation of the 3–4 termination hairpin. RNA polymerase is free to continue transcribing the entire operon. If tryptophan levels in the cell are high, the ribosome will translate the entire leader peptide without interruption and will only stall during translation termination at the stop codon. At this point the ribosome physically shields both sequences 1–2. Sequences 3–4 are thus free to form the 3–4 structure which terminates transcription.

The end result is that the operon will be transcribed only when tryptophan is unavailable for the ribosome, while the *trp*L transcript is constitutively expressed.

To ensure that the ribosome binds and begins translation of the leader transcript immediately following its synthesis, a pause site exists in the *trp*L sequence. Upon reaching this site, RNA polymerase pauses transcription and apparently waits for translation to begin. This mechanism allows for synchronisation of transcription and translation, a key element in attenuation. A similar attenuation mechanism regulates the synthesis of histidine, phenylalanine and threonine.

Mechanism in the trp operon

The proposed mechanism of how this mRNA secondary structure and the *trp* leader peptide could regulate transcription of the *trp* biosynthetic enzymes includes the following.

- RNAP initiates transcription of the *trp* promoter.
- RNAP pauses at about nucleotide 90 at a secondary structure.
- Ribosomes engage this nascent mRNA and initiate translation of the leader peptide.
  - o RNAP is then 'released' from its pause and continues transcription.
- When RNAP reaches the region of the potential terminator, whether it continues or not is dependent on the position of the ribosome 'trailing behind'.
  - o If the ribosome stalls at the tandem *Trp* codons, waiting for the appropriate tRNA, region 1 is sequestered within the ribosome and thus cannot base pair with region 2. This means that region 2 and 3 become based paired before region 4 can be transcribed. This forces region 4 when it is made to be single stranded, preventing the formation of the region 3/4 terminator structure. Transcription will then continue.
  - o If the ribosome translates the leader peptide with no hesitation, it then covers a portion of region 2 preventing it from base pairing with region 3. Then when region 4 is transcribed, it forms a stem and loop with region 3 and transcription is terminated, generating a ca. 140 base transcript.
- This mechanism of control measures the amount of available, charged *Trp*-tRNA.

The location of ribosomes determines which alternate secondary structures form.

Attenuation in Eukaryotes

Research conducted on microRNA processing showed an evidence of attenuation process in Eukaryotes. After co-transcriptional endonucleolitical cleavage by Drosha 5'->3' exonuclease XRN2 may terminate further transcription by torpedo mechanism.

TRANSCRIPTION ATTENUATION

As many of the features of gene expression and its regulation have been revealed, it has become apparent that every organism, from the simplest to the most complex, utilises an appreciable fraction of its resources in regulatory processes that control its functional genes and interrelate their various activities. The development of regulatory mechanisms optimal for each organism, in its environmental niche, is thus a major theme in evolution. Macromolecular interactions are the principal events of gene regulation, with small and large molecules serving as signals for these regulatory activities.

Most prokaryotic operons are regulated transcriptionally at or near a short promoter region that binds relatively few regulatory proteins. These interactions may activate or inhibit transcription initiation. Regulatory mechanisms also target molecular events that occur subsequent to transcription initiation.

These mechanisms include processes that influence transcript elongation and transcription termination. In most eukaryotes, regulation of gene expression is more complex, with each gene's promoter/regulatory region replete with regulatory sites, or elements, that allow recognition of, and response to, many different regulatory proteins. The state of these proteins reflects their identity, the cell's environment, the stage of development, and the metabolic and other activities that are proceeding in the cells in which these regulatory proteins reside. Transcription attenuation also occurs in eukaryotes, but features of such mechanisms are only beginning to emerge.

It was once thought that repression of transcription initiation was sufficiently adaptable as a regulatory mechanism to be principally responsible for most gene regulation in most organisms. It is now apparent that each organism uses a variety of regulatory strategies in modulating gene expression. Often a single gene or operon is regulated by multiple independent mechanisms. In view of the extensive use of gene regulation, an important consideration for each organism during the course of evolution must have been how much genetic information to devote to regulatory processes. In some organisms, notably bacteria, the need for effective gene regulation must have conflicted with the desire to maintain a relatively small genome. A small genome would limit the number of regulatory genes and events that could be devoted to control and probably would favour regulatory mechanisms that require minimal genetic information. These evolutionary pressures notwithstanding, it is evident that even organisms with small genomes, such as viruses, make extensive use of gene regulation.

Once organisms were committed to differential gene regulation, it would have been advantageous to sense all external and internal events relevant to each gene's expression and to couple these events in one or more regulatory circuits. The use of both gene-specific regulatory mechanisms and global regulatory mechanisms that interrelated gene activities clearly would have been beneficial. It is perhaps not surprising that so many regulatory processes exist and that cells can sense and respond in so many ways to the numerous events that influence their behaviour.

Objectives of Transcription Attenuation as a Regulatory Mechanism

Transcription attenuation allows an organism to regulate gene expression by exploiting RNA sequences and structures, as opposed to information contained in DNA. It also allows cells to sense availability of the precursors needed for RNA and protein synthesis. An RNA signal can direct a transcribing RNA polymerase molecule to pause during transcript elongation, to terminate transcription prematurely, or to transcribe through a potential termination sequence. RNA sequences also can provide binding sites for regulatory factors that can influence the aforementioned events. Mutually exclusive RNA structures can allow determination of whether transcription will or will not be terminated at a particular site. By exploiting RNA sequences and structures in regulatory decisions, nature has engaged RNAs in ways that are not appropriate to regulation of transcription initiation. Thus, we see that translation is often used to mediate attenuation decisions. Similarly, a transcribing or paused RNA polymerase molecule itself, its associated transcription factors, or the Rho termination factor can serve as a regulatory target, thereby influencing attenuation. Transcription attenuation mechanisms therefore increase the repertoire of molecular events that an organism can exploit in optimising gene expression. Also, in many instances transcription attenuation proceeds without the participation of a specific regulatory protein.

ATTENUATION MECHANISMS IN ENTERIC BACTERIA

The hallmark of transcription attenuation is control over the continuation of transcript elongation at sites that are encountered by RNA polymerase prior to a particular gene. A wide variety of attenuation mechanisms have been discovered in enteric bacteria, and many examples fall into classes that share certain features. The four principal classes of attenuation mechanisms are (i) a class in which the location of a ribosome controls formation of alternative secondary structures in the nascent transcript (ribosome stalling, alternative RNA structure-dependent attenuation), (ii) a class in which coupling between ribosome and RNA polymerase movement can directly preclude formation of a terminator RNA hairpin (ribosome coupling-dependent attenuation), (iii) a class in which a *trans*-acting factor governs formation of a terminator structure by interacting with the nascent transcript (regulatory factor-dependent attenuation), and (iv) a class in which the action of the Rho termination protein in the RNA segment preceding a structural gene is regulated (Rho-dependent attenuation). We will consider these classes individually in the fonowing sections.

Class I: Ribosome Stalling, Alternative RNA Structure Formation

As described above, transcription attenuation was discovered in regulatory studies with the *his* and *trp* amino acid biosynthetic operons in *E. coli* and *S. typhimurium.* Subsequent investigations revealed that closely related mechanisms control termination in the leader regions ofthe *leu, thr, pheA, ilvGMEDA,* and *ilvBN* amino acid biosynthetic operons, as well as in the leader region of the *pheST* operon, which encodes the small *(pluS)* and large *(pheT)* subunits of phenylalanyl-tRNA synthetase. The evidence underlying current knowledge of these attenuation mechanisms has been the subject of two recent reviews, which include a case-by-case account of the published information about each, the complete secondary structures of the alternative RNA structures that can form from each operon's leader transcript, and an up-to-date and detailed account of the different intermediates and events involved in *tiP* operon attenuation.

Class II: Ribosome-RNA Polymerase Coupling

The first several examples of attenuation control discovered in *E. coli* and *S. typhimurium* involved mechanisms that regulated the expression of amino acid biosynthetic operons. Each example employed ribosome stalling at control co dons as a regulatory signal and an alternative transcript secondary structure as a means of preventing terminator hairpin formation. These similarities raised the possibility that attenuation control was limited to amino acid biosynthetic operons and to a single mechanism for regulating transcription termination. The first clear indication to the contrary was the discovery of attenuation control of *pyrEl* operon expression in *E. coli.* The *pyrEl* operon encodes the pyrimidine biosynthetic enzyme aspartate transcarbamylase, which is not involved directly in amino acid metabolism. Elucidation of the *pyrEl* attenuation control mechanism revealed that transcription termination at the attenuator, a Rho-independent transcription terminator that precedes the *pyrEl* structural genes, was regulated in a way fundamentally different from that described for the amino acid biosynthetic operons, namely, transcription termination was controlled by the extent of coupling (i.e. movement and location) of a translating ribosome and a transcribing RNA polymerase within the *pyrEl* leader region. In this case, the ribosome directly controls the formation of the terminator RNA hairpin by steric hindrance.

Shortly after the discovery of attenuation control of *pyrEl* expression, a similar mechanism was described for the *pyrE* gene of *E. coli,* which also encodes a pyrimidine biosynthetic enzyme. Attenuation control mechanisms equivalent to their *E. coli* counterparts also appear to regulate *pyrEl* and *pyrE* expression in *S. typhimurium.* At present, the *pyrEl* operon and *pyrE* gene provide the only examples of this second class of attenuation control, which we designate the ribosome-RNA polymerase coupling mechanism, however, attenuation control of *E. coli ampC* expression could be considered a special case.

Class III: Regulatory Factor Dependent

In the two classes of attenuation control described so far, regulation of transcription attenuation is achieved by coupling transcription and translation within the regulatory leader region. In the third class, called regulatory factor-dependent attenuation, the regulatory role of translation is replaced by a *trans*-acting RNA-binding factor. This factor can be a protein or an antisense RNA that binds a specific sequence in the leader (or intercistronic) region of the regulated transcript. Factor binding can either directly block the formation of an attenuator-specified terminator hairpin or indirectly control its formation by favouring a particular RNA secondary structure.

bgl operon: In *E. coli,* the best studied example of regulatory factor-dependent attenuation is regulation of *bgl* operon expression. In this case, the regulatory factor is a specialised RNA-binding protein. The *bgl* operon contains three genes, *bglG, bglF*, and *bglB,* which enable cells to use certain aromatic β-glucosides such as salicin and arbutin as carbon sources. The *bglG* gene encodes a positive regulatory protein, BglG, which is required for operon expression. The *bglF* gene encodes the β-glucoside-specific enzyme of the phosphoenolpyruvate-dependent phosphotransferase system (designated enzyme nBg1 or BglF), which is present in the cytoplasmic membrane and transports β-glucosidic sugars into the cell with concomitant phosphorylation of the sugar. The *bglB* gene encodes phosphb-β-glucosidase B, which hydrolyses phosphorylated β-glucosides to yield glucose-6-phosphate. The *bgl* operon is cryptic in wild-type cells, but a variety of spontaneous mutations activate the operon by enhancement of transcription initiation from β pre-existing but silent promoter. Once the operon is activated, full expression requires a β-glucoside inducer and also cyclic AMP (cAMP) and the cAMP receptor protein (CRP).

β-Glucoside-mediated regulation of *bgl* operon expression occurs through an attenuation control mechanism. In the absence of a β-glucoside inducer, most transcripts initiated at the activated *bgl* promoter are terminated at a Rho-independent attenuator located just upstream of *bglG,* the first gene in the operon. A second Rho-independent attenuator is located between *bglG* and the adjacent *bglF* gene. The positive regulator BglG is required to prevent transcription termination at both attenuators. Low levels of BglG and BglF are synthesised in the absence of β-glucosides, but under these conditions, BglF inactivates BglG by phosphorylation. Phosphorylation of *BglG* prevents the formation of dimers, which are required for RNA binding and antitermination activity.

In the presence of β-glucosides, BglF dephosphorylates BglG, allowing it to dimerise and function as an antitermination factor. Non-phosphorylated dimers of BglG prevent transcription termination within the operon by binding to a sequence in the *bgl* mRNA that precedes and partially overlaps the terminator hairpin encoded by each attenuator. This binding blocks the formation of the terminator hairpins, allowing expression of the operon. Apparently, the BglG-binding site forms an alternative secondmy structure that is recognised by BglG dimers. At present, it is not known if *S. typhimurium* carries a *bgl* operon. Attempts to clone parts of the operon by PCR have been unsuccessful. *S. typhimurium* does not grow on aromatic β-glucosides, indicating that if the genome includes a *bgl* operon, it is silent. Antisense RNA-Mediated Control of Plasmid Replication. At present, there are no clear cases of antisense RNA-dependent attenuation in *E. coli,* but this type of regulation can be illustrated by examining the mechanism that controls replication of the staphylococcal plasmid pTl81. An analogous mechanism controls replication of the streptococcal plasmid pIP50 1. Replication of plasmid pTl81 is controlled by the level of the initiator protein RepC. Constitutive transcription of plasmid pTl81 produces an antisense RNA capable of base pairing with a target sequence near the 5′ end of the *repC* transcript. When this pairing occurs early during *repC* transcription, it promotes the formation of an RNA hairpin 5′ to the *repC* start codon.

This hairpin causes premature Rho-independent transcription termination, which precludes *RepC* synthesis. In the absence of the antisense RNA (i.e. when plasmid copy number is low), an upstream sequence in the *repC* leader transcript pairs with the 5′ segment of the terminator hairpin, thereby blocking the signal for transcription termination and allowing synthesis of the full-length *repC* transcript. In this case, *RepC* is synthesised and can direct another round of plasmid replication.

Class IV: Rho Factor Dependent

E. coli and *S. typhimurium,* and perhaps most bacteria, have two distinct classes of transcription termination sites. One class, discussed previously, is responsible for termination in many operons regulated by transcription attenuation. Sites of this class appear to be recognised by RNA polymerase acting alone, they are referred to as Rho-independent or intrinsic termination sites. Sites of the second class require the action of the protein factor Rho. Rho interacts with both transcript and RNA polymerase and directs polymerase to terminate transcription. The first example of the use of transcription termination and its relief in gene reguliltion ipvolved Rho factor and its role in regulating early gene transcription in bacteriophage lambda. The phage specified *N* protein was shown to be responsible for antitermination at Rho-dependent termination sites.

Much is known about Rho's structure and mechanism of action. The characteristics of many Rho-binding sites and Rho termination sites have been determined. Rho has been shown to be an ATP-dependent RNADNA helicase, helicase activity is required for termination. Rho causes terminatiop. by contacting a paused RNA polymerase molecule and altering its behaviour. Rho action requires accessory factors, such as NusG. Models that explain Rho's binding to RNA, its relative movement on RNA, and the mechanism by which it promotes termination have been proposed. The end of an operon is often defined by a Rho-dependent termination site. Occasionally Rho termination. sites are located preceding or within a structural gene, where they allow Rho to participate in regulatory events that control gene expression. Rho is involved in transcription attenuation regulation in the *tna* (15S), *livL*, and rRNA operons, and it also modulates its own synthesis.

TRANSCRIPTION ATTENUATION MECHANISMS IN OTHER ORGANISMS

Although this review deals with attenuation mechanisms in *E. coli* and S. *typhimurium,* we think it essential that the reader be aware of several recent discoveries of novel attenuation mechanisms in other organisms, including both gram-negative and gmm-positive bacteria. Similar mechanisms could well be found in future studies of gene regulation in *E. coli* and S. *typhimurium*. Interestingly, these examples are principally class III mechanisms (i.e. regulatory factor-dependent attenuation), and they involve some operons whose homologs in *E. coli* and S. *typhimurium* are regulated by class I and class II mechanisms.

Bacillus Subtilis trp Operon

Attenuation control of the *trp* operon in *Bacillus subtilis,* as in *E. coli,* involves formation in the leader transcript of alternative secondary structures that either include or exclude a terminator hairpin. However, in *B. subtilis,* formation of the transcript secondary structures is controlled not by the position of a translating ribosome but by the binding of a regulatory protein, TRAP *(tIP* RNA-binding attenuation protein), which is encoded by the *mtl'B* gene. Under conditions of abundant tryptophan, TRAP binds to a segment of the leader transcript upstream of the terminator hairpin. This binding blocks formation of an antiterminator secondary structure equivalent to the *E. coli* 2:3 hairpin, thereby promoting formation of the terminator hairpin and causing transcription termination. Recent studies indicate that TRAP consists of 11 identical8-kDa subunits and that each tryptophan-activated subunit binds one closely spaced G/UAG repeat in the leader transcript.

Bacillus Subtilis pyr Operon

A similar mechanism also appears to regulate the *pyr* operon in *B. subtilis*. This operon encodes the six pyrimidine nucleotide biosynthetic enzymes and includes two additional, S-proximal genes: *pyrR*, which encodes a 20-kDa regulatory RNA-binding protein that also can catalyse the conversion of uracil and phosphoribosylpyrophosphate to UMP, and *pyrP*, which encodes an integral membrane uracil permease. Distinct Rho-independent terminators (attenuators) occur in the leader region, the *pyrR -PyrR* intercistronic region, and the *pyrP-pyrB* intercistronic region. Recent studies suggest that when pyrimidines are abundant, the *PyrR* protein binds to target sequences in the nascent transcript and disrupts formation of antiterminator secondary structures that, when the pyrimidine pool is depleted, prevent formation of the terminator hairpins. An intriguing feature of this mechanism is the use of an enzyme involved in pyrimidine metabolism as the RNA-binding protein, perhaps allowing the binding site for UMP to be used both in the enzymatic reaction and as an allosteric site to regulate the RNA-binding activity of *PyrR*.

tRNA Directed Transcription Anti-termination

An exciting recent discovery is the finding that transcription attenuation can be directly controlled by binding of a cognate uncharged tRNA to the nascent leader transcripts of at least 12 aminoacyl-tRNA synthetase and 6 amino acid biosynthetic genes and operons in a variety of gram-positive bacteria. These leader RNAs each contain three conserved stem-loop structures (I, II, and III), followed by a highly conserved 14-base element (T box) and then the attenuator-specified terminator hairpin. An unpaired triplet sequence, which corresponds to a codon for the cognate amino acid, occurs in a bulge region of each stem I. For all genes, an antiterminator hairpin can be formed by base pairing of a segment of the T box with a conserved sequence in the upstream portion of the terminator hairpin. In the antiterminator hairpin, the central seven bases of the T box form a bulge. When uncharged cognate tRNA is abundant, it presumably binds to the specifier sequence in stem I through codon-anticodon interactions and, near its 3′ end, to the T-box bulge in the antiterminator hairpin. This stabilises the antiterminator hairpin and permits readthrough transcription into the downstream genes. When the cognate tRNA is charged, it either does not bind stably or is unavailable for interaction because it is complexed with aminoacyl-tRNA synthetase or elongation factors. This allows the terminator hairpin to form and cause transcription termination. Thus, limitation of a particular amino acid or aminoacyl-tRNA synthetase increases the level of uncharged cognate tRNA(s), which in turn increases transcription of the genes encoding the enzymes that synthesise this amino acid or that charge it to tRNA.

Possibility of Transcription Attenuation in Eukaryotes

This section focuses on bacterial attenuation mechanisms, it is worth mentioning the possibility that transcription attenuation occurs in eukaryotes. Although similarities of features in eukaryotic transcriptional units to those found for bacterial attenuatots have led to several suggestions of transcription attenuation in eukaryotes, to date there is no documented example of a eukaryotic gene whose expression is regulated at a discrete transcription termination site. However, in at least some cases (the human and murine *c*-mycproto-oncogenes, for instance), the susceptibility of RNA polymerase II to multiple, weak termination sites within or upstream from a gene appears to be controlled by events at or near the promoter. These mechanisms are most formally analogous to bacterial antitermination mechanisms, such as those found in rRNA operons or during growth of phage lambda. For example, the lambda N and Q proteins play roles somewhat similar to that of human immunodeficiency virus type 1 Tat protein, whose binding to a promoter-proximal RNA structure (the transactivation response region) is required for efficient synthesis of full-length mRNA. Although other types of attenuation mechanisms have not been found in eukaryotes, we caution against concluding they do not exist.

An important lesson from studies of bacterial attenuation is. that regulatory mechanisms evolve special features that uniquely couple transcription of a particular gene to the metabolic need for its gene product. Control of RNA chain elongation in eukaryotes is poorly understood, and these linkages may still be unrecognised. Both class III mechanisms and, as we have noted elsewhere, coupling of transcription by RNA polymerase II to assembly of the mRNA splicing machinery (in analogy to coupling to ribosome movement in bacteria) could plausibly occur in eukaryotes.

EVOLUTIONARY ASPECTS AND EXPECTATIONS

Thus, a variety of transcription attenuation mechanisms that are used by *E. coli* and/or *S. typhimurium* in regulating expression of specific operons. The diversity of these mechanisms and the variety of molecules and events involved lead us to suspect that there are many as yet undiscovered mechanisms of transcription attenuation used by bacteria. Potential targets for regulatory events that could modulate transcription termination are RNA polymerase, polymerase accessory proteins, RNA-binding proteins, ribosomal components, polypeptide and ribosome release factors, termination factors, and the transcripts themselves. Thus, as mentioned in the introduction, the many potertial targets for regulation by transcription attenuation probably offer cells options that are not available for regulation of transcription initiation. A second consideration is the impact of evolution on adoption of successful regulatory strategies. If RNA did serve as the sole genetic material during some early period, as some suggest, and if this RNA was translated by a primitive translational process, then some of the transcription attenuation mechanisms in use today could have evolved from regulatory mechanisms that were operating prior to the appearance of DNA. It seems likely that successful strategies would have been retained.

Thus, there are only a few well-documented examples of transcription attenuation in eukaryotes. The patterns of gene expression in higher organisms suggest that a common regulatory objective is to provide each genetic unit with a variety of *cis* regulatory sites or elements that allow an appropriate response to numerous regulatory proteins that are produced or modified during different stages of growth and development. Give the need for regulatory diversity, it seems likely that some forms of transcription attenuation will be found to be common in eukaryotes.

Chapter 7

RNA Splicing and RNA Silencing

INTRODUCTION

In molecular biology, splicing is a modification of an RNA after transcription, in which introns are removed and exons are joined. This is needed for the typical eukaryotic messenger RNA before it can be used to produce a correct protein through translation. For many eukaryotic introns, splicing is done in a series of reactions which are catalysed by the spliceosome, a complex of small nuclear ribonucleoproteins (snRNPs), but there are also self-splicing introns (Fig. 7.1).

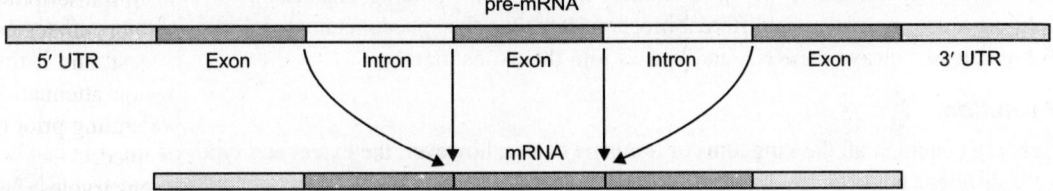

Fig. 7.1: Simple illustration of exons and introns in pre-mRNA and the formation of mature mRNA by splicing. The UTRs are non-coding parts of exons at the ends of the mRNA.

SPLICING PATHWAYS

Several methods of RNA splicing occur in nature: The type of splicing depends on the structure of the spliced intron and the catalysts required for splicing to occur.

Spliceosomal Introns

Spliceosomal introns often reside in eukaryotic protein-coding genes. Within the intron, a 3' splice site, 5' splice site, and branch site are required for splicing. The 5' splice site or splice donor site includes an almost invariant sequence GU at the 5' end of the intron, within a larger, less highly conserved consensus region. The 3' splice site or splice acceptor site terminates the intron with an almost invariant AG sequence. Upstream (5'-ward) from the AG there is a region high in pyrimidines (C and U), or polypyrimidine tract. Upstream from the polypyrimidine tract is the branch point, which includes an adenine nucleotide.

Point mutations in the underlying DNA or errors during transcription can activate a 'cryptic splice site' in part of the transcript that usually is not spliced. This results in a mature messenger RNA with a missing section of an exon. In this way a point mutation, which usually only affects a single amino acid, can manifest as a deletion in the final protein.

Spliceosome Formation and Activity

Splicing is catalysed by the spliceosome which is a large RNA-protein complex composed of five small nuclear ribonucleoproteins (snRNPs, pronounced 'snurps'). The RNA components of snRNPs interact with the intron and may be involved in catalysis.

Self-splicing

Self-splicing occurs for rare introns that form a ribozyme, performing the functions of the spliceosome by RNA alone. There are three kinds of self-splicing introns, Group I, Group II and Group III. Group I and II introns perform splicing similar to the spliceosome without requiring any protein. This similarity suggests that Group I and II introns may be evolutionarily related to the spliceosome. Self-splicing may also be very ancient, and may have existed in an RNA world present before protein. Although the two splicing mechanisms described below do not require any proteins to occur, 5 additional RNA molecules and over 50 proteins are used and hydrolyses many ATP molecules. The splicing mechanisms use ATP in order to accurately splice mRNAs. If the cell were to not use any ATPs, the process would be highly inaccurate and many mistakes would occur.

tRNA splicing

tRNA (also tRNA-like) splicing is another rare form of splicing that usually occurs in tRNA. The splicing reaction involves a different biochemistry than the spliceomsomal and self-splicing pathways. Ribonucleases cleave the RNA and ligases join the exons together.

Evolution

Splicing occurs in all the kingdoms or domains of life, however, the extent and types of splicing can be very different between the major divisions. Eukaryotes splice many protein-coding messenger RNAs and some non-coding RNAs. Prokaryotes, on the other hand, splice rarely and mostly non-coding RNAs. Another important difference between these two groups of organisms is that prokaryotes completely lack the correct spliceosomal pathway. Because spliceosomal introns are not conserved in all species, there is debate concerning when spliceosomal splicing evolved. Two models have been proposed: the intron late and intron early models (Table 7.1).

Table 7.1: Splicing diversity.

	Eukaryotes	*Prokaryotes*
Spliceosomal	+	–
Self-splicing	+	+
tRNA	+	+

Biochemical mechanism

Spliceosomal splicing and self-splicing involves a two-step biochemical process. Both steps involve transesterification reactions that occur between RNA nucleotides. tRNA splicing, however, is an exception and does not occur by transesterification (Fig. 7.2). Spliceosomal and self-splicing transesterification reactions occur via two sequential transesterification reactions. First, the 2'OH of a specific branch-point nucleotide within the intron that is defined during spliceosome assembly performs a nucleophilic attack on the first nucleotide of the intron at the 5' splice site forming the lariat intermediate. Second, the 3'OH of the released 5' exon then performs a nucleophilic attack at the last nucleotide of the intron at the 3' splice site thus joining the exons and releasing the intron lariat.

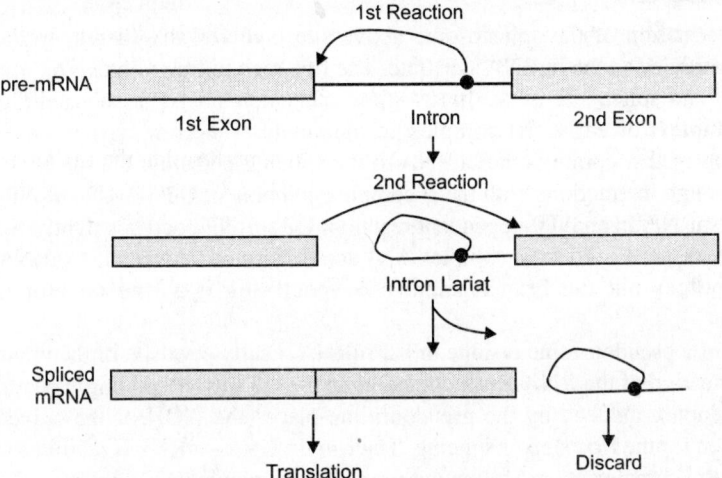

Fig. 7.2: Diagram illustrating the two-step biochemistry of splicing.

Alternative splicing

In many cases, the splicing process can create a range of unique proteins by varying the exon composition of the same messenger RNA. This phenomenon is then called alternative splicing. Alternative splicing can occur in many ways. Exons can be extended or skipped, or introns can be retained.

Experimental manipulation of splicing

Splicing events can be experimentally altered by binding steric-blocking antisense oligos such as morpholinos or peptide nucleic acids to snRNP binding sites, to the branch-point nucleotide that closes the lariat or to splice-regulatory element binding sites.

Splicing errors

Common errors are given below:
1. Mutation of a splice site resulting in loss of function of that site. Results in exposure of a premature stop codon, loss of an exon, or inclusion of an intron.
2. Mutation of a splice site reducing specificity. May result in variation in the splice location, causing insertion or deletion of amino acids or most likely, a loss of the reading frame.
3. Displacement of a splice site, leading to inclusion or exclusion of more RNA than expected, resulting in longer or shorter exons.

Many splicing errors are safeguarded by a cellular quality control mechanism termed nonsense mediated mRNA decay [NMD].

Protein splicing

Not only pre-mRNA but also proteins can undergo splicing. Although the biomolecular mechanisms are different, the principle is the same, that parts of the protein, called inteins instead of introns, are removed. The remaining parts, called exteins instead of exons, are fused together. Protein splicing has been observed in all sorts of organisms, including bacteria, archaea, plants, yeast and human.

Spliceosome Assembly

The model for formation of the spliceosome active site involves an ordered, stepwise assembly of discrete snRNP particles on the hnRNA substrate. The first recognition of hnRNAs involves U1 snRNP binding to the 5′ end splice site of the hnRNA and other non-snRNP associated factors to form the commitment complex, or early (E) complex in mammals. The commitment complex is an ATP-independent complex that commits the hnRNA to the splicing pathway. U2 snRNP is recruited to the branch region through interactions with the E complex component U2AF (U2 snRNP auxiliary factor) and possibly U1 snRNP. In an ATP-dependent reaction, U2 snRNP becomes tightly associated with the branch point sequence (BPS) to form complex A. A duplex formed between U2 snRNA and the hnRNA branch region bulges out the branch adenosine specifying it as the nucleophile for the first transesterification.

The presence of a pseudouridine residue in U2 snRNA, nearly opposite of the branch site, results in an altered conformation of the RNA-RNA duplex upon the U2 snRNP binding. Specifically, the altered structure of the duplex induced by the pseudouridine places the 2′OH of the bulged adenosine in a favourable position for the first step of splicing. The U4/U5/U6 tri-snRNP is recruited to the assembling spliceosome to form complex B, and following several rearrangements, complex C (the spliceosome) is activated for catalysis. It is unclear how the triple snRNP is recruited to complex A, but this process may be mediated through protein-protein interactions and/or base pairing interactions between U2 snRNA and U6 snRNA.

The U5 snRNP interacts with sequences at the 5′ and 3′ splice sites via the invariant loop of U5 snRNA and U5 protein components interact with the 3′ splice site region.

Upon recruitment of the triple snRNP, several RNA-RNA rearrangements precede the first catalytic step and further rearrangements occur in the catalytically active spliceosome. Several of the RNA-RNA interactions are mutually exclusive, however, it is not known what triggers these interactions, nor the order of these rearrangements. The first rearrangement is probably the displacement of U1 snRNP from the 5′ splice site and formation of a U6 snRNA interaction. It is known that U1 snRNP is only weakly associated with fully formed spliceosomes, and U1 snRNP is inhibitory to the formation of a U6-5′ splice site interaction on a model of substrate oligonucleotide containing a short 5′ exon and 5′ splice site. Binding of U2 snRNP to the branch point sequence (BPS) is one example of an RNA-RNA interaction displacing a protein-RNA interaction. Upon recruitment of U2 snRNP, the branch binding protein SF1 in the commitment complex is displaced since the binding site of U2 snRNA and SF1 are mutually exclusive events.

Within the U2 snRNA, there are other mutually exclusive rearrangements that occur between competing conformations. For example, in the active form, stem loop IIa is favoured, in the inactive form a mutually exclusive interaction between the loop and a downstream sequence predominates. It is unclear how U4 is displaced from U6 snRNAm, although RNA has been implicated in spliceosome assembly, and may function to unwind U4/U6 and promote the formation of a U2/U6 snRNA interaction. The interactions of U4/U6 stem loops I and II dissociate and the freed stem loop II region of U6 folds on itself to form an intramolecular stem loop and U4 is no longer required in further spliceosome assembly. The freed stem loop I region of U6 base pairs with U2 snRNA forming the U2/U6 helix I. However, the helix I structure is mutually exclusive with the 3′ half of an internal 5′ stem loop region of U2 snRNA.

Ribozyme

A ribozyme (from ribonucleic acid enzyme, also called RNA enzyme or catalytic RNA) is an RNA molecule possessing a well defined tertiary structure that enables it to catalyse a chemical reaction. Many natural ribozymes catalyse either the hydrolysis of one of their own phosphodiester bonds or the hydrolysis of bonds in other RNAs, but they have also been found to catalyse the aminotransferase activity of the ribosome (Fig. 7.3).

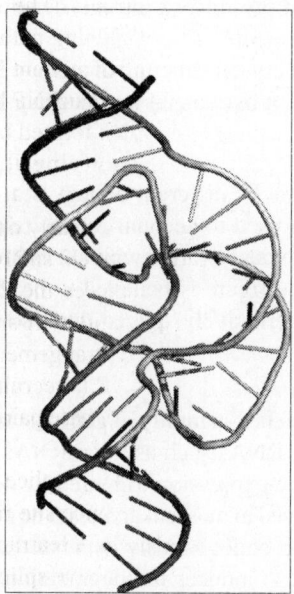

Fig. 7.3: Structure of hammerhead ribozyme.

Investigators studying the origin of life have produced ribozymes in the laboratory that are capable of catalysing their own synthesis under very specific conditions, such as an RNA polymerase ribozyme. Mutagenesis and selection has been performed resulting in isolation of improved variants of the 'Round-18' polymerase ribozyme from 2001. 'B6.61' is able to add up to 20 nucleotides to a primer template in 24 hr, until it decomposes by hydrolysis of its phosphodiester bonds.

Spliceosome

A spliceosome is a complex of specialised RNA and protein subunits that removes introns from a transcribed pre-mRNA (hnRNA) segment. This process is generally referred to as splicing. Each spliceosome is composed of five small nuclear RNA proteins, called snRNPs, (pronounced snurps) and a range of non-snRNP associated protein factors. The snRNPs that make up the nuclear spliceosome are named U1, U2, U4, U5, and U6, and participate in several RNA-RNA and RNA-protein interactions. The RNA component of the snRNP is rich in uridine (the nucleoside analog of the uracil nucleotide).

The canonical assembly of the spliceosome occurs a new on each hnRNA. The hnRNA contains specific sequence elements that are recognised and utilised during spliceosome assembly. These include the 5′ end splice, the branch point sequence, the polypyrimidine tract, and the 3′ end splice site. The spliceosome catalyses the removal of introns, and the ligation of the flanking exons.

Introns typically have a GU nucleotide sequence at the 5′ end splice site, and an AG at the 3′ end splice site. The 3′ splice site can be further defined by a variable length of polypyrimidines, called the polypyrimidine tract (PPT), which serves the dual function of recruiting factors to the 3′ splice site and possibly recruiting factors to the branch point sequence (BPS).

The BPS contains the conserved adenosine required for the first step of splicing. A group of less abundant snRNPs, U11, U12, U4atac, and U6atac, together with U5, are subunits of the so-called minor spliceosome that splices a rare class of pre-mRNA introns, denoted U12-type. These snRNPs form the U12 spliceosome are located in the cytosol.

New evidence derived from the first crystal structure of a group II intron suggests that the spliceosome is actually a ribozyme, and that it uses a two–metal ion mechanism for catalysis.

Alternative splicing

Alternative splicing (the recombination of different exons) is a major source of genetic diversity in eukaryotes. Splice variants have been used to account for the relatively small number of genes in the human genome. For years the estimate widely varied with top estimates reaching 100000 genes, but now, due to the Human Genome Project the figure is believed to be closer to 20000 genes. One particular *Drosophila* gene (DSCAM) can be alternatively spliced into 38000 different mRNA.

RNA SILENCING

RNA silencing or RNA interference refers to a family of gene silencing effects by which gene expression is negatively regulated by non-coding RNAs such as microRNAs. RNA silencing may also be defined as sequence-specific regulation of gene expression triggered by double-stranded RNA (dsRNA). RNA silencing mechanisms are highly conserved in most eukaryotes. The most common and well-studied example is RNA interference (RNAi), in which endogenously expressed microRNA (miRNA) or exogenously derived small interfering RNA (siRNA) induces the degradation of complementary messenger RNA. Other classes of small RNA have been identified, including piwi-interacting RNA (piRNA) and its subspecies repeat associated small interfering RNA (rasiRNA).

RNA silencing describes several mechanistically related pathways which are involved in controlling and regulating gene expression. RNA silencing pathways are associated with the regulatory activity of small non-coding RNAs (approximately 20–30 nucleotides in length) that function as factors involved in inactivating homologous sequences, promoting endonuclease activity, translational arrest, and/or chromatic or DNA modification. In the context in which the phenomenon was first studied, small RNA was found to play an important role in defending plants against viruses. For example, these studies demonstrated that enzymes detect double-stranded RNA (dsRNA) not normally found in cells and digest it into small pieces that are not able to cause disease.

While some functions of RNA silencing and its machinery are understood, many are not. For example, RNA silencing has been shown to be important in the regulation of development and in the control of transposition events. RNA silencing has been shown to play a role in antiviral protection in plants as well as insects. Also in yeast, RNA silencing has been shown to maintain heterochromatin structure. However, the varied and nuanced role of RNA silencing in the regulation of gene expression remains an ongoing scientific inquiry. A range of diverse functions have been proposed for a growing number of characterised small RNA sequences, e.g. regulation of developmental, neuronal cell fate, cell death, proliferation, fat storage, haematopoietic cell fate, insulin secretion.

RNA silencing functions by repressing translation or by cleaving messenger RNA (mRNA), depending on the amount of complementarity of base-pairing. RNA has been largely investigated within its role as an intermediary in the translation of genes into proteins. More active regulatory functions, however, only began to be addressed by researchers beginning in the late-1990s. The landmark study providing an understanding of the first identified mechanism was published in 1998 by Fire and others demonstrating that double-stranded RNA could act as a trigger for gene silencing. Since then, various other classes of RNA silencing have been identified and characterised. Presently, the therapeutic potential of these discoveries is being explored, for example, in the context of targeted gene therapy. While RNA silencing is an evolving class of mechanisms, a common theme is the fundamental relationship between small RNAs and gene expression. It has also been observed that the major RNA silencing pathways currently identified have mechanisms of action which may involve both post-transcriptional gene silencing (PTGS) as well as chromatin-dependent gene silencing (CDGS) pathways.CDGS involves the assembly of small RNA complexes on nascent transcripts and is regarded as encompassing mechanisms of action which implicate transcriptional gene silencing (TGS) and co-transcriptional gene silencing (CTGS) events. This is significant at least because the evidence suggests that small RNAs play a role in the modulation of chromatin structure and TGS.

Despite early focus in the literature on RNA interference (RNAi) as a core mechanism which occurs at the level of messenger RNA translation, others have since been identified in the broader family of conserved RNA silencing pathways acting at the DNA and chromatin level. RNA silencing refers to the silencing activity of a range of small RNAs and is generally regarded as a broader category than RNAi. While the terms have sometimes been used interchangeably in the literature, RNAi is generally regarded as a branch of RNA silencing. To the extent it is useful to craft a distinction between these related concepts, RNA silencing may be thought of as referring to the broader scheme of small RNA related controls involved in gene expression and the protection of the genome against mobile repetitive DNA sequences, retroelements, and transposons to the extent that these can induce mutations. The molecular mechanisms for RNA silencing were initially studied in plants but have since broadened to cover a variety of subjects, from fungi to mammals, providing strong evidence that these pathways are highly conserved. At least three primary classes of small RNA have currently been identified, namely: small interfering RNA (siRNA), microRNA (miRNA), and piwi-interacting RNA (piRNA).

small interfering RNA (siRNA)

siRNAs act in the nucleus and the cytoplasm and are involved in RNAi as well as CDGS. siRNAs come from long dsRNA precursors derived from a variety of single-stranded RNA (ssRNA) precursors, such as sense and antisense RNAs. siRNAs also come from hairpin RNAs derived from transcription of inverted repeat regions. siRNAs may also arise enzymatically from non-coding RNA precursors. The volume of literature on siRNA within the framework of RNAi is extensive.

microRNA (miRNA)

The majority of miRNAs act in the cytoplasm and mediate mRNA degradation or translational arrest. However, some plant miRNAs have been shown to act directly to promote DNA methylation. miRNAs come from hairpin precursors generated by the RNaseIII enzymes Drosha and Dicer. Both miRNA and siRNA form either the RNA-induced silencing complex (RISC) or the nuclear form of RISC known as RNA-induced transcriptional silencing complex (RITS). The volume of literature on miRNA within the framework of RNAi is extensive.

Three prime untranslated regions and microRNAs

Three prime untranslated regions (3'UTRs) of messenger RNAs (mRNAs) often contain regulatory sequences that post-transcriptionally cause RNA interference. Such 3'-UTRs often contain both binding sites for microRNAs (miRNAs) as well as for regulatory proteins. By binding to specific sites within the 3'-UTR, miRNAs can decrease gene expression of various mRNAs by either inhibiting translation or directly causing degradation of the transcript. The 3'-UTR also may have silencer regions that bind repressor proteins that inhibit the expression of a mRNA. The 3'-UTR often contains microRNA response elements (MREs). MREs are sequences to which miRNAs bind. These are prevalent motifs within 3'-UTRs. Among all regulatory motifs within the 3'-UTRs (e.g. including silencer regions), MREs make up about half of the motifs.

As of 2014, the miRBase web site, an archive of miRNA sequences and annotations, listed 28645 entries in 233 biologic species. Of these, 1881 miRNAs were in annotated human miRNA loci. miRNAs were predicted to have an average of about four hundred target mRNAs (affecting expression of several hundred genes). Freidman and others estimate that >45000 miRNA target sites within human mRNA 3'UTRs are conserved above background levels, and >60% of human protein-coding genes have been under selective pressure to maintain pairing to miRNAs.

Direct experiments show that a single miRNA can reduce the stability of hundreds of unique mRNAs. Other experiments show that a single miRNA may repress the production of hundreds of proteins, but that this repression often is relatively mild (less than 2-fold).

The effects of miRNA dysregulation of gene expression seem to be important in cancer. For instance, in gastrointestinal cancers, nine miRNAs have been identified as epigenetically altered and effective in down regulating DNA repair enzymes. The effects of miRNA dysregulation of gene expression also seem to be important in neuropsychiatric disorders, such as schizophrenia, bipolar disorder, major depression, Parkinson's disease, Alzheimer's disease and autism spectrum disorders.

piwi-interacting RNA (piRNA)

piRNAs represent the largest class of small non-coding RNA molecules expressed in animal cells, deriving from a large variety of sources, including repetitive DNA and transposons. However, the biogenesis of piRNAs is also the least well understood. piRNAs appear to act both at the post-transcriptional and chromatin levels. They are distinct from miRNA due to at least an increase in terms of size and complexity. Repeat associated small interfering RNA (rasiRNAs) are considered to be a subspecies of piRNA.

Mechanism

The most basic mechanistic flow for RNA Silencing is as follows:

(1) RNA with inverted repeats hairpin/panhandle constructs → (2) dsRNA → (3) miRNAs/siRNAs → (4) RISC → (5) Destruction of target mRNA.

1. It has been discovered that the best precursor to good RNA silencing is to have single stranded antisense RNA with inverted repeats which, in turn, build small hairpin RNA and panhandle constructs. The hairpin or panhandle constructs exist so that the RNA can remain independent and not anneal with other RNA strands.

2. These small hairpin RNAs and/or panhandles then get transported from the nucleus to the cytosol through the nuclear export receptor called exportin-5, and then get transformed into a dsRNA, a double stranded RNA, which, like DNA, is a double stranded series of nucleotides. If the mechanism didn't use dsRNAs, but only single strands, there would be a higher chance for it to hybridise to other 'good' mRNAs. As a double strand, it can be kept on call for when it is needed.

3. The dsRNA then gets cut up by a Dicer into small (21–28 nt = nucleotides long) strands of miRNAs (microRNAs) or siRNAs (short interfering RNAs.) A Dicer is an endoribonuclease RNase, which is a complex of a protein mixed with strand(s) of RNA.

4. Lastly, the double stranded miRNAs/siRNAs separate into single strands, the antisense RNA strand of the two will combine with another endoribonuclease enzyme complex called RISC (RNA-induced silencing complex), which includes the catalytic component Argonaute, and will guide the RISC to break up the 'perfectly complementary' target mRNA or viral genomic RNA so that it can be destroyed.

5. It means that based on a short sequence specific area, a corresponding mRNA will be cut. To make sure, it will be cut in many other places as well. (If the mechanism only worked with a long stretch, then there would be higher chance that it would not have time to match to its complementary long mRNA.) It has also been shown that the repeated-associated short interference RNAs (rasiRNA) have a role in guiding chromatin modification.

Biological Functions

Immunity against viruses or transposons

RNA silencing is the mechanism that our cells (and cells from all kingdoms) use to fight RNA viruses and transposons (which originate from our own cells as well as from other vehicles). In the case of RNA viruses, these get destroyed immediately by the mechanism cited above. In the case of transposons, it's a little more indirect. Since transposons are located in different parts of the genome, the different transcriptions from the different promoters produce complementary mRNAs that can hybridise with each other. When this happens, the RNAi machinery goes into action, debilitating the mRNAs of the proteins that would be required to move the transposons themselves.

Practical Applications

Growing understanding of small RNA gene-silencing mechanisms involving dsRNA-mediated sequence-specific mRNA degradation has directly impacted the fields of functional genomics, biomedicine, and experimental biology. The following section describes various applications involving the effects of RNA silencing. These include uses in biotechnology, therapeutics, and laboratory research. Bioinformatics techniques are also being applied to identify and characterise large numbers of small RNAs and their targets.

Biotechnology

Artificial introduction of long dsRNAs or siRNAs has been adopted as a tool to inactivate gene expression, both in cultured cells and in living organisms. Structural and functional resolution of small RNAs as the effectors of RNA silencing has had a direct impact on experimental biology. For example, dsRNA may be synthesised to have a specific sequence complementary to a gene of interest. Once introduced into a cell or biological system, it is recognised as exogenous genetic material and activates the corresponding

RNA silencing pathway. This mechanism can be used to effect decreases in gene expression with respect to the target, useful for investigating loss of function for genes relative to a phenotype. That is, studying the phenotypic and/or physiologic effects of expression decreases can reveal the role of a gene product. The observable effects can be nuanced, such that some methods can distinguish between 'knockdown' (decrease expression) and 'knockout' (eliminate expression) of a gene. RNA interference technologies have been noted recently as one of the most widely utilised techniques in functional genomics. Screens developed using small RNAs have been used to identify genes involved in fundamental processes such as cell division, apoptosis and fat regulation.

Biomedicine

Since at least the mid-2000s, there has been intensifying interest in developing short interfering RNAs for biomedical and therapeutic applications. Bolstering this interest is a growing number of experiments which have successfully demonstrated the clinical potential and safety of small RNAs for combatting diseases ranging from viral infections to cancer as well as neurodegenerative disorders. In 2004, the first Investigational New Drug applications for siRNA were filed in the United States with the Food and Drug Administration, it was intended as a therapy for age-related macular degeneration. RNA silencing *in vitro* and *in vivo* has been accomplished by creating triggers (nucleic acids that induce RNAi) either via expression in viruses or synthesis of oligonucleotides. Optimistically many studies indicate that small RNA-based therapies may offer novel and potent weapons against pathogens and diseases where small molecule/pharmacologic and vaccine/biologic treatments have failed or proved less effective in the past. However, it is also warned that the design and delivery of small RNA effector molecules should be carefully considered in order to ensure safety and efficacy.

The role of RNA silencing in therapeutics, clinical medicine, and diagnostics is a fast developing area and it is expected that in the next few years some of the compounds using this technology will reach market approval. A report has been summarised below to highlight the many clinical domains in which RNA silencing is playing an increasingly important role, chief among them are ocular and retinal disorders, cancer, kidney disorders, LDL lowering, and antiviral. The following table displays a listing of RNAi based therapy currently in various phases of clinical trials. The status of these trials can be monitored on the ClinicalTrials.gov website, a service of the National Institutes of Health (NIH). Of note are treatments in development for ocular and retinal disorders, that were among the first compounds to reach clinical development. AGN211745 (sirna027) (Allergan) and bevasiranib (Cand5) (Opko) underwent clinical development for the treatment of age-related macular degeneration, but trials were terminated before the compounds reached the market. Other compounds in development for ocular conditions include SYL040012 (Sylentis) and QPI-007 (Quark). SYL040012 (bamosinan) is a drug candidate under clinical development for glaucoma, a progressive optic neurdegeneration frequently associated to increased intraocular pressure, QPI-007 is a candidate for the treatment of angle-closure glaucoma and Non-arteritic anterior ischaemic optic neuropathy, both compounds are currently undergoing phase II clinical trials. Several compounds are also under development for conditions such as cancer and rare diseases.

SECTION IV

Cell Cycle Regulation, Genetics of Cancer, Cancer and the Environment

Chapter 8

Cell Cycle and Cancer

INTRODUCTION

The cell cycle, the process by which cells progress and divide, lies at the heart of cancer. In normal cells, the cell cycle is controlled by a complex series of signalling pathways by which a cell grows, replicates its DNA and divides. This process also includes mechanisms to ensure errors are corrected, and if not, the cells commit suicide (apoptosis). In cancer, as a result of genetic mutations, this regulatory process malfunctions, resulting in uncontrolled cell proliferation. Cell cycle, the ordered sequence of events that occur in a cell in preparation for cell division. The cell cycle is a four-stage process in which the cell increases in size (gap 1, or G1, stage), copies its DNA (synthesis, or S, stage), prepares to divide (gap 2, or G2, stage), and divides (mitosis, or M, stage). The stages G1, S, and G2 make up interphase, which accounts for the span between cell divisions. On the basis of the stimulatory and inhibitory messages a cell receives, it 'decides' whether or not it should enter the cell cycle and divide.

The proteins that play a role in stimulating cell division can be classified into four groups—growth factors, growth factor receptors, signal transducers, and nuclear regulatory proteins (transcription factors). For a stimulatory signal to reach the nucleus and 'turn on' cell division, four main steps must occur. First, a growth factor must bind to its receptor on the cell membrane. Second, the receptor must become temporarily activated by this binding event. Third, this activation must stimulate a signal to be transmitted, or transduced, from the receptor at the cell surface to the nucleus within the cell. Finally, transcription factors within the nucleus must initiate the transcription of genes involved in cell proliferation. (Transcription is the process by which DNA is converted into RNA. Proteins are then made according to the RNA blueprint, and therefore transcription is crucial as an initial step in protein production.)

Cells use special proteins and checkpoint signalling systems to ensure that the cell cycle progresses properly. Checkpoints at the end of G1 and at the beginning of G2 are designed to assess DNA for damage before and after S phase. Likewise, a checkpoint during mitosis ensures that the cell's spindle fibres are properly aligned in metaphase before the chromosomes are separated in anaphase. If DNA damage or abnormalities in spindle formation are detected at these checkpoints, the cell is forced to undergo programmed cell death, or apoptosis. However, the cell cycle and its checkpoint systems can be sabotaged by defective proteins or genes that cause malignant transformation of the cell, which can lead to cancer. For example, mutations in a protein called p53, which normally detects abnormalities in DNA at the G1 checkpoint, can enable cancer-causing mutations to bypass this checkpoint and allow the cell to escape apoptosis.

CELL CYCLE

Cell division occurs in defined stages, which together comprise the cell cycle. In terms of the genetic material, cells must replicate their chromosomal DNA once every cell cycle and segregate the sister chromatids produced by DNA replication to yield two genetically identical daughter cells (Fig. 8.1).

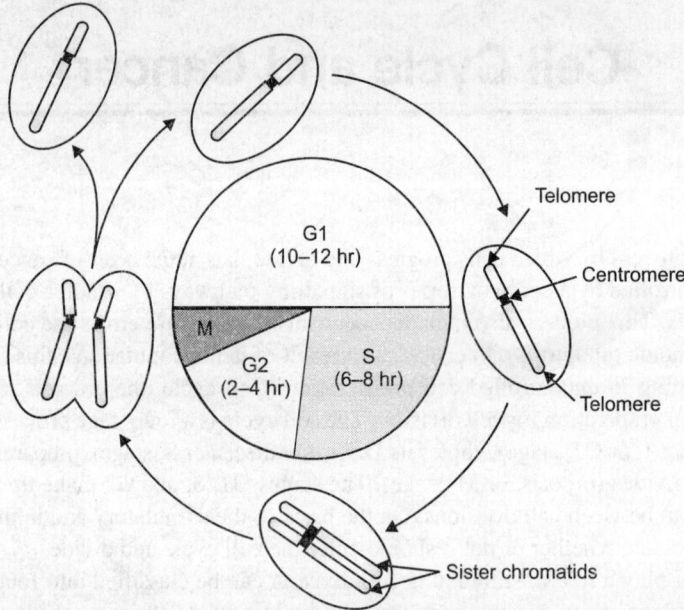

Fig. 8.1: The chromosome cycle. A key purpose of cell division is the duplication of the genetic material carried on chromosomes and its accurate segregation such that each daughter cell acquires one copy of each chromatid.

During DNA replication, cohesion proteins attach the replicated sister chromatids to each other, holding them together. This sister chromatid cohesion is critical for the subsequent alignment of each pair of sister chromatids on the mitotic spindle and it is therefore essential for the subsequent segregation of one (and only one) chromatid of each pair into each of the two daughter cells. The cell division cycle is broken up into four stages: G1, S, G2 and M (Fig. 8.2). DNA replication occurs during S ('synthesis') phase. DNA packaging, chromosome segregation and cell division (cytokinesis) occur in M (mitosis). S phase and M phase are separated by Gap phases. G1 is the gap between M and S. Cell growth is one of the important events of G1. The transition from G1 to S is the critical control point in the cell cycle. G2 is the gap between S and M and provides time for proofreading to ensure DNA is properly replicated and packaged prior to cell division. G0 or quiescence occurs when cells exit the cell cycle due to the absence of growth-promoting signals or presence of prodifferentiation signals. Ordered progression through each phase is intricately regulated through both positive and negative regulatory signalling molecules. The G1, S and G2 phases comprise interphase, which accounts for most of the time in each cell cycle.

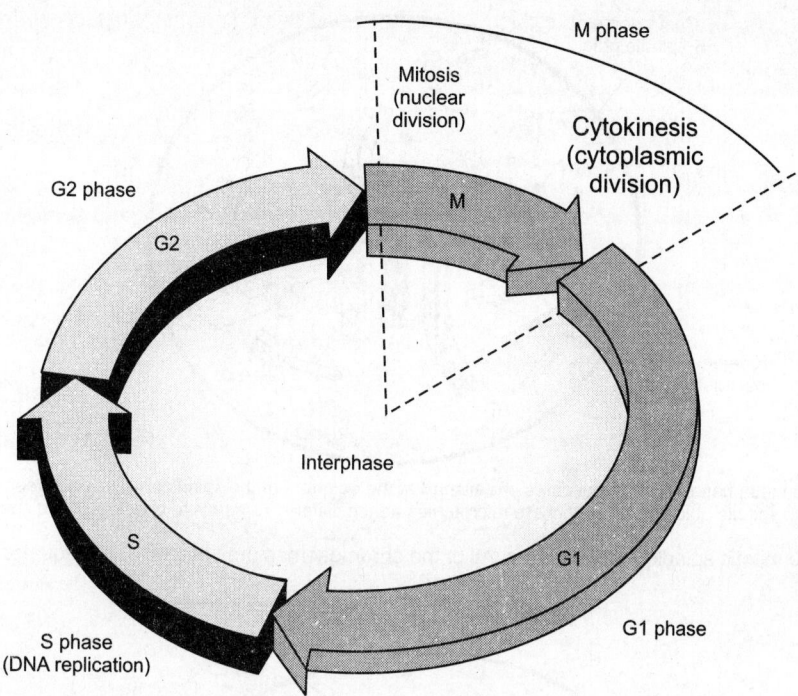

Fig. 8.2: The cell cycle.

The M phase, mitosis, is relatively short (approximately 1 hr of a 24 hr cell cycle). Mitosis is itself divided into several steps, described below.

Assembly of the mitotic spindle: At the very beginning of M phase (called prophase), the chromosomes condense while the cytoplasmic microtubules are being reorganised to build a bipolar mitotic spindle. Its purpose is to accurately segregate the two sister chromatids to opposite poles of the cell.

Steps leading to metaphase: The nuclear envelope then breaks down, allowing the sister chromatids, which are attached to each other through sister chromatid cohesion, to become linked to the micro-tubules via attachment sites on each chromatid called kinetochores. Kinetochores are protein-DNA complexes in which proteins that can capture microtubules are held tightly by DNA sequences at the centromere on each sister chromatid pair. The other end of a spindle microtubule is attached to a centrosome (the major microtubule organising center in the cell, also called the spindle pole body), which has duplicated by this time to form the two spindle poles. Because the two kinetochores on each pair of sister chromatids are attached to opposite spindle poles, they are under tension due to pulling forces that are attempting to move them to opposite poles. Eventually, the balance between these forces causes each chromosome to line up near the center of the spindle, which marks the metaphase stage of mitosis (Fig. 8.3).

Anaphase: After all the chromosomes achieve bipolar attachment to spindle micro-tubules in metaphase, sister chromatid cohesion is rapidly dissolved. As a result, the pulling forces of the microtubules cause the two sister chromatids to move rapidly to the opposite poles (Fig. 8.4).

Cytokinesis: After sister chromatids segregate to opposite poles, cells physically divide into two daughter cells through a process that involves pinching in of the plasma membrane (Fig. 8.5).

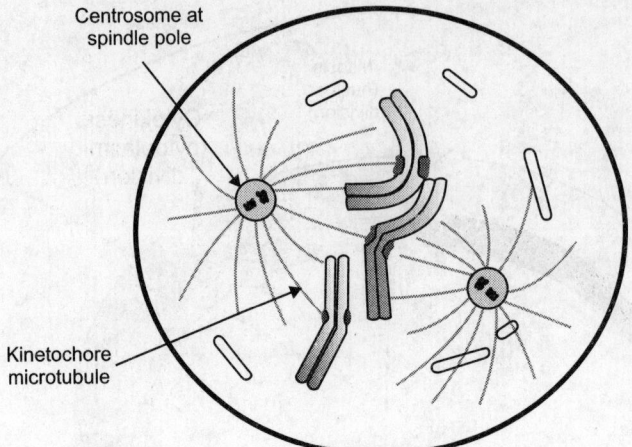

At metaphase, the chromosomes are aligned at the equators of the spindle, midway between the spindle poles. The kinetochore microtubles attach sister chromatids to opposite of the spindle

Fig. 8.3: The mitotic spindle at metaphase. All of the chromosomes are lined up at the equator of the spindle.

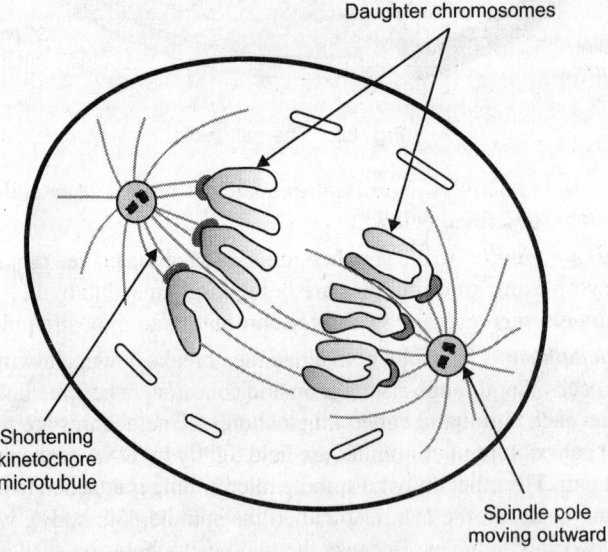

At anaphase, the sister chromatids synchronously separate to form two daughter chromosomes, and each is pulled slowly toward the spindle pole it faces. The kinetochore microtubles get shorter and the spindle poles also move apart, both processes contribute to chromosome segregation.

Fig. 8.4: Anaphase. Only three pairs of sister chromatids are shown, however, in a diploid cell, this occurs simultaneously for all 46 human chromosomes (that is, for 46 pairs of sister chromatids).

CELL CYCLE CONTROL: ACTIVATORS AND BRAKES

How is the cell cycle controlled? The mechanisms of regulation can be broken down into two parts: First, how is the cell cycle regulated so that the different phases occur in the correct order? Second, how

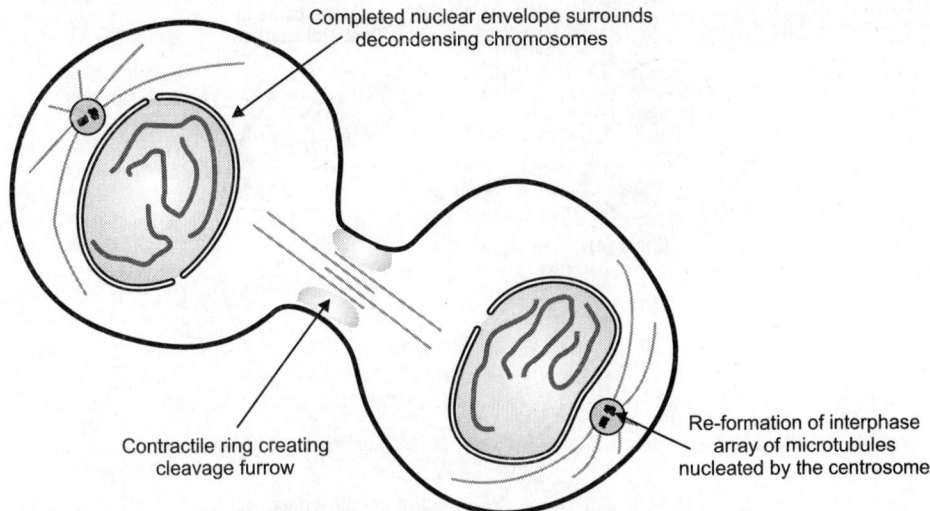

Completed nuclear envelope surrounds decondensing chromosomes

Contractile ring creating cleavage furrow

Re-formation of interphase array of microtubules nucleated by the centrosome

During cytokinesis, the cytoplasm is divided in two by a contractile ringe of actin and myosin filaments, which pinches the cell in two to create two daughters, each with one nucleus.

Fig. 8.5: Cytokinesis. After the two sister chromatids are segregated to opposite poles, cells undergo cytokinesis by an organised pinching in of the plasma membrane.

do extracellular signals activate or inhibit the cell cycle? This section addresses the first question, the next section addresses the second. Not until the 1980s was it discovered that a special regulatory system acts like the controller on a washing machine to drive the cell through each of its stages. This regulatory system is more than a billion years old and most of its central components are essentially the same in single-celled eukaryotes such as yeasts and humans. This has made it possible to use the readily accessible yeast cell to dissect many of the details that underlie the normal regulatory mechanisms that control the growth of the cells in our bodies.

Cyclin Dependent Kinases: The Core Activators of the Cell Cycle Control System

The events that occur in each part of the cell cycle are carried out by specific proteins and these proteins must be synthesised or activated at the correct time in the cycle. For example, before DNA synthesis can begin, the enzymes that produce the nucleotides used in DNA synthesis must be activated. This occurs late in G1 phase. Cell cycle progression is positively regulated by a family of protein kinases called cyclin-dependent kinases (Cdks), which function to turn specific proteins on and off at appropriate times in the cell cycle. Like other protein kinases, Cdks turn proteins on or off by phosphorylating them. Each cyclin-dependent kinase has two subunits-a kinase subunit (the Cdk catalytic subunit) and a cyclin subunit (Fig. 8.6). As a monomer, the Cdk has no enzymatic activity, activation requires association with a cyclin protein, which functions as an allosteric activator.

Cyclins were first identified as key cell-cycle regulators when it was observed that they undergo a cycle of synthesis and regulated destruction during each cell cycle. There are several different Cdks and a number of cyclins. The kinase subunits are present throughout the cell cycle, while the cyclin subunits are produced and degraded at specific times in the cell cycle, thus providing temporal regulation of the cyclin-Cdk complex. As the cyclin subunit is produced, it binds to the kinase subunit and activates it.

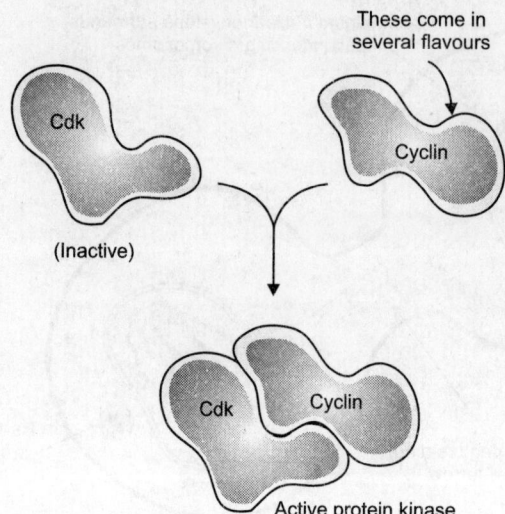

Fig. 8.6: Cyclin-dependent kinases (Cdks). Cdks are the key regulators of the cell division cycle in organisms as diverse as baker's yeast and humans. Cyclin-dependent kinases have two subunits, the kinase (often simply called the Cdk) and a regulatory protein called a cyclin.

The cyclin subunit also targets its kinase partner to specific protein substrates. The key cyclin-Cdk complexes that drive the human cell cycle are listed in Table 8.1.

Table 8.1: The four key cyclin-Cdks that drive the cell cycle.

Name of cyclin-Cdk complex	Name of component cyclin	Name of component Cdk partner
G1-Cdk	Cyclin D	Cdk4, Cdk6
G1/S-Cdk	Cyclin E	Cdk2
S-Cdk	Cyclin A	Cdk2
M-Cdk	Cyclin B	Cdk1

The cell cycle can be viewed as a Cdk cycle (Fig. 8.7). Activation of G1-Cdks by cyclin D turns on the events that occur in the early phase of G1. One of these is synthesis of cyclin E. As cyclin E is made, it binds to Cdk2, forming G1/S-Cdk. As the G1/S-Cdk activity accumulates to a critical threshold, it triggers the transition from late G1 into S phase. Cyclin A is made in S phase. It also binds to Cdk2, forming the S-Cdk that is required for DNA synthesis. Cyclin B is made during S phase and G2. As it is made, it binds to Cdk1 forming M-Cdk. When M-Cdk reaches a threshold activity, it triggers the transition from G2 into the prophase stage of mitosis.

G1 Regulation: How the G1-Cdk Turns on the G1/S Cdk

During G1, cells prepare for DNA replication. They must synthesise proteins necessary to replicate their genome and then assemble the various components of the DNA replication machinery onto the origins of replication. This is coordinated with nutrient and growth factor availability to ensure the cell is in an environment that supports cell division. The G1 phase of the cell cycle is unique in that it represents the only time where cells are sensitive to signals from their extracellular environment.

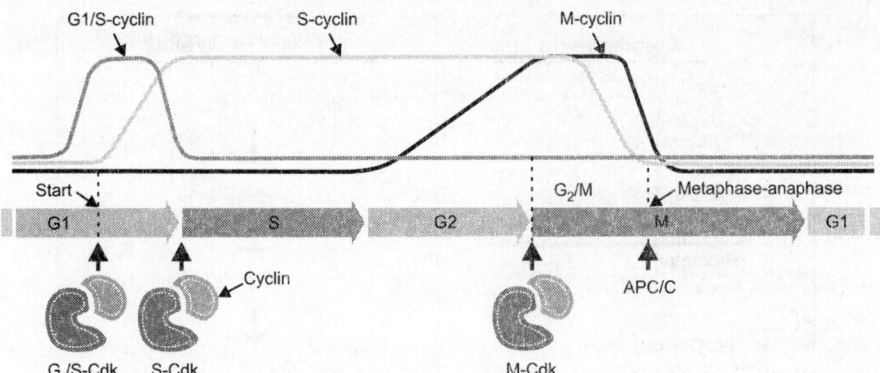

Fig. 8.7: The cell cycle as a Cdk cycle. Different phases of the cell cycle are driven by different cyclin-Cdk complexes. In this simplified view, only a G_1/S-Cdk, a S-Cdk and a M-Cdk are shown. These act in sequence, as each cyclin protein is produced, to program the following critical events: the G_1-S transition known as Start, S phase (DNA synthesis), and the start of M phase (mitosis). In addition, as described in the text, a G_1-Cdk activated by cyclin D phosphorylates the Rb protein to produce cyclin E, which is required for G_1/S-Cdk activity. Note that the activity of each Cdk disappears rapidly at a specific time in the cell cycle (as the specific cyclin protein is degraded). The APC/C is a large protein complex that controls a proteolytic process required for the separation of sister chromatids at anaphase.

Cells require growth factor-dependent signals up to a point in late G1, referred to as the 'restriction point' or start, after which the transition is made into S phase. The transition between early G1 and late G1 ('Start') illustrates one way that cyclin-dependent kinases regulate the progression of the cell around the cell cycle. This is a crucial control point that is often dysregulated in cancer.

In order to move from early G1 to late G1, the cell must synthesize cyclin E. Transcription of the cyclin E gene requires a transcription factor called E2F. In cells that are not proliferating and in cells that are in early G1, the E2F transcription factor is bound to the promoter for the cyclin E gene, but it is inhibited by a protein that binds it, called Rb. (Rb stands for Retinoblastoma, a childhood tumor of the retina—more on this in the Tumor Suppressor and Oncogene). Rb is a nuclear phospho-protein that plays a key role in regulating the cell cycle. It exists in an active underphos-phorylated state and an inactive hyperphosphorylated state. In its active state, Rb serves as a brake that prevents advancement of cells from G1 to S phase. When G1-Cdk activity increases near the middle of G1, G1-Cdk phosphorylates the Rb protein and inactivates it (Fig. 8.8). Inactive phosphorylated Rb releases from E2F and allows transcription of the cyclin E gene to take place. The cyclin E protein binds to the Cdk2 kinase to form the G1/S-Cdk. E2F also transcribes a number of other genes important for S phase, including the genes for DNA polymerase and thymidylate synthase. Importantly, the production of a cyclin E and thus CDK2-cyclin E activity, represents the transition from mitogen-dependent to mitogen–independent cell cycle progression (or passage through 'start'), irreversibly committing the cells to enter S phase. Once cells enter S phase, they are committed to divide without additional growth factor stimulation.

Brakes on the Cell Cycle: Cdk Inhibitors

The Rb protein can be viewed as a 'brake' on the cell cycle because it prevents the transcription of the gene for cyclin E by inhibiting E2F. Three other proteins that act as 'brakes' on the cell cycle are the Cdk inhibitors p16, p21 and p27.

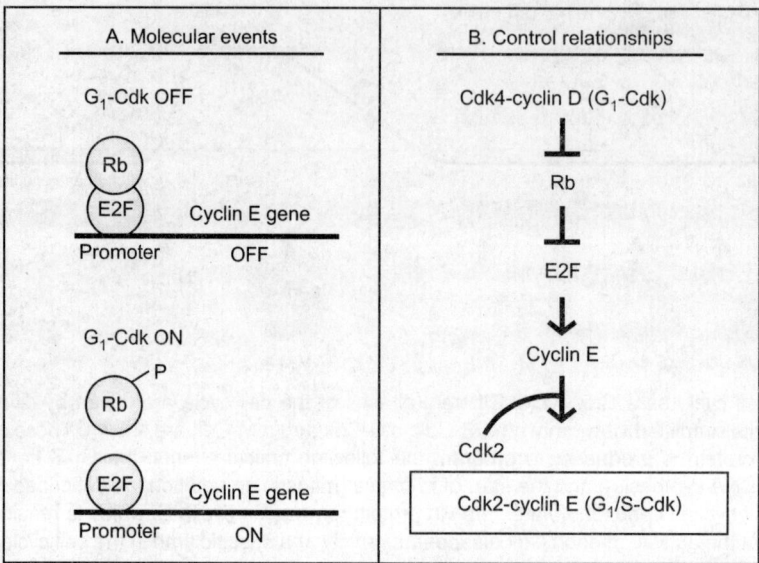

Fig. 8.8: How the G1-Cdk activates the G1/S-Cdk. The G1-Cdk (Cdk4-cyclin D) phos-phorylates the Rb (Retinoblastoma) protein releasing it from transcription factor E2F. E2F can now activate transcription of cyclin E, which in turn results in the production of cyclin E protein and formation of the G1/S Cdk. In describing signaling systems, it is common to use an arrow to indicate an activation and the T-shaped symbol to indicate an inhibition.

These act by binding directly to Cdk-cyclin complexes and blocking their protein kinase activity (Fig. 8.9). Cdk inhibitors fall into two classes: specific and general. The Ink4 (inhibitors of Cdk4) family of proteins, including p16, bind exclusively to and inhibit the G1 Cdks, Cdk4/6-cylin D. The Cip/Kip family of Cdk inhibitors, including p21 and p27, bind to a broad range of Cdk-cyclin complexes, shutting off the cell cycle at multiple points. Functionally, p21 and p27 appear to mainly inhibit Cdk2 complexes. The alterations in these inhibitor proteins play an important role in cancer.

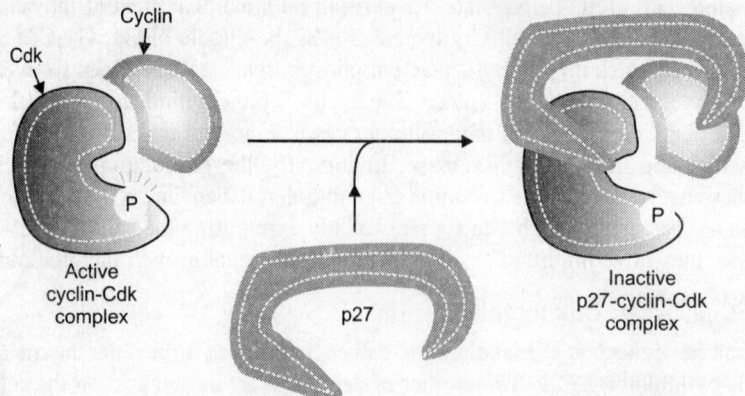

Fig. 8.9: How Cdk inhibitors bind to and inactivate Cdks.

Why is the cell cycle controlled by both activators (e.g. cyclins) and inhibitors (e.g. Rb, p16, p21, p27)? As we will see, it helps each cell to respond to multiple inputs, so that it enters the cell cycle only when the correct combination of conditions are present. The control of cycle entry by both growth activating and growth inhibiting signals is part of a 'fail-safe' system for insuring that cell proliferation only occurs when it is useful to a multicellular organism like ourselves.

Without a complex control system of this type, humans could not exist, because we would all get cancer at a very early age (probably in utero).

CONTROLLING PROLIFERATION: MITOGENS, ANTI-MITOGENS AND CELL SIGNALLING

General Principles of Cell Signalling

Cell signalling processes are central to all of human biology and medicine. Although the details of cell signalling pathways can become very complex, the big picture of cell signalling (e.g. transmitting information from the extra-cellular environment into the cell so it can respond appropriately) is straight-forward. Signalling pathways are built from a limited set of molecules and molecular mechanisms (e.g. phosphorylation or proteolysis) that allow for communication within and between cells.

The underlying molecular mechanisms used in signalling pathways show a number of common properties. In particular, they allow signalling proteins to undergo switch-like activation from an inactive to an active state (for example by receptor clustering, activation of the Epidermal Growth Factor (EGF) receptor tyrosine kinase. EGF binds to the EGF receptor through an extracellular ligand binding domain, leading to dimerisation of the receptor is shown in Fig. 8.10.

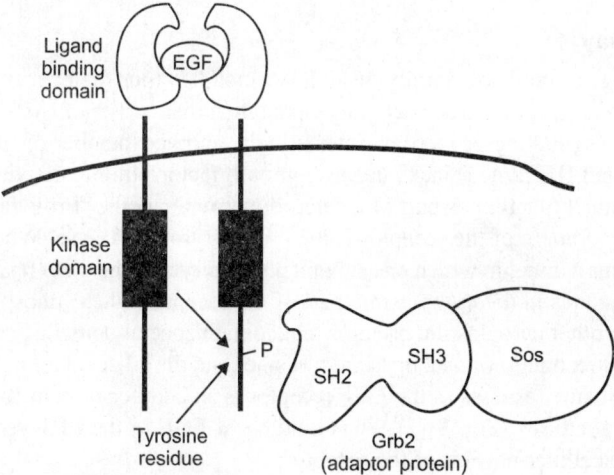

Fig. 8.10: Activation of the Epidermal Growth Factor (EGF) receptor tyrosine kinase. EGF binds to the EGF receptor through an extracellular ligand binding domain, leading to dimerisation of the receptor. Dimerisation causes one subunit to phosphorylate the other (transphosphorylation) on specific tyrosine residues. The SH2 domain of the Grb2 adaptor protein then binds to the region of the EGF receptor containing the phosphorylated tyrosines. Grb2 in turn, uses its second common protein domain, called SH3, to bind to another protein called Sos. Grp2 is known as an adapter protein, since it function to hold two other proteins together. Sos is a member of a large family of proteins that regulate G proteins (GTP-binding proteins) by causing the exchange of a tightly bound GDP molecule for GTP (see Fig. 8.13).

GTP-binding to Ras proteins and stabilisation of b catenin, as described below) and they can also be readily reversed (e.g. by receptor down-regulation, hydrolysis of bound GTP and b catenin degradation). The two major classes of cell surface receptor proteins present in all cells: the G-protein-linked receptor family. The other major class is referred to as the enzyme-linked receptor family. This class includes receptors linked to protein kinases, which fall into two subgroups: the receptor tyrosine kinases (RTKs) and the receptor serine/threonine kinases. An example of each is discussed below.

Mitogens and Anti-Mitogens

Non-dividing cells exist in phase called G0 (G zero). G0 cells can re-enter the cell cycle in G1 when stimulated by mitogens, which are extracellular proteins that stimulate cell proliferation by directly controlling the entry of cells into the cell cycle. (For historical reasons, mitogens are often loosely referred to as growth factors. Although it is best to reserve the latter term for those signalling molecules that actually induce cell growth, i.e. the increase in cell mass, these terms are often used interchangeably). Conversely, cells can be arrested in G1, via., the action of anti-mitogens (proteins that inhibit the activity of mitogens). Many mitogens and a smaller number of anti-mitogens are known. We will discuss one example of each: the mitogen epidermal growth factor (EGF) and the anti-mitogen transforming growth factor β (TGFβ). The receptors for these factors are both enzyme-linked receptors. The EGF receptor or EGFR, is an example of a receptor tyrosine kinase (RTK) and the TGFβ receptor is a receptor serine/threonine kinase, What are the normal functions of these factors? One function of EGF is to promote wound healing. After a wound is formed, epidermal and inflammatory cells secrete EGF and other growth factors. It signals cells at the margins of the wound to proliferate so that the wound may be healed. TGFβ acts as a brake to this process so that the proliferation is coordinated with other aspects of wound healing.

EGF Signalling Pathway

The EGF receptor belongs to the ErbB family of RTKs, which has four members capable of homo–or heterodimerisation. Each receptor heterodimer can respond to a distinct set of extracellular ligands and has different intracellular signalling properties. Interestingly, another member of the ErbB family, the ErbB2 receptor (also called HER2/neu) lacks intrinsic growth factor-binding activity. Consequently, in normal cells HER2/neu must function as part of a heterodimer with another ErbB family member, such as EGF. The cytoplasmic domain of the receptor is the protein tyrosine kinase. When EGF binds to its receptor, the receptor forms a dimer in which one subunit phosphorylates the other (transphosphorylation) on particular tyrosine residues in the cytoplasmic part of the receptor. These phosphorylated tyrosines serve as binding sites for other cytoplasmic proteins that contain special domains, called SH2 domains. SH2 domains specifically recognise phosphorylated tyrosines and the adjacent amino acids. One protein that binds to phos-photyrosine residues in the EGF receptor is an adaptor protein called Grb2. Grb2, in turn, recruits a protein called Sos (Fig. 8.11). Thus binding of EGF to the EGF receptor recruits both Grb2 and Sos to the intracellular portion of the receptor.

Sos is a guanine nucleotide exchange factor (GEF). It acts on a small monomeric GTP binding protein, Ras. The Ras protein is bound to the inner surface of the plasma membrane. Like the G-proteins discussed by Dr. Fulton in the Prologue, Ras can exist in two states: an inactive state in which GDP is bound and an active state in which GTP is bound. Sos activates Ras by promoting the release of its GDP and binding of GTP. Recruitment of Sos to the plasma membrane where Ras is located results in the activation of Ras. Ras can be returned to its inactive form through the hydrolysis of GTP to GDP. This step occurs when a GTPase-activating protein (GAP) binds Ras and induces the hydrolysis of its GTP

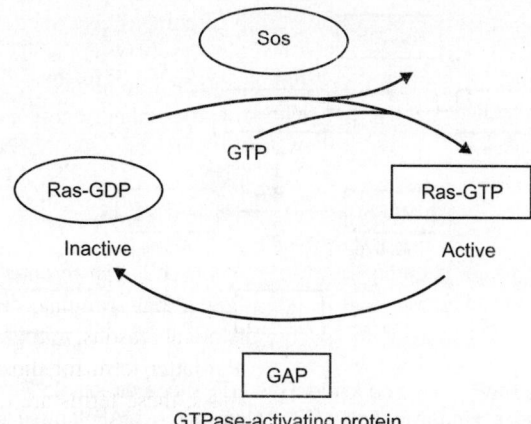

GTPase-activating protein

Fig. 8.11: Sos is a guanine nucleotide exchange protein (GEF) that activates the Ras protein. Ras is a monomeric GTP-binding protein that is only active in its GTP-bound form. In its GDP bound form, Ras is inactive. When Sos binds to Grb2 at the EGF receptor, it is brought close to membrane-bound Ras-GDP molecules, causing the Ras to release its GDP and bind a GTP in its place. A second common type of protein is a GTPase-activating protein (GAP), which inactivates Ras by promoting its GTP hydrolysis. The cell contains hundreds of monomeric GTP-binding proteins that serve to regulate many different functions. Each is regulated in a similar way by GEFs and GAPs.

(see Fig. 8.11). In its GTP-bound (active) state, Ras turns on a protein kinase cascade, in which protein kinases sequentially activate each other through phosphorylation (Fig. 8.12). Active Ras binds to and activates a protein kinase called Raf. In turn, Raf phosphorylates and activates another kinase called MEK (MAP kinase kinase). MEK in turn phospho-rylates and activates mitogen-activated protein kinase, MAP kinase. This chain of phosphorylation events is called the MAP kinase cascade. MAP kinase phosphorylates gene-specific transcription factors in the cell nucleus that bind to the promoters of genes and promote cell proliferation. One important transcription factor that is up-regulated by the MAP kinase cascade is Myc, which is the product of the c-MYC gene. One of the targets of transcription factors that are activated by the MAP kinase cascade is the cyclin D gene. Thus, a multi-tiered pathway connects the presence of a mitogen (EGF) outside the cell to increased expression of a key component of the cell cycle control machinery (the cyclin D gene) in the nucleus (Fig. 8.13). Increased expression of the cyclin D gene leads to the activation of G1-Cdk, pushing the cell to proliferate, as explained previously.

Wnt Signalling

The Wnt proteins are mitogens analogous to EGF. They function in a signalling pathway that regulates cell proliferation by controlling proteolysis of a key signalling protein (Fig. 8.14). The Wnt signalling pathway plays a central role during embryonic development and also serves important functions in adults. For example, Wnt signalling is necessary for the proliferation of stem cells in the proliferative zones in the gut epithelium (the crypts that lie between the microvilli of the epithelium) (Fig. 8.15). Colon cancer is almost invariably associated with the hyperactivation of this pathway in an early step of tumor evolution. As illustrated in Fig. 8.14, Wnt proteins bind to a cell surface receptor called Frizzled. Frizzled controls the stability of a protein called β-catenin, which functions together with a protein called TCF to form a transcription factor that activates the promoter of the cyclin D gene.

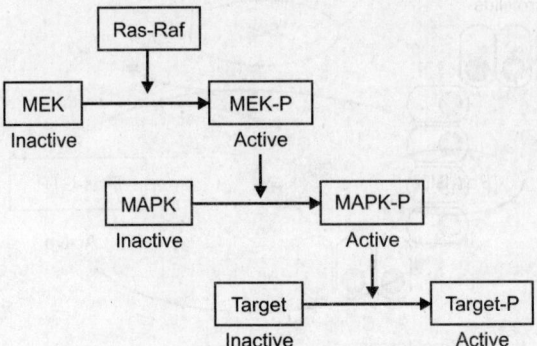

Fig. 8.12: Ras activates the MAP kinase cascade. Ras-GTP binds directly to Raf, which activates its kinase activity. Raf phosphorylates a kinase called MEK (also called MAP kinase kinase). After it has been phosphorylated by Raf, MEK phosphorylates MAP kinase (mitogen activated protein kinase, MAPK). Active MAPK then phosphorylates its target proteins, including transcription factors, stimulating the entry of the cell into the cell cycle.

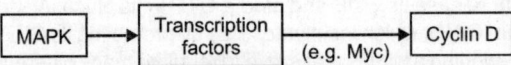

Fig. 8.13: Activation of MAP kinase leads to the transcription of cyclin D. MAPK phos-phorylates transcription factors. This in turn leads to the transcription of the Myc gene, which itself encodes a transcription factor for the cyclin D gene.

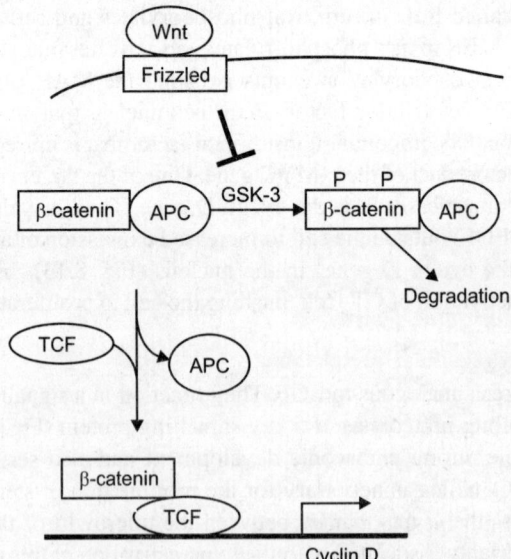

Fig. 8.14: The Wnt signalling pathway.

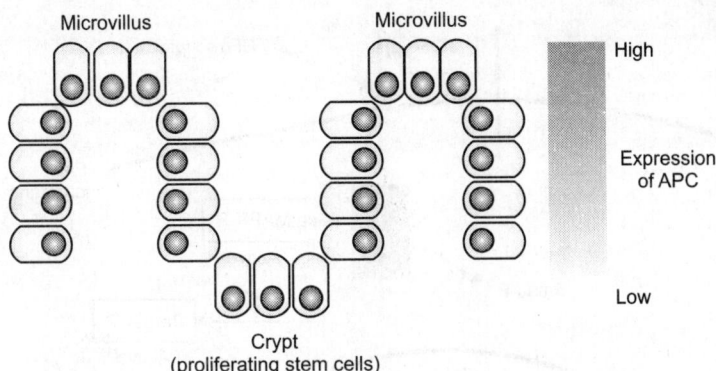

Fig. 8.15: Expression of the APC gene in the gut epithelium. Shown is a schematic of a microvillus in the gut epithelium showing the zone of proliferation (crypts) and the gradient of expression of the APC gene, whose protein product inhibits Wnt signalling.

When Wnt is bound, Frizzled turns off a protein kinase called GSK-3. GSK-3 normally functions to promote the degradation of β-catenin, thus preventing it from activating the cyclin D promoter. Phosphorylation of β-catenin by the protein kinase GSK-3 results in its degradation. However, GSK-3 can only phosphorylate β-catenin when β-catenin is bound to a protein called APC (adenomatous polyposis coli). Thus, APC is necessary to hold β-catenin in check and loss or inactivation of APC is associated with development of colorectal cancer.

(*Note:* This APC protein is not to be confused with APC/C, the anaphase promoting complex/cyclosome, to be described later in this chapter).

Once GSK-3 is inhibited by Frizzled, β-catenin is no longer degraded, allowing it to associate with TCF and activate the cyclin D promoter and promote cell proliferation. Thus, Wnt signalling promotes cell proliferation through the effect of β-catenin on cyclin D production. While Wnt proteins are the extracellular growth factors that activate this pathway, cells also control the pathway from within the cell by varying the transcription of the APC gene, whose protein product inhibits the Wnt signalling pathway. For example, in the epithelium of the colon, there exists a gradient of APC expression that is highest in the terminally differentiated nondividing cells in the microvilli and lowest in the proliferating stem cells in the crypts.

TGFb-Smad: An Anti-mitogenic Pathway

Like EGF, TGFβ is an extracellular protein that binds a cell surface receptor. However, instead of causing cell proliferation, this molecule causes cells to arrest their cell cycle and enter G0. How does this occur? The TGFβ receptor is a transmembrane serine/threonine kinase. Upon binding to TGFß, the receptor phosphorylates proteins in the cytoplasm called Smads (Fig. 8.16). Once phosphorylated, Smad proteins then enter the nucleus and function as transcription factors to turn on specific target genes. A key gene turned on by TGFβ is the Cdk inhibitor p21 discussed above. The activation of p21 blocks G1-S transition by inhibiting Cdk2-Cyclin E/A, leading to the arrest of the cell cycle. Thus, TGFβ arrests cell division by turning on transcription of the gene for a Cdk inhibitor.

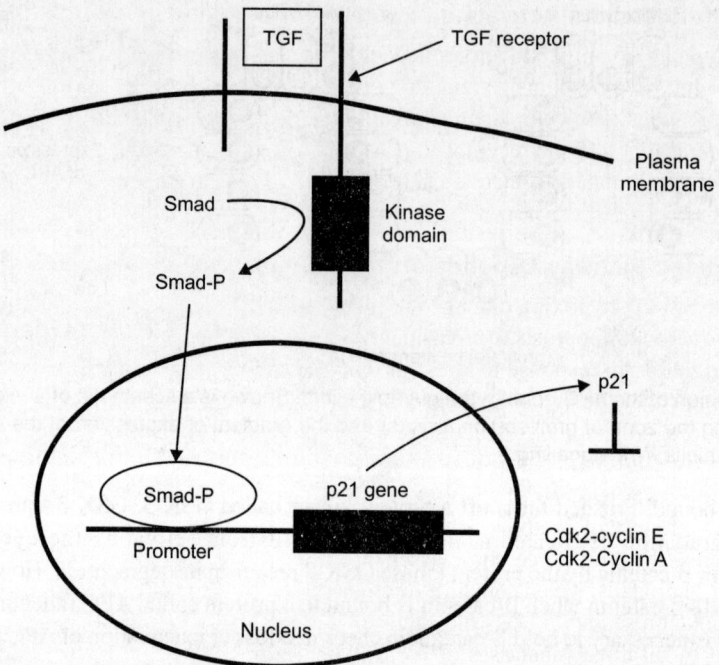

Fig. 8.16: How TGFβ arrests cell division. TGFβ binds to the TGFβ receptor. Binding of TGFβ activates the receptor's intracellular protein kinase domain, leading to phosphorylation of Smad proteins on serine and threonines. Phosphorylated smads enter the nucleus and bind to promoters of genes to control transcription. A key target is the p21 gene. The p21 protein in turn inhibits cyclin E/A- cdk2 complexes, thus leading to cell cycle arrests.

APOPTOSIS

As previously explained, the number of cells in a tissue is controlled not only by cell proliferation, but also by programmed cell death or apoptosis. For a tissue to stay the same size, cell proliferation and cell death must be perfectly balanced. Apoptosis plays important roles both during development and in mature tissues. For example, during development of a limb, tissue present between the digits must be removed. This occurs through localised apoptosis (Fig. 8.17). As described in the Prologue block, the process of apoptosis requires the activation of a special class of proteases inside the cell known as caspases. Caspase molecules normally exist as inactive procaspase molecules in the cell. Procaspase activation is carefully controlled, so that the cell only kills itself when this is appropriate for the success of the organism as a whole.

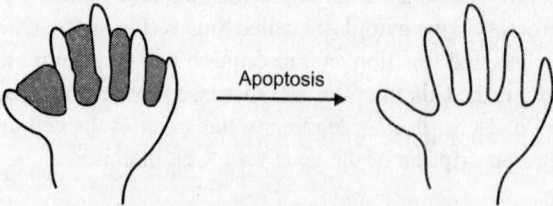

Fig. 8.17: Programmed cell death.

Cell-surface Death Receptors Activate an Extrinsic Apoptotic Pathway

Procaspase activation can be initiated from outside the cell, as happens in the immune system when T cells kill their target cells by producing a signalling protein called Fas ligand. The Fas ligand binds to its receptor, Fas, on target cells. The cytoplasmic domain of a 'death receptor' such as Fas is then triggered to bind adaptor proteins that link the receptor to procaspase-8 molecules. The aggregated procaspase-8 molecules are thereby stimulated to cleave each other, initiating a proteolytic cascade that leads to apoptosis (Fig. 8.18a).

An Intrinsic Apoptotic Pathway Depends on Mitochondria

When cells are stressed (e.g. hypoxia), damaged (e.g. unrepaired DNA damage) or become abnormal in other ways, they can activate apoptosis from inside the cell by triggering a similar process of procaspase aggregation and activation. In response to stress or damage, pro-apoptotic signals induce mitochondria to release cytochrome c into the cytosol, where it binds and activates an adaptor protein called Apaf-1. This causes Apaf-1 to aggregate into a wheel-like complex called an apoptosome. This aggregate then recruits a set of procaspase-9 molecules, which become activated to trigger a caspase cascade causing cell death (Fig. 8.18b). The release of cytochrome c from the mitochondria is tightly controlled by members of the Bcl-2 family of proteins, all of which contain at least one BH protein domain. Within this family of proteins, there are three sub-classes (Table 8.2): two subclasses promote apoptosis (the 'pro-apoptotic' BH123 proteins, which contain 3 different BH protein domains and the BH3-only proteins) and one subclass antagonises apoptosis (the 'anti-apoptotic' Bcl-2 proteins). The BH3 domain is the only domain shared by all three subclasses of proteins and it can mediate a direct binding interaction between one pro-apoptotic protein and one anti-apoptotic protein to form heterodimers.

Table 8.2: Three subclasses of proteins in the Bcl-2 family that control apoptosis by the intracellular (intrinsic) pathway.

Domains	BH 1,2,3	BH 1,2,3,4	BH 3 only
Function	Pro-apoptotic	Anti-apoptotic	Pro-apoptotic
Examples	Bak, Bax	Bcl-2	Bad, Bid, Puma

The central players are the BH123 family members, Bak and Bax, which can form channels in the mitochondrial outer membrane that cause cytochrome c and other proteins in the mitochondrion's intermembrane space to be released into the cytoplasm, thereby activating procaspase-9 via Apaf-1. The anti-apoptotic Bcl-2 proteins appear to bind directly to Bak and Bax to inhibit them, thereby serving to keep the cell alive. The remaining BH3-only pro-apoptotic subclass is composed of a large number of proteins that bind to various subsets of the anti-apoptotic Bcl-2 proteins, forming heterodimers with them. If large enough amounts of the BH3 proteins are present in the right combinations, they will dissociate all of these inhibitors from Bak and Bax, thereby permitting the channel formation and inducing cell death (Fig. 8.19). In summary, it is the balance between the activities of the set of anti-apoptotic Bcl-2 proteins and the two subclasses of pro-apoptotic proteins that determines whether a mammalian cell lives or dies by the intrinsic pathway of apoptosis. This balance is determined through a complex and poorly understood signalling network that continually monitors the state of the cell. For example, only if a cell is in its expected location in the organism will it receive the specific survival signals that it requires to prevent apoptosis. Thus it is not surprising that cancer cells often acquire mutations that allow them to alter the balance between pro- and anti-apoptotic proteins, making it less likely for them to commit suicide even under conditions when normal cells would.

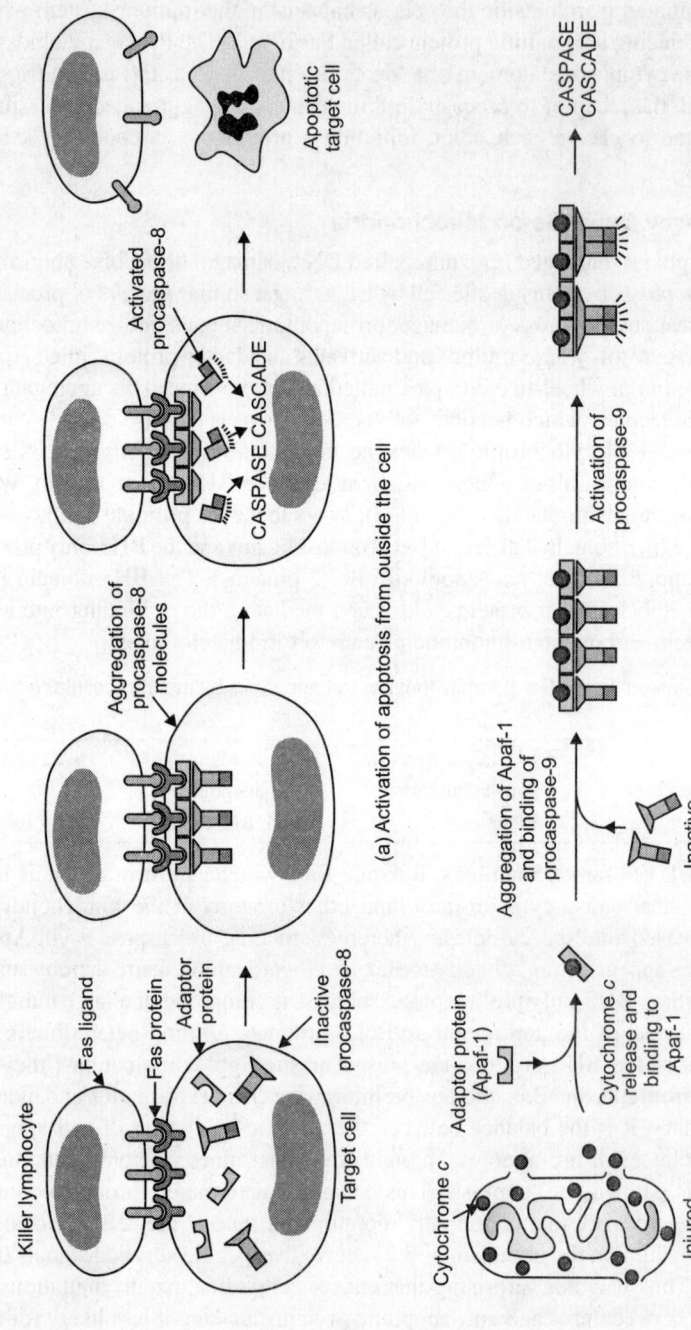

Fig. 8.18: Induction of apoptosis by either extracellular or intracellular signals. (a) Extracellular activation. Adaptor proteins bind the intracellular region of aggregated Fas proteins, causing the aggregation of procaspase-8 molecules. These then cleave one another to initiate the caspase cascade and (b) Intracellular activation. Mitochondria release cytochrome c, which binds to and causes the aggregation of the adaptor protein Apaf-1. Apaf-1 binds and aggregates procaspase-9 molecules, which are activated to trigger a caspase cascade, leading to apoptotic cell death.

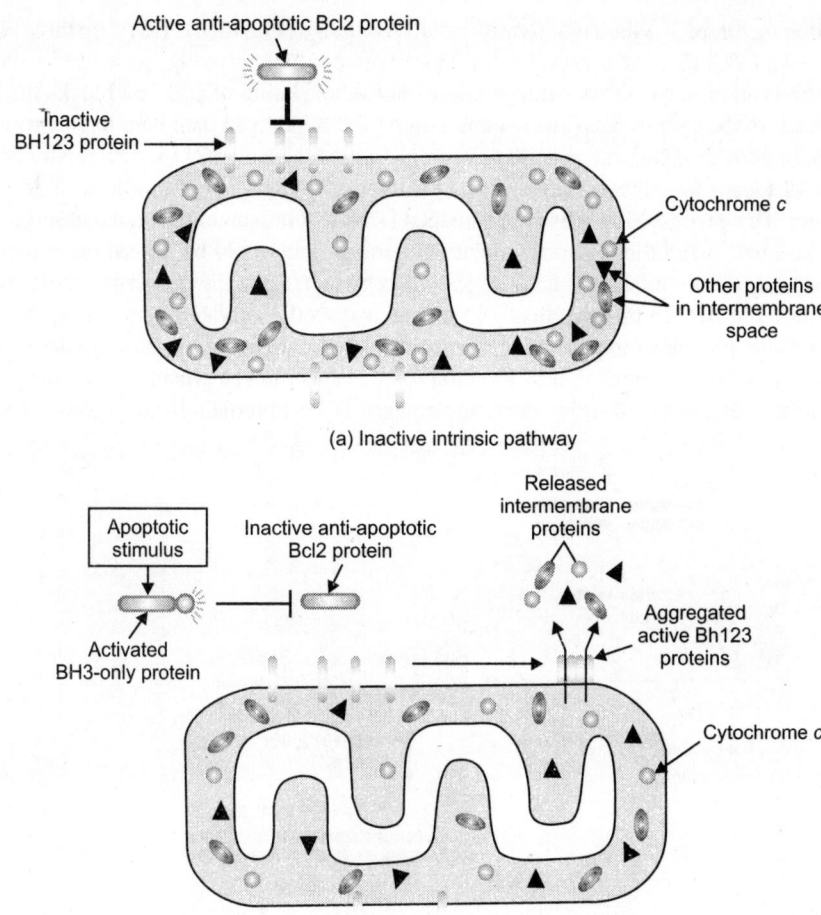

(a) Inactive intrinsic pathway

(b) Activation of intrinsic pathway

Fig. 8.19: How pro-apoptotic BH3-only and anti-apoptotic Bcl2 proteins regulate the intrinsic pathway of apoptosis. (a) In the absence of an apoptotic stimulus, anti-apoptotic Bcl2 proteins bind to and inhibit the BH123 proteins on the mitochondrial outer membrane (and in the cytosol-not shown) and (b) In the presence of an apoptotic stimulus, BH3-only proteins are activated and bind to the anti-apoptotic Bcl2 proteins so that they can no longer inhibit the BH123 proteins, which now become activated an aggregate in the outer mitochondrial membrane and promote the release of intermembrane mitochondrial proteins into the cytosol. Some activated BH3-only proteins may stimulate mitochondrial protein release more directly by binding to and activating the BH123 proteins. Although not shown, the anti-apoptotic Bcl2 protins are bound to the mitochondrial surface.

P53 THE CELL CYCLE AND APOPTOSIS

The cell cycle is controlled at certain stages by checkpoints. These are biochemical mechanisms that stop the cell cycle if certain conditions are not met. One checkpoint is the G1 DNA damage checkpoint. If cells contain unrepaired damage to their DNA, the cell cycle is arrested in G1. This arrest requires a key transcription factor, p53, which is activated by DNA damage (Fig. 8.20). There are three components to the system: (i) a DNA damage sensor, (ii) the Mdm2 protein that normally causes p53 to be degraded and (iii) the p53 protein itself. DNA damage causes phosphorylation of p53 and blocks the binding of Mdm2. This leads to the stabilisation and accumulation of p53. p53 can then bind to the promoter of the p21 Cdk inhibitor described earlier and activate its transcription, causing p21 to accumulate. The resulting inhibition of Cdks leads to cell cycle arrest. If p53 activation continues for a prolonged period of time, apoptosis ensues. This process kills cells with damaged DNA that remain unrepaired and serves to remove cells from tissues that may otherwise accumulate mutations that would be passed on to their daughter cells. High levels of p53 are thought to activate apoptosis by increasing the transcription of several genes. One target gene is the BH123 protein Bax, whose gene is directly activated by p53 (Fig. 8.21). In light of the important role p53 plays in preventing unrepaired DNA damage to be passed on to daughter cells, it is not surprising that p53 is found to play a central role in cancer development. In fact, the p53 pathway is mutated in nearly all cancers, thereby allowing damaged DNA to remain in cells as they proliferate.

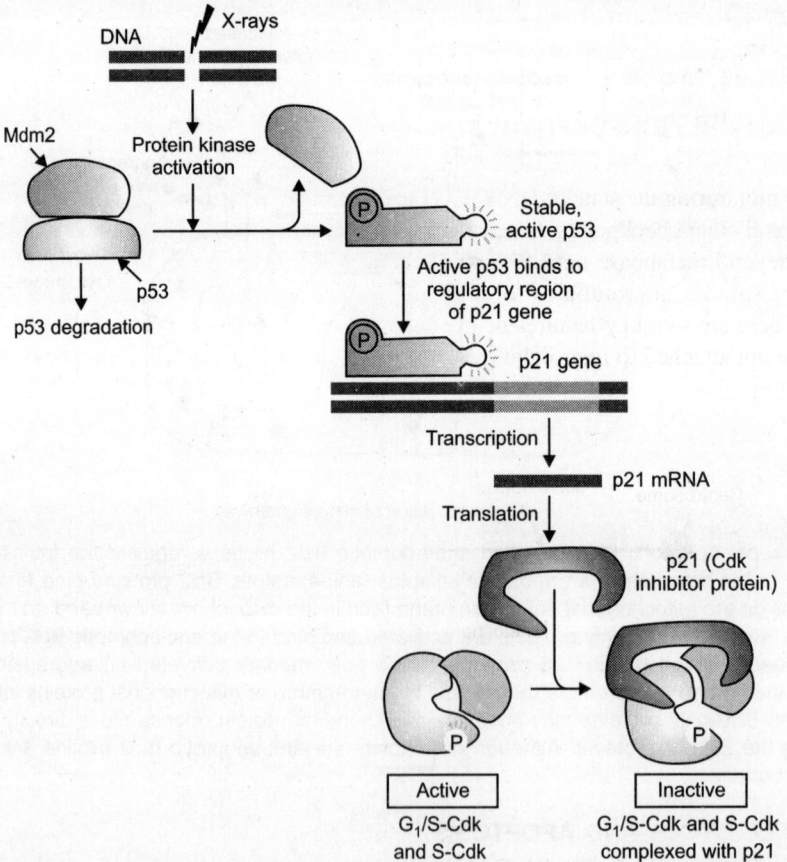

Fig. 8.20: How DNA damage activates p53 and causes cell-cycle arrest. DNA damage activates a protein kinase that phosphorylates p53, preventing its degradation. This leads to the production of high levels of the Cdk inhibitor p21.

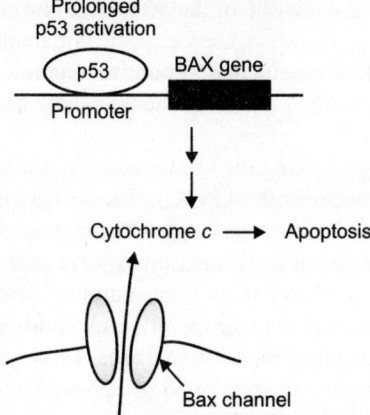

Fig. 8.21: DNA damage can lead to apoptosis. Prolonged activation of p53 in response to DNA damage results in apoptosis. p53 activates the transcription of several genes involved in apoptosis including that for the pro-apoptotic BH123 protein Bax shown here.

SPINDLE ASSEMBLY CHECKPOINT: THE IMPORTANCE OF REGULATED PROTEOLYSIS IN THE CELL

In addition to monitoring the state of DNA in G1 before entering S phase, cells also monitor the state of the cell at several other checkpoints. One, called spindle assembly checkpoint, ensures that mitosis does not proceed beyond metaphase until the spindle is properly assembled. This checkpoint monitors the attachment of spindle microtubules to each kinetochore through the action of the Mad2 protein (Fig. 8.22). There are two key features of the checkpoint: (i) Mad2 associates with kinetochores only when they are not attached to microtubules and (ii) Mad2 becomes activated for arresting mitosis only

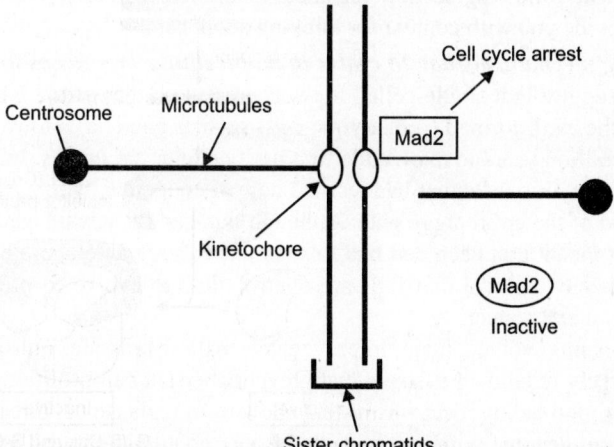

Fig. 8.22: Spindle assembly checkpoint. This checkpoint functions through the action of the Mad2 protein, which binds to kinetochores that have not attached to microtubules. When bound to kinetochores, Mad2 triggers cell cycle arrest. Once microtubules are attached to all of the kinetichores, Mad2 is no longer active and the cell cycle proceeds.

when bound to such kinetochores. If even one of the 46 human chromosomes is not attached correctly to microtubules, enough Mad2 is activated to keep the cell in metaphase. Only when the spindle has been properly assembled with all of the kinetochores bound to microtubules does Mad2 becomes inactive and allow anaphase to proceed. If there is a problem with spindle assembly, Mad2 will arrest the cell cycle until the problem is resolved.

Active Mad2 exerts its effects by blocking the key regulator of the metaphase-to-anaphase transition, the anaphase-promoting complex/cyclosome (APC/C). The APC/C is a member of a large family of important enzymes, called ubiquitin ligases, that trigger the regulated destruction of target proteins in the cell. The actual proteolysis is carried out by proteasomes, large protein complexes that pump selective proteins into their interior in order to cleave them into small fragments.

As a ubiquitin ligase, the APC/C marks proteins for uptake into proteasomes by covalently adding multiple copies of the small protein called ubiquitin to them. The polyubiquitin chain added to a protein is recognised by the proteasome, causing the protein to be destroyed. One of the destroyed proteins is an inhibitor of the protein that cuts the linkages holding the sister chromatid pairs together. The removal of the inhibitor allows the separation of sisters and unleashes anaphase. The S- and M-cyclins are the second major targets of the APC/C. The destruction of these cyclins inactivates the corresponding Cdks. As a result, the many proteins phosphorylated by Cdks from S phase to early mitosis are dephosphorylated by various protein phosphatases that are present in the anaphase cell. This dephosphorylation of Cdk targets is required for the completion of M phase, including the final steps in mitosis and the process of cytokinesis. Not surprisingly, cells defective in the spindle assembly checkpoint show high rates of aneuploidy because of errors in chromosome segregation during mitosis. Defects in the spindle-assembly check-point and specifically in Mad2, have been associated with tumorigenesis.

EVOLUTION OF CELL SIGNALLING AND CANCER

Now that we have explored the key aspects of normal cell proliferation, we can begin to consider what goes awry in cancer cells. The following section considers theoretical aspects of the evolution of cell signalling and cancer to provide you with context for thinking about cancer development and treatment.

Elaborate cell signalling mechanisms had to evolve in multicellular organisms to prevent cancer: Various types of evidence suggest that single-celled life was present on the earth 3.5 billion years ago, about a billion years after the earth formed (prokaryotic cells such as bacteria). However, it appears to have required another two billion years to evolve the first multicellular organisms. Initially these were very small aggregates of eukaryotic cells that had learned how to cooperate, with each cell restraining its own growth for the good of the entire aggregate. Although this had the advantage of allowing each type of cell to specialise, it meant that each cell had to send and receive an elaborate set of signals to determine its appropriate behaviour and that fail-safe controls had to evolve to prevent the type of selfish cell behaviour that we call cancer.

As larger and larger organisms evolved, major improvements to these fail-safe controls had to develop in the form of multiple, largely redundant systems that prevent aberrant cell proliferation. Why? Even with the overlapping set of proofreading mechanisms that allow us to replicate the three billion (3×10^9) nucleotide pairs in the human genome with an error rate of only about one in a billion (10^{-9}), the fact that humans are formed from about 10^{14} cells means that billions of cells experience mutations every day, potentially disrupting the normal controls on cell growth. Viewed from this perspective, the surprising thing about large multicellular organisms is how infrequently cells misbehave to create a tumor. As we shall see, the reason we do not all die of cancer is that, in general, many different mutations need to accumulate in a single line of cells to cause this disease–perhaps 10 to 20. Obtaining a better under-standing the multiple layers of control that are circumvented during tumorigenesis will be key to controlling cancer. Unfortunately, there is still much to learn in this critical area of research.

Cells integrate the many signals that they receive in deciding whether to survive, grow and divide (proliferate), differentiate or die (apoptosis): Every cell contains many different cell surface receptor molecules, each of which recognises a particular molecule at the cell exterior. Some of these bind to signalling molecules that have been secreted by neighbouring cells, others bind to protein molecules held in the plasma membrane of tightly opposed adjacent cells, while others bind to the extracellular matrix. All of these signal molecules work in combinations to regulate the behaviour of the cell, with each of the hundreds or thousands of different cell types in our bodies responding to this babble of signals differently. As shown in Fig. 8.23, an individual cell generally requires multiple signals just to survive. It requires additional signals to grow and divide and a different set of additional signals to differentiate. If deprived of its required survival signals, a cell will undergo cell suicide (apoptosis). The actual situation is even more complex than illustrated in Fig. 8.23, since some extracellular signal molecules act to inhibit these and other cell behaviours or even to induce apoptosis.

How exactly a cell makes each of the all-or-none decisions is illustrated in Fig. 8.23 is not understood in detail. Speaking metaphorically, the decision is analogous to 'cell thinking'. Cells integrate the many signals they receive through a 'cross-talk' between different intracellular events triggered by different cell surface receptors. Some of the cross talk depends on simple 'coincidence detectors', as in the example shown in Fig. 8.24. Here two different signalling events are needed to activate a single protein inside the cell, because the protein needs to be phosphorylated at two different sites to become active. Thus, the activation of this protein occurs if and only if, two specific extracellular signals are present simultaneously. But much of the cross talk is more complex and not yet decipherable.

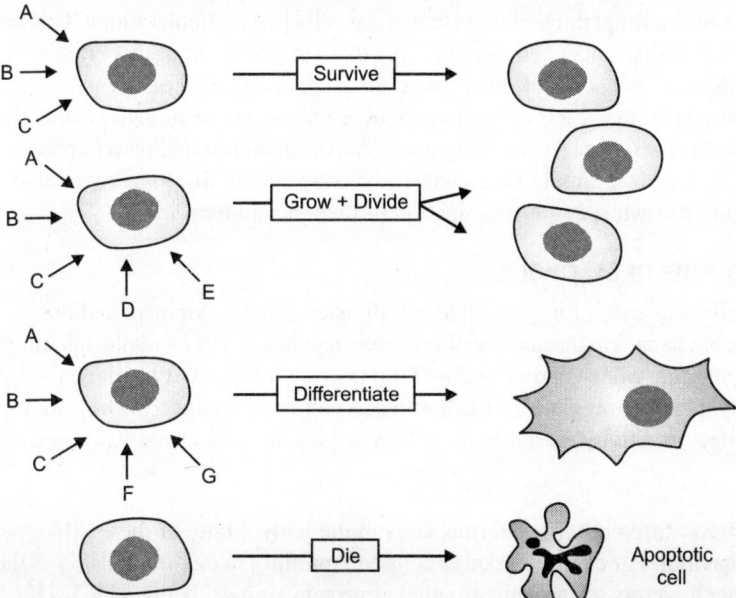

Fig. 8.23: How an animal cell depends on multiple extracellular signal molecules.

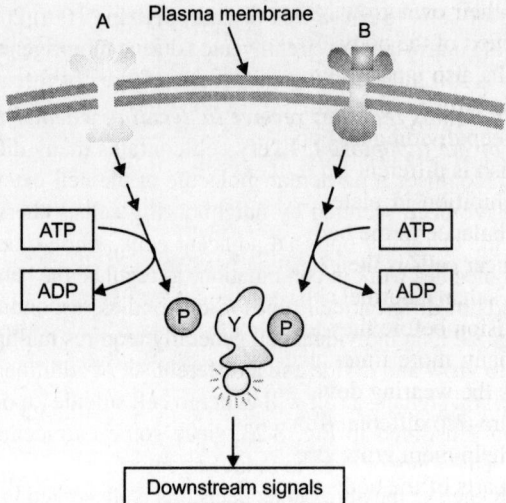

Fig. 8.24: Signal integration inside the cell. Here signals A and B each trigger a different intracellular signaling pathway. Both pathways involve the activation of a protein kinase that phosphorylates protein Y, but at a different site. Because both sites must be phosphorylated for protein Y to become activated, protein Y serves as a coincidence detector that indicates that both extracellular molecules A and B are present.

Cancer can be viewed as a disease in which a cell has accumulated so many changes in its intracellular processes that it has escaped from all of its normal requirements, thinking that it should proliferate and survive independent of its environment. The ideal cancer therapy would be based on an understanding of the exact, highly abnormal intracellular state of the cells in a particular tumor. One might then be able to induce apoptosis in the cancer cells by exposing them to a mixture of two or three specific signalling molecules (or inhibitors of such molecules), with no deleterious effect on normal cells. It is important to keep in mind, however, that each tumor has its own unique set of mutations and aberrant signalling pathways, resulting from a long evolutionary process of random mutation and natural selection during tumor progression. Thus, we should view cancer as a collection of different but related diseases, each of which may require its own specific combination of therapies to treat it.

CANCER AND THE CELL CYCLE

Cancer is basically a disease of uncontrolled cell division. Its development and progression are usually linked to a series of changes in the activity of cell cycle regulators. For example, inhibitors of the cell cycle keep cells from dividing when conditions aren't right, so too little activity of these inhibitors can promote cancer. Similarly, positive regulators of cell division can lead to cancer if they are too active. In most cases, these changes in activity are due to mutations in the genes that encode cell cycle regulator proteins.

Cancer Cells

Cancer cells behave differently than normal cells in the body. Many of these differences are related to cell division behaviour. For example, cancer cells can multiply in culture (outside of the body in a dish) without any growth factors, or growth-stimulating protein signals, being added. This is different from normal cells, which need growth factors to grow in culture.

Cancer cells may make their own growth factors, have growth factor pathways that are stuck in the 'on' position, or, in the context of the body, even trick neighbouring cells into producing growth factors to sustain them. Cancer cells also ignore signals that should cause them to stop dividing. For instance, when normal cells grown in a dish are crowded by neighbours on all sides, they will no longer divide. Cancer cells, in contrast, keep dividing and pile on top of each other in lumpy layers.

The environment in a dish is different from the environment in the human body, but scientists think that the loss of contact inhibition in plate-grown cancer cells reflects the loss of a mechanism that normally maintains tissue balance in the body.

Another hallmark of cancer cells is their 'replicative immortality,' a fancy term for the fact that they can divide many more times than a normal cell of the body. In general, human cells can go through only about 40–60 rounds of division before they lose the capacity to divide, 'grow old,' and eventually die. Cancer cells can divide many more times than this, largely because they express an enzyme called telomerase, which reverses the wearing down of chromosome ends that normally happens during each cell division. Cancer cells are also different from normal cells in other ways that aren't directly cell cycle related. These differences help them grow, divide, and form tumors. For instance, cancer cells gain the ability to migrate to other parts of the body, a process called metastasis, and to promote growth of new blood vessels, a process called angiogenesis (which gives tumor cells a source of oxygen and nutrients). Cancer cells also fail to undergo programmed cell death, or apoptosis, under conditions when normal cells would (e.g. due to DNA damage). In addition, emerging research shows that cancer cells may undergo metabolic changes that support increased cell growth and division.

How Cancer Develops

Cells have many different mechanisms to restrict cell division, repair DNA damage, and prevent the development of cancer. Because of this, it's thought that cancer develops in a multi-step process, in which multiple mechanisms must fail before a critical mass is reached and cells become cancerous. Specifically, most cancers arise as cells acquire a series of mutations (changes in DNA) that make them divide more quickly, escape internal and external controls on division, and avoid programmed cell death.

How might this process work? In a hypothetical example, a cell might first lose activity of a cell cycle inhibitor, an event that would make the cell's descendants divide a little more rapidly. It's unlikely that they would be cancerous, but they might form a benign tumor, a mass of cells that divide too much but don't have the potential to invade other tissues (metastasize).

Over time, a mutation might take place in one of the descendant cells, causing increased activity of a positive cell cycle regulator. The mutation might not cause cancer by itself either, but the offspring of this cell would divide even faster, creating a larger pool of cells in which a third mutation could take place. Eventually, one cell might gain enough mutations to take on the characteristics of a cancer cell and give rise to a malignant tumor, a group of cells that divide excessively and can invade other tissues.

As a tumor progresses, its cells typically acquire more and more mutations. Advanced-stage cancers may have major changes in their genomes, including large-scale mutations such as the loss or duplication of entire chromosomes. How do these changes arise? At least in some cases, they seem to be due to inactivating mutations in the very genes that keep the genome stable (that is, genes that prevent mutations from occurring or being passed on).

These genes encode proteins that sense and repair DNA damage, intercept DNA-binding chemicals, maintain the telomere caps on the ends of chromosomes, and play other key maintenance roles. If one of these genes is mutated and nonfunctional, other mutations can accumulate rapidly. So, if a cell has a nonfunctional genome stability factor, its descendants may reach the critical mass of mutations needed for cancer much faster than normal cells.

Cell Cycle Regulators and Cancer

Different types of cancer involve different types of mutations, and, each individual tumor has a unique set of genetic alterations. In general, however, mutations of two types of cell cycle regulators may promote the development of cancer: positive regulators may be overactivated (become oncogenic), while negative regulators, also called tumor suppressors, may be inactivated.

Oncogenes

Positive cell cycle regulators may be overactive in cancer. For instance, a growth factor receptor may send signals even when growth factors are not there, or a cyclin may be expressed at abnormally high levels. The overactive (cancer-promoting) forms of these genes are called oncogenes, while the normal, not-yet-mutated forms are called proto-oncogenes. This naming system reflects that a normal proto-oncogene can turn into an oncogene if it mutates in a way that increases its activity.

Mutations that turn proto-oncogenes into oncogenes can take different forms. Some change the amino acid sequence of the protein, altering its shape and trapping it in an 'always on' state. Others involve amplification, in which a cell gains extra copies of a gene and thus starts making too much protein. In still other cases, an error in DNA repair may attach a proto-oncogene to part of a different gene, producing a 'combo' protein with unregulated activity.

Many of the proteins that transmit growth factor signals are encoded by proto-oncogenes. Normally, these proteins drive cell cycle progression only when growth factors are available. If one of the proteins becomes overactive due to mutation, however, it may transmit signals even when no growth factor is around. The Ras protein, and the signalling enzyme Raf are all encoded by proto-oncogenes. Overactive forms of these proteins are often found in cancer cells. For instance, oncogenic Ras mutations are found in about 90% of pancreatic cancers. Ras is a G protein, meaning that it switches back and forth between an inactive form (bound to the small molecule GDP) and an active form (bound to the similar molecule GTP). Cancer-causing mutations often change Ras's structure so that it can no longer switch to its inactive form, or can do so only very slowly, leaving the protein stuck in the 'on' state.

Tumor suppressors

Negative regulators of the cell cycle may be less active (or even nonfunctional) in cancer cells. For instance, a protein that halts cell cycle progression in response to DNA damage may no longer sense damage or trigger a response. Genes that normally block cell cycle progression are known as tumor suppressors. Tumor suppressors prevent the formation of cancerous tumors when they are working correctly, and tumors may form when they mutate so they no longer work.

One of the most important tumor suppressors is tumor protein p53, which plays a key role in the cellular response to DNA damage. p53 acts primarily at the G1 checkpoint (controlling the G1 to S transition), where it blocks cell cycle progression in response to damaged DNA and other unfavorable conditions. When a cell's DNA is damaged, a sensor protein activates p53, which halts the cell cycle at the G1 checkpoint by triggering production of a cell-cycle inhibitor. This pause buys time for DNA repair, which also depends on p53, whose second job is to activate DNA repair enzymes. If the damage is fixed, p53 will release the cell, allowing it to continue through the cell cycle. If the damage is not fixable, p53 will play its third and final role: triggering apoptosis (programmed cell death) so that damaged DNA is not passed on. In cancer cells, p53 is often missing, nonfunctional, or less active than normal. For example, many cancerous tumors have a mutant form of p53 that can no longer bind DNA. Since p53 acts by binding to target genes and activating their transcription, the non-binding mutant protein is unable to do its job

When p53 is defective, a cell with damaged DNA may proceed with cell division. The daughter cells of such a division are likely to inherit mutations due to the unrepaired DNA of the mother cell. Over generations, cells with faulty p53 tend to accumulate mutations, some of which may turn proto-oncogenes to oncogenes or inactivate other tumor suppressors. p53 is the gene most commonly mutated in human cancers, and cancer cells without p53 mutations likely inactivate p53 through other mechanisms (e.g., increased activity of the proteins that cause p53 to be recycled).

CELL DIVISION AND CANCER

Cancer cells are cells gone wrong — in other words, they no longer respond to many of the signals that control cellular growth and death. Cancer cells originate within tissues and, as they grow and divide, they diverge ever further from normalcy. Over time, these cells become increasingly resistant to the controls that maintain normal tissue — and as a result, they divide more rapidly than their progenitors and become less dependent on signals from other cells. Cancer cells even evade programmed cell death, despite the fact that their multiple abnormalities would normally make them prime targets for apoptosis. In the late stages of cancer, cells break through normal tissue boundaries and metastasize (spread) to new sites in the body.

How Do Cancer Cells Differ from Normal Cells?

In normal cells, hundreds of genes intricately control the process of cell division. Normal growth requires a balance between the activity of those genes that promote cell proliferation and those that suppress it. It also relies on the activities of genes that signal when damaged cells should undergo apoptosis.

Cells become cancerous after mutations accumulate in the various genes that control cell proliferation. According to research findings from the Cancer Genome Project, most cancer cells possess 60 or more mutations. The challenge for medical researchers is to identify which of these mutations are responsible for particular kinds of cancer. This process is akin to searching for the proverbial needle in a haystack, because many of the mutations present in these cells have little to nothing to do with cancer growth.

Different kinds of cancers have different mutational signatures. However, scientific comparison of multiple tumor types has revealed that certain genes are mutated in cancer cells more often than others. For instance, growth-promoting genes, such as the gene for the signalling protein Ras, are among those most commonly mutated in cancer cells, becoming super-active and producing cells that are too strongly stimulated by growth receptors. Some chemotherapy drugs work to counteract these mutations by blocking the action of growth-signalling proteins. The breast cancer drug Herceptin, for example, blocks overactive receptor tyrosine kinases (RTKs), and the drug Gleevec blocks a mutant signalling kinase associated with chronic myelogenous leukemia. Other cancer-related mutations inactivate the genes that suppress cell proliferation or those that signal the need for apoptosis. These genes, known as tumor suppressor genes, normally function like brakes on proliferation, and both copies within a cell must be mutated in order for uncontrolled division to occur. For example, many cancer cells carry two mutant copies of the gene that codes for p53, a multifunctional protein that normally senses DNA damage and acts as a transcription factor for checkpoint control genes.

How Do Cancerous Changes Arise?

Gene mutations accumulate over time as a result of independent events. Consequently, the path to cancer involves multiple steps. In fact, many scientists view the progression of cancer as a microevolutionary process.

To understand what this means, consider the following: When a mutation gives a cancer cell a growth advantage, it can make more copies of itself than a normal cell can — and its offspring can outperform their noncancerous counterparts in the competition for resources. Later, a second mutation might provide the cancer cell with yet another reproductive advantage, which in turn intensifies its competitive advantage even more. And, if key checkpoints are missed or repair genes are damaged, then the rate of damage accumulation increases still further. This process continues with every new mutation that offers such benefits, and it is a driving force in the evolution of living things — not just cancer cells.

How Do Cancer Cells Spread to Other Tissues?

During the early stages of cancer, tumors are typically benign and remain confined within the normal boundaries of a tissue. As tumors grow and become malignant, however, they gain the ability to break through these boundaries and invade adjoining tissues. Invasive cancer cells often secrete proteases that enable them to degrade the extracellular matrix at a tissues boundary. Proteases also give cancer cells the ability to create new passageways in tissues. For example, they can break down the junctions that join cells together, thereby gaining access to new territories.

Metastasis — literally meaning 'new place' — is one of the terminal stages of cancer. In this stage, cancerous cells enter the bloodstream or the lymphatic system and travel to a new location in the body, where they begin to divide and lay the foundation for secondary tumors. Not all cancer cells can metastasize. In order to spread in this way, the cells must have the ability to penetrate the normal barriers of the body so that they can both enter and exit the blood or lymph vessels. Even traveling metastatic cancer cells face challenges when trying to grow in new areas.

Thus, cancer is unchecked cell growth. Mutations in genes can cause cancer by accelerating cell division rates or inhibiting normal controls on the system, such as cell cycle arrest or programmed cell death. As a mass of cancerous cells grows, it can develop into a tumor. Cancer cells can also invade neighboring tissues and sometimes even break off and travel to other parts of the body, leading to the formation of new tumors at those sites.

Chapter 9

Genetics of Cancer

INTRODUCTION

Cancer is a genetic disease—that is, cancer is caused by certain changes to genes that control the way our cells function, especially how they grow and divide. Genes carry the instructions to make proteins, which do much of the work in our cells. Certain gene changes can cause cells to evade normal growth controls and become cancer. For example, some cancer-causing gene changes increase production of a protein that makes cells grow. Others result in the production of a misshapen, and therefore nonfunctional, form of a protein that normally repairs cellular damage. Genetic changes that promote cancer can be inherited from our parents if the changes are present in germ cells, which are the reproductive cells of the body (eggs and sperm). Such changes, called germline changes, are found in every cell of the offspring. Cancer causing genetic changes can also be acquired during one's lifetime, as the result of errors that occur as cells divide or from exposure to carcinogenic substances that damage DNA, such as certain chemicals in tobacco smoke, and radiation, such as ultraviolet rays from the sun. Genetic changes that occur after conception are called somatic (or acquired) changes.

CELL NUMBERS, CELL DIVISION AND CELL DEATH

Cell numbers are a product of the rates of cell division (mitosis) and cell death (apoptosis). Cell numbers are precisely regulated in all multicellular organisms and this is achieved through controlling the rate of cell division, as well as death, of all cells within the organism. While not immediately obvious, with a little thought we know that this must be the case due to the remarkable consistency of size and form of individuals within a species (with some degree of deviation it has to be said but a squirrel always looks like a squirrel and a human like a human). So how are cell numbers in multicellular organisms regulated? New cells are produced through precise duplication of the contents of an existing cell, followed by division of this cell to form two daughter cells—a process known as mitosis. Cells are also eliminated in a similarly precise manner by triggering an internal cell suicide process known as apoptosis (or programmed cell death). The number of cells within a multicellular organism is thus a product of the rates of mitosis and apoptosis. Interference with the normal rate of mitosis or apoptosis can lead to increases (or decreases) in cell number. As we shall see, cancer represents a spectrum of conditions where normal controls on cell numbers have been lost. Cancer can arise as a result of gene mutations that affect the rate of mitosis as well as apoptosis, thereby leading to the accumulation of extra cells.

CANCER INCIDENCE VARIES BETWEEN TISSUES

Cancer is not a single disease but a diverse group of conditions that all share in common an increase in cell numbers within particular tissues. Cancers can either be benign (where the cancer fails to spread to other tissues and is, in most cases, non-life threatening) or malignant (where the cancer is invasive and spreads to other tissues within the body). Cancers can arise from practically any tissue in the body but are most commonly found to occur in epithelia—the sheets of cells that form the upper layer of the skin and that line the walls of cavities and tubes within the body. Cancers that arise from epithelia are called carcinomas and these tumours are responsible for more than 80% of all cancer-related deaths in the Western world.

The latter fact is probably related to two factors: (i) epithelia are at the highest risk of exposure to cancer-causing agents (carcinogens) because these cells line the surfaces of the body that are in direct contact with the environment (e.g. skin, lungs, mouth, esophagus, stomach, intestine, urinary tract, cervix) which is major source of carcinogens (as we shall see, carcinogens can be either chemical, physical or biological in nature), (ii) because epithelial cells are prone to damage (due to exposure to the environment or infectious agents) these cells have a high replacement rate and are therefore highly mitotic (i.e. these cells are constantly dividing).

Cancers arise more frequently in tissues that exhibit a high rate of mitosis probably because these cells are already dividing at a relatively high rate and the barriers to cell division are lower than in non-dividing tissues (post-mitotic tissues). This brings us to another important point, not all cells in the body divide at the same rate. Some tissues exhibit very low rates of cell division (brain and muscle tissue for example) and cancers rarely arise in such tissues as a result (although they may migrate there from other tissues). Some examples of common cancers that are epithelial in origin are given in Table 9.1.

Table 9.1: Carcinomas.

Tissue sites of more common types of adenocarcinoma	Tissue sites of more common types of squamous cell carcinoma	Others types of carcinoma
Lung	Skin	Small-cell lung carcinoma
Colon	Nasal cavity	Large-cell lung carcinoma
Breast	Oropharynx	Hepatocellular carcinoma
Pancrease	Larynx	Renal cell carcinoma
Stomach	Lung	Transitional-cell carcinoma
Esophagus	Esophagus	(of urinary bladder)
Prostate	Cervix	
Endometrium		
Ovary		

The remaining malignant tumours arise from non-epithelial tissues throughout the body. Those that arise from the various connective tissues, called sarcomas, account for 1% of the tumours encountered in cancer clinics. The second group of tumours of nonepithelial origin arise from the various cell types that constitute the blood-forming (hematopoietic) tissues and include the cells of the immune system. Such tumours (called hematopoietic malignancies) include the leukaemias and lymphomas and these account for approximately 17% of cancer-related deaths. The final group of nonepithelial tumours arise from various components of the central (i.e. brain) and peripheral nervous systems (i.e. spinal cord and outlying nerve tissue) and are termed neuroectodermal tumours. These account for approximately 2.5% of cancer-related deaths.

GOOD CORRELATION BETWEEN CELL DAMAGE OR INFECTION AND CANCER INCIDENCE

As we shall see, cancer most frequently arises as a result of mutations that affect genes that govern the rates of mitosis and/or apoptosis. Practically all carcinogens are mutagenic agents, that is, agents that cause genetic mutation. Thus, tissues that commonly experience the highest levels of exposure to carcinogens are also at the highest risk of mutation. Because epithelial tissues are continually exposed to high levels of substances that may contain carcinogens (in the air that we breath, the food we eat, the liquids we drink, the viruses we encounter) it follows that these cells are at the highest risk of acquiring mutations that may result in cancer. However, because of DNA damage detection and repair mechanisms, as well as mechanisms to limit the ability of abnormal cells to replicate (including the simple elimination of these cells by apoptosis, as well induction of a non-replicating state called senescence) it is important to note that the vast majority of mutations do not result in cancer. However, when cancers do arise, they are most commonly found in epithelial tissues since these are at the greatest risk of damage or infection (Table 9.2).

Table 9.2: Common human epithelial cancers.

Lung
Breast
Skin
Esophageal
Colon
Cervical
Stomach

As indicated above, viruses are also capable of causing cancer and, as we shall see below, cancer-causing viruses were instrumental in the discovery of the genetic basis of cancer. Viruses can provoke cancer through insertion into the genome of their hosts. This can result in cancer in two different ways: (i) the viral genome may carry a gene that enables the host cell to escape the normal controls placed upon it that restrict cell division and/or limit its lifespan, and (ii) the virus may integrate its genome close to a host gene that regulates proliferation and/or apoptosis and this can result in the aberrant expression of such genes.

CANCER IS A RELATIVELY RARE OCCURRENCE

The incidence of cancer is surprisingly low when one considers that the total number of cells in the human body is in the region of 10^{13} (that's 10 trillion!). In fact, the total number of cells produced in the lifetime of an average human is 1000-times this number (10^{16}) due to the fact that cells within many of our constituent tissues are undergoing relatively constant replacement (at a rate of 10^7 cells per second). When we consider the huge potential for mutations to occur in any one of these cells, either due to accidental mutation during replication of the genome during cell division or due to external mutagens, we have to conclude that cancer is a remarkably uncommon occurrence. This is most likely due to several layers of controls that have evolved to limit the uncontrolled division of cells due to the catastrophic consequences that this can have. Because of the relatively low incidence of tumours it might seem obvious that cancers typically arise from a single cell that eventually gives rise to a heterogenous tumour cell population. However, this fact was a matter of debate for quite some time because many tumours appear to be polyclonal upon diagnosis. This is because many of the mutations that promote the cancerous state can disable the normal DNA damage and repair systems that ensure the faithful transmission of DNA to daughter cells during cell division. Later in the course, we will discuss a particularly important gene product in this regard, p53. When such mutations do arise, they facilitate the accumulation of further mutations at a much more accelerated rate than would otherwise occur. Tumours typically undergo a sort of Darwinian selection process where a range of new genotypes are produced and the fittest of these survive in the face of factors that operate against the establishment of the tumour.

We now know that most tumours are monoclonal, that is, they have arisen from a single precursor cell that has become cancerous. Some of the evidence for this has come from studying tumours derived from B cells, the cells of the immune system that produce antibodies. The potential of our immune system to produce different antibodies is practically limitless, but only a single type of antibody is made by each individual B cell (this is due to the way in which antibody genes are shuffled to generate unique combinations and this occurs randomly during the maturation of each B cell). The main point to emphasise here is that B cell tumours (B cell lymphomas and multiple myelomas) would produce many different antibodies if they arose from multiple, independently transformed, B cells. Alternatively, such tumours will produce the same antibody if they arose from a single transformed B cell. So which is it? Analysis of the antibodies produced by B cell tumours revealed that they were monoclonal in nature, strongly suggesting that such tumours arose from a single cancerous progenitor.

Other evidence for the monoclonality of tumours comes from the analysis of chromosomal lesions that can be found in many cancers. Analysis of such lesions reveals that all cells of the tumour will typically display the same lesion. One of the most famous of these is the Philadelphia (or Ph) chromosome (named after its place of discovery) found in chronic myeloid leukaemia and results in the translocation of the BCR gene (and its associated promoter) upstream of the Abl gene to create a new fusion gene (Bcr-Abl), the protein product of which displays greatly increased kinase activity (Fig. 9.1).

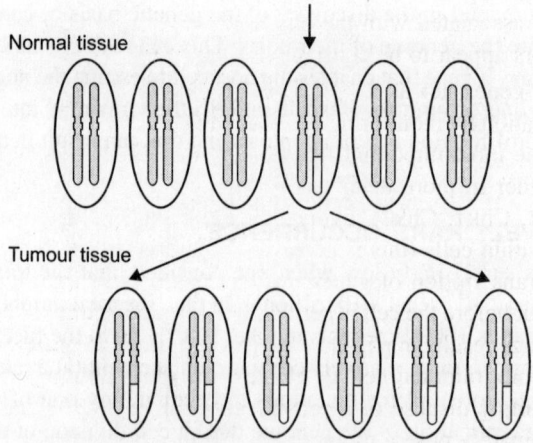

Fig. 9.1: Normal and tumour tissues.

CANCER IS A MULTI-STEP PROCESS

A single mutation is rarely, if ever, sufficient to cause cancer. This is due to mechanisms that have evolved over millennia to safeguard against such events. Multicellular organisms with specialised tissues can only prosper if their constituent cells work together to ensure the reproductive success and long-term survival of the organism. Should mutant cells arise that exhibit 'selfish' behaviour, by replicating themselves without regard to the needs of the organism, we can expect such cells to be treated harshly (death through apoptosis is the most common punishment). Therefore, it should be of little surprise to learn that practically all complex multicellular organisms have evolved a series of protective mechanisms that limit the potential for cancers to develop. For a cancer to develop therefore, the cell that gives rise to the cancer must overcome several factors that work against its survival. This is why cancers are a relatively rare occurrence. It has been estimated that 6–8 independent mutations are typically required for a tumour to occur.

Mutations in oncogenes and tumour suppressor genes contribute to the development of cancer. Mutations of host genes that enhance proliferation and/or other biological properties that increase the likelihood of cancer are called oncogenic mutat ions. An oncogene is a gene that, in mutated form, promotes cancer. Oncogenic mutations are typically gain-of-function mutations that increase the activity or expression level of the gene product. Conversely, tumour suppressor genes are genes that normally act to oppose the development of cancer. Such genes are frequently inactivated in cancers such that they no longer carry out their normal function. Such mutations are typically null mutations, or loss-of-function mutations, where the gene product has lost partial or total activity or expression. In certain circumstances, a genetic mutation may produce a dominant-interfering (also called dominant-negative) mutation that not only fails to carry out its normal function but can also interfere with the function of any remaining wild-type protein.

Some of the most important factors that prevent individual cells from proliferating in an uncontrolled manner include:

1. The requirement for growth factors: Cells require growth factors to enable them to divide and these factors are almost always provided by other cells (i.e. in a paracrine manner). Because the supply of growth factors is limiting, cancers need to find ways of either increasing the supply of such factors (by acquiring the ability to make these factors) or by mutating the downstream signalling molecules associated with the binding of growth factors to their membrane receptors such that the receptors appear to be constantly switched on.

2. Tumour suppressor genes act as a brake on proliferation: Certain proteins act to suppress uncontrolled proliferation by monitoring cells for signs of DNA damage or other signs of aberrant behaviour. One of the most important tumour suppressor genes is the p53 transcription factor, which we will consider in more detail later in the course. P53 operates by collaborating with proteins (ATM, ATR, Chk1, Chk2) involved in DNA damage detection and repair. When p53 becomes activated within cells (this is achieved through stabilisation of the normally-labile p53 protein) it induces transcription of genes that can block entry into mitosis. This enables DNA repair to be carried out before the cell is permitted to re-initiate mitosis. Perhaps more importantly, extensive DNA damage results in p53-dependent expression of genes (Noxa, Puma and Bax) that promote apoptosis (programmed cell death) and therefore eliminate the cell completely. It is probably better to simply dispose of a cell carrying damaged DNA rather than risk incomplete repair that could ultimately pose a threat to the viability of the whole organism. Because of the crucial role that p53 plays in monitoring the integrity of the genome, loss of p53 function can

greatly accelerate the progression to cancer. The p53 gene is found in mutant form in approximately 50% of all cancers.

3. The requirement for oxygen and nutrients: The supply of oxygen and nutrients is regulated by proximity to blood vessels. Because tumours are abnormal cell masses they require new blood vessels (neo-vascularisation) in order to grow beyond a certain size (1 cm^3). This is a major restraint upon the growth of solid tumours and, because of this, such tumours need to induce new blood vessels to grow (a process called angiogenesis) or cells of the tumour will die due to hypoxia (lack of oxygen) and nutrient deprivation. The ability to induce the growth of new blood vessels is thus a major step in cancer progression and is often linked to production of VEGF (vascular endothelial growth factor) by the tumour.

4. The immune system acts as a barrier to the development of cancer: Vertebrates and other higher organisms possess immune systems that are capable of recognising aberrant cells that may be expressing mutated proteins or cells that fail to express proteins that are normally expressed by healthy cells. Certain cells of the immune system (called cytotoxic T cells and natural killer cells) have evolved to patrol the body to weed out cells (by killing these cells via apoptosis) that are displaying mutant or 'foreign' proteins. Such cells serve an important defense against the development of cancer.

Because of these factors, a single mutagenic event is very unlikely to enable a cell to simultaneously escape all of the above growth controls. Instead, what typically happens is that a precancerous cell undergoes a process of progressive transformation from a relatively non-cancerous state to a progressively more transformed cancerous state. At each point along the way, further mutations occur (facilitated by previous mutations) that enable cells to progress to the next stage. Therefore, the development of cancer typically takes place over a relatively long time-frame and this is why cancers are more likely to arise (or become clinically-detectable) later in life. However, this can be accelerated if pre-existing mutations are inherited that already provide a fertile soil upon which further mutations can develop. Thus, cancer undoubtedly has an heritable component and this can have a significant impact upon the incidence of cancer in certain families or nationalities.

CELLULAR TRANSFORMATION

During the progression from a normal to a cancerous state, cells are often described to undergo 'transformation'. Cellular transformation is a term that is used to describe cells that are at various stages of the progression to cancer. Transformed cells display various properties that are not typically displayed by normal cells and these characteristics have been very useful for the discovery of genes that are involved in cancer development. Some of the characteristics of transformed cells will now be discussed.

Ability to grow in laboratory cultures (in vitro) for long periods of time: The ability to grow cells in the laboratory, *in vitro* (literally meaning 'in glass') as it is usually described, has greatly facilitated the study of normal cell function. However, in practice this is quite difficult to achieve as cells need to be supplied with all of the factors necessary for their survival, as well as factors that will stimulate cell division. While early studies managed to keep cells alive *in vitro* for various periods of time, it wasn't until the discovery of growth factors that it became possible to stimulate cells to undergo cell division in the laboratory setting. As mentioned earlier, growth factors are essential for cell division as these proteins bind to cell surface receptors and switch on signalling cascades that promote division of cells. Serum is a convenient source of such factors and when added to cells is able to promote division of most cell types. However, even in the presence of serum, untransformed cells will generally undergo a set number of cell divisions and will then become unresponsive. Thus, untransformed cells have a sort of inbuilt clock that limits the number of divisions that such cells can undergo before entering a state that is called replicative senescence. This limit (called the Hayflick limit after the scientist that discovered this phenomenon) varies somewhat from one cell type to another. Although it took many years to discover why this is, we now know that this relates to the shortening of chromosome ends (called telomeres) during each successive round of cell division. At some point the telomeres become so eroded (rather like the ends of a shoelace fraying with time) that further chromosomal duplication becomes impossible and cells can no longer undergo division. Such cells often display chromosomal fusions, breakages and other abberations. A hallmark of transformation is the ability to continue to divide well beyond the normal Hayflick limit and this appears to be related to the expression of an enzyme (called telomerase) that can repair telomeres and therefore greatly enhance the number of cell divisions that a cell expressing this enzyme can undertake. Telomerase expression is normally confined to embryonic cells or stem cells but many cancers display reactivation of telomerase gene expression which increases the number of cell divisions such cells can undergo.

Reduced requirement for growth factors: We have already mentioned growth factors several times as these proteins are critical for the initiation of cell division. Another hallmark of cellular transformation is a reduced requirement for such factors. This can be achieved in several ways. Some transformed cells acquire the ability to make their own growth factors (autocrine growth). Another way to achieve this is to greatly amplify the number of growth factor receptors expressed by the cell as this has the effect of mimicking growth factor receptor engagement. Yet another way to supplant the requirement for growth factors is to acquire mutations in genes that function in growth factor receptor signalling pathways, such that the signalling cascade is permanently switched on (examples of such mutations are the Ras and B-Raf mutations that are found in many cancers).

Anchorage-independence: Another feature of normal cells is that these cells (with the exception of blood cells) typically will not grow unless attached to a solid support or substratum. In the laboratory, this support is provided by the plastic cell culture vessel (petri dish or flask) that cells are grown in. However, normal cells will rapidly cease dividing when the flask is covered with a monolayer of cells. Transformed cells, on the other hand, will typically continue to divide by piling up on top of eachother and will even grow when completely detached from the flask (or when suspended in soft agar). Transformed cells will often betray their presence in a culture of otherwise healthy cells by forming disorganised clumps or foci where cells pile up into three-dimensional aggregates. Historically, such foci were important for the detection of cellular transformation.

Altered morphology: Transformed cells also exhibit abberant morphology. Whereas normal cells usually adopt a fully flattened conformation in culture, transformed cells often become more rounded or adopt a spindle morphology. This most likely relates to changes that occur to the cytoskeleton of such cells that result in a much more disorganised cytoskeleton and therefore a more flexible cell morphology. Thus, transformed cells aften look very different to their normal counterparts under the microscope and this feature is still exploited even today in the diagnosis of many cancers by histopathologists.

Loss of contact inhibition: Normal cells possess a property called contact inhibition. Such cells will cease to divide when they are in contact with other cells on all sides. This property results in the formation of ordered monolayers (layers of cells one cell thick) when untransformed cells are grown in culture. However, transformed cells do not display contact inhibition and will usually grow to much higher cell densities in culture as a result.

Ability to form tumours when introduced into immunocompromised mice: The ultimate test of the transformed state is whether such cells can form tumours when introduced into an animal host. In practice, this test is performed in immunocompromised mice that lack T cells due to a mutation that blocks the development of the thymus (the gland where T cells normally mature), this also has the knock on effect of blunting B-cell development. The use of immunocompromised mice dramatically reduces the likelyhood of rejection or elimination of the tumour that would normally result from an immune response to the tumour.

These mice also lose all of their hair and are called nude mice as a result. This also makes it convenient to track the growth of the tumour as the candidate tumour cells are frequently injected under the skin. It is important to note that cells displaying many of the hallmarks of the transformed phenotype often fail to establish tumours when introduced into nude mice, strongly suggesting that such cells are only partly, but not fully, transformed. Thus, the ability to form tumours *in vivo* is an important test of the fully-transformed state. This model has also proved very useful for pre-clinical testing (i.e. prior to testing in humans) of potential cancer therapies.

MUTANT GENES INTO NORMAL CELLS CAN RESULT IN FEATURES OF CELLULAR TRANSFORMATION

Because normal, untransformed, cells behave differently to transformed cells when placed into cell culture, many scientists began to look for ways to transform normal cells into cancerous cells by exposing such cells to mutagenic chemicals, viruses, or crucially, by introducing individual genes (often isolated from cancer cells) into such cells. This was made possible due to the discovery (in 1972) of a simple method for the introduction of DNA into cells. This method, called transfection, is still in everyday use in labs throughout the world and is used to test the function of individual genes upon expression in cells.

DNA transfection involves the formation of a complex between DNA and a calcium salt. This precipitates the DNA, which when added to cells, is then taken up by pinocytosis and escapes into the cell cytosol where it can then enter the nucleus and become expressed (and even integrated into the genome for permanent expression if a few experimental tricks are employed).

It is important to note that individual mutations may produce one or more of the features of transformed cells but may not fully transform cells. Several independent mutations are normally required to achieve a fully transformed state and this is why the development of cancer is a multi-step process. Cellular transformation assays have been of fundamental importance in unravelling the molecular basis of cancer as many cancer-causing mutations were discovered in the context of such assays. Typically, the assay is used in the following way.

Normal (i.e. untransformed) cells were treated with mutagenic chemicals in culture to introduce random mutations that initiated cellular transformation. But how could the mutant gene that provoked transformation be pinpointed? Note that this was well before the development of high through put sequencing methods so the challenge of isolating a mutant gene was a very formidable one (and still is, even using modern sequencing methods). However, by isolating DNA from the chemically-transformed cell population, followed by cutting it up into small pieces and reintroduction into normal cells using the transfection method, scientists could look for just those pieces of DNA that could reproduce the transformed state. Due to molecular tricks that we need not go into here, the pieces of DNA that were capable of transforming normal cells and indeed of forming tumours in nude mice (Fig. 9.2). This could then be isolated and sequenced to pinpoint the mutation that gave rise to the transformed state.

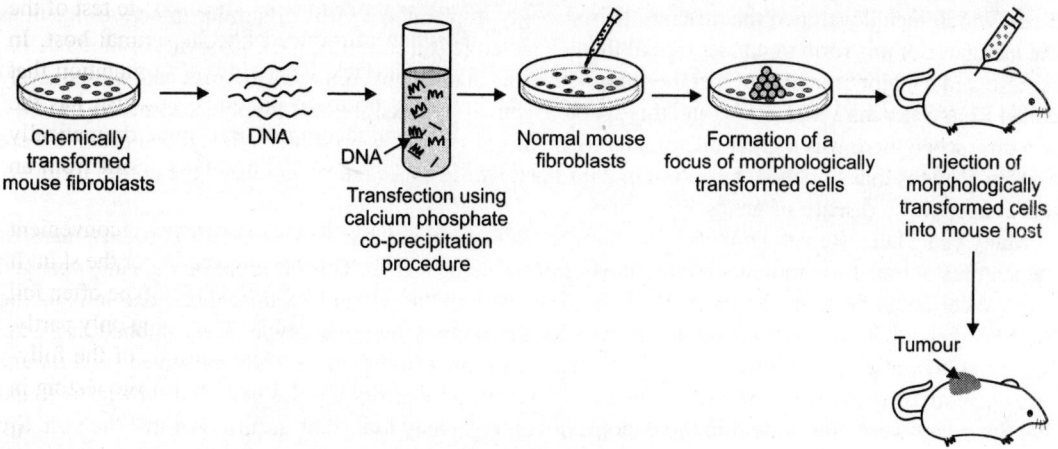

Fig. 9.2: Tumours in nude mice.

ONCOGENES AND TUMOUR SUPPRESSOR GENES

Oncogenes (Onco, from the Greek meaning 'bulk' or 'mass') are genes that, in their mutant forms, promote the development of cancer. Such genes are typically genes that normally promote cell division but, upon mutation, do this at an enhanced rate. Numerous oncogenes have been identified to date and many of these turn out to be growth factors, their receptors, or signalling proteins that act downstream of growth factor receptors. Some oncogenes are involved in the regulation of programmed cell death (apoptosis) and contribute to the development of cancer by greatly prolonging the lifespan of cells expressing mutant forms of such genes. Mutations that turn a gene into an oncogene are typically gain-of-function mutations that greatly increase the activity of the protein encoded by the gene. This can be achieved in a number of ways:

1. Through enhancing the stability of the protein.
2. Increasing the expression rate of the gene encoding this protein.
3. By altering the protein active site (if its an enzyme) such that it now functions at an enhanced rate or by some other conformational change that results in a more active protein.

Other Mechanisms

Other mechanisms are also possible such as tumour suppressor genes normally oppose cell proliferation or survival but, in their mutant forms, have lost the ability to do this. Thus, tumour suppressor genes normally suffer loss-of-function mutations in cancer and such mutations typically inactivate the normal function of such genes. In some cases, tumour suppressor genes may become mutated into dominant-interfering mutants that actually oppose the function of the wild-type protein these genes encode (we will see an example of this later when we discuss the p53 tumour suppressor gene).

DISCOVERY OF ONCOGENES

The study of tumour viruses introduced the notion that cancer was a disease of genes. In 1908 it was discovered that a filterable agent derived from chicken leukaemia cells could be transferred to other birds, which then developed the disease. This strongly implicated a virus or similar infectious agent as the instigator of this form of cancer (recall that a leukaemia is a cancer of the leukocytes or blood cells). represented a major breakthrough at the time. The virus that provoked these sarcomas was subsequently called Rous Sarcoma Virus (RSV) and this sparked a hunt for the viral genes involved. More importantly, at a time when there was a great uncertainty as to the cause of cancer (some believed that cancers were foreign growths that somehow took root in their hosts) these experiments solidified the notion for many that cancer was a disease of genes.

Many years later, Renato Dulbecco, working at Caltech, found that RSV could also produce many of the features of transformation upon infection of normal cells *in vitro*. This observation radically changed how cancer could be studied and, in 1974, Michael Bishop and Harold Varmus succeeded in isolating the RSV gene that was responsible for provoking the transformed phenotype. They dubbed this gene Src (an abbreviation of sarcoma) but quickly made a startling observation. They presumed (as did most other scientists) that normal untransformed cells would not express the Src gene but they soon found that Src genes were present within the genomes of all cells they looked at. It turns out that the viral Src gene (v-Src) they isolated is an example of a hijacked gene that became part of the viral genome due to the selective advantage it offered the virus upon entry into its host. Varmus and Bishop were subsequently awarded the Nobel Prize for Physiology or Medicine (in 1989) for their work, as Src was the first oncogene to be discovered.

But most cancers do not spread in an infectious way, so viruses were clearly not the only means of initiating cancer (although many scientists looked for evidence of viruses in many different cancers, generally with little success). However, some human cancers are caused by viral infection but the great majority of cancers are related to other factors (mainly environmental) that result in mutation of host genes. The search for other cancer causing oncogenes thus began and the notion that oncogenes were probably mutant forms of normal genes (dubbed proto-oncogenes) soon took hold. The transfection assay described earlier (where DNA prepared from tumours was fragmented into small pieces and introduced into normal cells) proved highly effective in identifying many additional oncogenes and such assays are still used for this purpose today.

RAS AND B-RAF ONCOGENES

Growth Factor Signalling Pathways and Cancer

Growth factors promote cell division through activating signalling cascades that switch on a battery of new genes that are required to replicate the contents of the cell (including its genome), culminating in the division of the duplicated cell contents into two new daughter cells. Clearly this is a massively complex process and cannot be embarked upon lightly. Therefore, the supply of growth factors is stringently controlled to ensure that cell numbers in target tissues are kept constant. Cells essentially compete for growth factors and, for cancers to develop, such cells must find a way of becoming independent of the requirement to receive growth factors to drive mitosis.

It turns out that different cancers solve the growth factor problem in slightly different ways. We have already mentioned that some cancers become growth factor independent by increasing the expression of growth factor receptors (for example, the Epidermal Growth Factor receptor, erbB, is upregulated in stomach, brain and breast cancer). This has the effect of making the cancer cell hyper-responsive to ambient levels of growth factor that would not normally stimulate cell division. In addition, enhanced expression of growth factor receptors can also increase the rate at which the receptors undergo spontaneous (i.e. ligand-independent) activation. Other tumours get around the requirement for growth factors by making their own. However, many other tumours dispense with the need for growth factors or their associated receptors altogether by acquiring mutations in key signalling molecules that act downstream of the growth factor receptor. A notable example of this type of mutation is found in the Ras and B-Raf proteins that play central roles in propagating mitogenic signals from many different growth factor receptors.

Ras Controls Raf Activation but only in its GTP-bound State

Ras is a GTP-binding protein that is normally tethered to the plasma membrane through a lipid modification that occurs during synthesis of this protein (Fig. 9.3). In its GTP bound state Ras is active but it soon hydrolyses GTP to GDP (by splitting off a phosphate group) to return to its inactive GDP-bound conformation. The primary job of Ras is to activate the downstream protein kinase, Raf, (in fact Raf comes in 3 flavours A-Raf, B-Raf and C-Raf).

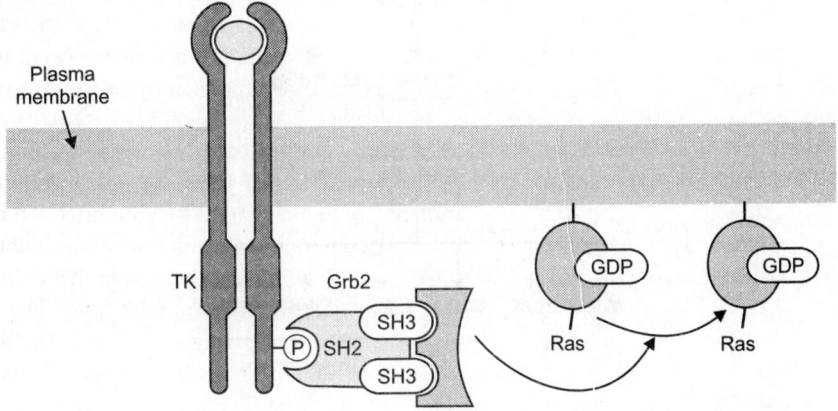

Fig. 9.3: Plasma membrane through a lipid modification that occurs during synthesis of this protein.

Ras-GTP drives Raf activation through recruitment of Raf to the plasma membrane

Ras activates Raf by recruiting the latter to the plasma membrane where Raf can now be phosphorylated by a membrane-associated kinase (thereby activating Raf). The nature of the kinase that activates Raf is still uncertain but Src (the first oncogene to be discovered) has been implicated in this process. But there is a problem. Ras cannot bind to Raf unless Ras is in a GTP-bound state and to bind a GTP molecule it needs help from a protein called a GDP/GTP exchange factor (commonly called a GEF) that will assist Ras in letting go of GDP, exchanging this for a GTP molecule.

Sos helps Ras to bind GTP

A major GEF for Ras is a protein called Sos (son of sevenless) but Sos does not normally live at the plasma membrane so it needs help to become recruited there. This help comes in the form of a protein called GRB2 (growth factor receptor-binding protein 2) which has a domain (called an SH3 domain) that Sos bind to. However, Grb2 does not normally live at the plasma membrane either, so how does it get there and bring Sos with it? The answer lies with growth factor receptors.

Growth factor receptor activation creates binding sites for Grb2 and associated Sos

Because many growth factors are dimeric in nature, engagement with their specific receptors results in aggregation of the receptor in the plasma membrane. Many growth factor receptors are kinases and aggregation of these molecules, as a result of ligand binding, typically results in the receptors phosphorylating eachother within their cytoplasmic tails (i.e. the part of the receptor that faces the cytoplasm). So, ligand-induced activation of the growth factor receptor creates binding sites for GRB2/Sos and this results in activation of Ras through Sos-mediated stimulation of GTP exchange on Ras. Ras then recruits Raf to the membrane, where it now becomes phosphorylated and active Raf propagates the signal further by activating the downstream kinase MEK, followed by ERK. Downstream processing of Ras (Fig. 9.4).

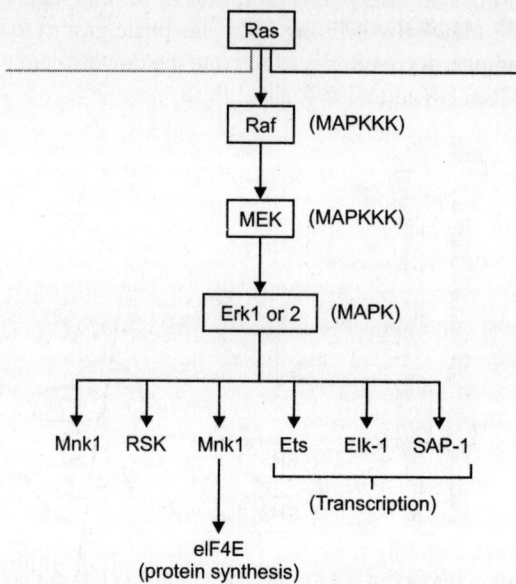

Fig. 9.4: Downstream processing of Ras.

Activation of the Ras/Raf/MEK/ERK Cascade Promotes the Expression of New Genes

As a result of this stepwise sequence of events, ERK (extracellular receptor-activated Kinase) becomes switched on and this kinase controls the activities of a battery of transcription factors that control the expression of numerous genes involved in cell division. Thus, activation of ERK, via Ras and Raf, promotes cell division through the action of ERK on transcription factors.

Mutation of Ras in Cancer

Because of its pivotal role in growth factor receptor signalling, Ras is very commonly mutated in cancer and these mutations typically increase the affinity of Ras for GTP such that Ras spends most of its time in the cells in the 'on' (i.e. GTP-bound) as opposed to the 'off' (i.e. GDP-bound) state. The pattern of Ras mutations in cancer is dictated by tissue type as well as Ras isoform (there are 3 Ras genes, H-Ras, K-Ras and N-Ras). 30% of cancers have Ras mutations and in most cases these mutations occur at poitions 12 and 13 of the Ras protein, right in the middle of the GTP-binding loop (called the P-loop

['P'= phosphate] region). In all cases, these mutations increase the activity of Ras and are therefore classified as gain-of-function mutations.

Mutant Ras can Transform Cells

Transfection of mutant Ras into many normal cell types is sufficient to partly transform these cells by increasing rates of proliferation and conferring growth-factor independence. However, in keeping with the notion that single mutations are rarely sufficient to cause cancer by themselves, mutant Ras transforms cells much more efficiently if these cells are also carrying a mutant p53 gene. This illustrates the synergistic interactions that occur between independent mutations to promote cell transformation.

B-Raf MUTATIONS AND MALIGNANT MELANOMA

Malignant melanoma is one of the most difficult to treat forms of human cancer (due to profound chemotherapeutic drug resistance) and the incidence of this condition in developed countries has risen faster than any other malignancy over the past 40 years. Melanoma occurs when the pigment-producing cells (melanocytes) within the basment membrane of the skin become transformed due to chromosomal lesions that frequently involve the B-Raf kinase.

Most melanomas arise on the exposed areas of the skin (limbs, face and trunk) and there is a strong correlation between intermittent high-intensity exposure to sunlight and development of melanoma. Unlike most other forms of cancer, melanoma incidence does not correlate with increasing age and melanoma is one of the most common causes of cancer and cancer-associated mortality within the 20–35 age group. While the majority (~85%) of individuals diagnosed with melanoma can be successfully treated with early intervention, late diagnosis has a very poor prognosis as malignant melanoma is highly invasive and is notoriously unresponsive to most conventional chemotherapeutic drugs. At present, only one US FDA-approved drug (Dacarbazine) demonstrates a degree of efficacy for the treatment of metastatic melanoma. Dacarbazine elicits a response in 15–25% of melanoma patients but complete response rates are very poor at around 5%. The mechanisms underlying this acute resistance to therapy remain unclear but are almost certainly related to dysregulation of the cell death (apoptosis) machinery within such cancers.

B-Raf is Mutated in the Majority of Melanomas

A major breakthrough in our understanding of the molecular basis of melanoma was the discovery, in 2002, that mutations in the B-Raf kinase are found in ~70% of melanomas. Significantly, mutations in B-Raf correlate with progression of melanoma from the early (radial growth phase) form of the disease which is treatable, to the more aggressive (vertical growth phase) metastatic phase, which is much more refractory to chemotherapy. Thus, mutation of B-Raf is very likely to be instrumental in the progression of melanoma and this protein is now considered to be a *bona fide* oncogene.

B-Raf Mutations Predominantly Alter a Single Amino Acid Residue

Approximately 80% of B-Raf mutations are found at position 600 of the B-Raf kinase where a valine is altered to a glutamic acid (V600E). The latter mutation produces a constitutively active kinase that is approximately 500 times more active than the wild type protein.

Mutation of B-Raf dramatically increases the levels of active MEK and of its downstream target, ERK. Similar to Ras mutations, B-Raf mutations therefore dramatically increase the levels of expression of genes that promote proliferation and, in addition, active B-Raf may also suppress the activation of the cell death machinery, thereby conferring a state of chemoresistance upon such cells.

B-Raf Mutations are Not Sufficient to Generate Cancers

Like Ras, mutations in B-Raf promote cellular transformation but additional genetic lesions are required to fully transform cells. We know this because B-Raf V600E mutations are commonly found in the benign lesions found on the skin of many individuals that are commonly called moles. Further mutations are required to allow these lesions to progress to a cancerous state and recent work suggests that mutations in the gene CDKN2a that encodes the ARF and p16 proteins (due to two alternative reading frames) cooperate with B-Raf to transform cells.

TUMOUR SUPPRESSOR GENES: P53 THE GUARDIAN OF THE GENOME

The monkey virus, SV40, is a DNA virus that can cause tumours largely due to a gene SV40 large T (for large Tumour) which encodes a protein that can neutralise the function of two key cellular proteins pRb (retinoblastoma protein) and p53. Upon infection of mouse cells with SV40, a strong immune response is generated against the SV40 large T antigen and antibodies specific for large T were subsequently used to look for the cellular targets of this viral protein. Large T antigen was thus immunoprecipitated from infected cells and these complexes were analysed by gel electrophoresis and were found to contain a protein of apparent molecular weight of 53 KDa—hence the designation of this protein as p53. This suggested that this protein may somehow be involved in the development of cancer (as it is bound to SV40 large T antigen upon infection by this virus).

Cloning of the p53 gene followed and it was initially found that co-transfection of p53 with the Ras oncogene into rat embryonic fibroblasts could transform these cells. This suggested that p53 might be an oncogene, but it later became apparent that the p53 clone used for these experiments was a mutant form of p53 (this clone had been isolated from a tumour cell line) that was acting as a dominant-negative mutant. Subsequent cloning of the wild-type p53 gene instead showed that the normal function of this gene is to suppress transformation. Comparison of the normal and mutant p53 genes revealed that the two genes differed by a single point mutation that converted p53 into an dominant-interfering mutant protein.

P53 Normally Functions to Suppress Proliferation in Response to DNA Damage and Other Forms of Cell Stress

In 1987 it became apparent that mutant p53 alleles are very common in a wide variety of human tumours (30–50%). So, how does mutant p53 contribute to the development of cancer? Experiments suggesting that even a single mutant p53 allele could contribute to the development of cancer implied that mutant p53 molecules may not be simple null mutations (i.e. mutations that result in a loss of function of the gene in question). Sequence analyses of mutant p53 alleles from various cancers revealed that the great majority of these were missense rather than nonsense mutations. To date, more than 15,000 tumour p53 alleles have been sequenced and 75% of these mutants carry missense mutations (these are mutations that change the gene coding sequence to result in a subtly different amino acid composition rather than disrupting expression of the protein completely), suggesting that tumours somehow benefit from mutant p53 rather than simple loss of p53 function.

P53 normally functions as a heterotetramer and it soon became obvious that a mutant p53 protein, when incorporated into the tetramer, could disrupt the function of the complex. If a single mutant p53 molecule can disrupt the function of a tetramer then only one sixteenth of p53 in a cell carrying a dominant-negative p53 allele will be functional.

P53 Normally has a Short Half-life

Staining of cells with anti-p53 antibodies revealed that p53 is normally a nuclear protein and this suggested that this protein might be a transcription factor. Other experiments revealed that this protein normally has a very short half-life of 20 minutes or so. This is because the stability of the p53 protein is controlled by another protein, Mdm2 (called Hdm2 in human cells). Mdm2 binds to p53 and targets this protein for degradation via the ubiquitin-proteasome protein destruction pathway. Mdm2 also exports p53 out of the nucleus thereby preventing access of p53 to DNA and blocking its transcriptional activity. Interestingly, the expression of Mdm2 is controlled by p53, therefore, p53 controls the synthesis of its own inhibitor.

In healthy cells, Mdm2 normally has the upper hand and p53 is constantly degraded as a result. However, upon damage of DNA by radiation or chemical mutagens, Mdm2 is phosphorylated by a kinase (ATM) involved in the detection of DNA strand breaks. This inactivates Mdm2 and results in the stabilisation of p53. There is some redundancy in the system because p53 can also be directly phosphorylated by ATM and also by other kinases (Chk1 and Chk2, Chk is an abbreviation of checkpoint) that are involved in the DNA damage response pathway. Phosphorylation of p53 by ATM, Chk1 or Chk2 can also stabilised p53. Thus, the half-life of p53 is greatly enhanced in response to DNA damage.

A Variety of Signals Cause the Stabilisation of p53

During the early 1990's it was discovered that in addition to UV radiation and X-rays, several other chemical DNA damaging agents and also agents that disrupt microtubule function could cause p53 accumulation. Thus, p53 accumulates in cells when there is evidence that some form of DNA damage has taken place.

Function of p53

As mentioned above, p53 is a transcription factor and controls the expression of genes that can arrest the cell division cycle–the p21 gene is the most notable gene controlled by p53 in this context. Therefore, upon stabilisation of p53, the p21 protein is rapidly expressed and this halts the cell cycle by inhibiting certain kinases that are crucial to cell division (the cyclin-dependent kinases).

P53 also induces the expression of DNA polymerase! that is involved in DNA repair. Therefore, upon detection of DNA damage (by ATM, Chk1, Chk2) p53 becomes stabilised, it halts cell division and induces proteins required for DNA repair.

But p53 also controls the expression of genes that can directly trigger apoptosis. The products of these genes, Bax, Noxa and Puma, can directly engage the apoptosis machinery and result in the rapid death of the cell. It is not clear how the decision between cell cycle arrest and repair, versus apoptosis is made, but this may relate to the levels of p53 that accumulate in the cell, and by extension, to the degree of DNA damage that a cell has suffered. Therefore, low levels of DNA damage may result in cell division arrest and repair while higher levels may trigger p53-dependent apoptosis.

P53 Mutations are Most Commonly Found within the DNA-binding Domain

Significantly, the great majority of mutations found within the p53 gene are found within the DNA-binding region of the protein. This results in the production of a mutant p53 protein that can still form part of the p53 tetramer but cannot properly bind to their target genes within DNA. This has the effect of creating a dominant-interfering mutant protein that can neutralise the function of wild-type p53 protein found in the same tetramers. Interestingly, because p53 controls the expression of its own inhibitor (Mdm2), cells carrying mutant p53 molecules often display greatly elevate levels of the p53 protein. Therefore, one of the hallmarks of cancer is often greatly increased levels of p53, which is unfortunately incapable of activating transcription of its target genes due to its mutant properties.

Some individuals inherit p53 mutations (Li-Fraumeni syndrome) and 60% of these individuals develop cancer by age 22.

In summary, mutation of p53 greatly facilitates the progression to cancer by disabling two important outcomes of DNA damage: cell cycle arrest and apoptosis.

Chapter 10

Cancer and the Environment

INTRODUCTION

Cancer is a generic term for a large group of diseases that can affect any part of the body. Other terms used are malignant tumours and neoplasms. One defining feature of cancer is the creation of abnormal cells that grow beyond their usual boundaries, and which can then invade adjoining parts of the body and spread to other organs. This process is referred to as metastasis. Cancer develops over several years and has many causes. Several factors both inside and outside the body contribute to the development of cancer. In this context, scientists refer to everything outside the body that interacts with humans as the environment.

FACTORS OUTSIDE THE BODY (ENVIRONMENTAL FACTORS)

Exposure to a wide variety of natural and man-made substances in the environment accounts for at least two-thirds of all the cases of cancer in the United States. These environmental factors include lifestyle choices like cigarette smoking, excessive alcohol consumption, poor diet, lack of exercise, excessive sunlight exposure, and sexual behaviour that increases exposure to certain viruses. Other factors include exposure to certain medical drugs, hormones, radiation, viruses, bacteria, and environmental chemicals that may be present in the air, water, food, and workplace. The cancer risks associated with many environmental chemicals have been identified through studies of occupational groups that have higher exposures to these chemicals than the general population.

The importance of the environment can be seen in the differences in cancer rates throughout the world and the change in cancer rates when groups of people move from one country to another. For example, when Asians, who have low rates of prostate and breast cancer and high rates of stomach cancer in their native countries, immigrate to the United States, their prostate and breast cancer rates rise over time until they are nearly equal to or greater than the higher levels of these cancers in the United States. Likewise, their rates of stomach cancer fall, becoming nearly equal to the lower US rates. Lifestyle factors such as diet, exercise, and being overweight are thought to play a major role in the trends for breast and prostate cancers, and infection with the *Helicobacter pylori* (Fig. 10.1) bacterium is an important risk factor for stomach cancer.

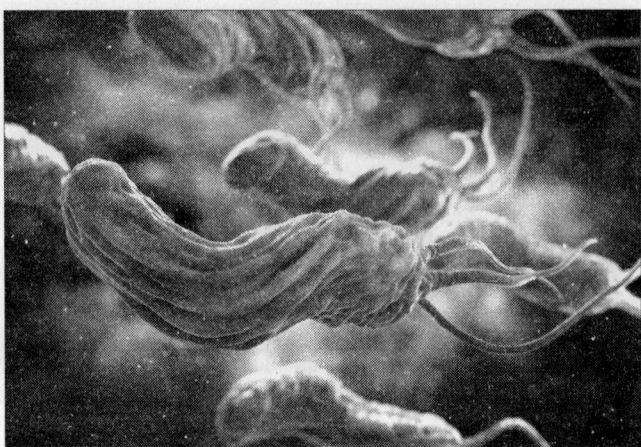

Fig. 10.1: *Helicobacter pylori.*

Recently, the rapid rise in the rates of *colorectal* cancer in Japan and China suggests an environmental cause such as lifestyle factors. Different environmental exposures are linked to specific kinds of cancer. For example, exposure to asbestos is linked primarily to lung cancer, whereas exposure to benzidine, a chemical found in certain dyes, is associated with bladder cancer. In contrast, smoking is linked to cancers of the lung, bladder, mouth, colon, kidney, throat, voice box, esophagus, lip, stomach, cervix, liver, and pancreas.

Factors Inside the Body

Certain factors inside the body make some people more likely to develop cancer than others. For instance, some people either inherit or acquire the following conditions: altered genes in the body's cells, abnormal hormone levels in the bloodstream, or a weakened immune system. Each of these factors may make an individual more susceptible to cancer. One of the ways scientists know that genes play an important role in the development of cancer is from studying certain rare families where family members over several generations develop similar cancers. It appears that these families are passing on an altered gene that carries with it a high chance of getting cancer. Several genes that greatly increase a person's chance of developing certain cancers (e.g. colon, breast, and ovary) have been identified. Only a very small percentage of people in the general population have abnormal copies of these genes. Cancers caused by these genes, known as familial cancers,account for only two to five percent of all cancers.

Gene alterations may also contribute to individual differences in susceptibility to environmental carcinogens (cancer-causing substances). For instance, people differ in their ability to eliminate cancer-causing agents from their body to which they have been exposed, or to repair *DNA* damage that was caused by such agents. These gene alterations may also be passed on in families and account for higher rates of cancer in these families. Higher rates of cancer in families may also be related to shared environmental exposures like diet or exposure to carcinogens at work.

Interaction of Environmental Factors and Genes

Environmental factors such as viruses, sunlight, and chemicals interact with cells throughout our lives. Mechanisms to repair damage to our genes and healthy lifestyle choices (wearing protective clothing for Sun exposure or not smoking) help to protect us from harmful exposures. However, over time, substances in the environment may cause gene alterations, which accumulate inside our cells. While many alterations have no effect on a person's health, permanent changes in certain genes can lead to cancer. The chance that an individual will develop cancer in response to a particular environmental agent depends on several interacting factors—how long and how often a person is exposed to a particular substance, his/her exposure to other agents, genetic factors, diet, lifestyle, health, age, and gender. For example, diet, alcohol consumption, and certain medications can affect the levels of chemicals in the body that break down cancer-causing substances. Because of the complex interplay of many factors, it is not possible to predict whether a specific environmental exposure will cause a particular person to develop cancer. We know that certain genetic and environmental factors increase the risk of developing cancer, but we rarely know exactly which combination of factors is responsible for a person's specific cancer. This also means that we usually don't know why one person gets cancer and another does not.

NATURE OF CANCER

There are more than 100 types of cancer. Cancer begins inside a cell, the basic building block of all living things. Normally, when the body needs more cells, older ones die off and younger cells divide to form new cells that take their place. When cancer develops, however, the orderly process of producing new cells breaks down. Cells continue to divide when new cells are not needed, and a growth or extra mass of cells called a tumour is formed. Over time, changes may take place in tumour cells that cause them to invade and interfere with the function of normal tissues.

It takes many years for the development of a tumour and even more years until detection of a tumour and its spread to other parts of the body. People exposed to carcinogens from smoking cigarettes, for example, generally do not develop detectable cancer for 20 to 30 years.

There is much evidence to suggest that permanent changes in our genes are responsible for tumour development. These can be inherited or acquired throughout one's lifetime. Scientists have identified more than 300 altered genes that can play a role in tumour development. An alteration in growth-promoting genes, known as oncogenes, for example, can signal the cell to divide out of control, similar to having a gas pedal stuck to the floorboard. On the other hand, an alteration in tumour suppressor genes, which normally serve as brakes for dividing cells, will allow cells with damaged DNA to continue dividing, rather than repairing the DNA or eliminating the injured cells. One explanation for the fact that cancer occurs more frequently in older people may be that, for a tumour to develop, a cell must acquire several gene alterations that accumulate as we age.

Types of Tumours

Tumours are classified as either benign or malignant. Benign tumours are not cancer and do not spread to other parts of the body. A malignant tumour can metastasise—a process during which cancer cells escape from the tumour, enter the bloodstream or lymphatic system, and spread to nearby parts of the body and eventually to sites far away from the original tumour. Some benign tumours may, over time, become malignant tumours. The development of malignant tumours involves many steps taking place over several years. The earlier a tumour is detected, the less likely it will have spread to other parts of the body. In the past 25 years, enormous progress has been made in defining the molecular events that take place as a normal cell becomes malignant and the critical genes thought to be involved. Most cancers are named for the organ or type of cell in which they begin to grow, such as lung, stomach, breast, or colon cancer. Some of the names for other cancers, however, are less clear. *Melanoma* is a cancer of cells in the skin, eyes, and some other tissues, known as melanocytes, that make pigment. Leukemias are cancers of the blood cells, and lymphomas are cancers that develop in the lymphatic system. The most common cancers in the US are carcinomas. Carcinomas are cancers that develop in the tissue that lines the surfaces of certain organs, such as the lung, liver, skin, or breast. This tissue is called epithelial tissue. Cancers that develop in the epithelial tissue of specific organs are called carcinoma of the lung, or carcinoma of the breast, for example. Another group of cancers is sarcomas: these arise from cells in bone, cartilage, fat, connective tissue, and muscle.

SUBSTANCES IN THE ENVIRONMENT KNOWN TO CAUSE CANCER IN HUMANS

Every two years, scientists from a wide range of government agencies and educational institutions collaborate with scientists from the National Toxicology Programme (NTP) in Research Triangle Park, NC, to publish the Report on Carcinogens. The report identifies substances that are either known to cause or suspected of causing cancer in humans and to which a significant number of people in the United States are exposed.

Tobacco

Exposure to the carcinogens in tobacco products accounts for about one-third of all cancer deaths in the United States each year. Cigarette, cigar, and pipe smoking, chewing tobacco, snuff, and exposure to environmental tobacco smoke (ETS or second hand smoke) are all linked to increased cancer risks. Cigarette, cigar, and pipe smoking have been associated with cancers of the lung, mouth, bladder, colon, kidney, throat, nasal cavity, voice box, esophagus, lip, stomach, cervix, liver, and pancreas, and with leukemia, smokeless tobacco has been linked to cancers of the mouth, and ETS has been implicated in lung cancer. Cigarette smoke contains more than 100 cancer-causing substances. The risk for cancers of the mouth, voice box, and esophagus is further increased among smokers who also drink more than two drinks/day.

Diet/Weight/Physical Inactivity

Because there are few definite relationships between food and cancer, the Report on Carcinogens does not refer to the cancer-related effects of specific foods. However, several studies show that heavy consumption of red and preserved meats, salt-preserved foods, and salt probably increase the risk of colorectal and stomach cancers. There is also evidence that a diet rich in fruits and vegetables may decrease the risks of esophageal, stomach, and colorectal cancers.

Being overweight or obese appears to be one of the most important modifiable causes of cancer, after tobacco. Large population studies show a consistent association between obesity and certain kinds of cancer. The strongest links are with breast cancer in older women, and cancers of the *endometrium*, kidney, colon, and esophagus. There is strong evidence that physical inactivity increases the risk for colon and breast cancer. The beneficial effect of exercise is greatest among very active people. Together, it is estimated that inactivity and obesity account for 25 to 30 per cent of the cases of several major cancers—colon, breast (postmenopausal), endometrial, kidney, and cancer of the esophagus.

Alcoholic Drinks

Heavy drinkers (more than two drinks/day) have an increased risk of cancer, particularly among those who also smoke. Cancers associated with heavy drinking include cancers of the mouth, throat, voice box, liver, and esophagus. There is also some evidence linking alcohol and cancer of the breast.

Ultraviolet Radiation

Ultraviolet (UV) radiation from the Sun, sunlamps, or tanning beds causes premature aging of the skin and DNA damage that can lead to melanoma and other forms of skin cancer. The incidence of skin cancers is rapidly increasing.

Viruses and Bacteria

Infectious agents such as viruses and bacteria clearly contribute to the development of several types of cancer. A sexually transmitted virus called human papillomavirus (HPV) is the primary cause of cervical and anal cancer. Women who begin sexual intercourse at age 16 or younger or have many sexual partners have an increased risk of infection. Infection with HPV is increasingly common. However, even though infection with HPV is the primary cause of cervical cancer, most infections do not result in cancer.

Hepatitis B (HBV) and hepatitis C (HCV) viral infections are major causes of liver cancer. In Asia and Africa, HBV is usually acquired in childhood and it carries a high risk of liver cancer. HBV infection is less common in the United States. Risk factors for HBV include occupational exposure to blood products, injection drug use, and high-risk sexual behaviour (unprotected sex with multiple partners). A vaccine is available to prevent infection with HBV. The rising incidence of liver cancer in the United States is thought to be due to HCV. The strongest risk factor for HCV infection is injection drug use, but sexual transmission is also possible. People who received a blood transfusion prior to 1989 may also be infected with this virus. Currently, there is no vaccine for HCV.

Almost all adults are infected with Epstein-Barr virus (EBV), which is linked to some types of lymphoma. EBV is the virus that causes mononucleosis. Another type of virus called Kaposi's sarcoma-associated herpesvirus (KSHV), also known as human herpesvirus 8 (HHV-8), is linked to a particular type of sarcoma called Kaposi's sarcoma. KSHV infection only occurs through close person-to-person contacts. In Mediterranean and African countries, KSHV infection in childhood is common. In the US, KSHV infection is most common in homosexual men. The risk of cancer for people infected with either KSHV or EBV is low, except for those whose immune systems are weakened, such as people infected with the human immunodeficiency virus (HIV), the virus that causes AIDS.

Infection with *Helicobacter pylori*, a bacterium, is widespread and is the primary cause of peptic ulcers and chronic gastritis (inflammation of the stomach). *H. pylori* contributes to the development of stomach cancer. Most *H. pylori* infections, however, result in neither symptoms nor cancer.

Ionising Radiation

Ionising radiation is invisible, high-frequency radiation that can damage the DNA or genes inside the body. Everyone is exposed to very small doses of ionising radiation from cosmic rays (rays that enter the earth's atmosphere from outer space). Radiation from this source may account for a very small percentage (about 1 per cent) of our total cancer risk.

Some homes have elevated levels of radon, a naturally occurring radioactive gas found at low levels in most soil. Radon is produced by the breakdown of uranium, which naturally releases low levels of ionising radiation. Higher levels of radon can be found in certain types of rocky soil. The health effects of radon were first seen in the elevated levels of lung cancer found in underground uranium miners in the United States and around the world. Radon gas seeps into homes from the surrounding soil through cracks and other openings in the foundation. About 1 out of 20 homes has elevated levels of radon. Even though the cancer risks for radon exposure in the home are much lower than for radon-exposed miners, it is estimated that about 20000 lung cancer deaths every year are caused by radon exposure in homes.

There are various strategies for reducing residential radon exposure. Another source of ionising radiation is the radioactive substances released by atomic bombs or nuclear weapons known as 'fallout.' The doses of ionising radiation received by the atomic bomb survivors in Japan resulted in increased risks of leukemia and cancers of the breast, thyroid, lung, stomach, and other organs.

People are also exposed to ionising radiation during certain medical procedures. Some patients who receive radiation to treat cancer or other conditions may be at increased cancer risk. For example, persons treated with radiation in childhood to treat acne, ringworm, and other head and neck conditions have been shown to be at increased risk for thyroid cancer and other tumours of the head and neck.

X-rays used to diagnose or screen for a disease are also forms of ionising radiation. The dose of radiation from procedures used to diagnose or screen for a disease is much lower than the dose received to treat a disease. Most studies on the long-term effects of exposure to radiation used to diagnose or screen for cancers or other diseases have not shown an elevated cancer risk, but it is possible that there is a small risk associated with this exposure.

One exception is children whose mothers received diagnostic X-rays during pregnancy. These children were found to have increased risks of childhood leukemia and other types of cancer, which led to the current ban on diagnostic X-rays in pregnant women. Several other studies of women who received small weekly X-ray doses to the chest over extended periods to monitor treatment for tuberculosis showed a radiation-related increased risk of breast cancer.

Pesticides

In the United States, a number of pesticides have been banned or their use has been restricted. These include ethylene oxide, amitrole, some chlorophenoxy herbicides, DDT, dimethylhydrazine, hexachloro-benzene, hexamethylphosphoramide, chlordecone, lead acetate, lindane, mirex, nitrofen, and toxaphene. Studies of people with high exposures to pesticides, such as farmers, pesticide applicators, crop duster pilots, and manufacturers, have found high rates of blood and lymphatic system cancers, cancers of the lip, stomach, lung, brain, and prostate, as well as melanoma and other skin cancers. So far, human studies do not allow researchers to sort out exactly which pesticides are linked to which cancers.

Medical Drugs

Some drugs used to treat cancer (e.g. cyclophosphamide, chlorambucil, melphalan) have been shown to increase the occurrence of second cancers, including leukemia. Others that are used as immuno-suppressants, such as cyclosporin and azathioprine for patients having organ transplants, also are associated with increased cancer risks, especially lymphoma. However, the Food and Drug Administration has determined that the life-saving benefits of these drugs outweigh the additional cancer risks years later. It is recommended that people weigh the risks and benefits concerning the use of a drug with the help of a physician or other health care specialist.

Some medicines have been linked to reduced risk of cancer. For example, some studies find a reduced risk of colon cancer in persons who regularly take aspirin or other nonsteroidal anti-inflammatory medicines. Evidence for protection of other cancers such as breast cancer or prostate cancer is inconsistent.

Estrogens used to treat symptoms of menopause and other gynecological conditions have been shown to increase the incidence of endometrial cancer. In addition, some studies have shown an increased risk of breast cancer with estrogen use, but a reduced risk of colon cancer. Progesterone, another hormone now taken in combination with estrogen for hormone replacement therapy in older women, helps to protect against the increased endometrial cancer risk with estrogen alone. However, increased risks of breast cancer, heart disease, stroke, and blood clots have recently been shown to be associated with the use of estrogen plus progestin, a synthetic form of progesterone. Long-term users of combination oral contraceptives have substantially reduced risks of endometrial and ovarian cancers, but may experience increases in early-onset breast cancers and liver cancer. The amount of estrogen and progesterone in oral contraceptives is substantially less than in previous years, which means that the risk of the current formulations is likely to be less than those used in the past.

Increased risks of endometrial cancer as well as increased risks of stroke and blood clots are also associated with tamoxifen use. Tamoxifen is a synthetic hormone used to prevent the recurrence of breast cancer after breast cancer surgery. It is also used to prevent breast cancer in women at high risk for the disease because of family history or other factors. Again, it is recommended that people weigh the risks and benefits concerning the use of a drug with the help of a physician or other health care specialist.

Diethylstilbestrol (DES) is a synthetic form of estrogen prescribed to pregnant women from the early 1940s to 1971. It was found that their daughters who were exposed to DES before birth have an increased chance of developing a rare type of cervical and vaginal cancer. In addition, women who took DES during pregnancy may have a slightly higher risk for developing breast cancer. Based on these findings, DES is no longer prescribed, and its use as a cattle feed additive has been banned.

Solvents

Several solvents used in paint thinners, paint and grease removers, and in the dry cleaning industry are known or suspected of being cancer-causing in animal studies. These include benzene, carbon tetrachloride, chloroform, dichloromethane (methylene chloride), tetrachloroethylene, and trichloroethylene. Human studies are suggestive, but not conclusive, except for benzene. Therefore, with the exception of benzene, these substances are listed as likely to be cancer-causing in humans.

Benzene is known to cause leukemia in humans. It has widespread use as a solvent in the chemical and drug industries and as a gasoline component. After 1997, its use as an ingredient in pesticides was banned. Workers employed in the petrochemical industry, pharmaceutical industry, leather industry, rubber industry, gas stations, and in the transportation industry are exposed to benzene. Inhaling contaminated air is the primary method of exposure. Because benzene is present in gasoline, air contamination occurs around gas stations and in congested areas with automobile exhaust. It is also present in cigarette smoke. It is estimated that half of the exposure to benzene in the United States is from cigarette smoking. About half of the US population is exposed to benzene from industrial sources, and virtually everyone in the country is exposed to benzene in gasoline.

Fibres, Fine Particles, and Dust

Exposures to various fibers, fine particles, and dust occur in several industrial settings and are associated with increased cancer risks. Exposure can also occur in nonindustrial settings. Asbestos fibers and all commercial forms of asbestos are human carcinogens. Increased rates of mesothelioma, a rare cancer of the lining of the lung and abdominal cavity, and cancer of the lung have been consistently observed in a variety of occupations involving asbestos exposure. Asbestos exposures account for the largest percent of occupational cancer, with the greatest risks among workers who smoke. Asbestos fibers are released into the environment from the use and deterioration of more than 5000 asbestos products, including roofing, thermal, and electrical insulation, cement pipe and sheet, flooring, gaskets, plastics, and textile and paper products. Workers in asbestos insulation, brake maintenance and repair, and building demolition jobs are exposed to high levels of asbestos. The entire population may have been exposed to some degree because asbestos has been so widely used. Because the use of asbestos has been greatly restricted in the United States, exposure to the general population has decreased. Nonetheless, workers employed in construction trades, electricians, and carpenters can still experience high levels of asbestos exposures through renovations, repairs, and demolitions. Ceramic fibers are now used as insulation materials and are a replacement for asbestos. Because they can withstand high temperatures, they are used to line furnaces and kilns. These fibers cause lung cancer in experimental animals.

Silica dusts are associated with an excess risk of lung cancer in humans and are found in industrial and occupational settings such as coal mines, mills, granite quarrying and processing, crushed stone and related industries, and sandblasting operations. Wood dust, associated with cancers of the nasal cavities and sinuses, is a known carcinogen for unprotected workers who are exposed regularly from sanding operations and furniture manufacturing.

Dioxins

Dioxins are unwanted by-products of chemical processes that contain chlorine and hydrocarbons (substances that contain both hydrogen and carbon). There are at least 100 different kinds of dioxins. They are not intentionally manufactured by industry. They are produced by paper and pulp bleaching, incineration of municipal, toxic, and hospital wastes, certain electrical fires, and smelters (plants where metal is extracted from ores). They are also found as a contaminant in some insecticides, herbicides, and wood preservatives. Dioxins are widespread environmental contaminants. They accumulate in fats and break down slowly. A particular dioxin that is likely to be carcinogenic to humans is called TCDD (2,3,7,8-tetrachlorodibenzo-pdioxin). TCDD is highly carcinogenic in animals, and, in highly exposed workers, increased overall cancer death rates have been reported. Fortunately, modifications of industrial processes such as bleaching and incineration have resulted in reduced dioxin emissions and have lowered dioxin levels in people. The general population is exposed to low levels of TCDD primarily from eating dairy products, fish, and meat, including poultry.

Polycyclic Aromatic Hydrocarbons (PAHs)

A number of studies show increased incidence of cancer (lung, skin, and urinary cancers) in humans exposed to mixtures of polycyclic aromatic hydrocarbons (PAHs). The primary source of PAHs is from burning carbon-containing compounds. PAHs in air are produced by burning wood and fuel for homes. They are also contained in gasoline and diesel exhaust, soot, coke, cigar and cigarette smoke, and charcoal-broiled foods. In addition, they are the by-products of open fires, waste incinerators, coal gasification, and coke oven emissions. Foods that contain small amounts of PAHs include smoked, barbecued, or charcoal-broiled foods, roasted coffees, and sausages.

Metals Arsenic compounds are associated with many forms of skin, lung, bladder, kidney, and liver cancers, particularly when high levels are consumed in drinking water. In addition, occupational exposure to inhaled arsenic, especially in mining and copper smelting, has been consistently associated with an increased risk of lung cancer. Arsenic is also used in wood preservatives, glass, herbicides, insecticides (ant killers), and pesticides, and it is a general environmental contaminant of air, food, and water.

Beryllium compounds are known to cause lung cancer based primarily on studies of workers in beryllium production facilities. These compounds are used as metals for aerospace and defense industries, for electrical components, X-ray tubes, nuclear weapons, aircraft brakes, rocket fuel additives, light aircraft construction, and the manufacture of ceramics, and as an additive to glass and plastics, dental applications, and golf clubs. Industry is also increasingly using beryllium for fibre optics and cellular network communication systems. Workers can be exposed through jobs related to the above activities, as well as through recycling of computers, cell phones, and other high-tech products. Outside of these industries, beryllium exposure occurs primarily through the burning of coal and fuel oil. The general population can be exposed to trace amounts of beryllium by inhaling air and consuming food contaminated with beryllium residues. Small concentrations have been reported in drinking water, food, and tobacco.

Studies of groups of workers show that cadmium metal and cadmium compounds are associated with an increased risk of lung cancer. Workers with the highest exposures are those involved in removing zinc and lead from minerals, producing cadmium powders, welding cadmium-coated steel, and working with solders that contain cadmium.

Cadmium metal is primarily used to coat metals to prevent corrosion. Other uses are in plastic and synthetic products, in batteries, as stabilisers for polyvinyl chloride, and in fungicides. The industrial processes involved in making these products release cadmium into the air, surface water, ground water, and topsoil where it can be taken up by both land and water plants and, in turn, transferred to animals. Contaminated topsoil that allows uptake into tobacco plants may be indirectly responsible for the greatest nonoccupational human exposure to cadmium—smoking. Food is the main source of human exposure to cadmium for nonsmokers.

Some chromium compounds are known to cause lung cancer. The steel industry is the major consumer of chromium. It is used for protection against corrosion of metal accessories, including automotive parts, as well as for electroplating, layering one metal over another. Electroplating converts chromium, the carcinogenic form, to a noncarcinogenic form of chromium. This means that workers who handle chromium are at greater risk than the general population. Other uses include nuclear and high-temperature research, the textile and leather-tanning industry, pigments for floor covering products, paper, cement, and asphalt roofing, and creating an emerald colour in coloured glass. Chromium is widely distributed in the air, water, soil, and food, and the entire population is probably exposed to some of these compounds. The highest exposure occurs in occupations related to stainless steel production, welding, chrome plating, and leather tanning. Typical levels in most fresh foods are low.

Lead acetate and lead phosphate are likely to be human carcinogens based on the evidence of kidney and brain tumours in animal studies. Lead acetate is used in cotton dyes, as a coating for metals, as a drier in paints, varnishes, and pigment inks, as a colorant in certain permanent hair dyes (progressive dyes), in explosives, and in washes to treat poison ivy. Lead phosphate is used as a stabiliser in certain plastics and specialty glass. Primary exposures are through skin contact, eating, and inhaling.

Nickel and nickel compounds are associated with several kinds of cancers in rats and mice. Studies in human populations link nickel exposure to cancers of the nasal cavity, lung, and possibly the larynx (voice box). Nickel is used in steel, dental fillings, copper and brass, permanent magnets, storage batteries, and glazes. Because nickel is present in the air, water, soil, food, and consumer products in the United States, we are exposed through eating, breathing, and skin contact.

Diesel Exhaust Particles

The particles in diesel exhaust are suspected of being carcinogens because of the elevated lung cancer rates found in occupational groups exposed to diesel exhaust, such as railroad workers, mine workers, bus garage workers, trucking company workers, car mechanics, and people who work around diesel generators. Cancer risks from lower exposures in day-to-day living are not known.

Toxins from Fungi

Aflatoxins are cancer-causing substances produced by certain types of fungi growing on food. Grains and peanuts are the most common foods on which these fungi grow. Meat, eggs, and milk from animals that eat aflatoxincontaminated feed are other sources of exposure. Agricultural workers are potentially at risk if they inhale contaminated airborne grain dust. Exposure to high levels of aflatoxins increases the risk of liver cancer. Peanuts are screened for aflatoxin in most countries, including the United States, before processing. The risk of aflatoxin exposure is higher in developing countries where there is no screening for the fungus.

Vinyl Chloride

Vinyl chloride, a colourless gas, is a human carcinogen associated with lung cancers and angiosarcomas (blood vessel tumours) of the liver and brain. It is used almost exclusively in the United States by the plastics industry in manufacturing many consumer products, including containers, wrapping film, electrical insulation, water and drain pipes, hosing, flooring, windows, and credit cards. Human exposure can occur primarily in workers in the plastic industry, not by using the end products such as vinyl siding or hosing. The major source of releases of vinyl chloride into the environment is believed to be from the plastics industries.

People living near a plastics plant are exposed by breathing contaminated air, but the exposure of the general population away from the plant is essentially zero.

Benzidine

Benzidine was one of the first chemicals recognised as being associated with increased cancer risk in humans. As early as 1921, increased cases of bladder cancer were reported to be associated with benzidine, a compound used in the production of more than 250 benzidine-based dyes for textiles, paper, and leather products.

Human exposure to either benzidine or benzidine-based dyes is now known to be carcinogenic. The dyes break down into benzidine once inside the body. In most cases, dyes that metabolise to benzidine are hazards only in the vicinity of dye and pigment plants where wastes may escape or be discharged.

WAYS TO REDUCE THE RISK OF DEVELOPING CANCER OR DETECT CANCER AT AN EARLY STAGE

At least two-thirds of the cases of cancer are caused by environmental factors. Many of these cancers are linked to lifestyle factors that can be modified, such as cigarette smoking, excessive alcohol consumption, poor diet, physical inactivity, and being overweight or obese.

For example, one-third of all the cancer deaths in this country could be prevented by eliminating the use of tobacco products. After tobacco, being overweight or obese appears to be the most important preventable cause of cancer.

In addition to lifestyle choices, precautions can be taken in the home and workplace to reduce exposure to other harmful exposures. Here are some rules you can follow to reduce your risk of developing cancer:

- Don't smoke cigarettes, pipes, or cigars. Don't chew tobacco or dip snuff. Avoid smoke-filled rooms. The use of tobacco products is linked to many cancers.
- Lose weight if you are overweight. Obesity is strongly linked to breast cancer in older women and cancers of the endometrium, kidney, colon, and esophagus.

- Exercise regularly, at least 30 minutes per day for most days of the week. There is strong evidence that exercise by itself reduces the risk of colon and breast cancer. Risk is decreased the most among very active people.
- Avoid high-calorie, high-fat food. The chief causes of obesity are a lack of physical activity and eating too much high-calorie food.
- Avoid consuming large amounts of red and preserved meats, salt, and salt-preserved foods. These may increase the risk of colorectal and stomach cancers.
- Eat a daily diet that includes a variety of foods from plant sources, such as fresh fruits, vegetables, whole grains, and whole grain breads and cereals. Fruits and vegetables contain substances (e.g. antioxidants) that help defend against toxic agents and disease.
- Drink alcohol in moderation, if at all, especially if you smoke. (One or two alcoholic drinks a day is considered moderate.) Heavy drinking is linked to cancers of the mouth, throat, esophagus, voice box, liver, and breast.
- Avoid too much sunlight, particularly if you are fair skinned, by avoiding Sun exposure at midday (10 am–4 pm, when Sun exposure is strongest), wearing protective clothing, and using sunscreen. Many of the more than one million skin cancers diagnosed every year can be prevented by protection from the Sun rays. Avoid tanning beds and other artificial Sun or UV exposure.
- Avoid viral or bacterial infections:
  o Do not engage in unprotected or otherwise unsafe sexual intercourse that may result in HIV, HPV, hepatitis B, or hepatitis C infection.
  o Do not use recreational injection drugs, such as heroin or cocaine, that may result in HIV, hepatitis B, or hepatitis C infection.
  o Get vaccinated against hepatitis B infection, an easy and safe procedure if you are 18 years of age or younger. Also, get vaccinated if you are over 18 and at risk of infection. At-risk people include health care workers, IV drug users, and homosexual men. Currently, there is no vaccine for hepatitis C. (For vaccination information, visit: www.cdc.gov.)
  o Seek medical attention for chronic stomach problems because they might be caused by *H. pylori* infection, which can be treated.
- Seek medical attention and adhere to recommended treatments if you have HIV or hepatitis C infection. These infections increase your risk of developing certain cancers.
- Because repeated exposure to diagnostic X-rays could be harmful, talk to your doctor about the need for each X-ray and the use of shields to protect other parts of the body.
- Check your home for high levels of radon. Radon levels in a home can be greatly reduced by a professionally installed ventilation system in the basement.
- Avoid contact with pesticides. Exposure to pesticides comes largely through the skin. If contact occurs, wash up quickly.
- Make sure the room is well ventilated when working with solvents. Work outside, if possible, or open the windows.
- If you work in an environment with high exposures to fine particles, fibers, or dusts, wear the appropriate protective mask over your nose and mouth and make sure it fits properly and does not obstruct your view.

- Use good work practices when handling chemicals in the home or workplace. Wear proper personal protective equipment, keep protective equipment well maintained, clean spills immediately, keep work surfaces as free of dust and chemicals as possible, and use wet cleaning methods to avoid generating dust.
- Be aware that certain occupations are known to be associated with high cancer risks. Some of these include painters, furniture makers, workers in the iron, steel, coal, and rubber industries, and workers involved in boot and shoe manufacture or repair.
- Inquire at your workplace about Material Safety Data Sheets (MSDSs). A MSDS is a document that manufacturers of chemical products are required to develop for any product that contains hazardous substances. The MSDS contains information on the toxicity of a substance, whether it is considered to be cancer-causing, the recommended exposure levels of the ingredients in the product, and appropriate precautions to take or appropriate recommended personal protective equipment to wear. Employers are required to make the MSDSs accessible to employees and to inform/train employees about the information.
- Make sure your employer has put in place appropriate engineering controls such as local exhaust ventilation.

Detecting Cancers at an Early Stage

Sometimes exposures to toxic substances cannot be avoided. Certain diagnostic procedures will not reduce the exposure to substances in the environment but may detect cancers at an early stage before they spread to other parts of the body.

- Tell your health care provider about the chemicals you use at work or at home. With this information, your health care provider can perform appropriate medical screening tests for early detection of cancer.
- Ask your physician if there are increased cancer risks associated with your family or personal medical history or medical drugs you are taking. Appropriate screening procedures may be advised.
- Get a screening test on a regular basis for these cancers:
  o Breast: A mammogram, an X-ray of the breast, is the best method of finding breast cancer before symptoms appear. Several organisations recommend mammography screening every one to two years after age 40. Women at higher than average risk of breast cancer should seek expert advice about screening before age 40 and about the frequency of screening.
  o Cervix: The Pap test or Pap smear is the most successful screening tool used to screen for cancer of the cervix. Cells are collected from the cervix and examined under a microscope to detect cancer or changes that may lead to cancer. Many doctors recommend yearly Pap tests. Less frequent screening is recommended by some organisations for women with at least three consecutive negative exams.
  o Colon and Rectum: A number of screening tests are used to find colon and rectal cancer. If a person has a family medical history of colorectal cancer or is over the age of 50, a doctor may suggest one or more of these tests: the fecal occult blood test checks for small amounts of blood in the stool, a sigmoidoscopy is the use of a lighted tube to examine the rectum and lower colon, a colonoscopy is performed to see the entire colon and rectum. With either a sigmoidoscopy or a colonoscopy, abnormal tissue can be removed and examined under a microscope.

- Be alert for changes in your body. Cancer may cause a variety of symptoms. Here are some:
  - o Thickening or lump in any part of body: Obvious change in a wart or mole, a sore that does not heal, nagging cough or hoarseness, changes in bowel or bladder habits, indigestion or difficulty swallowing, unexplained changes in weight, unusual bleeding or discharge.

  These symptoms are NOT always caused by cancer. It is important to see a doctor about these or other physical changes that continue for some time. However, certain cancers have no obvious symptoms, so routine physical exams are recommended.
- Stay informed and be proactive.
  - o Ask your doctor questions.
  - o If you suspect that you are exposed to a carcinogen in your work or home environment, try to find out more. Use the resources at the end of the booklet to contact the agencies responsible for protecting the environment.
  - o Get involved in activities aimed at reducing our exposure to cancer-causing substances. Government agencies, industries, health professionals, and individuals can all contribute to reducing the risks in the environment. For example, in order to control the obestiy epidemic, efforts to increase physical activity and promote healthy eating are needed in many parts of society, including families, schools, day care centers, food companies, restaurants, work sites, health care systems, and departments of transportation and city-planning.

IDENTIFICATION OF CANCER CAUSING SUBSTANCES

Over the last 30 years scientists have worked hard to identify substances in the home, workplace, and general environment that cause cancer. This is a challenging task because there are more than 100,000 chemicals commonly used by Americans in household cleaners, solvents, pesticides, food additives, lawn care, and other products. Every year, another 1,000 or so are introduced.

Furthermore, these are single substances and do not take into account the mixtures and various combinations of commercial and consumer products that Americans are exposed to every day. In addition, many chemicals may be changed to different substances by the atmosphere, water, plants, and by incineration or combustion.

Adding to the complexity, scientists know that cancer-causing substances are sometimes created during the synthesis or combustion of other chemicals. Dioxin is an example of this kind of unwanted contaminant. Further complicating the problem is the fact that besides man-made chemicals, many natural products can also cause cancer.

Evidence for identifying cancer-causing substances comes from three sources: human studies, animal studies, and laboratory experiments with human cells. Evidence from each of these sources is important in helping public health officials make decisions about whether exposure to certain substances needs to be reduced or eliminated. The more information available, the more likely it is that they will be able to identify which substances are carcinogens.

Human Studies

The most certain method of identifying cancer-causing substances is to observe whether they have caused cancer in people. Epidemiologists design studies that follow certain populations over time to observe whether a specific agent (e.g. arsenic or benzene) or exposure (e.g. sunlight or smoking) is likely to cause cancer. Environmental causes of cancer have frequently been first noticed in the workplace. This is because workers in certain occupations have higher exposures to particular chemicals and for longer periods of time than the general population. The International Agency for Research on Cancer, an agency of the World Health Organisation, classified certain occupations as associated with cancer-causing exposures because of the increased incidence of cancers in these settings. Some of these include painters, furniture makers, workers in the iron, steel, coal, and rubber industries, and workers involved in boot and shoe manufacture or repair. This knowledge has helped these industries and public health specialists develop processes and safety procedures designed to minimise worker exposure to cancer-causing substances. So the risk is less now than in previous years.

However, health agencies would fail in their responsibility to prevent cancer if they merely document workplace-related cancers, because they would find out about cancer risks only after many people developed symptoms of the disease, sometimes as long as 20 to 30 years after the exposure. Other epidemiology studies compare the exposure histories of people who have developed cancer to comparison groups of people who have not developed cancer at a particular point in time.

Such studies allow researchers to look at a wide range of exposures that may have occurred in the past in a variety of settings, not just at those that occurred in a particular occupational setting. However, these studies may miss some important links between exposures and cancer.

It is often difficult to determine what chemicals people were exposed to many years earlier, to what degree they were exposed, and which specific ones are harmful. But because we cannot test potential cancer-causing agents with people, observational epidemiological studies are the best source of data on real world exposures and often do provide important clues.

Other testing methods involving animals and laboratory experiments are also important. They allow scientists to anticipate potential cancer-causing exposures before they cause large numbers of human cancers.

Animal Studies

Mice or rats are most commonly used to test for cancer-causing substances because they are smaller, easier to handle, and more economical than larger animals. Also, they are generally similar to humans in their response to carcinogens. Most major forms of human cancer have been reproduced in such animals through exposure to chemical carcinogens. Because the lifetime of rodents is only two to three years, they generally provide information about the cancer-causing potential of test materials relatively quickly. Special strains of mice and rats have been developed to be particularly suitable for cancer testing. However, differences in animal and human digestive physiology complicate the relevance of diet studies in animals.

Laboratory Experiments

As part of an ongoing effort to reduce the use of animals in testing for cancer, researchers are using human cells grown in the laboratory. Cells exposed to potential carcinogens are monitored to see whether molecular changes characteristic of cancer cells develop. Besides reducing the use of animals, these kinds of studies can be done more quickly and economically and can be useful in evaluating whether to perform the studies in rats and mice. Results from laboratory experiments also provide clues to epidemiologists about which hypotheses to test in human population studies (e.g. human observational studies evaluating the effect of exposure to formaldehyde and methylene chloride were initiated because of data from laboratory and animal studies)

In a few cases, the evidence from laboratory experiments, along with knowledge of the behaviour of related compounds known to be carcinogenic, was strong enough to classify a chemical as a known or probable human carcinogen. For example, experiments using human cells were used to classify more than 200 benzidine-based dyes as human carcinogens. Benzidine had already been classified as a known human carcinogen and scientists suspected that any dye that released benzidine inside the human body would also be a human carcinogen. When human cells grown in the laboratory were exposed to a particular dye, they were able to test whether benzidine was released. Those that did were classified as human carcinogens.

In another example, one piece of data that led to the classification of ethylene oxide (used as a starting material in the production of other chemicals and as a disinfectant and sterilant) as a known human carcinogen was from laboratory experiments showing that it caused DNA damage in blood cells from exposed workers.

Although these kinds of studies reduce our reliance on animals in toxicology research, the testing of potential carcinogens in rodents remains an important part of cancer prevention strategies. However, all scientific data available for a potential carcinogen are important. The combination of human studies, animal studies, and laboratory experiments provides scientists with the most complete understanding of chemical risks of cancer.

SUBSTANCES TO TEST IN ANIMALS AND HUMAN LABORATORY CELLS

Strategies for Testing in Animals or Human Laboratory Cells

Because resources are limited, scientists must decide which substances out of thousands of candidates should be selected for testing in animals or human cells. The tests are costly and time-consuming. For example, determining whether a chemical causes cancer in rats or mice can cost several million dollars and take several years to complete. Three factors generally guide the decision to test a substance:

Number of people exposed

Scientist test those chemicals that affect a large number of people or those for which the exposure levels have been unusually high. Pesticides, for example, fit both categories: they potentially affect a large number of people because of trace amounts on foods and their use in or around the home, and exposure levels are high in farming-related occupations.

Previous data

This could be a report that a chemical causes alterations in human DNA in laboratory cells, or a report that people exposed to a particular chemical in the workplace or at a specific geographical location are getting cancer at higher rates than expected. This kind of information provides important clues for decisions about animal testing. Before testing in animals was done, dioxins and polycyclic aromatic hydrocarbons were first suspected to be carcinogenic based on studies on human and animal cells.

Public concern

Chromium and some pesticides are examples of chemicals that were first brought to the attention of public health officials by a group of concerned citizens. The National Toxicology Programme has a Web site available to the public to suggest agents suspected of causing cancer: http://ntp-server.niehs.nih.gov, click on 'How to Nominate Compounds.'

Strategies for Carrying Out Large Population Studies

Similar considerations guide epidemiologists as to whether to begin large population studies. Some of these factors include:

- Data from animal studies suggesting a cancer-exposure link (e.g. vinyl chloride) or a related agent, which raises suspicion (e.g. acrylonitrile was studied because of its structural similarity to vinyl chloride).
- Suggestive results from other epidemiologic studies (large population studies).
- Biological mechanisms of an exposure that suggest a possible link to cancer.
- Pockets of cancer that cluster in a particular town or place or unusual case reports.
- Cancer trends—rates that change over time or with location.
- Changes in cancer rates within a population upon migration to new area.
- Introduction of a new exposure or technology for which epidemiologic data are needed, or an unusual exposure pattern that needs evaluation.

FACTORS SCIENTISTS CONSIDER IN DETERMINING THE RISK ASSOCIATED WITH DIFFERENT CANCER-CAUSING SUBSTANCES

Exposures to some substances are associated with high risks for getting cancer, while exposures to other substances carry very little risk. It is important to know that just being exposed to a chemical agent does not mean that you will get cancer. Risk assessment is the term used to determine the relationship between exposure to a substance and the likelihood of developing disease from that exposure.

Risk assessment is a critical tool used by public health agencies in making decisions about whether exposure to certain substances needs to be reduced or eliminated. Three factors are important to consider in risk assessment:

Potency

Potency is a measure of the capacity of a given amount of the substance to cause cancer. In some cases, exposures to small amounts are sufficient, whereas for others much higher exposures are needed. One potent carcinogen is the solvent benzene, which increases the risk for leukemia from small amounts in the air. Others, like DDT and chloroform, require higher exposures to increase the cancer risk by the same amount.

Type of Exposure

Public health agencies classify substances as known or suspected human carcinogens based on evidence of cancer from at least one type of exposure, such as:

- Workplace exposures—either high short-term or long-term exposures.
- Continuous low-level exposure or occasional exposure to carcinogens in air, food, water, drugs, or consumer products.
- Single, acute exposures following industrial accidents or similar incidents.

Dose Response

It is important to know whether the cancer risk increases as the exposure levels increase. This is known as a dose-response trend. Some dose-response trends are linear, which is often considered strong evidence for cancer risk. For example, if 10 units of a substance causes cancer in 1 out of 1000 people, then 1 unit of exposure would cause cancer in 1 out of 10000 people. In a linear dose response, the risk would continue to decrease as the exposure decreased all the way to zero. This means that a tiny risk of cancer is predicted for any exposure, no matter how small.

However, for some carcinogens, there may be an exposure level below which there is no detectable increase in risk. This type of dose response is sometimes called threshold dose response.

Some exposures cause cancer only among susceptible individuals. Factors such as age, gender, general health, state of the immune system, smoking history, diet, childhood exposures, and patterns of genetic alterations may play a role in susceptibility.

A chemical may be harmless unless a person has one or more factors that allow the chemical to be changed in the body to a more hazardous form. Risk assessment involves understanding the interactions of many susceptibility factors.

ACCEPTABLE EXPOSURE LEVELS FOR ENVIRONMENTAL CHEMICALS

Linear Dose Response

One of the first considerations by regulatory agencies such as the Environmental Protection Agency, Food and Drug Administration, and Occupational Safety and Health Administration is to determine whether a carcinogen exhibits linear or threshold-like dose-response behaviour. Even though government scientists conduct rigorous scientific reviews to evaluate everything that is known about a cancer-causing substance, there is frequently not enough information to distinguish between these two kinds of dose responses. Unless there is compelling evidence for a threshold-like mechanism, agencies assume, to protect the public health, that the dose response is linear. This means that they assume that any exposure, no matter how small, would have some risk.

Threshold-Like Dose Response

In the case of carcinogens exhibiting threshold-like dose responses, other factors such as age, gender, genetic makeup, and diet are taken into consideration. For example, the potentially greater health effects on children of pesticide residues on food are taken into consideration when setting acceptable exposure levels of pesticides.

Moreover, if the cancer testing is done in rats and mice, scientists consider the possibility that people are more sensitive than rats or mice to the cancer-causing effects of a particular chemical. These factors can result in setting acceptable levels of exposure as much as 1000 times below the level that causes a substantial increase in cancer in rodents. This approach gives more confidence that the acceptable level of exposure set by a regulatory agency will indeed protect the public health.

Risks Versus Benefits

Another factor adding to the difficulty of regulating the exposure to environmental chemicals is that many substances that may cause cancer in people also have some benefits.

Pharmaceuticals represent the best example of when benefit/risk analyses are routinely conducted. In the case of cancer chemotherapy drugs, we know that while they may be effective in treating or preventing cancer, they also may increase the risk of second cancers developing years after the treatment. However, since cancer is often immediately life-threatening, the benefits usually outweigh the risks. Tamoxifen, for example, which is effective in preventing the recurrence of breast cancer in many women, also increases the risk of uterine cancer, blood clots, and strokes. The benefits and risks were rigorously analysed by the Food and Drug Administration, the National Cancer Institute, and the World Health Organisation, and they all concluded that the benefits of tamoxifen for women who have had breast cancer or for a relatively small number of women who are at high risk of developing breast cancer strongly outweigh the serious risks associated with the drug.

Another example is pesticides. The use of pesticides has increased crop yields and has significantly benefited agricultural production. Yet there is concern over potential health effects of pesticide residues on foods consumed by humans. These potential risks are reduced by setting maximum residue levels on fruits, vegetables, and other produce and by using pesticides that are not carcinogenic.

SECTION V

Recombinant DNA, Methods of Creating DNA Molecules, Genomic Library and DNA Sequencing

Chapter 11

Recombinant DNA and Gene Cloning

INTRODUCTION

Recombinant DNA, which is often shortened to rDNA, is an artificially made DNA strand that is formed by the combination of two or more gene sequences. This new combination may or may not occur naturally, but is engineered specifically for a purpose to be used in one of the many applications of recombinant DNA. By combining two or more different strands of DNA, scientists are able to create a new strand of DNA. The most common recombinant process involves combining the DNA of two different organisms. Structure of DNA is given in Fig. 11.1. Recombinant DNA is possible because DNA molecules from all organisms share the same chemical structure. They differ only in the nucleotide sequence within that identical overall structure (Fig. 11.2). Recombinant DNA molecules are sometimes called chimeric DNA, because they are usually made of material from two different species, like the mythical chimera. rDNA technology uses palindromic sequences and leads to the production of sticky and blunt ends. The DNA sequences used in the construction of recombinant DNA molecules can originate from any species. For example, plant DNA may be joined to bacterial DNA, or human DNA may be joined with fungal DNA. In addition, DNA sequences that do not occur any where in nature may be created by the chemical synthesis of DNA and incorporated into recombinant molecules. Using recombinant DNA technology and synthetic DNA, literally any DNA sequence may be created and introduced into any of a very wide range of living organisms. Proteins that can result from the expression of recombinant DNA within living cells are termed recombinant proteins. When recombinant DNA encoding a protein is introduced into a host organism, the recombinant protein is not necessarily produced.

Expression of foreign proteins requires the use of specialised expression vectors and often necessitates significant restructure by foreign coding sequence. Recombinant DNA differs from genetic recombination in that the former results from artificial methods in the test tube, while the latter is a normal biological process that results in the remixing of existing DNA sequences in essentially all organisms.

CREATING RECOMBINANT DNA

Molecular cloning is the laboratory process used to create recombinant DNA. It is one of two widely used methods (along with polymerase chain reaction, abbreviation PCR) used to direct the replication

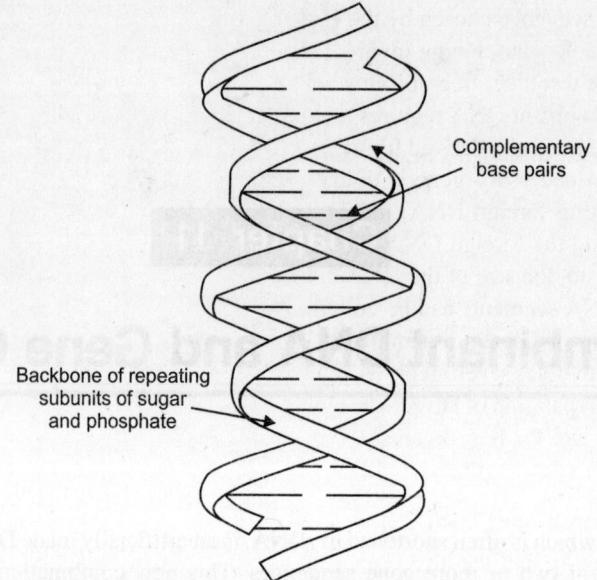

Fig. 11.1: Structure of DNA.

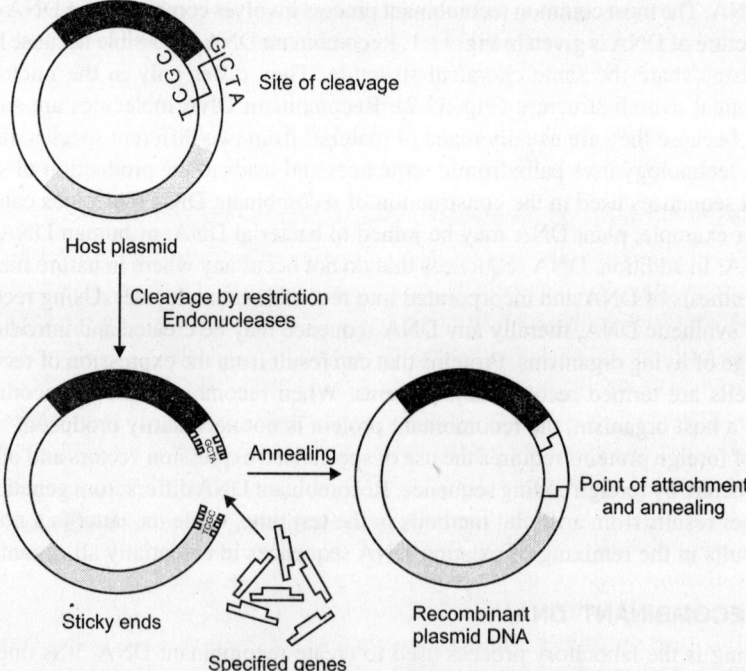

Fig. 11.2: Construction of recombinant DNA, in which a foreign DNA fragment is inserted into a plasmid vector. In this example, the gene indicated by the white colour is inactivated upon insertion of the foreign DNA fragment.

of any specific DNA sequence chosen by the experimentalist. The fundamental difference between the two methods is that molecular cloning involves replication of the DNA within a living cell, while PCR replicates DNA in the test tube, free of living cells.

Formation of recombinant DNA requires a cloning vector, a DNA molecule that replicates within a living cell. Vectors are generally derived from plasmids or viruses and represent relatively small segments of DNA that contain necessary genetic signals for replication, as well as additional elements for convenience in inserting foreign DNA, identifying cells that contain recombinant DNA, and, where appropriate, expressing the foreign DNA. The choice of vector for molecular cloning depends on the choice of host organism, the size of the DNA to be cloned and whether and how the foreign DNA is to be expressed. The DNA segments can be combined by using a variety of methods, such as restriction enzyme/ligase cloning or Gibson assembly. In standard cloning protocols, the cloning of any DNA fragment essentially involves seven steps: (i) choice of host organism and cloning vector, (ii) preparation of vector DNA, (iii) preparation of DNA to be cloned, (iv) creation of recombinant DNA, (v) introduction of recombinant DNA into the host organism, (vi) selection of organisms containing recombinant DNA and (vii) screening for clones with desired DNA inserts and biological properties.

Expression of Recombinant DNA

Following transplantation into the host organism, the foreign DNA contained within the recombinant DNA construct may or may not be expressed. That is, the DNA may simply be replicated without expression, or it may be transcribed and translated so that a recombinant protein is produced. Generally speaking, expression of a foreign gene requires restructuring the gene to include sequences that are required for producing an mRNA molecule that can be used by the host's translational apparatus (e.g. promoter, translational initiation signal and transcriptional terminator). Specific changes to the host organism may be made to improve expression of the ectopic gene. In addition, changes may be needed to the coding sequences as well, to optimise translation, make the protein soluble, direct the recombinant protein to the proper cellular or extracellular location and stabilise the protein from degradation.

Properties of Organisms Containing Recombinant DNA

In most cases, organisms containing recombinant DNA have apparently normal phenotypes. That is, their appearance, behaviour and metabolism are usually unchanged and the only way to demonstrate the presence of recombinant sequences is to examine the DNA itself, typically using a polymerase chain reaction (PCR) test. Significant exceptions exist and are discussed below.

If the rDNA sequences encode a gene that is expressed, then the presence of RNA and/or protein products of the recombinant gene can be detected, typically using RT-PCR or western hybridisation methods. Gross phenotypic changes are not the norm, unless the recombinant gene has been chosen and modified so as to generate biological activity in the host organism. Additional phenotypes that are encountered include toxicity to the host organism induced by the recombinant gene product, especially if it is over-expressed or expressed within inappropriate cells or tissues. In some cases, recombinant DNA can have deleterious effects even if it is not expressed. One mechanism by which this happens is insertional inactivation, in which the rDNA becomes inserted into a host cell's gene. In some cases, researchers use this phenomenon to 'knock out' genes to determine their biological function and importance. Another mechanism by which rDNA insertion into chromosomal DNA can affect gene expression is by inappropriate activation of previously unexpressed host cell genes. This can happen, for example, when a recombinant DNA fragment containing an active promoter becomes located next to a previously silent host cell gene, or when a host cell gene that functions to restrain gene expression undergoes insertional inactivation by recombinant DNA. There are three different methods by which Recombinant DNA is made. They are transformation, non-bacterial transformation and phage introduction and are described separately below.

Transformation: The first step in transformation is to select a piece of DNA to be inserted into a vector. The second step is to cut that piece of DNA with a restriction enzyme and then ligate the DNA insert into the vector with DNA Ligase. The insert contains a selectable marker which allows for identification of recombinant molecules. An antibiotic marker is often used so a host cell without a vector dies when exposed to a certain antibiotic and the host with the vector will live because it is resistant. The vector is inserted into a host cell, in a process called transformation. One example of a possible host cell is *E. coli.* The host cells must be specially prepared to take up the foreign DNA. Selectable markers can be for antibiotic resistance, colour changes, or any other characteristic which can distinguish transformed hosts from untransformed hosts. Different vectors have different properties to make them suitable to different applications. Some properties can include symmetrical cloning sites, size and high copy number.

Non-bacterial transformation: This is a process very similar to Transformation, which was described above. The only difference between the two is non-bacterial does not use bacteria such as *E. coli* for the host. In microinjection, the DNA is injected directly into the nucleus of the cell being transformed. In biolistics, the host cells are bombarded with high velocity microprojectiles, such as particles of gold or tungsten that have been coated with DNA.

Phage introduction: Phage introduction is the process of transfection, which is equivalent to transformation, except a phage is used instead of bacteria. *In vitro* packagings of a vector is used. This uses lambda or MI3 phages to produce phage plaques which contain recombinants. The recombinants that are created can be identified by differences in the recombinants and non-recombinants using various selection methods.

How does rDNA work?

Recombinant DNA works when the host cell expresses protein from the recombinant genes. A significant amount of recombinant protein will not be produced by the host unless expression factors are added. Protein expression depends upon the gene being surrounded by a collection of signals which provide instructions for the transcription and translation of the gene by the cell. These signals include the promoter, the ribosome binding site and the terminator. Expression vectors, in which the foreign DNA is inserted, contain these signals. Signals are species specific. In the case of *E. coli,* these signals must be *E. coli* signals as *E. coli* is unlikely to understand the signals of human promoters and terminators.

Problems are encountered if the gene contains introns or contains signals which act as terminators to a bacterial host. This results in premature termination and the recombinant protein may not be processed correctly, be folded correctly, or may even be degraded. Production of recombinant proteins in eukaryotic systems generally takes place in yeast and filamentous fungi. The use of animal cells is difficult due to the fact that many need a solid support surface, unlike bacteria and have complex growth needs. However, some proteins are too complex to be produced in bacterium, so eukaryotic cells must be used.

Importance of DNA

Recombinant DNA has been gaining in importance over the last few years and recombinant DNA will only become more important in the 21st century as genetic diseases become more prevelant and agricultural area is reduced.

Below are some of the areas where recombinant DNA will have an impact.

1. Better crops (drought and heat resistance).
2. Recombinant vaccines (i.e. Hepatitis B).
3. Prevention and cure of sickle cell anemia.
4. Prevention and cure of cystic fibrosis.
5. Production of clotting factors.
6. Production of insulin.
7. Production of recombinant pharmaceuticals.
8. Plants that produce their own insecticides.
9. Germ line and somatic gene therapy.

TOOLS AND TECHNIQUES OF RECOMBINANT DNA TECHNOLOGY

Recombinant DNA technology, which is also called gene cloning or molecular cloning, is an umbrella term that encompasses a number of experimental protocols, leading to the transfer of genetic information (DNA fragments, i.e. gene) from one organism to another. There are no single set of methods that can be used to meet this objective, however, a recombinant DNA experiment often follows the following steps.

Step 1: A foreign DNA fragment (gene) from a donor organism is extracted, enzymatically cleaved (cut/digested) and joined (ligated) to another DNA entity (a cloning vector) to form a new, recombinant DNA molecule (cloning vector – insert DNA construct).

Step 2: This cloning vector-insert DNA construct is transferred into and maintained within a host cell by a desired method. This process is called transformation.

Step 3: Those host cells, which have successfully inserted the new DNA fragment in their genome (transformed cells), are identified and selected (separated/isolated), from those who have not been transformed by this effort.

Step 4: The integration of foreign DNA in the host cells are ensured by various methods, e.g. amplification by polymerase chain reaction (PCR), southern blotting of DNA against a known probe, etc. and blotting of the protein product that is encoded by the cloned DNA sequence by the western blotting, etc. It is also confirmed by northern blotting techniques which elucidate synthesis of mRNA to ensure the expression on the introduced foreign genes in the transformed host cells.

Step 5: The modification in the character of the transgenic plant (produced from the transformed cells), which is an outcome of the genetic engineering is verified and steps for the application /use of new product with its commercial, social, environmental health risk assessments and ethical aspects are established.

GENE CLONING

Recombinant DNA technology or gene cloning is a new born discipline of science which aims to alter the heredity apparatus of a living cell. It is also popularly known as genetic engineering which is performed under highly controllable laboratory conditions so that the cell can form completely new functions.

A recombinant DNA molecule is produced in joining together two or more DNA segments usually originating from different organisms. This is achieved by using specific enzymes for cutting the DNA (by the help of restriction enzymes) into suitable fragments and then joining together the appropriate fragments (by, ligase enzyme). It is now possible to isolate a desired piece of DNA (out of millions of nucleotide pairs in a chromosome) and join this isolated piece with another DNA molecule to create a new DNA molecule in test tube (*in vitro*). This molecule is now introduced back into living organisms (such as bacteria) to produce large number of copies (gene cloning). These developments called 'recombinant DNA technique' or 'gene splicing' or 'genetic engineering' have made possible to produce chromosomes with gene combination that is never formed naturally.

Recombinant DNA technology involves several steps in specific sequence such as:

1. Isolation of genetic material.
2. Cutting of DNA at specific locations.
3. Recombinant DNA formation.
4. Cloning of DNA.

Isolation of genetic material (DNA): In majority of organisms deoxynobo-nucleic acid or DNA is the genetic material. It is present in chromosomes within the cell. To isolate DNA, the cell at first is to be broken open by treating cell with enzyme so that DNA with other macromolecules are released. To get pure DNA the other necessary macro molecules such as RNA, protein, polysaccharides are removed by treating with appropriate enzymes. This is often called foreign DNA. It is then incorporated into bacterial plasmid.

Cutting of DNA: To cut DNA at specific location restriction endonuclease enzyme is used. These enzymes are called as molecular scissor or molecular scalpel and found in bacteria. These enzymes can cut the, DNA at any known point. The enzymes can cut DNA of the plasmid as well as foreign DNA at specific sites. These sites or points are mostly 8 palindromic, i.e. the sequences which read the same both backward and forward.

Formation of recombinant DNA: As stated earlier a desired piece of DNA or a gene is first isolated. This is generally called as foreign DNA. It is then incorporated into bacterial plasmid (plasmids are rings of DNA other than main ring shaped DNA of a bacterium which can replicate independent of main DNA). For this DNA of the plasmid is cut open by endonuclease enzyme leaving the sticky ends. The foreign DNA is also cut out (by the same restriction endonuclease) and allowed to join the sticky ends of plasmid DNA. Such a plasmid DNA is now known as recombinant DNA.

Cloning of DNA: The recombinant plasmid DNA obtained above is allowed to multiply to form a clone of recombinant DNA. To achieve this recombinant plasmid DNA is introduced into a rapidly dividing bacterium. Each time the bacterium divides and replicates its DNA, it also copies the introduced recombinant plasmid and also the foreign DNA. This method of introducing plasmid DNA into a bacterium (usually *E. coli*) is known as transformation. In this process bacterial cell takes up pieces of naked DNA from the surrounding medium.

These bacteria with recombinant plasmid DNA are grown in nutrient medium where these double in number in every 20–30 minutes, producing millions of cells. In this way millions of copies of recombinant plasmid DNA are formed.

To recover the foreign DNA from recombinant plasmid DNA, the bacterial cells are broken. The foreign DNA is cut out of the recombinant plasmid DNA by appropriate restriction enzyme and separated by gel electrophoresis.

Important steps in recombinant DNA technology:

1. Isolation of DNA from the selected organism and preparation of DNA fragments (foreign DNA) to be cloned.

2. Insertion of the DNA fragments (foreign DNA) into a suitable vector (such as plasmid DNA) to produce recombinant DNA.

3. Introduction of the recombinant DNA into a suitable organism (such as bacteria) called host. This process is called transformation. Generally *E. coli* is used for cloning.

4. Multiplication of host cells and also multiplication of recombinant DNA and cloning of desired gene.

Molecular Cloning

Through several discoveries in the areas of molecular biology, nucleic acid enzymology and the molecular genetics of bacterial, virus and bacterial extra chromosomal DNA elements (plasmids), as well as of the other eukaryotic organisms, made it possible to develop recombinant DNA technology as such a revolutionary technique in the manipulating living organisms in desired manner. This technology would have not existed without the availability of enzymes (restriction enzyme, restriction endonucleases) that recognise specific double-stranded DNA sequences and cleave the DNA in both strands at these sequences.

Restriction endonucleases

For molecular cloning of a foreign gene into a cloning vector, it is necessary to cut the DNA fragment at a specific site containing the target sequences, both in the source DNA that contain the largest sequences and in the cloning vector. The cut sites in the both kinds of DNA must be consistent for each time into discrete and reproductive fragments. Subjecting isolated DNA to passage through a small-bore needle or to sonication produces double stranded pieces of DNA that may range from 0.3 to 5 kilo basepair (Kb), in length, but these fragments are produced by the random breaking of DNA and each time we may end up with DNA with different sequences. So by these simple procedures we can't cut the DNA at desired site with the targeted sequences.

The discovery of bacterial enzymes, that cut DNA molecules internally at the specific base pair sequences, called type II restriction endonucleases, made it feasible to obtain DNA sequences of desired nature from a source DNA and to insert it in the genome of another organism between the enzymatic cut sizes which can accommodate the new insert/foreign DNA. One of the first of these type II restriction endonucleases characterised from the bacterium *Escherichia coli* and it was designated *Eco* RI.

This enzyme binds to a DNA region with a specific palindromic sequence (the two strands are identical in this region when either is read in the same polarity, i.e. 5′ to 3′) of 6 base pairs (bp) and cuts between the guanine and adenine residues on each strand.

Eco RI enzyme specifically cleaves the internucleotide bond between the oxygen of the 3′ carbon of the sugar of one nucleotide and the phosphate group attached to 5′ carbon of the sugar of the adjacent nucleotide. The symmetrical staggered cleavage of DNA by *Eco* RI produces two single-stranded, complementary cut ends, each with extensions of four nucleotides. Each single-stranded extension, in this case, ends in a 5′-phosphate group and the 3′ – hydroxyl group from the opposite strand is recessed.

Eco RI type enzymes are not the only restriction endonucleases, which have been isolated and used for gene isolation and cloning. Hundred of other type II restriction endonucleases are known which have been isolated from the various bacteria. For naming them, as in *Eco* RI, genus of the source bacteria is the capitalised letter and the first two letters of the species name are in lowercase letters. The strain designation is often omitted from the name and roman numerals are used to designate the order of characterisation of different restriction endonucleases from the same organisms. For example, *Hpa* I and *Hpa* II are the first and second type II restriction endonucleases that were isolated from *Haemophilus parainfluenzae*.

Plant Genomes, Genomic and cDNA Libraries

The genetic information which controls the entire function of a plant is stored in the form of a polymer called deoxyribonucleic acid (DNA), in the cells as in the other eukaryotes. The instructions that control all the activities of a plant are stored in the DNA as genes, which are the DNA sequences making the functional ribonucleic acid (RNA) and proteins. In plants, each gene codes for one protein or functional RNA, so each plant contain a large number of gene which vary species to species and genus to genus. The total amount of DNA in the nucleus of a cell, or in organelles, is called 'the genome'.

In plant cells the genes may be organised in nuclei, mitochondria and chloroplasts. The nuclear genome is contained in large linear DNA molecules called chromosomes, which varies in size and number in different plant species, consequently the size of the genome also varies between the plant species (Table 11.1). The mitochondrial and chloroplast genome are, on the other hand, contained in the circular DNA in multiple copies in each organelle.

Table 11.1: Genome size of various plants.

Plant	Genome size (Mb)	Relative genome size compared with Arabidopsis
Arabidopsis	120–130	1
Rice	389–430	3.0
Maize	2500	20
Barley	5000	38
Wheat	15000–16960	128
Oilseed rape	1200	10
Garden pea	3947	33
Soyabean	1115	9
Potato	840	14
Tomato	950	8

Though the majority of genetic informations in green plants are contained in the nuclear genome, the mitochondria and the chloroplasts also share a significant amount of the genetic information that controls the functional biology of plants.

Significance of Genome Size and Organisation

The size of nuclear genome which represents an unreplicated DNA content (C-value) in the cells of organisms reflects the complexity of the organism. The genome of higher order organisms are generally bigger than those of lower order organism, for example, the C- value vary from $\sim 10^7$ to 10^{11} bp in eukaryotic organisms, having a trend of bigger size of genome in order of fungi, animals and plants as compared to bacteria. However, this simple relationship does not always hold true, a situation known as 'the C-value paradox'. We can see that in higher plants, for example, plants of similar size and similar groups can have a genome size that vary by several orders of magnitudes (see rice and wheat in Table 11.1) and many amphibian have C-values much larger than that of humans. Surprisingly only a small percentage of the genome is known to actually encode proteins which lead to the development of a character in terms of function or structure. It means a vast majority of DNA components in a genome in certain organisms are either non-coding and apparently function less or unrevealed yet by the known tools and techniques of plant biology and biotechnology.

CLONING VECTORS

DNA cloning is a technique to produce large quantities of a specific DNA segment. The DNA segment to be cloned is first linked to a vector DNA, which is a vehicle for carrying foreign DNA into a suitable host cell, such as the bacterium *E. coli*. The vector contains sequences that allow it to be replicated within the host cell.

The rDNA technology allows the cloning of random DNA or cDNA segments, often used as probes as well as cloning of the specific genes, which has either been isolated from the genome or synthesised in laboratory or obtained as cDNA from specific mRNA sequences.

Vectors for Genetic Engineering

Genetic engineering become possible because vectors like plasmids and phages reproduce in a host (e.g. *E. coli*) in their usual manner even after insertion of foreign DNA, the inserted DNA also replicate faithfully with the parent DNA (The technique is called gene cloning and the vectors used for this purpose are called cloning vectors). Using a variety of cloning, gene can be isolated, cloned and characterised and new characters can be inserted vector beyond the taxonomic boundaries. The vectors can also manipulate the expression of the inserted genes in the host, expression vactors.

Various kinds of vectors are available, e.g. plasmids, (often used for cloning DNA segments of small size (upto 10 kilobases), phages (20–25 Kbp), cosmids (40–50 Kbp DNA segment), bacteriophage P1 system and F-factor based vectors (BACs = bacterial artificial chromosomes), YACs, MACs, etc. can allow cloning of DNA segments, as large as 100 to 1000 Kbp (or 1 Mp = 10^6 bp) length (preferred when fragments bigger than 50–100 Kbp are to be cloned), phagemids (combine desirable features of both plasmids and bacteriophases), BACs and PACs (100–300 Kbp), YACs (100–2000 Kbp), MACs (mammalian artificial chromosomes (> 1000 Kbp).

Plasmids and Vectors

Plasmids are self replicating circular (rarely linear) duplex DNA molecules, which are maintained in a bacterial cell, yeast cell or eukaryotic cell organelles, e.g. chloroplasts and mitochondria in a definite number of copies (characteristic to the specific organism or organelle). The number can range from as small as 1 to as large as 1000 copies per cell. Plasmids are a preferable source as cloning vectors, due to their increased yield potential.

The concept of cloning a foreign DNA segment in plasmid is discussed below.

A plasmid (pBR322) confers resistance to both ampicillin and tetracycline. The restriction endonuclease enzyme can cut it at ampicillin site at which a foreign DNA can get inserted.

After insertion this foreign gene ampicillin resistance will be ineffective, whereas the tetracycline resistance will be maintained intact. By the differential resistance capability of the plasmids wild type and recombinant type can be separated.

Plasmid vectors are often used for cloning segments of small size (upto 10 kilobases). Commonly used *E. coli* plasmid vectors are pBR322 and pBR 327 vectors. Some details of *Agrobacterium* plasmid vectors which are most widely used in plant transformation are discussed below.

Lamda phage (λ) vectors

For preparing genomic libraries of the eukaryotes, cloning of larger DNA segments are required. Phase lambda (λ) vectors can permit cloning of 20–25 Kbp long segments. Working with phage lambda considered easier and more efficient for making genomic and cDNA libraries.

Cosmids as vectors

Cosmid vectors can also permit cloning of DNA segments upto 45 Kbp long. They are plasmid particles with *cos* sites, allow the packing of DNA into phage particles *in vitro*. Certain specific DNA sequences, those for *cos* sites are inserted easily into cosmids. It is highly efficient vector to produce a complete genomic library of 10^6–10^7 clones from a mere 1 µg of insert DNA.

Mammalian Artificial Chromosomes (MACs)

To clone large DNA segments in mammalian cells MACs, have been produced with the isolation of mammalian telomere and centromere. MACs are designed to be replicate, segregate and express in a mammalian cell like any other mammalian chromosome along with other chromosomes. Since it will be an independent chromosome, with all the functional elements (telomeres, origins of replication, centromere, etc.) MAC will not be integrated with the genome and can be used as a vector maintaining a single copy per cell. It could carry large fragments of DNA (upto 1000 Kbp) representing an intact eukaryotic split gene with exons and introns permitting its normal expression regulated by the associated promoter sequences.

Plant and Animal Viruses as Vectors

Cauliflower mosaic virus (CAMV), Tobacco mosaic virus (TMV) and Gemini viruses are those groups of plant viruses which have been used as vectors for cloning DNA segments. Due to their high potential of fast replication in the appropriate hosts, they can multiply the inserted foreign DNA very fast and in very large numbers of copies. A number of animal viruses are also used as vectors, either for the delivery of DNA into the host genome or for the fast and higher level amplification of foreign genes using the virus based promoters.

Transposons as Vectors

Transposons are mobile DNA segments that are able to move and integrate throughout an organism's genome. Certain transposons of higher plants (e.g. Ac/Ds or Mn1 of maize) and P-element of *Drosophila* are the common transposons used as cloning vectors. Transposons possess short terminal reports enclosing along DNA segment containing the gene for transposase enzyme responsible for transposition. Part of this region can be deleted and the transposon can be used for cloning of foreign DNA segments as it occur in other cases.

Genomic and cDNA Libraries

Genomic DNA is the genetic material of an organism stored in its genetic pool, whereas cDNA is DNA sequence derived from mRNA isolated from a specific metabolically active tissue of an organism. A mixture of clones each carrying DNA sequences derived either from the genomic DNA or from cDNA are called as gnomic or cDNA libraries respectively. These libraries are constructed and used for various steps involved in rDNA technology.

Genomic Library

Cloning of a complete genome as library of random genomic clones is also called as a shotgun experiment. In this protocol, genomic DNA is extracted and then broken into fragments of reasonable size by restriction endonucleases and subsequently inserted into a cloning vector to generate a population of chimeric vector molecule. The DNA fragments cloned in this manner are known as genomic library. Once prepared, the clones can be put into the plasmid vector and retrieved whenever required for various purposes, e.g. identification and isolation of genes, source genes for genetic engineering, genetic studies, etc.

Various restriction endonucleases can cut the fragments of varying sizes, which facilitate the fragmentation of genome for library making depending on the genome size and vector type. For a probability level of 99% that all the sequences are present in a genomic library of a species about 1500 cloned fragments are needed for *E. coli*, 4600 for yeast, 48000 for *Drosophila melanogaster* and 800000 for human being.

cDNA Library from mRNAs

cDNA (complementary DNA) libraries are prepared by the help of activated mRNA, isolated from the cells actively synthesising proteins (for example meristems, roots and leaves in plants). The cDNA is obtained as a reverse transcriptase induced copy of mRNA. Though cDNA molecules can be made double stranded (Fig. 11.3) it differ from genomic clones in lacking the introns present in split genes. The advantage of cDNA libraries is being capable to be expressed in bacteria, which do not have the machinery to process the eukaryotic split gene Hn RNA into mRNA. These libraries can be processed with colony hybridisation technique (Fig. 11.4) for isolation of a gene sequence.

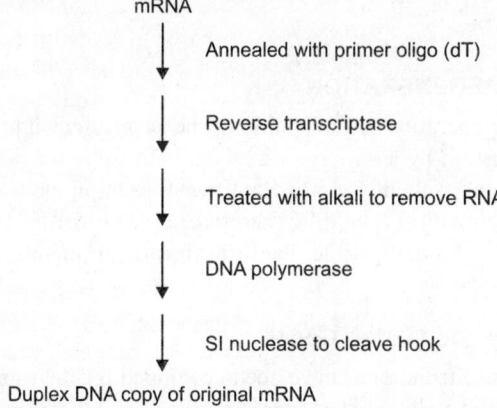

mRNA

↓   Annealed with primer oligo (dT)

↓   Reverse transcriptase

↓   Treated with alkali to remove RNA

↓   DNA polymerase

↓   SI nuclease to cleave hook

Duplex DNA copy of original mRNA

Fig. 11.3: Schematic presentation synthesis of cDNA from mRNA, using reverse transcriptase enzyme.

Transposable Elements and Gene Walking

A transposable element (TE) is a DNA sequence that is able to move and integrate throughout an organisms genome. In contrast to homologous recombination processes that require at least some degree of sequence homology. Thus, the mechanism of integration of TE into chromosomes are considered as non homologous recombination and is highly useful in rDNA technology.

Discovery of transposable elements began in the 1940s with the experimental work of Marcus Roades and Barabara McClintok during their classical work on maize genetics. They indicated that genomes may contain unstable and possibly mobile components as they found the appearance of unexpected phenotypes amongst the progeny of certain strains of maize. Later it was confirmed in bacteria and higher organisms that such unusual genetic results are consequence of the insertion of mobile DNA pieces, known a transposable elements (also called as jumping genes).

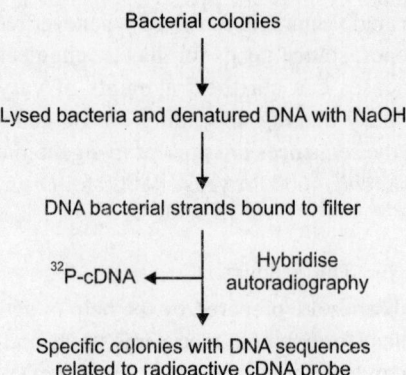

Fig. 11.4: Colony hybridisation technique for selection and isolation of DNA fragment having sequence complimentary to a radioactively labelled probe.

Though the findings of Roades and McClintock was the first clear indication that movable DNA sequences existed in any genome, the first evidence for occurrence existed in any genome, isolation and characterisation of transposable element was obtained from *E. coli* after development of molecular techniques up to the late 1970s.

VECTORS FOR PLANT REGENERATION

Various methods of plant regeneration are available to the plant biotechnologist. Some plant species may be amenable to regeneration by a variety of methods, but some may only be regenerated by one method. Not all plant tissues are suited to every plant transformation method and not all plant species can be regenerated by every method. There is, therefore, a need to find both a suitable plant tissue culture/regeneration regime and a compatible plant transformation methodology for biotechnological improvement of plants.

Vectors for Gene Delivery and Marker Genes

In last one decade, a number of techniques have been developed for the transfer of genes into plants.

These techniques can be divided into two broad groups:

1. Those employing a vector, such as *agrobacterium* or cauliflower mosaic virus or gemini virus.
2. Non-biological techniques- which employ physical or chemical means of transferring genes into cells/protoplasts or intact plants.

Biology of *agrobacterium*

Agrobacterium are gram negative ubiquitous soil phytopathogen that genetically transforms plant cells. In nature this transformation results in crown gall tumours (cancerous growth) or hairy roots (prolific root formation) at the infection sites in a range the consequence of transfer, integration and expression of a particular segment of DNA, the t-DNA (transfer dNA) from the tumour inducing (*ti*) or root inducing (*ri*) plasmid within the bacterium to plant cell genome. Over the last one decade, the basic principle involved in this transformation process has led to the design of modified non-oncogenic *agrobacterium* strains that can be used to transfer any DNA of interest to plant cells without interfering with their normal growth and regeneration property.

ti plasmid and t-DNA

1. All tumour forming (virulent) strains of *agrobacterium* harbour a large plasmid (140–235 kb) called *ti* or *ri* plasmid. A discrete segment (t-DNA) of this plasmid which is bordered by 25 bp conserved repeats and ranges in size from 14–24 kb (approximately 1/10th of plasmid) is transferred to the plant cell and stably integrated to plant nuclear DNA (Fig. 11.5).

2. Most of the genes that are located within t-dNA do not express in bacteria, but express only after t-dNA is inserted into the plant genome, because these genes possess typical eukaryotic promoter and polyadenylation signals. The products of t-DNA are responsible for oncogenicity (crown gall) formation. The three genes of t-DNA region *tms1 (iaam), tms2 (iaah)* and *tmr (ipt)* direct the constitutive synthesis of the phytohormones, auxin and cytokinins which are responsible for rapid proliferation of plant cells resulting into tumerous growth such as crown gall. The first two genes (*tms1* and *tms2*) encode enzymes that synthesise the plant hormone auxin (indole-3- acetic acid). Specially *tms1* codes for the enzyme tryptophan-2-mono-oxygenase which converts tryptophan to indole-3-acetamide and gene *tms 2* contains the information for indole-3-acetamide hydrolase, which converts indole-3-acetamide to indole-3-acetic acid, in addition, the third gene *tmr* encodes isopentenyl transferase enzyme, which adds 5'-amp to an isoprenoid side chain to form the cytokinin isopentenyl adenine and isopentenyl adenosine.

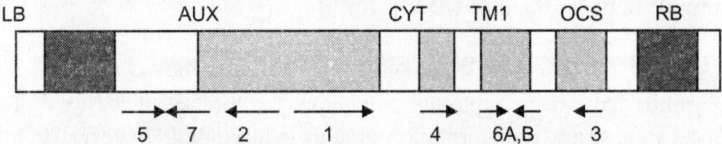

Fig. 11.5: The genetic organisation of the *t1* t-DNA of an octopine-type *ti* plasmid. only the *t1* region is shown as this ha homology with the t-DNA of nopaline-type *ti* plasmids.eight open reading frames (orfs) are indicated (1–7), although orfs 5 and 7 are not discussed in this text. Regions of import are shaded light grey and include the aux genes (which encode enzymes involced in auxin biosynthesis), cyt which encodes isopentyl transferase (an enzyme involved in cytokinin production, *tm1* which is involved in regulating tumour size and ocs (octopine synthase) which encodes opine synthesis.

T-DNA Transfer

Extensive genetic and molecular biology studies have revealed that three genetic components of *agrobacterium* are involved in t-DNA transfer.

Agrobacterium chromosomal genes: The initial step toward gene transfer by *agrobacterium* is the attachment of bacterium to plant cell at wound sites. The nature of plant cell receptors to which *agrobacterium* binds is unknown. Four different bacterial chromosomal virulence loci *chv, cel, psc a* and *att* are involved in the binding of bacteria to plant cells.

Now it is believed that the bacteria respond to certain low molecular weight phenolic compounds such as acetosyringone and hydroxyacetosyringone which are secreted by susceptible wounded plants. These wound -response compounds resemble some of the products of phenylpropanoid metabolism, which is the major plant pathway for the synthesis of plant secondary metabolites such as lignins and flavanoids. These small molecules (i.e. acetosyringone, hydroxyl acetosyringone) act to induce the activity of the virulence (*vir*) genes.

T-DNA BORDER SEQUENCES

The structure and organisation of the integrated t-DNA in tumour cells has been studied in detail. The main conclusions of these studies are listed below.

1. None of the t-DNA encoded genes are required for t-DNA transfer.
2. t-DNA does not influence the site of insertion since t-DNA inserts were found to be at random locations in the genome and present at a range of copy numbers (averaging 2–3) within individual transformed cell lines.
3. t-DNA is a discrete unit which is inserted into the plant genome without modification.
4. t-DNA regions on all *ti* or *ri* plasmids are flanked by almost 25 bp direct repeat or border sequences. These 25 bp repeat sequences particularly those on the right border to t-DNA are absolutely required for t-DNA transfer and that they function in a *cis*-acting and polar fashion. Any DNA sequence placed between these borders can be transferred into plant cell.
5. Detection of the first 6 bp or the last 10 bp of the 25 bp sequence blocks t-DNA transfer.

T-DNA Transfer Process

Two proteins encoded by the *vird* operon, *vird1* and *vird2*, act as a site specific endonuclease which produce nicks between 3 or 4 base pairs on the bottom strand of each 25 bp repeat. The *vird2* protein attaches to the 5′ terminus of the nicked right border t-DNA and replicative process synthesises a single stranded DNA from the bottom strand of t-DNA.

AGROBACTERIUM AS A VECTOR SYSTEM

Agrobacterium plasmids have been exploited as vectors for biological delivery of foreign DNA to plants, this is the most wide spread transformation strategy in use today. However, (wild type *ti* plasmids) have several serious limitations as routine cloning vector.

The phytohormone biosynthetic genes encoded on t-DNA of wild-type *ti* plasmids interfere with the regeneration of transformed cells growing in culture. Therefore, the phytohormone (auxin and cytokinin) genes completely removed (disarmed plasmid) for t-DNA to regenerate complete plants from transformed plant cells. A gene encoding opine synthesis is not useful to a transgenic plant and may lower the final plant yield by diverting plant resources into opine production. Therefore, the opine synthesis gene should be removed. For recombinant DNA experiments, however, a much smaller version is preferred, so large segments of DNA that are not essential for a cloning vector must be removed. Because *ti* plasmid does not replicate in *E. coli*, the convenience of perpetuating and manipulating *ti* plasmids carrying inserted DNA sequences in this bacterium does not exist. Therefore, in developing *ti* plasmid - based vectors, an origin of replication that can be used in *E. coli* must be added.

To overcome these constraints, many non-oncogenic transformation vectors with different features have been constructed. They fall into two broad categories, the *cis* and the *trans* vectors.

cis vectors contain both the border sequences and the *vir* region on the same replicon (co-integration) whereas in *trans* vectors both the border and *vir* functions are on two replicons (binary vectors).

Co-integrate Vectors and Other Vectors for Gene Transfer to Plants

The co-integrating system involves two independent plasmids. (i) a non-oncogenic (disarmed) *ti* plasmid (in which majority of t-DNA is removed and replaced by a section of DNA homologous to small *E. coli* cloning vector) in *agrobacterium* and (ii) an intermediate vector which can't replicate in *agrobacterium*, is used for cloning and manipulation of the gene which are to be introduced in *E. coli*. Since both the plasmids have a region of homology which undergoes recombination to form a large, co-integrated plasmid after conjugation between *agrobacterium* and *E. coli*.

The main advantage of the co-integrate vectors is their high stability in *agrobacterium*. However, two disadvantages are the detailed knowledge required of the *ti* plasmid before it can be manipulated and the relatively low rates of co-integrate formation (about 10^{-5}).

Binary Vector

The binary vectors are based on the principle that *vir* gene products can function in trans configuration. These vectors (binary vectors) contain t-DNA border repeats as well as both *E. coli* and *agrobacterium* origin of replication but no *vir* genes, it is actually an *E. coli agrobacterium* shuttle vector. All the cloning steps are carried out in *E. coli* before the vector conjugatively transferred into *agrobacterium* which contains a disarmed *ti* plasmid lacking the entire t-DNA region, but an intact *vir* region (helper *ti* plasmid, e.g. *pal4404*).

Many binary vectors have been developed which differ in size, source of 25 bp repeat sequence, plant selection marker, bacterial selection marker and cloning sites for the insertion of DNA for transfer to plants. Unlike co-integrative vectors, binary vectors need not have any homology with the resident *ti* plasmid and are capable of autonomous replication, usually in multiple copies within *agrobacterium*. This gives the binary a considerable advantage over the co-integrative system since any binary can be used in conjunction with any *vir* helper strain even with wild type oncogenic strains of *agrobacterium*.

The presence of genes encoded in the t-DNA of a binary plasmid in *agrobacterium* is confirmed easily by plasmid restriction digests, rather than by southern hybridisation or PCR, which is required to detect large co-integrated plasmids. As a result of these features, binary vectors have virtually excluded co-integrate vectors.

CAMV as Vector

One feature of CAMV which makes it attractive as a vector is that viruses spread systematically throughout the plant. In order for CAMV to be transmitted through the vascular system of plant, the DNA must be assembled within virion. The strategy for delivering foreign genes using CAMV has to replace a small section of genome, not required for virus propagation, with foreign DNA small enough not to interfere with packing of genome into the virion particle.

Direct Gene Transfer Methods

Table 11.2 in addition to the vector mediated gene transfer methods, these are certain direct gene transfer methods has been used for genetic transformation a brief account of these methods.

Table 11.2: Direct gene transfer method.

Direct gene transfer method	Comments
Particle bombardment	Very successful method. Risk of gene rearrangements and high copy number. Useful for transient expression assays
Electroporation	Transgenic plants obtained from a range of cereal crops low efficiency. Requires careful optimisation
DNA uptake into protoplasts	Used for all major cereal crops. Requires optimisation with a regenerable cell suspension that may not be available
Silicon carbide fibres	Requires regenerable cell suspensions. Transgenic plants obtained from a number of species

Promoters and terminators

An obvious requirement for any gene that is to be expressed as transgene in plants is that it is expressed correctly (or at least in a predictable fashion). It is known that the major determinant of gene expression (level, location and timing) is the region upstream of the coding region. This region, termed 'the promoter', is therefore of vital importance. Any gene, that is to be expressed in the transformed plant must has to possess an eukaryotic promoter that will function in plants. This is an important consideration as many of the genes that are to be expressed in plants, *Bt* gene, reporter genes and selectable marker genes, etc. are bacterial in origin. They, therefore, have to be cloned with a promoter that will drive their expression in plants. Transgenes also need to have suitable terminator sequences at their 3′ terminus to ensure that transcription ceases at the correct position. Failure to stop transcription can lead to the production of aberrant transcripts and can result in a range of deleterious effects, including inactivation of gene products and increased gene silencing. In additions to the basic need for the promoter to be capable of driving expression of the gene in plants, there are other considerations that need to be taken into account, such as promoter strength, tissue specificity and developmental regulations, etc.

Agrobacterium derived promoter and terminator sequences: The genes from the *ti* plasmid of *Agrobacterium* that code for opine synthesis and in particular the nopaline synthase (*nos*) gene, are widely used as a source of both promoters and terminators in plant transformation vectors. Although derived from bacterial genes, their presence on the T-DNA means they are adapted to function in plants. The *nos* promoter is usually considered to be constitutive.

The 35 S promoter

The most widely used promoter used to drive expression of genes in plant transformation vectors is the promoter of the cauliflower mosaic virus 35 S RNA gene (35 S promoter). This promoter is considered to be expressed in all tissues of transgenic plants (though not necessarily in all cell types). In dicots it drives expression at high levels, although in monocots the level of expression is not so high. This makes the 35 S promoter ideal for driving the expression of selectable marker genes and in some cases of reporter genes, as expression is more or less guaranteed. In monocots, alternatives, such as the maize *ubiquitin I* promoter or the rice actin promoter/first intron sequence, are often used to drive the high level expression of transgenes.

Tissue specific promoters

Considerable effort has been made in isolating promoters that can be used to drive expression in a tissue specific manner. The expression of any potentially harmful substances can be limited to tissues that are not consumed by animals or humans and genes involved in specific processes can be limited to tissues in which that process occurs. In certain cases the promoters have been found not to function, or not to drive expression in the predicted pattern, in heterologous systems. Therefore considerable care has been taken with the use of promoters.

Inducible promoters

Inducible expression systems can be divided into three categories: (i) non-plant-derived systems, (ii) plant derived systems, (iii) plant-derived systems based on developmental control of gene expression.

Non-plant-derived systems are independent of the normal plant processes, requiring use of inducers on agricultural scale. While the plant derived systems do not have the advantage of independence from normal plant processes. This makes their use potentially simpler as the application of an inducer is not required.

Marker genes

During the genetic transformation of plants, often the success in integration of introduced foreign genes is a very-low frequency event. It will be, otherwise wastage of time, energy and resources to maintain a large number of regenerants (shoots or somatic embryos) obtained from the initial transformation efforts. Therefore it is vital that some means for selecting the transformed tissue/plantlets at initial stages should be deviced. To achieve the above target some marker genes are also cloned along with the 'gene of interest' in the cloning vectors. The marker genes are broadly of two types: (i) selectable markers and (ii) reporter genes.

Selectable markers

The selectable marker gene cloned within the vector confers resistance that is toxic to plants. The selection in such cases is based on the inclusion of a substance toxic to the plants in the culture media. The transformed cells/tissues/plants expressing the bacterial genes showing resistance to such toxic substances are survived onto such culture media, whereas other normal (wild type) non transformed cells/tissues/plants get die. Table 11.3 list certain selectable markers often used in plant genetic engineering.

Table 11.3: Selectable markers used in plant transformation.

Selectable marker gene	Abbreviation	Source of gene	Selection mechanism	Selective agent
Hygromycin phosphotransferase	hpt/aphiv/byg	E. coli	Antibiotic resistance	Hygromycin
Neomycin phosphotransferase II	nptII/neo	E. coli	Antibiotic resistance	Kanamycin Geneticin (G 418)
Neomycin phosphotransferase III	nptII	Streptococcus faecalis	Antibiotic resistance	Kanamycin Geneticin (G 418)
Glyphosphate oxidoreductase	gox	Achromobacter	LBAA resistance	Herbicide Glyphosate
Phophinothricin acetyltransferase	bar/pat	Streptomyces hygroscopicus	Herbicide resistance	Bialophos Glufosinate
Mannose-6-phosphate isomerase	bmi/man A	E. coli	Alternative carbon source	Mannose
Betaine aldehyde dehydrogenase	badh	Spinach	Detoxication	Betain aldehyde

Reporter genes

In addition to the selectable markers or as an alternative to them, reporter genes (Table 11.4) are used as markers in many plant transformation vectors. At present, only a small number of reporter genes in widespread use in plant transformation vectors the reporter genes should be, ideally, easy to assay, preferably with a non-destructive assay system and there should be little or no endogenous activity in the plant to be transformed.

MONITORING PLANT DIVERSITY THROUGH DNA

The living world is a complex combination of different levels of organisms. The key components of life are at one extreme and communities of species at the other extreme.

Table 11.4: Reporter genes used in plant transformation.

Reporter gene	Abbreviation	Source of gene	Detection/assay
β-glucuronidase	gus/uid A	E. coli	Fluorimetric (quantitative) or historical (*in situ*), non-radioactive
Green fluorescent protein	gfp	Aequorea victoria (jelly fish)	Fluorescence, non-destructive
Chloromphenicol	cat	E. coli	Radioactive assay of plant extract, sensitive, acetyltransferase semi-quantitative
Luciferase	luç	Photinus pyralis (firefly)	Luminscence
Luciferase	Lux A, Lux B	Vibrio barveyi	Luminscence

The manifestations of all types of diversities are found at all these levels of organisms. Biodiversity is the shorter form of word biological diversity which means diversity in the biological world. Thus one can define biodiversity as the degree of variety in nature with regards to biological species.

TYPES OF BIODIVERSITY

Genetic Diversity

It is the variation of genes within the species. This results distinct population of one, even same species. It gives genetic variation within a population or varieties within one species. There are two reasons for differences between individual organisms. One is variation in the gene which all organisms possess which is passed from one to its offsprings. The other is the influence of environment on each individual organism. The variation in the sequence of four base pairs in DNA chain forms the genetic variation in the organism. The recombination of genetic material during cell division makes it an imperative for genetic diversity within a species. Loss of genetic diversity within a species is called genetic erosion.

The whole area of agricultural productivity and development depend on genetic diversity. The plant as well as animal genetic resources play important role in the economy of a country. Genetic diversity is the whole basis for a sustainable life system in the earth.

Assessment of Genetic Diversity in Crop Plants

The assessment of genetic diversity within and between plant populations is routinely performed using various techniques such as: (i) morphological, (ii) biochemical characterisation/evaluation (allozyme), in the pregenomic era and (iii) DNA (or molecular) marker analysis especially single nucleotide polymorphism (SNPs) in postgenomic era.

Markers can exhibit similar modes of inheritance, as we observe for any other traits, that is, dominant/recessive or codominant. If the genetic pattern of homozygotes can be distinguished from that of heterozygotes, then a marker is said to be codominant. Generally codominant markers are more informative than the dominant markers. Morphological markers are based on visually accessible traits such as flower colour, seed shape, growth habits and pigmentation and it does not require expensive technology but large tracts of land area are often required for these field experiments, making it possibly more expensive than molecular assessment in western (developed) countries and equally expensive in Asian and Middle East (developing) countries considering the labour cost and availability. These marker traits are often susceptible to phenotypic plasticity, conversely, this allows assessment of diversity in the presence of environmental variation which cannot be neglected from the genotypic variation. These types of markers are still having advantage and they are mandatory for distinguishing the adult plants from their genetic contamination in the field, for example, spiny seeds, bristled panicle and flower/leaf colour variants. Second type of genetic marker is called biochemical markers, allelic variants of enzymes called isozymes that are detected by electrophoresis and specific staining. Isozyme markers are codominant in nature. They detect diversity at functional gene level and have simple inheritance. It requires only small amounts of plant material for its detection. However, only a limited number of enzymes markers are available and these enzymes are not alone but it has complex structural and special problems, thus, the resolution of genetic diversity is limited to explore. The third and most widely used genetic marker type is molecular markers, comprising a large variety of DNA molecular markers, which can be employed for analysis of genetic and molecular variation. These markers can detect the variation that arises from deletion, duplication, inversion and/or insertion in the chromosomes. Such markers themselves do not affect the phenotype of the traits of interest because they are located only near or linked to genes controlling the traits. These markers are inherited both in dominant and codominant patterns. Different markers have different genetic qualities (they can be dominant or codominant, can amplify anonymous or characterised loci, can contain expressed or nonexpressed sequences, etc.).

A molecular marker can be defined as a genomic locus, detected through probe or specific starter (primer) which, in virtue of its presence, distinguishes unequivocally the chromosomic trait which it represents as well as the flanking regions at the 3′ and 5′ extremity. Molecular markers (MM) may or may not correlate with phenotypic expression of a genomic trait. They offer numerous advantages over conventional, phenotype-based alternatives as they are stable and detectable in all tissues regardless of growth, differentiation, development, or defense status of the cell. Additionally, they are not confounded by environmental, pleiotropic and epistatic effects.

Species Diversity

Species diversity is defined as the number of species and abundance of each species that live in a particular location. The number of species that live in a certain location is called species richness. If you were to measure the species richness of a forest, you might find 20 bird species, 50 plant species and 10 mammal species. Abundance is the number of individuals of each species. This refers to the variety of species within a particular region. The number of species in a region is a measure for such diversity. The richness of species in a given region provides a yard stick for species diversity. Species diversity depends as much on the genetic diversity as on the environmental condition. Colder regions support less than the warmer regions for species diversity. The good climate with good physical geography supports a better species diversity. Species richness is a term which is used to measure the biodiversity of a given site. In addition to species richness, species endemism is a term used to measure biodiversity by way of assessing the magnitude of differences between species. In the taxonomic system similar species are grouped together in general, similar genera in families, families in orders and so on till in the level of kingdom. This process is a genuine attempt to find relationships between organisms. The higher taxa have thousands of species. Species that are very different from one another contributes more to overall biodiversity.

Importance of Species Diversity

There are numerous reasons why species diversity is essential. Each species has a role in the ecosystem. For example, bees are primary pollinators. Imagine what would happen if bees went extinct. Fruits and vegetables could be next and subsequently the animals that feed off them - this chain links all the way to humans. Various species provide us not only with food but also contribute to clean water, breathable air, fertile soils, climate stability, pollution absorption, building materials for our homes, prevention of disease outbreaks, medicinal resources and more. Species diversity contributes to ecosystem health. Each species is like a thread holding together an ecosystem. If a species disappears, an entire ecosystem can start to unravel. Species diversity is crucial for ecosystem health. For example, in the Pacific Northwest, salmon holds together the entire ecosystem. Salmon carry rich nutrients from the ocean back to the stream environment. When salmon die, those nutrients are gobbled up by insects, plants, mammals and birds. If salmon were to disappear, the impacts would be felt through the entire food chain.

Species diversity also contributes to medicine. Scientists have discovered that over 3000 plants have cancer-fighting properties. For example, a plant called rosy periwinkle has natural chemicals that help treat childhood leukemia. Also, the fruit of a tree called the Chinese star anise is an ingredient in flu vaccines. The list goes on: aspirin, codeine and pseudoephedrine all are sourced from plants. There are medicinal treasures still yet to be discovered. Perhaps hidden in some forest is the cure to cancer.

Ecological Diversity

Ecological diversity relates to the different forms of life which are present in a particular site, in a more precise sense, it concerns the different species of a particular genus which are present in an ecological community. The measures, or indices, of ecological diversity, are statistical summaries of the abundance vector, that is, the frequencies or proportions of each species in the community. As a concept, diversity relates both to the number of species (richness) and to their apportionment within the community (evenness or equitability), other things being equal, there is greater diversity when the number of species grows and when all the species are fairly represented.

In other words ecological diversity is the number of species in a community of organisms. Maintaining both types of diversity is fundamental to the functioning of ecosystems and hence to human welfare. Relationships between plant diversity and ecosystem properties can be explored by classifying component species into three categories – dominants, subordinates and transients. Dominants recur in particular vegetation types, are relatively large, exhibit coarse-grained foraging for resources and, as individual species, make a substantial contribution to the plant biomass. Subordinates also show high fidelity of association with particular vegetation types but they are smaller in stature, forage on a more restricted scale and tend to occupy microhabitats delimited by the architecture and phenology of their associated dominants. Transients comprise a heterogeneous assortment of species of low abundance and persistence, a high proportion are juveniles of species that occur as dominants or subordinates in neighbouring ecosystems.

Components of Biodiversity

Thus, while discussing biodiversity as a whole these three components are tackled together. Genetic diversity is the first step in the process where a base mutation, in a suitable locus, could lead to a new species. Continuous inbreeding often unbalances the genetic make-up of a species by promoting admixture of genes. Accumulated knowledge by population genetics indicates that each species has its own inherent gene diversity that diverges through natural selection. The species diversity and ecosystem diversity then follow. In ecosystem, even soil microbes can determine diversity within plants and animals—by their interactions with them. So, biodiversity is the total gene pool or genetic polymorphism in an area and ecosystems have the collection of all organisms within a particular area each differing in physical structure, genome composition and gene function. Along a latitudinal gradient, species diversity tends to increase toward tropical areas. Within tropical areas, species diversity increases along a longitudinal gradient. Availability of nutrients is also another main factor for species diversity. The picture is the same on land, rivers and delta. Therein sunlight, nutrients and biotic interferences determine diversity. It ultimately leads to evolution.

Land and aquatic ecosystems are highly dynamic—though they are often disturbed by biotic interferences. Coral reef though has an entirely different ecosystem, it is also subjected to outside interferences. On the other hand, deep-sea ecosystem has less outside interferences. It may be noted that a minimum amount of genetic diversity within a population is essential for a species survival. Healthy ecosystem supports high biological diversity, on the other hand, stressed, unhealthy, or highly disturbed ecosystems do not. By recent DNA techniques these can be monitored.

CONSEQUENCES OF THREATENED ECOSYSTEM

The factors which threat biodiversity would change the environment and humans would be in danger, because humans (a small segment of earth's germplasm) exploit the majority of Earth's, resources. At present, scientists, media, public and governmental agencies worldwide have begun to recognise the danger from large-scale human interferences that lead to species extinctions.

The rate of this extinction on this globe—particularly in developing and under-developed countries—is occurring on an enormous scale—at a rate that had rivalled or even surpassed those of the Cretaceous period when many species including the dinosaurs became extinct.

At present, every nation is conscious about its natural resources and is trying to catalogue local flora and fauna, especially endemic species by looking at their DNA profiles because unlike other characters DNA is less susceptible to environment and biotic factors.

However, the change at species level first comes at DNA level of an individual. That change is manifested in the phenotypic appearance and adaptability of that individual within a population. Better forms diverge quickly. Even within highly diverse ecosystems, species elements can differ widely—bringing the incompatibility barrier between two or more populations.

SUSTAINABLE USE OF PLANT DIVERSITY

At present, it is of paramount importance to note the threats to plant biodiversity and to device methodology to counteract them, because plants provide medicine, food and materials for the industries. The situation will remain unchanged, as long Homo sapiens would survive. If the species richness vanishes from this globe, the very survival of Homo sapiens would be problematical.

Moreover, maintenance of the biological diversity of marine and estuarine systems is largely overlooked, all over the world even though it is generally accepted that marine systems are far more species rich and have greater ecosystem diversity than terrestrial systems.

So, maintenance or sustainability of plant resources on land, ponds, lakes, river and oceans is essential. Sustainable use of plant biodiversity (of course entire biodiversity) is the need of today's world because bio-prospecting is the new terminology for the use of microbes, wild flora and fauna.

MONITORING DNA DIVERSITY

The best way to measure the degree of genetic diversity and measuring genome polymorphism, within a population, species, genus, or higher-level taxon, is a resolution by molecular markers, particularly the DNA and protein marker. The advantage of a molecular marker over morphological markers is its superior quality and environment has no effect on these markers during the growth and differentiation of an organism.

DNA MARKERS

The important properties of a good marker are given below:

1. Easy recognition of all phenotypes (homo-or heterozygotes).
2. Early expression during plant development.
3. No effect on alternate alleles on plant morphology.
4. No or low interaction among markers, etc.

Unlike morphological markers, genetic (molecular) markers can fulfill these criteria because rate of evolution could be measured by looking into genetic molecules of related or unrelated taxa. Amongst the two types of molecular markers (DNA and proteins), DNA is superior over protein markers as they are least affected by the environmental fluctuations. Gene sequences are useful to develop molecular markers. Often arbitrary sequences are also used successfully to measure genetic diversity. Works of many scientists, who are currently using DNA markers in plant genetics and plant evolution, was timely from the standpoint that this is a rapidly developing technology that can be compared with the nuclear science in mid-twentieth century. Moreover, repetitive DNAs often may be highly mobile (transposon). So, often they control gene function. By doing so, repetitive DNAs provide tools to mother nature to play—to evolve different life forms. So, for an attempt to measure biological diversity, the best bet would be to look into gene-control elements sequence-diversity.

The absolute amount of single copy appears to remain meagre in large plant genome where genome replication is the rule rather than an exception. In maize, broad bean, lily and in many other plants, no more than a very small percentage of genome appears to consist of single-copy DNA sequences.

It is important to note that many kinetic measurements, with single-copy DNAs, are overestimates because the re-association kinetics was performed at criteria where extensively diverged 'fossil' repeats displayed single-copy kinetics. An additional complication is that extensive short-repeat sequence interspersion makes it difficult to find single-copy sequences much larger than several kbp (kilo basepairs) in all but small genomes, e.g. *Arabidopsis*.

At present, any genome structure can be investigated with DNA markers. Restriction fragment length polymorphism analysis is the first technique widely used to detect variation even at the gene sequence level. It is a DNA-DNA hybridisation technique where a labelled DNA probe is used to identify the level of base sequence diversity by hybridising that probe with template DNA strand. Another aspect of RFLP is the use of restriction endonucleases that could detect sequence diversity in allied genomes. A probe (marker)-enzyme combination is used to resolute the differences between individual genomes.

The application of RFLP as molecular markers has proven to be a powerful tool for studies in both basic and applied plant genetics and also to study genome evolution. The principal difficulty with RFLP is its reliance on cloning (to produce marker), Southern blotting and Southern hybridisation. For this, one must aim at the development, optimisation and validation of methodologies with special emphasis on high-throughput procedures right from the beginning (e.g. homogenisation of material and DNA extraction). Methods thus developed are to use the probes (markers) to detect the presence or absence of a gene, pedigree analysis, expression of a particular trait, etc. Therefore it is not only time-consuming but costly too.

PCR-based techniques: DNA replication protocol that is known as polymerase chain reaction (PCR). This protocol can be recognised as 'Photocopying of a DNA molecule' by repeated DNA polymerisation reactions. It could replace the requirement of cloning for multiplying DNA probes (DNA fragments, marker). In recent years, use of PCR-based markers could solve some of the limitations of earlier RFLP protocols.

Chapter 12

Method of Creating Recombinant DNA Molecules

INTRODUCTION

Recombinant DNA is the term applied to chimeric DNA molecules that are constructed in vitro, then propagated in a host cell or organism. The basic recombinant DNA consists of a vector and an insert (Fig. 12.1). The vector is a replicon (see Replicon) capable of replicating in the cells of choice. It is endowed with a functional replication origin, usually carries a selectable marker, and typically has been engineered to accommodate inserts conveniently.

Vectors are based on naturally occurring replicons, such as bacterial plasmids, viruses, or cellular chromosomes. Inserts can be of any sort – long or short segments of DNA, from natural or synthetic sources. The resulting recombinant DNAs are often referred to as clones, which is shorthand for chimeric DNAs that are isolated in cellular or viral clones, and the process of producing these recombinants is frequently called DNA cloning or gene cloning.

Recombinant DNA technology is a major DNA-based tool that opens a new age for modern biotechnology. With this technology, a gene or multiple genes can be identified, cut, and inserted into the genome of another organism. Using this technology, the first drugs of medical biotechnology were produced, namely human insulin.

METHOD OF CREATING RECOMBINANT DNA MOLECULES

- Single chimeric DNA formed by combining two or more different fragments of DNA from diverse organisms is generally called as recombinant DNA and the method applied to create recombinant DNA is called recombinant DNA technology.
- The organism, from which the candidate DNA is isolated, is called Donor organism. The organism which will accept the foreign gene is called Host organism.
- Genetic material from one organism is selected and then artificially introduced to a host organism. if the foreign recombinant DNA integrates into the host genome, it gets replicated along with the genome and then express the foreign protein.

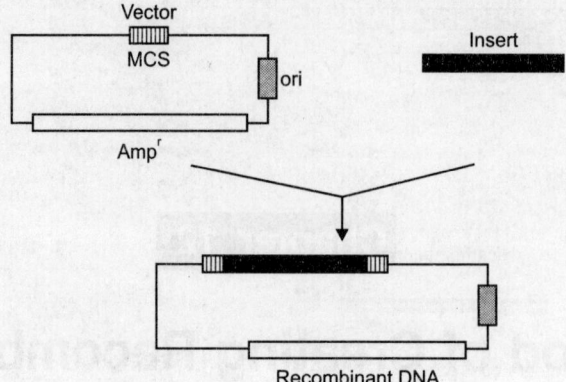

Fig. 12.1: The structure of a recombinant DNA. The vector illustrated here is a bacterial plasmid that has an origin of replication (ori), a selectable marker in the form of a gene conferring resistance to the antibiotic ampicillin (Amp^r), and a multiple cloning site (MCS). The insert can be any type of DNA sequence. The recombinant DNA is created by joining the vector and insert.

• Paul Berg, Herbert W. Boyer and Stanley N. Cohen are the pioneers of recombinant DNA technology.
• A hybrid of the SV40 mammalian DNA virus genome and phage λ was one of the recombinant DNA molecules to be first engineered.

There are three approaches to make recombinant DNA:

1. Transformation.
2. Non-bacterial transformation/transfection.
3. Phage introduction/transduction.

Transformation

Transformation is direct uptake of exogenous DNA via cell membrane leading to incorporation into the host DNA. It is commonly occurred in bacteria. Transformation requires different tools of molecular biology to insert foreign DNA into the host. For example, vector to carry the foreign DNA to the host, restriction enzymes to cut the DNA in specific site, ligase to join two DNA molecule, etc.

Non-bacterial Transformation/Transfection

The process of foreign DNA uptake by host cell driven by mechanical or chemical factors is classified under non-bacterial transformation, also termed as transfection. Different methods of non-bacterial transformation are microinjection, liposome mediated transformation, biolistics, etc.

Phage Introduction/Transduction

Phage vector is used to carry and replicate foreign DNA inside the bacterial host system. The phage DNA inserts into the host chromosome by recombination. Phage λ had short regions of single-stranded DNA with complementary base sequences called 'cohesive' (*Cos*) sites. Base pairing between the complementary cos sites allows the linear genome to form a circle within the host bacterium. Circularised viral genome can be integrated into the bacterial genome by homologous recombination between attP site of viral genome and attB site of bacterial genome (Fig. 12.2).

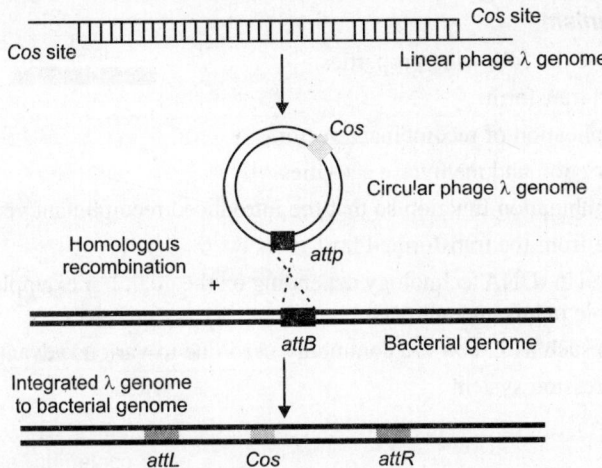

Fig 12.2: Bacteriophage λ genome circularisation and recombination with bacterial genome.

Methods involved in recombinant DNA technology

Molecular cloning is a process for creating recombinant DNA and generally involves the following steps :

1. Selection of a cloning vector.
2. Selection of a host organism.
3. Preparation of a vector DNA.
4. Preparation of DNA to be cloned.
5. Creation of recombinant DNA vector (having foreign DNA).
6. Introduction of recombinant vector into host organism.
7. Selection of clones having insert vector.
8. Screening and multiplication of recombinant clones with desired DNA inserts (Fig. 12.3).

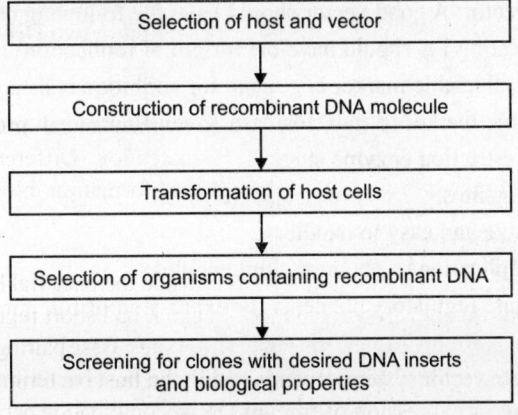

Fig 12.3: Steps in gene cloning.

Choice of host organism

A good host should have the following properties:
- Easy to grow and transform.
- Do not hinder replication of recombinant vector.
- Do not have restriction and methylase activities.
- Deficient in recombination function so that the introduced recombinant vector is not altered.
- Easily retrievable from the transformed host.

Various hosts are used in rDNA technology depending on the goal: For example bacteria, yeast, plant cells, animal cells, whole plants and animals.

Prokaryotic systems such as *E. coli* are commonly used due to various advantages like:
- Well studied expression system
- Compact genome
- Versatile
- Easy to transform
- Widely available
- Rapid growth of recombinant organisms with minimal equipment.

Only disadvantage is that they lack post-translational modification (PTMs) machinery required for eukaryotic proteins. Eukaryotic systems are difficult to handle in contrast to bacterial hosts. They are favoured for expression of recombinant proteins which require post translational modification and only if they can grow easily in continuous culture.

Choice of vector

Vector is an autonomously replicating (inside a host cell) DNA molecule designed from a plasmid or phage DNA to carry a foreign DNA inside the host cell. Transformation vectors are of two types:
- Cloning vector is used increasing the number of copies of a cloned DNA fragment.
- Expression vector is used for expression of foreign gene into a protein.
- If a vector is designed to perform equally in two different hosts, it is called a shuttle vector.

Properties of an ideal vector: A good vector should have the following characteristics:
- Autonomously replicating i.e. should have *ori* (origin of replication) region.
- Contain at least one selectable marker e. g. gene for antibiotic resistance.
- May contain a scorable marker (β-galactosidase, green fluorescent protein, etc.)
- Presence of unique restriction enzyme site.
- Have multiple cloning sites.
- Preferably small in size and easy to handle.
- Relaxed control of replication to obtain multiple copies.
- Presence of appropriate regulatory elements for expression of foreign gene.
- High copy number

The selection of a suitable vector system depends mainly on the size limit of insert DNA and the type of host intended for cloning or expression of foreign DNA.

List of different vectors

- Plasmids are circular DNA molecules that exist independently of chromosomal DNA and can replicate autonomously. Plasmids carry one or more genes which mostly code for useful characteristic of host. All plasmids have sequence that can act as origin of replication. Plasmids of different sizes and possessing different copy number are present.
- Phage vectors are consist of mainly DNA molecule (sometimes RNA), that carrys large number of genes and are surrounded by a protein coat called as capsid. They can be used as vehicles for carrying DNA insert after modification to remove pathogenic genes and minimising the size.
- Cosmids are hybrid between a phage DNA and bacterial plasmid. They have cos sites which are essentially required for packaging lambda (λ) into phage protein coat. They can carry large DNA insert.
- Fosmids are cosmid like plasmid but they are based on F-plasmid.
- Phagemids are plasmids having a part of M13 genome.
- Artificial chromosomes are artificially constructed DNA construct used for transferring DNA.

Preparation of vector DNA

The vector DNA is cleaved by restriction endonucleases at the site where foreign DNA is desired to be inserted. The restriction enzyme is selected to generate a configuration at the cleavage site compatible with the ends of the foreign DNA. This can be achieved either by cleaving the foreign DNA and vector DNA with the same restriction enzyme or by adding adaptors/ linkers to both the ends of the insert DNA.

Preparation of DNA to be cloned

DNA to be cloned can be obtained by:

1. Cutting using restriction enzyme from genomic or organellar DNA.
2. PCR based amplification.
3. Chemical synthesis.

The DNA to be cloned is isolated and treated with restriction enzymes to generate random fragments with ends capable of being linked to those of the vector. While choosing the restriction enzyme to cut the desired gene, care should be taken so that the restriction enzyme does not cut in the middle of the gene, but only at the ends. PCR based methods are used to obtain DNA segments, using either genomic DNA or mRNA as template sequences through reverse transcription. Short length sequences can be artificially synthesised *in vitro*. If necessary, linkers or adapters containing desired restriction sites are added to create the ends which are compatible with the vector. The complementary sticky ends result in an efficient ligation due to the formation a stable structure.

Creation of recombinant DNA by ligation

- The vector DNA, foreign DNA and DNA ligase enzyme are added together at appropriate concentrations which results in the covalent linkage between the ends of DNA fragments.
- DNA ligase recognises the ends of linear DNA molecules and gives a complex mixture of DNA molecules with randomly joined ends (Fig. 12.4).
- The resulting recombinant DNA vector is then introduced into the host organism.

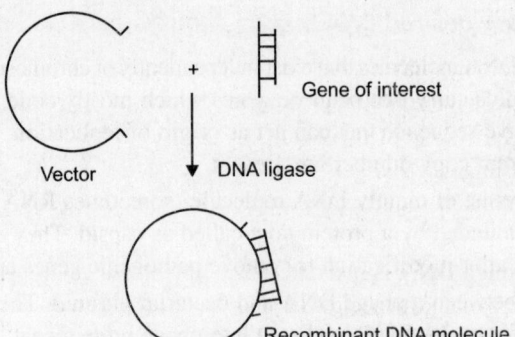

Fig 12.4: Preparation of recombinant DNA.

- In addition to desired recombinant DNA, complex mixture containing self ligated vector DNA, foreign DNA linked with other sequences and several other combinations of vector and foreign DNA also appear in the reaction mixture.
- Sorting of the complex mixture is done by agarose gel electrophoresis based on size of the recombinant vector.

Introduction of recombinant DNA into host organism

- For the propagation of a cloned gene, the recombinant DNA molecules have to be introduced into a host.
- Numerous methods of gene transfer are available to meet the diverse requirement and compatibility with the host (e.g. transformation, transduction, transfection, electroporation, etc.).
- Transformation is the process in which microorganisms are able to take up the DNA from their surrounding via plasma membrane and express it. Cells should be competent to take up the foreign DNA.
- DNA transfer into mammalian cells cultured *in vitro* using non-viral vectors is termed as transfection.
- Transduction is the process of transfer of DNA molecule using viruses.
- Both transformation and transfection requires preparation of the cells through a specific growth condition and chemical treatment process that varies with the specific species and cell types to be used. For example – Calcium chloride is used for preparation of competent *E. coli* cells.
- Electroporation uses electrical pulses to create transient holes in the cell membrane through which DNA is translocated across the cell membrane. Cell wall has to be previously removed in plants to increase the rate of transfer. Electroporation is usually done by two methods: (i) high voltage for short time, and (ii) low voltage for long time.
- Electroporation and transduction are very efficient methods to transfer DNA into cells.

Selection of host cells/organism containing vector sequences

Selection of the transformed cells from the non-transformed population is done by using selectable marker genes that confers resistance to antibiotics. Hence, cells only having the vector with the resistance gene for the antibiotic would grow in the selection media containing the antibiotic (ampicillin, tetracycline, etc.), while the non-transformed cells would die.

Screening clones having desired DNA inserts with the help of biological properties

- After selection of colonies having the vector, the next step is to screen the colonies having the recombinant vector (vector containing foreign DNA insert).
- Bacterial cloning vectors (e.g. pUC19, pGEM vectors) use the blue-white screening system based on lacZ system to distinguish transgenic cells from those that contain the parental vector (i.e. vector DNA with no recombinant sequence inserted). The recombinant colonies are grown in presence of X-gal.
- In these vectors, foreign DNA is inserted into a sequence that encodes an essential part of beta-galactosidase (an enzyme which cleaves galactose). Its activity results in formation of a blue colour colony on the culture medium (Fig. 12.5).
- Insertion of the foreign DNA into the beta-galactosidase coding sequence disrupts the function of the enzyme, and colonies containing recombinant plasmids give no blue colour (white).
- Using this colour phenotype, transgenic bacterial clones can be easily identified from those that do not contain recombinant DNA.

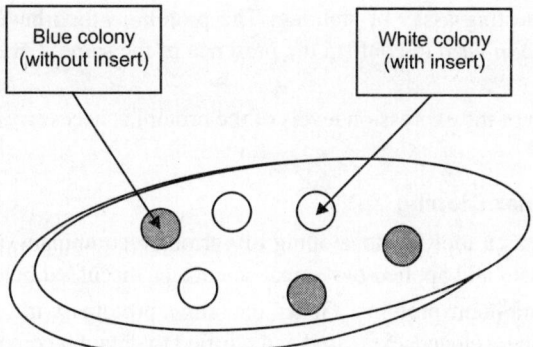

Fig. 12.5: Screening for clones with desired DNA inserts.

Insertional inactivation of antibiotic gene can also be used for the selection of recombinant cells:

- A vector is chosen where restriction sites are available for cloning within the antibiotic gene. Insertion of a foreign gene in the restriction site will lead to the loss of activity of the selectable marker (antibiotic) gene. For example-pBR322 have several restriction sites. BamH1 cuts at a one position within genes that code for tetracycline resistance. Thus recombinant pBR322 carrying foreign DNA at BamH1 site will not confer resistance to tetracycline, but are still resistant to ampicillin, which remains elsewhere.
- These recombinant cells are selected by replica plating method. The transformed cells are first plated on ampicillin containing medium and after the selection of transformed from non-transformed, the colonies are replica plated on medium containing tetracycline for screening of recombinant clones. After incubation, the viable colonies carrying pBR322 without DNA insert will appear and the positions in plate where the non-viable recombinant clones are present can be easily identified. Using the original master plate, these recombinant clones are picked up and subcultured using the same procedure to obtain a pure recombinant clone.

Screening for expression

Gene expression involves the synthesis of mRNA through transcription followed by synthesis of protein through translation. If the purpose of cloning is to express a foreign gene, it is necessary to check the expression both at the mRNA and protein level in terms of quality and quantity.

Screening for foreign gene mRNA transcript can be done by:

- Northern blotting: It involves the electrophoresis for the separation of RNA on the basis of size, and then transfer of RNA from the electrophoresis gel to the blotting membrane. It is then detected by a hybridization probe complementary to target sequence.
- Reverse transcriptase PCR: The RNA strand is reverse transcribed into its DNA complement (cDNA) using the enzyme reverse transcriptase and the resulting cDNA are then amplified using routine PCR method.

Screening for foreign protein is done by:

- Western blotting: It involves the process of electrophoretic separation of cellular proteins followed by transfer to a blotting membrane, incubation with a complimentary primary antibody probe and detection with a labelled secondary antibody.
- Activity/functional testing assay or staining: The proteins which have specific functionality or activity can be tested *in vitro* to confirm the presence of the same. For example, protease activity testing or staining.

Quantitative evaluation of the expression levels of the protein is necessary to achieve desired amount of protein.

Applications of Molecular Cloning

Molecular cloning serves as a tool for developing of various recombinant cells and organisms which has application both in basic and applied biological science as discussed below.

- Production of recombinant proteins: Genes encoding proteins with diagnostic, therapeutic or commercial value can be cloned, expressed and purified to obtain recombinant proteins in bulk with limited space and lesser time. Examples include Humulin – the human insulin expressed in *E. coli*.
- Gene therapy is used for correcting a disorder or deficiency.
- To study the structure and function of a particular gene using a model host organism.
- To study the regulation of gene expression during developmental stages.
- Complete genome sequence of an organism having large genome size can be facilitated by BAC or YAC library formation using rDNA technology.

POLYMERASE CHAIN REACTION

The polymerase chain reaction (PCR) is a technique in molecular biology to amplify a single or few copies of a piece of DNA across several orders of magnitude, generating thousands to millions of copies of a particular DNA sequence. The method relies on thermal cycling, consisting of cycles of repeated heating and cooling of the reaction for DNA melting and enzymatic replication of the DNA. Primers (short DNA fragments) containing sequences complementary to the target region along with a DNA polymerase (after which the method is named) are key components to enable selective and repeated amplification. As PCR progresses, the DNA generated is itself used as a template for replication, setting in motion a chain reaction in which the DNA template is exponentially amplified. PCR can be extensively modified to perform a wide array of genetic manipulations. Almost all PCR applications employ a heat-stable DNA polymerase, such as Taq polymerase, an enzyme originally isolated from the bacterium *Thermus aquaticus*. This DNA polymerase enzymatically assembles a new DNA strand from DNA building blocks, the nucleotides, by using single-stranded DNA as a template and DNA oligonucleotides (also called DNA primers), which are required for initiation of DNA synthesis.

The vast majority of PCR methods use thermal cycling, i.e. alternately heating and cooling the PCR sample to a defined series of temperature steps. These thermal cycling steps are necessary first to physically separate the two strands in a DNA double helix at a high temperature in a process called DNA melting. At a lower temperature, each strand is then used as the template in DNA synthesis by the DNA polymerase to selectively amplify the target DNA. The selectivity of PCR results from the use of primers that are complementary to the DNA region targeted for amplification under specific thermal cycling conditions. PCR is now a common and often indispensable technique used in medical and biological research labs for a variety of applications. These include DNA cloning for sequencing, DNA-based phylogeny, or functional analysis of genes, the diagnosis of hereditary diseases, the identification of genetic fingerprints (used in forensic sciences and paternity testing), and the detection and diagnosis of infectious diseases.

PCR Principles and Procedure

PCR is used to amplify a specific region of a DNA strand (the DNA target). Most PCR methods typically amplify DNA fragments of up to ~10 kilo base pairs (kb), although some techniques allow for amplification of fragments up to 40 kb in size.

A basic PCR set up requires several components and reagents. These components include:

1. DNA template that contains the DNA region (target) to be amplified.
2. Two primers that are complementary to the 3′ (three prime) ends of each of the sense and anti-sense strand of the DNA target.
3. Taq polymerase or another DNA polymerase with a temperature optimum at around 70°C.
4. Deoxynucleoside triphosphates (dNTPs, also very commonly and erroneously called deoxynucleotide triphosphates), the building blocks from which the DNA polymerases synthesises a new DNA strand.
5. Buffer solution, providing a suitable chemical environment for optimum activity and stability of the DNA polymerase.
6. Divalent cations, magnesium or manganese ions, generally Mg^{2+} is used, but Mn^{2+} can be utilised for PCR-mediated DNA mutagenesis, as higher Mn^{2+} concentration increases the error rate during DNA synthesis.
7. Monovalent cation potassium ions.

The PCR is commonly carried out in a reaction volume of 10–200 μl in small reaction tubes (0.2–0.5 ml volumes) in a thermal cycler. The thermal cycler heats and cools the reaction tubes to achieve the temperatures required at each step of the reaction. Many modern thermal cyclers make use of the Peltier effect which permits both heating and cooling of the block holding the PCR tubes simply by reversing the electric current. Thin-walled reaction tubes permit favourable thermal conductivity to allow for rapid thermal equilibration. Most thermal cyclers have heated lids to prevent condensation at the top of the reaction tube. Older thermocyclers lacking a heated lid require a layer of oil on top of the reaction mixture or a ball of wax inside the tube.

Procedure

Typically, PCR consists of a series of 20–40 repeated temperature changes, called cycles, with each cycle commonly consisting of 2–3 discrete temperature steps. Most protocols call for cycles that have three temperature steps (Fig. 12.6). The cycling is often preceded by a single temperature step (called *hold*) at a high temperature (>90°C), and followed by one hold at the end for final product extension or brief storage. The temperatures used and the length of time they are applied in each cycle depend on a variety of parameters. These include the enzyme used for DNA synthesis, the concentration of divalent ions and dNTPs in the reaction, and the melting temperature (T_m) of the primers.

1. Initialisation step: This step consists of heating the reaction to a temperature of 94°–96°C (or 98 °C if extremely thermostable polymerases are used), which is held for 1–9 minutes. It is only required for DNA polymerases that require heat activation by hot-start PCR.

2. Denaturation step: This step is the first regular cycling event and consists of heating the reaction to 94°–98°C for 20–30 seconds. It causes DNA melting of the DNA template by disrupting the hydrogen bonds between complementary bases, yielding single-stranded DNA molecules.

3. Annealing step: The reaction temperature is lowered to 50°–65°C for 20–40 seconds allowing annealing of the primers to the single-stranded DNA template. Typically the annealing temperature is about 3–5 degrees Celsius below the T_m of the primers used. Stable DNA-DNA hydrogen bonds are only formed when the primer sequence very closely matches the template sequence. The polymerase binds to the primer-template hybrid and begins DNA synthesis.

4. Extension/elongation step: The temperature at this step depends on the DNA polymerase used, Taq polymerase has its optimum activity temperature at 75°–80°C, and commonly a temperature of 72°C is used with this enzyme. At this step the DNA polymerase synthesises a new DNA strand complementary to the DNA template strand by adding dNTPs that are complementary to the template in 5′ to 3′ direction, condensing the 5′-phosphate group of the dNTPs with the 3′-hydroxyl group at the end of the nascent (extending) DNA strand. The extension time depends both on the DNA polymerase used and on the length of the DNA fragment to be amplified. As a rule-of-thumb, at its optimum temperature, the DNA polymerase will polymerise a thousand bases per minute. Under optimum conditions, i.e. if there are no limitations due to limiting substrates or reagents, at each extension step, the amount of DNA target is doubled, leading to exponential (geometric) amplification of the specific DNA fragment.

5. Final elongation: This single step is occasionally performed at a temperature of 70°–74°C for 5–15 minutes after the last PCR cycle to ensure that any remaining single-stranded DNA is fully extended.

6. Final hold: This step at 4°–15°C for an indefinite time may be employed for short-term storage of the reaction.

To check whether the PCR generated the anticipated DNA fragment (also sometimes referred to as the amplimer or amplicon), agarose gel electrophoresis is employed for size separation of the PCR products. The size(s) of PCR products is determined by comparison with a DNA ladder (a molecular weight marker), which contains DNA fragments of known size, run on the gel alongside the PCR products.

PCR Stages

The PCR process can be divided into three stages:

1. Exponential amplification: At every cycle, the amount of product is doubled (assuming 100 per cent reaction efficiency). The reaction is very sensitive: Only minute quantities of DNA need to be present.

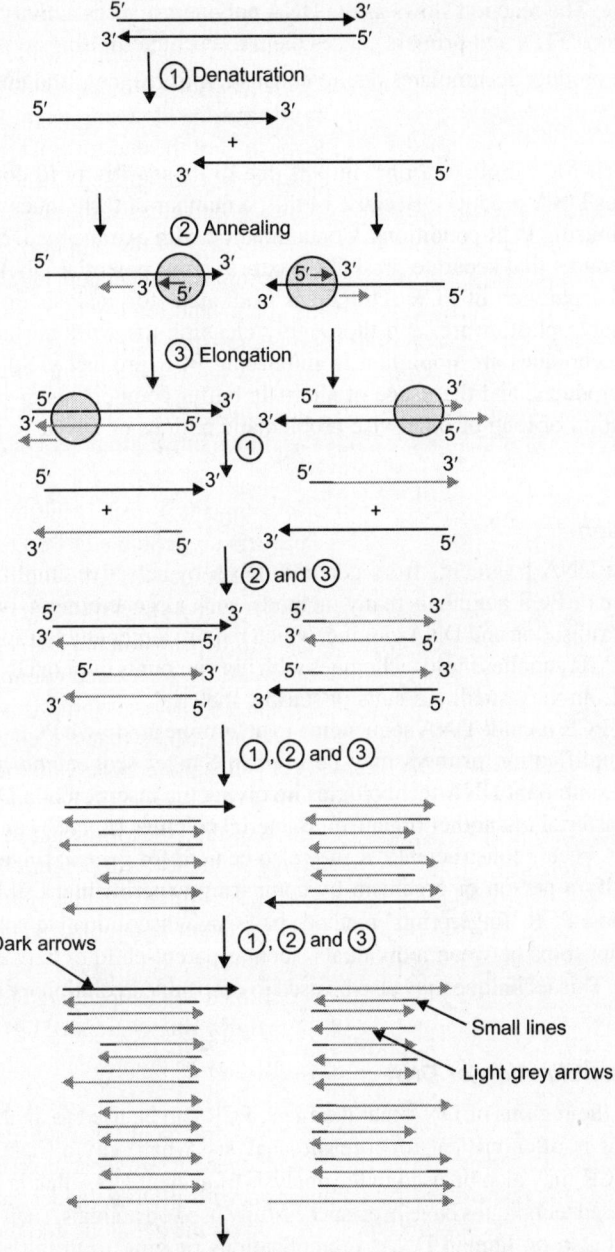

Fig. 12.6: Schematic drawing of the PCR cycle. (1) Denaturing at 94°–96°C. (2) Annealing at ~65°C. (3) Elongation at 72°C. Four cycles are shown here. The dark arrows represent the DNA template to which primers (smal lines) anneal that are extended by the DNA polymerase (light grey circles), to give shorter DNA products (light grey arrows), which themselves are used as templates as PCR progresses.

2. Levelling off stage: The reaction slows as the DNA polymerase loses activity and as consumption of reagents such as dNTPs and primers causes them to become limiting.

3. Plateau: No more product accumulates due to exhaustion of reagents and enzyme.

PCR optimisation

In practice, PCR can fail for various reasons, in part due to its sensitivity to contamination causing amplification of spurious DNA products. Because of this, a number of techniques and procedures have been developed for optimising PCR conditions. Contamination with extraneous DNA is addressed with lab protocols and procedures that separate pre-PCR mixtures from potential DNA contaminants. This usually involves spatial separation of PCR-setup areas from areas for analysis or purification of PCR products, use of disposable plasticware, and thoroughly cleaning the work surface between reaction setups. Primer-design techniques are important in improving PCR product yield and in avoiding the formation of spurious products, and the usage of alternate buffer components or polymerase enzymes can help with amplification of long or otherwise problematic regions of DNA.

Application of PCR

Selective DNA isolation

PCR allows isolation of DNA fragments from genomic DNA by selective amplification of a specific region of DNA. This use of PCR augments many methods, such as generating hybridisation probes for southern or northern hybridisation and DNA cloning, which require larger amounts of DNA, representing a specific DNA region. PCR supplies these techniques with high amounts of pure DNA, enabling analysis of DNA samples even from very small amounts of starting material.

Other applications of PCR include DNA sequencing to determine unknown PCR-amplified sequences in which one of the amplification primers may be used in Sanger sequencing, isolation of a DNA sequence to expedite recombinant DNA technologies involving the insertion of a DNA sequence into a plasmid or the genetic material of another organism. Bacterial colonies (*E. coli*) can be rapidly screened by PCR for correct DNA vector constructs. PCR may also be used for genetic fingerprinting, a forensic technique used to identify a person or organism by comparing experimental DNAs through different PCR-based methods. Some PCR 'fingerprints' methods have high discriminative power and can be used to identify genetic relationships between individuals, such as parent-child or between siblings, and are used in paternity testing. This technique may also be used to determine evolutionary relationships among organisms.

Amplification and quantification of DNA

Because PCR amplifies the regions of DNA that it targets, PCR can be used to analyse extremely small amounts of sample. This is often critical for forensic analysis, when only a trace amount of DNA is available as evidence. PCR may also be used in the analysis of ancient DNA that is tens of thousands of years old. These PCR-based techniques have been successfully used on animals, such as a forty-thousand-year-old mammoth, and also on human DNA, in applications ranging from the analysis of Egyptian mummies to the identification of a Russian tsar. Quantitative PCR methods allow the estimation of the amount of a given sequence present in a sample — a technique often applied to quantitatively determine levels of gene expression. Real-time PCR is an established tool for DNA quantification that measures the accumulation of DNA product after each round of PCR amplification.

PCR in diagnosis of diseases

PCR permits early diagnosis of malignant diseases such as leukemia and lymphomas, which is currently the highest developed in cancer research and is already being used routinely. PCR assays can be performed directly on genomic DNA samples to detect translocation-specific malignant cells at a sensitivity which is at least 10,000 fold higher than other methods. PCR also permits identification of non-cultivatable or slow-growing micro-organisms such as mycobacteria, anaerobic bacteria, or viruses from tissue culture assays and animal models. The basis for PCR diagnostic applications in microbiology is the detection of infectious agents and the discrimination of non-pathogenic from pathogenic strains by virtue of specific genes. Viral DNA can likewise be detected by PCR.

The primers used need to be specific to the targeted sequences in the DNA of a virus, and the PCR can be used for diagnostic analyses or DNA sequencing of the viral genome. The high sensitivity of PCR permits virus detection soon after infection and even before the onset of disease. Such early detection may give physicians a significant lead in treatment. The amount of virus ('viral load') in a patient can also be quantified by PCR-based DNA quantitation techniques.

Variations on the Basic PCR Technique

1. Allele-specific PCR: A diagnostic or cloning technique which is based on single-nucleotide polymorphisms (SNPs) (single-base differences in DNA). It requires prior knowledge of a DNA sequence, including differences between alleles, and uses primers whose 3' ends encompass the SNP. PCR amplification under stringent conditions is much less efficient in the presence of a mismatch between template and primer, so successful amplification with an SNP-specific primer signals presence of the specific SNP in a sequence.

2. Assembly PCR or polymerase cycling assembly (PCA): Artificial synthesis of long DNA sequences by performing PCR on a pool of long oligonucleotides with short overlapping segments. The oligonucleotides alternate between sense and antisense directions, and the overlapping segments determine the order of the PCR fragments, thereby selectively producing the final long DNA product.

3. Asymmetric PCR: Preferentially amplifies one DNA strand in a double-stranded DNA template. It is used in sequencing and hybridisation probing where amplification of only one of the two complementary strands is required. PCR is carried out as usual, but with a great excess of the primer for the strand targeted for amplification. Because of the slow (arithmetic) amplification later in the reaction after the limiting primer has been used up, extra cycles of PCR are required. A recent modification on this process, known as Linear-after-the-exponential-PCR (LATE-PCR), uses a limiting primer with a higher melting temperature (T_m) than the excess primer to maintain reaction efficiency as the limiting primer concentration decreases mid-reaction.

4. Helicase-dependent amplification: Similar to traditional PCR, but uses a constant temperature rather than cycling through denaturation and annealing/extension cycles. DNA helicase, an enzyme that unwinds DNA, is used in place of thermal denaturation.

5. Hot-start PCR: A technique that reduces non-specific amplification during the initial set up stages of the PCR. It may be performed manually by heating the reaction components to the melting temperature (e.g. 95°C) before adding the polymerase. Specialised enzyme systems have been developed that inhibit the polymerase's activity at ambient temperature, either by the binding of an antibody or by the presence of covalently bound inhibitors that only dissociate after a high-

temperature activation step. Hot-start/cold-finish PCR is achieved with new hybrid polymerases that are inactive at ambient temperature and are instantly activated at elongation temperature.

6. Intersequence-specific PCR (ISSR): A PCR method for DNA fingerprinting that amplifies regions between simple sequence repeats to produce a unique fingerprint of amplified fragment lengths.

7. Inverse PCR: Inverse PCR is commonly used to identify the flanking sequences around genomic inserts. It involves a series of DNA digestions and self ligation, resulting in known sequences at either end of the unknown sequence.

8. Ligation-mediated PCR: Uses small DNA linkers ligated to the DNA of interest and multiple primers annealing to the DNA linkers, it has been used for DNA sequencing, genome walking, and DNA footprinting.

9. Methylation-specific PCR (MSP): Developed by Stephen Baylin and Jim Herman at the Johns Hopkins School of Medicine, and is used to detect methylation of CpG islands in genomic DNA. DNA is first treated with sodium bisulphite, which converts unmethylated cytosine bases to uracil, which is recognised by PCR primers as thymine. Two PCRs are then carried out on the modified DNA, using primer sets identical except at any CpG islands within the primer sequences. At these points, one primer set recognises DNA with cytosines to amplify methylated DNA, and one set recognises DNA with uracil or thymine to amplify unmethylated DNA. MSP using qPCR can also be performed to obtain quantitative rather than qualitative information about methylation.

10. Miniprimer PCR: Uses a thermostable polymerase (S-Tbr) that can extend from short primers ('smalligos') as short as 9 or 10 nucleotides. This method permits PCR targeting to smaller primer binding regions, and is used to amplify conserved DNA sequences, such as the 16S (or eukaryotic 18S) rRNA gene.

11. Multiplex ligation-dependent probe amplification (MLPA): Permits multiple targets to be amplified with only a single primer pair, thus avoiding the resolution limitations of multiplex PCR.

12. Multiplex-PCR: Consists of multiple primer sets within a single PCR mixture to produce amplicons of varying sizes that are specific to different DNA sequences. By targeting multiple genes at once, additional information may be gained from a single test run that otherwise would require several times the reagents and more time to perform. Annealing temperatures for each of the primer sets must be optimised to work correctly within a single reaction, and amplicon sizes, i.e. their base pair length, should be different enough to form distinct bands when visualised by gel electrophoresis.

13. Nested PCR: Increases the specificity of DNA amplification, by reducing background due to non-specific amplification of DNA. Two sets of primers are used in two successive PCRs. In the first reaction, one pair of primers is used to generate DNA products, which besides the intended target, may still consist of non-specifically amplified DNA fragments. The product(s) are then used in a second PCR with a set of primers whose binding sites are completely or partially different from and located 3′ of each of the primers used in the first reaction. Nested PCR is often more successful in specifically amplifying long DNA fragments than conventional PCR, but it requires more detailed knowledge of the target sequences.

14. Overlap-extension PCR: A genetic engineering technique allowing the construction of a DNA sequence with an alteration inserted beyond the limit of the longest practical primer length.

15. Quantitative PCR (Q-PCR): Used to measure the quantity of a PCR product (commonly in real-time). It quantitatively measures starting amounts of DNA, cDNA or RNA. Q-PCR is commonly used to determine whether a DNA sequence is present in a sample and the number of its copies in

the sample. Quantitative real time PCR has a very high degree of precision. QRT-PCR methods use fluorescent dyes, such as Sybr Green, EvaGreen or fluorophore-containing DNA probes, such as TaqMan, to measure the amount of amplified product in real time. It is also sometimes abbreviated to RT-PCR (real time PCR) or RQ-PCR. QRT-PCR or RTQ-PCR are more appropriate contractions, since RT-PCR commonly refers to reverse transcription PCR, often used in conjunction with Q-PCR.

16. Reverse transcription PCR (RT-PCR): For amplifying DNA from RNA. Reverse transcriptase reverse transcribes RNA into cDNA, which is then amplified by PCR. RT-PCR is widely used in expression profiling, to determine the expression of a gene or to identify the sequence of an RNA transcript, including transcription start and termination sites. If the genomic DNA sequence of a gene is known, RT-PCR can be used to map the location of exons and introns in the gene. The 5′ end of a gene (corresponding to the transcription start site) is typically identified by RACE-PCR (Rapid Amplification of cDNA Ends).

17. Solid phase PCR: Encompasses multiple meanings, including Polony Amplification (where PCR colonies are derived in a gel matrix, for example), Bridge PCR (primers are covalently linked to a solid-support surface), conventional Solid Phase PCR (where Asymmetric PCR is applied in the presence of solid support bearing primer with sequence matching one of the aqueous primers) and enhanced solid phase PCR (where conventional Solid Phase PCR can be improved by employing high T_m and nested solid support primer with optional application of a thermal 'step' to favour solid support priming).

18. Thermal asymmetric interlaced PCR (TAIL-PCR): For isolation of an unknown sequence flanking a known sequence. Within the known sequence, TAIL-PCR uses a nested pair of primers with differing annealing temperatures, a degenerate primer is used to amplify in the other direction from the unknown sequence.

19. Touchdown PCR (Step-down PCR): A variant of PCR that aims to reduce nonspecific background by gradually lowering the annealing temperature as PCR cycling progresses. The annealing temperature at the initial cycles is usually a few degrees (3°–5°C) above the T_m of the primers used, while at the later cycles, it is a few degrees (3°–5°C) below the primer T_m. The higher temperatures give greater specificity for primer binding, and the lower temperatures permit more efficient amplification from the specific products formed during the initial cycles.

20. PAN-AC: Uses isothermal conditions for amplification, and may be used in living cells.

21. Universal fast walking: For genome walking and genetic fingerprinting using a more specific 'two-sided' PCR than conventional 'one-sided' approaches (using only one gene-specific primer and one general primer-which can lead to artefactual 'noise') by virtue of a mechanism involving lariat structure formation. Streamlined derivatives of UFW are LaNe RAGE (lariat-dependent nested PCR for rapid amplification of genomic DNA ends), 5′RACE LaNe and 3′RACE LaNe.

Chapter 13

Genomic Library and DNA Sequencing

INTRODUCTION

A genomic library is an organism specific collection of DNA covering the entire genome of an organism. It contains all DNA sequences such as expressed genes, non-expressed genes, exons and introns, promoter and terminator regions and intervening DNA sequences.

CONSTRUCTION OF GENOMIC LIBRARY

Construction of a genomic DNA library involves isolation, purification and fragmentation of genomic DNA followed by cloning of the fragmented DNA using suitable vectors. The eukaryotic cell nuclei are purified by digestion with protease and organic (phenol-chloroform) extraction. The derived genomic DNA is too large to incorporate into a vector and needs to be broken up into desirable fragment sizes. Fragmentation of DNA can be achieved by physical method and enzymatic method. The library created contains representative copies of all DNA fragments present within the genome.

Mechanisms for Cleaving DNA

Physical method

It involves mechanical shearing of genomic DNA using a narrow-gauge syringe needle or sonication to break up the DNA into suitable size fragments that can be cloned. Typically, an average DNA fragment size of about 20 kb is desirable for cloning into λ based vectors. DNA fragmentation is random which may result in variable sized DNA fragments. This method requires large quantities of DNA.

Enzymatic method

- It involves use of restriction enzyme for the fragmentation of purified DNA.
- This method is limited by distribution probability of site prone to the action of restriction enzymes which will generate shorter DNA fragments than the desired size.
- To overcome this problem, partial digestion of the DNA molecule is usually carried out using known quantity of restriction enzyme to obtain fragments of ideal size.

- If, a gene to be cloned contains multiple recognition sites for a particular restriction enzyme, the complete digestion will generate fragments that are generally too small to clone. As a consequence, the gene may not be represented within a library (Fig. 13.1).
- The two factors which govern the selection of the restriction enzymes are- type of ends (blunt or sticky) generated by the enzyme action and susceptibility of the enzyme to chemical modification of bases like methylation which can inhibit the enzyme activity.
- The fragments of desired size can be recovered by either agarose gel electrophoresis or sucrose gradient technique and ligated to suitable vectors.

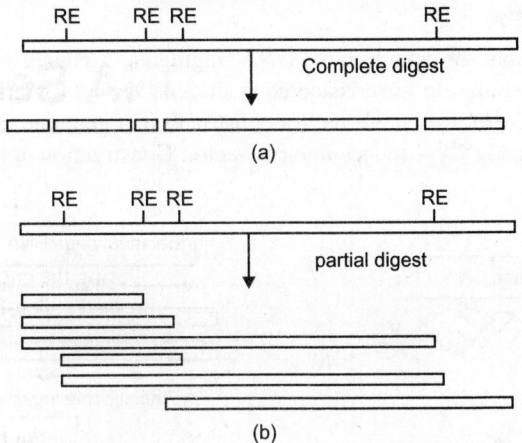

Fig. 13.1: The complete (a) and partial (b) digestion of a DNA fragment using restriction enzymes.

Partial restriction digestion is achieved using restriction enzymes that produce blunt or sticky ends as described below:

1. Restriction enzymes generating blunt ends: The genomic DNA can be digested using restriction enzymes that generate blunt ends, e.g. *HaeIII* and *AluI*.

Hae III: 5' - GG | CC - 3'   Alu I: 5' - AG | CT - 3'

3' - CC | GG - 5'   3' - TC | GA - 5'

Blunt ends are converted into sticky ends prior to cloning. These blunt ended DNA fragments can be ligated to oligonucleotides that contain the recognition sequence for a restriction enzyme called linkers or possess an overhanging sticky end for cloning into particular restriction sites called adaptors.

- Linkers: Linkers are short stretches of double stranded DNA of length 8–14 bp that have recognition site for restriction enzymes. Linkers are ligated to blunt end DNA by ligase enzyme. The linker ligation is more efficient as compared to blunt-end ligation of larger molecules because of the presence of high concentration of these small molecules in the reaction. The ligated DNA can be digested with appropriate restriction enzyme generating cohesive ends required for cloning in a vector. The restriction sites for the enzyme used to generate cohesive ends may be present within the target DNA fragment which may limit their use for cloning.

- Adapters: These are short stretches of oligonucleotide with cohesive ends or a linker digested with restriction enzymes prior to ligation. Addition of adaptors to the ends of a DNA converts the blunt ends into cohesive ends.

2. Restriction enzymes that generate sticky ends: Genomic DNA can be digested with commonly available restriction enzymes that generate sticky ends. For example, digestion of genomic DNA with the restriction enzyme *Sau3AI* (recognition sequence 5'-GATC-3') generates DNA fragments that are compatible with the sticky end produced by *BamHI* (recognition sequence 5'-GGATCC-3') cleavage of a vector. Once the DNA fragments are produced, they are cloned into a suitable vector.

Cloning of Genomic DNA

Various vectors are available for cloning large DNA fragments. λ phage, yeast artificial chromosome, bacterial artificial chromosome, etc. are considered as suitable vectors for larger DNA and λ replacement vectors like λ*DASH* and *EMBL3* are preferred for construction of genomic DNA library. T4 DNA ligase is used to ligate the selected DNA sequence into the vector. Construction of genomic library is shown in Fig. 13.2.

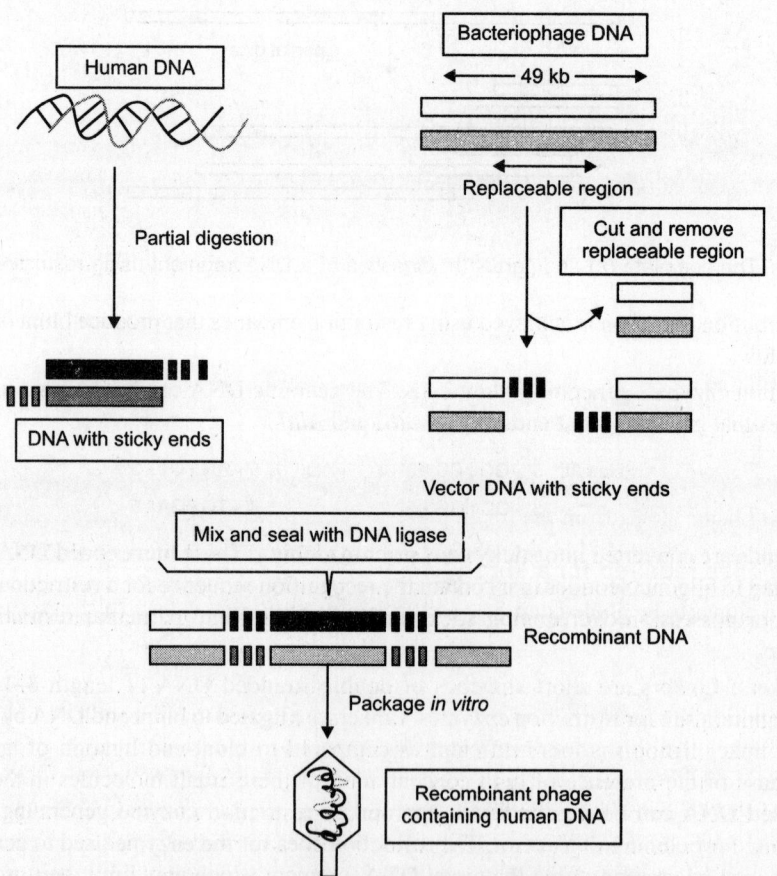

Fig. 13.2: Construction of genomic library

λ *replacement vectors*

The λ*EMBL* series of vectors are widely used for genomic library construction. The multiple cloning sites of these vectors flanking the stuffer fragment contain opposed promoters for the T3 and T7 RNA polymerases. The restriction digestion of the recombinant vector generates short fragments of insert DNA left attached to these promoters. This generates RNA probes for the ends of the DNA insert. These vectors can be made conveniently, directly from the vector, without recourse to sub-cloning.

High-capacity vectors

The high capacity cloning vectors used for the construction of genomic libraries are cosmids, bacterial artificial chromosomes (BACs), P1-derived artificial chromosomes (PACs) and yeast artificial chromosomes (YACs). They are designed to handle longer DNA inserts, much larger than for λ replacement vectors. So they require lower number of recombinantsto be screened for identification of a particular gene of interest. Vectors used for cloning genomic libraries is shown in Table 13.1.

Table 13.1: Vectors used for cloning genomic libraries.

Vector	*Insert size*	*Features*
λ phages	Up to 20–30 kb	Genome size-47 kb, efficient packaging system, replacement vectors usually employed, used to study individual genes
Cosmids	Up to 40 kb	Contains *cos* site of λ phage to allow packaging, propagate in *E. coli* as plasmids, useful for sub-cloning of DNA inserts from YAC, BAC, PAC, etc.
Fosmids	35-45 kb	Contains F plasmid origin of replication and λ*cos* site, low copy number, stable
Bacterial artificial chromosomes (BACs)	Up to 300kb	Based on F-plasmid, relatively large and high capacity vectors
P1 artificial chromosomes (PACs)	Up to 300 kb	Derived from DNA of P1 bacteriophage, combines the features of P1 and BACs, used to clone larger genes and in physical mapping, chromosome walking as well as shotgun sequencing of complex genomes.
Yeast artificial chromosomes (YACs)	Up to 2000kb	Allow identification of successful transformants (BAC clones are highly stable and highly efficient)

The recombinant vectors and insert combinations are grown in *E. coli* such that a single bacterial colony or viral plaque arises from the ligation of a single genomic DNA fragment into the vector.

Number of clones required for a library

The number of clones to be pooled depends upon the size of the genome *f* and average size of the cloned DNA.

Let (*f*) be the fraction of the genome size compared to the average individual cloned fragment size, would represent the lowest possible number of clones that the library must contain.

The minimum number of clones required can be calculated as- *f* = genome size/fragment size.

For the *E. coli* genome (4.6 Mb) with an average cloned fragment size of 5 kb, *f* will be 920.

The number of independent recombinants required in the library must be greater than *f*, as sampling variation leads to the several times inclusion and exclusion of some sequences in a library of just *f* recombinants. In 1976, Clarke and Carbon derived a formula to calculate probability (P) of including any DNA sequence in a random library of *N* independent recombinants.

The actual number of clones required can be calculated as:

$$N = \frac{\ln (1 - P)}{\ln (1 - 1/f)}$$

where, N = number of clones and P = probability that a given gene will be present.

Bigger the library better will be the chance of finding the gene of interest. The pooling together of either recombinant plaques or bacterial colonies generates a primary library.

Amplified Library

- The primary library created is usually of a low titer and unstable. The stability and titer can be increased by amplification. For this, the phages or bacterial colonies are plated out several times and the resulting progenies are collected to form an amplified library.
- The amplified library can then be stored almost indefinitely due to longshelf-life of phages.
- It usually has a much larger volume than the primary library, and consequently may be screened several times.
- It is possible that the amplification process will result in the composition of the amplified library not truly reflecting the primary one.
- Certain DNA sequences may be relatively toxic to *E. coli* cells. As a consequence bacteria harboring such clones will grow more slowly than other bacteria harboring non-toxic DNA sequences. Such problematic DNA sequences present in the primary library may be lost or under-represented after the growth phase required to produce the amplified library.

Subgenomic Library

Subgenomic library is a library which represents only a fraction of the genome. Enhancing the fold of purification of target DNA is crucial for subgenomic DNA libraries which can be achieved by multiple, sequential digestion when information of the restriction map of the sequences of interest is known. After initial purification of a given fragment, the purification can further be increased by redigestion with another enzyme generating a smaller (clonable) fragment relative to original DNA.

Advantages of Genomic Libraries

- Identification of a clone encoding a particular gene of interest.
- It is useful for prokaryotic organisms having relatively small genomes.
- Genomic libraries from eukaryotic organisms are very important to study the genome sequence of a particular gene, including its regulatory sequences and its pattern of introns and exons.

Disadvantages of Genomic Library

- Genome libraries from eukaryotes having very large genomes contain a lot of DNA which does not code for proteins and also contain non-coding DNA such as repetitive DNA and regulatory regions which makes them less than ideal.
- Genomic library from a eukaryotic organism will not work if the screening method requires the expression of a gene.

Applications of Genomic Library

- To determine the complete genome sequence of a given organism.
- To study and generate transgenic animals through genetic engineering, serving as a source of genomic sequence.
- To study the function of regulatory sequences *in vitro*.
- To study the genetic mutations.
- Used for genome mapping, sequencing and the assembly of clone contigs.

Comparison of Genomic and cDNA Libraries

cDNA library has revolutionised the field of molecular genetics and recombinant DNA technology. It consists of a population of bacterial transformants or phage lysates in which each mRNA isolated from an organism is represented as its cDNA insertion in a vector. cDNA libraries are used to express eukaryotic genes in prokaryotes. In addition, cDNAs are used to generate expressed sequence tags (ESTs) and splices variant analysis. Some of the differences of cDNA library with genomic library are presented in Table 13.2.

Table 13.2: Features of genomic and cDNA library.

Feature	Genomic library	cDNA library
Sequences present	Ideally, all genomic sequences	Only structural genes that are transcribed
Contents affected by:		
(a) Developmental stage	No	Yes
(b) Cell type	No	Yes
Features of DNA inserts representing a gene:		
(a) Size	As present in genome	Ordinarily, much smaller
(b) Introns	Present	Absent
(c) 5'- and 3'-regulatory sequences	Present	Absent
As compared to the genome		
(a) Enrichment of sequences	In amplified genomic libraries	For abundant mRNAs
(b) Redundancy in frequency	In amplified libraries	For rare mRNA species
(c) Variant forms of a gene	Not possible	For such genes, whose RNA transcripts are alternatively spliced

DNA SEQUENCES

Deoxyribonucleic acid (DNA) contains genetic information of an organism that is unique for each organism. The entire cellular DNA of any organism, bacteria, plant or animal is known as its genome, as is the entire genetic material of a virus. A DNA sequence is considered to be unique if it is present in only one copy in a haploid genome. A haploid genome contains only a single copy of each chromosome. In humans, for example, a haploid number of chromosomes is 23. However, not all of the DNA contained in the genome is considered as unique, there are also various repetitive sequences present.

DNA and Genome Structure

A DNA strand is composed of a strand of nucleotides (nitrogen-based building blocks of DNA and RNA). Each nucleotide contains a phosphate attached to a sugar molecule (deoxiribose) and one of four bases, guanine (G), cytosine (C), adenine (A) or thymine (T). It is the arrangement of the bases in a sequence, for example ATTGCCAT, that determines the encoded gene. This sequence allows scientists to identify organisms, genes, or fragments of genes. One of the main characteristics of DNA is the fact that it forms double stranded molecules (helices) by forming hydrogen bonds between the complementary strands inside the helix and a sugar-phosphate backbone outside. This pairing is not random, A always pairs with T, and C pairs with G, therefore, a sequence complementary to ATTCCGAT will be TAAGGCTA.

Genes are the sequences of encoded proteins, and together with the surrounding regulatory sequences are, considered as unique genomic sequences, because they are present as single copies in a haploid genome. In contrast, some sequences are present in multiple copies and are known as repetitive fragments. The simplest genomes of viruses and bacteria contain mostly unique sequences with only a few repetitive regions. However, the proportion of repetitive DNA increases in higher organisms, for example sea urchins have only 38% unique sequences and human just over 50%.

The genes encoding the same protein in bacteria, plants, and humans show some similarity as the majority of the encoded proteins perform the same or similar function across the species. Such homology between the sequences allows scientists to identify the genes in humans by using fragments of mouse or yeast genes to search for similar DNA fragments. Although most of the genes show some species-dependent differences, not all of them can be used to discriminate between organisms. Only a few genes can be used for this purpose. The two main groups are ribosomal (16S in bacteria and 18S in animals) and mitochondrial genes.

Ribosomal genes are useful for tracing evolution and relationships, especially in bacteria. However, mitochondrial genes have an advantage over the ribosomal genes as they are not encoded by the nuclear DNA, but are present as circular molecules in the cells. As such they are less likely to be degraded with time, therefore bones, teeth, or tissue fragments can be identified even after a long time.

Exploiting Unique DNA Sequences

The presence of unique DNA sequences allows scientists to identify signature sequences that can be later used as probes to detect individual organisms or to detect a particular gene. Changes of even one base pair can be readily detected by most hybridisation techniques and by sequencing. Signature sequences are particularly important for diagnosis of viruses, which are the pathogens that lack ribosomal or mitochondrial genes. Their detection and identification is greatly simplified by using these sequences, as traditional methods can take up to a few weeks.

The unique DNA sequences can also be used to design primers (short DNA fragments needed to initiate DNA amplification) for polymerase chain reaction (PCR). There is adequate difference between all the genes within one organism, as well as between organisms from different species, to ensure that the selected primers will only amplify the target sequence even if a mixture of different DNA molecules is present. This allows scientists to design diagnostic and identification tests for the common pathogens and diseases and for parts of the pathogen's genome.

Identification of people: Although every person has unique DNA (except for the identical twins), identification of people is not based on the sequencing of someone's genome. Instead, analysis of mitochondrial DNA in a region of a displacement-loop (D-loop or control region) or of short tandem repeats (STRs) is used for identification purposes. D-loop analysis is used for individual identification in forensic analysis. This is possible due to the polymorphisms of such sequences resulting from substitutions of base pairs during DNA replication process (for example, instead of A, DNA polymerase incorporates T).

The D-loop region is 1274 base pairs long and is located between the genes encoding transfer RNA (tRNA) for proline and tRNA for phenylalanine and contains the regulatory regions of the for replication other genes.

The main method used for the identification of the changes in this region is PCR amplification and sequencing. However, new microarray approaches are under development.

Encoding secret messages: DNA sequences offer a unique method of encrypting messages or concealing information. A DNA sequence encoding a message is flanked on the sites by primers that will be later used to amplify if by PCR and sequence. An encryption code is selected by a group that is using the system, for example, each letter and number might be assigned three base pairs. The DNA strand with a message is prepared and mixed with human genomic DNA fractionated to the same size as the message. To further conceal the DNA from an enemy, DNA from another species can be added. An intended recipient of the message can decode it by PCR amplification and sequencing. Sending such as message is as simple as writing a letter and enclosing the DNA coded message as a microdot. Once the DNA mix is prepared, it is spotted over a dot on paper from which the microdots are cut out and attached to the full stops in the letter. If such a letter falls into the wrong hands finding a message will be extremely difficult, as it will be buried among millions of others, and reading it without the primer sequences and encryption code will be impossible.

DNA encrypted messages can be used for safekeeping important information, but also to pass on espionage information. Although the method is simple, it requires molecular biology equipment to decode and can be too troublesome for everyday use.

Use of Unique DNA Sequences

Unique DNA sequences are already used as security tools. The ability to synthetically create DNA molecules allows the generation not only of spy messages, but more importantly, unique signatures that would protect consumers from product fakes. Similar methods were used at the Sydney Olympic Games in 2000 to mark all of the official merchandise. In this case, an invisible ink mixed with DNA obtained from one of the athletes was used. Protection is not limited to manufacturers. Unique DNA sequences are also used by artists such as Thomas Kinkade and cartoon creator Joseph Barbera, who protect their artwork by DNA signatures.

The major use of unique DNA sequences for security, however, is in the area of environmental surveillance and identification of agents of biological warfare. The sequences used for these purposes are often kept secret. Most of the producers of DNA recognition instruments use such sequences to design their products.

Finally, forensic science relies in many cases on the use of unique sequences for identification of biological traces and individual identification.

Repeated Sequence (DNA)

Repeated sequences (aka. repetitive elements, or repeats) are patterns of nucleic acids (DNA or RNA) that occur in multiple copies throughout the genome. The functions and descriptions of these sequences are currently being characterised by scientists. Repetitive DNA was first detected because of its rapid reassociation kinetics.

Types

There are 3 major categories of repeated sequence or repeats:

- Terminal repeats.
- Tandem repeats: Copies which lie adjacent to each other, either directly or inverted.
  - o Satellite DNA: Typically found in centromeres and heterochromatin.
  - o Minisatellite: Tepeat units from about 10 to 60 base pairs, found in many places in the genome, including the centromeres.
  - o Microsatellite: Repeat units of less than 10 base pairs, this includes telomeres, which typically have 6 to 8 base pair repeat units.
- Interspersed repeats (aka. interspersed nuclear elements).
  - o Transposable elements.
    - » DNA transposons.
    - » Retrotransposons.
      LTR-retrotranposons (HERVs)
      Non LTR-retrotranposons
      SINEs (Short Interspersed Nuclear Elements)
      LINEs (Long Interspersed Nuclear Elements)
      SVAs

In primates, the majority of LINEs are LINE-1 and the majority of SINEs are Alu's. SVAs are hominoid specific. In prokaryotes, CRISPR are arrays of alternating repeats and spacers.

Other types repeated sequences

- Direct repeats:
  - o Global direct repeat.
  - o Local direct simple repeats.
  - o Local direct repeats.
  - o Local direct repeats with spacer.
- Inverted repeats:
  - o Global inverted repeat.
  - o Local inverted repeat.
  - o Inverted repeat with spacer.
  - o Palindromic repeat.
- Mirror and everted repeats.

SECTION VI

Genomics, Proteomics, Genome Annotation, Bacterial and Eukaryotic Genomes, Comparative and Minimal Genomics and Genome Mapping

Chapter 14

Genomics, Proteomics and Genome Annotation

INTRODUCTION

Bioinformatics is basically database mining—the extraction, sorting and analysing of sequence information about genes, genomes and proteins. Genes have to be sequenced, in order to do that, they must be isolated and cloned into the appropriate form which will allow them to be manipulated in the laboratory. Therefore, cloning and sequencing are not part of bioinformatics per second. Cloning and sequencing, combined with bioinformatics, however, are interwoven activities. The technical advancement of one activity greatly impacts the other two. The increasing numbers of sequences improve the quality of statistical analysis, while the development of new bioinformatics software allows for the identification of biological functions associated with sequence patterns, thus allowing faster detection and cloning of novel genes.

DNA CLONING AND PCR

DNA sequences are often found based on predictive tools, meaning that sequence similarities of newly discovered genes yield information about their physiological functions and structures, PCR (polymerase chain reaction), finding sequence fragments of significance (how is significance judged? By predictive biology, once again), finding distribution of genes or mRNAs (often an indicator of gene activity in an organism) and amplifying the amount of DNA for purification, sequencing and mutational analysis.

Analysing the rapidly accumulating sequence and structure information must be done with accuracy if the underlying methods of obtaining this information are to be evaluated in a critical and timely manner. Therefore, it is helpful to understand the biological background of how DNA and protein sequences are obtained.

DNA Cloning

Cloning is commonly known as the process of asexually producing a group of cells (clones), all genetically identical, from a single ancestor. Here, it refers to the use of DNA manipulation procedures to produce multiple copies of a single gene or segment of DNA through recombinant DNA technology. A desired gene or DNA fragment is cut out of its chromosomal location and inserted into vector DNA that is used for replication (amplification) in a host organism. Such cloning vectors are DNA molecules originating from viruses, bacteria or yeast that contain proper strings of promoter sequences to control gene expression independently of DNA amplification in the host cell. Thus, a bacterial promoter is used on vectors for mammalian expression systems (cell lines). The bacterial RNA polymerase will specifically control the vector DNA, while the cell's genome is unaffected. Unrelated DNA fragments are integrated without loss of the vector's capacity for self-replication in its natural cellular environment, allowing foreign or recombinant DNA to be reproduced in large quantities in host cells. Examples of cloning vectors are plasmids (bacterial origin), cosmids (viral origin), yeast and bacterial artificial chromosomes. Vectors are also called expression vectors when they contain the elements necessary for gene regulation. This feature is used to synthesise large quantities of mRNA or proteins in host organisms that normally do not contain or express these genes.

Behind every sequence stored electronically in a computer database (electronic sequencing) is a physical library of tissue samples and cloned DNA. When originating from genome projects, they are often random collections of genomic DNA obtained through shotgun techniques such as mechanical shearing or *in vitro* radiation-induced chromosome fragmentation. Chromosomal fragments are recombined into expression vectors. The collection of those cloned fragments constitutes a library. A vector DNA contains genes that make possible their functional expression and transformation into cell lines.

Transcriptional Profiling

How is a gene of interest selected? A gene is a sequence of base pairs and despite the ability to predict a protein's function, experimental work to study the biochemistry and physiology of the actual protein is necessary. Yet before proceeding to laborious cell biology and biochemistry, the activity pattern of a gene (i.e. within which cells in a body and at what time of development or life stage a gene is expressed and a protein synthesised) is often the first piece of information used to select an 'interesting' project or to identify a useful 'target' for drug discovery. Specifically, some genes may be restricted to certain cell types, tissues or organs, their activity patterns may change from healthy to diseased (like tumours) or may differ among young and old people. How can the functional significance of a gene for a specific cell type, tissue or organism be evaluated? First, cells where a gene is expressed (Northern blotting) must be found. This is done by finding the corresponding messenger RNA that serves as the intermediary template for protein synthesis (the m in mRNA stands for messenger, meaning that the RNA sequence is used to translate or forward the DNA sequence information into an amino acid sequence). Cytoplasmic levels (concentrations) of mRNA are good indicators for gene activity. High levels of mRNA are in many, but not all, cases indicative of the presence of a protein. The presence of protein levels must be demonstrated independently, if it is to be established as fact.

Identifying mRNA is done by hybridising (binding) radio-active labelled oligonucleotides in a sequence-specific manner to isolate target mRNA. Obviously, some sequence information must be obtained in advance. This information could have been derived from short amino acid sequences obtained from protein fragments or peptides or by searching the DNA databases for sequences with desired properties such as a human homolog to a known gene from a mouse or rat or simply a similar, but not homologous sequence representing a potential novel gene and so forth. Comparing the hybridisation pattern of different samples at varying times during the life cycle of an organism or cell, before or after differentiation during development or under varying conditions (resting vs. hormone-induced state), can be used to construct a time-space map of where in the body a specific gene or groups of genes are actively expressed. Once the presence of a gene of interest has been verified, DNA fragments containing the gene need to be isolated and amplified. One strategy is to use enzyme reverse transcriptase (RT) which produces a DNA copy of the mRNA fragment. The gene that codes for the mRNA can be synthesised *in vitro* and is known as complementary DNA or cDNA. The cDNA represents the coding sequence of a gene including short noncoding or flanking, regions on either side that contain regulatory sequences. It is imperative to understand the importance of the coding sequence of eukaryotic genes because of the particularity of how most eukaryotic genes are organised on the chromosomes in the cell nucleus, which differs from the sequence found on the mRNA. A cDNA sequence of an eukaryotic gene is normally shorter than the genomic version due to the organisation of genes into coding (exons) and noncoding (introns) regions. Although the entire gene (intron plus exon plus control sequences) is transcribed into an mRNA, the mRNA will be catalytically modified in order to eliminate the introns or intervening sequences. This leaves a shortened mRNA—a combination of all exon fragments found at the genome level. This is why the use of mRNA for the synthesis of cDNA yields synthetic genes that differ from their genomic origin and can be cloned into vector DNA for easier use in the laboratory (such as *in vitro* biosynthesis of proteins, transformation of DNA into new cell lines and transgenic animals).

Positional Cloning

An alternative strategy used for the detection of hereditary disease genes is positional cloning. Here, a gene that causes a disease or contributes to the development of one, is first located on the chromosome using genetic markers, which are short, easily detectable sequences preferentially on noncoding parts of the genome. For this method, family histories must be available for analysis of the population genetics for those genes that contain mutations and appear at a specific frequency in the human population (alleles). An allele refers to a particular gene within the genome of every individual in a population. The actual sequence of the gene, however, may vary from individual to individual due to the random occurrence of mutations. While many mutations have no visible effect on the phenotype (i.e. the function of the protein), occasional mutations can cause the malfunctioning of this protein. Once a chromosomal location has been identified, clones with large inserts are identified by physical mapping, with subsequent identification of the gene(s) by sequencing. Finally, a mutation analysis compares the identified gene(s) in affected and unaffected members of a population.

Once the entire genome sequence is known, the human genome projects promise much faster identification of mutations related to diseases. Of course, the chosen sequence representing the human genome contains only one of two loci of any given gene within a population. The human genome sequence will, in fact, be the sequence of an individual revealing little information about allelic variants in a population. This will be achieved by a phenotypically selective partial genome comparison. Thus, mutation analysis of different members of the population is still a necessary step in the positional cloning approach, since no individual's genome can possibly be sequenced in its entirety. Polymorphism databases are specifically constructed to yield this information.

In addition, medical databases for every disease, susceptibility for infection, cancer and possibly psychological traits can be envisioned for the future.

Polymerase Chain Reaction (PCR)

The technique that revolutionised DNA amplification is polymerase chain reaction (PCR). This technique is used in virtually every biomedical laboratory in the world. The process has been automated and machines that amplify DNA from small quantities into large ones are commercially available. The process, from template design (oligonucleotide to find a target gene sequence in the genome library) to mapping an organ for gene expression, is done by computer programme. The increasing numbers of sequences allow the search for functional units of unknown genes. Large-scale identification of gene expression by measuring messenger RNA levels allows researchers to keep pace with the sequencing results of genome projects (public and proprietary libraries and databases). DNA sequences can be used to generate short search sequences to screen for mRNA. In an effort to increase the efficiency of finding good drug targets, the pharmaceutical industry is developing multiarray plate and microchip assays where hundreds, even thousands, of gene fragments or cell types can be screened in a single assay.

DNA chip technology developed by Affymetrix in Santa Clara, California is leading the technology push to determine tissue distribution of expressed genes and so-called expression sequence tags (ESTs). The importance of PCR to bioinformatics—and the genome projects in particular—is its ability to amplify DNA without any biological information attached. This means that both coding and noncoding regions can be analysed as long as short stretches of sequence (between 10 and 20 nucleotides long) are known. The technique is also extremely sensitive to initial sample quantity because of the enzymatically controlled DNA amplification process in noncellular test tube solutions.

GENOME ANALYSIS

Genome analysis can determine locations of genes on chromosomes and give information on heritability and linkage to other genes, genetics (classical), medical importance, gene therapy, tracking autosomal mutations and X-linked diseases. The yeast protein database (YPD) links information of DNA sequences, protein structure and function, cellular localisation and pathways and cell-cycle information into one coherent database with links to literature information, a commercial approach with the intention of selling database access to companies, proteomics as compared to genomics, 2-D gel electrophoresis, image processing, storage, retrieval and pattern recognition.

Genome Organisation

Bioinformatics tools and databases are slowly becoming an integrated system that reflects the complexity of organisms. With genome projects of small organisms being completed one by one, an understanding of the differences of genomes from the three urkingdoms (eubacteria, archaea and eukaryotes) and the relationship of genome organisation to the form and function of an organism may be just around the corner. Prokaryotes have very different genome structures compared to eukaryotes. While their names refer to the absence or presence of a nuclear compartment within the cell, the differences do not stop there. The relative frequency of coding vs. noncoding regions differs as do the arrangements of genes on the chromosomes. While bacteria have a compact genome with little noncoding DNA, eukaryotic chromosomes are often extremely large and found in great numbers, especially in plants. The genes of eukaryotes and the prokaryotic archaea are often fragmented into noncontinuous 'exons'.

Special databases containing entire genomes of organisms provide information such as relatedness of genes within the genome, closeness in space, coregulation, etc. For example, metabolic pathways in different bacterial species may vary because of an additional enzymatic step in one species but not another. The way to find out is to see if specific proteins belong to a cluster of genes (this structure is an operon) that is often aligned along the micro-organism's genome such that an entire pathway for the synthesis of an amino acid is upregulated in a coordinated fashion, avoiding the individual regulation of every enzyme needed for a pathway. The existence of pathways and multiple genes coding for the enzymes of pathways has important consequences on how mutations affect cellular physiology. Mutations affecting an enzyme that is part of a pathway may affect this entire pathway because it, as such, constitutes a phenotype. The progress in sequencing entire genomes of both prokaryotic and eukaryotic organisms will undoubtedly help in determining the physiological role of organisational structures of genomes and its importance for metabolic processes.

Although genes are important because they code for all the proteins and RNA existing in a cell, these structural genes often constitute a fraction of genomes, particularly in eukaryotic organisms—fungi, plants and animals. For example, an estimated 90 per cent of the human genome constitutes noncoding regions. It was not that long ago that these noncoding regions were casually dismissed as junk DNA, reflecting a lack of understanding and knowledge of their function. More and more, the DNA that does not code for proteins or RNA (regulatory, structural and enzymatic) is being recognised as important in how cells have access to the coding 10 per cent of DNA. Essentially, this noncoding DNA is important in replication and control of cell-specific gene expression. It seems to contain information that is 'read only' (short sequences that function as specific binding sites for proteins involved in gene expression and replication). Such proteins are growth factor or hormone receptors. These protein-binding elements are crucial for cells and play a role in cell differentiation, morphogenesis and pattern formation during embryogenesis.

The implications of noncoding regions in DNA on evolution is tremendous. Because mutations are random events, the noncoding parts of chromosomes absorb most of these changes in base composition and serve as a 'playground' for chromosomal recombination and accumulation of silent mutations. Polymorphic markers (the markers used in DNA fingerprinting technology) are found in this portion of the DNA. A surprising finding of genetic analysis of clusters of genes from different individuals reflects the high frequency of nucleotide sequence differences between individuals (restriction fragment length polymorphism: reflects sequence variations in DNA sites that can be cleaved by DNA restriction enzymes). This genetic polymorphism has recently been used in forensic science. This so-called genetic 'fingerprinting' yields information unique to one individual in several billion. Genetic fingerprinting has changed our court system. The use of PCR has been successful in identification since very tiny tissue samples from blood stains, dead skin or a single hair found at a crime scene are enough to amplify DNA for analysis.

To understand the relationship between the 'blueprint' of life and life itself requires information about the relative position of genes within the genome, as well as the relationship between sequence and structure in proteins. Since proteins are not isolated entities and multiple protein-protein interactions are the basis of cellular activity, selection pressure on individual genes is likely to be coupled over several genes whose proteins work together. This makes sequence-to-structure and structure-to-function relationships extremely complex. The multitude of interactions is too complex. New technologies such as genomics and proteomics, where the simultaneous expression levels of RNA or proteins are determined, are starting points to address the complex molecular interactions involved in cells.

How do we measure independence and interdependence of inheritable properties? We can refer to Gregor Mendel and his study of independently inherited traits on the colour and consistency of peas. At the molecular level, two independent traits (phenotype) are coded for by genes (or alleles) located on physically separated chromosomes. If they are located on the same chromosome they are regularly—but not necessarily—inherited together (because the distance between genes on the same chromosome is also crucial), i.e. they are said not to segregate.

The importance of genome structures and chromosomal stability can be demonstrated in studies of the molecular evolution of histone proteins—the proteins responsible for the packing and storage of DNA into high-density forms of our chromosomes. During cell division, chromosomes condense into the well-known, double-arm structures (pairs of chromosomes, see karyotype), but during the normal resting state of a cell, these chromosomes are loosely packed and amenable to the proteins that transcribe genes into RNA (polymerase) and others which control access to DNA (transcription factors). This is the essence of gene regulation (transcription or expression). It is a balance of access to DNA strands among structural proteins (or histones), the nucleic acid synthesising proteins (or polymerases) and DNA binding proteins (or transcription factors) which control accessibility of polymerases to the DNA molecule.

The importance of gene transcription in the viability of organisms is obvious, since genes code for proteins and proteins control every process within a cell. The importance of chromosome structure, however, is less clear, but evidence indicates that interfering with the structure of chromosomes is lethal for cells. Analysing the amino acid sequence of histone proteins has provided one line of evidence. Histone genes are highly conserved across all species within the eukaryotic kingdom. They are a key feature of the genetics of animals, plants and fungi. Their conserved sequences also indicate a single evolutionary ancestor cell or organism from which all modern eukaryotes are derived. Indeed, histone proteins are used as molecular docks, molecular rulers to measure the phylogenetic distance (time since separation of two species) between distantly related organisms. The survival of an organism (or a population) is linked to its phenotype and hereditary changes in phenotype (mutations) occur and are stored exclusively at the DNA level by random changes in the base composition (DNA sequence). Mutations are 'rejected' if the phenotype confers a lethal trait. The organism either dies before reaching reproductive age or becomes infertile, thus losing the chance to pass its genome to the next generation. The rate of mutations accumulating in a gene (nucleotide sequences which are not rejected) over time is a direct measure of the importance of the phenotype (the protein) to the viability of the individual, but not of the population. Allelic variations within a population, however, are indicators of the susceptibility of specific genes to mutations. Histone genes show an extremely low mutation rate over hundreds of millions of years indicating that the structure of these proteins is essential for all eukaryotic organisms. This means that besides gene replication and transcription, differential DNA packing in chromosomes during different states of the cell cycle is crucial for survival.

Genomics, the attempt to catalog the gene content, organisation and temporal expression patterns of a genome, will give detailed information about the evolution of cellular function. It is therefore not surprising that the Internet has become an essential tool for scientists because of the many databases containing information about the genomes of thousands of species, their taxonomy and evolutionary relationship in the form of phylogenetic trees or 'the tree of life'. Phylogenetic trees are visual ways of understanding evolutionary relationships.

The tree of life is a figurative representation of the diversifying life forms on earth originating from a common ancestor. It is believed that there is only one such tree (e.g. a single progenitor 'cell') and that life is not of multiple origin. Although reasonable and consistent with the findings of molecular biologists, this is speculative and corroborates the notion of the slim chance of life having arisen by chance out of nonliving matter. That this event happened is not disputed here, but it is astounding since scientists agree that the spontaneous generation of new life from (in-) organic material is highly unlikely.

The tree of life project provides a visual overview of the phylogeny of all life on earth. It is not a molecular evolution type of tree, but a classical taxonomy tree. This is a very useful tool for molecular biologists who often have no formal training in evolution, zoology, botany and ecology. The project contains information about the diversity of organisms on Earth, their history and characteristics. It is a multi-authored website coordinated and created by David R. Maddison at the University of Arizona.

Proteins can be found as part of larger protein complexes and only within the context of these complexes can the activity of these proteins be studied. They are not independent, thus their genes cannot be independent, yet some proteins linked through functional complex formation are coded by genes found randomly, without any apparent linkage on different chromosomes. Is there significance for such an apparent lack of organisation of certain groups of genes in the human genome? The red blood cell protein haemoglobin, the transport molecule in our blood that helps carry oxygen from the lungs to target muscles or organs like the brain, is made of four tightly packed protein subunits coded for by two different genes. The genes are called alpha and beta globin genes and the functional haemoglobin protein complex contains two copies of each gene product. Although these two genes always need to be expressed together for the proper complex formation (there is no functional haemoglobin made of four alpha subunits or four beta subunits), the globin gene coding for the alpha subunit is actually a cluster of alpha globin genes with slightly different sequences and is differentially expressed during subsequent embryonic stages. Thus, only one gene copy of the alpha cluster is expressed at any given time during development. While clusters are located close to each other, the alpha subunit cluster is found on chromosome 16, while the cluster for beta globin subunits is found on chromosome 11.

Anatomical and physiological phenotypes are multi-trait phenotypes, meaning that several gene products constitute the genotype. Besides the obvious visual characteristics of an individual's appearance, cellular metabolism is the best example for studying multi-enzyme pathways. The synthesis and degradation of metabolites such as sugars, fats, amino acids and lipids are part of these complex, interdependent pathways. The organisation of genes that constitute a pathway for individual metabolites in genomes is different for different organisms. As a rule, there is no strict correlation between proteins that functionally and structurally interact with each other and the position of their genes on chromosomes. Sometimes such genes are closely grouped into functional units in gene expression and are often loosely scattered all over the genome. Functional genomics may help shed some light on this problem.

There is a definite relationship between a particular DNA sequence and the chromosomal morphology of the organism. The following distinct morphological (structural) features have been established:

1. Telomeric regions (tandemly repeated sequences, ageing related).
2. Centromeric regions (tandemly repeated sequences).
3. Nucleolar organiser (genes for ribosomal RNA, relate to Fig. 14.1 of metacentric chromosome pair).

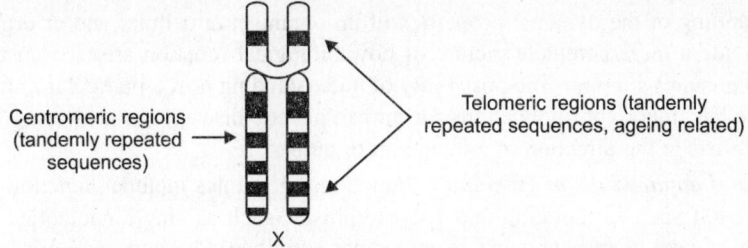

Centromeric regions (tandemly repeated sequences)

Telomeric regions (tandemly repeated sequences, ageing related)

X

Fig. 14.1: Chromosome pair, G-banding and chromosome identification.

Because of the relationship between gene function and chromosome structure, the physical mapping of genomes is essential to gaining an understanding of the uniqueness of an organism and its developmental plan (stages of life cycle). The uniqueness of an organism lies not only in its gene composition, but also its chromosome structure. Mammalian chromosomes come in metacentric and acrocentric form. It has been shown that one reason members of different species (although closely related in their gene sequences) are reproductively incompatible is that their chromosomal structures (the superstructure of DNA which is also dependent on histone proteins) are incompatible during cell fusion and division (mitosis, meiosis). Here we can see the emergence of a loop where genes coding for histone proteins are regulated by how these proteins interact with each other and DNA to form the superstructure of chromosomes and which determines the viability of the cell because of its importance during cell division. Nucleotide changes (mutations) in histone genes affect their amino acid composition, which affects chromosome structure, which affects histone gene inheritance (replication) and expression (transcription).

FUNCTIONAL GENOMICS

Functional genomics is a field of molecular biology that attempts to make use of the vast wealth of data produced by genomic projects (such as genome sequencing projects) to describe gene (and protein) functions and interactions. Unlike genomics, functional genomics focuses on the dynamic aspects such as gene transcription, translation, and protein–protein interactions, as opposed to the static aspects of the genomic information such as DNA sequence or structures. Functional genomics attempts to answer questions about the function of DNA at the levels of genes, RNA transcripts, and protein products. A key characteristic of functional genomics studies is their genome-wide approach to these questions, generally involving high-throughput methods rather than a more traditional 'gene-by-gene' approach.

Goals of functional genomics: The goal of functional genomics is to understand the relationship between an organisms genome and its phenotype. The term functional genomics is often used broadly to refer to the many possible approaches to understanding the properties and function of the entirety of an organisms genes and gene products. This definition is somewhat variable, Gibson and Muse define it as 'approaches under development to ascertain the biochemical, cellular, and/or physiological properties of each and every gene product', while Pevsner includes the study of nongenic elements in his definition: 'the genome-wide study of the function of DNA (including genes and nongenic elements), as well as the nucleic acid and protein products encoded by DNA'. Functional genomics involves studies of natural variation in genes, RNA, and proteins over time (such as an organisms development) or space (such as its body regions), as well as studies of natural or experimental functional disruptions affecting genes, chromosomes, RNA, or proteins.

The promise of functional genomics is to expand and synthesise genomic and proteomic knowledge into an understanding of the dynamic properties of an organism at cellular and/or organismal levels. This would provide a more complete picture of how biological function arises from the information encoded in an organisms genome. The possibility of understanding how a particular mutation leads to a given phenotype has important implications for human genetic diseases, as answering these questions could point scientists in the direction of a treatment or cure.

Techniques and applications of Genomics: Functional genomics includes function-related aspects of the genome itself such as mutation and polymorphism (such as single nucleotide polymorphism (SNP) analysis), as well as measurement of molecular activities. The latter comprise a number of '-omics' such as transcriptomics (gene expression), proteomics (protein expression), and metabolomics. Functional genomics uses mostly multiplex techniques to measure the abundance of many or all gene products such as mRNAs or proteins within a biological sample. Together these measurement modalities endeavor to quantitate the various biological processes and improve our understanding of gene and protein functions and interactions.

STRUCTURAL GENOMICS

Structural genomics seeks to describe the 3-dimensional structure of every protein encoded by a given genome. This genome-based approach allows for a high-throughput method of structure determination by a combination of experimental and modelling approaches. The principal difference between structural genomics and traditional structural prediction is that structural genomics attempts to determine the structure of every protein encoded by the genome, rather than focusing on one particular protein. With full-genome sequences available, structure prediction can be done more quickly through a combination of experimental and modelling approaches, especially because the availability of large number of sequenced genomes and previously solved protein structures allows scientists to model protein structure on the structures of previously solved homologs. Because protein structure is closely linked with protein function, the structural genomics has the potential to inform knowledge of protein function. In addition to elucidating protein functions, structural genomics can be used to identify novel protein folds and potential targets for drug discovery. Structural genomics involves taking a large number of approaches to structure determination, including experimental methods using genomic sequences or modelling-based approaches based on sequence or structural homology to a protein of known structure or based on chemical and physical principles for a protein with no homology to any known structure.

As opposed to traditional structural biology, the determination of a protein structure through a structural genomics effort often (but not always) comes before anything is known regarding the protein function. This raises new challenges in structural bioinformatics, i.e. determining protein function from its 3D structure. Structural genomics emphasises high throughput determination of protein structures. This is performed in dedicated centers of structural genomics.

While most structural biologists pursue structures of individual proteins or protein groups, specialists in structural genomics pursue structures of proteins on a genome wide scale. This implies large-scale cloning, expression and purification. One main advantage of this approach is economy of scale. On the other hand, the scientific value of some resultant structures is at times questioned. One advantage of structural genomics, such as the Protein Structure Initiative, is that the scientific community gets immediate access to new structures, as well as to reagents such as clones and protein. A disadvantage is that many of these structures are of proteins of unknown function and do not have corresponding publications. This requires new ways of communicating this structural information to the broader research community. The Bioinformatics core of the Joint center for structural genomics (JCSG) has recently developed a wiki-based approach namely Open protein structure annotation network (TOPSAN) (link) for annotating protein structures emerging from high-throughput structural genomics centers.

Goals of structural genomics: One goal of structural genomics is to identify novel protein folds. Experimental methods of protein structure determination require proteins that express and/or crystallise well, which may inherently bias the kinds of proteins folds that this experimental data elucidate. A genomic, modelling-based approach such as *ab initio* modelling may be better able to identify novel protein folds than the experimental approaches because they are not limited by experimental constraints.

Protein function depends on 3-D structure and these 3-D structures are more highly conserved than sequences. Thus, the high-throughput structure determination methods of structural genomics have the potential to inform our understanding of protein functions. This also has potential implications for drug discovery and protein engineering. Furthermore, every protein that is added to the structural database increases the likelihood that the database will include homologous sequences of other unknown proteins. The Protein Structure Initiative (PSI) is a multifaceted effort funded by the National Institutes of Health with various academic and industrial partners that aims to increase knowledge of protein structure using a structural genomics approach and to improve structure-determination methodology.

Methods of structural genomics: Structural genomics takes advantage of completed genome sequences in several ways in order to determine protein structures. The gene sequence of the target protein can also be compared to a known sequence and structural information can then be inferred from the known protein's structure. Structural genomics can be used to predict novel protein folds based on other structural data. Structural genomics can also take modelling-based approach that relies on homology between the unknown protein and a solved protein structure.

de novo methods: Completed genome sequences allow every open reading frame (ORF), the part of a gene that is likely to contain the sequence for the mRNA and protein, to be cloned and expressed as protein. These proteins are then purified and crystallised, and then subjected to one of two types of structure determination: X-ray crystallography and Nuclear Magnetic Resonance (NMR). The whole genome sequence allows for the design of every primer required in order to amplify all of the ORFs, clone them into bacteria, and then express them. By using a whole-genome approach to this traditional method of protein structure determination, all of the proteins encoded by the genome can be expressed at once. This approach allows for the structural determination of every protein that is encoded by the genome.

Modelling-based methods: ab initio modelling: This approach uses protein sequence data and the chemical and physical interactions of the encoded amino acids to predict the 3-D structures of proteins with no homology to solved protein structures. One highly successful method for *ab initio* modelling is the Rosetta programme, which divides the protein into short segments and arranges short polypeptide chain into a low-energy local conformation. Rosetta is available for commercial use and for non-commercial use through its public programme, Robetta.

Sequence-based modelling: This modelling technique compares the gene sequence of an unknown protein with sequences of proteins with known structures. Depending on the degree of similarity between the sequences, the structure of the known protein can be used as a model for solving the structure of the unknown protein. Highly accurate modelling is considered to require at least 50% amino acid sequence identity between the unknown protein and the solved structure. 30–50% sequence identity gives a model of intermediate-accuracy, and sequence identity below 30% gives low-accuracy models. It has been predicted that at least 16,000 protein structures will need to be determined in order for all structural motifs to be represented at least once and thus allowing the structure of any unknown protein to be solved accurately through modelling. One disadvantage of this method, however, is that structure is more conserved than sequence and thus sequence-based modelling may not be the most accurate way to predict protein structures.

Threading: Threading bases structural modelling on fold similarities rather than sequence identity. This method may help identify distantly related proteins and can be used to infer molecular functions.

PROTEOMICS

Proteomics is the large-scale study of proteins, particularly their structures and functions. Proteins are vital parts of living organisms, as they are the main components of the physiological metabolic pathways of cells. The proteome is the entire set of proteins, produced or modified by an organism or system. This varies with time and distinct requirements, or stresses, that a cell or organism undergoes. Proteomics is an interdisciplinary domain formed on the basis of the research and development of the Human Genome

Project, it is also emerging scientific research and exploration of proteomes from the overall level of intracellular protein composition, structure, and its own unique activity patterns. It is an important component of functional genomics. While proteomics generally refers to the large-scale experimental analysis of proteins, it is often specifically used for protein purification and mass spectrometry.

Proteomics and Biological Systems

After genomics and transcriptomics, proteomics is the next step in the study of biological systems. It is more complicated than genomics because an organisms genome is more or less constant, whereas the proteome differs from cell to cell and from time to time. Distinct genes are expressed in different cell types, which means that even the basic set of proteins that are produced in a cell needs to be identified. In the past this phenomenon was done by mRNA analysis, but it was found not to correlate with protein content. It is now known that mRNA is not always translated into protein, and the amount of protein produced for a given amount of mRNA depends on the gene it is transcribed from and on the current physiological state of the cell. Proteomics confirms the presence of the protein and provides a direct measure of the quantity present.

Post-translational modifications

Not only does the translation from mRNA cause differences, but many proteins are also subjected to a wide variety of chemical modifications after translation. Many of these post-translational modifications are critical to the proteins function.

Phosphorylation: One such modification is phosphorylation, which happens to many enzymes and structural proteins in the process of cell signalling. The addition of a phosphate to particular amino acids—most commonly serine and threonine mediated by serine/threonine kinases, or more rarely tyrosine mediated by tyrosine kinases—causes a protein to become a target for binding or interacting with a distinct set of other proteins that recognise the phosphorylated domain. Because protein phosphorylation is one of the most-studied protein modifications, many 'proteomic' efforts are geared to determining the set of phosphorylated proteins in a particular cell or tissue-type under particular circumstances. This alerts the scientist to the signalling pathways that may be active in that instance.

Ubiquitination: Ubiquitin is a small protein that can be affixed to certain protein substrates by enzymes called E3 ubiquitin ligases. Determining which proteins are poly-ubiquitinated helps understand how protein pathways are regulated. This is, therefore, an additional legitimate 'proteomic' study. Similarly, once a researcher determines which substrates are ubiquitinated by each ligase, determining the set of ligases expressed in a particular cell type is helpful.

Additional modifications: Listing all the protein modifications that might be studied in a 'proteomics' project would require a discussion of most of biochemistry. Therefore, a short list illustrates the complexity of the problem. In addition to phosphorylation and ubiquitination, proteins can be subjected to (among others) methylation, acetylation, glycosylation, oxidation and nitrosylation. Some proteins undergo all these modifications, often in time-dependent combinations. This illustrates the potential complexity of studying protein structure and function.

Distinct proteins are made under distinct settings

Even studying a particular cell type, that cell may make different sets of proteins at different times, or under different conditions. Furthermore, as mentioned, any one protein can undergo a wide range of post-translational modifications.

Therefore a 'proteomics' study can become complex, even if the topic of the study is restricted. In more ambitious settings, such as when a biomarker for a tumour is sought–when the proteomics scientist is obliged to study sera samples from multiple cancer patients–the amount of complexity that must be dealt with is as great as in any modern biological project.

Proteomics is the large scale of study of proteins, particularly their function and structure. Proteomics is an excellent approach for studying changes in metabolism in response to different stress conditions.

Protein, highly complex substance that is present in all living organisms. Proteins are the polymers of amino acids. Proteins play an important role in metabolic activities. Primary structure of protein is determined by the sequence of specific amino acids, encoded by the mRNA, which directs the proper folding of the polypeptide chain into the secondary structure. One type of secondary structure is the alpha helix, a region of the polypeptide that folds into a corkscrew shape. Beta strands are linear structures of polypeptides, bonding together to form a flat beta sheet. Turns and coils interact chemically with each other to form the unique three dimensional shape of the proper three dimensional structure creates the final protein. Many proteins, however, have several different polypeptide subunits that make the final active protein. For these proteins, the interactions between the different subunits form the quaternary structure. One of the most promising developments to come from the study of human genes and proteins has been the identification of potential new drugs for the treatments of disease. This relies on genome and proteome information to identify proteins associated with a disease. The term 'proteomics' was first coined in 1995 and was defined as the large-scale characterisation of the entire protein complement of a cell line, tissue, or organism. Proteomics is the large-scale study of proteins particularly their composition, structures, functions, and interactions of the proteins directing the activities of cell. The main theme of interest proteomics it gives a much better understanding of an organism than genomics. Genomics can give a rough estimation of expression of a protein. Most of the proteins function in collaboration with other proteins, and the main goal of proteomics are to identify which proteins interact. After genomics, proteomics is often considered as the advanced step in the study of biological systems. It is much more complicated than genomics, mostly because while an organism's genome is more or less constant, the total protein expression profile always changes with time, micro and macro environmental conditions.

Mass spectrometry (MS) has been widely used in forensic science in the identification of compounds, particularly illicit drugs. MS is a technique that allows the detection of compounds by separating ions by their unique mass (mass-to-charge ratios) using a mass spectrometer. The method relies on the fact that every compound has a unique fragmentation pattern (mass spectrum). The sample is ionised, the sample ions are separated based on their differing masses and relative abundance.

Types of Proteomics

Based on the protein response under stress conditions proteomics are classified into different groups.

Expression proteomics

Expression proteomics is used to study the qualitative and quantitative expression of total proteins under two different conditions. Like the normal cell and treated or diseased cell can be compared to understand the protein that is responsible for the stress or diseased state or the protein that is expressed due to disease. Typically, expression proteomics studies are addressed to the investigation of the expression protein patterns in abnormal cells. For example, compare tumour tissue sample and the normal tissue can be analysed for differential protein expression. 2-D gel electrophoresis, mass spectrometry technique were used to observed the protein expressional changes, which is present and absent in tumour tissue, when compared with normal tissue. These are over expressed and under expressed can be identified and characterised protein activities multi-protein complexes, and signalling pathways. Identification of these proteins will give valuable information about molecular biology of tumour formation and disease-specific manner for use as diagnostic markers or therapeutic targets.

Structural proteomics

Structural proteomics helps to understand three dimensional shape and structural complexities of functional proteins. Structural prediction of a protein when its amino acid sequence is determined directly by sequencing or from the gene with a method called homology modelling. Structural proteomics can give detailed information about the structure and function of protein complexes present in a specific cellular organelle. It is possible to identify all the proteins present in a complex system such as membranes, ribosomes, and cell organelles and to characterise all the protein interactions that can be possible between these proteins and protein complexes. Different technologies such as X-ray crystallography and NMR spectroscopy were mainly used for structure determination.

Functional proteomics

Functional proteomics explains understanding the protein functions as well as unravelling molecular mechanisms within the cell then depend on the identification of the interacting protein partners. The association of an unknown protein with partners belonging to a specific protein complex involved in a particular mechanism would in fact, be strongly suggestive of its biological function. Furthermore detailed description of the cellular signalling pathways might greatly benefit from the elucidation of protein-protein interactions *in vivo*.

Techniques involved in proteomics

In proteomic analysis both analytical and bioinformatics tools were used to characterise protein structure and functions. Analytical techniques 2-D gel electrophoresis, MALDI-TOF MS were used. In case of bioinformatics numbers of software tools were used.

2-D gel electrophoresis

In 2-D gel electrophoresis, protein samples are resolved based on charge, in a step called isoelectric focusing, and then based on molecular weight in second step 13. The result is an image in thousands of small spots, each representing a protein. A good 2-D gel can resolve one thousand to two thousand protein spots, which appear after staining, as dots in the gel. 2-D gel electrophoresis technique is mainly used to compare two similar samples to find specific protein differences.

2-D electrophoresis workflow chart

2-D Electrophoresis workflow chart are shown in Fig. 14.2. Prepare the protein at a concentration and in a solution suitable for IEF. Choose a method that maintains the native charge, solubility, and relative abundance of proteins of interest. Separate proteins according to pI by IEF. Select the appropriate IPG strip length and pH gradient for the desired resolution and sample load. Select appropriate sample loading and separation conditions.

Separate proteins according to size by SDS-PAGE. Select the appropriate gel size and composition and separation conditions. Visualise proteins using either a total protein stain or fluorescent protein tags.

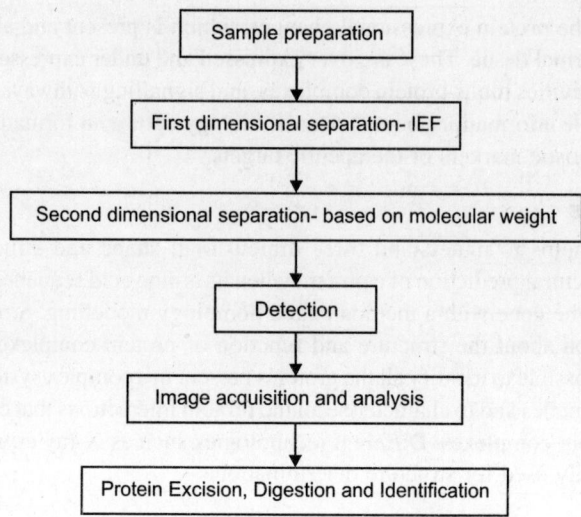

Fig. 14.2: 2-D Electrophoresis workflow chart.

Select a staining technique that matches sensitivity requirements and available imaging equipment. Capture digital images of the 2-D patterns using appropriate imaging equipment and software. Then analyse the patterns using 2-D software. Excise protein spots of interest from the gel digest the proteins, and the digests by MS.

MS analysis

Mass spectrometry is an analytical technique that produces spectra of the masses of the atoms or molecules comprising a sample of material. The spectra are used to determine the elemental or isotopic signature of a sample, the masses of particles and of molecules, and to elucidate the chemical structures of molecules, such as peptides and other chemical compounds. Mass spectrometry works by ionising chemical compounds to generate charged molecules or molecule fragments and measuring their mass to charge ratios. MALDI-TOF is the most useful technique for protein identification.

MALDI-TOF-MS

Matrix Assisted Laser Desorption/Ionisation is a soft ionisation technique used in spectrometry, allowing to analysis the biomolecules like DNA, protein, peptides. Biomolecules and synthetic polymers have low volatility and are thermally unstable, which has limited the use of MS as a means of characterisation. These problems have been minimised through the development of MALDI-TOF MS (Fig. 14.3), which allows for the mass determination of biomolecules by ionisation and vapourisation without degradation, a Laser beam used to ionise the sample.

Protein sample have been characterised by HPLC or SDS PAGE by generating peptide maps. These peptide maps have been used as fingerprints of protein or as a tool to know the purity of a known protein in a known sample. Mass spectrometry gives a peptide map when proteins are digested with proteolytic enzymes like trypsin. This peptide map can be used to search a sequence database to find a good match from the existing database.

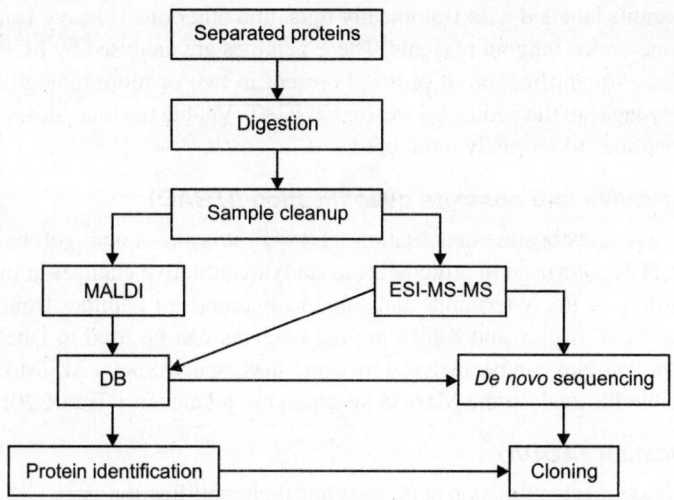

Fig. 14.3: MALDI-TOF MS analysis representing image.

Sample preparation

MALDI-TOF MS is used to characterise, biomolecules like proteins, peptides and polymers of organic compounds. Sample preparation for MALDI-TOF is very interesting and important step. Purify the protein sample before going MALDI-TOF analysis because it is more tolerant to sample contaminants but contaminants can seriously disturb incorporation of sample molecules with growing matrix crystals. Sample can mix with matrix in 1:2 ratio. Different types of matrices are used based on sample, some of matrix are 2-(4-hydroxy phenylazo benzoic acid, 2,4,6-trihydroxyacetophenone, 3-aminoquinolone, cinnamic acid, etc.). Dried droplet technique is predominantly applied for MALDI-TOF analysis, protein sample, mixed with matrix on a metal plate. The combination of matrices yielded slightly performance. Small volumes should be used for standard metal plates. On the other hand, hydrophilic sample anchors are efficient for the generation of small spots.

Matrix

A good matrix consist the following properties, i.e. Matrix must be able to absorb UV wavelength of usually 237 nm, being easily exited and ability to transfer of proton to the sample molecules. Main role of the matrix is adsorption of energy from laser pulse, and then transfer to sample this energy can causes the vapourisation of the sample. For protein samples typical MALDI matrix consist of hydroxylated benzoic acid and cinnamic acid derivatives.

Advanced Methods in Proteomics

Isotope-coded affinity tags (ICAT)

It is a gel- free method for quantitative proteomics that relies on chemical labelling reagents. These chemical probes consist of three general elements, i.e. defined amino acid side chain, an isotopically coded linker, and a tag for the affinity isolation of labelled proteins/peptides. For quantitative comparison of two proteomes, sample labelled with isotopically light, and other one is heavy version. Both samples combined with isotope-coded tagging reagents. These peptides are analysed by LC-MS. The technique mainly used the relative quantification of proteins present in two or more biological samples. Visible isotope-coded affinity tags are the additional method in ICAT- Visible tag that allows the electrophoresis position of tagged peptides to be easily monitored.

Isobaric tags for relative and absolute quantification (iTRAQ)

Isobaric tags for relative and absolute quantitation (iTRAQ), it is also a non- gel- based technique used to quantify proteins. iTRAQ is used in proteomics to study quantitative changes in the proteome. Based on the covalent labelling of the N-terminus and side chain amines of peptides from protein digestions with tags of varying mass, 4-plex and 8-plex are the reagents can be used to label all peptides from different samples. The samples can be analysed by using mass spectrometry MS/MS. Different types of software's are available for analyse the MS/MS spectras, i.e. j-Tracker, j-TraqX 20.

Absolute quantification (AQUA)

AQUA, studies the absolute quantification of proteins and their modification sates. Covalent modifications can be used to prepare synthetic proteins. These modifications are chemically identical to naturally occurring post-translational modifications. These types of peptides used to quantify the post translational modified proteins after proteolysis with the help of tandem mass spectrometer.

ESI-Q-IT-MS

Micro electrospray ionisation (ESI)-Quadrupole ion trap (QIT) Time of flight (TOF) mass spectrometer (MS) has a very good resolution. In ESI ionisation proteins are ionised in solution and carry multiple charge state. The advantage of using ESI-QTOF analysis for protein mass determination is that due to the high charge state of proteins their m/z measurements is typically less than 2000 and the TOF detector has a very good mass accuracy in this scan range. This result is more accurate mass measurements for proteins in ESI-QTOF.

SELDI-TOF-MS

The technique Surface-enhanced laser desorption/ionisation (SELDI) is used for the analysis of protein mixtures, it is an ionisation method in mass spectrometry. SELDI is typically used with time-of-flight mass spectrometers and is used to detect proteins in clinical samples, to compare protein levels with and without a disease can be used for biomarker discovery.

Applications of Proteomics

Proteomics is widely used technique in biological fields, mainly applied in Oncology (Tumour biology), Bio-medicine, Agriculture and Food Microbiology.

Oncology

Oncology refers study of Tumour cell, Tumour metastasis, is the process spread of cancer from one organ to another non-adjacent organ cause death in patients. The major challenge in medicine to describe the molecular and cellular mechanisms underlying tumour metastasis. Analyse the protein expressions correlated to the metastatic process which help to understand the mechanism of metastasis and thus facilitate the development of strategies for the therapeutic interventions and clinical management of cancer. Proteomics is a systematic research, the main aim of this research is to characterise the protein expressions, functions of tumour cells and widely used in biomarker discovery.

Bio-medical applications

The study of interactions between microbial pathogens and their hosts is called 'infectomics'. It is very interesting area in proteomics. It deals with the fundamentals of the infections origin and their effect on organs. The main aim of this research is to prevent or cure disease at starting level. Advanced diagnostic issues related to emerging infections, increasing of fastidious bacteria, and generation of patient- tailored phenotypes.

Agricultural applications

The applications of plant proteomics scientific research is still in budding stage. Proteomics is also used to know plant-insect interactions that help identify candidate genes involved in the defensive response of plants to herbivore. Population growth and effect of global climate changes imposing severe limits on the sustainability of agricultural crop production.

Food Microbiology

The use of proteomics in food technology is presented especially for characterisation and standardisation of raw materials, process development, and detection of batch-to batch variations and quality control of the final product. Further attention is paid to the aspects of food safety, especially regarding biological and microbial safety and the use of genetically modified foods.

Based on the above findings the present review was concluded that the applications for proteomics are relevant to all of the biological process and provides a means to utilise the expressed protein data in a more effective way.

Limitations of Genomics and Proteomics Studies

Proteomics gives a different level of understanding than genomics for many reasons:

- The level of transcription of a gene gives only a rough estimate of its level of translation into a protein. An mRNA produced in abundance may be degraded rapidly or translated inefficiently, resulting in a small amount of protein.
- As mentioned above many proteins experience post-translational modifications that profoundly affect their activities, for example some proteins are not active until they become phosphorylated. Methods such as phosphoproteomics and glycoproteomics are used to study post-translational modifications.
- Many transcripts give rise to more than one protein, through alternative splicing or alternative post-translational modifications.
- Many proteins form complexes with other proteins or RNA molecules, and only function in the presence of these other molecules.
- Protein degradation rate plays an important role in protein content.

Reproducibility: Proteomics experiments conducted in one laboratory are not easily reproduced in another. For instance, Peng and others have identified 1504 yeast proteins in a proteomics experiment of which only 858 were found in a similar previous study. Further, the previous study identified 607 proteins that were not found by Peng and others. This translates to a reproducibility of 57 to 59%.

GENOME ANNOTATION

DNA annotation or genome annotation is the process of identifying the locations of genes and all of the coding regions in a genome and determining what those genes do. An annotation (irrespective of the context) is a note added by way of explanation or commentary. Once a genome is sequenced, it needs to be annotated to make sense of it. For DNA annotation, a previously unknown sequence representation of genetic material is enriched with information relating genomic position to intron-exon boundaries, regulatory sequences, repeats, gene names and protein products.

This annotation is stored in genomic databases such as Mouse Genome Informatics, FlyBase, and WormBase. Educational materials on some aspects of biological annotation from the 2006 Gene Ontology annotation camp and similar events are available at the Gene Ontology website. The National Center for Biomedical Ontology develops tools for automated annotation of database records based on the textual descriptions of those records. As a general method, dcGO has an automated procedure for statistically inferring associations between ontology terms and protein domains or combinations of domains from the existing gene/protein-level annotations.

Process of Genome Annotation

Genome annotation consists of three main steps:

1. Identifying portions of the genome that do not code for proteins.
2. Identifying elements on the genome, a process called gene prediction.
3. Attaching biological information to these elements.

Automatic annotation tools attempt to perform these steps via computer analysis, as opposed to manual annotation which involves human expertise. Ideally, these approaches co-exist and complement each other in the same annotation pipeline.

A simple method of gene annotation relies on homology based search tools, like BLAST, to search for homologous genes in specific databases, the resulting information is then used to annotate genes and genomes. However, as information is added to the annotation platform, manual annotators become capable of deconvoluting discrepancies between genes that are given the same annotation. Some databases use genome context information, similarity scores, experimental data, and integrations of other resources to provide genome annotations through their Subsystems approach. Other databases (e.g. Ensembl) rely on curated data sources as well as a range of different software tools in their automated genome annotation pipeline.

Structural annotation consists of the identification of genomic elements:

- ORFs and their localisation
- Gene structure
- Coding regions
- Location of regulatory motifs

Functional annotation consists of attaching biological information to genomic elements.

- Biochemical function
- Biological function
- Involved regulation and interactions
- Expression

These steps may involve both biological experiments and in silico analysis. Proteogenomics based approaches utilise information from expressed proteins, often derived from mass spectrometry, to improve genomics annotations. A variety of software tools have been developed to permit scientists to view and share genome annotations, example maker.

Genome annotation remains a major challenge for scientists investigating the human genome, now that the genome sequences of more than a thousand human individuals (The 100000 Genomes Project, UK) and several model organisms are largely complete. Identifying the locations of genes and other genetic control elements is often described as defining the biological 'parts list' for the assembly and normal operation of an organism. Scientists are still at an early stage in the process of delineating this parts list and in understanding how all the parts 'fit together'.

Genome annotation is an active area of investigation and involves a number of different organisations in the life science community which publish the results of their efforts in publicly available biological databases accessible via the web and other electronic means.

The most time consuming and costliest aspect of the early stages of a genome project is the collecting the DNA sequence of a genome. This is a linear collection of all the sequences that define the species. But as a dataset, this sequence itself is devoid of content. The genome must be annotated, or described, in a manner that can be of use to biologists of all types. Given the wealth of information that is found within the sequence, it is not too much of a stretch to consider the possibility that in the years following the publication of the sequence much more time and money will be spent on deciphering all the nuances and subtleties.

When genome annotation is first mentioned, what typically comes to mind is the description of the genes that are distributed throughout the genome. The genes themselves contain a wealth of information that helps to describe the species. It is these genes whose collective expression define what the species will look like through out its life cycle, how it will reproduce, and the manner it will respond to its environment. Individually, the coding region of a gene contains the information that defines the nature of an expressed protein or a functional RNA molecule. In the controlling regions of a gene, sequences can be discovered that define where, when, and the degree to which the gene will be expressed. As you can imagine defining genes and their control regions is one aspect of the genome sequence that is of interest to many researchers. But this is not the only information that is important.

Complex eukaryotes also contain a repetitive class of sequences. The best know and well described repetitive sequences are the transposable elements. These include the DNA elements similar to those first described in corn by McClintock. But these are not the most abundant transposable element class. The distinction is held by the retrotransposons class of elements that move via an RNA intermediate. The shear fact that nearly half of the human genome consists of transposable elements makes them a significant research topic.

Simple sequence repeats, or SSRs, are another major repetitive class found in genomes. These repeats, that consist of localized repetitions of di- or tri-nucleotides, have been well described in many species and currently are widely used as markers linked to other genes in the genome. Using *in silico* approaches to uncover the proximity relationship of SSRs to all genes has tremendous potential for diagnostic purposes. Genomes have long histories involving many different types of events that lead to the construction of the current genomic landscape. We are now beginning to appreciate the extent to which genomes evolved by large scale, or segmental duplications. Take the case of *Arabidopsis*. It was chosen as a model organism because it was considered to be essentially devoid of gene duplications. Early studies suggested that the genome was essentially single copy. But the final sequence of the *Arabidopsis* genome revealed that nearly all of the genome had undergone duplications on a large scale. Similar patterns of local (intrachromosomal) and distal (interchromosomal) duplications were also noted for the human, but to a lesser degree in the mouse genome.

A final non-gene description of a genome characterizes single nucleotide polymorphisms (SNPs). Allelic differences between genes underlie the variation in gene expression. These can be large scale deletions that render a gene essentially useless, or a triplet deletion that causes the loss of a key amino acid and a subsequent loss of function. A famous example is the triplet nucleotide deletion in the cystic fibrosis gene that leads to the loss of an important phenylalanine amino acid. Other differences, though are much more subtle such as the single nucleotide difference in the β-hemaglobin gene that generates the sickle cell anemia allele. Such differences between the two alleles is called a SNP. If a genome project uses multiple individuals as there DNA source, SNPs can be uncovered. These can then be used in association mapping studies to determine if a particular allelic difference is responsible for an unusual phenotype. The public human genome project uncovered 1.4 million SNPs, and other projects are searching for more. The current estimate is that the human genome contains 10 million SNPs.

Annotation Approaches

Nucleotide annotation

The first step of nucleotide annotation is to find a sequence that has the features of a gene. Many eukaryotic genes contain specific features, such as introns that separate exons, that can serve are markers for the discovery process. Therefore, it is important to develop a software programme that properly recognizes such features. A number of programmes are available that perform these searches. A key feature of each of these programmes are *sensor* algorithms that identifies the key structural features. For genes, these would include, for example, introns that are defined by the consensus splice site junctions (GT...AG). The programme might also include other sensors that detect a transcriptional start site or recognize specific GC content. Collectively, potential genes are discovered by scanning the DNA sequence in all six possible reading frames to ensure all possible genes are recognized for further analysis.

Once a sequence has been defined as a gene, the next step is to name it. The naming of genes relies upon the significant amount of research that predated genome projects. This research was historically done on a gene-by-gene approach to clone and characterize individual genes that were of interest to a specific research group. For example, many of the proteins involved in the housekeeping processes of a cell have been characterized at the nucleotide and protein levels. This information is stored in large databases such as GenBank and Swiss-Prot. Therefore with a specific sequence highlighted as a potential gene, the next step is to determine if that sequence indeed is like some other gene or protein.

Naming the genes

The software tool most often used to annotate (or name) a gene is BLAST. This stands for Basic Local Alignment Search Tool. This series of computer programmes looks for sequence similarities. Basically, it consists of a query (the sequence to which you are looking for a match) and a database. Typically, a database such as GenBank or Swiss-Prot is used to uncover sequences that are similar to the query. The query can be either a protein or nucleotide sequence. The database can be either a nucleotide or protein database. It is also possible to use a translated version of a nucleotide query, or to search a translated version of a database when the input query is an amino acid sequence. The more recent versions of BLAST can incorporate gaps to discover homologies.

A critical database used to determine if a sequence is indeed a gene contains EST (Expressed Sequence Tags) sequences. ESTs are DNA sequences of expressed genes that are represented in a cDNA library. The data is collected by end sequencing (usually the 3′ end) a large collection of clones representing transcripts expressed under a specific developmental or environmental condition. Because they are expressed, then they clearly were transcribed from functioning gene. Therefore, the predicted genes are also used as a BLAST query against an EST database

Non-gene RNA sequences

Programmes are also available that searce for non-gene RNA sequences that are important components of the genome. These sequences include the ribosomal RNAs and tRNAs that are essential for protein translation. In addition, the small nuclear RNAs important to processes such as RNA splicing are necessarily components of the gneome. These sequences exhibit a high degree of conservation, and therefore, are easily recognizable. Finally, the recent discovery of microRNAs has added another sequence class. These RNAs act as suppressors of gene expression by binding to the mRNA of specific genes.

The abundance of research that targets the discovery of regulatory regions in the genome has described many short sequences (motifs) that are target sites to which proteins that regulate gene expression bind. Similarity searches of these short motifs are relatively straightforward. The success of this process, though, depends on experiments that define these and other motifs. Using the concept of conserved orthology among species, scanning sequences in the promoter region upstream of the transcriptional start site for several related species may uncover previously unknown conserved motifs that can later be tested experimentally.

Repetitive elements can populate genomes to large degrees. Because of the conserved nature of these sequences, it is fairly straightforward to discover these. For example, full (or nearly full) retrotransposon elements encode a reverse transcriptase protein. Similarity searches for these are fairly powerful. Once these are discovered, they can be used for subsequent nucleotide searchs for other elements that have diverged over time. Cataloging the repetitive elements is a critical first annotation step because it greatly reduces the amount of sequence that must be searched during the gene discovery process described above. To discover segmental gene duplications, the repetitive class of sequences is first removed by a process called repeat masking. Then each gene is compared against the genome sequence itself to discover if it represented again in the genome. In this manner, blocks of genes that have undergone duplication can be uncovered. When looking for SNPs, researchers have a number of resources. The basic reference gene can be from the individual used in the initial sequencing. That gene sequence can then be compared to other databases representing sequences derived from other individuals. A good comparison would involve the reference gene with the sequences found in an EST database. The source mRNA for EST projects is typically not from the original source used for genomic sequencing. Therefore variability between the reference and EST sequence is a SNP.

A novel search for controlling element motifs

All genes are controlled by sequences upstream of the transcriptional start site. A number of the sequences are important because they represent the site to which transcription factor, proteins that control gene expression, bind. A major goal of annotation would be to describe those sequences, and eventually determine how universal those sequences are in the promoter of specific genes. The first step is to describe such sequences in a reference species and use that information for further comparative analyses. A recent report describes a sequence-based approach to uncovering these sequence motifs.

The yeast (*Saccharomyces cerevisiae*) genome has been sequenced and many members of the total gene array (6331 genes) have been named. Each of these genes contains an upstream controlling region. These controlling sequences, by their very nature, must reside in the 'intergenic' region that lies between each gene. For yeast, these regions are rather small and average about 500 nucleotides. Over evolutionary time, these regions tend to diverge to a greater extent than the coding regions. This divergence actually offers a means to uncover important sequences because these would be under selection pressure and would maintain sequence continuity overtime to ensure the gene can still be properly expressed in the evolved species.

Cliften and others applied a *phylogenetic footprinting* method to uncover these conserved motifs. They chose five additional *Saccharomyces* species to analyse. Three of these are closely related to the standard yeast speices (*S. mikatae*, *S. kundriavzevii*, and *S. bayanus*). and two more distant species (*S. castelli* and *S. kluyveri*). The closely related species average 59 to 67% sequence identity, whereas the distant species are 33.9% identical. Each of these five species were sequenced to a 2–3X genome coverage using the whole genome shotgun approach. This provided an 85–95% coverage of the genome sequence of each species. With five species in hand, the group reannotated the genomes. This lead to a reduction in the number of 'real' gene to a value of 5773.

With each gene annotated, the researchers took the shared intergenic sequences upstream of each gene and aligned them using CLUSTALW, a programme that aligns multiple sequences. They aligned the four related sequences and then performed the alignment with all six species. With the four species, alignment over 50% of the intergenic regions were shared, whereas with all species this number was reduced to 40%. Sequence identity among the four species averaged 37.1% over all of the promoters. Peak identity was located at 125–250 nt upstream of the ATG translational start site. This suggests (i) this region is enriched for regulatory sequences, (ii) regulatory sequences are close to ATG site in yeast, and (iii) phylogenomics might uncover controlling elements by looking for conserved sequence elements.

These experiments discovered the following. First, only 15.7% of the integenic regions contain one of the seven sequence motifs that define a TATA box. This is a striking result since TATA boxes are considered essential elements for transcription initiation. Several motifs were shared among genes with similar biological functions. Other motifs were common to genes expressed during similar expression conditions such as stress, cell cycling or meiosis. This provides a new catalog of potential sequences that can later be studied experimentally to determine their biological significance and to uncover the factors which interact with these sequence to control gene expression.

Chapter 15

Bacterial and Eukaryotic Genomes

INTRODUCTION

Bacterial genomes are generally smaller and less variant in size between species when compared with genomes of animals and single cell eukaryotes. Bacterial genomes can range in size anywhere from about 130 kbp to over 14 Mbp. Recent advances in sequencing technology led to the discovery of a high correlation between the number of genes and the genome size of bacteria, suggesting that bacteria have relatively small amounts of noncoding DNA. A striking discovery by Cole and others described massive amounts of gene decay when comparing Leprosy *bacillus* to ancestral bacteria. Studies have since shown that a large number of bacterial species have undergone genomic degradation resulting in a decrease in genome size from their ancestral state. Over the years, researchers have proposed several theories to explain the general trend of bacterial genome decay and the relatively small size of bacterial genomes. Compelling evidence indicates that the apparent degradation of bacterial genomes is owed to a deletional bias. Bacterial genomes are generally smaller and less variant in size between species when compared with genomes of animals and single cell eukaryotes. Bacterial genomes can range in size anywhere from 139 kbp to 13000 kbp. Recent advances in sequencing technology led to the discovery of a high correlation between the number of genes and the genome size of bacteria, suggesting that bacteria have relatively small amounts of noncoding DNA. A striking discovery by Cole and others described massive amounts of gene decay when comparing Leprosy *bacillus* to ancestral bacteria.

Studies have since shown that a large number of bacterial species have undergone genomic degradation resulting in a decrease in genome size from their ancestral state. Over the years, researchers have proposed several theories to explain the general trend of bacterial genome decay and the relatively small size of bacterial genomes. Compelling evidence indicates that the apparent degradation of bacterial genomes is owed to a deletional bias.

METHODS AND TECHNIQUES OF BACTERIAL GENOMES

As of 2014, there are over 30,000 sequenced bacterial genomes publicly available and thousands of metagenome projects. Projects such as the Genomic Encyclopedia of Bacteria and *Archaea* (GEBA) intend to add more genomes. The single gene comparison is now being supplanted by more general methods.

These methods have resulted in novel perspectives on genetic relationships that previously have only been estimated. A significant achievement in the second decade of bacterial genome sequencing was the production of metagenomic data, which covers all DNA present in a sample. Previously, there were only two metagenomic projects published.

BACTERIAL GENOMES

Bacteria possess a compact genome architecture distinct from eukaryotes in two important ways: bacteria show a strong correlation between genome size and number of functional genes in a genome, and those genes are structured into operons. The main reason for the relative density of bacterial genomes compared to eukaryotic genomes (especially multicellular eukaryotes) is the presence of noncoding DNA in the form of intergenic regions and introns. Some notable exceptions include recently formed pathogenic bacteria. Furthermore, amongst species of bacteria, there is relatively little variation in genome size when compared with the genome sizes of other major groups of life. Genome size is of little relevance when considering the number of functional genes in eukaryotic species. In bacteria however, the strong correlation between the number of genes and the genome size makes the size of bacterial genomes an interesting topic for research and discussion. The general trends of bacterial evolution indicate that bacteria started as free-living organisms. Evolutionary paths led some bacteria to become pathogens and symbionts.

The lifestyles of bacteria play an integral role in their respective genome sizes. Free-living bacteria have the largest genomes out of the three types of bacteria, however, they have fewer pseudogenes than bacteria that have recently acquired pathogenicity. Facultative and recently evolved pathogenic bacteria exhibit a smaller genome size than free-living bacteria, yet they have more pseudogenes than any other form of bacteria. Obligate bacterial symbionts or pathogens have the smallest genomes and the fewest pseudogenes of the three groups. The relationship between life-styles of bacteria and genome size raises questions as to the mechanisms of bacterial genome evolution. Researchers have developed several theories to explain the patterns of genome size evolution amongst bacteria.

Genome Comparisons and Phylogeny

As single-gene comparisons have largely given way to genome comparisons, phylogeny of bacterial genomes have improved in accuracy. The Average Nucleotide Identity method quantifies genetic distance between entire genomes by taking advantage of regions of about 10,000 bp. With enough data from genomes of one genus, algorithms are executed to categorise species. This has been done for the Pseudomonas avellanae species in 2013. To extract information about bacterial genomes, core- and pan-genome sizes have been assessed for several strains of bacteria. In 2012, the number of core gene families was about 3000. However, by 2015, with an over tenfold increased in available genomes, the pan-genome has increased as well. There is roughly a positive correlation between the number of genomes added and the growth of the pan-genome. On the other hand, the core genome has remain static since 2012. Currently, the E. coli pan-genome is composed of about 90000 gene families. About one-third of these exist only in a single genome. Many of these, however, are merely gene fragments and the result of calling errors. Still, there are probably over 60000 unique gene families in E. coli.

Theories of Bacterial Genome Evolution

Bacteria lose a large amount of genes as they transition from free-living or facultatively parasitic life cycles to permanent host-dependent life. Towards the lower end of the scale of bacterial genome size are the mycoplasmas and related bacteria. Early molecular phylogenetic studies revealed that mycoplasmas represented an evolutionary derived state, contrary to prior hypotheses. Furthermore, it is now known that mycoplasmas are just one instance of many of genome shrinkage in obligately host-associated bacteria. Other examples are *Rickettsia*, *Buchnera aphidicola*, and *Borrelia burgdorferi*.

Small genome size in such species is associated with certain particularities, such as rapid evolution of polypeptide sequences and low GC content in the genome. The convergent evolution of these qualities in unrelated bacteria suggests that an obligate association with a host promotes genome reduction.

Given that over 80% of almost all of the fully sequenced bacterial genomes consist of intact ORFs, and that gene length is nearly constant at ~1 kb per gene, it is inferred that small genomes have few metabolic capabilities. While free-living bacteria, such as *E. coli*, *Salmonella species*, or *Bacillus* species, usually have 1500 to 6000 proteins encoded in their DNA, obligately pathogenic bacteria often have as few as 500 to 1000 such proteins. Collin and others explanation that reduced genomes maintain genes that are necessary for vital processes pertaining to cellular growth and replication, in addition to those genes that are required to survive in the bacterias ecological niche. However, sequence data contradicts this hypothesis. The set of universal orthologs amongst eubacteria comprises only 15% of each genome. Thus, each lineage has taken a different evolutionary path to reduced size. Because universal cellular processes require over 80 genes, variation in genes imply that the same functions can be achieved by exploitation of nonhomologous genes.

Host-dependent bacteria are able to secure many compounds required for metabolism from the host's cytoplasm or tissue. They can, in turn, discard their own biosynthetic pathways and associated genes. This removal explains many of the specific gene losses. For example, the *Rickettsia* species, which relies on specific energy substrate from its host, has lost many of its native energy metabolism genes. Similarly, most small genomes have lost their amino acid biosynthesising genes, as these are found in the host instead. One exception is the *Buchnera*, an obligate maternally transmitted symbiont of aphids. It retains 54 genes for biosynthesis of crucial amino acids, but no longer has pathways for those amino acids that the host can synthesise. Pathways for nucleotide biosynthesis are gone from many reduced genomes. Those anabolic pathways that evolved through niche adaptation remain in particular genomes.

The hypothesis that unused genes are eventually removed does not explain why many of the removed genes would indeed remain helpful in obligate pathogens. For example, many eliminated genes code for products that are involved in universal cellular processes, including replication, transcription, and translation. Even genes supporting DNA recombination and repair are deleted from every small genome. In addition, small genomes have fewer tRNAs, utilising one for several amino acids. So, a single codon pairs with multiple codons, which likely yields less-than-optimal translation machinery. It is unknown why obligate intracellular pathogens would benefit by retaining fewer tRNAs and fewer DNA repair enzymes. Another factor to consider is the change in population that corresponds to an evolution towards an obligately pathogenic life. Such a shift in lifestyle often results in a reduction in the genetic population size of a lineage, since there is a finite number of hosts to occupy. This genetic drift may result in fixation of mutations that inactivate otherwise beneficial genes, or otherwise may decrease the efficiency of gene products. Hence, not will only useless genes be lost (as mutations disrupt them once the bacteria has settled into host dependency), but also beneficial genes may be lost if genetic drift enforces ineffective purifying selection.

The number of universally maintained genes is small and inadequate for independent cellular growth and replication, so that small genome species must achieve such feats by means of varying genes. This is done partly through nonorthologous gene displacement. That is, the role of one gene is replaced by another gene that achieves the same function. Redundancy within the ancestral, larger genome is eliminated. The descendant small genome content depends on the content of chromosomal deletions that occur in the early stages of genome reduction. The very small genome of *M. genitalium* possesses dispensable genes. In a study in which single genes of this organism were inactivated using transposon-mediated mutagenesis, at least 129 of its 484 ORGs were not required for growth. A much smaller genome than that of the *M. genitalium* is therefore feasible.

Doubling time

One theory predicts that bacteria have smaller genomes due to a selective pressure on genome size to ensure faster replication. The theory is based upon the logical premise that smaller bacterial genomes will take less time to replicate. Subsequently, smaller genomes will be selected preferentially due to enhanced fitness. A study done by Collin and others indicated little to no correlation between genome size and doubling time. The data indicates that selection is not a suitable explanation for the small sizes of bacterial genomes. Still, many researchers believe there is some selective pressure on bacteria to maintain small genome size.

Deletional bias

Selection is but one process involved in evolution. Two other major processes (mutation and genetic drift) can be used to explain the genome sizes of various types of bacteria. A study done by Collin and others examined the size of insertions and deletions in bacterial pseudogenes. Results indicated that mutational deletions tend to be larger than insertions in bacteria in the absence of gene transfer or gene duplication. Insertions caused by horizontal or lateral gene transfer and gene duplication tend to involve transfer of large amounts of genetic material. Assuming a lack of these processes, genomes will tend to reduce in size in the absence of selective constraint. Evidence of a deletional bias is present in the respective genome sizes of free-living bacteria, facultative and recently derived parasites and obligate parasites and symbionts.

Free-living bacteria tend to have large population sizes and are subject to more opportunity for gene transfer. As such, selection can effectively operate on free-living bacteria to remove deleterious sequences resulting in a relatively small number of pseudogenes. Continually, further selective pressure is evident as free-living bacteria must produce all gene-products independent of a host. Given that there is sufficient opportunity for gene transfer to occur and there are selective pressures against even slightly deleterious deletions, it is intuitive that free-living bacteria should have the largest bacterial genomes of all bacteria types. Recently formed parasites undergo severe bottlenecks and can rely on host environments to provide gene products. As such, in recently formed and facultative parasites, there is an accumulation of *pseudogenes* and transposable elements due to a lack of selective pressure against deletions.

The population bottlenecks reduce gene transfer and as such, deletional bias ensures the reduction of genome size in parasitic bacteria. Obligatory parasites and symbionts have the smallest genome sizes due to prolonged effects of deletional bias. Parasites which have evolved to occupy specific niches are not exposed to much selective pressure. As such, genetic drift dominates the evolution of niche specific bacteria. Extended exposure to deletional bias ensures the removal of most superfluous sequences. Symbionts occur in drastically lower numbers and undergo the most severe bottlenecks of any bacterial type. There is almost no opportunity for gene transfer for endosymbiotic bacteria and as such, genome compaction can be extreme. One of the smallest bacterial genomes ever to be sequenced is that of the endosymbiont *Carsonella rudii*. At 160 kbp, the genome of *Carsonella* is one of the most streamlined examples of a genome examined to date.

Genomic Reduction

Molecular phylogenetics has revealed that every clade of bacteria with genome sizes under 2 Mb was derived from ancestors with much larger genomes, thus refuting the hypothesis that bacteria evolved by the successive doubling of small-genomed ancestors. Recent studies performed by Nilsson and others examined the rates of bacterial genome reduction of obligate bacteria. Bacteria were cultured introducing frequent bottlenecks and growing cells in serial passage to reduce gene transfer so as to mimic conditions of endosymbiotic bacteria. The data predicted that bacteria exhibiting a one-day generation time lose as many as 1000 kbp in as few as 50000 years (a relatively short evolutionary time period). Furthermore, after deleting genes essential to the methyl-directed DNA mismatch repair (MMR) system, it was shown that bacterial genome size reduction increased in rate by as much as 50 times. These results indicate that genome size reduction can occur relatively rapidly, and loss of certain genes can speed up the process of bacterial genome compaction. This is not to suggest that all bacterial genomes are reducing in size and complexity. While many types of bacteria have reduced in genome size from an ancestral state, there are still a huge number of bacteria that maintained or increased genome size over ancestral states. Free-living bacteria experience huge population sizes, fast generation times and a relatively high potential for gene transfer. While deletional bias tends to remove unnecessary sequences, selection can operate significantly amongst free-living bacteria resulting in evolution of new genes and processes.

Horizontal Gene Transfer

Unlike eukaryotes, which evolve mainly through the modification of existing genetic information, bacteria have acquired a large percentage of their genetic diversity by the horizontal transfer of genes. This creates quite dynamic genomes, in which DNA can be introduced into and removed from the chromosome.

Bacteria have more variation in their metabolic properties, cellular structures, and lifestyles than can be accounted for by point mutations alone. For example, none of the phenotypic traits that distinguish *E. coli* from *Salmonella enterica* can be attributed to point mutation. On the contrary, evidence suggests that horizontal gene transfer has bolstered the diversification and speciation of many bacteria.

Horizontal gene transfer is often detected via DNA sequence information. DNA segments obtained by this mechanism often reveal a narrow phylogenetic distribution between related species. Furthermore, these regions sometimes display an unexpected level of similarity to genes from taxa that are assumed to be quite divergent.

Although gene comparisons and phylogenetic studies are helpful in investigating horizontal gene transfer, the DNA sequences of genes are even more revelatory of their origin and ancestry within a genome. Bacterial species differ widely in overall GC content, although the genes in any one species genome are roughly identical with respect to base composition, patterns of codon usage, and frequencies of di- and trinucleotides. As a result, sequences that are newly acquired through lateral transfer can be identified via their characteristics, which remains that of the donor. For example, many of the *S. enterica* genes that are not present in *E. coli* have base compositions that differ from the overall 52% GC content of the entire chromosome. Within this species, some lineages have more than a megabase of DNA that is not present in other lineages. The base compositions of these lineage-specific sequences imply that at least half of these sequences were captured through lateral transfer. Furthermore, the regions adjacent to horizontally obtained genes often have remnants of translocatable elements, transfer origins of plasmids, or known attachment sites of phage integrases. In some species, a large proportion of laterally transferred genes originate from plasmid-, phage-, or transposon-related sequences.

Although sequence-based methods reveal the prevalence of horizontal gene transfer in bacteria, the results tend to be underestimates of the magnitude of this mechanism, since sequences obtained from donors whose sequence characteristics are similar to those of the recipient will avoid detection.

Comparisons of completely sequenced genomes confirm that bacterial chromosomes are amalgams of ancestral and laterally acquired sequences. The hyperthermophilic Eubacteria Aquifex aeolicus and Thermotoga maritima each has many genes that are similar in protein sequence to homologues in thermophilic *Archaea*. 24% of Thermotoga's 1877 ORFs and 16% of Aquifex's 1512 ORFs show high matches to an *Archaeal* protein, while mesophiles such as *E. coli* and *B. subtilis* have far lesser proportions of genes that are most like Archaeal homologues.

Mechanisms of lateral transfer

The genesis of new abilities due to horizontal gene transfer has three requirements. First, there must exist a possible route for the donor DNA to be accepted by the recipient cell. Additionally, the obtained sequence must be integrated with the rest of the genome. Finally, these integrated genes must benefit the recipient bacterial organism. The first two steps can be achieved via three mechanisms: transformation, transduction and conjugation. Transformation involves the uptake of named DNA from the environment. Through transformation, DNA can be transmitted between distantly related organisms. Some bacterial species, such as *Haemophilus influenzae* and *Neisseria gonorrhoeae*, are continuously competent to accept DNA. Other species, such as *Bacillus subtilis* and *Streptococcus pneumoniae*, become competent when they enter a particular phase in their lifecycle.

Transformation in *N. gonorrhoeae* and *H. influenzae* is effective only if particular recognition sequences are found in the recipient genomes (5'-GCCGTCTGAA-3' and 5'-AAGTGCGGT-3'. respectively). Although the existence of certain uptake sequences improve transformation capability between related species, many of the inherently competent bacterial species, such as *B. subtilis* and *S. pneumoniae*, do not display sequence preference.

New genes may be introduced into bacteria by a bacteriophage that has replicated within a donor through generalised transduction or specialised transduction. The amount of DNA that can be transmitted in one event is constrained by the size of the phage capsid (although the upper limit is about 100 kilobases). While phages are numerous in the environment, the range of micro-organisms that can be transduced depends on receptor recognition by the bacteriophage. Transduction does not require both donor and recipient cells to be present simultaneously in time nor space. Phage-encoded proteins both mediate the transfer of DNA into the recipient cytoplasm and assist integration of DNA into the chromosome.

Conjugation involves physical contact between donor and recipient cells and is able to mediate transfers of genes between domains, such as between bacteria and yeast. DNA is transmitted from donor to recipient either by self-transmissible or mobilisable plasmid. Conjugation may mediate the transfer of chromosomal sequences by plasmids that integrate into the chromosome.

Despite the multitude of mechanisms mediating gene transfer among bacteria, the process's success is not guaranteed unless the received sequence is stably maintained in the recipient. DNA integration can be sustained through one of many processes. One is persistence as an episome, another is homologous recombination, and still another is illegitimate incorporation through lucky double-strand break repair.

Traits introduced through lateral gene transfer

Antimicrobial resistance genes grant an organism the ability to grow its ecological niche, since it can now survive in the presence of previously lethal compounds. As the benefit to a bacterium earned from receiving such genes are time- and space-independent, those sequences that are highly mobile are selected for. Plasmids are quite mobilizable between taxa and are the most frequent way by which bacteria acquire antibiotic resistance genes. Adoption of a pathogenic lifestyle often yields a fundamental shift in an organism's ecological niche. The erratic phylogenetic distribution of pathogenic organisms implies that bacterial virulence is a consequence of the presence, or obtainment of, genes that are missing in avirulent forms. Evidence of this includes the discovery of large 'virulence' plasmids in pathogenic *Shigella* and *Yersinia*, as well as the ability to bestow pathogenic properties onto *E. coli* via experimental exposure to genes from other species.

EUKARYOTIC GENOMES

Eukaryotic genomes are composed of one or more linear DNA chromosomes. The number of chromosomes varies widely from Jack jumper ants and an asexual nemotode, which each have only one pair, to a fern species that has 720 pairs. A typical human cell has two copies of each of 22 autosomes, one inherited from each parent, plus two sex chromosomes, making it diploid. Gametes, such as ova, sperm, spores, and pollen, are haploid, meaning they carry only one copy of each chromosome.

In addition to the chromosomes in the nucleus, organelles such as the chloroplasts and mitochondria have their own DNA. Mitochondria are sometimes said to have their own genome often referred to as the 'mitochondrial genome'. The DNA found within the chloroplast may be referred to as the 'plastome'. Like the bacteria they originated from, mitochondria and chloroplasts have a circular chromosome.

Unlike prokaryotes, eukaryotes have exon-intron organisation of protein coding genes and variable amounts of repetitive DNA. In mammals and plants, the majority of the genome is composed of repetitive DNA. Two features of eukaryotic genomes present a major information-processing challenge:

1. The typical multicellular eukaryotic genome is much larger than that of a prokaryotic cell.
2. Cell specialisation limits the expression of many genes to specific cells.

The estimated 25000 genes in the human genome include an enormous amount of DNA that does not code for RNA or protein. This DNA is elaborately organised. Not only is the DNA associated with protein, but also this DNA-protein complex called chromatin is organised into higher structural levels than the DNA-protein complex in prokaryotes.

Chromatin Structure is based on Successive Levels of DNA Packing

- While the single circular chromosome of bacteria is coiled and looped in a complex but orderly manner, eukaryotic chromatin is far more complex.
- Eukaryotic DNA is precisely combined with large amounts of protein. The resulting chromatin undergoes striking changes in the course of the cell cycle.
  o During interphase of the cell cycle, chromatin fibers are usually highly extended within the nucleus.
- As a cell prepares for meiosis, its chromatin condenses, forming a characteristic number of short, thick chromosomes that can be distinguished with a light microscope.
- Eukaryotic chromosomes contain an enormous amount of DNA relative to their condensed length.
  o Each human chromosome averages about 1.5×10^8 nucleotide pairs.
  o If extended, each DNA molecule would be about 4 cm long, thousands of times longer than the cell diameter.
  o This chromosome and 45 other human chromosomes fit into the nucleus.

o This occurs through an elaborate, multilevel system of DNA packing.
- Histone proteins are responsible for the first level of DNA packaging.
o The mass of histone in chromatin is approximately equal to the mass of DNA.
o Their positively charged amino acids bind tightly to negatively charged DNA.
o The five types of histones are very similar from one eukaryote to another, and similar proteins are found in prokaryotes.
o The conservation of histone genes during evolution reflects their pivotal role in organising DNA within cells.
- Unfolded chromatin has the appearance of beads on a string.
o In this configuration, a chromatin fiber is 10 nm in diameter (the 10-nm fiber).
- Each bead of chromatin is a nucleosome, the basic unit of DNA packing.
o The 'string' between the beads is called linker DNA.
- A nucleosome consists of DNA wound around a protein core composed of two molecules each of four types of histone: H2A, H2B, H3, and H4.
o The amino acid (N-terminus) of each histone protein (the histone tail) extends outward from the nucleosome.
o A molecule of a fifth histone, H1, attaches to the DNA near the nucleosome.
- The beaded string seems to remain essentially intact throughout the cell cycle.
- Histones leave the DNA only transiently during DNA replication.
- They stay with the DNA during transcription.
o By changing shape and position, nucleosomes allow RNA-synthesising polymerases to move along the DNA.
- The next level of packing is due to the interactions between the histone tails of one nucleosome and the linker DNA and nucleosomes to either side.
o With the aid of histone H1, these interactions cause the 10-nm to coil to form the 30-nm chromatin fiber.
- This fiber forms looped domains attached to a scaffold of nonhistone proteins to make up a 300-nm fiber.
- In a mitotic chromosome, the looped domains coil and fold to produce the characteristic metaphase chromosome.
- These packing steps are highly specific and precise, with particular genes located in the same places on metaphase chromosomes.
- Interphase chromatin is generally much less condensed than the chromatin of mitotic chromosomes, but it shows several of the same levels of higher-order packing.
o Much of the chromatin is present as a 10-nm fiber, and some is compacted into a 30-nm fiber, which in some regions is folded into looped domains.
o An interphase chromosome lacks an obvious scaffold, but its looped domains seem to be attached to the nuclear lamina on the inside of the nuclear envelope, and perhaps also to fibers of the nuclear matrix.
- The chromatin of each chromosome occupies a specific restricted area within the interphase nucleus.

- Interphase chromosomes have highly condensed areas, heterochromatin, and less compacted areas, euchromatin.
- Heterochromatin DNA is largely inaccessible to transcription enzymes.
  - o Looser packing of euchromatin makes its DNA accessible to enzymes and available for transcription.

Gene Expression can be regulated at any Stage, but the Key Step is Transcription

- Like unicellular organisms, the tens of thousands of genes in the cells of multicellular eukaryotes are continually turned on and off in response to signals from their internal and external environments.
- Gene expression must be controlled on a long-term basis during cellular differentiation, the divergence in form and function as cells in a multicellular organism specialise.
  - o A typical human cell probably expresses about 20% of its genes at any given time.
  - o Highly specialised cells, such as nerves or muscles, express only a tiny fraction of their genes.
    Although all the cells in an organism contain an identical genome, the subset of genes expressed in the cells of each type is unique.
    The differences between cell types are due to differential gene expression, the expression of different genes by cells with the same genome.
- The genomes of eukaryotes may contain tens of thousands of genes.
  - o For quite a few species, only a small amount of the DNA—1.5% in humans—codes for protein.
  - o Of the remaining DNA, a very small fraction consists of genes for rRNA and tRNA.
  - o Most of the rest of the DNA seems to be largely noncoding, although researchers have found that a significant amount of it is transcribed into RNAs of unknown function.
- Problems with gene expression and control can lead to imbalance and diseases, including cancers.
- Our understanding of the mechanisms controlling gene expression in eukaryotes has been enhanced by new research methods, including advances in DNA technology.
- In all organisms, the expression of specific genes is most commonly regulated at transcription, often in response to signals coming from outside the cell.
  - o The term gene expression is often equated with transcription.
  - o With their greater complexity, eukaryotes have opportunities for controlling gene expression at additional stages.
- Each stage in the entire process of gene expression provides a potential control point where gene expression can be turned on or off, sped up or slowed down.
  - o A web of control connects different genes and their products.
- These levels of control include chromatin packing, transcription, RNA processing, translation, and various alterations to the protein product. Chromatin modifications affect the availability of genes for transcription.
- In addition to its role in packing DNA inside the nucleus, chromatin organisation regulates gene expression.
  - o Genes of densely condensed heterochromatin are usually not expressed, presumably because transcription proteins cannot reach the DNA.

- o A genes location relative to nucleosomes and to attachment sites to the chromosome scaffold or nuclear lamina can affect transcription.
- Chemical modifications of chromatin play a key role in chromatin structure and gene expression.
- Chemical modifications of histones play a direct role in the regulation of gene transcription.
- The *N*-terminus of each histone molecule in a nucleosome protrudes outward from the nucleosome.
  - o These histone tails are accessible to various modifying enzymes, which catalyse the addition or removal of specific chemical groups.
- Histone acetylation (addition of an acetyl group —$COCH_3$) and deacetylation appear to play a direct role in the regulation of gene transcription.
  - o Acetylated histones grip DNA less tightly, providing easier access for transcription proteins in this region.
  - o Some of the enzymes responsible for acetylation or deacetylation are associated with or are components of transcription factors that bind to promoters.
  - o Thus histone acetylation enzymes may promote the initiation of transcription not only by modifying chromatin structure, but also by binding to and recruiting components of the transcription machinery.
- DNA methylation is the attachment by specific enzymes of methyl groups (—CH_3) to DNA bases after DNA synthesis.
- Inactive DNA is generally highly methylated compared to DNA that is actively transcribed.
  - o For example, the inactivated mammalian X chromosome in females is heavily methylated.
- Genes are usually more heavily methylated in cells where they are not expressed.
  - o Demethylating certain inactive genes turns them on.
  - o However, there are exceptions to this pattern.
- DNA methylation proteins recruit histone deacetylation enzymes, providing a mechanism by which DNA methylation and histone deacetylation cooperate to repress transcription.
- In some species, DNA methylation is responsible for long-term inactivation of genes during cellular differentiation.
  - o Once methylated, genes usually stay that way through successive cell divisions.
  - o Methylation enzymes recognise sites on one strand that are already methylated and correctly methylate the daughter strand after each round of DNA replication.
- This methylation patterns accounts for genomic imprinting in which methylation turns off either the maternal or paternal alleles of certain genes at the start of development.
- The chromatin modifications just discussed do not alter DNA sequence, and yet they may be passed along to future generations of cells.
  - o Inheritance of traits by mechanisms not directly involving the nucleotide sequence is called epigenetic inheritance.
- Researchers are amassing more and more evidence for the importance of epigenetic information in the regulation of gene expression.
  - o Enzymes that modify chromatin structure are integral parts of the cell's machinery for regulating transcription.

Transcription initiation is controlled by proteins that interact with DNA and with each other

- Chromatin-modifying enzymes provide initial control of gene expression by making a region of DNA either more available or less available for transcription.
- A cluster of proteins called a transcription initiation complex assembles on the promoter sequence at the 'upstream' end of the gene.
  - o One component, RNA polymerase II, transcribes the gene, synthesising a primary RNA transcript or pre-mRNA.
  - o RNA processing includes enzymatic addition of a 5' cap and a poly-A tail, as well as splicing out of introns to yield a mature mRNA.
- Multiple control elements are associated with most eukaryotic genes.
  - o Control elements are noncoding DNA segments that regulate transcription by binding certain proteins.
  - o These control elements and the proteins they bind are critical to the precise regulation of gene expression in different cell types.
- To initiate transcription, eukaryotic RNA polymerase requires the assistance of proteins called transcription factors.
  - o General transcription factors are essential for the transcription of all protein-coding genes.
  - o Only a few general transcription factors independently bind a DNA sequence such as the TATA box within the promoter.
  - o Others in the initiation complex are involved in protein-protein interactions, binding each other and RNA polymerase II.
- The interaction of general transcription factors and RNA polymerase II with a promoter usually leads to only a low rate of initiation and production of few RNA transcripts.
- In eukaryotes, high levels of transcription of particular genes depend on the interaction of control elements with specific transcription factors.
- Some control elements, named proximal control elements, are located close to the promoter.
- Distant control elements, enhancers, may be thousands of nucleotides away from the promoter or even downstream of the gene or within an intron.
- A given gene may have multiple enhancers, each active at a different time or in a different cell type or location in the organism.
- An activator is a protein that binds to an enhancer to stimulate transcription of a gene.
  - o Protein-mediated bending of DNA brings bound activators in contact with a group of mediator proteins that interact with proteins at the promoter.
  - o This helps assemble and position the initiation complex on the promoter.
- Eukaryotic genes also have repressor proteins to inhibit expression of a gene.
  - o Eukaryotic repressors can cause inhibition of gene expression by blocking the binding of activators to their control elements or to components of the transcription machinery or by turning off transcription even in the presence of activators.
- Some activators and repressors act indirectly to influence chromatin structure.
  - o Some activators recruit proteins that acetylate histones near the promoters of specific genes, promoting transcription.

- o Some repressors recruit proteins that deacetylate histones, reducing transcription or silencing the gene.
- o Recruitment of chromatin-modifying proteins seems to be the most common mechanism of repression in eukaryotes.
- The number of nucleotide sequences found in control elements is surprisingly small.
- For many genes, the particular combination of control elements associated with the gene may be more important than the presence of a single unique control element in regulating transcription of the gene.
- Even with only a dozen control element sequences, a large number of combinations are possible.
- A particular combination of control elements will be able to activate transcription only when the appropriate activator proteins are present, such as at a precise time during development or in a particular cell type.
- o The use of different combinations of control elements allows fine regulation of transcription with a small set of control elements.
- In prokaryotes, coordinately controlled genes are often clustered into an operon with a single promoter and other control elements upstream.
- o The genes of the operon are transcribed into a single mRNA and translated together.
- In contrast, very few eukaryotic genes are organised this way.
- Recent studies of the genomes of several eukaryotic species have found that some coexpressed genes are clustered near each other on the same chromosome.
- o Each eukaryotic gene in these clusters has its own promoter and is individually transcribed.
- o The coordinate regulation of clustered genes in eukaryotic cells is thought to involve changes in the chromatin structure that makes the entire group of genes either available or unavailable for transcription.
- More commonly, genes coding for the enzymes of a metabolic pathway are scattered over different chromosomes.
- Coordinate gene expression in eukaryotes depends on the association of a specific control element or combination of control elements with every gene of a dispersed group.
- A common group of transcription factors binds to all the genes in the group, promoting simultaneous gene transcription.
- o For example, a steroid hormone enters a cell and binds to a specific receptor protein in the cytoplasm or nucleus, forming a hormone-receptor complex that serves as a transcription activator.
- o Every gene whose transcription is stimulated by that steroid hormone has a control element recognised by that hormone-receptor complex.
- o Other signal molecules control gene expression indirectly by triggering signal-transduction pathways that lead to activation of transcription.
- Systems for coordinating gene regulation probably arose early in evolutionary history and evolved by the duplication and distribution of control elements within the genome.

Post-transcriptional mechanisms play supporting roles in the control of gene expression

- Gene expression may be blocked or stimulated by any posttranscriptional step.
- By using regulatory mechanisms that operate after transcription, a cell can rapidly fine-tune gene expression in response to environmental changes without altering its transcriptional patterns.
- RNA processing in the nucleus and the export of mRNA to the cytoplasm provide opportunities for gene regulation that are not available in bacteria.
- In alternative RNA splicing, different mRNA molecules are produced from the same primary transcript, depending on which RNA segments are treated as exons and which as introns.
  - o Regulatory proteins specific to a cell type control intron-exon choices by binding to regulatory sequences within the primary transcript.
- The life span of an mRNA molecule is an important factor in determining the pattern of protein synthesis.
- Prokaryotic mRNA molecules may be degraded after only a few minutes.
- Eukaryotic mRNAs typically last for hours, days, or weeks.
  - o In red blood cells, mRNAs for hemoglobin polypeptides are unusually stable and are translated repeatedly.
- A common pathway of mRNA breakdown begins with enzymatic shortening of the poly-A tail.
  - o This triggers the enzymatic removal of the 5' cap.
  - o This is followed by rapid degradation of the mRNA by nucleases.
- Nucleotide sequences in the untranslated trailer region at the 3' end affect mRNA stability.
  - o Transferring such a sequence from a short-lived mRNA to a normally stable mRNA results in quick mRNA degradation.
- During the past few years, researchers have found small single-stranded RNA molecules called microRNAs, or miRNAs, that bind to complementary sequences in mRNA molecules.
  - o miRNAs are formed from longer RNA precursors that fold back on themselves, forming a long hairpin structure stabilised by hydrogen bonding.
  - o An enzyme called Dicer cuts the double-stranded RNA into short fragments.
  - o One of the two strands is degraded. The other miRNA strand associates with a protein complex and directs the complex to any mRNA molecules with a complementary sequence.
  - o The miRNA-protein complex then degrades the target mRNA or blocks its translation.
- The phenomenon of inhibition of gene expression by RNA molecules is called RNA interference (RNAi).
  - o Small interfering RNAs (siRNAs) are similar in size and function to miRNAs and are generated by similar mechanisms in eukaryotic cells.
- Cellular RNAi pathways lead to the destruction of RNAs and may have originated as a natural defense against infection by RNA viruses.
  - o Whatever their origin, RNAi plays an important role in regulating gene expression in the cell.
- Translation of specific mRNAs can be blocked by regulatory proteins that bind to specific sequences or structures within the 5' leader region of mRNA.

- o This prevents attachment of ribosomes.
- mRNAs may be stored in egg cells without poly-A tails of sufficient size to allow translation initiation.
- o At the appropriate time during development, a cytoplasmic enzyme adds more A residues, allowing translation to begin.
- Protein factors required to initiate translation in eukaryotes offer targets for simultaneously controlling translation of all mRNAs in a cell.
- o This allows the cell to shut down translation if environmental conditions are poor (for example, shortage of a key constituent) or until the appropriate conditions exist (for example, after fertilisation in an egg or during daylight in plants).
- Finally, eukaryotic polypeptides must often be processed to yield functional proteins.
- o This may include cleavage, chemical modifications, and transport to the appropriate destination.
- The cell limits the lifetimes of normal proteins by selective degradation.
- o Many proteins, like the cyclins in the cell cycle, must be short-lived to function appropriately.
- Proteins intended for degradation are marked by the attachment of ubiquitin proteins.
- Giant protein complexes called proteasomes recognise the ubiquitin and degrade the tagged protein.
- o Mutations making cell cycle proteins impervious to proteasome degradation can lead to cancer.

Cancer Results from Genetic Changes that affect Cell Cycle Control

- Cancer is a disease in which cells escape the control methods that normally regulate cell growth and division.
- o The gene regulation systems that go wrong during cancer are the very same systems that play important roles in embryonic development, the immune response, and other biological processes.
- The genes that normally regulate cell growth and division during the cell cycle include genes for growth factors, their receptors, and the intracellular molecules of signaling pathways.
- o Mutations altering any of these genes in somatic cells can lead to cancer.
- The agent of such changes can be random spontaneous mutations or environmental influences such as chemical carcinogens, X-rays, or certain viruses.
- In 1911, Peyton Rous discovered a virus that causes cancer in chickens.
- o Since then, scientists have recognised a number of tumor viruses that cause cancer in various animals, including humans.
- o All tumor viruses transform cells into cancer cells through the integration of viral nucleic acid into host cell DNA.
- Cancer-causing genes, oncogenes, were initially discovered in retroviruses, but close counterparts, proto-oncogenes, have been found in other organisms.
- The products of proto-oncogenes are proteins that stimulate normal cell growth and division and play essential functions in normal cells.
- A proto-oncogene becomes an oncogene following genetic changes that lead to an increase in the proto-oncogene's protein production or the activity of each protein molecule.
- o These genetic changes include movements of DNA within the genome, amplification of the proto-oncogene, and point mutations in the control element of the proto-oncogene.

- Cancer cells frequently have chromosomes that have been broken and rejoined incorrectly.
  - o This may translocate a fragment to a location near an active promoter or other control element.
  - o Movement of transposable elements may also place a more active promoter near a proto-oncogene, increasing its expression.
- Amplification increases the number of copies of the proto-oncogene in the cell.
- A point mutation in the promoter or enhancer of a proto-oncogene may increase its expression.
  - o A point mutation in the coding sequence may lead to translation of a protein that is more active or longer-lived.
- Mutations to tumor-suppressor genes, whose normal products inhibit cell division, also contribute to cancer.
- Any decrease in the normal activity of a tumor-suppressor protein may contribute to cancer.
  - o Some tumor-suppressor proteins normally repair damaged DNA, preventing the accumulation of cancer-causing mutations.
  - o Others control the adhesion of cells to each other or to an extracellular matrix, crucial for normal tissues and often absent in cancers.
  - o Still others are components of cell-signaling pathways that inhibit the cell cycle.

Oncogene proteins and faulty tumor-suppressor proteins interfere with normal signaling pathways

- The proteins encoded by many proto-oncogenes and tumor-suppressor genes are components of cell-signaling pathways.
- Mutations in the products of two key genes, the ras proto-oncogene, and the p53 tumour suppressor gene occur in 30% and 50% of human cancers, respectively.
- Both the Ras protein and the p53 protein are components of signal-transduction pathways that convey external signals to the DNA in the cells nucleus.
- Ras, the product of the ras gene, is a G protein that relays a growth signal from a growth factor receptor on the plasma membrane to a cascade of protein kinases.
  - o At the end of the pathway is the synthesis of a protein that stimulates the cell cycle.
  - o Many ras oncogenes have a point mutation that leads to a hyperactive version of the Ras protein that can issue signals on its own, resulting in excessive cell division.
- The p53 gene, named for its 53000-dalton protein product, is often called the 'guardian angel of the genome.'
- Damage to the cell's DNA acts as a signal that leads to expression of the p53 gene.
- The p53 protein is a transcription factor for several genes.
  - o It can activate the p21 gene, which halts the cell cycle.
  - o It can turn on genes involved in DNA repair.
  - o When DNA damage is irreparable, the p53 protein can activate 'suicide genes' whose protein products cause cell death by apoptosis.
- A mutation that knocks out the p53 gene can lead to excessive cell growth and cancer.

Multiple mutations underlie the development of cancer

- More than one somatic mutation is generally needed to produce the changes characteristic of a full-fledged cancer cell.
- If cancer results from an accumulation of mutations, and if mutations occur throughout life, then the longer we live, the more likely we are to develop cancer.
- Colorectal cancer, with 135000 new cases and 60000 deaths in the United States each year, illustrates a multistep cancer path.
- The first sign is often a polyp, a small benign growth in the colon lining.
  - o The cells of the polyp look normal but divide unusually frequently.
- Through gradual accumulation of mutations that activate oncogenes and knock out tumor-suppressor genes, the polyp can develop into a malignant tumor.
- About a half dozen DNA changes must occur for a cell to become fully cancerous.
- These usually include the appearance of at least one active oncogene and the mutation or loss of several tumor-suppressor genes.
  - o Since mutant tumour-suppressor alleles are usually recessive, mutations must knock out both alleles.
  - o Most oncogenes behave as dominant alleles and require only one mutation.
- In many malignant tumours, the gene for telomerase is activated, removing a natural limit on the number of times the cell can divide.
- Viruses, especially retroviruses, play a role in about 15% of human cancer cases worldwide.
  - o These include some types of leukemia, liver cancer, and cancer of the cervix.
- Viruses promote cancer development by integrating their DNA into that of infected cells.
  - o By this process, a retrovirus may donate an oncogene to the cell.
- Alternatively, insertion of viral DNA may disrupt a tumor-suppressor gene or convert a protooncogene to an oncogene.
- Some viruses produce proteins that inactivate p53 and other tumor-suppressor proteins, making the cell more prone to becoming cancerous.
- The fact that multiple genetic changes are required to produce a cancer cell helps explain the predispositions to cancer that run in some families.
  - o An individual inheriting an oncogene or a mutant allele of a tumor-suppressor gene will be one step closer to accumulating the necessary mutations for cancer to develop.
- Geneticists are devoting much effort to finding inherited cancer alleles so that predisposition to certain cancers can be detected early in life.
  - o About 15% of colorectal cancers involve inherited mutations, especially to DNA repair genes or to the tumor-suppressor gene adenomatous polyposis coli, or APC.
    Normal functions of the APC gene include regulation of cell migration and adhesion.
    Even in patients with no family history of the disease, APC is mutated in about 60% of colorectal cancers.
  - o Between 5–10% of breast cancer cases show an inherited predisposition.
    This is the second most common type of cancer in the United States, striking more than 180000 women annually and leading to 40000 annual deaths.

Mutations to one of two tumor-suppressor genes, BRCA1 and BRCA2, increase the risk of breast and ovarian cancer.

o   A woman who inherits one mutant BRCA1 allele has a 60% probability of developing breast cancer before age 50 (versus a 2% probability in an individual with two normal alleles).

o   BRCA1 and BRCA2 are considered tumor-suppressor genes because their wild-type alleles protect against breast cancer and because their mutant alleles are recessive.

o   Recent evidence suggests that the BRCA2 protein is directly involved in repairing breaks that occur in both strands of DNA.

Eukaryotic genomes can have many noncoding DNA sequences in addition to genes

*   Several trends are evident when we compare the genomes of prokaryotes to those of eukaryotes.

*   There is a general trend from smaller to larger genomes, but with fewer genes in a given length of DNA.

o   Humans have 500 to 1500 times as many base pairs in their genome as most prokaryotes, but only 5 to 15 times as many genes.

*   Most of the DNA in a prokaryote genome codes for protein, tRNA, or rRNA.

o   The small amount of noncoding DNA consists mainly of regulatory sequences.

*   In eukaryotes, most of the DNA (98.5% in humans) does not code for protein or RNA.

o   Gene-related regulatory sequences and introns account for 24% of the human genome.

  Introns account for most of the difference in average length of eukaryotic (27000 base pairs) and prokaryotic genes (1000 base pairs).

o   Most intergenic DNA is repetitive DNA, present in multiple copies in the genome.

  Transposable elements and related sequences make up 44% of the entire human genome.

*   The first evidence for transposable elements came from geneticist Barbara McClintock's breeding experiments with Indian corn (maize) in the 1940s and 1950s.

*   Eukaryotic transposable elements are of two types: transposons, which move within a genome by means of a DNA intermediate, and retrotransposons, which move by means of an RNA intermediate, a transcript of the retrotransposon DNA.

o   Transposons can move by a 'cut and paste' mechanism, which removes the element from its original site, or by a 'copy and paste' mechanism, which leaves a copy behind.

o   Retrotransposons always leave a copy at the original site, since they are initially transcribed into an RNA intermediate.

*   Most transposons are retrotransposons, in which the transcribed RNA includes the code for an enzyme that catalyses the insertion of the retrotransposon and may include a gene for reverse transcriptase.

o   Reverse transcriptase uses the RNA molecule originally transcribed from the retrotransposon as a template to synthesise a double-stranded DNA copy.

*   Multiple copies of transposable elements and related sequences are scattered throughout eukaryotic genomes.

o   A single unit is hundreds or thousands of base pairs long, and the dispersed 'copies' are similar but not identical to one another.

- o Some of the copies are transposable elements and some are related sequences that have lost the ability to move.
- o Transposable elements and related sequences make up 25–50% of most mammalian genomes, and an even higher percentage in amphibians and angiosperms.
- In primates, a large portion of transposable element–related DNA consists of a family of similar sequences called Alu elements.
- o These sequences account for approximately 10% of the human genome.
- o Alu elements are about 300 nucleotides long, shorter than most functional transposable elements, and they do not code for protein.
- o Many Alu elements are transcribed into RNA molecules.
- o However, their cellular function is unknown.
- Repetitive DNA that is not related to transposable elements probably arose by mistakes that occurred during DNA replication or recombination.
- o Repetitive DNA accounts for about 15% of the human genome.
- o Five percent of the human genome consists of large-segment duplications in which 10,000 to 300000 nucleotide pairs seem to have been copied from one chromosomal location to another.
- Simple sequence DNA contains many copies of tandemly repeated short sequences of 15–500 nucleotides.
- o There may be as many as several hundred thousand repetitions of a nucleotide sequence.
- o Simple sequence DNA makes up 3% of the human genome.
- o Much of the genome's simple sequence DNA is located at chromosomal telomeres and centromeres, suggesting that it plays a structural role.
- o The DNA at centromeres is essential for the separation of chromatids in cell division and may also help to organise the chromatin within the interphase nucleus.
- o Telomeric DNA prevents gene loss as DNA shortens with each round of replication and also binds proteins that protect the ends of a chromosome from degradation or attachment to other chromosomes.

Gene families have evolved by duplication of ancestral genes

- Sequences coding for proteins and structural RNAs compose a mere 1.5% of the human genome.
- o If introns and regulatory sequences are included, gene-related DNA makes up 25% of the human genome.
- In humans, solitary genes present in one copy per haploid set of chromosomes make up only half of the total coding DNA.
- The rest occurs in multigene families, collections of identical or very similar genes.
- Some multigene families consist of identical DNA sequences that may be clustered tandemly.
- o These code for RNA products or for histone proteins.
- o For example, the three largest rRNA molecules are encoded in a single transcription unit that is repeated tandemly hundreds to thousands of times.
- o This transcript is cleaved to yield three rRNA molecules that combine with proteins and one other kind of rRNA to form ribosomal subunits.

- Two related families of nonidentical genes encode globins, a group of proteins that include the α (alpha) and β (beta) polypeptide sequences of hemoglobin.
- The different versions of each globin subunit are expressed at different times in development, allowing hemoglobin to function effectively in the changing environment of the developing animal.
  - o Within both the α and β families are sequences that are expressed during the embryonic, fetal, and/or adult stage of development.
  - o In humans, the embryonic and fetal hemoglobins have higher affinity for oxygen than do adult forms, ensuring transfer of oxygen from mother to developing fetus.
  - o Also found in the globin gene family clusters are several pseudogenes, DNA sequences similar to real genes that do not yield functional proteins.

Duplications, Rearrangements, and Mutations of DNA Contribute to Genome Evolution

- The earliest forms of life likely had a minimal number of genes, including only those necessary for survival and reproduction.
- The size of genomes has increased over evolutionary time, with the extra genetic material providing raw material for gene diversification.
- An accident in meiosis can result in one or more extra sets of chromosomes, a condition known as polyploidy.
  - o In a polyploid organism, one complete set of genes can provide essential functions for the organism.
  - o The genes in the extra set may diverge by accumulating mutations.
    These variations may persist if the organism carrying them survives and reproduces.
  - o In this way, genes with novel functions may evolve.
- Errors during meiosis due to unequal crossing over during Prophase I can lead to duplication of individual genes.
- Slippage during DNA replication can result in deletion or duplication of DNA regions.
  - o Such errors can lead to regions of repeats, such as simple sequence DNA.
- Major rearrangements of at least one set of genes occur during immune system differentiation.
- Duplication events can lead to the evolution of genes with related functions, such as the α-globin and β-globin gene families.
  - o A comparison of gene sequences within a multigene family indicates that they all evolved from one common ancestral globin gene, which was duplicated and diverged about 450–500 million years ago.
- After the duplication events, the differences between the genes in the d family arose from mutations that accumulated in the gene copies over many generations.
  - o The necessary function provided by an α-globin protein was fulfilled by one gene, while other copies of the β-globin gene accumulated random mutations.
  - o Some mutations may have altered the function of the protein product in ways that were beneficial to the organism without changing its oxygen-carrying function.
- The similarity in the amino acid sequences of the various α-globin and β-globin proteins supports this model of gene duplication and mutation.

o Random mutations accumulating over time in the pseudogenes have destroyed their function.

o In other gene families, one copy of a duplicated gene can undergo alterations that lead to a completely new function for the protein product.

o The genes for lysozyme and α-lactalbumin are good examples.

Lysozyme is an enzyme that helps prevent infection by hydrolysing bacterial cell walls.

α-lactalbumin is a nonenzymatic protein that plays a role in mammalian milk production.

• Both genes are found in mammals, while only lysozyme is found in birds.

o The two proteins are similar in their amino acids sequences and 3-D structures.

• These findings suggest that at some time after the bird and mammalian lineage had separated, the lysozyme gene underwent a duplication event in the mammalian lineage but not in the avian lineage.

o Subsequently, one copy of the duplicated lysozyme gene evolved into a gene encoding α-lactalbumin, a protein with a completely different function.

• Rearrangement of existing DNA sequences has also contributed to genome evolution.

o The presence of introns in eukaryotic genes may have promoted the evolution of new and potentially useful proteins by facilitating the duplication or repositioning of exons in the genome.

o A particular exon within a gene could be duplicated on one chromosome and deleted from the homologous chromosome.

o The gene with the duplicated exon would code for a protein with a second copy of the encoded domain.

• This change in the proteins structure could augment its function by increasing its stability or altering its ability to bind a particular ligand.

• Mixing and matching of different exons within or between genes owing to errors in meiotic recombination is called exon shuffling and could lead to new proteins with novel combinations of functions.

• The persistence of transposable elements as a large percentage of eukaryotic genomes suggests that they play an important role in shaping a genome over evolutionary time.

• These elements can contribute to evolution of the genome by promoting recombination, disrupting cellular genes or control elements, and carrying entire genes or individual exons to new locations.

• The presence of homologous transposable element sequences scattered throughout the genome allows recombination to take place between different chromosomes.

o Most of these alterations are likely detrimental, causing chromosomal translocations and other changes in the genome that may be lethal to the organism.

o Over the course of evolutionary time, an occasional recombination may be advantageous.

o The movement of transposable elements around the genome can have several direct consequences.

If a transposable element 'jumps' into the middle of a coding sequence of a protein-coding gene, it prevents the normal functioning of that gene.

If a transposable element inserts within a regulatory sequence, it may increase or decrease protein production.

o During transposition, a transposable element may transfer genes to a new position on the genome or may insert an exon from one gene into another gene.

o Transposable elements can lead to new coding sequences when an Alu element hops into introns to create a weak alternative splice site in the RNA transcript.

   Splicing will usually occur at the regular splice sites, producing the original protein.

   Occasionally, splicing will occur at the new weak site.

o In this way, alternative genetic combinations can be 'tried out' while the function of the original gene product is retained.

o These processes produce no effect or harmful effects in most individual cases.

o However, over long periods of time, the generation of genetic diversity provides more raw material for natural selection to work on during evolution.

Chapter 16

Comparative and Minimal Genomics

INTRODUCTION

Because all modern genomes have arisen from common ancestral genomes, the relationships between genomes can be studies with this fact in mind. This commonality means that information gained in one organism can have application in other even distantly related organisms. Comparative genomics enables the application of information gained from facile model systems to agricultural and medical problems. The nature and significance of differences between genomes also provides a powerful tool for determining the relationship between genotype and phenotype through comparative genomics and morphological and physiological studies.

COMPARATIVE GENOMICS

Comparative genomics is a field of biological research in which the genomic features of different organisms are compared. The genomic features may include the DNA sequence, genes, gene order, regulatory sequences, and other genomic structural landmarks. In this branch of genomics, whole or large parts of genomes resulting from genome projects are compared to study basic biological similarities and differences as well as evolutionary relationships between organisms.

The major principle of comparative genomics is that common features of two organisms will often be encoded within the DNA that is evolutionary conserved between them. Therefore, comparative genomic approaches start with making some form of alignment of genome sequences and looking for orthologous sequences (sequences that share a common ancestry) in the aligned genomes and checking to what extent those sequences are conserved. Based on these, inference on genome and molecular evolution are made and this may in turn be put in the context of, for example, phenotypic evolution or population genetics. Virtually started as soon as the whole genomes of two organisms became available (that is, the genomes of the bacteria *Haemophilus influenzae* (Fig. 16.1) and *Mycoplasma genitalium* (Fig. 16.2) in 1995, comparative genomics is now a standard component of the analysis of every new genome sequence. With the explosion in the number of genome project due to the advancements in DNA sequencing technologies, particularly the next-generation sequencing methods in late 2000s, this field has become more sophisticated, making it possible to deal with many genomes in a single study.

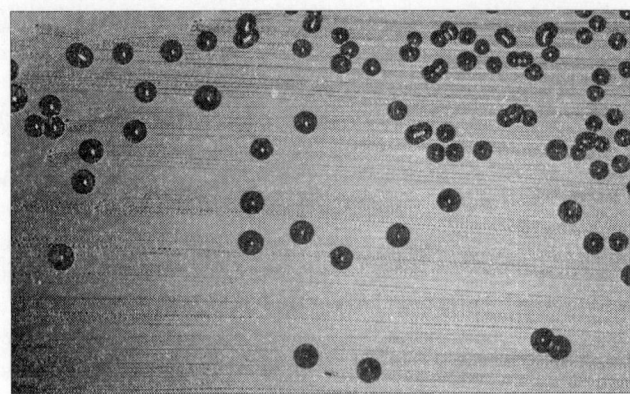

Fig. 16.1: *Haemophilus influenzae.*

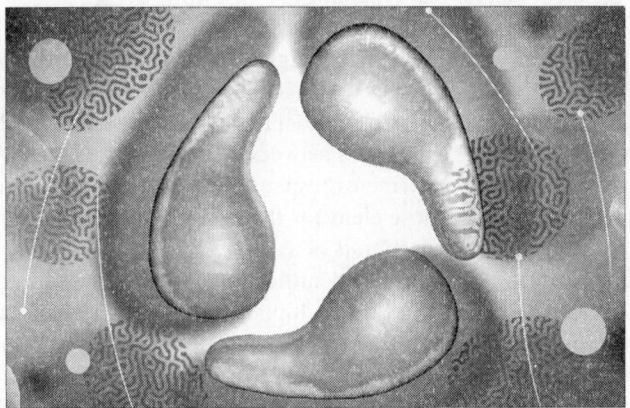

Fig. 16.2: *Mycoplasma genitalium.*

Comparative genomics has revealed high levels of similarity between closely related oganisms, such as humans and chimpanzees, and, more surprisingly, similarity between seemingly distantly related organisms, such as humans and the yeast *Saccharomyces cerevisiae*. It has also showed the extreme diversity of the gene composition in different evolutionary lineages.

Evolutionary Principles

One character of Biology is evolution, evolutionary theory is also the theoretical foundation of comparative genomics, and at the same time the results of comparative genomics unprecedentedly enriched and developed the theory of evolution. When two or more of the genome sequence compared, in essence get the evolutionary relationships of the sequence in the phylogenetic tree. Increased genome information of study makes molecular evolution, gene function at the genome level possible. Based on a variety of biological genome data and the study of vertical and horizontal evolution process, can understand vital parts of gene structure and its regulation function for life. But as a result in biological genome about 1.5~14.5% of the genes related to 'lateral migration phenomenon', namely the gene transfer between populations which can exist at the same time, the differences in sequence result has nothing to do with the evolution. So in the system analysis, it needs to establish a relatively complete evolution model, in order to avoid gene transfer and the influence of the lack of more appropriate species which are conserved sequence. Similarity of related genomes is the basis of comparative genomics.

Two creatures which have a recent common ancestor, the species difference genomes between them were evolved from ancestors genome, the closer the two organisms on the evolutionary stages, the higher their genome correlated. If there is close relationship between them, then their genome will behave like linear (synteny), namely some or all of the genetic sequences are conservative. So scientists can use the homology of the sequence and structure of encoding between mode genomes, by known genome mapping information to locate other genes in the genome, so as to reveal the potential function of the genes, clarify evolutionary relationship and the inner structure of the genome.

Orthologous sequences are separate because of speciation: A gene exists in the original species, the species divided into two species, so genes in new species are orthologous. Paralogy sequences are separate by gene cloning (gene duplication): if a particular gene in the biology is copied, then the copy of the two sequences is paralogy. A pair of orthologous sequences is called orthologous pairs (orthologs), a pair of paralogy sequence is called collateral pairs (paralogs).

Orthologous pairs usually have the same or similar function, but not necessarily on collateral pairs: due to the lack of the power of natural selection, the original duplicate copy of the genes are variation and get free new functions. Comparative genomics exploits both similarities and differences in the proteins, RNA, and regulatory regions of different organisms to infer how selection has acted upon these elements. Those elements that are responsible for similarities between different species should be conserved through time (stabilising selection), while those elements responsible for differences among species should be divergent (positive selection). Finally, those elements that are unimportant to the evolutionary success of the organism will be unconserved (selection is neutral).

One of the important goals of the field is the identification of the mechanisms of eukaryotic genome evolution. It is however often complicated by the multiplicity of events that have taken place throughout the history of individual lineages, leaving only distorted and superimposed traces in the genome of each living organism. For this reason comparative genomics studies of small model organisms (for example the model Caenorhabditis elegans and closely related Caenorhabditis briggsae) are of great importance to advance our understanding of general mechanisms of evolution.

Methods

Computational approaches to genome comparison have recently become a common research topic in computer science. A public collection of case studies and demonstrations is growing, ranging from whole genome comparisons to gene expression analysis. This has increased the introduction of different ideas, including concepts from systems and control, information theory, strings analysis and data mining. It is anticipated that computational approaches will become and remain a standard topic for research and teaching, while multiple courses will begin training students to be fluent in both topics.

Tools

Computational tools for analysing sequences and complete genomes are developed quickly due to the availability of large amount of genomic data. At the same time, comparative analysis tools are progressed and improved. In the challenges about these analyses, it is very important to visualise the comparative results. Visualisation of sequence conservation is a tough task of comparative sequence analysis. As we know, it is highly inefficient to examine the alignment of long genomic regions manually. Internet-based genome browsers provide many useful tools for investigating genomic sequences due to integrating all sequence-based biological information on genomic regions. When we extract large amount of relevant biological data, they can be very easy to use and less time-consuming.

- UCSC Browser: This site contains the reference sequence and working draft assemblies for a large collection of genomes.
- Ensembl: The Ensembl project produces genome databases for vertebrates and other eukaryotic species, and makes this information freely available online.
- MapView: The Map Viewer provides a wide variety of genome mapping and sequencing data.
- VISTA is a comprehensive suite of programs and databases for comparative analysis of genomic sequences. It was built to visualise the results of comparative analysis based on DNA alignments. The presentation of comparative data generated by VISTA can easily suit both small and large scale of data.

An advantage of using online tools is that these websites are being developed and updated constantly. There are many new settings and content can be used online to improve efficiency.

Applications

Agriculture: Agriculture is a field that reaps the benefits of comparative genomics. Identifying the loci of advantageous genes is a key step in breeding crops that are optimised for greater yield, cost-efficiency, quality, and disease resistance. For example, one genome wide association study conducted on 517 rice landraces revealed 80 loci associated with several categories of agronomic performance, such as grain weight, amylose content and drought tolerance. Many of the loci were previously uncharacterised. Not only is this methodology powerful, it is also quick. Previous methods of identifying loci associated with agronomic performance required several generations of carefully monitored breeding of parent strains, a time consuming effort that is unnecessary for comparative genomic studies.

Medicine: The medical field also benefits from the study of comparative genomics. Vaccinology in particular has experienced useful advances in technology due to genomic approaches to problems. In an approach known as reverse vaccinology, researchers can discover candidate antigens for vaccine development by analysing the genome of a pathogen or a family of pathogens. Applying a comparative genomics approach by analysing the genomes of several related pathogens can lead to the development of vaccines that are multiprotective. A team of researchers employed such an approach to create a universal vaccine for Group B *Streptococcus*, a group of bacteria responsible for severe neonatal infection. Comparative genomics can also be used to generate specificity for vaccines against pathogens that are closely related to commensal microorganisms. For example, researchers used comparative genomic analysis of commensal and pathogenic strains of *E. coli* to identify pathogen specific genes as a basis for finding antigens that result in immune response against pathogenic strains but not commensal ones.

Research: Comparative genomics also opens up new avenues in other areas of research. As DNA sequencing technology has become more accessible, the number of sequenced genomes has grown. With the increasing reservoir of available genomic data, the potency of comparative genomic inference has grown as well. A notable case of this increased potency is found in recent primate research. Comparative genomic methods have allowed researchers to gather information about genetic variation, differential gene expression, and evolutionary dynamics in primates that were indiscernible using previous data and methods. The Great Ape Genome Project used comparative genomic methods to investigate genetic variation with reference to the six great ape species, finding healthy levels of variation in their gene pool despite shrinking population size. Another study showed that patterns of DNA methylation, which are a known regulation mechanism for gene expression, differ in the prefrontal cortex of humans versus chimps, and implicated this difference in the evolutionary divergence of the two species.

MINIMAL GENOME

The concept of minimal genome assumes that genomes can be reduced to a bare minimum, given that they contain many non-essential genes of limited or situational importance to the organism. Therefore, if a collection of all the essential genes were put together, a minimum genome could be created artificially in a stable environment. By adding more genes, the creation of an organism of desired properties is possible. The concept of minimal genome arose from the observations that many genes do not appear to be necessary for survival.

In order to create a new organism a scientist must determine the minimal set of genes required for metabolism and replication. This can be achieved by experimental and computational analysis of the biochemical pathways needed to carry out basic metabolism and reproduction. A good model for a minimal genome is Mycoplasma genitalium, the organism with the smallest known genome. Most genes that are used by this organism are usually considered essential for survival, based on this concept a minimal set of 256 genes has been proposed.

Genome Reduction in Nature

Bacteria

Many naturally occurring bacteria have reduced genomes even though they may not be reduced to the bare minimum. Although these genomes are thus not 'minimal', they are good models for genome reduction and thus 'minimal genomes'. Genome reduction occurs most commonly in endosymbiotic, parasitic or pathogenic bacteria that live in their hosts. The host provides most of the nutrients such bacteria require, hence the bacteria do not need the genes for producing such compounds themselves. Examples include species of Buchnera, Chlamydia, Treponema, Mycoplasma, and many others. One of the most reduced genomes in free-living bacteria has been found in Pelagibacter ubique which encodes 1354 proteins. *Mycoplasma genitalium* has been used as a prime model for minimal genomes. It is a human urogenital pathogen which has the smallest genome of size 580 kb and it consists of only 482 protein-coding genes.

Viruses

Viruses have the smallest genomes in nature. For instance, bacteriophage MS2 consists of only 3569 nucleotides (single-stranded RNA) and encodes just four proteins. Similarly, among eukaryotic viruses, porcine circoviruses are among the smallest. They encode only 2–3 open reading frames.

Rise of the minimal genome and construction of synthetic mycoplasma

It was a collaborative effort by the National Aeronautics and Space Administration (NASA) and the two scientists: Morowitz and Tourtellote that this concept arose. NASA in the 1960s was searching for extraterrestrial life forms, assuming that if they existed they may be simple creatures. While Morowitz, to attract people's attention published about mycoplasmas as being the smallest and simplest self-replicating creatures. The two grouped together and came up with an idea to assemble a living cell from the components of mycoplasmas. Since, mycoplasmas are built with a minimum set of organelles such as: a plasma membrane, ribosomes and a circular double stranded DNA, it was selected as the best candidate for cell reassembly. Morowitz' major idea was to define the entire machinery of mycoplasmas cell in molecular level. He announced that an international effort would help him accomplish this main objective.

The main plan consisted of:

1. Physical and functional mapping with complete sequencing of the mycoplasma.
2. Determine the open reading frames (ORFs).
3. Determining the encoded amino acids.
4. Understanding the functions of genes.
5. Reassemble mycoplasma's machinery cell.

This entire process was hard work, meanwhile even when papers were being published on the construction of minimal genome, by the 1980s Richard Herrmann's laboratory had successfully managed to fully sequence and genetically characterise the 800kb genome of *M. pneumoniae*. That small of a genome itself took close to three years of hard work. Later in the 1995s another laboratory located in Maryland the Institute for Genomic Research (TIGR) collaborated with the teams of Johns Hopkins and University of North Carolina.

Their organism for genome sequencing was Mycoplasma genitalium consisting of only 580 kb genome, the sequencing of which was done in 6 months.

The sequencing data revealed many interesting facts about *M. genitalium* such as discovery of some conserved genes, which ultimately helped in defining essentiality to life, of a minimal self-replicating cell. By far *M. genitalium* has become the prime candidate for minimal genome project. In fact these organisms are closest to minimal genome capable of self-replicating.

Minimal set of essential genes are typically found by selective inactivation or deletions of genes and then testing the effect of each under a given set conditions. The discovery of essential genes have been done by the J. Craig Venter institute, they claim *M. genitalium* consists of 381 essential genes.

The next venture that the J.Craig Venter institute landed upon was creating a synthetic organism named Mycoplasma laboratorium, through minimal set genes of *M. genitalium*. This project opens new doors for synthetic biology because this impressive creation is being built upon by bringing together chemical synthesis and recombination cloning methodology.

How to begin reconstructing

Reconstruction of a minimal genome is possible by using the knowledge of existing genomes via which the sets of genes, essential for living can also be determined. Once the set of essential genetic elements are known, one can proceed to define the key pathways and core-players by modelling simulations and wet lab genome engineering. The two organisms upon which the 'minimal gene set for cellular life' was applied were: Haemophilus influenzae, and *M. genitalium*. A list of orthologous proteins were compiled in hope that it would contain protein necessary for cell survival, as orthologous analysis determines how two organisms evolved and shed away any non-essential genes. Since, H. influenza and *M. genitalium* are Gram negative and Gram positive bacteria and due to their vast evolution it was expected that these organisms would be enriched genes that were of universal importance.

However, 244 detected orthologs discovered contained no parasitism-specific proteins. The conclusion of this analysis was that similar biochemical functions might be performed by non- orthologous proteins. Even when biochemical pathways of these two organisms were mapped, several pathways were present but many were incomplete. Proteins determined to be common between the two organisms were non-orthologous to each other. Much of the research mainly focuses on the ancestral genome and less on the minimal genome. Studies of these existing genomes have helped determine that orthologous genes found in these two species are not necessarily essential for survival, in fact non-orthologous genes were found to be more important. Also, it was determined that in order for proteins to share same functions they do not need to have same sequence or common three dimensional folds.

Distinguishing between orthologs and paralogs and detecting displacements of orthologs have been quiet beneficial in reconstructing evolution and determining the minimal gene set required for a cellular life. Instead, of conducting a strict orthology study, comparing groups of orthologs and occurrence in most clades instead of every species helped encounter genes lost or displaced. Only genomes that have been completely sequenced have enabled in studying orthologs among group of organisms. Without a fully sequenced genome it would not be possible to determine the essential minimal gene set required for survival.

Essential genes of M. genitalium

J. Craig Venter Institute (JCVI) conducted a study to find all the essential genes of *M. genitalium* through global transposon mutagenesis. As a result they found that 382 out of 482 protein coding genes were essential. Genes encoding proteins of unknown function constitute 28% of the essential protein coding genes set. Before conducting this study the JCVI had performed another study on the non-essential genes, genes not required for growth, of M.genitalium, where they reported the use of transposon mutagenesis. Despite figuring out the non-essential genes, it is not confirmed that the products that these genes make have any important biological functions. It was only through gene essentiality studies of bacteria that JCVI have been able to compose a hypothetical minimal gene sets.

Number of Essential Genes

The number of essential genes is different for each organism. In fact, each organism has a different number of essential genes, depending on which strain (or individual) is tested. In addition, the number depends on the conditions under which an organism is tested. In several bacteria (or other microbes such as yeast) all or most genes have been deleted individually to determine which genes are 'essential' for survival. Such tests are usually carried out on rich media which contain all nutrients. However, if all nutrients are provided, genes required for the synthesis of nutrients are not 'essential'. When cells are grown on minimal media, many more genes are essential as they may be needed to synthesise such nutrients (e.g. vitamins). The numbers provided in Table 16.1 typically have been collected using rich media.

Table 16.1: Organisms and essential genes collected from rich media.

Organism	Essential genes
Escherichia coli	1617
Haemophilus influenzae	642
Streptococcus pneumoniae	244
Mycoplasma genitalium	381
Vibrio cholerae	779
Staphylococcus aureus	653
Saccharomyces cerevisiae	1110

The number of essential genes were collected from the Database of Essential Genes (DEG). The organisms listed in this table have been systematically tested for essential genes.

First self replicating synthetic cell

May 20, 2010- Researchers at the JCVI have successfully created a synthetic bacterial cell that is capable of replicating itself. The team has synthesised a 1.08 million base pair chromosome of a modified *Mycoplasma mycoides*. The synthetic cell is called: Mycoplasma mycoides JCVI-syn1.0. One of the remarkable thing about this cell is that its DNA was built in the computer and then brought to life in the laboratory. The original proteins and biological materials of the converted cell use the new artificially DNA to generate daughter cells. These daughter cells are of synthetic origin and capable of further replication. This proves that genomes can be designed on computers. The steps they applied to build this was first they simulated a model of this genome computationally, they identified DNA via watermarks, next, they chemically produced this genome in the laboratory and finally, transplanted this genome into a recipient cell to produce a synthetic cell solely controlled by this synthetic genome.

Just the first half of the project has taken 15 years to complete and there is still more to come. The team designed an accurate, digitised genome of *M. mycoides*. A total of 1078 cassettes all 1080 base pair long were built. These cassettes were designed in a way that the end of each DNA cassette overlapped by 80 base pairs. The whole assembled genome was transplanted in yeast cells and grown as yeast artificial chromosome. This synthetic cell will be now able to show scientists how truly a cell works.

Now that they have synthetic cells growing in their laboratory, the JCVI group can focus on their ultimate goal of synthesising a minimal cell containing just the essential genes necessary for life.

Future direction and uses of minimal genome

Based on JCVI's progress in the field of synthetic biology, it is possible that in near future scientists will be able to propagate *M. genitalium*s genome in the form of naked DNA, into recipient mycoplasmas cells and replace their original genome with a synthetic genome. Since, mycoplasmas have no cell wall, the transfer of a naked DNA into their cell is possible. The only requirement now is the technique to include the synthetic genome of *M. genitalium* into mycoplasma cells. To some extent this has become possible, the first replicating synthetic cell has already been developed by the JCVI and they are now on to creating their first synthetic life, consisting of minimal number of essential genes. This new breakthrough in synthetic biology will certainly bring in a new approach to understand biology, and this redesigning and prototyping genomes will later become beneficial to biotechnology companies, enabling them to produce synthetic microbes that produce new, cheaper and better bio-products.

Uses of minimal genome:
1. Identification of essential genes.
2. Reduced genetic complexity that allows greater predictability of engineered strains.
3. Engineer plants to resist herbicides or harsh environmental conditions.
4. Synthetically produce pharmaceuticals
5. Large scale benefits: clean energy
6. Renewable chemicals
7. Sequestering carbon from the atmosphere.
8. Create beneficial microbes to make them produce bio-products.

Chapter 17

Genome Mapping

INTRODUCTION

Gene mapping, also called genome mapping, is the creation of a genetic map assigning DNA fragments to chromosomes. When a genome is first investigated, this map is nonexistent. The map improves with the scientific progress and is perfect when the genomic DNA sequencing of the species has been completed. During this process, and for the investigation of differences in strain, the fragments are identified by small tags. These may be genetic markers (PCR products) or the unique sequence-dependent pattern of DNA-cutting enzymes.

The ordering is derived from genetic observations (recombinant frequency) for these markers or in the second case from a computational integration of the fingerprinting data. The term 'mapping' is used in two different but related contexts.

Two different ways of mapping are distinguished. Genetic mapping uses classical genetic techniques (e.g. pedigree analysis or breeding experiments) to determine sequence features within a genome. Using modern molecular biology techniques for the same purpose is usually referred to as physical mapping.

Physical mapping: In physical mapping, the DNA is cut by a restriction enzyme. Once cut, the DNA fragments are separated by electrophoresis. The resulting pattern of DNA migration (i.e. its genetic fingerprint) is used to identify what stretch of DNA is in the clone. By analysing the fingerprints, contigs are assembled by automated (FPC) or manual means (Pathfinders) into overlapping DNA stretches. Now a good choice of clones can be made to efficiently sequence the clones to determine the DNA sequence of the organism under study.

Macrorestriction is a type of physical mapping wherein the high molecular weight DNA is digested with a restriction enzyme having a low number of restriction sites.

There are alternative ways to determine how DNA in a group of clones overlap without completely sequencing the clones. Once the map is determined, the clones can be used as a resource to efficiently contain large stretches of the genome. This type of mapping is more accurate than genetic maps.

Genes can be mapped prior to the complete sequencing by independent approaches like *in situ* hybridisation.

WHOLE GENOME SEQUENCING

Whole genome sequencing (also known as full genome sequencing, complete genome sequencing, or entire genome sequencing) is a laboratory process that determines the complete DNA sequence of an organisms genome at a single time. This entails sequencing all of an organisms chromosomal DNA as well as DNA contained in the mitochondria and, for plants, in the chloroplast.

Whole genome sequencing should not be confused with DNA profiling, which only determines the likelihood that genetic material came from a particular individual or group, and does not contain additional information on genetic relationships, origin or susceptibility to specific diseases. Also unlike full genome sequencing, SNP genotyping covers less than 0.1% of the genome. Almost all truly complete genomes are of microbes, the term 'full genome' is thus sometimes used loosely to mean greater than 95%. The remainder of this section focuses on nearly complete human genomes.

In general, knowing the complete DNA sequence of an individual's genome does not, on its own, provide useful clinical information, but this may change over time as a large number of scientific studies continue to be published detailing clear associations between specific genetic variants and disease.

The tool of gene sequencing at SNP level enables scientists to pinpoint functional variants from association studies and improve the knowledge available to researchers interested in evolutionary biology, and hence may lay the foundation for predicting disease susceptibility and drug response. An image of the 46 chromosomes, making up the diploid genome of human male in shown in Fig. 17.1.

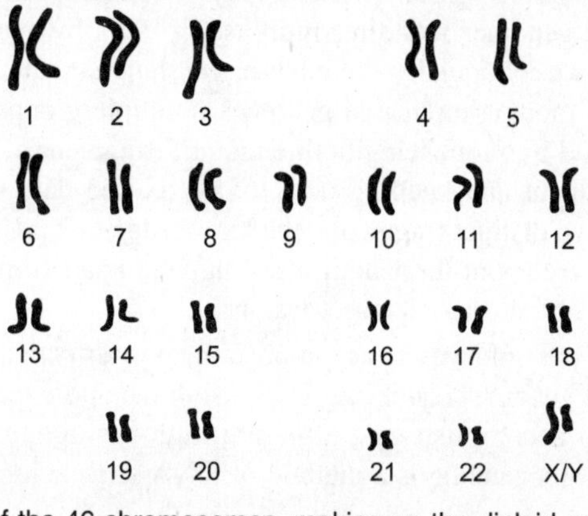

Fig. 17.1: An image of the 46 chromosomes, making up the diploid genome of human male.

Cells used for Sequencing

Almost any biological sample containing a full copy of the DNA—even a very small amount of DNA or ancient DNA—can provide the genetic material necessary for full genome sequencing. Such samples may include saliva, epithelial cells, bone marrow, hair (as long as the hair contains a hair follicle), seeds, plant leaves, or anything else that has DNA-containing cells.

The genome sequence of a single cell selected from a mixed population of cells can be determined using techniques of single cell genome sequencing. This has important advantages in environmental microbiology in cases where a single cell of a particular micro-organism species can be isolated from a mixed population by microscopy on the basis of its morphological or other distinguishing characteristics. In such cases the normally necessary steps of isolation and growth of the organism in culture may be omitted, thus allowing the sequencing of a much greater spectrum of organism genomes.

Single cell genome sequencing is being tested as a method of preimplantation genetic diagnosis, wherein a cell from the embryo created by *in vitro* fertilisation is taken and analysed before embryo transfer into the uterus. After implantation, cell-free fetal DNA can be taken by simple venipuncture from the mother and used for whole genome sequencing of the fetus.

Mutation Frequencies in Cancers

Whole genome sequencing has established the mutation frequency for whole human genomes. The mutation frequency in the whole genome between generations for humans (parent to child) is about 70 new mutations per generation. An even lower level of variation was found comparing whole genome sequencing in blood cells for a pair of monozygotic (identical twins) 100 year old centenarians. Only 8 somatic differences were found, though somatic variation occurring in less than 20% of blood cells would be undetected.

In the specifically protein coding regions of the human genome, it is estimated that there are about 0.35 mutations that would change the protein sequence between parent/child generations (less than one mutated protein per generation). Cancers, however, have much higher mutation frequencies. The particular frequency depends on tissue type, whether there is a mis-match DNA repair deficiency, and exposure to DNA damaging agents such as UV-irradiation or components of tobacco smoke.

Early techniques: Sequencing of nearly an entire human genome was first accomplished in 2000 partly through the use of shotgun sequencing technology. While full genome shotgun sequencing for small (4000–7000 base pair) genomes was already in use in 1979, broader application benefited from pairwise end sequencing, known colloquially as double-barrel shotgun sequencing. As sequencing projects began to take on longer and more complicated genomes, multiple groups began to realise that useful information could be obtained by sequencing both ends of a fragment of DNA. Although sequencing both ends of the same fragment and keeping track of the paired data was more cumbersome than sequencing a single end of two distinct fragments, the knowledge that the two sequences were oriented in opposite directions and were about the length of a fragment apart from each other was valuable in reconstructing the sequence of the original target fragment.

Current techniques: One possible way to accomplish the cost-effective high-throughput sequencing necessary to accomplish full genome sequencing is by using nanopore technology.

Another possible way to accomplish cost-effective high-throughput sequencing is by utilising fluorophore technology. Pyrosequencing is a method of DNA sequencing based on the sequencing by synthesis principle.

Commercialisation: A number of public and private companies are competing to develop a full genome sequencing platform that is commercially robust for both research and clinical use.

Disruption to DNA Array Market

Full genome sequencing provides information on a genome that is orders of magnitude larger than that provided by the previous leader in genotyping technology, DNA arrays. For humans, DNA arrays currently provide genotypic information on up to one million genetic variants, while full genome sequencing will provide information on all six billion bases in the human genome, or 3000 times more data. Because of this, full genome sequencing is considered a disruptive innovation to the DNA array markets as the accuracy of both range from 99.98% to 99.999% (in non-repetitive DNA regions). Agilent, another established DNA array manufacturer, is working on targeted (selective region) genome sequencing technologies. It is thought that Affymetrix, the pioneer of array technology in the 1990s, has fallen behind due to significant corporate and stock turbulence and is currently not working on any known full genome sequencing approach. It is unknown what will happen to the DNA array market once full genome sequencing becomes commercially widespread, especially as companies and laboratories providing this disruptive technology start to realise economies of scale. It is postulated, however, that this new technology may significantly diminish the total market size for arrays and any other sequencing technology once it becomes common place for individuals and newborns to have their full genomes sequenced.

Sequencing versus Analysis

In principle, full genome sequencing can provide raw data on all six billion nucleotides in an individual's DNA. However, it does not provide an analysis of what that information means or how it might be utilised in various clinical applications, such as in medicine to help prevent disease. As of 2010 the companies that are working on providing full genome sequencing provide clinical CLIA certified data (Illumina) and analytical services for the interpretation of the full genome data, with only one institution offering sequencing and analysis in a clinical setting. Nevertheless there is plenty of room for researchers or companies to improve such analyses and make it useful to physicians and patients.

Societal Impact

Inexpensive, time-efficient full genome sequencing will be a major accomplishment not only for the field of genomics, but for the entire human civilisation because, for the first time, individuals will be able to have their entire genome sequenced. Utilising this information, it is speculated that health care professionals, such as physicians and genetic counselors, will eventually be able to use genomic information to predict what diseases a person may get in the future and attempt to either minimise the impact of that disease or avoid it altogether through the implementation of personalised, preventive medicine. Full genome sequencing will allow health care professionals to analyse the entire human genome of an individual and therefore detect all disease-related genetic variants, regardless of the genetic variant's prevalence or frequency. This will enable the rapidly emerging medical fields of predictive medicine and personalised medicine and will mark a significant leap forward for the clinical genetic revolution. Full genome sequencing is clearly of great importance for research into the basis of genetic disease and has shown significant benefit to a subset of individuals with rare disease in the clinical setting. The traditional guidelines for genetic testing have been developed over the course of several decades since it first became possible to test for genetic markers associated with disease, prior to the advent of cost-effective, comprehensive genetic screening. It is established that norms, such as in the sciences and the field of genetics, are subject to change and evolve over time. It is unknown whether traditional norms practiced in medical genetics today will be altered by new technological advancements such as full genome sequencing.

Today, parents have the legal authority to obtain testing of any kind for their children. Currently available newborn screening for childhood diseases allows detection of rare disorders that can be prevented or better treated by early detection and intervention.

ETHICAL CONCERNS

The majority of ethicists insist that the privacy of individuals undergoing genetic testing must be protected under all circumstances. Data obtained from whole genome sequencing cannot only reveal a lot of information about the individual who is the source of DNA, but it can also reveal a lot of probabilistic information about the DNA sequence of close genetic relatives. Furthermore, the data obtained from whole genome sequencing can also reveal a lot of useful predictive information about the relatives present and future health risks. This raises important questions about what obligations, if any, are owned to the family members of the individuals who are undergoing genetic testing.

SEQUENCE ASSEMBLY

Sequence assembly refers to aligning and merging fragments of a much longer DNA sequence in order to reconstruct the original sequence. This is needed as DNA sequencing technology cannot read whole genomes in one go, but rather reads small pieces of between 20 and 30000 bases, depending on the technology used. Typically the short fragments, called reads, result from shotgun sequencing genomic DNA, or gene transcript (ESTs).

The problem of sequence assembly can be compared to taking many copies of a book, passing each of them through a shredder with a different cutter, and piecing the text of the book back together just by looking at the shredded pieces. Besides the obvious difficulty of this task, there are some extra practical issues: the original may have many repeated paragraphs, and some shreds may be modified during shredding to have typos. Excerpts from another book may also be added in, and some shreds may be completely unrecognisable.

Genome Assemblers

The first sequence assemblers began to appear in the late 1980s and early 1990s as variants of simpler sequence alignment programs to piece together vast quantities of fragments generated by automated sequencing instruments called DNA sequencers. As the sequenced organisms grew in size and complexity (from small viruses over plasmids to bacteria and finally eukaryotes), the assembly programs used in these genome projects needed increasingly sophisticated strategies to handle:

- Terabytes of sequencing data which need processing on computing clusters.
- Identical and nearly identical sequences (known as repeats) which can, in the worst case, increase the time and space complexity of algorithms exponentially.
- Errors in the fragments from the sequencing instruments, which can confound assembly.

Faced with the challenge of assembling the first larger eukaryotic genomes—the fruit fly *Drosophila melanogaster* in 2000 and the human genome just a year later,—scientists developed assemblers like Celera Assembler and Arachne able to handle genomes of 100–300 million base pairs. Subsequent to these efforts, several other groups, mostly at the major genome (Fig. 17.2) sequencing centers, built large-scale assemblers, and an open source effort known as AMOS was launched to bring together all the innovations in genome assembly technology under the open source framework.

EST assemblers: Expressed Sequence Tag or EST assembly differs from genome assembly in several ways. The sequences for EST assembly are the transcribed mRNA of a cell and represent only a subset of the whole genome. At a first glance, underlying algorithmical problems differ between genome and EST assembly. For instance, genomes often have large amounts of repetitive sequences, mainly in the inter-genic parts. Since ESTs represent gene transcripts, they will not contain these repeats. On the other hand, cells tend to have a certain number of genes that are constantly expressed in very high numbers, which again leads to the problem of similar sequences present in high numbers in the data set to be assembled.

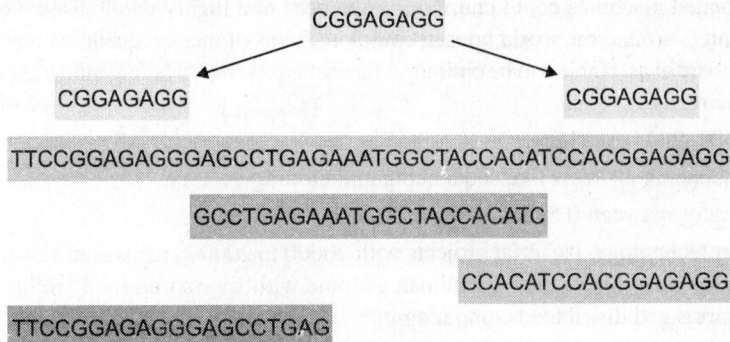

Fig. 17.2: Sample sequence showing how a sequence assembler would take fragments and match by overlaps. Image also shows the potential problem of repeats in the sequence.

Furthermore, genes sometimes overlap in the genome (sense-antisense transcription), and should ideally still be assembled separately. EST assembly is also complicated by features like (*cis-*) alternative splicing, trans-splicing, single-nucleotide polymorphism, recoding, and post-transcriptional modification.

De novo vs Mapping Assembly

In sequence assembly, two different types can be distinguished:

1. *De novo*: Assembling short reads to create full-length (sometimes novel) sequences.
2. Mapping: Assembling reads against an existing backbone sequence, building a sequence that is similar but not necessarily identical to the backbone sequence.

In terms of complexity and time requirements, *de novo* assemblies are orders of magnitude slower and more memory intensive than mapping assemblies. This is mostly due to the fact that the assembly algorithm needs to compare every read with every other read (an operation that has a naive time complexity of $O(n^2)$, using a hash this can be reduced significantly). Referring to the comparison drawn to shredded books in the introduction: while for mapping assemblies one would have a very similar book as template (perhaps with the names of the main characters and a few locations changed), the *de novo* assemblies are more hardcore in a sense as one would not know before hand whether this would become a science book, a novel, a catalogue, or even several books. Also, every shred would be compared with every other shred.

Influence of Technological Changes

The complexity of sequence assembly is driven by two major factors: the number of fragments and their lengths. While more and longer fragments allow better identification of sequence overlaps, they also pose problems as the underlying algorithms show quadratic or even exponential complexity behaviour to both number of fragments and their length. And while shorter sequences are faster to align, they also complicate the layout phase of an assembly as shorter reads are more difficult to use with repeats or near identical repeats. In the earliest days of DNA sequencing, scientists could only gain a few sequences of short length (some dozen bases) after weeks of work in laboratories. Hence, these sequences could be aligned in a few minutes by hand. In 1975, the Dideoxy termination method (also known as Sanger sequencing) was invented and until shortly after 2000, the technology was improved up to a point where fully automated machines could churn out sequences in a highly parallelised mode 24 hr a day. Large genome centers around the world housed complete farms of these sequencing machines, which in turn led to the necessity of assemblers to be optimised for sequences from whole-genome shotgun sequencing projects where the reads:

- Are about 800–900 bases long.
- Contain sequencing artifacts like sequencing and cloning vectors.
- Have error rates between 0.5 and 10%.

With the Sanger technology, bacterial projects with 20000 to 200000 reads could easily be assembled on one computer. Larger projects, like the human genome with approximately 35 million reads, needed large computing farms and distributed computing.

Greedy Algorithm

Given a set of sequence fragments the object is to find the shortest common super sequence.

1. Calculate pairwise alignments of all fragments.
2. Choose two fragments with the largest overlap.
3. Merge chosen fragments.
4. Repeat step 2 and 3 until only one fragment is left.

The result is a suboptimal solution to the problem.

SEQUENCE ALIGNMENT

In bioinformatics, a sequence alignment is a way of arranging the sequences of DNA, RNA, or protein to identify regions of similarity that may be a consequence of functional, structural, or evolutionary relationships between the sequences. Aligned sequences of nucleotide or amino acid residues are typically represented as rows within a matrix. Gaps are inserted between the residues so that identical or similar characters are aligned in successive columns.

Interpretation

If two sequences in an alignment share a common ancestor, mismatches can be interpreted as point mutations and gaps as indels (that is, insertion or deletion mutations) introduced in one or both lineages in the time since they diverged from one another. In sequence alignments of proteins, the degree of similarity between amino acids occupying a particular position in the sequence can be interpreted as a rough measure of how conserved a particular region or sequence motif is among lineages. The absence of substitutions, or the presence of only very conservative substitutions (that is, the substitution of amino acids whose side chains have similar biochemical properties) in a particular region of the sequence, suggest that this region has structural or functional importance. Although DNA and RNA nucleotide bases are more similar to each other than are amino acids, the conservation of base pairs can indicate a similar functional or structural role.

Alignment Methods

Very short or very similar sequences can be aligned by hand. However, most interesting problems require the alignment of lengthy, highly variable or extremely numerous sequences that cannot be aligned solely by human effort. Instead, human knowledge is applied in constructing algorithms to produce high-quality sequence alignments, and occasionally in adjusting the final results to reflect patterns that are difficult to represent algorithmically (especially in the case of nucleotide sequences). Computational approaches to sequence alignment generally fall into two categories: global alignments and local alignments. Calculating a global alignment is a form of global optimisation that 'forces' the alignment to span the entire length of all query sequences. By contrast, local alignments identify regions of similarity within long sequences that are often widely divergent overall. Local alignments are often preferable, but can be more difficult to calculate because of the additional challenge of identifying the regions of similarity. A variety of computational algorithms have been applied to the sequence alignment problem. These include slow but formally correct methods like dynamic programming. These also include efficient, heuristic algorithms or probabilistic methods designed for large-scale database search, that do not guarantee to find best matches.

Representations

Alignments are commonly represented both graphically and in text format. In almost all sequence alignment representations, sequences are written in rows arranged so that aligned residues appear in successive columns. In text formats, aligned columns containing identical or similar characters are indicated with a system of conservation symbols. As in the image above, an asterisk or pipe symbol is used to show identity between two columns, other less common symbols include a colon for conservative substitutions and a period for semiconservative substitutions. Many sequence visualisation programs also use colour to display information about the properties of the individual sequence elements, in DNA and RNA sequences, this equates to assigning each nucleotide its own colour. In protein alignments, such as the one in the image above, colour is often used to indicate amino acid properties to aid in judging the conservation of a given amino acid substitution. For multiple sequences the last row in each column is often the consensus sequence determined by the alignment, the consensus sequence is also often represented in graphical format with a sequence logo in which the size of each nucleotide or amino acid letter corresponds to its degree of conservation.

Sequence alignments can be stored in a wide variety of text-based file formats, many of which were originally developed in conjunction with a specific alignment program or implementation. Most web-based tools allow a limited number of input and output formats, such as FASTA format and GenBank format and the output is not easily editable. Several conversion programs that provide graphical and/or command line interfaces are available, such as READSEQ and EMBOSS. There are also several programming packages which provide this conversion functionality, such as BioPerl and BioRuby.

Global and Local Alignments

Global alignments, which attempt to align every residue in every sequence, are most useful when the sequences in the query set are similar and of roughly equal size. (This does not mean global alignments cannot end in gaps.) A general global alignment technique is the Needleman–Wunsch algorithm, which is based on dynamic programming. Local alignments are more useful for dissimilar sequences that are suspected to contain regions of similarity or similar sequence motifs within their larger sequence context. The Smith–Waterman algorithm is a general local alignment method also based on dynamic programming.

Hybrid methods, known as semiglobal or 'glocal' (short for global-local) methods, attempt to find the best possible alignment that includes the start and end of one or the other sequence. This can be especially useful when the downstream part of one sequence overlaps with the upstream part of the other sequence. In this case, neither global nor local alignment is entirely appropriate: a global alignment would attempt to force the alignment to extend beyond the region of overlap, while a local alignment might not fully cover the region of overlap. Another case where semiglobal alignment is useful is when one sequence is short (for example a gene sequence) and the other is very long (for example a chromosome sequence). In that case, the short sequence should be globally aligned but only a local alignment is desired for the long sequence.

Pairwise Alignment

Pairwise sequence alignment methods are used to find the best-matching piecewise (local) or global alignments of two query sequences. Pairwise alignments can only be used between two sequences at a time, but they are efficient to calculate and are often used for methods that do not require extreme precision (such as searching a database for sequences with high similarity to a query). The three primary methods of producing pairwise alignments are dot-matrix methods, dynamic programming, and word methods, however, multiple sequence alignment techniques can also align pairs of sequences. Although each method has its individual strengths and weaknesses, all three pairwise methods have difficulty with highly repetitive sequences of low information content- especially where the number of repetitions differ in the two sequences to be aligned. One way of quantifying the utility of a given pairwise alignment is the 'maximum unique match' (MUM), or the longest subsequence that occurs in both query sequences. Longer MUM sequences typically reflect closer relatedness.

Dot-matrix methods

The dot-matrix approach, which implicitly produces a family of alignments for individual sequence regions, is qualitative and conceptually simple, though time-consuming to analyse on a large scale. In the absence of noise, it can be easy to visually identify certain sequence features—such as insertions, deletions, repeats, or inverted repeats—from a dot-matrix plot. To construct a dot-matrix plot, the two sequences are written along the top row and leftmost column of a two-dimensional matrix and a dot is placed at any point where the characters in the appropriate columns match—this is a typical recurrence plot.

Some implementations vary the size or intensity of the dot depending on the degree of similarity of the two characters, to accommodate conservative substitutions. The dot plots of very closely related sequences will appear as a single line along the matrixs main diagonal.

Problems with dot plots as an information display technique include: noise, lack of clarity, non-intuitiveness, difficulty extracting match summary statistics and match positions on the two sequences. There is also much wasted space where the match data is inherently duplicated across the diagonal and most of the actual area of the plot is taken up by either empty space or noise, and, finally, dot-plots are limited to two sequences. Dot plots can also be used to assess repetitiveness in a single sequence. A sequence can be plotted against itself and regions that share significant similarities will appear as lines off the main diagonal. This effect can occur when a protein consists of multiple similar structural domains.

Dynamic programming

The technique of dynamic programming can be applied to produce global alignments via the Needleman-Wunsch algorithm, and local alignments via the Smith-Waterman algorithm. In typical usage, protein alignments use a substitution matrix to assign scores to amino-acid matches or mismatches, and a gap penalty for matching an amino acid in one sequence to a gap in the other. DNA and RNA alignments may use a scoring matrix, but in practice often simply assign a positive match score, a negative mismatch score, and a negative gap penalty. (In standard dynamic programming, the score of each amino acid position is independent of the identity of its neighbours, and therefore base stacking effects are not taken into account. However, it is possible to account for such effects by modifying the algorithm.) A common extension to standard linear gap costs, is the usage of two different gap penalties for opening a gap and for extending a gap. Typically the former is much larger than the latter, e.g. -10 for gap open and -2 for gap extension. Thus, the number of gaps in an alignment is usually reduced and residues and gaps are kept together, which typically makes more biological sense. The Gotoh algorithm implements affine gap costs by using three matrices.

Dynamic programming can be useful in aligning nucleotide to protein sequences, a task complicated by the need to take into account frameshift mutations (usually insertions or deletions). The framesearch method produces a series of global or local pairwise alignments between a query nucleotide sequence and a search set of protein sequences, or vice versa. Its ability to evaluate frameshifts offset by an arbitrary number of nucleotides makes the method useful for sequences containing large numbers of indels, which can be very difficult to align with more efficient heuristic methods. In practice, the method requires large amounts of computing power or a system whose architecture is specialised for dynamic programming.

The BLAST and EMBOSS suites provide basic tools for creating translated alignments (though some of these approaches take advantage of side-effects of sequence searching capabilities of the tools). More general methods are available from both commercial sources, such as FrameSearch, distributed as part of the Accelrys GCG package, and Open Source software such as Genewise.

The dynamic programming method is guaranteed to find an optimal alignment given a particular scoring function, however, identifying a good scoring function is often an empirical rather than a theoretical matter. Although dynamic programming is extensible to more than two sequences, it is prohibitively slow for large numbers of sequences or extremely long sequences.

Word methods

Word methods, also known as k-tuple methods, are heuristic methods that are not guaranteed to find an optimal alignment solution, but are significantly more efficient than dynamic programming. These methods are especially useful in large-scale database searches where it is understood that a large proportion of the candidate sequences will have essentially no significant match with the query sequence. Word methods are best known for their implementation in the database search tools FASTA and the BLAST family. Word methods identify a series of short, nonoverlapping subsequences in the query sequence that are then matched to candidate database sequences. The relative positions of the word in the two sequences being compared are subtracted to obtain an offset, this will indicate a region of alignment if multiple distinct words produce the same offset. Only if this region is detected do these methods apply more sensitive alignment criteria, thus, many unnecessary comparisons with sequences of no appreciable similarity are eliminated.

In the FASTA method, the user defines a value k to use as the word length with which to search the database. The method is slower but more sensitive at lower values of k, which are also preferred for searches involving a very short query sequence. The BLAST family of search methods provides a number of algorithms optimised for particular types of queries, such as searching for distantly related sequence matches. BLAST was developed to provide a faster alternative to FASTA without sacrificing much accuracy, like FASTA, BLAST uses a word search of length k, but evaluates only the most significant word matches, rather than every word match as does FASTA. Most BLAST implementations use a fixed default word length that is optimised for the query and database type, and that is changed only under special circumstances, such as when searching with repetitive or very short query sequences. Implementations can be found via a number of web portals, such as EMBL FASTA and NCBI BLAST.

Multiple Sequence Alignment

Multiple sequence alignment is an extension of pairwise alignment to incorporate more than two sequences at a time. Multiple alignment methods try to align all of the sequences in a given query set. Multiple alignments are often used in identifying conserved sequence regions across a group of sequences hypothesised to be evolutionarily related. Such conserved sequence motifs can be used in conjunction with structural and mechanistic information to locate the catalytic active sites of enzymes. Alignments are also used to aid in establishing evolutionary relationships by constructing phylogenetic trees.

Multiple sequence alignments are computationally difficult to produce and most formulations of the problem lead to NP-complete combinatorial optimisation problems. Nevertheless, the utility of these alignments in bioinformatics has led to the development of a variety of methods suitable for aligning three or more sequences.

Dynamic programming

The technique of dynamic programming is theoretically applicable to any number of sequences, however, because it is computationally expensive in both time and memory, it is rarely used for more than three or four sequences in its most basic form. This method requires constructing the n-dimensional equivalent of the sequence matrix formed from two sequences, where n is the number of sequences in the query. Standard dynamic programming is first used on all pairs of query sequences and then the 'alignment space' is filled in by considering possible matches or gaps at intermediate positions, eventually constructing an alignment essentially between each two-sequence alignment. Although this technique is computationally expensive, its guarantee of a global optimum solution is useful in cases where only a few sequences need to be aligned accurately. One method for reducing the computational demands of dynamic programming, which relies on the 'sum of pairs' objective function, has been implemented in the MSA software package.

Progressive methods

Progressive, hierarchical, or tree methods generate a multiple sequence alignment by first aligning the most similar sequences and then adding successively less related sequences or groups to the alignment until the entire query set has been incorporated into the solution. The initial tree describing the sequence relatedness is based on pairwise comparisons that may include heuristic pairwise alignment methods similar to FASTA. Progressive alignment results are dependent on the choice of 'most related' sequences and thus can be sensitive to inaccuracies in the initial pairwise alignments. Most progressive multiple sequence alignment methods additionally weight the sequences in the query set according to their relatedness, which reduces the likelihood of making a poor choice of initial sequences and thus improves alignment accuracy. Many variations of the Clustal progressive implementation are used for multiple sequence alignment, phylogenetic tree construction, and as input for protein structure prediction.

Iterative methods

Iterative methods attempt to improve on the heavy dependence on the accuracy of the initial pairwise alignments, which is the weak point of the progressive methods. Iterative methods optimise an objective function based on a selected alignment scoring method by assigning an initial global alignment and then realigning sequence subsets. The realigned subsets are then themselves aligned to produce the next iteration's multiple sequence alignment. Various ways of selecting the sequence subgroups and objective function are reviewed in.

Motif finding

Motif finding, also known as profile analysis, constructs global multiple sequence alignments that attempt to align short conserved sequence motifs among the sequences in the query set. This is usually done by first constructing a general global multiple sequence alignment, after which the highly conserved regions are isolated and used to construct a set of profile matrices. The profile matrix for each conserved region is arranged like a scoring matrix but its frequency counts for each amino acid or nucleotide at each position are derived from the conserved region's character distribution rather than from a more general empirical distribution. The profile matrices are then used to search other sequences for occurrences of the motif they characterise. In cases where the original data set contained a small number of sequences, or only highly related sequences, pseudocounts are added to normalise the character distributions represented in the motif.

Techniques inspired by computer science

A variety of general optimisation algorithms commonly used in computer science have also been applied to the multiple sequence alignment problem. Hidden Markov models have been used to produce probability scores for a family of possible multiple sequence alignments for a given query set, although early HMM-based methods produced underwhelming performance, later applications have found them especially effective in detecting remotely related sequences because they are less susceptible to noise created by conservative or semiconservative substitutions. Genetic algorithms and simulated annealing have also been used in optimising multiple sequence alignment scores as judged by a scoring function like the sum-of-pairs method.

Structural Alignment

Structural alignments, which are usually specific to protein and sometimes RNA sequences, use information about the secondary and tertiary structure of the protein or RNA molecule to aid in aligning the sequences. These methods can be used for two or more sequences and typically produce local alignments, however, because they depend on the availability of structural information, they can only be used for sequences whose corresponding structures are known (usually through X-ray crystallography or NMR spectroscopy). Because both protein and RNA structure is more evolutionarily conserved than sequence, structural alignments can be more reliable between sequences that are very distantly related and that have diverged so extensively that sequence comparison cannot reliably detect their similarity.

Structural alignments are used as the 'gold standard' in evaluating alignments for homology-based protein structure prediction because they explicitly align regions of the protein sequence that are structurally similar rather than relying exclusively on sequence information. However, clearly structural alignments cannot be used in structure prediction because at least one sequence in the query set is the target to be modelled, for which the structure is not known. It has been shown that, given the structural alignment between a target and a template sequence, highly accurate models of the target protein sequence can be produced, a major stumbling block in homology-based structure prediction is the production of structurally accurate alignments given only sequence information.

DALI

The DALI method, or distance matrix alignment, is a fragment-based method for constructing structural alignments based on contact similarity patterns between successive hexapeptides in the query sequences. It can generate pairwise or multiple alignments and identify a query sequence's structural neighbours in the Protein Data Bank (PDB). It has been used to construct the FSSP structural alignment database (Fold classification based on Structure-Structure alignment of Proteins, or Families of Structurally Similar Proteins). A DALI webserver can be accessed at EBI DALI and the FSSP is located at The Dali Database.

SSAP

SSAP (sequential structure alignment program) is a dynamic programming-based method of structural alignment that uses atom-to-atom vectors in structure space as comparison points. It has been extended since its original description to include multiple as well as pairwise alignments, and has been used in the construction of the CATH (Class, Architecture, Topology, Homology) hierarchical database classification of protein folds. The CATH database can be accessed at CATH Protein Structure Classification.

Combinatorial extension

The combinatorial extension method of structural alignment generates a pairwise structural alignment by using local geometry to align short fragments of the two proteins being analysed and then assembles these fragments into a larger alignment. Based on measures such as rigid-body root mean square distance, residue distances, local secondary structure, and surrounding environmental features such as residue neighbour hydrophobicity, local alignments called 'aligned fragment pairs' are generated and used to build a similarity matrix representing all possible structural alignments within predefined cutoff criteria. A path from one protein structure state to the other is then traced through the matrix by extending the growing alignment one fragment at a time. The optimal such path defines the combinatorial-extension alignment. A web-based server implementing the method and providing a database of pairwise alignments of structures in the Protein Data Bank is located at the Combinatorial Extension website.

Phylogenetic Analysis

Phylogenetics and sequence alignment are closely related fields due to the shared necessity of evaluating sequence relatedness. The field of phylogenetics makes extensive use of sequence alignments in the construction and interpretation of phylogenetic trees, which are used to classify the evolutionary relationships between homologous genes represented in the genomes of divergent species. The degree to which sequences in a query set differ is qualitatively related to the sequences' evolutionary distance from one another. Thus, high sequence identity suggests that the sequences in question have a comparatively young most recent common ancestor, while low identity suggests that the divergence is more ancient.

This approximation, which reflects the 'molecular clock' hypothesis that a roughly constant rate of evolutionary change can be used to extrapolate the elapsed time since two genes first diverged (that is, the coalescence time), assumes that the effects of mutation and selection are constant across sequence lineages. Therefore it does not account for possible difference among organisms or species in the rates of DNA repair or the possible functional conservation of specific regions in a sequence. (In the case of nucleotide sequences, the molecular clock hypothesis in its most basic form also discounts the difference in acceptance rates between silent mutations that do not alter the meaning of a given codon and other mutations that result in a different amino acid being incorporated into the protein.) More statistically accurate methods allow the evolutionary rate on each branch of the phylogenetic tree to vary, thus producing better estimates of coalescence times for genes.

Progressive multiple alignment techniques produce a phylogenetic tree by necessity because they incorporate sequences into the growing alignment in order of relatedness. Other techniques that assemble multiple sequence alignments and phylogenetic trees score and sort trees first and calculate a multiple sequence alignment from the highest-scoring tree. Commonly used methods of phylogenetic tree construction are mainly heuristic because the problem of selecting the optimal tree, like the problem of selecting the optimal multiple sequence alignment, is NP-hard.

Assessment of significance

Sequence alignments are useful in bioinformatics for identifying sequence similarity, producing phylogenetic trees, and developing homology models of protein structures. However, the biological relevance of sequence alignments is not always clear. Alignments are often assumed to reflect a degree of evolutionary change between sequences descended from a common ancestor, however, it is formally possible that convergent evolution can occur to produce apparent similarity between proteins that are evolutionarily unrelated but perform similar functions and have similar structures.

In database searches such as BLAST, statistical methods can determine the likelihood of a particular alignment between sequences or sequence regions arising by chance given the size and composition of the database being searched. These values can vary significantly depending on the search space. In particular, the likelihood of finding a given alignment by chance increases if the database consists only of sequences from the same organism as the query sequence. Repetitive sequences in the database or query can also distort both the search results and the assessment of statistical significance, BLAST automatically filters such repetitive sequences in the query to avoid apparent hits that are statistical artifacts.

Assessment of credibility

Statistical significance indicates the probability that an alignment of a given quality could arise by chance, but does not indicate how much superior a given alignment is to alternative alignments of the same sequences. Measures of alignment credibility indicate the extent to which the best scoring alignments for a given pair of sequences are substantially similar.

Scoring functions

The choice of a scoring function that reflects biological or statistical observations about known sequences is important to producing good alignments. Protein sequences are frequently aligned using substitution matrices that reflect the probabilities of given character-to-character substitutions. A series of matrices called PAM matrices (Point Accepted Mutation matrices, originally defined by Margaret Dayhoff and sometimes referred to as 'Dayhoff matrices') explicitly encode evolutionary approximations regarding the rates and probabilities of particular amino acid mutations. Another common series of scoring matrices, known as BLOSUM (Blocks Substitution Matrix), encodes empirically derived substitution probabilities. Variants of both types of matrices are used to detect sequences with differing levels of divergence, thus allowing users of BLAST or FASTA to restrict searches to more closely related matches or expand to detect more divergent sequences. Gap penalties account for the introduction of a gap on the evolutionary model, an insertion or deletion mutation in both nucleotide and protein sequences, and therefore the penalty values should be proportional to the expected rate of such mutations. The quality of the alignments produced therefore depends on the quality of the scoring function.

It can be very useful and instructive to try the same alignment several times with different choices for scoring matrix and/or gap penalty values and compare the results. Regions where the solution is weak or non-unique can often be identified by observing which regions of the alignment are robust to variations in alignment parameters.

Other Biological Uses

Sequenced RNA, such as expressed sequence tags and full-length mRNAs, can be aligned to a sequenced genome to find where there are genes and get information about alternative splicing and RNA editing. Sequence alignment is also a part of genome assembly, where sequences are aligned to find overlap so that contigs (long stretches of sequence) can be formed. Another use is SNP analysis, where sequences from different individuals are aligned to find single basepairs that are often different in a population.

Non-biological Uses

The methods used for biological sequence alignment have also found applications in other fields, most notably in natural language processing and in social sciences, where the Needleman-Wunsch algorithm is usually referred to as Optimal matching. Techniques that generate the set of elements from which words will be selected in natural-language generation algorithms have borrowed multiple sequence alignment techniques from bioinformatics to produce linguistic versions of computer-generated mathematical proofs. In the field of historical and comparative linguistics, sequence alignment has been used to partially automate the comparative method by which linguists traditionally reconstruct languages. Business and marketing research has also applied multiple sequence alignment techniques in analysing series of purchases over time.

Software

A more complete list of available software categorised by algorithm and alignment type is available at sequence alignment software, but common software tools used for general sequence alignment tasks include ClustalW2 and T-coffee for alignment, and BLAST and FASTA3x for database searching. Commercial tools such as Geneious and PatternHunter are also available. Alignment algorithms and software can be directly compared to one another using a standardised set of benchmark reference multiple sequence alignments known as BAliBASE.

The data set consists of structural alignments, which can be considered a standard against which purely sequence-based methods are compared. The relative performance of many common alignment methods on frequently encountered alignment problems has been tabulated and selected results published online at BAliBASE. A comprehensive list of BAliBASE scores for many (currently 12) different alignment tools can be computed within the protein workbench STRAP.

GENOME ANNOTATION

Genome annotation is the process of attaching biological information to sequences.

It consists of three main steps:

1. Identifying portions of the genome that do not code for proteins.
2. Identifying elements on the genome, a process called gene prediction.
3. Attaching biological information to these elements.

Automatic annotation tools try to perform all this by computer analysis, as opposed to manual annotation which involves human expertise. Ideally, these approaches co-exist and complement each other in the same annotation pipeline. The basic level of annotation is using BLAST for finding similarities, and then annotating genomes based on that. However, now-a-days more and more additional information is added to the annotation platform. The additional information allows manual annotators to deconvolute discrepancies between genes that are given the same annotation.

Some databases use genome context information, similarity scores, experimental data, and integrations of other resources to provide genome annotations through their subsystems approach. Other databases (e.g. *Ensembl*) rely on both curated data sources as well as a range of different software tools in their automated genome annotation pipeline.

Structural annotation consists of the identification of genomic elements such as:

- ORFs and their localisation.
- Gene structure.
- Coding regions.
- Location of regulatory motifs.

Functional annotation consists of attaching biological information to genomic elements such as:

- Biochemical function.
- Biological function.
- Involved regulation and interactions.
- Expression.

These steps may involve both biological experiments and in silico analysis. Proteo-genomics based approaches utilise information from expressed proteins, often derived from mass spectrometry, to improve genomics annotations. A variety of software tools have been developed to permit scientists to view and share genome annotations.

Genome annotation remains a major challenge for scientists investigating the human genome, now that the genome sequences of more than a thousand human individuals and several model organisms are largely complete. Identifying the locations of genes and other genetic control elements is often described as defining the biological 'parts list' for the assembly and normal operation of an organism. Scientists are still at an early stage in the process of delineating this parts list and in understanding how all the parts 'fit together'. Genome annotation is an active area of investigation and involves a number of different organisations in the life science community which publish the results of their efforts in publicly available biological databases accessible via the web and other electronic means.

VARIATION AND ITS CAUSES

Variation, in biology, any difference between cells, individual organisms, or groups of organisms of any species caused either by genetic differences (genotypic variation) or by the effect of environmental factors on the expression of the genetic potentials (phenotypic variation). Variation may be shown in physical appearance, metabolism, fertility, mode of reproduction, behaviour, learning and mental ability, and other obvious or measurable characters.

Genotypic variations are caused by differences in number or structure of chromosomes or by differences in the genes carried by the chromosomes. Eye colour, body form, and disease resistance are genotypic variations. Individuals with multiple sets of chromosomes are called polyploid, many common plants have two or more times the normal number of chromosomes, and new species may arise by this type of variation. A variation cannot be identified as genotypic by observation of the organism, breeding experiments must be performed under controlled environmental conditions to determine whether or not the alteration is inheritable.

Environmentally caused variations may result from one factor or the combined effects of several factors, such as climate, food supply, and actions of other organisms. Phenotypic variations also include stages in an organism's life cycle and seasonal variations in an individual. These variations do not involve any hereditary alteration and in general are not transmitted to future generations, consequently, they are not significant in the process of evolution.

Variations are classified either as continuous, or quantitative (smoothly grading between two extremes, with the majority of individuals at the centre, as height in human populations), or as discontinuous, or qualitative (composed of well-defined classes, as blood groups in man). A discontinuous variation with several classes, none of which is very small, is known as a polymorphic variation. The separation of most higher organisms into males and females and the occurrence of several forms of a butterfly of the same species, each coloured to blend with a different vegetation, are examples of polymorphic variation.

GENOTYPIC AND PHENOTYPIC VARIATIONS

In this section studies of the relation between genotype and phenotype, especially of the motility of the soil nematode *Caenorhabditis elegans*, are described. First, the background of the study of motility is briefly reviewed. Thus, we can focus on the results of the isolation of mutants that are useful for understanding the gene function of other animals.

A brief overview of recent research follows. As details on *C. elegans* have already appeared in two monographs, the principal approach to the study of this animal is explained only briefly. A typical genetic analysis of the motility mutant gene known as *unc* (uncoordinated) is described. More than one hundred *unc*-genes have been isolated and classified into five groups. *unc* genes are related in various ways to muscle and other proteins like cytoskeleton proteins, transcription factors, ion channels of *trans*-membrane proteins, kinases or enzymes, and neuron-related proteins. Interestingly, these proteins are known to be abundant in the multicellular organisms from the results of genome sequencing. Other mutant genes are also described. Strategies for the genetic analysis of genes involved in heterochronicity, vulva formation, chemotaxis, and cell death are briefly presented. Finally, an overview of the post genome research is discussed. The reasons why *C. elegans* research has progressed so rapidly and the strategy for experiments in progress are also explained.

Brief Introduction to the Genetics of the Nematode Caenorhabditis

Sydney Brenner first used the soil nematode *Caenorhabditis elegans* to study development and the nervous system in 1967. *C. elegans* feeds bacteria and grows on nutrient growth medium at 20°C. The hermaphrodite grows into an adult in three days and lays about 200 eggs after self-fertilization. Genes can be transferred from rare arising males to the hermaphrodite by mating. This is probably the most convenient animal model for genetics and biochemistry. In *C. elegans*, mutant phenotypes include Unc (uncoordinated), Sma (small), Lon (long), and Dpy (dpy).

Changes in morphology and other visible characteristics also arise from mutant genes. Bacterial motility is observed only by an indirect approach: swarm formation in semi-solid agar medium on a petri dish. Worm motility can be observed directly by dissecting microscopy, which is an advantage when isolating a mutant. Worms have muscle tissues: a pharynx for feeding, a body wall for locomotion, a vulva for laying eggs, and an anus for defecation.

Interestingly, the pharynx is similar to the heart muscle of vertebrates. The analysis of worm muscle genes is therefore applicable to vertebrates. Molecular biology can provide an understanding of one organism through study of another by comparing amino acid sequence homology or cell proliferation. Two monographs are available for *C. elegans*: 'The nematode *Caenorhabditis elegans*' and '*C. elegans* II.'

Cell Lineage and Genome Sequence

How fertilised eggs divide and cells proliferate is fundamental to our understanding of development. The use of a dissecting microscope and visible light easily reveals the cell division in *C. elegans* without any pretreatment. In 1983, after seven years of study, John Sulston reported the process of cell proliferation. There are 959 cells after the programmed cell death of 131 cells. This is made clear by recording the position of the nucleus. This information is available at the web site AceDB. The most important conclusion from completing the cell lineage is that cell proliferation is divided into two stages: cell division and morphogenesis. Most of the cell division is complete by the 500-cell stage, with only a limited number of cells continuing to undergo asymmetrical division to form special muscle, cuticle, neurons, and vulva. This indicates that, even in higher animals, characteristic appearances come from a limited cell lineage. Thus, it should be noted that many genes are conserved in species from the nematode and *Drosophila* to mice, and even humans. This conclusion is also true for genome analysis. Higher organisms have transcription factors, a cytoskeleton, signal transduction molecules, and kinase/phosphatase. These molecules specialise the cells of multi-cellular organisms. This means that the conclusions drawn from a simple model like the nematode or *Drosophila* are also true for mice and humans, as is known from molecular genetic studies on bacteria. Genome structure and gene numbers are discussed in more detail in the next section.

Genetics and Mutants

The nematode *Caenorhabditis elegans* grows as a hermaphrodite and lays eggs after self-fertilization. It is therefore easy to isolate a mutant from a single worm that has a heterozygous chromosome. In 1974, Sydney Brenner established the genetics of the nematode, and since then many mutants have been isolated from numerous phenotypes. The first mutants to be identified were Sma (small body), Lon (long body), and Mab (male abnormal), together with *Unc* (uncoordinated), these phenotypes being easy to recognise. It is also possible to isolate a mutant that has no phenotypic variation under normal conditions but a novel phenotype under a specific set of conditions. Drug or temperature sensitivity is used as a conditional marker. It is possible to isolate a mutant that has a novel phenotype under specific conditions after treatment of some mutagens, which is why so many important mutations have phenotypic variations. Recently, another genetic approach has been used to isolate mutations based on motility in the genome, applying transposons such as Tc1 in the nematode and P-element in *Drosophila*. The insertion of a transposon into a gene disrupts its function. Knock-out of the gene by inserting Tc1 in *C. elegans* produces an increase in genomic size, as detected by Southern analysis. If a mutant is isolated by a transposon insertion, a mutant gene can be isolated by the transposon fused fragment. Designed transposons are also used in *Drosophila* for studying promoter activity. When a P-element is inserted into downstream of a gene's promoter, lac-Z gene activity can be detected by staining the mutant fly. This approach allows one to know where the gene was expressed and which gene was disrupted by transposon insertion. These transposon functions are essentially similar from bacteria to maize.

HERITABILITY

Heritability is a statistic used in breeding and genetics works that estimates how much of the genetic diversity of a phenotypic trait in a population is due to genetic differences in that population. Other causes of measured variation in a trait are characterised as environmental factors, including measurement error. In human studies of heritability these are often apportioned into factors from 'shared environment' and 'non-shared environment' based on whether they tend to result in persons brought up in the same household more or less similar to persons who were not.

Some humans in a population are taller than others, heritability attempts to identify how much genetics play a role in part of the population being taller. Heritability is estimated by comparing individual phenotypic variation among differently related individuals in a population. Heritability is an important concept in quantitative genetics, particularly in selective breeding and behaviour genetics (for instance, twin studies), but is less widely used in population genetics.

Geoffrey Miller, an evolutionary psychologist, has said, writing about sexual selection and biological fitness, 'The concept of heritability applies only to traits that differ between individuals. If a trait exists in precisely the same form across all individuals, it may be inherited, but it cannot be heritable.'

Heritability measures the fraction of phenotype variability that can be attributed to genetic variation. This is not the same as saying that this fraction of an individual phenotype is caused by genetics. In addition, heritability can change without any genetic change occurring, such as when the environment starts contributing to more variation. A case in point, consider that both genes and environment have the potential to influence intelligence. Heritability could increase if genetic variation increases, causing individuals to show more phenotypic variation, like showing different levels of intelligence. On the other hand, heritability might also increase if the environmental variation decreases, causing individuals to show less phenotypic variation, like showing more similar levels of intelligence. Heritability increases when genetics are contributing more variation or because non-genetic factors are contributing less variation, what matters is the relative contribution. Heritability is specific to a particular population in a particular environment.

The extent of dependence of phenotype on environment can also be a function of the genes involved. Matters of heritability are complicated because genes may canalize a phenotype, making its expression almost inevitable in all occurring environments. Individuals with the same genotype can also exhibit different phenotypes through a mechanism called phenotypic plasticity, which makes heritability difficult to measure in some cases. Recent insights in molecular biology have identified changes in transcriptional activity of individual genes associated with environmental changes. However, there are a large number of genes whose transcription is not affected by the environment.

Estimating Heritability

Thus, heritability can be observed or measured directly, heritability must be estimated from the similarities observed in subjects varying in their level of genetic or environmental similarity. The statistical analyses required to estimate the genetic and environmental components of variance depend on the sample characteristics. Briefly, better estimates are obtained using data from individuals with widely varying levels of genetic relationship such as twins, siblings, parents and offspring, rather than from more distantly related (and therefore less similar) subjects. The standard error for heritability estimates is improved with large sample sizes.

In non-human populations it is often possible to collect information in a controlled way. For example, among farm animals it is easy to arrange for a bull to produce offspring from a large number of cows and to control environments. Such experimental control is impossible when gathering human data, relying on naturally occurring relationships and environments.

Studies of human heritability often utilise adoption study designs, often with identical twins who have been separated early in life and raised in different environments. Such individuals have identical genotypes and can be used to separate the effects of genotype and environment. A limit of this design is the common prenatal environment and the relatively low numbers of twins reared apart. A second and more common design is the twin study in which the similarity of identical and fraternal twins is used to estimate heritability. These studies can be limited by the fact that identical twins are not completely genetically identical, potentially resulting in an underestimation of heritability. Studies of twins also examine differences between twins and non-twin siblings, for instance to examine phenomena such as intrauterine competition (for example, twin-to-twin transfusion syndrome).

Heritability estimates are always relative to the genetic and environmental factors in the population, and are not absolute measurements of the contribution of genetic and environmental factors to a phenotype. Heritability estimates reflect the amount of variation in genotypic effects compared to variation in environmental effects.

Heritability can be made larger by diversifying the genetic background, e.g. by using only very out bred individuals (which increases VarG) and/or by minimising environmental effects (decreasing VarE). The converse also holds. Due to such effects, different populations of a species might have different heritabilities for the same trait.

In observational studies, or because of evokative effects (where a genome evokes environments by its effect on them), G and E may covary: gene environment correlation. Depending on the methods used to estimate heritability, correlations between genetic factors and shared or non-shared environments may or may not be confounded with heritability.

Common misunderstandings of heritability estimates

A common estimate of heritability is called the Heritability Index (HI), which ranges from 0 – 1. A HI index of 0 means that none of the variability between people in the study sample on the trait under investigation is due to genetic factors, an HI of 1 indicates the opposite.

Heritability estimates are often misinterpreted if it is not understood that they refer to the proportion of variation between individuals on a trait that is due to genetic factors. It does not indicate the degree of genetic influence on the development of a trait of an individual. For example, it is incorrect to say that since the heritability of personality traits is about 0.6, that means that 60% of your personality is inherited from your parents and 40% comes from the environment.

Even a highly heritable trait (such as eye colour) assumes environmental inputs which are required for development: for instance temperatures and an atmosphere supporting life, etc. A more useful distinction than 'nature vs. nurture' is 'obligate vs. facultative'—under typical environmental ranges, what traits are more 'obligate' (e.g. the nose—everyone has a nose) or more 'facultative' (sensitive to environmental variations, such as specific language learned during infancy). Another useful distinction is between traits that are likely to be adaptations (such as the umbilical cord) vs. those that are byproducts of adaptations (such as the belly button), or are due to random variation (non-adaptive variation in belly button shape, e.g. convex or concave).

Estimation methods

There are essentially two schools of thought regarding estimation of heritability. One school of thought was developed by Sewall Wright at The University of Chicago, and further popularised by C. C. Li (University of Chicago) and J. L. Lush (Iowa State University). It is based on the analysis of correlations and, by extension, regression. Path Analysis was developed by Sewall Wright as a way of estimating heritability. The second was originally developed by R. A. Fisher and expanded at The University of Edinburgh, Iowa State University, and North Carolina State University, as well as other schools. It is based on the analysis of variance of breeding studies, using the intraclass correlation of relatives. Various methods of estimating components of variance (and, hence, heritability) from ANOVA are used in these analyses.

PROTEIN-BASED DRUGS

The future of pharmacy belongs to a special category of therapeutics and diagnostics referred to as protein-based drugs. To date, modern medicine has relied heavily on synthetically or chemically produced drugs to treat or prevent diseases and conditions.

However, developments in the field of molecular biology have led to an increase in our knowledge of biological systems and their interactions. For example, scientists know more about the sources of many diseases and how the human body fights diseases. They are now focussing on using the body's own tools to fight diseases by developing therapeutics that mimic the actions of the body's arsenal.

Proteins are biomolecules that are essential in determining the structure and carrying out most of the functions in living cells that make up all living organisms. They are made up of individual units called amino acids, which although similar in structure, have different characteristics. There are about 20 different amino acids in nature and these assemble in chains of varying lengths to form proteins. The order of amino acids determines the structure and function of the protein. This order is specified by genes. Proteins in living organisms are classified according to their biological roles.

These include:

1. Enzymatic: Proteins that trigger all the chemical reactions that occur in the cells of living organisms.
2. Transport: Proteins that carry other substances throughout the body or molecules across cell membranes. For instance, the protein haemoglobin carries oxygen from the lungs to other parts of the body.
3. Structural: Proteins that help in supporting functions in the body. For instance, Keratin is the protein that is important for supporting hair and other skin parts.
4. Storage: Proteins that store amino acids. For instance, casein is the protein in milk that provides a source of amino acids for baby mammals.
5. Hormonal: Proteins that coordinate bodily activities. For instance, insulin is the protein hormone secreted by the pancreas that regulates the level of sugar in the blood.
6. Receptor: Proteins that are built into the membrane of a cell and detect chemical signals released by other cells. They contribute to the cell's response to the chemical stimuli.
7. Contractile: Proteins that help in movement. For example, actin and myosin are responsible for the movement of muscles.
8. Defensive: Protect the body against diseases. For example, antibodies are proteins that protect the body against viruses and harmful bacteria.

Protein-based drugs are any substance that uses the different proteins that occur naturally in any living organism, to diagnose, prevent and treat diseases and conditions or to restore or maintain normal body functions. Humans have traditionally used animal and plant sources to obtain proteins (such as hormones and clotting factors) in order to treat different diseases and conditions. Many of these were extracted from human and animal corpses. Revolutionary discoveries in science and modern medicine propelled the large scale production of chemical drugs to be used in human health care.

However, today, advances in biotechnology have led to the increased use of living organisms and biological substances in the production of protein drugs for human health care. Specifically, the use of recombinant DNA (rDNA) technology has enabled the production of large quantities of protein drugs.

Types of Protein-Based Drugs

Cytokines: These drugs regulate the immune system. That is, they are proteins that activate the immune system cells to carry out different immune functions.

Hormones: Protein drugs that regulate functions in the body. As drugs, these proteins can be used to elevate levels of certain hormones, such as estrogen during menopause or growth deficiency. They can also be used to treat certain diseases such as diabetes, or conditions such as infertility.

Clotting factors: Proteins that regulate the clotting of blood. These drugs are used to treat blood clotting disorders such as haemophilia.

Vaccines: Proteins that stimulate the immune system to produce specific antibodies used to prevent or treat diseases.

Monoclonal antibodies: Proteins that mark a specific foreign material (such as cancer cells, disease-causing bacteria and viruses), for removal or destruction by other components of the immune system. These are also used as effective diagnostic tools for many specific genetic diseases and other conditions such as pregnancy.

The science – How do protein-based drugs work?

Protein-based drugs are developed by cloning the genes responsible for specific proteins naturally produced by the human body. The genes are cloned using vectors such as bacteria. The gene of interest is first isolated and then incorporated into the bacteria, which are multiplied in bioreactors to produce many copies of the gene. The cloned genes are then genetically engineered into micro-organisms or animals to produce the proteins. When the protein is used as a drug (for preventative or therapeutic purposes), it performs the same function as the already naturally-occurring protein in the body.

Biotechnology and protein-based drugs

Prior to advances in biotechnology such as rDNA technology, the few protein drugs available were taken directly from human and animal corpses. For instance, the human growth hormone was taken from human corpses and insulin required to treat diabetes was collected from slaughtered pigs. These drugs were available in limited supply and they were expensive, given their sources. Biotechnology has boosted the production of protein-based drugs in two significant ways.

Hybridoma cell technology

Hybridomas are the fusion of tumour cells with certain white blood cells. They replicate endlessly and can be used to produce specific protein-based drugs called monoclonal antibodies which are effective in treating cancers and other conditions.

Recombinant DNA technology

The introduction of rDNA technology or genetic engineering, has provided a large and cost-efficient source of protein-based drugs. Using genetic engineering, the gene that encodes for the required protein is transferred from one organism into another, which is capable of producing large amounts of the drug.

Genes determine what proteins do. If the gene encoding for a certain protein is known, it is possible to produce this protein. Biotechnology has enabled scientists to identify the different genes that encode for certain proteins. The human genome project has increased our knowledge of genes responsible for many diseases. The identified genes can be used to produce proteins and administer them to prevent and treat diseases. Production of protein-based drugs through rDNA technology can be achieved through two common ways: through transgenic animals (pharming), micro-organisms such as *E. coli* bacteria or through hybridomas.

Transgenic animals for protein drug production

Transgenic Animals in health care are animals that have been genetically modified to produce a particular protein drug. The DNA gene for the desired protein is coupled with a DNA signal directing its production in the mammary glands. The new gene functions in the mammary glands so that the protein drug is made only in the milk. The coupled DNA is injected into fertilised cow, sheep, goat or mouse embryo's. The injected embryos are implanted into surrogate mothers. The surviving embryos are then born normally and after these have been raised to maturity and bred, they produce the protein during lactation. The protein is then harvested from the milk and formulated into a protein based drug.

To sum up the eventual objective of producing a desired protein in an economical heterologous host is influenced by a variety of factors. However, maximising production of heterologous proteins for commercial application is still an art. We have begun to understand factors influencing the eventual production. These factors, described in detail in this section are varied and at times poorly understood. Largely the approach remains empirical. However, our collective experience will permit us to rationalise our approach in designing heterologous production of commercially important proteins in a variety of expression systems. Subsequent to production, stabilisation and formulation of proteins will pose significant hurdles in utilising the natural biological catalysts and other proteins for therapeutic and industrial purposes.

SECTION VII

Developmental Genetics and Genetic Control of Development

Chapter 18

Developmental Genetics

INTRODUCTION

Developmental genetics is the study of the way in which genes control the growth and development of an organism throughout its life-cycle. A newly fertilised egg cell - or zygote - contains a unique collection of genes that will control its development from a single cell into an embryo through patterns of differential gene expression in the process of embryogenesis.

Creating an organism from a single cell involves three processes:

- Cell division through mitosis.
- Cell differentiation through gene activation and inactivation.
- Morphogenesis pattern formation through the combined effects of cell division, cell differentiation and cell death.

Genes control patterns of cell division and cell death (apoptosis) in the developing embryo. Genes also control the differentiation of cells from an original totipotent state (able to make all cell types) through a pluripotent state (able to make some cells types, like stem cells) to their final destination as specific cell types or cell lineages (cell determination). Cells differentiate into different types of cells because of differential patterns of gene expression. Genes may be activated or inactivated (silenced) by regulation of the processes of transcription and translation.

Genes are activated by proteins called transcription factors, which bind to promoters at the start of the gene and regulate the process of transcription. Transcription factors are the products of other genes that, in turn, may have been activated by other transcription factors. This cascade of genes and transcription factors is initiated by control genes that are activated by autonomous, conditional or syncytial specification.

- Autonomous specification (especially common in invertebrates). Some chemicals and structures in the fertilised egg cell are inherited unevenly by subsequent cell populations. These cytoplasmic, or morphogenetic, determinants include RNA molecules, which code for transcription factors, as well as other proteins and organelles in the cytoplasm. Different concentrations of these factors in different cell populations cause different patterns of gene expression and subsequent cell differentiation.

- Conditional specification (found in all vertebrates and some invertebrates). Cells are differentiated by interactions with neighbouring cells. In some cases, cells, or groups of cells, in the developing embryo release proteins, including transcription factors. These morphogens act on the control genes of other cells, starting cascades of gene activation and inactivation. In some cases, the morphogens set up concentration gradients as they diffuse through the embryo, and the differentiation of cells is dependent on their position along the gradient.

- Syncytial specification: In many insects, cell differentiation is the result of interactions within cells, not between cells. Incomplete cell divisions after fertilisation result in a cell containing many nuclei (a syncytium). Morphogens diffuse through the syncytium to set up concentration gradients that give cells information about their position: for example, along the anterior-posterior axis.

The basic three-dimensional layout of the body plan is established early in development: Anterior and posterior, dorsal and ventral. A group of very similar genes - homeobox genes - have been found to regulate the process in fungi, plants and animals. Homeobox genes contain a specific nucleotide sequence, the homeobox region, which is about 180 nucleotides long. The homeobox produces a collection of transcription factor proteins (the homeodomain) that acts with other transcription factors to produce a cascade of gene activation and inactivation.

The homeobox genes responsible for segment identity during the formation of metazoan organisms are called homeotic genes, and mutations in these genes (homeotic mutations) can cause large disruptions to the body plan. For example, the Antennapedia mutation in the fruit fly (*Drosophila melanogaster*) causes legs - not antennae - to develop on the fly's head. In vertebrates, one particular subgroup of homeobox genes - the Hox genes - control the development of the limbs and other body parts.

BASIC TOOLS OF DEVELOPMENTAL GENETICS

DNA Analysis

Embryologist Theodor Boveri (1904) wrote that to discover the mechanisms of development, it was 'not cell nuclei, not even individual chromosomes, but certain parts of certain chromosomes from certain cells that must be isolated and collected in enormous quantities for analysis.' This analysis was finally made possible by the techniques of gene cloning, DNA sequencing, Southern blotting, gene knockouts, and enhancer traps. In addition, techniques for showing which enhancers and promoters are methylated and which are unmethylated have become more important, as investigations of differential gene transcription have focused on these elements.

RNA Analysis

Differential gene transcription is critical in development. In order to know the time of gene expression and the place of gene expression, one has to be able to have procedures that actually locate a particular type of messenger RNA. These techniques include northern blots, RT-PCR, *in situ* hybridisation, and array technology. To ascertain the function of these mRNAs, new techniques have been formulated, which include antisense and RNA interference (which destroy messages), Cre-lox analysis (which allows the message to be made or destroyed in particular cell types) and ChIP-on-Chip techniques.

Bioinformatics

Modern developmental genetics often involves comparing DNA sequences (especially regulatory units such as enhancers and 3′ UTRs) and looking at specific genomes to determine how genes are being regulated. 'Highthroughput' RNA analysis by microand macroarrays enables researchers to compare thousands of mRNAs, and computer-aided synthetic techniques can predict interactions between proteins and mRNAs. Various free websites enable researchers to use the tools that allow such comparisons. Other sites are organism- or organspecific and are used by researchers studying that particular organ or organism.

HOMEOTIC GENE

In evolutionary developmental biology, homeotic genes are genes which regulate the development of anatomical structures in various organisms such as echinoderms, insects, mammals, and plants. This regulation is done via the programming of various transcription factors by the homeotic genes, and these factors affect genes through regulatory genetic pathways. Mutations in homeotic genes cause displaced body parts (homeosis), such as antennae growing at the posterior of the fly instead of at the head. Mutations that lead to such ectopic placements are usually lethal.

Types of Homeotic Gene

There are several subsets of homeotic genes. They include many of the Hox and ParaHox genes that are important for segmentation. Hox genes are found in bilateral animals, including *Drosophila* (in which they were first discovered) and humans. Hox genes are a subset of the homeobox genes. The Hox genes are often conserved across species, so some of the Hox genes of *Drosophila* are homologous to those in humans. In general, Hox genes play a role of regulating expression of genes as well as aiding in development and assignment of specific structures during embryonic growth. This can range from segmentation in *Drosophila* to central nervous system (CNS) development in vertebrates. Both Hox and ParaHox are grouped as HOX-Like (HOXL) genes, a subset of the ANTP class (named after the *Drosophila* gene, Antennapedia).

They also include the MADS-box-containing genes involved in the ABC model of flower development. Besides flower-producing plants, the MADS-box motif is also present in other organisms such as insects, yeasts, and mammals. They have various functions depending on the organism including flower development, proto-oncogene transcription, and gene regulation in specific cells (such as muscle cells).

Despite the terms being commonly interchanged, not all homeotic genes are Hox genes, the MADS-box genes are homeotic but not Hox genes. Thus, the Hox genes are a subset of homeotic genes.

Drosophila melanogaster

Homeotic selector gene complexes in the fruit fly *Drosophila melanogaster*. One of the most commonly studied model organisms in regards to homeotic genes is the fruit fly *Drosophila melanogaster*. Its homeotic genes occur in either the Antennapedia complex (ANT-C) or the Bithorax complex (BX-C) discovered by Edward B. Lewis. Each of the complexes focuses on a different area of development. The antennapedia complex consists of five genes, including proboscipedia, and is involved in the development of the front of the embryo, forming the segments of the head and thorax. The bithorax complex consists of three main genes and is involved in the development of the back of the embryo, namely the abdomen and the posterior segments of the thorax. During development (starting at the blastoderm stage of the embryo), these genes are constantly expressed to assign structures and roles to the different segments of the fly's body. For *Drosophila*, these genes can be analysed using the Flybase database. Much research has been done on homeotic genes in different organisms, ranging from basic understanding of how the molecules work to mutations to how homeotic genes affect the human body. Changing the expression levels of homeotic genes can negatively impact the organism. For example, in one study, a pathogenic phytoplasma caused homeotic genes in a flowering plant to either be significantly upregulated or down-regulated. This led to severe phenotypic changes including dwarfing, defects in the pistils, hypopigmentation, and the development of leaf-like structures on most floral organs. In another study, it was found that the homeotic gene Cdx2 acts as a tumour suppressor. In normal expression levels, the gene prevents tumorgenesis and colorectal cancer when exposed to carcinogens, however, when Cdx2 was not well expressed, carcinogens caused tumour development. These studies, along with many others, show the importance of homeotic genes even after development.

Expression of the Homeotic Genes

Molecular cloning of the homeotic genes makes it possible to study their spatial and temporal pattern of expression during development. The two major techniques used are the localisation of homeotic gene transcripts by *in situ* hybridisation, and detection of homeotic proteins using antibodies raised against polypeptides made in bacteria. The expression pattern of homeotic genes is rather complex because it changes rapidly with time, and also because many homeotic genes produce multiple transcripts, which may have different spatial or temporal distributions. However, the most important aspect of the expression is that the homeotic selector genes are expressed in a segment-specific manner during embryogenesis and during larval development.

Regulation of Homeotic Genes

How the segment-specific spatial pattern of expression is achieved is one of the central questions relevant to the understanding of homeotic genes. There is some evidence suggesting that a common mechanism exists for controlling the expression of most, if not all, of the homeotic genes. First, there is a set of genes that appears to affect the expression of many homeotic genes simultaneously as judged from the mutant phenotype. Second, as discussed above, similarities exist between the patterns of expression of different homeotic genes during development.

MATERNAL TO ZYGOTIC TRANSITION

Maternal to zygotic transition (MZT, also known as Embryonic Genome Activation) is the stage in embryonic development during which development comes under the exclusive control of the zygotic genome rather than the maternal (egg) genome. The egg contains stored maternal genetic material mRNA which controls embryo development until the onset of MZT. After MZT the diploid embryo takes over genetic control. This requires both zygotic genome activation (ZGA) and degradation of maternal products. This process is important because it is the first time that the new embryonic genome is utilised and the paternal and maternal genomes are used in combination (i.e. different alleles will be expressed). The zygotic genome now drives embryo development. MZT is often thought to be synonymous with midblastula transition (MBT), but these processes are, in fact, distinct.

However, the MBT roughly coincides with ZGA in many metazoans, and thus may share some common regulatory features. For example, both processes are proposed to be regulated by the nucleocytoplasmic ratio. MBT strictly refers to changes in the cell cycle and cell motility that occur just prior to gastrulation. In the early cleavage stages of embryogenesis, rapid divisions occur synchronously and there are no 'gap' stages in the cell cycle. During these stages, there is also little to no transcription of mRNA from the zygotic genome, but zygotic transcription is not required for MBT to occur. Cellular functions during early cleavage are carried out primarily by maternal products – proteins and mRNAs contributed to the egg during oogenesis.

Zygotic Genome Activation

To begin transcription of zygotic genes, the embryo must first overcome the silencing that has been established. The cause of this silencing could be due to several factors: chromatin modifications leading to repression, lack of adequate transcription machinery, or lack of time in which significant transcription can occur due to the shortened cell cycles. Evidence for the first method was provided by Newport and Kirschner's experiments showing that nucleocytoplasmic ratio plays a role in activating zygotic transcription. They suggest that a defined amount of repressor is packaged into the egg, and that the exponential amplification of DNA at each cell cycle results in titration of the repressor at the appropriate time. Indeed, in Xenopus embryos in which excess DNA is introduced, transcription begins earlier. More recently, evidence has been shown that transcription of a subset of genes in Xenopus is delayed by one cell cycle in haploid embryos. The second mechanism of repression has also been addressed experimentally. Prioleau and others show that by introducing TATA binding protein (TBP) into Xenopus oocytes, the block in transcription can be partially overcome. The hypothesis that shortened cell cycles can cause repression of transcription is supported by the observation that mitosis causes transcription to cease. The generally accepted mechanism for the initiation of embryonic gene regulatory networks in mammals is that there are multiple waves of MZT. In mouse, the first of these occurs in the zygote, where expression of a few pioneering transcription factors gradually increases the expression of target genes downstream. This induction of genes leads to a second major MZT event.

Clearing of Maternal Transcripts

To eliminate the contribution of maternal gene products to development, maternally-supplied mRNAs must be degraded in the embryo. Studies in *Drosophila* have shown that sequences in the 3′ UTR of maternal transcripts mediate their degradation (reviewed by Tadros and Lipshitz) These sequences are recognised by regulatory proteins that cause destabilisation or degradation of the transcripts. Recent studies in both zebrafish and Xenopus have found evidence of a role for microRNAs in degradation of maternal transcripts. In zebrafish, the microRNA miR-430 is expressed at the onset of zygotic transcription and targets several hundred mRNAs for deadenylation and degradation. Many of these targets are genes that are expressed maternally. Similarly, in Xenopus, the miR-430 ortholog miR-427 has been shown to target maternal mRNAs for deadenylation. Specifically, miR-427 targets include cell cycle regulators such as Cyclin A1 and Cyclin B2.

DROSOPHILA EMBRYOGENESIS

Ventral view of repeating denticle bands on the cuticle of a 22-hr-old embryo (Fig. 18.1). The head is on the left. *Drosophila embryogenesis*, the process by which *Drosophila* (fruit fly) embryos form, is a favourite model system for genetics and developmental biology. The study of its embryogenesis unlocked the century-long puzzle of how development was controlled, creating the field of evolutionary developmental biology. The small size, short generation time, and large brood size make it ideal for genetic studies. Transparent embryos facilitate developmental studies. *Drosophila melanogaster* was introduced into the field of genetic experiments by Thomas Hunt Morgan in 1909.

Life Cycle

Drosophila display a holometabolous method of development, meaning that they have three distinct stages of their post-embryonic life cycle, each with a radically different body plan: larva, pupa and finally, adult. The machinery necessary for the function and smooth transition between these three phases develops

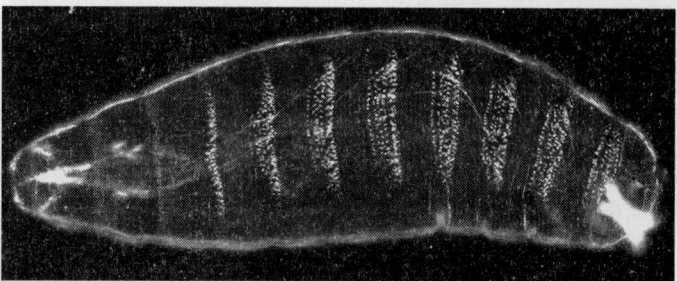

Fig. 18.1: Ventral view of repeating denticle bands on the cuticle of a 22-hr-old embryo. The head is on the left.

during embryogenesis. During embryogenesis, the larval stage fly will develop and hatch at a stage of its life known as the first larval instar. Cells that will produce adult structures are put aside in imaginal discs. During the pupal stage, the larval body breaks down as the imaginal disks grow and produce the adult body. This process is called complete metamorphosis. About 24 hr after fertilisation, an egg hatches into a larva, which undergoes three molts taking about 5.5 to 6 days, after which it is called a pupa. The pupa metamorphoses into an adult fly, which takes about 3.5 to 4.5 days. The entire growth process from egg to adult fly takes an estimated 10 to 12 days to complete at 25°C.

The mother fly produces oocytes that already have anterior-posterior and dorsal-ventral axes defined by maternal activities.

Embryogenesis in *Drosophila* is unique among model organisms in that cleavage occurs in a multinucleate syncytium (strictly a coenocyte). Early on, 256 nuclei migrate to the perimeter of the egg, creating the syncytial blastoderm. The germ line segregates from the somatic cells through the formation of pole cells at the posterior end of the embryo. After thirteen mitotic divisions and about 4 hr after fertilisation, an estimated 6000 nuclei accumulate in the unseparated cytoplasm of the oocyte before they migrate to the surface and are encompassed by plasma membranes to form cells surrounding the yolk sac producing a cellular blastoderm.

Like other triploblastic metazoa, gastrulation leads to the formation of three germ layers: the endoderm, mesoderm, and ectoderm. The mesoderm invaginates from the ventral furrow (VF), as does the ectoderm that will give rise to the midgut. The pole cells are internalised by a different route. Germ band elongation involves many rearrangements of cells, and the appearance of distinct differences in the cells of the three germ bands and various regions of the embryo. The posterior region (including the hindgut) expands and extends towards the anterior pole along the dorsal side of the embryo. At this time, segments of the embryo become visible, creating a striped arrangement along the anterior-posterior axis. The earliest signs of segmentation appear during this phase with the formation of parasegmental furrows. This is also when the tracheal pits form, the first signs of structures for breathing.

Germ band retraction returns the hindgut to the dorsal side of the posterior pole and coincides with overt segmentation. The remaining stages involve the internalisation of the nervous system (ectoderm) and the formation of internal organs (mainly mesoderm).

Anterior-posterior Axis Patterning in *Drosophila*

One of the best understood examples of pattern formation is the patterning along the future head to tail (antero-posterior) axis of the fruit fly *Drosophila melanogaster*. There are three fundamental types of genes that give way to the developmental structure of the fly: maternal effect genes, segmentation genes, and homeotic genes. The development of *Drosophila* is particularly well studied, and it is representative of a major class of animals, the insects or insecta. Other multicellular organisms sometimes use similar mechanisms for axis formation, although the relative importance of signal transfer between the earliest cells of many developing organisms is greater than in the example described here.

Maternal effect genes

The building-blocks of anterior-posterior axis patterning in *Drosophila* are laid out during egg formation (oogenesis), well before the egg is fertilised and deposited. The maternal effect genes are responsible for the polarity of the egg and of the embryo. The developing egg (oocyte) is polarised by differentially localised mRNA molecules (Fig. 18.2).

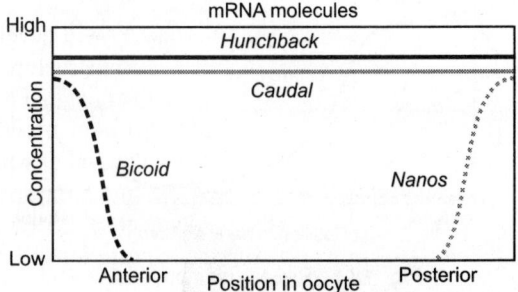

Fig. 18.2: mRNA distributions.

The genes that code for these mRNAs, called maternal effect genes, encode for proteins that get translated upon fertilisation to establish concentration gradients that span the egg. *Bicoid* and *Hunchback* are the maternal effect genes that are most important for patterning of anterior parts (head and thorax) of the *Drosophila* embryo. *Nanos* and *Caudal* are maternal effect genes that are important in the formation of more posterior abdominal segments of the *Drosophila* embryo.

In embryos from *bicoid* mutant mothers, the head and thoracic structures are converted to the abdomen making the embryo with posterior structures on both ends, a lethal phenotype. Cytoskeletal elements such as microtubules are polarised within the oocyte and can be used to allow the localisation of mRNA molecules to specific parts of the cell. Maternally synthesised bicoid mRNAs attach to microtubules and are concentrated at the anterior ends of forming *Drosophila* eggs. In unfertilised eggs, transcripts are still strictly localised at the tip, but immediately after fertilisation, a small mRNA gradient is formed in the anterior 20% of the eggs. Another report documents a mRNA gradient up to 40%. nanos mRNA also attaches to a *Drosophila* eggs cytoskeleton but is concentrated at the posterior end of the egg. *hunchback* and *caudal* mRNAs lack special location control systems and are fairly evenly spread throughout the entire interior of the egg cells.

It has been shown that the dsRNA-binding protein STAUFEN (STAU1) is responsible for guiding bicoid, nanos and other proteins, which play a role in forming the anterior-posterior axis, to the correct regions of the embryo to build gradients. When the mRNAs from the maternal effect genes are translated into proteins, a Bicoid protein gradient forms at the anterior end of the egg. Nanos protein forms a gradient at the posterior end. The Bicoid protein blocks translation of caudal mRNA so Caudal protein is of lower concentration at the anterior part of the embryo and at higher concentration at the posterior part of the embryo. This is of opposite direction of the Bicoid protein. The caudal protein then activates later to turn genes on to form the posterior structures during the segmentation phase. Nanos protein creates a posterior-to-anterior slope and is a morphogen that helps in abdomen formation. Nanos protein, in complex with Pumilio protein, binds to the hunchback mRNA and blocks its translation in the posterior end of *Drosophila* embryos (Fig. 18.3). The Bicoid, Hunchback, and Caudal proteins are transcription factors. The Bicoid protein is a morphogen as well. The Nanos protein is a translational repressor protein. Bicoid has a DNA-binding homeodomain that binds both DNA and the nanos mRNA. Bicoid binds a specific RNA sequence in the 3′ untranslated region, called the Bicoid 3′-UTR regulatory element, of caudal mRNA and blocks translation.

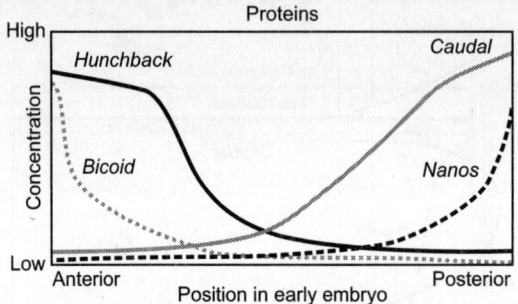

Fig. 18.3: Protein distributions.

Hunchback protein levels in the early embryo are significantly augmented by new hunchback gene transcription and translation of the resulting zygotically produced mRNA. During early *Drosophila embryogenesis*, there are nuclear divisions without cell division. The many nuclei that are produced distribute themselves around the periphery of the cell cytoplasm. Gene expression in these nuclei is regulated by the Bicoid, Hunchback, and Caudal proteins. For example, Bicoid acts as a transcriptional activator of hunchback gene transcription. In order for development to continue, Hunchback is needed in an area that is declining in amount from anterior to posterior. This is created by the Nanos protein whose existence is at a declining slope from posterior to anterior ends.

Gap genes

The other important function of the gradients of Bicoid, Hunchback, and Caudal proteins is in the transcriptional regulation of other zygotically expressed proteins. Many of these are the protein products derived from members of the 'gap' family of developmental control genes. giant, huckebein, hunchback, knirps, Krüppel and tailless are all gap genes. Their expression patterns in the early embryo are determined by the maternal effect gene products. The gap genes are part of a larger family called the segmentation genes. These genes establish the segmented body plan of the embryo along the anterior-posterior axis. The segmentation genes specify 14 parasegments that are closely related to the final anatomical segments. The gap genes are the first layer of a hierarchical cascade of the segmentation control genes.

Additional segmentation genes

Two additional classes of segmentation genes are expressed after the gap gene products. The pair-rule genes are expressed in striped patterns of seven bands perpendicular to the anterior-posterior axis. These patterns of expression are established within the syncytial blastoderm. After these initial patterning events, cell membranes form around the nuclei of the syncytial blastoderm converting it to a cellular blastoderm.

The expression patterns of the final class of segmentation genes, the segment polarity genes, are then fine-tuned by interactions between the cells of adjacent parasegments with genes such as engrailed. The Engrailed protein is a transcription factor that is expressed in one row of cells at the edge of each parasegment. This expression pattern is initiated by the pair-rule genes (like even-skipped) that code for transcription factors that regulate the engrailed genes transcription in the syncytial blastoderm (Fig. 18.4).

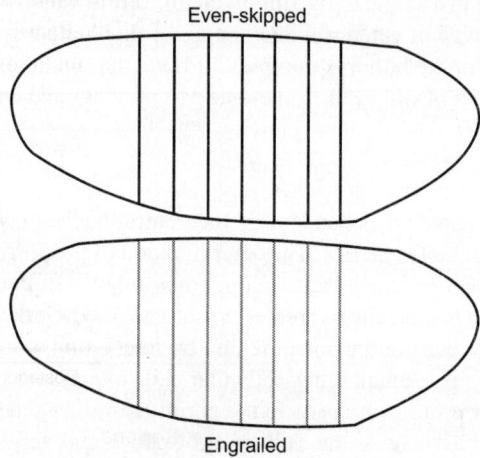

Even-skipped

Engrailed

Fig. 18.4: Pair rule.

Cells that make Engrailed can make the cell-to-cell signalling protein Hedgehog. The motion of Hedgehog is limited by its lipid modification, and so Hedgehog activates a thin stripe of cells anterior to the Engrailed-expressing cells. Only cells to one side of the Engrailed-expressing cells are competent to respond to Hedgehog because they express the receptor protein Patched. Cells with activated Patched receptor make the Wingless protein. Wingless is a secreted protein that acts on the adjacent rows of cells by activating its cell surface receptor, Frizzled.

Wingless acts on Engrailed-expressing cells to stabilise Engrailed expression after the cellular blastoderm forms. The Naked cuticle protein is induced by Wingless to limit the number of rows of cells that express Engrailed. The short-range, reciprocal signalling by Hedgehog and Wingless, held in check by the Patched and Naked proteins, stabilises the boundary between each segment. The Wingless protein is called 'wingless' because of the phenotype of some wingless mutants. Wingless and Hedgehog also function in multiple tissues later in embryogenesis and also during metamorphosis.

The transcription factors that are coded for by segmentation genes regulate yet another family of developmental control genes, the homeotic selector genes. These genes exist in two ordered groups on *Drosophila* chromosome 3. The order of the genes on the chromosome reflects the order that they are expressed along the anterior-posterior axis of the developing embryo. The Antennapedia group of homeotic selector genes includes labial, antennapedia, sex combs reduced, deformed, and proboscipedia. Labial and Deformed proteins are expressed in head segments where they activate the genes that define head features. Sex-combs-reduced and Antennapedia specify the properties of thoracic segments. The bithorax group of homeotic selector genes control the specialisations of the third thoracic segment and the abdominal segments. Mutations in some homeotic genes can often be lethal and the cycle of life will end at embryogenesis.

In 1995, the Nobel Prize for Physiology or Medicine was awarded for studies concerning the genetic control of early embryonic development to Christiane Nüsslein-Volhard, Edward B. Lewis and Eric Wieschaus. Their research on genetic screening for embryo patterning mutants revealed the role played in early embryologic development by homeobox genes like bicoid. An example of a homeotic mutation is the so-called Antennapedia mutation. In *Drosophila*, antennae and legs are created by the same basic 'programme', they only differ in a single transcription factor. If this transcription factor is damaged, the fly grows legs on its head instead of antennae. See images of this 'antennapedia' mutant and others, at FlyBase. Another example is in the bithorax complex. If nonlethal mutations occur in this complex, it can cause the fly to have two sets of wings, instead of one pair of wings and one pair of halteres, which aid in balance in flight.

Dorsal-ventral Axis

Formation of the dorsal-ventral axis is dependent on the ventral nuclear concentration of a maternally synthesised transcription factor called Dorsal. The determination of the dorsal side of the embryo occurs during oogenesis when the oocyte nucleus moves along microtubules from the posterior to the anterior-dorsal margin of the oocyte. The nucleus expresses a protein called Gurken which is secreted locally and thus only activates follicle cells in the dorsal region by interacting with the Torpedo receptor. This inhibits the production of Pipe protein and thus follicular cells expressing Pipe are on the ventral side. Pipe activates an extracellular protease cascade in the perivitelline space between the follicle cells and the egg which results in the cleavage of the Toll-ligand Spätzle and activation of the Toll signalling cascade on the ventral side. Dorsal protein is present throughout embryonic cytoplasm but bound to Cactus which prevents it from translocating to the nucleus. Toll signalling results in the degradation of Cactus which allows Dorsal to enter the nuclei on the ventral side of the blastoderm. Overall, a difference in the localisation of the oocyte nucleus becomes a difference in the signalling state of the surrounding follicle cells which then signal to the resulting blastoderm nuclei. Once in the nucleus, Dorsal activates different genes depending upon its nuclear concentration. This process sets up a gradient between the ventral and dorsal side of the blastoderm embryo with the repression or induction of Dorsal target genes being differentially regulated. At the ventral end of the embryo, blastoderm nuclei exposed to high concentrations of dorsal protein induce the transcription of the transcription factors twist and snail while repressing zerknüllt and decapentaplegic. This results in the formation of the mesoderm. In the lateral regions of the embryo, low nuclear concentrations of Dorsal lead to the expression of rhomboid which identifies future neuroectoderm. More dorsally, active Dpp signalling represses rhomboid thus confining it to the lateral blastoderm nuclei. At the dorsal side of the embryo, blastoderm nuclei where this is little or no nuclear dorsal protein express zerknüllt, tolloid, and decapentaplegic (Dpp). This leads to the specification of non-neural ectoderm and later in the blastula stage to anmioserosa. The ventral activity of the TGF-β family signalling protein Dpp is maintained by the expression of the secreted Dpp-antagonist Sog (short gastrulation) in the neuroectoderm. Sog binds to and prevents Dpp from diffusing to the ventral side of the embryo and through the cleavage of Sog by Tolloid also enables a sharpening of the Dpp gradient on the dorsal side. The DV axis of *Drosophila* is due to the interaction of two gradients – a ventral concentration of nuclear Dorsal and a dorsal concentration of Dpp activity.

CELL–CELL INTERACTION

Cell–cell interaction refers to the direct interactions between cell surfaces that play a crucial role in the development and function of multicellular organisms. These interactions allow cells to communicate with each other in response to changes in their microenvironment. This ability to send and receive signals is essential for the survival of the cell. Interactions between cells can be stable such as those made through cell junctions. These junctions are involved in the communication and organisation of cells within a particular tissue. Others are transient or temporary such as those between cells of the immune system or the interactions involved in tissue inflammation. These types of intercellular interactions are distinguished from other types such as those between cells and the extracellular matrix. The loss of communication between cells can result in uncontrollable cell growth and cancer.

Stable Interactions

Stable cell-cell interactions are required for cell adhesion within a tissue and controlling the shape and function of cells.These stable interactions involve cell junctions which are multiprotein complexes that provide contact between neighboring cells. Cell junctions allow for the preservation and proper functioning of epithelial cell sheets. These junctions are also important in the organisation of tissues where cells of one type can only adhere to cells of the same tissue rather than to a different tissue.

Tight junctions

Tight junctions are multi-protein complexes that hold cells of a same tissue together and prevent movement of water and water-soluble molecules between cells. In epithelial cells, they function also to separate the extracellular fluid surrounding their apical and basolateral membranes. These junctions exist as a continuous band located just below the apical surface between the membranes of neighboring epithelial cells. The tight junctions on adjacent cells line up so as to produce a seal between different tissues and body cavities. For example, the apical surface of gastrointestinal epithelial cells serve as a selective permeable barrier that separates the external environment from the body. The permeability of these junctions is dependent on a variety of factors including protein makeup of that junction, tissue type and signaling from the cells.

Tight junctions are made up of many different proteins. The four main transmembrane proteins are occludin, claudin, junctional adhesion molecules (JAMs) and tricellulins. The extracellular domains of these proteins form the tight junction barrier by making homophilic (between proteins of the same kind) and heterophilic interactions (between different types of proteins) with the protein domains on adjacent cells. Their cytoplasmic domains interact with the cell cytoskeleton to anchor them.

Anchoring junctions

Of the three types of anchoring junctions, only two are involved in cell-cell interactions: adherens junctions and desmosomes. Both are found in many types of cells. Adjacent epithelial cells are connected by adherens junctions on their lateral membranes. They are located just below tight junctions. Their function is to give shape and tension to cells and tissues and they are also the site of cell-cell signaling. Adherens junctions are made of cell adhesion molecules from the cadherin family. There are over 100 types of cadherins, corresponding to the many different types of cells and tissues with varying anchoring needs. The most common are E-, N- and P-cadherins. In the adherens junctions of epithelial cells, E-cadherin is the most abundant.

Desmosomes also provide strength and durability to cells and tissues and are located just below adherens junctions. They are sites of adhesion and do not encircle the cell. They are made of two specialised cadherins, desmoglein and desmocollin. These proteins have extracellular domains that interact with each other on adjacent cells. On the cytoplasmic side, plakins form plaques which anchor the desmosomes to intermediate filaments composed of keratin proteins. Desmosomes also play a role in cell-cell signalling.

Gap junctions

Gap junctions are the main site of cell-cell signaling or communication that allow small molecules to diffuse between adjacent cells. In vertebrates, gap junctions are composed of transmembrane proteins called connexins. They form hexagonal pores or channels through which ions, sugars, and other small molecules can pass. Each pore is made of 12 connexin molecules, 6 form a hemichannel on one cell membrane and interact with a hemichannel on an adjacent cell membrane. The permeability of these junctions is regulated by many factors including pH and Ca^{2+} concentration.

Receptor proteins in direct-contact signalling

Receptor proteins on the cell surface have the ability to bind specific signaling molecules secreted by other cells. Cell signaling allows cells to communicate with adjacent cells, nearby cells (paracrine) and even distant cells (endocrine). This binding induces a conformational change in the receptor which, in turn, elicits a response in the corresponding cell. These responses include changes in gene expression and alterations in cytoskeleton structure. The extracellular face of the plasma membrane has a variety of proteins, carbohydrates, and lipids which project outward and act as signals. Direct contact between cells allows the receptors on one cell to bind the small molecules attached to the plasma membrane of different cell. In eukaryotes, many of the cells during early development communicate through direct contact.

Synaptic signaling, an integral part of nervous system activity, occurs between neurons and target cells. These target cells can also be neurons or other cell types (i.e. muscle or gland cells). Protocadherins, a member of the cadherin family, mediate the adhesion of neurons to their target cells at synapses otherwise known as synaptic junctions. In order to for communication to occur between a neuron and its target cell, a wave of depolarisation travels the length of the neuron and causes neurotransmitters to be released into the synaptic junction. These neurotransmitters bind and activate receptors on the post-synaptic neuron thereby transmitting the signal to the target cell. Thus, a post-synaptic membrane belongs to the membrane receiving the signal, while a pre-synaptic membrane is the source of the neurotransmitter. In a neuromuscular junction, a synapse is formed between a motor neuron and muscle fibers. In vertebrates, acetylcholine released from the motor neuron acts as a neurotransmitter which depolarises the muscle fiber and causes muscle contraction. A neuron's ability to receive and integrate simultaneous signals from the environment and other neurons allows for complex animal behaviour.

Plant cell-cell interactions

Plant cells are surrounded by cell walls which are barriers for cell-cell communication. This barrier is overcome by specialised junctions called plasmodesmata. They are similar to gap junctions, connecting the cytosol of adjacent cells. Small molecules (<1000 Da), such as ions, amino acids, and sugars, can diffuse freely through plasmodesmata. These small molecules include signaling molecule and transcription factors. The size of the channel is also regulated to allow molecules up to 10,000 Da in size. The permeability of these channels is dependent on many factors, including Ca^{2+} concentration. An increase in cytosolic Ca^{2+} concentration will reversibly limit passage through the plasmodesmata. Unlike gap junctions, the cell membranes of adjacent cells merge to form a continuous channel called an annulus. Additionally, within the channel, there is an extension of the endoplasmic reticulum, called a desmotubule, which spans between the cells. The cell-cell interactions facilitated by plasmodesmata play an important role in development of plant cells and tissues and defense against viral infection.

Transient Interactions

Immune system

Leukocytes or white blood cells destroy abnormal cells and also provide protection against bacteria and other foreign matter. These interactions are transitory in nature but are crucial as an immediate immune response. To fight infection, leukocytes must move from the blood into the affected tissues. This movement into tissues is called extravasation. It requires successive forming and breaking of cell-cell interactions between the leukocytes and the endothelial cells that line blood vessels. These cell-cell interactions are mediated mainly by a group of Cell Adhesion Molecules (CAMs) called selectins.

T helper cells, central to the immune system, interact with other leukocytes by releasing signals known as cytokines which activate and stimulate the proliferation of B cells and killer T cells. T helper cells also directly interact with macrophages, cells that engulf foreign matter and display antigens on its surface. T-helper cells that possess the appropriate receptors can bind to these antigens and proliferate resulting in T-helper cells that have the ability to identify the same antigens.

Coagulation

Coagulation or blood clotting relies on, in addition to the production of fibrin, interactions between platelets. When the endothelium or the lining of a blood vessel is damaged, connective tissue including collagen fibers is locally exposed. Initially, platelets stick to the exposed connective tissue through specific cell-surface receptors. This is followed by platelet activation and aggregation in which platelets become firmly attached and release chemicals that recruit neighboring platelets to the site of vascular injury. A meshwork of fibrin then forms around this aggregation of platelets to increase the strength of the clot.

Cell interactions between bacteria

Bacterial populations interact in a similar manner to cells in tissue. They communicate through physical interactions and signaling molecules such as homoserine lactones and peptides as a means to control metabolism and regulate growth. A common example and one of the most studied forms of bacterial cell interactions is biofilm. Biofilm is a cell aggregate that can be attached to biological or abiotic surfaces. Bacteria form biofilms to adapt to various environments such as changes in substrate availability. For example, the formation of biofilm increases a bacterial cells resistance to antibiotics compared to cells which are not part of the aggregate.

Pathological Implications

Cancer

Cancer can result from the loss of cell-cell interaction. In normal cells, growth is controlled by contact inhibition in which contact with neighboring cells causes a stunt in cell growth. Contact inhibition is thought to be mediated by cadherins, proteins that play an important role in cell adhesion. This inhibition prevents cells from piling up on top of one another and forming mounds. However, in cancerous cells where expression of E-cadherin is lost, contact inhibition is lost and results in uncontrolled growth or proliferation, tumor formation, and metastasis.

Bacterial pathogens

In order for pathogenic bacteria to invade a cell, communication with the host cell is required. The first step for invading bacteria is usually adhesion to host cells. Strong anchoring, a characteristic that determines virulence, prevents the bacteria from being washed away before infection occurs. Bacterial cells can bind to many host cell surface structures such as glycolipids and glycoproteins which serve as attachment receptors. Once attached, the bacteria begin to interact with the host to disrupt its normal functioning and disrupt or rearrange its cytoskeleton. Proteins on the bacteria surface can interact with protein receptors on the host thereby affecting signal transduction within the cell. Alterations to signaling are favorable to bacteria because these alterations provide conditions under which the pathogen can invade. Many pathogens have Type III secretion systems which can directly inject protein toxins into the host cells. These toxins ultimately lead to rearrangement of the cytoskeleton and entry of the bacteria.

Disease

Cell–cell interactions are highly specific and are tightly regulated. Genetic defects and dysregulation of these interactions can cause many different diseases. Dysregulation that leads to leukocyte migration into healthy tissues can cause conditions such as acute respiratory distress syndrome and some types of arthritis. The autoimmune disease pemphigus vulgaris results from autoantibodies to desmoglein and other normal body proteins. The autoantibodies disrupt the adhesion between epithelial cells. This causes blisters of the skin and mucous membranes. Mutations in the connexin genes cause 8 human diseases including heart malformations and neurosensory deafness.

Chapter 19

Genetic Control of Development

INTRODUCTION

Development is the process through which a multicellular organism arises from a single cell. During development, cells become specialised, or differentiated, taking on different functions and forms. The organism develops a characteristic three-dimensional shape, the parts of which (such as limbs and organs) continue to maintain the same relationship to each other even as the organism grows. How the genes in a single fertilised egg dictate the creation of a complex multicellular creature is the central question in the genetic control of development. While we are often most curious about human developmental processes, very little is known about the genetics of human development specifically, because experimentation on human embryos is forbidden by law and ethics. Instead, the details of genetic control are best understood in several model organisms, including the roundworm (*Caenorhabditis elegans*), the fruit fly (*Drosophila melanogaster*), the zebrafish, and the mouse.

Each organism differs in the details, and in some cases the overall logic, of genetic control. The understanding of developmental control is not complete for any of these organisms, but scientists have come to understand several mechanisms that contribute to, but do not entirely explain, development.

GENETIC DETERMINISM

Genetic determinism is the mechanism by which genes, along with environmental conditions, determine morphological and behavioural phenotypes.

Alternative Use

The term genetic determinism has sometimes been mistakenly applied to the unscientific belief that genes determine, to the exclusion of environmental influence, how an organism turns out. Such views have sometimes been attributed to opponents, or forwarded in hypothetical arguments, without having been actually held by anyone: as CH Waddington wrote in 1957, 'It is of course a truism which has long been recognised that the development of any individual is affected both by the hereditary determinants which come into the fertilised egg from the two parents and also by the nature of the environment in which the development takes place.' The use of genetic determinism in this sense of an accusation of holding unscientific beliefs originates in the historical 'nature versus nurture' dispute, especially during the 1970s and 1980s. A related error is the supposed misconception holding that geneticists and molecular biologists have only recently come to the realisation that environment is essential in the development of the organism from egg to adult.

EMBRYONIC DIFFERENTIATION IN ANIMALS

Embryonic differentiation is the process of development during which embryonic cells specialise and diverse tissue structures arise. Animals are made up of many different cell types, each with specific functions in the body. However, during early embryonic development, the embryo does not yet possess these varied cells; this is where embryonic differentiation comes into play. The differentiation of cells during embryogenesis is the key to cell, tissue, organ, and organism identity. Once an egg is fertilised by a sperm, a zygote is formed. The zygote divides into multiple cells in a process known as cleavage, triggering the beginning of embryonic differentiation. During cleavage, the zygote divides but maintains its size in the process.

This zygotic division produces blastomeres which later make up the hollow sphere known as the blastula. Cells migrate within the blastula to locations that will later define the structure of the embryo and consequent organism. In this process, called gastrulation, three germ layers arise: the endoderm, mesoderm, and ectoderm. Cells in these three layers will give rise to different parts of the organism. The endoderm eventually becomes the gut. The mesoderm develops into muscle, the skeletal system, some organs, and connective tissue. The ectoderm differentiates into the nervous system and skin. As the embryo continues to develop, individual cells continue to differentiate.

These differentiated cell types are made from what were initially the same types of pluripotent embryonic stem cells. An assortment of physiological mechanisms guides certain cells towards particular developmental pathways, creating varying cell types. This is made possible by the cells inherent ability to control what genes are expressed and translated into proteins. Every cell contains DNA within the nucleus, containing the blueprint to build many different proteins in the cell. Different signals can cause embryonic cells to select specific parts of the DNA which can then be used to synthesise proteins, eventually building different cell types. Differentiation of cells in the embryo is brought about by both internal cellular factors as well as extracellular factors that act on the cell from the outside. Much remains to be understood about the exact molecular interactions that govern cellular differentiation. It is understood, however, diversifying the ratio of and types of internal and external influences on certain cells, allows many divergent cell types to arise.

There are two main types of cellular development that pertain to embryos: mosaic development or regulative development. In mosaic development (which is not characteristic of mammals, but of organisms such as annelids) differentiation occurs in steps that are set in order and progression, without input occurring between neighbouring cells. On the other hand, regulative development involves the interaction of adjacent cells, within what is known as embryonic fields.

The advantage of regulative development is the flexibility that it confers to differentiation. For example, a cells pathway may change depending on the cellular environment in which it is placed, not merely by its internal mechanisms. The process of embryonic differentiation is crucial to proper animal development. The processes involved in embryonic differentiation continue to be explored and have relevance to studies involving embryonic stem cells and *in vitro* cell differentiation. As scientists continue to study the physiological mechanisms of embryonic development the process of embryonic differentiation should continue to be understood in greater and greater detail.

CELL SIGNALLING

Cell signalling is part of a complex system of communication that governs basic cellular activities and coordinates cell actions. The ability of cells to perceive and correctly respond to their microenvironment is the basis of development, tissue repair, and immunity as well as normal tissue homeostasis. Errors in cellular information processing are responsible for diseases such as cancer, autoimmunity, and diabetes. By understanding cell signalling, diseases may be treated effectively and, theoretically, artificial tissues may be created. Traditional work in biology has focused on studying individual parts of cell signalling pathways. Systems biology research helps us to understand the underlying structure of cell signalling networks and how changes in these networks may affect the transmission and flow of information. Such networks are complex systems in their organisation and may exhibit a number of emergent properties including bistability and ultrasensitivity. Analysis of cell signalling networks requires a combination of experimental and theoretical approaches including the development and analysis of simulations and modelling. Long-range allostery is often a significant component of cell signalling events.

Signalling between Cells of One Organism and Multiple Organisms

Cell signalling has been most extensively studied in the context of human diseases and signalling between cells of a single organism. However, cell signalling may also occur between the cells of two different organisms. In many mammals, early embryo cells exchange signals with cells of the uterus. In the human gastrointestinal tract, bacteria exchange signals with each other and with human epithelial and immune system cells. For the yeast *Saccharomyces* cerevisiae during mating, some cells send a peptide signal (mating factor pheromones) into their environment. The mating factor peptide may bind to a cell surface receptor on other yeast cells and induce them to prepare for mating.

Classification of cell signalling

Signalling within, between, and among cells is subdivided into the following classifications:

- Intracrine signals are produced by the target cell that stay within the target cell.
- Autocrine signals are produced by the target cell, are secreted, and affect the target cell itself via receptors. Sometimes autocrine cells can target cells close by if they are the same type of cell as the emitting cell. An example of this are immune cells.
- Juxtacrine signals target adjacent (touching) cells. These signals are transmitted along cell membranes via protein or lipid components integral to the membrane and are capable of affecting either the emitting cell or cells immediately adjacent.
- Paracrine signals target cells in the vicinity of the emitting cell. Neurotransmitters represent an example.
- Endocrine signals target distant cells. Endocrine cells produce hormones that travel through the blood to reach all parts of the body.

Cells communicate with each other via direct contact (juxtacrine signalling), over short distances (paracrine signalling), or over large distances and/or scales (endocrine signalling).

Cell signalling in multicellular organisms

In a multicellular organism, signalling between cells occurs either through release into the extracellular space, divided in paracrine signalling (over short distances) and endocrine signalling (over long distances), or by direct contact, known as juxtacrine signalling. Autocrine signalling is a special case of paracrine signalling where the secreting cell has the ability to respond to the secreted signalling molecule. Synaptic signalling is a special case of paracrine signalling (for chemical synapses) or juxtacrine signalling (for electrical synapses) between neurons and target cells. Signalling molecules interact with a target cell as a ligand to cell surface receptors, and/or by entering into the cell through its membrane or endocytosis for intracrine signalling. This generally results in the activation of second messengers, leading to various physiological effects.

Receptors for cell motility and differentiation

Cells receive information from their neighbours through a class of proteins known as receptors. Notch is a cell surface protein that functions as a receptor. Animals have a small set of genes that code for signalling proteins that interact specifically with Notch receptors and stimulate a response in cells that express Notch on their surface. Molecules that activate (or, in some cases, inhibit) receptors can be classified as hormones, neurotransmitters, cytokines, and growth factors, but all of these are called receptor ligands. The details of ligand-receptor interactions are fundamental to cell signalling.

The notch acts as a receptor for ligands that are expressed on adjacent cells. While some receptors are cell surface proteins, others are found inside cells. For example, estrogen is a hydrophobic molecule that can pass through the lipid bilayer of the membranes. As part of the endocrine system, intracellular estrogen receptors from a variety of cell types can be activated by estrogen produced in the ovaries.

Signalling Pathways

In some cases, receptor activation caused by ligand binding to a receptor is directly coupled to the cell's response to the ligand. For example, the neurotransmitter GABA can activate a cell surface receptor that is part of an ion channel. GABA binding to a GABAA receptor on a neuron opens a chloride-selective ion channel that is part of the receptor. GABAA receptor activation allows negatively charged chloride ions to move into the neuron, which inhibits the ability of the neuron to produce action potentials. However, for many cell surface receptors, ligand-receptor interactions are not directly linked to the cell's response. The activated receptor must first interact with other proteins inside the cell before the ultimate physiological effect of the ligand on the cell's behaviour is produced. Often, the behaviour of a chain of several interacting cell proteins is altered following receptor activation. The entire set of cell changes induced by receptor activation is called a signal transduction mechanism or pathway.

IMMORTALISED CELL LINE

An immortalised cell line is a population of cells from a multicellular organism which would normally not proliferate indefinitely but, due to mutation, have evaded normal cellular senescence and instead can keep undergoing division. The cells can therefore be grown for prolonged periods *in vitro*. The mutations required for immortality can occur naturally or be intentionally induced for experimental purposes. Immortal cell lines are a very important tool for research into the biochemistry and cell biology of multicellular organisms. Immortalised cell lines have also found uses in biotechnology. There are various immortal cell lines. Some of them are normal cell lines e.g. derived from stem cells. Other immortalised cell lines are the *in vitro* equivalent of cancerous cells. Cancer occurs when a somatic cell which normally cannot divide undergoes mutations which cause de-regulation of the normal cell cycle controls leading to uncontrolled proliferation. Immortalised cell lines have undergone similar mutations allowing a cell type which would normally not be able to divide to be proliferated *in vitro*. The origins of some immortal cell lines, for example HeLa human cells, are from naturally occurring cancers.

Role and Uses of Immortalised Cell Lines

Immortalised cell lines are widely used as a simple model for more complex biological systems, for example for the analysis of the biochemistry and cell biology of mammalian (including human) cells. The main advantage of using an immortal cell line for research is its immortality; the cells can be grown indefinitely in culture. This simplifies analysis of the biology of cells which may otherwise have a limited lifetime. Immortalised cell lines can also be cloned giving rise to a clonal population which can, in turn, be propagated indefinitely. This allows an analysis to be repeated many times on genetically identical cells which is desirable for repeatable scientific experiments. The alternative, performing an analysis on primary cells from multiple tissue donors, does not have this advantage.

Immortalised cell lines find use in biotechnology where they are a cost-effective way of growing cells similar to those found in a multicellular organism *in vitro*. The cells are used for a wide variety of purposes, from testing toxicity of compounds or drugs to production of eukaryotic proteins.

Methods for generating immortalised cell lines

There are several methods for generating immortalised cell lines:

1. Isolation from a naturally occurring cancer. This is the original method for generating an immortalised cell line.

2. Spontaneous or induced random mutagenesis and selection for cells which are able to undergo division.

3. Introduction of a viral gene that partially deregulates the cell cycle.

4. Artificial expression of key proteins required for immortality, for example telomerase which prevents degradation of chromosome ends during DNA replication in eukaryotes

5. Hybridoma technology, specifically used for the generation of immortalised antibody-producing B cell lines, where an antibody-producing B cell is fused with a myeloma (B cell cancer) cell.

NEMATODE

The nematodes or roundworms (phylum Nematoda) are the most diverse phylum of pseudocoelomates, and one of the most diverse of all animals. It has been estimated that the total number of nematode species might be approximately 1000000. Unlike cnidarians or flatworms, roundworms have a digestive system that is like a tube with openings at both ends. Nematodes have successfully adapted to nearly every ecosystem from marine to freshwater, from the polar regions to the tropics, as well as the highest to the lowest of elevations. They are ubiquitous in freshwater, marine, and terrestrial environments, where they often outnumber other animals in both individual and species counts, and are found in locations as diverse as mountains, deserts and oceanic trenches. They represent, for example, 90 per cent of all life on the seafloor of the earth. Their many parasitic forms include pathogens in most plants and animals (including humans). Some nematodes can undergo cryptobiosis. One group of carnivorous fungi, the nemato-phagous fungi, are predators of soil nematodes.

Reproduction

Most nematode species are dioecious, with separate male and female individuals. Both sexes possess one or two tubular gonads. In males, the sperm are produced at the end of the gonad, and migrate along its length as they mature. The testes each open into a relatively wide sperm duct and then into a glandular and muscular ejaculatory duct associated with the cloaca. In females, the ovaries each open into an oviduct and then a glandular uterus. The uteri both open into a common vagina, usually located in the middle of the ventral surface.

Reproduction is usually sexual. Males are usually smaller than females (often much smaller) and often have a characteristically bent tail for holding the female for copulation. During copulation, one or more chitinised spicules move out of the cloaca and are inserted into genital pore of the female. Amoeboid sperm crawl along the spicule into the female worm. Nematode sperm is thought to be the only eukaryotic cell without the globular protein G-actin.

Eggs may be embryonated or unembryonated when passed by the female, meaning that their fertilised eggs may not yet be developed. A few species are known to be ovoviviparous. The eggs are protected by an outer shell, secreted by the uterus. In free-living roundworms, the eggs hatch into larvae, which appear essentially identical to the adults, except for an underdeveloped reproductive system; in parasitic round-worms, the life cycle is often much more complicated.

Free-living species

In free-living species, development usually consists of four molts of the cuticle during growth. Different species feed on materials as varied as algae, fungi, small animals, fecal matter, dead organisms and living tissues. Free-living marine nematodes are important and abundant members of the meiobenthos. They play an important role in the decomposition process, aid in recycling of nutrients in marine environments and are sensitive to changes in the environment caused by pollution.

Parasitic species

Nematodes commonly parasitic on humans include ascarids (*Ascaris*), filarias, hookworms, pinworms (*Enterobius*) and whipworms (*Trichuris trichiura*). The species *Trichinella spiralis*, commonly known as the trichina worm, occurs in rats, pigs, and humans, and is responsible for the disease trichinosis.

OOCYTE

An oocyte, oöcyte, ovocyte, or rarely ocyte, is a female gametocyte or germ cell involved in reproduction. In other words, it is an immature ovum, or egg cell. An oocyte is produced in the ovary during female gametogenesis. The female germ cells produce a primordial germ cell (PGC), which then undergoes mitosis, forming oogonia. During oogenesis, the oogonia become primary oocytes.

Formation

The formation of an oocyte is called oocytogenesis, which is a part of oogenesis. Oogenesis results in the formation of both primary oocytes before birth, and of secondary oocytes after it as part of ovulation.

Maternal Contributions

Because the fate of an oocyte is to become fertilised and ultimately grow into a fully functioning organism, it must be ready to regulate multiple cellular and developmental processes. The oocyte, a large and complex cell, must be supplied with numerous molecules that will direct the growth of the embryo and control cellular activities. As the oocyte is a product of female gametogenesis, the maternal contribution to the oocyte and consequently the newly fertilised egg is enormous. There are many types of molecules that are maternally supplied to the oocyte, which will direct various activities within the growing zygote.

Paternal Contributions

The spermatozoon that fertilises an oocyte will contribute its pronucleus, the other half of the zygotic genome. In some species, the spermatozoon will also contribute a centriole, which will help make up the zygotic centrosome required for the first division. However, in some species, such as in the mouse, the entire centrosome is acquired maternally. Currently under investigation is the possibility of other cytoplasmic contributions made to the embryo by the spermatozoon.

During fertilisation, the sperm provides three essential parts to the oocyte: (i) a signalling or activating factor, which causes the metabolically dormant oocyte to activate, (ii) the haploid paternal genome and (iii) the centrosome, which is responsible for maintaining the microtubule system.

GERMLINE MUTATION

A germline mutation is any detectable and heritable variation in the lineage of germ cells. Mutations in these cells are transmitted to offspring, while, on the other hand, those in somatic cells are not. A germline mutation gives rise to a constitutional mutation in the offspring, that is, a mutation that is present in virtually every cell. A constitutional mutation can also occur very soon after fertilisation, or continue from a previous constitutional mutation in a parent.

This distinction is most important in animals, where germ cells are distinct from somatic cells. However, in plants, the reproductive cells in a particular flower will be derived from the same meristem as the cells in that flower and on the stem leading to the flower, which is a different population of cells than those that give rise to the other flowers on the plant. Single-celled organisms have no distinction between germline and somatic tissues.

In animals, mutations are more likely to occur in sperm than in ova, because a larger number of cell divisions are involved in the production of sperm. Mutations that are not germline are somatic mutations, which are also called acquired mutations.

GENE DUPLICATION

Gene duplication (or chromosomal duplication or gene amplification) is a major mechanism through which new genetic material is generated during molecular evolution. It can be defined as any duplication of a region of DNA that contains a gene. Gene duplications can arise as products of several types of errors in DNA replication and repair machinery as well as through fortuitous capture by selfish genetic elements. Common sources of gene duplications include ectopic homologous recombination, retrotransposition event, aneuploidy, polyploidy, and replication slippage.

Mechanisms of Duplication

Ectopic recombination

Duplications arise from an event termed unequal crossing-over that occurs during meiosis between misaligned homologous chromosomes. The chance of this happening is a function of the degree of sharing of repetitive elements between two chromosomes. The product of this recombination are a duplication at the site of the exchange and a reciprocal deletion. Ectopic recombination is typically mediated by sequence similarity at the duplicate breakpoints, which form direct repeats. Repetitive genetic elements such as transposable elements offer one source of repetitive DNA that can facilitate recombination, and they are often found at duplication breakpoints in plants and mammals.

Replication slippage

Replication slippage is an error in DNA replication that can produce duplications of short genetic sequences. During replication DNA polymerase begins to copy the DNA. At some point during the replication process, the polymerase dissociates from the DNA and replication stalls. When the polymerase reattaches to the DNA strand, it aligns the replicating strand to an incorrect position and incidentally copies the same section more than once. Replication slippage is also often facilitated by repetitive sequence, but requires only a few bases of similarity.

Retrotransposition

During cellular invasion by a replicating retroelement or retrovirus, viral proteins copy their genome by reverse transcribing RNA to DNA. If viral proteins aberrantly attach to cellular mRNA, they can reverse transcribe copies of genes to create retrogenes. Retrogenes usually lack intronic sequence, and often contain poly A sequences that are also integrated into the genome. Many retrogenes display changes in gene regulation in comparison to their parental gene sequences, which sometimes results in novel functions.

Aneuploidy

Aneuploidy occurs when nondisjunction at a single chromosome results in an abnormal number of chromosomes. Aneuploidy is often harmful and in mammals regularly leads to spontaneous abortions (miscarriages). Some aneuploid individuals are viable, for example trisomy 21 in humans which leads to Down syndrome. Aneuploidy often alters gene dosage in ways that are detrimental to the organism, and therefore is unlikely to spread through populations.

Whole genome duplication

Whole genome duplication, or polyploidy is a product of nondisjunction during meiosis which results in additional copies of the entire genome. Polyploidy is common in plants, but historically has also occurred in animals, with two rounds of whole genome duplication in the vertebrate lineage leading to humans. After whole genome duplications many sets of additional genes are eventually lost, returning to singleton state. However, retention of many genes, most notably Hox genes, has led to adaptive innovation. Polyploid is also a well known source of speciation, as offspring, which have different numbers of chromosomes compared to parent species, are often unable to interbreed with non-polyploid organisms. Whole genome duplications are thought to be less detrimental than aneuploidy as the relative dosage of individual genes should be the same.

Identifying Duplications in Sequenced Genomes

Criteria and single genome scans

The two genes that exist after a gene duplication event are called paralogs and usually code for proteins with a similar function and/or structure. By contrast, orthologous genes present in different species which are each originally derived from the same ancestral sequence.

It is important (but often difficult) to differentiate between paralogs and orthologs in biological research. Experiments on human gene function can often be carried out on other species if a homolog to a human gene can be found in the genome of that species, but only if the homolog is orthologous. If they are paralogs and resulted from a gene duplication event, their functions are likely to be too different. One or more copies of duplicated genes that constitutes a gene family may be affected by an insertion of transposable elements that causes significant variation between them in their sequence and finally may become responsible for divergent evolution. This may also render the chances and the rate of gene conversion between the homologs of gene duplicates due to less or no similarity in their sequences.

Paralogs can be identified in single genomes through a sequence comparison of all annotated gene models to one another. Such a comparison can be performed on translated amino acid sequences (e.g. BLASTp, tBLASTx) to identify ancient duplications or on DNA nucleotide sequences (e.g. BLASTn, megablast) to identify more recent duplications. Most studies to identify gene duplications require reciprocal-best-hits or fuzzy reciprocal-best-hits, where each paralog must be the others single best match in a sequence comparison. Most gene duplications exist as low copy repeats (LCRs) rather highly repetitive sequences like transposable elements. They are mostly found in pericentronomic, subtelomeric and interstitial regions of a chromosome. Many LCRs, due to their size (>1Kb), similarity, and orientation, are highly susceptible to duplications and deletions.

Genomic microarrays detect duplications

Technologies such as genomic microarrays, also called array comparative genomic hybridisation (array CGH), are used to detect chromosomal abnormalities, such as microduplications, in a high throughput fashion from genomic DNA samples. In particular, DNA microarray technology can simultaneously monitor the expression levels of thousands of genes across many treatments or experimental conditions, greatly facilitating the evolutionary studies of gene regulation after gene duplication or speciation.

Next generation sequencing

Gene duplications can also be identified through the use of next-generation sequencing platforms. The simplest means to identify duplications in genomic resequencing data is through the use of paired-end sequencing reads. Tandem duplications are indicated by sequencing read pairs which map in abnormal orientations. Through a combination of increased sequence coverage and abnormal mapping orientation, it is possible to identify duplications in genomic sequencing data.

Gene Duplication as Amplification

Gene duplication doesn't necessarily constitute a lasting change in a species genome. In fact, such changes often don't last past the initial host organism. From the perspective of molecular genetics, amplification is one of many ways in which a gene can be overexpressed. Genetic amplification can occur artificially, as with the use of the polymerase chain reaction technique to amplify short strands of DNA *in vitro* using enzymes, or it can occur naturally, as described above. If it's a natural duplication, it can still take place in a somatic cell, rather than a germline cell (which would be necessary for a lasting evolutionary change).

Role in cancer

Duplications of oncogenes are a common cause of many types of cancer. In such cases the genetic duplication occurs in a somatic cell and affects only the genome of the cancer cells themselves, not the entire organism, much less any subsequent offspring.

PATTERN FORMATION

The science of pattern formation deals with the visible, (statistically) orderly outcomes of self-organisation and the common principles behind similar patterns in nature. In developmental biology, pattern formation refers to the generation of complex organisations of cell fates in space and time. Pattern formation is controlled by genes. The role of genes in pattern formation is well seen in the anterior-posterior patterning of embryos from the model organism *Drosophila melanogaster* (a fruit fly).

Examples of Pattern Formation

Examples of pattern formation can be found in Biology, Chemistry, Physics and Mathematics, and can readily be simulated with Computer graphics, as described in turn below.

Biology

Animal markings, segmentation of animals, phyllotaxis, neuronal activation patterns like tonotopy, and predator-prey equations' trajectories are all examples of how natural patterns are formed. In developmental biology, pattern formation describes the mechanism by which initially equivalent cells in a developing tissue in an embryo assume complex forms and functions. The process of embryogenesis involves coordinated cell fate control. Pattern formation is genetically controlled, and often involves each cell in a field sensing and responding to its position along a morphogen gradient, followed by short distance cell-to-cell communication through cell signalling pathways to refine the initial pattern. In this context, a field of cells is the group of cells whose fates are affected by responding to the same set positional information cues. This conceptual model was first described as the French flag model in the 1960s.

Anterior-posterior axis patterning in Drosophila

One of the best understood examples of pattern formation is the patterning along the future head to tail (antero-posterior) axis of the fruit fly *Drosophila melanogaster*. The development of this fly is particularly well studied, and it is representative of a major class of animals, the insects. Other multicellular organisms sometimes use similar mechanisms for axis formation, although signal transfer between the earliest cells of many developing organisms is often more important than in *Drosophila*.

Growth of colonies

Bacterial colonies show a large variety of beautiful patterns formed during colony growth. The resulting shapes depend on the growth conditions. In particular, stresses (hardness of the culture medium, lack of nutrients, etc.) enhance the complexity of the resulting patterns. Other organisms such as slime moulds display remarkable patterns caused by the dynamics of chemical signalling.

Vegetation patterns

Vegetation patterns such as tiger bush and fir waves form for different reasons. Tiger bush consists of stripes of bushes on arid slopes in countries such as Niger where plant growth is limited by rainfall. Each roughly horizontal stripe of vegetation absorbs rainwater from the bare zone immediately above it. In contrast, fir waves occur in forests on mountain slopes after wind disturbance, during regeneration. When trees fall, the trees that they had sheltered become exposed and are in turn more likely to be damaged, so gaps tend to expand downwind. Meanwhile, on the windward side, young trees grow, protected by the wind shadow of the remaining tall trees.

PIGMENT DISPERSING FACTOR

Pigment dispersing factor (PDF) is a gene that encodes for the protein PDF, which is part of a large family of neuropeptides. Its hormonal product, pigment dispersing hormone (PDH), was named for the diurnal pigment movement effect it has in crustacean retinal cells, and was initially discovered in the central nervous system of arthropods. The movement and aggregation of the pigments in retina cells and extra-retinal cells is hypothesised to be under a split hormonal control mechanism. One hormonal set is responsible for concentrating chromatophoral pigment and responds to changes in the length of darkness presented to the organism whereas another set is responsible for dispersion and responds to the light cycle. However, insect PDF genes do not function in such pigment migration since they lack the chromatophore. The gene was first isolated and studied in *Drosophila* by Jeffrey C. Hall's laboratory at Brandeis University in 1998, and has been found to function as a neuromodulator in controlling circadian rhythms.

Gene Characteristics

In *Drosophila*, the pdf gene is intronless and is located at 97B on the third chromosome. It exists in a single copy per haploid genome and the approximately 0.8 kb transcript is expressed in the *Drosophila*s head. The cDNA clone in flies has 1080 base pairs with a single exon. Six alleles of this gene have been reported and are found in dorsal lateral neurons and the ventral lateral neurons in the *Drosophila* brain.

Pdf role in the circadian pathways

In the *Drosophila* brain, a group of cells called the lateral ventral neurons is thought to be the principle pacemaker regulating the circadian rhythm of *Drosophila* locomotion. Variation in PDF levels, which is expressed by some of these specialised cells, is believed to be the primary output of oscillations within these cells, coordinating fly circadian behavior.

Study on E and M cells

The 150 pacemaker neurons in *Drosophila* are organised into two groups of cells called M (morning) and E (evening) oscillators in the small and large lateral neurons (LNvs). These two groups of cells were first observed by Colin Pittendrigh in 1976. As indicated by their names, the two oscillators control circadian rhythm at different times of the day, yet the two must coordinate to synchronise circadian activity. PDF synchronises phase of M oscillators, while in E oscillators PDF delays their cycling and increases their amplitude. Stoleru and others. used mosaic (genetics) transgenic animals with different circadian periods to study the two oscillators.

Their study showed that M-cells periodically send a 'reset' signal which determines the oscillations of the E-cells. It is believed that the reset signal is PDF, because it is M-cell specific and plays a large role in maintaining normal rhythmicity.

PDF from s-LNv is responsible for the maintenance of a free-running rhythm, while PDF from large lateral ventral neurons is not required for normal behavior. Experiments at Brandeis University have shown that PDF neuropeptide is localised in small lateral ventral neurons (s-LNv) that specifically control morning anticipatory behavior. However, it has been found that large LNv working with other circadian neurons is sufficient to rescue the morning anticipation behavior and startle response in s-LNv-ablated flies. Thus, PDF's role in setting the free-running rhythm and the timing of light-dark cycles comes from both types of lateral ventral neurons.

Further evidence of distinct E and M peaks in *Drosophila* was provided by Grima and others This work confirmed that the small lateral ventral neurons, which express PDF, are necessary for the morning peak in *Drosophila* circadian rhythms. Flies lacking functional s-LNv did not possess a lights-on anticipatory activity for the morning peak.

Other behavioural aspects of *Drosophila* such as eclosion activity have been monitored with ectopic expression of pdf, which in this case is concentrated in the dorsal central brain. These alterations in expression caused severely altered rhythmic behavior in eclosion of larvae, further substantiating the evidence that PDF modulates the rhythmic control of *Drosophila* behaviour.

Chemistry

- Belousov-Zhabotinsky reaction.
- Liesegang rings.

Physics

Bénard cells, Laser, cloud formations in stripes or rolls. Ripples in icicles. Washboard patterns on dirtroads. Dendrites in solidification, liquid crystals. Solitons.

Mathematics

Sphere packings and coverings. Mathematics underlies the other pattern formation mechanisms listed.

Computer graphics

Some types of automata have been used to generate organic-looking textures for more realistic shading of 3d objects. A popular photoshop plugin, KPT 6, included a filter called 'KPT reaction'. Reaction produced reaction-diffusion style patterns based on the supplied seed image.

A similar effect to the 'KPT reaction' can be achieved with convolution functions in digital image processing, with a little patience, by repeatedly sharpening and blurring an image in a graphics editor. If other filters are used, such as emboss or edge detection, different types of effects can be achieved.

Computers are often used to simulate the biological, physical or chemical processes that lead to pattern formation, and they can display the results in a realistic way. Calculations using models like Reaction-diffusion or MClone are based on the actual mathematical equations designed by the scientists to model the studied phenomena.

GAP GENE

A gap gene is a type of gene involved in the development of the segmented embryos of some arthropods. Gap genes are defined by the effect of a mutation in that gene, which causes the loss of contiguous body segments, resembling a gap in the normal body plan. Each gap gene, therefore, is necessary for the development of a section of the organism. Gap genes were first described by Christiane Nüsslein-Volhard and Eric Wieschaus in 1980. They used a genetic screen to identify genes required for embryonic development in the fruit fly *Drosophila* melanogaster. They found three genes–knirps, Krüppel and hunchback–where mutations caused deletion of particular stretches of segments.

Later work identified more gap genes in the *Drosophila* early embryo–giant, huckebein and tailless. Further gap genes including orthodenticle and buttonhead are required for the development of the *Drosophila* head. Once the gap genes had been identified at the molecular level it was found that each gap gene is expressed in a band in the early embryo generally correlated with the region that is absent in the mutant. In *Drosophila* the gap genes encode transcription factors, and they directly control the expression of another set of genes involved in segmentation, the pair-rule genes. The gap genes themselves are expressed under the control of maternal effect genes such as bicoid and nanos, and regulate each other to achieve their precise expression patterns.

Gene Activation

Expression of tailless is activated by torso protein in the poles of the embryo. Tailless is also regulated in a complex manner by the maternal-effect gene bicoid. Both embryonically-transcribed hunchback and maternally-transcribed hunchback are activated by bicoid protein in the anterior and is inhibited in the posterior by nanos protein. Embryonically-transcribed hunchback protein is able to exhibit the same effects on Krüppel and knirps as maternally-transcribed hunchback.

The Krüppel gene is activated when the bicoid protein gradient declines steeply, at the central part of the embryo. Krüppel is regulated by five regulatory proteins: bicoid, hunchback, tailless, knirps and giant. Krüppel is inhibited by high levels of hunchback, high levels of giant, and tailless, which establishes the anterior boundary of Krüppel expression. Krüppel is also inhibited by knirps and activated by low levels of bicoid and low levels of hunchback, which establishes the posterior boundary of Krüppel expression. The knirps gene appears to be spontaneously activated.

It is repressed by hunchback. Hunchback repression thus defines the anterior boundary of the knirps gene. Due to more efficient inhibition of the knirps gene by hunchback, knirps is expressed more posterially in the embryo compared to Krüppel. Tailless protein inhibits knirps gene expression in the posterior part of the embryo, allowing the knirps protein to be expressed only in the central part of the embryo (but more posterior compared to Krüppel). This is due to the ability of both hunchback and tailless to bind to the enhancer regions of knirps.

Mechanism of action

The gap gene proteins code for transcription factors that regulate the expression of pair-rule genes and homeotic genes by competing for binding to their enhancer regions. It has been demonstrated that gap gene expression in the *Drosophila* blastoderm exhibit a property called as canalisation, a property of developing organisms to produce a consistent phenotype despite variations in genotype or environment. It has been recently proposed that canalisation is a manifestation of cross regulation of gap genes expression and can be understood as arising from the actions of attractors in the gap gene dynamical system.

Pair-rule Gene

A pair-rule gene is a type of gene involved in the development of the segmented embryos of insects. Pair-rule genes are defined by the effect of a mutation in that gene, which causes the loss of the normal developmental pattern in alternating segments.

Pair-rule genes were first described by Christiane Nüsslein-Volhard and Eric Wieschaus in 1980. They used a genetic screen to identify genes required for embryonic development in the fruit fly *Drosophila* melanogaster. In normal unmutated *Drosophila*, each segment produces bristles called denticles in a band arranged on the side of the segment closer to the head (the anterior). They found five genes–even-skipped, hairy, odd-skipped, paired and runt–where mutations caused the deletion of a particular region of every alternate segment.

For example, in even-skipped, the denticle bands of alternate segments are missing, which results in an embryo having half the number of denticle bands. Later work identified more pair-rule genes in the *Drosophila* early embryo–fushi tarazu, odd-paired, sloppy paired, and tenm.

Once the pair-rule genes had been identified at the molecular level it was found that each gene is expressed in alternate parasegments–regions in the embryo that are closely related to segments, but are slightly out of register. Each parasegment includes the posterior part of one (future) segment, and an anterior part of the next (more posterior) segment. The bands of expression of the pair-rule genes correspond to the regions missing in the mutant. The expression of the pair-rule genes in bands is dependent both upon direct regulation by the gap genes and on regulatory interactions between the pair-rule genes themselves.

Segment Polarity Gene

A segmentation gene is a generic term for a gene whose function is to specify tissue pattern in each repeated unit of a segmented organism. In the fruit fly *Drosophila melanogaster*, segment polarity genes help to define the anterior and posterior polarities within each embryonic parasegment by regulating the transmission of signals via the Wnt signalling pathway and Hedgehog signalling pathway. Segment polarity genes are expressed in the embryo following expression of the gap genes and pair-rule genes. The most commonly cited examples of these genes are engrailed and gooseberry in *D. melanogaster*.

SECTION VIII

Quantitative and Population Genetics

Chapter 20

Quantitative Genetics

INTRODUCTION

Quantitative genetics is a branch of population genetics that deals with phenotypes that vary continuously (in characters such as height or mass)—as opposed to discretely identifiable phenotypes and gene-products (such as eye-colour, or the presence of a particular biochemical).

Both branches use the frequencies of different alleles of a gene in breeding populations (gamodemes), and combine them with concepts from simple Mendelian inheritance to analyse inheritance patterns across generations and descendant lines. While population genetics can focus on particular genes and their subsequent metabolic products, quantitative genetics focuses more on the outward phenotypes, and summaries only of the underlying genetics.

This, however, can be viewed as its strength, because it facilitates an interface with the biological macrocosm, including micro-evolution and artificial selection in plant and animal breeding. Both branches share some common history, and some mathematics: for example, they use expansion of the quadratic equation to represent the fertilisation of gametes to form the zygote.

However, because of the continuous distribution of phenotypic values, quantitative genetics must employ many other statistical methods (such as the effect, the mean and the variance) to link the phenotype to underlying genetics principles. Some phenotypes (attributes) may be analysed either as discrete categories or as continuous phenotypes, depending on the definition of cut-off points, or on the metric used to quantify them. Analysis of quantitative trait loci, or QTL, is a more recent addition to quantitative genetics, linking it more directly to molecular genetics.

BASIC PRINCIPLES OF QUANTITATIVE GENETICS

Gene Effects

In diploid organisms, the average genotypic 'value' (locus value) may be defined by the allele 'effect' together with a dominance effect, and also by how genes interact with genes at other loci (epistasis). The founder of quantitative genetics Sir Ronald Fisher perceived much of this when he proposed the first mathematics of this branch of genetics.

Being a statistician, he defined the gene effects as deviations from a central value—enabling the use of statistical concepts such as mean and variance, which use this idea. The central value he chose for the gene was the midpoint between the two opposing homozygotes at the one locus. The deviation from there to the 'greater' homozygous genotype can be named '+a' , and therefore it is '−a' from that same midpoint to the 'lesser' homozygote genotype. This is the 'allele' effect mentioned above. The heterozygote deviation from the same midpoint can be named 'd', this being the 'dominance' effect referred to above. Figure 20.1 gives details of gene effects and phenotype values. However, in reality we measure phenotypes, and the figure also shows how observed phenotypes relate to the gene effects. Formal definitions of these effects recognise this phenotypic focus. Epistasis has been approached statistically as interaction (i.e. inconsistencies), but epigenetics suggests a new approach may be needed.

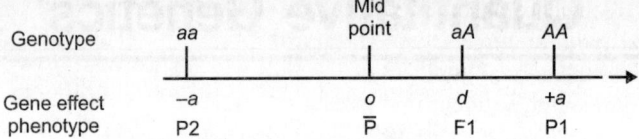

Fig. 20.1: Gene effects and Phenotype values.

Allele and Genotype Frequencies

To obtain means, variances and other statistics, both quantities and their occurrences are required. The gene effects (above) provide the framework for quantities: and the frequencies of the contrasting alleles in the fertilisation gamete-pool provide the information on occurrences.

Self fertilisation an alternative

Having noticed that the pea is naturally self-pollinated, we cannot continue to use it as an example for illustrating random fertilisation properties. Self-fertilisation ('selfing') is a major alternative to random fertilisation, especially within Plants. Most of the Earths cereals are naturally self-pollinated (rice, wheat, barley, for example), as well as the pulses. Considering the millions of individuals of each of these on Earth at any time, it's obvious that self-fertilisation is at least as significant as random fertilisation. Self-fertilisation is the most intensive form of inbreeding, which arises whenever there is restricted independence in the genetical origins of gametes.

Population Mean

The population mean shifts the central reference point from the homozygote midpoint (mp) to the mean of a sexually reproduced population. This is important not only to relocate the focus into the natural world, but also to use a measure of central tendency used by Statistics/Biometrics. In particular, the square of this mean is the correction factor, which is used to obtain the genotypic variances later. For each genotype in turn, its allele effect is multiplied by its genotype frequency, and the products are accumulated across all genotypes in the model. Some algebraic simplification usually follows to reach a succinct result.

Environmental Variance

The environmental variance is phenotypic variability, which cannot be ascribed to genetics. This sounds simple, but the experimental design needed to separate the two needs very careful planning. Even the 'external' environment can be divided into spatial and temporal components, as well as partitions such as 'litter' or 'family' and 'culture' or 'history'. Where does epigenetic variance get placed?

Is it embedded within epistasis: or is it 'internal environment'? These components are very dependent upon the actual experimental model used to do the research.

VARIATION AND ITS CAUSES

Variation, in biology, any difference between cells, individual organisms, or groups of organisms of any species caused either by genetic differences (genotypic variation) or by the effect of environmental factors on the expression of the genetic potentials (phenotypic variation). Variation may be shown in physical appearance, metabolism, fertility, mode of reproduction, behaviour, learning and mental ability, and other obvious or measurable characters.

Genotypic variations are caused by differences in number or structure of chromosomes or by differences in the genes carried by the chromosomes. Eye colour, body form, and disease resistance are genotypic variations. Individuals with multiple sets of chromosomes are called polyploid, many common plants have two or more times the normal number of chromosomes, and new species may arise by this type of variation. A variation cannot be identified as genotypic by observation of the organism, breeding experiments must be performed under controlled environmental conditions to determine whether or not the alteration is inheritable.

Environmentally caused variations may result from one factor or the combined effects of several factors, such as climate, food supply, and actions of other organisms. Phenotypic variations also include stages in an organism's life cycle and seasonal variations in an individual. These variations do not involve any hereditary alteration and in general are not transmitted to future generations, consequently, they are not significant in the process of evolution.

Variations are classified either as continuous, or quantitative (smoothly grading between two extremes, with the majority of individuals at the centre, as height in human populations), or as discontinuous, or qualitative (composed of well-defined classes, as blood groups in man). A discontinuous variation with several classes, none of which is very small, is known as a polymorphic variation. The separation of most higher organisms into males and females and the occurrence of several forms of a butterfly of the same species, each coloured to blend with a different vegetation, are examples of polymorphic variation.

Genotypic and Phenotypic Variations

In this section studies of the relation between genotype and phenotype, especially of the motility of the soil nematode *Caenorhabditis elegans*, are described. First, the background of the study of motility is briefly reviewed. We focus on the results of the isolation of mutants that are useful for understanding the gene function of other animals.

A brief overview of recent research follows. As details on *C. elegans* have already appeared in two monographs, the principal approach to the study of this animal is explained only briefly. A typical genetic analysis of the motility mutant gene known as *unc* (uncoordinated) is described. More than one hundred *unc*-genes have been isolated and classified into five groups. *unc* genes are related in various ways to muscle and other proteins like cytoskeleton proteins, transcription factors, ion channels of *trans*-membrane proteins, kinases or enzymes, and neuron-related proteins. Interestingly, these proteins are known to be abundant in the multicellular organisms from the results of genome sequencing. Other mutant genes are also described. Strategies for the genetic analysis of genes involved in heterochronicity, vulva formation, chemotaxis, and cell death are briefly presented. Finally, an overview of the post genome research is discussed. The reasons why *C. elegans* research has progressed so rapidly and the strategy for experiments in progress are also explained.

Genetics of the Nematode Caenorhabditis

Sydney Brenner first used the soil nematode *Caenorhabditis elegans* to study development and the nervous system in 1967. *C. elegans* feeds bacteria and grows on nutrient growth medium at 20°C. The hermaphrodite grows into an adult in three days and lays about 200 eggs after self-fertilisation. Genes can be transferred from rare arising males to the hermaphrodite by mating. This is probably the most convenient animal model for genetics and biochemistry. In *C. elegans*, mutant phenotypes include Unc (uncoordinated), Sma (small), Lon (long), and Dpy (dpy).

Changes in morphology and other visible characteristics also arise from mutant genes. Bacterial motility is observed only by an indirect approach: swarm formation in semi-solid agar medium on a petri dish. Worm motility can be observed directly by dissecting microscopy, which is an advantage when isolating a mutant. Worms have muscle tissues: a pharynx for feeding, a body wall for locomotion, a vulva for laying eggs, and an anus for defecation.

Interestingly, the pharynx is similar to the heart muscle of vertebrates. The analysis of worm muscle genes is therefore applicable to vertebrates. Molecular biology can provide an understanding of one organism through study of another by comparing amino acid sequence homology or cell proliferation. Two monographs are available for *C. elegans*: 'The nematode *Caenorhabditis elegans*' and '*C. elegans* II.'

These describe conventional methods for handling and basic knowledge developed through many research studies. In the later monograph, more recent studies into subjects such as cell death and signal transduction are explained more precisely. Completion of the genome sequencing of *C. elegans* in 1998 accelerated study of the relation between genes and functions by using transposon insertion, RNA interference, and transgene techniques.

Cell Lineage and Genome Sequence

How fertilised eggs divide and cells proliferate is fundamental to our understanding of development. The use of a dissecting microscope and visible light easily reveals the cell division in *C. elegans* without any pretreatment. In 1983, after seven years of study, John Sulston reported the process of cell proliferation. There are 959 cells after the programmed cell death of 131 cells. This is made clear by recording the position of the nucleus. This information is available at the web site AceDB. The most important conclusion from completing the cell lineage is that cell proliferation is divided into two stages: cell division and morphogenesis. Most of the cell division is complete by the 500-cell stage, with only a limited number of cells continuing to undergo asymmetrical division to form special muscle, cuticle, neurons, and vulva. This indicates that, even in higher animals, characteristic appearances come from a limited cell lineage. We should note that many genes are conserved in species from the nematode and *Drosophila* to mice, and even humans. This conclusion is also true for genome analysis. Higher organisms have transcription factors, a cytoskeleton, signal transduction molecules, and kinase/phosphatase. These molecules specialise the cells of multi-cellular organisms. This means that the conclusions drawn from a simple model like the nematode or *Drosophila* are also true for mice and humans, as is known from molecular genetic studies on bacteria. Genome structure and gene numbers are discussed in more detail in the next section.

Genetics and Mutants

The nematode Caenorhabditis elegans grows as a hermaphrodite and lays eggs after self-fertilisation. It is therefore easy to isolate a mutant from a single worm that has a heterozygous chromosome. In 1974, Sydney Brenner established the genetics of the nematode, and since then many mutants have been isolated from numerous phenotypes. The first mutants to be identified were Sma (small body), Lon (long body), and Mab (male abnormal), together with Unc (uncoordinated), these phenotypes being easy to recognise. It is also possible to isolate a mutant that has no phenotypic variation under normal conditions but a novel phenotype under a specific set of conditions. Drug or temperature sensitivity is used as a conditional marker. It is possible to isolate a mutant that has a novel phenotype under specific conditions after treatment of some mutagens, which is why so many important mutations have phenotypic variations. Recently, another genetic approach has been used to isolate mutations based on motility in the genome, applying transposons such as Tc1 in the nematode and P-element in *Drosophila*. The insertion of a transposon into a gene disrupts its function. Knock-out of the gene by inserting Tc1 in *C. elegans* produces an increase in genomic size, as detected by Southern analysis. If a mutant is isolated by a transposon insertion, a mutant gene can be isolated by the transposon fused fragment. Designed transposons are also used in *Drosophila* for studying promoter activity. When a P-element is inserted into downstream of a gene's promoter, lac-Z gene activity can be detected by staining the mutant fly. This approach allows one to know where the gene was expressed and which gene was disrupted by transposon insertion. These transposon functions are essentially similar from bacteria to maize.

GENE–ENVIRONMENT INTERACTION

Gene–environment interaction (or genotype–environment interaction or G×E) is when two different genotypes respond to environmental variation in different ways. A norm of reaction is a graph that shows the relationship between genes and environmental factors when phenotypic differences are continuous. They can help illustrate G×E interactions. When the norm of reaction is not parallel, as shown in the Fig. 20.2, there is a gene by environment interaction. This indicates that each genotype responds to environmental variation in a different way.

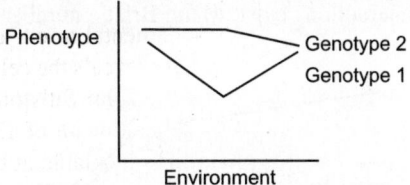

Fig. 20.2: This norm of reaction shows lines that are not parallel indicating a gene by environment interaction. Each genotype is responding to environmental variation in a different way.

Gene–environment interactions are studied to gain a better understanding of various phenomena. In genetic epidemiology, gene-environment interactions are useful for understanding some diseases. Sometimes, sensitivity to environmental risk factors for a disease are inherited rather than the disease itself being inherited. Individuals with different genotypes are affected differently by exposure to the same environmental factors, and thus gene-environment interactions can result in different disease phenotypes. For example, sunlight exposure has a stronger influence on skin cancer risk in fair-skinned humans than in individuals with darker skin.

Nature versus nurture debates assume that variation in a trait is primarily due to either genetic differences or environmental differences. However, the current scientific opinion holds that neither genetic differences nor environmental differences are solely responsible for producing phenotypic variation, and that virtually all traits are influenced by both genetic and environmental differences. Statistical analysis of the genetic and environmental differences contributing to the phenotype would have to be used to confirm these as gene-environment interactions. There are two different conceptions of gene–environment interaction. Tabery has labelled them biometric and developmental interaction, while Sesardic uses the terms statistical and commonsense interaction.

The biometric (or statistical) conception has its origins in research programmes that seek to measure the relative proportions of genetic and environmental contributions to phenotypic variation within populations. Biometric gene–environment interaction has particular currency in population genetics and behavioural genetics. Any interaction results in the breakdown of the additivity of the main effects of heredity and environment, but whether such interaction is present in particular settings is an empirical question. Biometric interaction is relevant in the context of research on individual differences rather than in the context of the development of a particular organism. Developmental gene–environment interaction is a concept more commonly used by developmental geneticists and developmental psychobiologists. Developmental interaction is not seen merely as a statistical phenomenon. Whether statistical interaction is present or not, developmental interaction is in any case manifested in the causal interaction of genes and environments in producing an individual's phenotype.

Examples

In Drosophila: A classic example of gene–environment interaction was performed on *Drosophila* by Lewontin in 1981. In their experiment they demonstrated that the mean bristle number on *Drosophila* could vary with changing temperatures. As seen in the graph to the right, different genotypes reacted differently to the changing environment. Each line represents a given genotype, and the slope of the line reflects the changing phenotype (Bristle number) with changing temperature. Some individuals had an increase in bristle number with increasing temperature while others had a sharp decrease in bristle number with increasing temperature. This showed that the norms of reaction were not parallel for these flies, proving that gene-environment interactions exist. Mean Bristle number by °C is shown in Fig. 20.3.

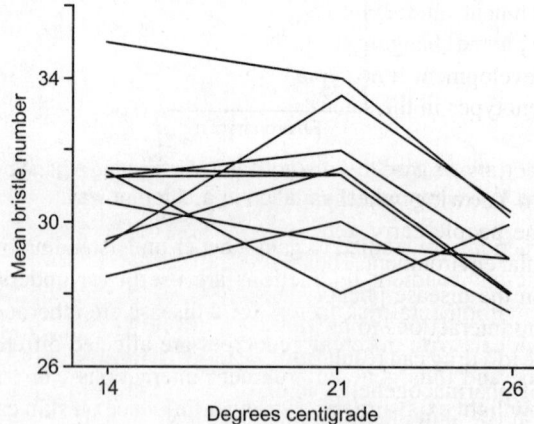

Fig. 20.3: Mean Bristle number by °C.

In plants: Seven genetically distinct yarrow plants were collected and three cuttings taken from each plant. One cutting of each genotype was planted at low, medium, and high elevations, respectively. When the plants matured, no one genotype grew best at all altitudes, and at each altitude the seven genotypes fared differently. For example, one genotype grew the tallest at the medium elevation but attained only middling height at the other two elevations. The best growers at low and high elevation grew poorly at medium elevation. The medium altitude produced the worst overall results, but still yielded one tall and two medium-tall samples. Altitude had an effect on each genotype, but not to the same degree nor in the same way. Phenylketonuria (PKU) is a human genetic condition caused by mutations to a gene coding for a particular liver enzyme. In the absence of this enzyme, an amino acid known as phenylalanine does not get converted into the next amino acid in a biochemical pathway, and therefore too much phenylalanine passes into the blood and other tissues. This disturbs brain development leading to mental retardation and other problems. PKU affects approximately 1 out of every 15000 infants in the US However, most affected infants do not grow up impaired because of a standard screening programme used in the US and other industrialised societies. Newborns found to have high levels of phenylalanine in their blood can be put on a special, phenylalanine-free diet. If they are put on this diet right away and stay on it, these children avoid the severe effects of PKU. This example shows that a change in environment (lowering Phenylalanine consumption) can affect the phenotype of a particular trait, demonstrating a gene-environment interaction.

A functional polymorphism in the monoamine oxidase A (MAOA) gene promoter can moderate the association between early life trauma and increased risk for violence and antisocial behaviour. Low MAOA activity is a significant risk factor for aggressive and antisocial behaviour in adults who report victimisation as children. Persons who were abused as children but have a genotype conferring high levels of MAOA expression are less likely to develop symptoms of antisocial behaviour. These findings must be interpreted with caution, however, because gene association studies on complex traits are notorious for being very difficult to confirm.

In Drosophila eggs: Contrary to the aforementioned examples, length of egg development in *Drosophila* as a function of temperature demonstrates the lack of gene-environment interactions. The attached graph shows parallel reaction norms for a variety of individual *Drosophila* flies, showing that there is not a gene-environment interaction present between the two variables. In other words, each genotype responds similarly to the changing environment producing similar phenotypes. For all individual genotypes, average egg development time decreases with increasing temperature. The environment is influencing each of the genotypes in the same predictable manner.

Medical significance

Doctors are interested in knowing whether disease can be prevented by reducing exposure to environmental risks. Some people carry genetic factors that confer susceptibility or resistance to a certain disorder in a particular environment. The interaction between the genetic factors and environmental stimulus is what results in the disease phenotype. There may be significant public health benefits in using gene by environment interactions to prevent or cure disease.

An individuals response to a drug can result from various gene by environment interactions. Therefore, the clinical importance of pharmacogenetics and gene by environment interactions comes from the possibility that genomic, along with environmental information, will allow more accurate predictions of an individual's drug response. This would allow doctors to more precisely select a certain drug and dosage to achieve therapeutic response in a patient while minimising side effects and adverse drug reactions. This information could also help to prevent the health care costs associated with adverse drug reactions and inconveniently prescribing drugs to patients who likely won't respond to them. In a similar manner, an individual can respond to other environmental stimuli, factors or challenges differently according to specific genetic differences or alleles. These other factors include the diet and specific nutrients within the diet, physical activity, alcohol and tobacco use, sleep (bed time, duration), and any of a number of exposures (or exposome), including toxins, pollutants, sunlight (latitude north/south of the equator), among any number of others. The diet, for example, is modifiable and has significant impact on a host of cardiometabolic diseases, including cardiovascular disease, coronary artery disease, coronary heart disease, type 2 diabetes, hypertension, stroke, myocardial infarction, and non-alcoholic fatty liver disease. In the clinic, typically assessed risks of these conditions include blood lipids (triglyceride, and HDL, LDL and total cholesterol), glycemic traits (plasma glucose and insulin, HOMA-IR, beta cell function as HOMA-BC), obesity anthropometrics (BMI/obesity, adiposity, body weight, waist circumference, waist-to-hip ratio), vascular measures (diastolic and systolic blood pressure), and biomarkers of inflammation. Gene-Environment interactions can modulate the adverse effects of an allele that confers increased risk of disease, or can exacerbate the genotype-phenotype relationship and increase risk, in a manner often referred to as nutrigenetics. A catalog of genetic variants that associate with these and related cardiometabolic phenotypes and modified by common environmental factors is available. Such could be used to aid in constructing an individualised diet, as has been undertaken by the EU-funded Food4Me project.

QUANTITATIVE TRAIT LOCUS

A quantitative trait locus (QTL) is a section of DNA (the locus) that correlates with variation in a phenotype (the quantitative trait). The QTL typically is linked to, or contains, the genes that control that phenotype. QTLs are mapped by identifying which molecular markers (such as SNPs or AFLPs) correlate with an observed trait. This is often an early step in identifying and sequencing the actual genes that cause the trait variation. Quantitative traits are phenotypes (characteristics) that vary in degree and can be attributed to polygenic effects, i.e. the product of two or more genes, and their environment.

Quantitative Traits

Polygenic inheritance refers to inheritance of a phenotypic characteristic (trait) that is attributable to two or more genes and can be measured quantitatively. Multifactorial inheritance refers to polygenic inheritance that also includes interactions with the environment. Unlike monogenic traits, polygenic traits do not follow patterns of Mendelian inheritance (discrete categories). Instead, their phenotypes typically vary along a continuous gradient depicted by a bell curve. An example of a polygenic trait is human skin colour variation. Several genes factor into determining a person's natural skin colour, so modifying only one of those genes can change skin colour slightly or in some cases, such as for SLC24A5, moderately. Many disorders with genetic components are polygenic, including autism, cancer, diabetes and numerous others. Most phenotypic characteristics are the result of the interaction of multiple genes. Examples of disease processes generally considered to be results of multifactorial etiology:

Congenital malformation

- Cleft palate
- Congenital dislocation of the hip
- Congenital heart defects
- Neural tube defects
- Pyloric stenosis
- Talipes

Adult onset diseases

- *Diabetes Mellitus*
- Cancer
- Epilepsy
- Glaucoma
- Hypertension
- Ischaemic heart disease
- Manic depression
- Schizophrenia
- Psoriasis
- Thyroid diseases
- Alzheimer's disease

Multifactorially inherited diseases are said to constitute the majority of genetic disorders affecting humans which will result in hospitalisation or special care of some kind.

Multifactorial Traits in General

Trait controlled by the both environment and genetic factor. Usually, multifactorial traits outside of illness result in what we see as continuous characteristics in organisms, especially human organisms such as: height, skin colour, and body mass. All of these phenotypes are complicated by a great deal of give-and-take between genes and environmental effects. The continuous distribution of traits such as height and skin colour described above, reflects the action of genes that do not manifest typical patterns of dominance and recessiveness. Instead the contributions of each involved locus are thought to be additive. Writers have distinguished this kind of inheritance as polygenic, or quantitative inheritance.

Thus, due to the nature of polygenic traits, inheritance will not follow the same pattern as a simple monohybrid or dihybrid cross. Polygenic inheritance can be explained as Mendelian inheritance at many loci, resulting in a trait which is normally-distributed. If n is the number of involved loci, then the coefficients of the binomial expansion of $(a + b)^{2n}$ will give the frequency of distribution of all n allele combinations. For a sufficiently high n, this binomial distribution will begin to resemble a normal distribution. From this viewpoint, a disease state will become apparent at one of the tails of the distribution, past some threshold value. Disease states of increasing severity will be expected the further one goes past the threshold and away from the mean.

Heritable disease and multifactorial inheritance

A mutation resulting in a disease state is often recessive, so both alleles must be mutant in order for the disease to be expressed phenotypically. A disease or syndrome may also be the result of the expression of mutant alleles at more than one locus. When more than one gene is involved, with or without the presence of environmental triggers, we say that the disease is the result of multifactorial inheritance.

The more genes involved in the cross, the more the distribution of the genotypes will resemble a normal, or Gaussian distribution. This shows that multifactorial inheritance is polygenic, and genetic frequencies can be predicted by way of a polyhybrid Mendelian cross. Phenotypic frequencies are a different matter, especially if they are complicated by environmental factors. The paradigm of polygenic inheritance as being used to define multifactorial disease has encountered much disagreement. Turnpenny discusses how simple polygenic inheritance cannot explain some diseases such as the onset of Type I diabetes mellitus, and that in cases such as these, not all genes are thought to make an equal contribution. The assumption of polygenic inheritance is that all involved loci make an equal contribution to the symptoms of the disease. This should result in a normal curve distribution of genotypes. When it does not, the idea of polygenetic inheritance cannot be supported for that illness.

Examples of such diseases

Examples of such diseases are not new to medicine. The above examples are well-known examples of diseases having both genetic and environmental components. Other examples involve atopic diseases such as eczema or dermatitis, spina bifida (open spine), and anencephaly (open skull). While schizophrenia is widely believed to be multifactorially genetic by biopsychiatrists, no characteristic genetic markers have been determined with any certainty.

If it is shown that the brothers and sisters of the patient have the disease, then there is a strong chance that the disease is genetic and that the patient will also be a genetic carrier. This is not quite enough as it also needs to be proven that the pattern of inheritance is non-Mendelian. This would require studying dozens, even hundreds of different family pedigrees before a conclusion of multifactorial inheritance is drawn. This often takes several years.

If multifactorial inheritance is indeed the case, then the chance of the patient contracting the disease is reduced only if cousins and more distant relatives have the disease. It must be stated that while multi-factorially-inherited diseases tend to run in families, inheritance will not follow the same pattern as a simple monohybrid or dihybrid cross. If a genetic cause is suspected and little else is known about the illness, then it remains to be seen exactly how many genes are involved in the phenotypic expression of the disease. Once that is determined, the question must be answered: if two people have the required genes, why are there differences in expression between them? Generally, what makes the two individuals different are likely to be environmental factors. Due to the involved nature of genetic investigations needed to determine such inheritance patterns, this is not usually the first avenue of investigation one would choose to determine etiology.

Typically, QTLs underlie continuous traits (those traits that vary continuously, e.g. height) as opposed to discrete traits (traits that have two or several character values, e.g. red hair in humans, a recessive trait, or smooth vs. wrinkled peas used by Mendel in his experiments). Moreover, a single phenotypic trait is usually determined by many genes. Consequently, many QTLs are associated with a single trait.

A quantitative trait locus (QTL) is a region of DNA that is associated with a particular phenotypic trait. These QTLs are often found on different chromosomes. Knowing the number of QTLs that explains variation in the phenotypic trait tells us about the genetic architecture of a trait. It may tell us that plant height is controlled by many genes of small effect, or by a few genes of large effect.

Another use of QTLs is to identify candidate genes underlying a trait. Once a region of DNA is identified as contributing to a phenotype, it can be sequenced. The DNA sequence of any genes in this region can then be compared to a database of DNA for genes whose function is already known. In a recent development, classical QTL analyses are combined with gene expression profiling, i.e. by DNA microarrays.

Such expression QTLs (eQTLs) describe *cis*- and *trans*-controlling elements for the expression of often disease-associated genes. Observed epistatic effects have been found beneficial to identify the gene responsible by a cross-validation of genes within the interacting loci with metabolic pathway- and scientific literature databases.

QTL mapping

For organisms whose genomes are known, one might now try to exclude genes in the identified region whose function is known with some certainty not to be connected with the trait in question. If the genome is not available, it may be an option to sequence the identified region and determine the putative functions of genes by their similarity to genes with known function, usually in other genomes. This can be done using BLAST, an online tool that allows users to enter a primary sequence and search for similar sequences within the BLAST database of genes from various organisms. It is often not the actual gene underlying the phenotypic trait, but rather a region of DNA that is closely linked with the gene. Another interest of statistical geneticists using QTL mapping is to determine the complexity of the genetic architecture underlying a phenotypic trait. For example, they may be interested in knowing whether a phenotype is shaped by many independent loci, or by a few loci, and do those loci interact. This can provide information on how the phenotype may be evolving.

Analysis of variance

The simplest method for QTL mapping is analysis of variance (ANOVA, sometimes called 'marker regression') at the marker loci. In this method, in a backcross, one may calculate a t-statistic to compare the averages of the two marker genotype groups. For other types of crosses (such as the intercross), where there are more than two possible genotypes, one uses a more general form of ANOVA, which provides a so-called F-statistic. The ANOVA approach for QTL mapping has three important weaknesses. First, we do not receive separate estimates of QTL location and QTL effect. QTL location is indicated only by looking at which markers give the greatest differences between genotype group averages, and the apparent QTL effect at a marker will be smaller than the true QTL effect as a result of recombination between the marker and the QTL. Second, we must discard individuals whose genotypes are missing at the marker. Third, when the markers are widely spaced, the QTL may be quite far from all markers, and so the power for QTL detection will decrease.

Interval mapping

Lander and Botstein developed interval mapping, which overcomes the three disadvantages of analysis of variance at marker loci. Interval mapping is currently the most popular approach for QTL mapping in experimental crosses. The method makes use of a genetic map of the typed markers, and, like analysis of variance, assumes the presence of a single QTL. In interval mapping, each locus is considered one at a time and the logarithm of the odds ratio (LOD score) is calculated for the model that the given locus is a true QTL. The odds ratio is related to the Pearson correlation coefficient between the phenotype and the marker genotype for each individual in the experimental cross. The term 'interval mapping' is used for estimating the position of a QTL within two markers (often indicated as 'marker-bracket'). Interval mapping is originally based on the maximum likelihood but there are also very good approximations possible with simple regression.

The principle for QTL mapping is: (i) The Likelihood can be calculated for a given set of parameters (particularly QTL effect and QTL position) given the observed data on phenotypes and marker genotypes, (ii) The estimates for the parameters are those where the likelihood are highest and (iii) A significance threshold can be established by permutation testing.

Conventional methods for the detection of quantitative trait loci (QTLs) are based on a comparison of single QTL models with a model assuming no QTL. For instance in the 'interval mapping' method the likelihood for a single putative QTL is assessed at each location on the genome. However, QTLs located elsewhere on the genome can have an interfering effect. As a consequence, the power of detection may be compromised, and the estimates of locations and effects of QTLs may be biased. Even nonexisting so-called 'ghost' QTLs may appear. Therefore, it is obvious that multiple QTLs could be mapped more efficiently and more accurately by using multiple QTL models. One popular approach to handle QTL mapping where multiple QTL contribute to a trait is to iteratively scan the genome and add known QTL to the regression model as QTLs are identified. This method, termed composite interval mapping determine both the location and effects size of QTL more accurately than single-QTL approaches, especially in small mapping populations where the effect of correlation between genotypes in the mapping population may be problematic.

Composite interval mapping (CIM)

In this method, one performs interval mapping using a subset of marker loci as covariates. These markers serve as proxies for other QTLs to increase the resolution of interval mapping, by accounting for linked QTLs and reducing the residual variation. The key problem with CIM concerns the choice of suitable marker loci to serve as covariates, once these have been chosen, CIM turns the model selection problem into a single-dimensional scan. The choice of marker covariates has not been solved, however. Not surprisingly, the appropriate markers are those closest to the true QTLs, and so if one could find these, the QTL mapping problem would be complete anyway.

Family-pedigree based mapping

Family based QTL mapping, or Family-pedigree based mapping (Linkage and association mapping), involves multiple families instead of a single family. Family based QTL mapping has been the only way for mapping of genes where experimental crosses are difficult to make. However, due to some advantages, now plant geneticists are attempting to incorporate some of the methods pioneered in human genetics. Using family-pedigree based approach has been discussed. Family-based linkage and association has been successfully implemented.

HERITABILITY

Heritability is a statistic used in breeding and genetics works that estimates how much of the genetic diversity of a phenotypic trait in a population is due to genetic differences in that population. Other causes of measured variation in a trait are characterised as environmental factors, including measurement error. In human studies of heritability these are often apportioned into factors from 'shared environment' and 'non-shared environment' based on whether they tend to result in persons brought up in the same household more or less similar to persons who were not.

Some humans in a population are taller than others, heritability attempts to identify how much genetics play a role in part of the population being taller. Heritability is estimated by comparing individual phenotypic variation among differently related individuals in a population. Heritability is an important concept in quantitative genetics, particularly in selective breeding and behaviour genetics (for instance, twin studies), but is less widely used in population genetics.

Geoffrey Miller, an evolutionary psychologist, has said, writing about sexual selection and biological fitness, 'The concept of heritability applies only to traits that differ between individuals. If a trait exists in precisely the same form across all individuals, it may be inherited, but it cannot be heritable.' Heritability measures the fraction of phenotype variability that can be attributed to genetic variation. This is not the same as saying that this fraction of an individual phenotype is caused by genetics. In addition, heritability can change without any genetic change occurring, such as when the environment starts contributing to more variation. A case in point, consider that both genes and environment have the potential to influence intelligence. Heritability could increase if genetic variation increases, causing individuals to show more phenotypic variation, like showing different levels of intelligence. On the other hand, heritability might also increase if the environmental variation decreases, causing individuals to show less phenotypic variation, like showing more similar levels of intelligence. Heritability increases when genetics are contributing more variation or because non-genetic factors are contributing less variation, what matters is the relative contribution. Heritability is specific to a particular population in a particular environment.

The extent of dependence of phenotype on environment can also be a function of the genes involved. Matters of heritability are complicated because genes may canalise a phenotype, making its expression almost inevitable in all occurring environments. Individuals with the same genotype can also exhibit different phenotypes through a mechanism called phenotypic plasticity, which makes heritability difficult to measure in some cases. Recent insights in molecular biology have identified changes in transcriptional activity of individual genes associated with environmental changes. However, there are a large number of genes whose transcription is not affected by the environment.

Estimates of heritability use statistical analyses to help to identify the causes of differences between individuals. Since heritability is concerned with variance, it is necessarily an account of the differences between individuals in a population. Heritability can be univariate–examining a single trait–or multivariate– examining the genetic and environmental associations between multiple traits at once. This allows a test of the genetic overlap between different phenotypes: for instance hair colour and eye colour. Environment and genetics may also interact, and heritability analyses can test for and examine these interactions (GxE models).

A prerequisite for heritability analyses is that there is some population variation to account for. This last point highlights the fact that heritability cannot take into account the effect of factors which are invariant in the population. Factors may be invariant if they are absent and do not exist in the population, such as no one having access to a particular antibiotic, or because they are omni-present, like if everyone is drinking coffee. In practice, all human behavioural traits vary and almost all traits show some heritability.

Any particular phenotype can be modelled as the sum of genetic and environmental effects:

Phenotype (P) = Genotype (G) + Environment (E).

Likewise the variance in the trait – $Var(P)$ – is the sum of effects as follows:

$Var(P) = Var(G) + Var(E) + 2 Cov(G,E)$.

In a planned experiment $Cov(G,E)$ can be controlled and held at 0. In this case, heritability is defined as:

$$H^2 = \frac{Var(G)}{Var(P)}$$

H^2 is the broad-sense heritability. This reflects all the genetic contributions to a population's phenotypic variance including additive, dominant, and epistatic (multi-genic interactions), as well as maternal and paternal effects, where individuals are directly affected by their parents' phenotype, such as with milk production in mammals.

A particularly important component of the genetic variance is the additive variance, $Var(A)$, which is the variance due to the average effects (additive effects) of the alleles. Since each parent passes a single allele per locus to each offspring, parent-offspring resemblance depends upon the average effect of single alleles. Additive variance represents, therefore, the genetic component of variance responsible for parent-offspring resemblance. The additive genetic portion of the phenotypic variance is known as Narrow-sense heritability and is defined as:

$$h^2 = \frac{\text{Var}(A)}{\text{Var}(P)}$$

An upper case H^2 is used to denote broad sense, and lower case h^2 for narrow sense.

Additive variance is important for selection. If a selective pressure such as improving livestock is exerted, the response of the trait is directly related to narrow-sense heritability. The mean of the trait will increase in the next generation as a function of how much the mean of the selected parents differs from the mean of the population from which the selected parents were chosen. The observed response to selection leads to an estimate of the narrow-sense heritability (called realised heritability). This is the principle underlying artificial selection or breeding.

Estimating Heritability

Since only P can be observed or measured directly, heritability must be estimated from the similarities observed in subjects varying in their level of genetic or environmental similarity. The statistical analyses required to estimate the genetic and environmental components of variance depend on the sample characteristics. Briefly, better estimates are obtained using data from individuals with widely varying levels of genetic relationship such as twins, siblings, parents and offspring, rather than from more distantly related (and therefore less similar) subjects. The standard error for heritability estimates is improved with large sample sizes.

In non-human populations it is often possible to collect information in a controlled way. For example, among farm animals it is easy to arrange for a bull to produce offspring from a large number of cows and to control environments. Such experimental control is impossible when gathering human data, relying on naturally occurring relationships and environments.

Studies of human heritability often utilise adoption study designs, often with identical twins who have been separated early in life and raised in different environments. Such individuals have identical genotypes and can be used to separate the effects of genotype and environment. A limit of this design is the common prenatal environment and the relatively low numbers of twins reared apart. A second and more common design is the twin study in which the similarity of identical and fraternal twins is used to estimate heritability. These studies can be limited by the fact that identical twins are not completely genetically identical, potentially resulting in an underestimation of heritability. Studies of twins also examine differences between twins and non-twin siblings, for instance to examine phenomena such as intrauterine competition (for example, twin-to-twin transfusion syndrome). Heritability estimates are always relative to the genetic and environmental factors in the population, and are not absolute measurements of the contribution of genetic and environmental factors to a phenotype. Heritability estimates reflect the amount of variation in genotypic effects compared to variation in environmental effects.

Heritability can be made larger by diversifying the genetic background, e.g. by using only very out bred individuals (which increases VarG) and/or by minimising environmental effects (decreasing VarE). The converse also holds. Due to such effects, different populations of a species might have different heritabilities for the same trait. In observational studies, or because of evokative effects (where a genome evokes environments by its effect on them), G and E may covary: gene environment correlation. Depending on the methods used to estimate heritability, correlations between genetic factors and shared or non-shared environments may or may not be confounded with heritability.

Common misunderstandings of heritability estimates

A common estimate of heritability is called the Heritability Index (HI), which ranges from 0–1. A HI index of 0 means that none of the variability between people in the study sample on the trait under investigation is due to genetic factors, an HI of 1 indicates the opposite.

Heritability estimates are often misinterpreted if it is not understood that they refer to the proportion of variation between individuals on a trait that is due to genetic factors. It does not indicate the degree of genetic influence on the development of a trait of an individual. For example, it is incorrect to say that since the heritability of personality traits is about 0.6, that means that 60% of your personality is inherited from your parents and 40% comes from the environment.

Even a highly heritable trait (such as eye colour) assumes environmental inputs which are required for development: for instance temperatures and an atmosphere supporting life, etc. A more useful distinction than 'nature vs. nurture' is 'obligate vs. facultative'—under typical environmental ranges, what traits are more 'obligate' (e.g. the nose—everyone has a nose) or more 'facultative' (sensitive to environmental variations, such as specific language learned during infancy). Another useful distinction is between traits that are likely to be adaptations (such as the umbilical cord) vs. those that are byproducts of adaptations (such as the belly button), or are due to random variation (non-adaptive variation in belly button shape, e.g. convex or concave).

Estimation methods

There are essentially two schools of thought regarding estimation of heritability. One school of thought was developed by Sewall Wright at The University of Chicago, and further popularised by C. C. Li (University of Chicago) and J. L. Lush (Iowa State University). It is based on the analysis of correlations and, by extension, regression. Path Analysis was developed by Sewall Wright as a way of estimating heritability. The second was originally developed by R. A. Fisher and expanded at The University of Edinburgh, Iowa State University, and North Carolina State University, as well as other schools. It is based on the analysis of variance of breeding studies, using the intraclass correlation of relatives. Various methods of estimating components of variance (and, hence, heritability) from ANOVA are used in these analyses.

TWIN STUDY

Twin studies reveal the absolute and relative importance of environmental and genetic influences on individuals in a sample. Twin research is considered a key tool in behavioural genetics and in content fields, from biology to psychology. Twin studies are part of the methods used in behaviour genetics, which includes all data that are genetically informative–siblings, adoptees, pedigree data, etc. Twins are a valuable source for observation because they allow the study of varying family environments (across pairs) and widely differing genetic makeup: 'identical' or monozygotic (MZ) twins share nearly 100% of their genes, which means that most differences between the twins (such as height, susceptibility to boredom, intelligence, depression, etc.) is due to experiences that one twin has but not the other twin. 'Fraternal' or dizygotic (DZ) twins share only about 50% of their genes. Thus powerful tests of the effects of genes can be made. Twins share many aspects of their environment (e.g. uterine environment, parenting style, education, wealth, culture, community) by virtue of being born in the same time and place. The presence of a given genetic trait in only one member of a pair of identical twins (called discordance) provides a powerful window into environmental effects. The classical twin design compares the similarity of monozygotic (identical) and dizygotic (fraternal) twins. If identical twins are considerably more similar than fraternal twins (which is found for most traits), this implicates that genes play an important role in these traits. By comparing many hundreds of families of twins, researchers can then understand more about the roles of genetic effects, shared environment, and unique environment in shaping behaviour.

Modern twin studies have shown that almost all traits are in part influenced by genetic differences, with some characteristics showing a strong influence (e.g. height), others an intermediate level (e.g. personality traits) and some more complex heritabilities, with evidence for different genes affecting different aspects of the trait—as in the case of autism.

Methods

The power of twin designs arises from the fact that twins may be either monozygotic (identical (MZ): developing from a single fertilised egg and therefore sharing all of their alleles)–or dizygotic (DZ: developing from two fertilised eggs and therefore sharing on average 50% of their polymorphic alleles, the same level of genetic similarity as found in non-twin siblings). These known differences in genetic similarity, together with a testable assumption of equal environments for identical and fraternal twins creates the basis for the twin design for exploring the effects of genetic and environmental variance on a phenotype. The basic logic of the twin study can be understood with very little mathematics beyond an understanding of correlation and the concept of variance.

Like all behaviour genetic research, the classic twin study begins from assessing the variance of a behaviour (called a phenotype by geneticists) in a large group, and attempts to estimate how much of this is due to:

- Genetic effects (heritability).
- Shared environment-events that happen to both twins, affecting them in the same way.
- Unshared, or unique, environment-events that occur to one twin but not the other, or events that affect either twin in a different way.

Typically these three components are called A (additive genetics) C (common environment) and E (unique environment), hence the acronym 'ACE'. It is also possible to examine non-additive genetics effects (often denoted D for dominance (ADE model), see below for more complex twin designs).

The ACE model indicates what proportion of variance in a trait is heritable, versus the proportions which are due to shared environment or unshared environment. Research is carried out using SEM programmes such as OpenMx, however the core logic of the twin design is the same, as described below:

Monozygotic (identical-MZ) twins raised in a family share both 100% of their genes, and all of the shared environment. Any differences arising between them in these circumstances are random (unique). The correlation between identical twins provides an estimate of $A + C$. Dizygotic (DZ) twins also share C, but share on average 50% of their genes: so the correlation between fraternal twins is a direct estimate of $\frac{1}{2} A + C$. If r is correlation, then r_{mz} and r_{dz} are simply the correlations of the trait in identical and fraternal twins respectively. For any particular trait, then:

$$r_{mz} = A + C$$

$$r_{dz} = \frac{1}{2} A + C$$

A, therefore, is twice the difference between identical and fraternal twin correlations : the additive genetic effect (Falconer's formula). C is simply the MZ correlation minus this estimate of A. The random (unique) factor E is $1 - r_{mz}$: i.e. MZ twins differ due to unique environments only. Stated again, the difference between these two sums, then, allows us to solve for A, C, and E. As the difference between the identical and fraternal correlations is due entirely to a halving of the genetic similarity, the additive genetic effect 'A' is simply twice the difference between the identical and fraternal correlations:

$$A = 2\ (r_{mz} - r_{dz})$$

As the identical correlation reflects the full effect of A and C, E can be estimated by subtracting this correlation from 1

$$E = 1 - r_{mz}$$

Finally, C can be derived:

$$C = r_{mz} - A$$

Sex Differences

Genetic factors may differ between the sexes, both in gene expression and in the range of gene × environment interactions. Fraternal opposite sex twin pairs are invaluable in explicating these effects. In an extreme case, a gene may only be expressed in one sex (qualitative sex limitation). More commonly, the effects of gene-alleles may depend on the sex of the individual. A gene might cause a change of 100 g in weight in males, but perhaps 150g in females a quantitative gene effect. Such effects are Environments may impact on the ability of genes to express themselves and may do this via sex differences. For instance genes affecting voting behaviour would have no effect in females if females are excluded from the vote. More generally, the logic of sex-difference testing can extend to any defined sub-group of individuals. In cases such as these, the correlation for same and opposite sex DZ twins will differ, betraying the effect of the sex difference.

For this reason, it is normal to distinguish three types of fraternal twins. A standard analytic workflow would involve testing for sex-limitation by fitting models to five groups, identical male, identical female, fraternal male, fraternal female, and fraternal opposite sex. Twin modelling thus goes beyond correlation to test causal models involving potential causal variables, such as sex.

Selective breeding

Selective breeding (also called artificial selection) is the process by which humans use animal breeding and plant breeding to selectively develop particular phenotypic traits (characteristics) by choosing which typically animal or plant males and females will sexually reproduce and have offspring together. Domesticated animals are known as breeds, normally bred by a professional breeder, while plants are known as varieties, cultigens, or cultivars in plants. Two purebred animals of different breeds produce a crossbreed, and crossbred plants are called hybrids.

There are two approaches or types of artificial selection, or selective breeding. First is the traditional 'breeder's approach' in which the breeder or experimenter applies 'a known amount of selection to a single phenotypic trait' by examining the chosen trait and choosing to breed only those that exhibit higher or 'extreme values' of that trait. The second is called 'controlled natural selection,' which is essentially natural selection in a controlled environment. In this, the breeder does not choose which individuals being tested 'survive or reproduce,' as he or she could in the traditional approach. There are also 'selection experiments,' which is a third approach and these are conducted in order to determine the 'strength of natural selection in the wild.' However, this is more often an observational approach as opposed to an experimental approach.

In animal breeding, techniques such as inbreeding, linebreeding, and outcrossing are utilised. In plant breeding, similar methods are used. The deliberate exploitation of selective breeding to produce desired results has become very common in agriculture and experimental biology.

Selective breeding can be unintentional, e.g. resulting from the process of human cultivation, and it may also produce unintended–desirable or undesirable–results. For example, in some grains, an increase in seed size may have resulted from certain ploughing practices rather than from the intentional selection of larger seeds. Most likely, there has been an interdependence between natural and artificial factors that have resulted in plant domestication.

Animal breeding

Animals with homogeneous appearance, behaviour, and other characteristics are known as particular breeds, and they are bred through culling animals with particular traits and selecting for further breeding those with other traits. Purebred animals have a single, recognizable breed, and purebreds with recorded lineage are called pedigreed. Crossbreeds are a mix of two purebreds, whereas mixed breeds are a mix of several breeds, often unknown. Animal breeding begins with breeding stock, a group of animals used for the purpose of planned breeding. When individuals are looking to breed animals, they look for certain valuable traits in purebred stock for a certain purpose, or may intend to use some type of crossbreeding to produce a new type of stock with different, and, it is presumed, superior abilities in a given area of endeavor. For example, to breed chickens, a typical breeder intends to receive eggs, meat, and new, young birds for further reproduction. Thus, the breeder has to study different breeds and types of chickens and analyse what can be expected from a certain set of characteristics before he or she starts breeding them. Therefore, when purchasing initial breeding stock, the breeder seeks a group of birds that will most closely fit the purpose intended.

Plant breeding

Plant breeding has been used for thousands of years, and began with the domestication of wild plants into uniform and predictable agricultural cultigens. High-yielding varieties have been particularly important in agriculture. Selective plant breeding is also used in research to produce transgenic animals that breed 'true' (i.e. are homozygous) for artificially inserted or deleted genes.

Selective breeding in aquaculture

Selective breeding in aquaculture holds high potential for the genetic improvement of fish and shellfish. Unlike terrestrial livestock, the potential benefits of selective breeding in aquaculture were not realised until recently. This is because high mortality led to the selection of only a few broodstock, causing inbreeding depression, which then forced the use of wild broodstock. This was evident in selective breeding programmes for growth rate, which resulted in slow growth and high mortality.

Control of the reproduction cycle was one of the main reasons as it is a requisite for selective breeding programmes. Artificial reproduction was not achieved because of the difficulties in hatching or feeding some farmed species such as eel and yellowtail farming. A suspected reason associated with the late realisation of success in selective breeding programmes in aquaculture was the education of the concerned people – researchers, advisory personnel and fish farmers. The education of fish biologists paid less attention to quantitative genetics and breeding plans. Another was the failure of documentation of the genetic gains in successive generations. This in turn led to failure in quantifying economic benefits that successful selective breeding programmes produce. Documentation of the genetic changes was considered important as they help in fine tuning further selection schemes.

Advantages and disadvantages of breeding

Selective breeding is a direct way to determine if a specific trait can 'evolve in response to selection.' A single-generation method of breeding is not as accurate or direct. The process is also more practical and easier to understand than sibling analysis. The former tests 'differences between line means' while the latter is dependent upon 'variance and covariance components.' Essentially, selective breeding is better for traits such as physiology and behaviour that are hard to measure because it requires fewer individuals to test than single-generation testing. However, there are disadvantages to this process. Because a single experiment done in selective breeding cannot be used to assess an entire group of 'genetic variances and covariances,' individual experiments must be done for every individual trait. Also, because of the necessity of selective breeding experiments to require maintaining the organisms tested in a lab or greenhouse, it is impractical to use this breeding method on many organisms. Controlled mating instances are difficult to carry out in this case and this is a necessary component of selective breeding.

HETEROSIS

Heterosis hybrid vigor, or outbreeding enhancement, is the improved or increased function of any biological quality in a hybrid offspring. The adjective derived from heterosis is heterotic. A mixed-breed dog is shown in Fig. 20.4. An offspring exhibits heterosis if its traits are enhanced as a result of mixing the genetic contributions of its parents. These effects can be due to Mendelian or non-Mendelian inheritance. Heterosis is often discussed as the opposite of inbreeding depression although differences in these two concepts can be seen in evolutionary considerations such as the role of genetic variation or the effects of genetic drift in small populations on these concepts. Inbreeding depression occurs when related parents have children with traits that negatively influence their fitness largely due to homozygosity. In such instances, outcrossing should result in heterosis. Not all outcrosses result in heterosis. For example, when a hybrid inherits traits from its parents that are not fully compatible, fitness can be reduced. This is a form of outbreeding depression.

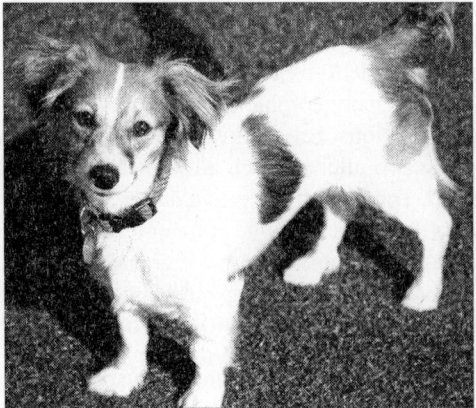

Fig. 20.4: A mixed-breed dog.

Dominance Versus Overdominance

Dominance versus overdominance is a scientific controversy in the field of genetics that has persisted for more than a century. These two alternative hypotheses were first stated in 1908.

Genetic basis

When a population is small or inbred, it tends to lose genetic diversity. Inbreeding depression is the loss of fitness due to loss of genetic diversity. Inbred strains tend to be homozygous for recessive alleles that are mildly harmful (or produce a trait that is undesirable from the standpoint of the breeder). Heterosis or hybrid vigor, on the other hand, is the tendency of outbred strains to exceed both inbred parents in fitness. Selective breeding of plants and animals, including hybridisation, began long before there was an understanding of underlying scientific principles. In the early 20th century, after Mendel's laws came to be understood and accepted, geneticists undertook to explain the superior vigor of many plant hybrids. Two competing hypotheses, which are not mutually exclusive, were developed:

Genetic and epigenetic bases of heterosis

The genetic dominance hypothesis attributes the superiority of hybrids to the masking of expression of undesirable (deleterious) recessive alleles from one parent by dominant (usually wild-type) alleles from the other. It attributes the poor performance of inbred strains to the expression of homozygous deleterious recessive alleles. The genetic overdominance hypothesis states that some combinations of alleles (which can be obtained by crossing two inbred strains) are especially advantageous when paired in a heterozygous individual. This hypothesis is commonly invoked to explain the persistence of some alleles (most famously the Sickle cell trait allele) that are harmful in homozygotes. In normal circumstances, such harmful alleles would be removed from a population through the process of natural selection. Like the dominance hypothesis, it attributes the poor performance of inbred strains to expression of such harmful recessive alleles. In any case, outcross matings provide the benefit of masking deleterious recessive alleles in progeny. This benefit has been proposed to be a major factor in the maintenance of sexual reproduction among eukaryotes.

MHC in animals

One example of where particular genes may be important in vertebrate animals for heterosis is the major histocompatibility complex. Vertebrates inherit several copies of both MHC class I and MHC class II from each parent, which are used in antigen presentation as part of the adaptive immune system. Each different copy of the genes is able to bind and present a different set of potential peptides to T-lymphocytes. These genes are highly polymorphic throughout populations, but will be more similar in smaller, more closely related populations. Breeding between more genetically distant individuals will decrease the chance of inheriting two alleles which are the same or similar, allowing a more diverse range of peptides to be presented. This therefore gives a decreased chance that any particular pathogen will not be recognised, and means that more antigenic proteins on any pathogen are likely to be recognised, giving a greater range of T-cell activation and therefore a greater response. This will also mean that the immunity acquired to the pathogen will be against a greater range of antigens, meaning that the pathogen must mutate more before immunity is lost. Thus hybrids will be less likely to be succumb to pathogenic disease and will be more capable of fighting off infection.

In plants

Crosses between inbreds from different heterotic groups result in vigorous F1 hybrids with significantly more heterosis than F1 hybrids from inbreds within the same heterotic group or pattern. Heterotic groups are created by plant breeders to classify inbred lines, and can be progressively improved by reciprocal recurrent selection.

Heterosis is used to increase yields, uniformity, and vigor. Hybrid breeding methods are used in maize, sorghum, rice, sugar beet, onion, spinach, sunflowers, broccoli and to create a more psychoactive cannabis.

Hybrid livestock

The concept of heterosis is also applied in the production of commercial livestock. In cattle, hybrids between Black Angus and Hereford produce a hybrid known as a 'Black Baldy'. In swine, 'blue butts' are produced by the cross of Hampshire and Yorkshire. Other, more exotic hybrids such as 'beefalo' are also used for specialty markets.

Heterosis in dogs

In 2013, a study found that mixed breeds live on average 1.2 years longer than pure breeds, and that increasing body-weight was negatively correlated with longevity (i.e. the heavier the dog the less its lifespan). John Scott and John Fuller performed a detailed study of purebred cocker spaniels, purebred basenjis, and hybrids between them. They found that hybrids ran faster than either parent, perhaps due to heterosis. Other characteristics, such as basal heart rate, did not show any heterosis–the dog's basal heart rate was close to the average of its parents–perhaps due to the additive effects of multiple genes. Sometimes people working on a dog breeding programme find no useful heterosis.

Humans

Human beings are all extremely genetically similar to one another, but less similar, than for instance dogs. Michael Mingroni has proposed heterosis, in the form of hybrid vigor associated with historical reductions of the levels of inbreeding, as an explanation of the Flynn effect, the steady rise in IQ test scores around the world during the twentieth century. However, James R. Flynn has pointed out that even if everyone mated with a sibling in 1900, subsequent increases in heterosis would not be a sufficient explanation of the observed IQ gains. Correlation between Relatives on the Supposition of Mendelian Inheritance 'The Correlation between Relatives on the Supposition of Mendelian Inheritance' is a scientific paper by Ronald Fisher which was published in the Philosophical Transactions of the Royal Society of Edinburgh in 1918. In it, Fisher puts forward a genetics conceptual model that shows that continuous variation amongst phenotypic traits could be the result of Mendelian inheritance. The paper also contains the first use of the statistical term variance.

Genetic correlation

Genetic correlation is the proportion of variance that two traits share due to genetic causes. Outside the theoretical boundary case of traits with zero heritability (the proportion of observable differences in a trait between individuals within a population that is due to genetic differences), the genetic correlation of traits is independent of their heritability: i.e. two traits can have a very high genetic correlation even when the heritability of each is low and *vice versa*.

The genetic correlation, then, tells us how much of the genetic influence on two traits is common to both: if it is above zero, this suggests that the two traits are influenced by common genes. This can be an important constraint on conceptualisations of the two traits: traits which seem different phenotypically but which share a common genetic basis require an explanation for how these genes can influence both traits. For example, consider two traits dark skin and black hair. These two traits may individually have a very high heritability (most of the population-level variation in the trait due to genetic differences, or in simpler terms, genetics contributes significantly to these two traits), however, they may still have a very low genetic correlation if, for instance, these two traits were being controlled by different, non-overlapping, non-linked genetic loci.

GENETIC ARCHITECTURE

Genetic architecture refers to the underlying genetic basis of a phenotypic trait. A synonymous term is the 'genotype-phenotype map', the way that genotypes lead to the phenotypes.

- The genotype-phenotype map has been analysed in terms of several principal axes: Epistasis, polygeny, pleiotropy, quasi-continuity, modularity, phenotypic plasticity, robustness, and evolvability.

- Epistasis: when the alleles at one locus change the phenotypic effects of genetic variation at another locus, the two genes are said to exhibit 'epistasis' in their interactions.

- Polygeny: When multiple genes contribute to a particular phenotypic character, the map is said to possess 'polygeny'. The genetic architecture in cases of polygeny can be further characterised by the spectrum of contributions of the genes, e.g. many genes of small effect vs. few genes of large effect.

- Pleiotropy: When multiple phenotypic characters are affected by a single genetic variation, the map is said to possess 'pleiotropy'.

- Quasi-continuity: When small genetic changes map to small phenotypic changes, the map is said to possess 'quasi-continuity' (Lewontin).

- Modularity: When two different phenotypic characters can be mapped to mostly non-overlapping sets of genes, the map is said to possess 'modularity', though this concept is still in flux in the scientific literature.

- Plasticity: When a single genotype gives rise to a spectrum of phenotypes, the phenotype is said to have 'plasticity'. The plasticity may occur as different phenotypes among different individuals of the same genotype, or different phenotypes within the lifetime of a single individual, or different phenotypes in response to specific environmental conditions.

- Mutational robustness: When the same phenotype occurs in an organism despite a variety of environmental perturbations, it is said to be 'robust'. When the same phenotype is produced despite mutations in the genes involved it its production, it is said to possess 'mutational robustness'.

- Evolvability: When there is a significant chance that genetic variation can be produced which produces a net increase in adaptation in an organism, the genotype-phenotype map is said to have 'evolvability'.

- Transgressive phenotype: When a phenotype is more extreme than the phenotype displayed by either of the parental lines.

Chapter 21

Population Genetics

INTRODUCTION

Population genetics is the study of the distributions and changes of allele frequency in a population, as the population is subject to the four main evolutionary processes: natural selection, genetic drift, mutation and gene flow. It also takes into account the factors of recombination, population subdivision and population structure. Studies in this branch of biology examine such phenomena as adaptation and speciation. *Biston betularia f. typica* is the white-bodied form of the peppered moth is shown in Fig. 21.1. Population genetics is the study of the frequency and interaction of alleles and genes in populations. A sexual population is a set of organisms in which any pair of members can breed together. This implies that all members belong to the same species and live near each other. For example, all of the moths of the same species living in an isolated forest are a population. A gene in this population may have several alternate forms, which account for variations between the phenotypes of the organisms. An example might be a gene for colouration in moths that has two alleles: black and white. A gene pool is the complete set of alleles for a gene in a single population, the allele frequency for an allele is the fraction of the genes in the pool that is composed of that allele (for example, what fraction of moth colouration genes are the black allele). Evolution occurs when there are changes in the frequencies of alleles within a population, for example, the allele for black colour in a population of moths becoming more common.

FOUR PROCESSES OF POPULATION GENETICS

Natural Selection

Natural selection is the fact that some traits make it more likely for an organism to survive and reproduce. Population genetics describes natural selection by defining fitness as a propensity or probability of survival and reproduction in a particular environment. The fitness is normally given by the symbol $w = 1-s$ where s is the selection coefficient. Natural selection acts on phenotypes, or the observable characteristics of organisms, but the genetically heritable basis of any phenotype which gives a reproductive advantage will become more common in a population. In this way, natural selection converts differences in fitness into changes in allele frequency in a population over successive generations. Before the advent

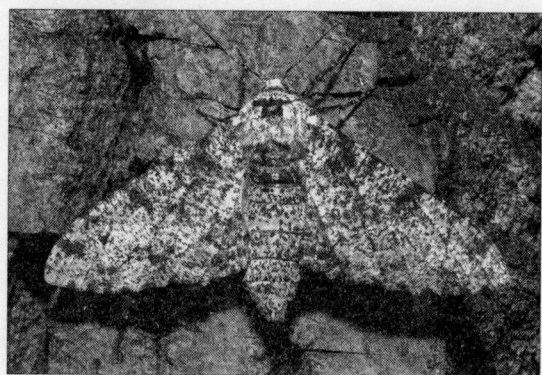

Fig. 21.1: *Biston betularia f. typica* is the white-bodied form of the peppered moth.

of population genetics, many biologists doubted that small differences in fitness were sufficient to make a large difference to evolution. Population geneticists addressed this concern in part by comparing selection to genetic drift. Selection can overcome genetic drift when s is greater than 1 divided by the effective population size. When this criterion is met, the probability that a new advantageous mutant becomes fixed is approximately equal to $2s$. The time until fixation of such an allele depends little on genetic drift, and is approximately proportional to $\log(sN)/s$.

Genetic Drift

Genetic drift is a change in allele frequencies caused by random sampling. That is, the alleles in the offspring are a random sample of those in the parents. Genetic drift may cause gene variants to disappear completely, and thereby reduce genetic variability. In contrast to natural selection, which makes gene variants more common or less common depending on their reproductive success, the changes due to genetic drift are not driven by environmental or adaptive pressures, and may be beneficial, neutral, or detrimental to reproductive success. Genomic drift in ebola could interfere with sequence based drug development (Fig. 21.2).

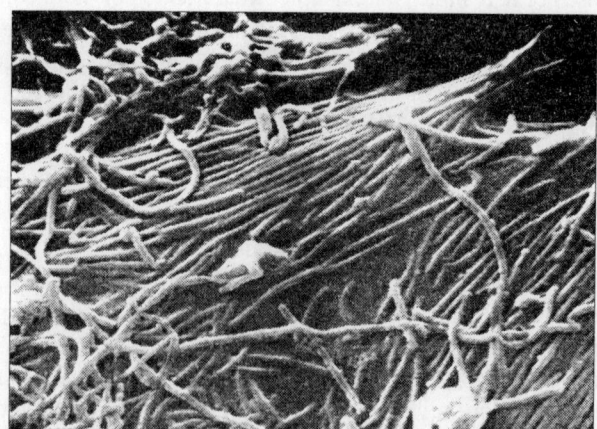

Fig. 21.2: Genomic drift in ebola based drug development.

The effect of genetic drift is larger for alleles present in few copies than when an allele is present in many copies. Scientists wage vigorous debates over the relative importance of genetic drift compared with natural selection. Ronald Fisher held the view that genetic drift plays at the most a minor role in evolution, and this remained the dominant view for several decades. Motoo Kimura rekindled the debate with his neutral theory of molecular evolution which claims that most of the changes in the genetic material are caused by neutral mutations and genetic drift. The role of genetic drift by means of sampling error in evolution has been criticised by John H Gillespie and Will Provine, who argue that selection on linked sites is a more important stochastic force. The population genetics of genetic drift are described using either branching processes or a diffusion equation describing changes in allele frequency. These approaches are usually applied to the Wright-Fisher and Moran models of population genetics. Assuming genetic drift is the only evolutionary force acting on an allele, after t generations in many replicated populations, starting with allele frequencies of p and q, the variance in allele frequency across those populations is:

$$V_t \approx pq\left(1 - \exp\left\{-\frac{t}{2N_e}\right\}\right)$$

Mutation

Mutation is the ultimate source of genetic variation in the form of new alleles. Mutation can result in several different types of change in DNA sequences, these can either have no effect, alter the product of a gene, or prevent the gene from functioning. Studies in the fly *Drosophila* melanogaster suggest that if a mutation changes a protein produced by a gene, this will probably be harmful, with about 70 per cent of these mutations having damaging effects, and the remainder being either neutral or weakly beneficial. Mutations can involve large sections of DNA becoming duplicated, usually through genetic recombination. These duplications are a major source of raw material for evolving new genes, with tens to hundreds of genes duplicated in animal genomes every million years. Most genes belong to larger families of genes of shared ancestry. Novel genes are produced by several methods, commonly through the duplication and mutation of an ancestral gene, or by recombining parts of different genes to form new combinations with new functions. Here, domains act as modules, each with a particular and independent function, that can be mixed together to produce genes encoding new proteins with novel properties. For example, the human eye uses four genes to make structures that sense light: three for colour vision and one for night vision, all four arose from a single ancestral gene. Another advantage of duplicating a gene (or even an entire genome) is that this increases redundancy, this allows one gene in the pair to acquire a new function while the other copy performs the original function. Other types of mutation occasionally create new genes from previously noncoding DNA.

In addition to being a major source of variation, mutation may also function as a mechanism of evolution when there are different probabilities at the molecular level for different mutations to occur, a process known as mutation bias. If two genotypes, for example one with the nucleotide G and another with the nucleotide A in the same position, have the same fitness, but mutation from G to A happens more often than mutation from A to G, then genotypes with A will tend to evolve. Different insertion vs. deletion mutation biases in different taxa can lead to the evolution of different genome sizes. Developmental or mutational biases have also been observed in morphological evolution. For example, according to the phenotype-first theory of evolution, mutations can eventually cause the genetic assimilation of traits that were previously induced by the environment. Mutation can cause garden mossrose to produce flowers of different colours.

Mutation bias effects are superimposed on other processes. If selection would favour either one out of two mutations, but there is no extra advantage to having both, then the mutation that occurs the most frequently is the one that is most likely to become fixed in a population. Mutations leading to the loss of function of a gene are much more common than mutations that produce a new, fully functional gene. Most loss of function mutations are selected against. But when selection is weak, mutation bias towards loss of function can affect evolution. For example, pigments are no longer useful when animals live in the darkness of caves, and tend to be lost. This kind of loss of function can occur because of mutation bias, and/or because the function had a cost, and once the benefit of the function disappeared, natural selection leads to the loss. Loss of sporulation ability in a bacterium during laboratory evolution appears to have been caused by mutation bias, rather than natural selection against the cost of maintaining sporulation ability. When there is no selection for loss of function, the speed at which loss evolves depends more on the mutation rate than it does on the effective population size, indicating that it is driven more by mutation bias than by genetic drift.

Evolution of mutation rate

Due to the damaging effects that mutations can have on cells, organisms have evolved mechanisms such as DNA repair to remove mutations. Therefore, the optimal mutation rate for a species is a trade-off between costs of a high mutation rate, such as deleterious mutations, and the metabolic costs of maintaining systems to reduce the mutation rate, such as DNA repair enzymes. Viruses that use RNA as their genetic material have rapid mutation rates, which can be an advantage since these viruses will evolve constantly and rapidly, and thus evade the defensive responses of, e.g. the human immune system.

Gene flow and transfer

Gene flow is the exchange of genes between populations, which are usually of the same species. Examples of gene flow within a species include the migration and then breeding of organisms, or the exchange of pollen. Gene transfer between species includes the formation of hybrid organisms and horizontal gene transfer. Migration into or out of a population can change allele frequencies, as well as introducing genetic variation into a population. Immigration may add new genetic material to the established gene pool of a population. Conversely, emigration may remove genetic material. Population genetic models can be used to reconstruct the history of gene flow between populations.

Reproductive isolation

As barriers to reproduction between two diverging populations are required for the populations to become new species, gene flow may slow this process by spreading genetic differences between the populations. Gene flow is hindered by mountain ranges, oceans and deserts or even man-made structures such as the Great Wall of China, which has hindered the flow of plant genes. Depending on how far two species have diverged since their most recent common ancestor, it may still be possible for them to produce offspring, as with horses and donkeys mating to produce mules. Such hybrids are generally infertile, due to the two different sets of chromosomes being unable to pair up during meiosis. In this case, closely related species may regularly interbreed, but hybrids will be selected against and the species will remain distinct. However, viable hybrids are occasionally formed and these new species can either have properties intermediate between their parent species, or possess a totally new phenotype. The importance of hybridisation in creating new species of animals is unclear, although cases have been seen in many types of animals, with the gray tree frog being a particularly well-studied example.

Hybridisation is, however, an important means of speciation in plants, since polyploidy (having more than two copies of each chromosome) is tolerated in plants more readily than in animals. Polyploidy is important in hybrids as it allows reproduction, with the two different sets of chromosomes each being able to pair with an identical partner during meiosis. Polyploids also have more genetic diversity, which allows them to avoid inbreeding depression in small populations.

Genetic structure

Because of physical barriers to migration, along with limited tendency for individuals to move or spread (vagility), and tendency to remain or come back to natal place (philopatry), natural populations rarely all interbreed as convenient in theoretical random models (panmixy). There is usually a geographic range within which individuals are more closely related to one another than those randomly selected from the general population. This is described as the extent to which a population is genetically structured. Genetic structuring can be caused by migration due to historical climate change, species range expansion or current availability of habitat.

Horizontal gene transfer

Horizontal gene transfer (Fig. 21.3) is the transfer of genetic material from one organism to another organism that is not its offspring, this is most common among bacteria. In medicine, this contributes to the spread of antibiotic resistance, as when one bacteria acquires resistance genes it can rapidly transfer them to other species. Horizontal transfer of genes from bacteria to eukaryotes such as the yeast *Saccharomyces cerevisiae* and the adzuki bean beetle Callosobruchus chinensis may also have occurred. An example of larger-scale transfers are the eukaryotic bdelloid rotifers, which appear to have received a range of genes from bacteria, fungi, and plants. Viruses can also carry DNA between organisms, allowing transfer of genes even across biological domains. Large-scale gene transfer has also occurred between the ancestors of eukaryotic cells and prokaryotes, during the acquisition of chloroplasts and mitochondria.

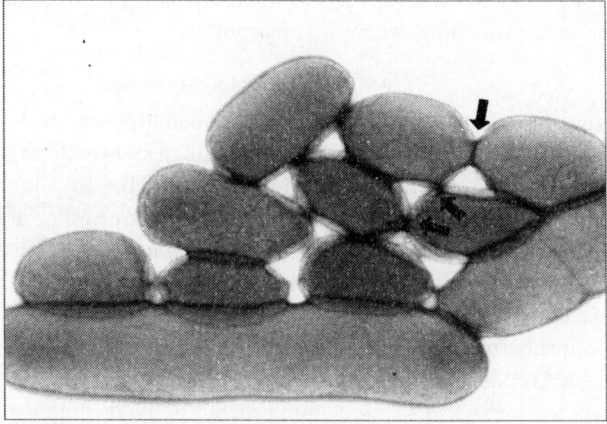

Fig. 21.3: Horizontal gene transfer.

Complications

Basic models of population genetics consider only one gene locus at a time. In practice, epistatic and linkage relationships between loci may also be important.

Epistasis

Because of epistasis, the phenotypic effect of an allele at one locus may depend on which alleles are present at many other loci. Selection does not act on a single locus, but on a phenotype that arises through development from a complete genotype.

According to Lewontin, the theoretical task for population genetics is a process in two spaces: a 'genotypic space' and a 'phenotypic space'. The challenge of a complete theory of population genetics is to provide a set of laws that predictably map a population of genotypes (G_1) to a phenotype space (P_1), where selection takes place, and another set of laws that map the resulting population (P_2) back to genotype space (G_2) where Mendelian genetics can predict the next generation of genotypes, thus completing the cycle. Even leaving aside for the moment the non-Mendelian aspects of molecular genetics, this is clearly a gargantuan task. Visualising this transformation schematically:

$$G_1 \xrightarrow{T_1} P_1 \xrightarrow{T_2} P_2 \xrightarrow{T_3} G_2 \xrightarrow{T_4} G_1' \to \ldots$$

T_1 represents the genetic and epigenetic laws, the aspects of functional biology, or development, that transform a genotype into phenotype. We will refer to this as the 'genotype-phenotype map'. T_2 is the transformation due to natural selection, T_3 are epigenetic relations that predict genotypes based on the selected phenotypes and finally T_4 the rules of Mendelian genetics. In practice, there are two bodies of evolutionary theory that exist in parallel, traditional population genetics operating in the genotype space and the biometric theory used in plant and animal breeding, operating in phenotype space.

The missing part is the mapping between the genotype and phenotype space. This leads to a 'sleight of hand' (as Lewontin terms it) whereby variables in the equations of one domain, are considered parameters or constants, where, in a full-treatment they would be transformed themselves by the evolutionary process and are in reality functions of the state variables in the other domain.

The 'sleight of hand' is assuming that we know this mapping. Proceeding as if we do understand it is enough to analyse many cases of interest. For example, if the phenotype is almost one-to-one with genotype (sickle-cell disease) or the time-scale is sufficiently short, the 'constants' can be treated as such, however, there are many situations where it is inaccurate.

Linkage

If all genes are in linkage equilibrium, the effect of an allele at one locus can be averaged across the gene pool at other loci. In reality, one allele is frequently found in linkage disequilibrium with genes at other loci, especially with genes located nearby on the same chromosome. Recombination breaks up this linkage disequilibrium too slowly to avoid genetic hitchhiking, where an allele at one locus rises to high frequency because it is linked to an allele under selection at a nearby locus. This is a problem for population genetic models that treat one gene locus at a time. It can, however, be exploited as a method for detecting the action of natural selection via selective sweeps.

In the extreme case of primarily asexual populations, linkage is complete, and different population genetic equations can be derived and solved, which behave quite differently from the sexual case. Most microbes, such as bacteria, are asexual. The population genetics of micro-organisms lays the foundations for tracking the origin and evolution of antibiotic resistance and deadly infectious pathogens. Population genetics of micro-organisms is also an essential factor for devising strategies for the conservation and better utilisation of beneficial microbes.

ALLELE FREQUENCY

Allele frequency, or gene frequency, is the proportion of a particular allele (variant of a gene) among all allele copies being considered. It can be formally defined as the percentage of all alleles at a given locus in a population gene pool represented by a particular allele. In other words, it is the number of copies of a particular allele divided by the number of copies of all alleles at the genetic place (locus) in a population. It is usually expressed as a percentage. In population genetics, allele frequencies are used to depict the amount of genetic diversity at the individual, population, and species level. It is also the relative proportion of all alleles of a gene that are of a designated type.

Given the following:

1. A particular locus on a chromosome and the gene occupying that locus.

2. A population of N individuals carrying n loci in each of their somatic cells (e.g. two loci in the cells of diploid species, which contain two sets of chromosomes).

3. Different alleles of the gene exist.

4. One allele exists in a copies.

Then the allele frequency is the fraction or percentage of all the occurrences of that locus that is occupied by a given allele and the frequency of one of the alleles is $i/(nN)$.

For example, if the frequency of an allele is 20% in a given population, then among population members, one in five chromosomes will carry that allele. Four out of five will be occupied by other variants of the gene.

Note that for diploid genes the fraction of individuals that carry this allele may be nearly two in five (36%). The reason for this is that if the allele distributes randomly, then the binomial theorem will apply: 32% of the population will be heterozygous for the allele (i.e. carry one copy of that allele and one copy of another in each somatic cell) and 4% will be homozygous (carrying two copies of the allele). Together, this means that 36% of diploid individuals would be expected to carry an allele that has a frequency of 20%. However, alleles distribute randomly only under certain assumptions, including the absence of selection. When these conditions apply, a population is said to be in Hardy–Weinberg equilibrium. The frequencies of all the alleles of a given gene often are graphed together as an allele frequency distribution histogram, or allele frequency spectrum. Population genetics studies the different 'forces' that might lead to changes in the distribution and frequencies of alleles—in other words, to evolution. Besides selection, these forces include genetic drift, mutation and migration.

Calculation of Allele Frequencies from Genotype Frequencies

The actual frequency calculations depend on the ploidy of the species for autosomal genes.

Monoploids

The frequency of an allele a is the quotient of the number of copies of the allele and the population or sample size.

Diploids

If $f(AA)$, $f(Aa)$, and $f(aa)$ are the frequencies of the three genotypes at a locus with two alleles, then the frequency p of the A-allele and the frequency q of the a-allele are obtained by counting alleles.

Because each homozygote *AA* consists only of *A*-alleles, and because half of the alleles of each heterozygote *Aa* are *A*-alleles, the total frequency *p* of *A*-alleles in the population is calculated as:

$$p = f(AA) + \frac{1}{2}f(Aa) = \text{frequency of } A$$

Similarly, the frequency *q* of the *a*-allele is given by:

$$p = f(aa) + \frac{1}{2}f(Aa) = \text{frequency of } a$$

It would be expected that *p* and *q* sum to 1, since they are the frequencies of the only two alleles present. Indeed they do:

$$p + q = f(AA) + f(aa) + f(Aa) = 1$$

and from this we get:

$$q = 1 - p \text{ and } p = 1 - q$$

If there are more than two different allelic forms, the frequency for each allele is simply the frequency of its homozygote plus half the sum of the frequencies for all the heterozygotes in which it appears.

Allele frequency can always be calculated from genotype frequency, whereas the reverse requires that the Hardy–Weinberg conditions of random mating apply. This is partly due to the three genotype frequencies and the two allele frequencies. It is easier to reduce from three to two.

An example population

Consider a population of ten individuals and a given locus with two possible alleles, *A* and *a*. Suppose that the genotypes of the individuals are as follows:

AA, *Aa*, *AA*, *aa*, *Aa*, *AA*, *AA*, *Aa*, *Aa*, and *AA*

Then the allele frequencies of allele *A* and allele *a* are:

$$p = prob_A = \frac{2+1+2+0+1+2+2+1+1+2}{2 \times 10} = 0.7$$

$$q = prob_a = \frac{0+1+0+2+1+0+0+1+1+0}{2 \times 10} = 0.3$$

so if a locus is chosen at random there is a 70% chance it will be the *A* allele, and a 30% chance it will be the a allele.

Allele frequency dynamics

The dynamics of allele and gene frequencies are affected by several factors such as migration, mutation, drift, population size, mating and others. The Hardy-Weinberg law describes an equilibrium for diploids genes.

GENOTYPE FREQUENCY

Genetic variation in populations can be analysed and quantified by the frequency of alleles. Two fundamental calculations are central to population genetics: allele frequencies and genotype frequencies. Genotype frequency in a population is the number of individuals with a given genotype divided by the total number of individuals in the population. In population genetics, the genotype frequency is the frequency or proportion (i.e. $0 < f < 1$) of genotypes in a population.

Although allele and genotype frequencies are related, it is important to clearly distinguish them. Genotype frequency may also be used in the future (for 'genomic profiling') to predict someone's having a disease or even a birth defect. It can also be used to determine ethnic diversity.

Numerical Example

As an example, let's consider a population of 100 four-o'clock plants (Mirabilis jalapa) with the following genotypes:

- 49 red-flowered plants with the genotype *AA*.
- 42 pink-flowered plants with genotype *Aa*.
- 9 white-flowered plants with genotype *aa*.

When calculating an allele frequency for a diploid species, remember that homozygous individuals have two copies of an allele, whereas heterozygotes have only one. In our example, each of the 42 pink-flowered heterozygotes has one copy of the a allele, and each of the 9 white-flowered homozygotes has two copies. Therefore, the allele frequency for a (the white colour allele) equals:

$$f(a) = \frac{(Aa) + 2 \times (aa)}{2 \times (AA) + 2 \times (Aa) + 2 \times (aa)} = \frac{42 + 2 \times 9}{2 \times 49 + 2 \times 42 + 2 \times 9} = \frac{60}{200} = 0.3$$

This result tells us that the allele frequency of a is 0.3. In other words, 30% of the alleles for this gene in the population are the a allele.

Compare genotype frequency: let's now calculate the genotype frequency of *aa* homozygotes (white-flowered plants).

$$f(aa) = \frac{9}{49 + 42 + 9} = \frac{9}{10} = 0.09 = 9\%$$

Allele and genotype frequencies always sum to less than or equal to one (in other words, less than or equal to 100%). The Hardy–Weinberg law describes the relationship between allele and genotype frequencies when a population is not evolving. Let's examine the Hardy–Weinberg equation using the population of four-o'clock plants that we considered above:

If the allele *A* frequency is denoted by the symbol p and the allele *a* frequency denoted by q, then $p + q = 1$. For example, if $p = 0.7$, then q must be 0.3. In other words, if the allele frequency of A equals 70%, the remaining 30% of the alleles must be a, because together they equal 100%.

For a gene that exists in two alleles, the Hardy–Weinberg equation states that:

$$(p^2) + (2pq) + (q^2) = 1$$

If we apply this equation to our flower colour gene, then

$f(AA) = p^2$ (genotype frequency of homozygotes)

$f(Aa) = 2pq$ (genotype frequency of heterozygotes)

$f(aa) = q^2$ (genotype frequency of homozygotes)

If $p = 0.7$ and $q = 0.3$, then

$f(AA) = p^2 = (0.7)^2 = 0.49$

$f(Aa) = 2pq = 2 \times (0.7) \times (0.3) = 0.42$

$f(aa) = q^2 = (0.3)^2 = 0.09$

This result tells us that, if the allele frequency of *A* is 70% and the allele frequency of *a* is 30%, the expected genotype frequency of *AA* is 49%, *Aa* is 42%, and aa is 9%.

POLYMORPHISM (BIOLOGY)

Polymorphism in biology is said to occur when two or more clearly different phenotypes exist in the same population of a species—in other words, the occurrence of more than one form or morph. In order to be classified as such, morphs must occupy the same habitat at the same time and belong to a panmictic population (one with random mating). Figure 21.4 shows light-morph jaguar and dark-morph or melanistic jaguar is shown in Fig. 21.5.

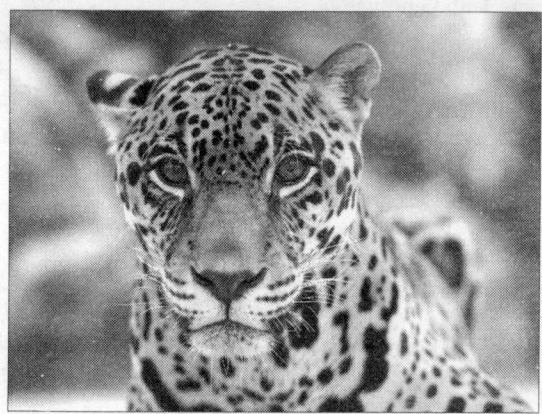

Fig. 21.4: Light-morph jaguar.

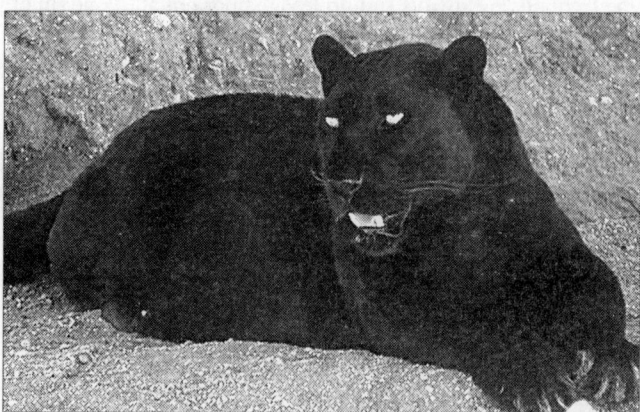

Fig. 21.5: Dark-morph or melanistic jaguar (about 6% of the South American population).

Polymorphism as described here involves morphs of the phenotype. The term is also used somewhat differently by molecular biologists to describe certain point mutations in the genotype, such as SNPs (see also RFLPs). Polymorphism is common in nature, it is related to biodiversity, genetic variation and adaptation, it usually functions to retain variety of form in a population living in a varied environment.

The most common example is sexual dimorphism, which occurs in many organisms. Other examples are mimetic forms of butterflies (see mimicry), and human hemoglobin and blood types.

According to the theory of evolution, polymorphism results from evolutionary processes, as does any aspect of a species. It is heritable and is modified by natural selection. In polyphenism, an individual's genetic make-up allows for different morphs, and the switch mechanism that determines which morph is shown is environmental. In genetic polymorphism, the genetic make-up determines the morph. Ants exhibit both types in a single population. Polymorphism also refers to the occurrence of structurally and functionally more than two different types of individuals, called zooids within the same organism. It is a characteristic feature of Cnidarians. For example, in Obelia there are feeding individuals, the gastrozooids, the individuals capable of asexual reproduction only, the gonozooids, blastostyles and free-living or sexually reproducing individuals, the medusae.

Although in general use polymorphism is quite a broad term, in biology it has been given a specific meaning, being distinguishable from monomorphism (having only one form). A more specific term, when there are only two forms, is dimorphism. The term omits characters showing continuous variation (such as weight), even though this has a heritable component. Polymorphism deals with forms in which the variation is discrete (discontinuous) or strongly bimodal or polymodal.

Morphs must occupy the same habitat at the same time: this excludes geographical races and seasonal forms. The use of the words morph or polymorphism for what is a visibly different geographical race or variant is common, but incorrect. The significance of geographical variation is in that it may lead to allopatric speciation, whereas true polymorphism takes place in panmictic populations. The term was first used to describe visible forms, but nowadays it has been extended to include cryptic morphs, for instance blood types, which can be revealed by a test. Rare variations are not classified as polymorphisms, and mutations by themselves do not constitute polymorphisms. To qualify as a polymorphism there has to be some kind of balance between morphs underpinned by inheritance. The criterion is that the frequency of the least common morph is too high simply to be the result of new mutations or, as a rough guide, that it is greater than 1 per cent (though that is far higher than any normal mutation rate for a single allele).

Various synonymous terms exist for the various polymorphic forms of an organism. The most common are morph and morpha, while a more formal term is morphotype. Form and phase are sometimes also used, but are easily confused in zoology with, respectively, 'form' in a population of animals, and 'phase' as a colour or other change in an organism due to environmental conditions (temperature, humidity, etc.). Phenotypic traits and characteristics are also possible descriptions, though that would imply just a limited aspect of the body.

Ecology

Selection, whether natural or artificial, changes the frequency of morphs within a population, this occurs when morphs reproduce with different degrees of success. A genetic (or balanced) polymorphism usually persists over many generations, maintained by two or more opposed and powerful selection pressures. Diver found banding morphs in Cepaea nemoralis could be seen in pre-fossil shells going back to the Mesolithic Holocene. Apes have similar blood groups to humans, this suggests rather strongly that this kind of polymorphism is quite ancient, at least as far back as the last common ancestor of the apes and man, and possibly even further. Figure 21.6 shows the white morph of the monarch in Hawaii.

The relative proportions of the morphs may vary, the actual values are determined by the effective fitness of the morphs at a particular time and place. The mechanism of heterozygote advantage assures the population of some alternative alleles at the locus or loci involved. Only if competing selection

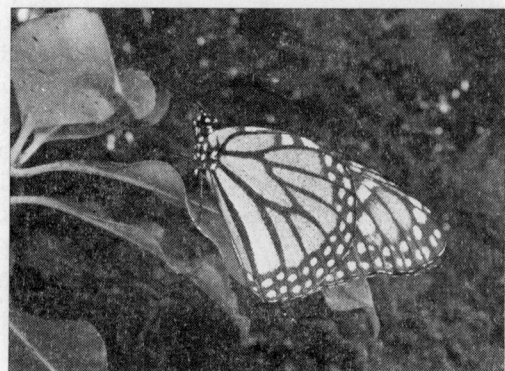

Fig. 21.6: The white morph of the monarch in Hawaii is partly a result of apostatic selection.

disappears will an allele disappear. However, heterozygote advantage is not the only way a polymorphism can be maintained. Apostatic selection, whereby a predator consumes a common morph whilst overlooking rarer morphs is possible and does occur. This would tend to preserve rarer morphs from extinction. Polymorphism has a lot to do with the adaptation of a species to its environment, which may vary in colour, food supply, predation and in many other ways. Polymorphism is one good way the opportunities get to be used, it has survival value, and the selection of modifier genes may reinforce the polymorphism. In addition, polymorphism seems to be associated with a higher rate of speciation.

Polymorphism and niche diversity

G. Evelyn Hutchinson, a founder of niche research, commented 'It is very likely from an ecological point of view that all species, or at least all common species, consist of populations adapted to more than one niche'. He gave as examples sexual size dimorphism and mimicry. In many cases where the male is short-lived and smaller than the female, he does not compete with her during her late pre-adult and adult life. Size difference may permit both sexes to exploit different niches. In elaborate cases of mimicry, such as the African butterfly Papilio dardanus, female morphs mimic a range of distasteful models, often in the same region. The fitness of each type of mimic decreases as it becomes more common, so the polymorphism is maintained by frequency-dependent selection. Thus the efficiency of the mimicry is maintained in a much increased total population.

Investigative methods

Investigation of polymorphism requires use of both field and laboratory techniques. In the field:
- Detailed survey of occurrence, habits and predation.
- Selection of an ecological area or areas, with well-defined boundaries.
- Capture, mark, release, recapture data.
- Relative numbers and distribution of morphs.
- Estimation of population sizes.

And in the laboratory:
- Genetic data from crosses.
- Population cages.

- Chromosome cytology if possible.
- Use of chromatography or similar techniques if morphs are cryptic (for example, biochemical).

Both types of work are equally important. Without proper field-work, the significance of the polymorphism to the species is uncertain, without laboratory breeding, the genetic basis is obscure. Even with insects, the work may take many years, examples of Batesian mimicry noted in the nineteenth century are still being researched.

Genetics

Genetic polymorphism

Since all polymorphism has a genetic basis, genetic polymorphism has a particular meaning:

Genetic polymorphism is the simultaneous occurrence in the same locality of two or more discontinuous forms in such proportions that the rarest of them cannot be maintained just by recurrent mutation or immigration, originally defined by Ford. The later definition by Cavalli-Sforza and Bodmer is currently used: 'Genetic polymorphism is the occurrence in the same population of two or more alleles at one locus, each with appreciable frequency', where the minimum frequency is typically taken as 1%.

The definition has three parts: (i) sympatry: one interbreeding population, (ii) discrete forms and (iii) not maintained just by mutation.

In simple words, the term polymorphism was originally used to describe variations in shape and form that distinguish normal individuals within a species from each other. These days, geneticists use the term genetic polymorphisms to describe the inter-individual, functionally silent differences in DNA sequence that make each human genome unique.

Genetic polymorphism is actively and steadily maintained in populations by natural selection, in contrast to transient polymorphisms where a form is progressively replaced by another. By definition, genetic polymorphism relates to a balance or equilibrium between morphs. The mechanisms that conserve it are types of balancing selection.

Mechanisms of balancing selection

- Heterosis (or heterozygote advantage): 'Heterosis: the heterozygote at a locus is fitter than either homozygote'.
- Frequency dependent selection: The fitness of a particular phenotype is dependent on its frequency relative to other phenotypes in a given population. Example: prey switching, where rare morphs of prey are actually fitter due to predators concentrating on the more frequent morphs.
- Fitness varies in time and space: Fitness of a genotype may vary greatly between larval and adult stages, or between parts of a habitat range.
- Selection acts differently at different levels: The fitness of a genotype may depend on the fitness of other genotypes in the population: this covers many natural situations where the best thing to do (from the point of view of survival and reproduction) depends on what other members of the population are doing at the time.

Pleiotropism

Most genes have more than one effect on the phenotype of an organism (pleiotropism). Some of these effects may be visible, and others cryptic, so it is often important to look beyond the most obvious effects of a gene to identify other effects. Cases occur where a gene affects an unimportant visible character, yet a change in fitness is recorded. In such cases the gene's other (cryptic or 'physiological') effects may be responsible for the change in fitness. 'If a neutral trait is pleiotropically linked to an advantageous one, it may emerge because of a process of natural selection. It was selected but this doesn't mean it is an adaptation. The reason is that, although it was selected, there was no selection for that trait.'

Epistasis

Epistasis occurs when the expression of one gene is modified by another gene. For example, gene A only shows its effect when allele B1 (at another Locus) is present, but not if it is absent. This is one of the ways in which two or more genes may combine to produce a coordinated change in more than one characteristic (for instance, in mimicry). Unlike the supergene, epistatic genes do not need to be closely linked or even on the same chromosome. Both pleiotropism and epistasis show that a gene need not relate to a character in the simple manner that was once supposed.

Origin of supergenes

Although a polymorphism can be controlled by alleles at a single locus (e.g. human ABO blood groups), the more complex forms are controlled by supergenes consisting of several tightly linked genes on a single chromosome. Batesian mimicry in butterflies and heterostyly in angiosperms are good examples. There is a long-standing debate as to how this situation could have arisen, and the question is not yet resolved.

Relevance for Evolutionary Theory

Polymorphism was crucial to research in ecological genetics by E. B. Ford and his co-workers from the mid-1920s to the 1970s (similar work continues today, especially on mimicry). The results had a considerable effect on the mid-century evolutionary synthesis, and on present evolutionary theory. The work started at a time when natural selection was largely discounted as the leading mechanism for evolution, continued through the middle period when Sewall Wright's ideas on drift were prominent, to the last quarter of the 20th century when ideas such as Kimura's neutral theory of molecular evolution was given much attention.

The significance of the work on ecological genetics is that it has shown how important selection is in the evolution of natural populations, and that selection is a much stronger force than was envisaged even by those population geneticists who believed in its importance, such as Haldane and Fisher.

Examples

Sexual dimorphism: Most eukaryotes species use sexual reproduction, the division into two sexes is a dimorphism. The question of evolution of sex from asexual reproduction has engaged the attentions of biologists such as Charles Darwin, August Weismann, Ronald Fisher, George C. Williams, John Maynard Smith and W. D. Hamilton, with varied success.

Human polymorphisms: Apart from sexual dimorphism, there are many other examples of human genetic polymorphisms. Infectious disease has been a major factor in human mortality, and so has affected the evolution of human populations. Evidence is now strong that many polymorphisms are maintained in human populations by balancing selection.

Human blood groups: All the common blood types, such as the ABO blood group system, are genetic polymorphisms. Here we see a system where there are more than two morphs: the phenotypes A, B, AB and O are present in all human populations, but vary in proportion in different parts of the world. The phenotypes are controlled by multiple alleles at one locus. These polymorphisms are seemingly never eliminated by natural selection, the reason came from a study of disease statistics.

Sickle-cell anaemia: Such a balance is seen more simply in sickle-cell anaemia, which is found mostly in tropical populations in Africa and India. An individual homozygous for the recessive sickle hemoglobin, HgbS, has a short expectancy of life, whereas the life expectancy of the standard hemoglobin (HgbA) homozygote and also the heterozygote is normal (though heterozygote individuals will suffer periodic problems).

Duffy system

The Duffy antigen is a protein located on the surface of red blood cells, encoded by the FY (DARC) gene. The protein encoded by this gene is a non-specific receptor for several chemokines, and is the known entry-point for the human malarial parasites Plasmodium vivax and Plasmodium knowlesi. Polymorphisms in this gene are the basis of the Duffy blood group system.

Human taste morphisms

A famous puzzle in human genetics is the genetic ability to taste phenylthiocarbamide (phenylthiourea or PTC), a morphism which was discovered in 1931. This substance, which to some of us is bitter, and to others tasteless, is of no great significance in itself, yet it is a genetic dimorphism. Because of its high frequency (which varies in different ethnic groups) it must be connected to some function of selective value.

Lactose tolerance and intolerance

The ability to metabolise lactose, a sugar found in milk and other dairy products, is a prominent dimorphism that has been linked to recent human evolution.

MHC molecules

The genes of the major histocompatibility complex (MHC) are highly polymorphic, and this diversity plays a very important role in resistance to pathogens. This is true for other species as well.

Cuckoo

Over fifty species in this family of birds practice brood parasitism, the details are best seen in the Common cuckoo (Cuculus canorus). In a season the female lays one egg in 15–20 other bird nests. She removes some or all of the host's clutch of eggs, and lays an egg which closely matches the host eggs. In Britain the cuckoo lays small eggs that match the size of the smaller host's. The eggs are thick-shelled as a defense to protect the egg if the host detects the fraud. Reed warbler feeding a cuckoo chick (Cuculus canorus) is shown in Fig. 21.7. The intruded egg develops exceptionally quickly, when the newly hatched cuckoo is only ten hours old, and still blind, it exhibits an urge to eject the other eggs or nestlings. It rolls them into a special depression on its back and heaves them out of the nest. The cuckoo nestling is apparently able to pressure the host adults for feeding by mimicking the cries of the host nestlings. The diversity of the cuckoos eggs is extraordinary, the forms resembling those of its most usual hosts.

Grove snail

The grove snail, Cepaea nemoralis, is famous for the rich polymorphism of its shell. The system is controlled by a series of multiple alleles. The shell colour series is brown (genetically the top dominant trait), dark pink, light pink, very pale pink, dark yellow and light yellow (the bottom or universal recessive trait). Bands may be present or absent, and if present from one to five in number

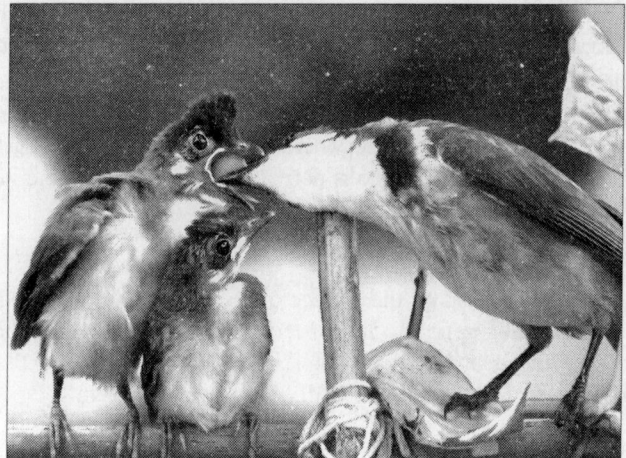

Fig. 21.7: Reed warbler feeding a cuckoo chick (Cuculus canorus).

Scarlet tiger moth

The scarlet tiger moth Callimorpha (Panaxia) dominula (family Arctiidae) occurs in continental Europe, western Asia and southern England. It is a day-flying moth, noxious-tasting, with brilliant warning colour in flight, but cryptic at rest. The moth is colonial in habit, and prefers marshy ground or hedgerows. The preferred food of the larvae is the herb Comfrey (Symphytum officinale). In England it has one generation per year.

Peppered moth

The peppered moth, Biston betularia, is justly famous as an example of a population responding in a heritable way to a significant change in their ecological circumstances. E.B. Ford described peppered moth evolution as 'one of the most striking, though not the most profound, evolutionary changes ever actually witnessed in nature'.

Two-spotted ladybird beetle

Adalia bipunctata, the two-spotted ladybird, is highly polymorphic. Its basic form is red with two black spots, but it has many other forms, the most important being melanic, with black elytra and red spots.

Mid-dorsal stripe in frogs

Some frog species display polymorphism by presence/absence of a light stripe going along the central part of their back. A light mid-dorsal stripe has been shown to be determined by a simple dominant gene in Rana limnocharis, Rana ridibunda, Rana sylvatica and Rana arvalis, that means the individuals both homozygtes by allele determining the presence of stripe and heterozygotes have the stripe, whereas only the individuals homozygotic by recessive allele are non-striped.

Ants

Ants exhibit a range of polymorphisms. First, there is their characteristic haplodiploid sex determination system, whereby all males are haploid, and all females diploid. Second, there is differentiation between both the females and males based mostly on feeding of larvae, which determines, for example, whether the imago is capable of reproduction. Lastly, there is differentiation of size and 'duties' (particularly of females), which are usually controlled by feeding and/or age, but which may sometimes be genetically controlled.

Reindeer and caribou

Genetic polymorphism of serum transferrins in reindeer is used in population and genetic studies. Gene concentrations of alleles in populations of reindeer of the North-East of Siberia were compared with those in reindeer inhabiting Norway, the northern regions of the European part of the USSR and from North American caribou.

Hoverfly polymorphism

Hoverfly mimics can be seen in almost any garden in the temperate zone. The Syrphidae are a large (5600+ species) family of flies, their imagos feed on nectar and pollen, and are well known for their mimicry of social hymenoptera. The mimicry is Batesian in nature: hoverflies are palatable but hymenoptera are generally unpalatable and may also be protected by stingers and/or armour.

Chromosome polymorphism in Drosophila

In the 1930s Dobzhansky and his co-workers collected *Drosophila* pseudoobscura and D. persimilis from wild populations in California and neighbouring states. Using Painter's technique they studied the polytene chromosomes and discovered that the wild populations were polymorphic for chromosomal inversions. All the flies look alike whatever inversions they carry: this is an example of a cryptic polymorphism. Accordingly, Dobzhansky favoured the idea that the morphs became fixed in the population by means of Sewall Wright's drift.

Chromosomal polymorphism in general

In 1973, M. J. D. White, then at the end of a long career investigating karyotypes, gave an interesting summary of the distribution of chromosome polymorphism. 'It is extremely difficult to get an adequate idea as to what fraction of the species of eukaryote organisms actually are polymorphic for structural rearrangements of the chromosomes. In Dipterous flies with polytene chromosomes... the figure is somewhere between 60 and 80 per cent. In grasshoppers pericentric inversion polymorphism is shown by only a small number of species. But in this group polymorphism for super-numerary chromosomes and chromosome regions is very strongly developed in many species.'

Heterostyly

An example of a botanical genetic polymorphism is heterostyly, in which flowers occur in different forms with different arrangements of the pistils and the stamens. The system is called heteromorphic self-incompatibility, and the general 'strategy' of stamens separated from pistils is known as herkogamy.

White-throated sparrows

The white-throated sparrow (Zonotrichia albicollis), a passerine bird of the American sparrow family Emberizidae, shows a clear dimorphism in both sexes throughout its large range. Their heads are either white-striped or tan-striped. These differences in plumage result from a balanced chromosomal inversion polymorphism, in white-striped (WS) birds, one copy of chromosome 2 is partly inverted, while in tan-striped (TS) birds, both copies are uninverted.

Darwin's finches

Whereas Darwin spent just five weeks in the Galápagos, and David Lack spent three months, Peter and Rosemary Grant and their colleagues have made research trips to the Galápagos for about thirty years, particularly studying Darwin's finches. Here we look briefly at the case of the large cactus finch, Geospiza conirostris, on Isla Genovesa (formerly Tower Island) which is formed from a shield volcano, and is home to a variety of birds. These birds, like all well-studied groups, show various kinds of morphism.

Common side-blotched lizards

Male common side-blotched lizards (Uta stansburiana) exhibit polymorphism in their throat pigmentation, and these different phenotypes are correlated with different mating strategies. Orange-throated males are the largest and most aggressive, defending large territories and keeping harems of females. Blue-throated males are of intermediate size, and guard smaller territories containing only a single female. Yellow-throated males are the smallest, and instead of holding territories they mimic females in order to sneak matings away from the other two morphs. The balance between these three morphs is maintained by frequency-dependent selection.

SINGLE-NUCLEOTIDE POLYMORPHISM

A single nucleotide polymorphism, also known as simple nucleotide polymorphism, (SNP, pronounced snip, plural snips) is a DNA sequence variation occurring commonly within a population (e.g. 1%) in which a single nucleotide — A, T, C or G — in the genome (or other shared sequence) differs between members of a biological species or paired chromosomes. For example, two sequenced DNA fragments from different individuals, AAGCCTA to AAGCTTA, contain a difference in a single nucleotide. In this case we say that there are two alleles. Almost all common SNPs have only two alleles. The genomic distribution of SNPs is not homogenous, SNPs occur in non-coding regions more frequently than in coding regions or, in general, where natural selection is acting and 'fixing' the allele (eliminating other variants) of the SNP that constitutes the most favourable genetic adaptation. Other factors, like genetic recombination and mutation rate, can also determine SNP density.

SNP density can be predicted by the presence of microsatellites: AT microsatellites in particular are potent predictors of SNP density, with long $(AT)(n)$ repeat tracts tending to be found in regions of significantly reduced SNP density and low GC content.

Within a population, SNPs can be assigned a minor allele frequency—the lowest allele frequency at a locus that is observed in a particular population. This is simply the lesser of the two allele frequencies for single-nucleotide polymorphisms. There are variations between human populations, so a SNP allele that is common in one geographical or ethnic group may be much rarer in another.

These genetic variations between individuals (particularly in non-coding parts of the genome) are sometimes exploited in DNA fingerprinting, which is used in forensic science. Also, these genetic variations underlie differences in our susceptibility to disease. The severity of illness and the way our body responds to treatments are also manifestations of genetic variations. For example, a single base mutation in the APOE (apolipoprotein E) gene is associated with a higher risk for Alzheimer disease.

Types of SNP

Single-nucleotide polymorphisms may fall within coding sequences of genes, non-coding regions of genes, or in the intergenic regions (regions between genes). SNPs within a coding sequence do not necessarily change the amino acid sequence of the protein that is produced, due to degeneracy of the genetic code.

SNPs in the coding region are of two types, synonymous and nonsynonymous SNPs. Synonymous SNPs do not affect the protein sequence while nonsynonymous SNPs change the amino acid sequence of protein. The nonsynonymous SNPs are of two types: missense and nonsense. SNPs that are not in protein-coding regions may still affect gene splicing, transcription factor binding, messenger RNA degradation, or the sequence of non-coding RNA. Gene expression affected by this type of SNP is referred to as an eSNP (expression SNP) and may be upstream or downstream from the gene.

Use

SNPs are studied, in biomedical research for comparing regions of the genome between cohorts (such as with matched cohorts with and without a disease) in genome-wide association studies. SNPs are studied in crop and livestock breeding programmes. SNPs are studied in genome-wide association studies (GWAS), e.g. as high-resolution markers in gene mapping related to diseases or normal traits.

Importance

Variations in the DNA sequences of humans can affect how humans develop diseases and respond to pathogens, chemicals, drugs, vaccines, and other agents. SNPs are also critical for personalised medicine. However, their greatest importance in biomedical research is for comparing regions of the genome between cohorts (such as with matched cohorts with and without a disease) in genome-wide association studies.

The study of SNPs is also important in crop and livestock breeding programmes. See SNP genotyping for details on the various methods used to identify SNPs.

SNPs are usually biallelic and thus easily assayed. A single SNP may cause a Mendelian disease. For complex diseases, SNPs do not usually function individually, rather, they work in coordination with other SNPs to manifest a disease condition as has been seen in Osteoporosis.

As of 8 June 2015, dbSNP listed 149,735,377 SNPs in humans.

SNPs have been used in genome-wide association studies (GWAS), e.g. as high-resolution markers in gene mapping related to diseases or normal traits. The knowledge of SNPs will help in understanding pharmacokinetics (PK) or pharmacodynamics, i.e. how drugs act in individuals with different genetic variants. A wide range of human diseases, e.g. sickle-cell anemia, ß-thalassemia and cystic fibrosis result from SNPs. Diseases with different SNPs may become relevant pharmacogenomic targets for drug therapy. Some SNPs are associated with the metabolism of different drugs.

SNPs without an observable impact on the phenotype (so called silent mutations) are still useful as genetic markers in genome-wide association studies, because of their quantity and the stable inheritance over generations.

On the other site, all types of SNPs can have observable phenotype or can result in disease:

- SNPs in non-coding regions can manifest in higher risk of cancer.
- SNPs in coding regions:
  - o Synonymous substitutions by the definition do not trigger amino acid change in the protein, but still can affect its function, e.g. seemingly silent mutation in the multidrug resistance gene 1 (MDR1), which codes for a cellular membrane pump that expels drugs from the cell, can slow down translation to allow the peptide chain to fold into an unusual conformation causing the mutant pump be less functional.
  - o Nonsynonymous substitutions:
    - › missense-single change in the base results in change in amino acid of protein and its malfunction which leads to disease (e.g. c.1580G>T SNP in LMNA gene-position 1580

(nt) in the DNA sequence (CGT codon) causing the guanine to be replaced with the thymine, yielding CTT codon in the DNA sequence, results at the protein level in the replacement of the arginine by the leucine in the position 527, at phenotype level this manifest with overlapping mandibuloacral dysplasia and progeria syndrome)

› nonsense-point mutation in a sequence of DNA that results in a premature stop codon, or a nonsense codon in the transcribed mRNA, and in a truncated, incomplete, and usually nonfunctional protein product (e.g. Cystic fibrosis caused by the G542X mutation in the cystic fibrosis transmembrane conductance regulator gene).

Examples

- rs6311 and rs6313 are SNPs in the Serotonin 5-HT2A receptor gene on human chromosome 13.
- A SNP in the F5 gene causes Factor V Leiden thrombophilia.
- rs3091244 is an example of a triallelic SNP in the CRP gene on human chromosome 1.
- TAS2R38 codes for PTC tasting ability, and contains 6 annotated SNPs.
- rs148649884 and rs138055828 in the FCN1 gene encoding M-ficolin crippled the ligand-binding capability of the recombinant M-ficolin.

Databases

As there are for genes, bioinformatics databases exist for SNPs. dbSNP is a SNP database from the National Center for Biotechnology Information (NCBI). Kaviar is a compendium of SNPs from multiple data sources including dbSNP. SNPedia is a wiki-style database supporting personal genome annotation, interpretation and analysis. The OMIM database describes the association between polymorphisms and diseases (e.g. gives diseases in text form), the Human Gene Mutation Database provides gene mutations causing or associated with human inherited diseases and functional SNPs, and GWAS Central allows users to visually interrogate the actual summary-level association data in one or more genome-wide association studies. The International SNP Map working group mapped the sequence flanking each SNP by alignment to the genomic sequence of large-insert clones in Genebank.

Nomenclature

The nomenclature for SNPs can be confusing: several variations can exist for an individual SNP and consensus has not yet been achieved. One approach is to write SNPs with a prefix, period and 'greater than' sign showing the wild-type and altered nucleotide or amino acid, for example, c.76A>T. SNPs are frequently referred to by their dbSNP rs number, as in the examples above.

SNP analysis

Analytical methods to discover novel SNPs and detect known SNPs include:

- DNA sequencing.
- Capillary electrophoresis.
- Mass spectrometry.
- Single-strand conformation polymorphism (SSCP).
- Single-base extension.
- Electrochemical analysis.
- Denaturing HPLC and gel electrophoresis.

- Restriction fragment length polymorphism.
- Hybridisation analysis.

MATING SYSTEM

A mating system is a way in which a group is structured in relation to sexual behaviour. The precise meaning depends upon the context. With respect to animals, the term describes which males and females mate, under which circumstances, recognised systems include monogamy, polygamy (which includes polygyny, polyandry, and polygynandry), and promiscuity, all of which lead to different mate choice outcomes and thus these systems affect how sexual selection works in the species which practice them. In plants, the term refers to the degree and circumstances of outcrossing. In human sociobiology, the terms have been extended to encompass the formation of relationships such as marriage.

In Plants

The primary mating systems in plants are outcrossing (cross-fertilisation), autogamy (self-fertilisation) and apomixis (asexual reproduction without fertilisation, but only when arising by modification of sexual function). Mixed mating systems, in which plants use two or even all three mating systems, are not uncommon.

A number of models have been used to describe the parameters of plant mating systems. The basic model is the mixed mating model, which is based on the assumption that every fertilisation is either self-fertilisation or completely random cross-fertilisation. More complex models relax this assumption, for example, the effective selfing model recognises that mating may be more common between pairs of closely related plants that between pairs of distantly related plants.

In Animals

The following are some of the mating systems generally recognised in animals:

- Monogamy: One male and one female have an exclusive mating relationship. The term 'pair bonding' often implies this. This is associated with one-male, one-female group compositions.
- Polygamy: Three types are recognised:
- Polygyny (the most common polygamous mating system in vertebrates so far studied): One male has an exclusive relationship with two or more females. This is associated with one-male, multi-female group compositions. Many perennial Vespula squamosa (southern Yellowjacket) colonies are polygynous.
- Polyandry: One female has an exclusive relationship with two or more males. This is very rare and is associated with multi-male, multi-female group compositions.
- Polygynandry: Polygynandry is a slight variation of this, where two or more males have an exclusive relationship with two or more females, the numbers of males and females don't have to be equal, and in vertebrate species studied so far, the number of males is usually less. This is associated with multi-male, multi-female group compositions.
- Promiscuity: A member of one sex within the social group mates with any member of the opposite sex. This is associated with multi-male, multi-female group compositions.

These mating relationships may or may not be associated with social relationships, in which the sexual partners stay together to become parenting partners. As the alternative term 'pair bonding' implies, this is usual in monogamy. In many polyandrous systems, the males and the female stay together to rear the young. In polygynous systems where the number of females paired with each male is low and the male will often stay with one female to help rear the young, while the other females rear their young on their own. In polygynandry, each of the males may assist one female, if all adults help rear all the young, the system is more usually called 'communal breeding'. In highly polygynous systems, and in promiscuous systems, paternal care of young is rare, or there may be no parental care at all.

These descriptions are idealised, and the social partnerships are often easier to observe than the mating relationships. In particular:

- The relationships are rarely exclusive for all individuals in a species. DNA fingerprinting studies have shown that even in pair-bonding, matings outside the pair (extra-pair copulations) occur with fair frequency, and a significant minority of offspring result from them.
- Some species show different mating systems in different circumstances, for example in different parts of their geographical range, or under different conditions of food availability
- Mixtures of the simple systems described above may occur.

In Humans

Compared to other vertebrates, where a species usually has a single mating system, human display great variety. Humans also differ by having formal marriages which in many cultures involve negotiation and arrangement between elder relatives. Regarding sexual dimorphism (see the section about animals above), humans falls in the intermediate group with moderate sex differences in body size but with relatively large testes. This indicates relatively frequent sperm competition which is supported by reports of extrapair paternity of 2–22% in socially monogamous and polygynous human societies. One estimate is that 83% of human societies are polygynous, 0.05% are polyandrous, and the rest are monogamous. Even the last group may at least in part be genetically polygynous.

Polygyny is associated with an increased sharing of subsistence provided by women. This is consistent with the theory that if women raise the children alone, men can concentrate on the mating effort. Polygyny is also associated with greater environmental variability in the form of variability of rainfall. This may increase the differences in the resources available to men. An important association is that polygyny is associated with a higher pathogen load in an area which may make having good genes in a male increasingly important. A high pathogen load also decreases the relative importance of sororal polygyny which may be because it becomes increasingly important to have genetic variability in the offspring (See Major histocompatibility complex and sexual selection).

Virtually all the terms used to describe animal mating systems were adopted from social anthropology, where they had been devised to describe systems of marriage. This shows that human sexual behavior is unusually flexible since, in most animal species, one mating system dominates. While there are close analogies between animal mating systems and human marriage institutions, these analogies should not be pressed too far, because in human societies, marriages typically have to be recognised by the entire social group in some way, and there is no equivalent process in animal societies. The temptation to draw conclusions about what is 'natural' for human sexual behavior from observations of animal mating systems should be resisted: a socio-biologist observing the kinds of behavior shown by humans in any other species would conclude that all known mating systems were natural for that species, depending on the circumstances or on individual differences.

- As culture increasingly affects human mating choices, ascertaining what is the 'natural' mating system of the human animal from a zoological perspective becomes increasingly difficult. Some clues can be taken from human anatomy, which is essentially unchanged from the prehistoric past.

- Humans have a large relative size of testes to body mass in comparison to most primates,
- Humans have a large ejaculate volume and sperm count in comparison to other primates,
- As compared to most primates, humans spend more time in copulation,
- As compared to most primates, humans copulate with greater frequency,
- The outward signs of estrous in women (i.e. higher body temperature, breast swelling, sugar cravings, etc.), are often perceived to be less obvious in comparison to the outward signs of ovulation in most other mammals,
- For most mammals, the estrous cycle and its outward signs bring on mating activity, the majority of female-initiated matings in humans coincides with estrous, but humans copulate throughout the reproductive cycle,
- After ejaculation/orgasm in males and females, humans release a hormone that has a sedative effect, however human females may remain sexually receptive and may remain in the plateau stage of orgasm if their orgasm has not been completed.

Some have suggested that these anatomical factors signify some degree of sperm competition, though as levels of genetic and societal promiscuity are highly varied across cultures, this evidence is far from conclusive.

MATING SYSTEMS IN SEXUAL ANIMALS

One of the most fascinating aspects of human life is how we choose our mates. Animals also choose their mates, sometimes with a great deal of care. Mating systems are important to understand because they reflect the result of natural selection on mate choice, and ultimately on strategies for maximising individual reproductive success. A mating system describes how males and females pair when choosing a mate. Males and females differ greatly in the investment each makes to reproduce, and may therefore approach mating with differing strategies. To study these differences, scientists observe mating systems and describe how males and females come together. When choosing mates, animals evolve species-typical strategies for maximising their reproductive success—this results in considerable diversity among animal species in their mating patterns.

Evolution of Sex

Asexually reproducing animals pass on all of their chromosomes, and consequently all copies of each gene, to their offspring. In contrast, due to meiosis, diploid sexually reproducing animals have two copies of each chromosome but only pass one copy of each chromosome on to an egg or sperm cell. This means that a sexually reproducing diploid animal only passes half of its total genes on to its offspring. Despite the cost of losing half of the potential passage of genes to the next generation, sexual reproduction is much more common than asexual reproduction among animals because it provides several evolutionary advantages. The major advantage of sexual reproduction comes from genetic recombination. Genetic recombination allows an organisms offspring to be genetically diverse. Sexual reproduction increases the chances of acquiring favourable mutations and is unlikely to propagate deleterious ones. Genetic diversity within a group of offspring is advantageous as the local environment changes. This idea becomes clear when we examine organisms that can reproduce both sexually and asexually. Aphids, for example, will favour asexual reproduction when their environment is stable. When the environment is going to turn cold, most species of aphids reproduce sexually, because sexual reproduction produces eggs that are freeze tolerant and can diapause during the winter. Genetic diversity may also lead to evolved defenses against parasites and disease. The mud snail, Potamopyrgus antipodarum, is host to several trematode parasites. Sexual individuals of this species are more common in areas where risk of trematode infection is high. In areas where the risk of infection is low, asexual individuals have displaced sexual ones. This suggests that the genetic diversity acquired from sexual reproduction is necessary for this species to defend against parasites, as asexual individuals may not easily survive in areas where parasites are high. A male bighorn sheep is shown in Fig. 21.8.

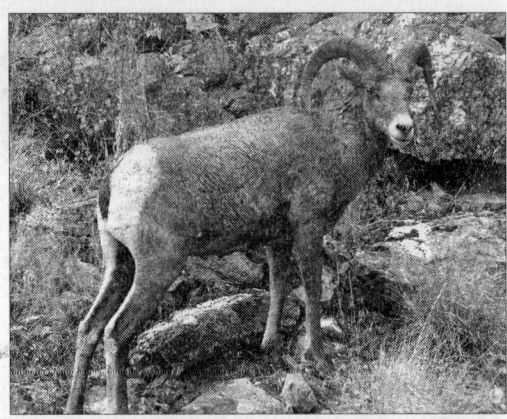

Fig. 21.8: A male bighorn sheep. The large horns are used in combat between males during mating season, and likely evolved as a result of intrasexual selection.

Sexual reproduction often involves evolutionary differentiation of males and females. Females typically produce significantly fewer gametes (eggs) than males and invest heavily in each one. On the other hand, males produce many gametes (sperm) and invest little into each one. These strong differences in gamete investment between the sexes leads to reproductive strategies between the sexes that, in some cases, conflict. Females may spend more care than males selecting a mate due to the high cost of their gametes.

Variance in Mating Success and Bateman's Principle

A key element of the study of mating systems is understanding how many mates an animal has in its lifetime. Bateman's principle helps to make predictions about mating success and number of mates. Bateman's principle postulates that variance among females in mating success is low, whereas variance among males in mating success is high. This stems from the fact that one mating in females should be enough to fertilise all their eggs whereas in males reproductive success is based on the number of times they have mated. In other words, nearly all females in a population mate and have offspring, but relatively few males mate successfully (Fig. 21.9). Those males that do mate tend to mate with many females-thus a few males have very high reproductive output, but many males have little or no reproductive output. This leads to the prediction that sexual selection should act more strongly on males, leading to greater elaboration of behavior and structures used in attracting mates in males than in females. Criticisms of Bateman's theory focus on the generality of the predictions. Contrary to the predictions of Bateman's principle, there are several possible advantages to female multiple matings. The female cichlid fish *Pseudotropheus spiliopterus* mates with any male they meet because they have a high risk of getting predated and a small population. This often leads to multiple matings by a single female. Mating with any male that is seen ensures that these cichlids have a chance at producing offspring. The female Malawi blue cichlid

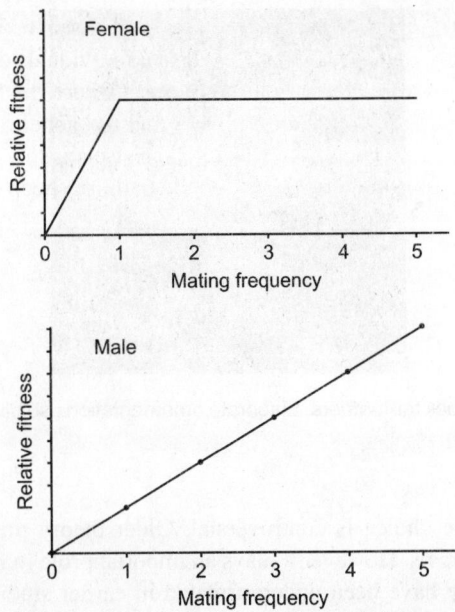

Fig. 21.9: Bateman's principle. These figures illustrate Bateman's principle—after one mating, female mating frequency increases and relative fitness remains constant, as the sperm from one mating is adequate to fertilise all the female's eggs. In males, as mating frequency increases relative fitness also increases proportionally.

has a high population but still participates in multiple matings. In this case multiple matings occur to avoid inbreeding and increase genetic diversity among the offspring. Additionally, multiple matings by females may increase the likelihood that they will find a compatible mate, one that is not sterile, or even help prevent infanticide.

Female Mate Choice

Mate choice is also a key element of mating systems. In most species, females are choosier when picking a mate than males. A significant reason for this is the higher investment females make in each gamete than males. Females may prefer certain males for a variety of reasons, including 'good genes', meaning that the male has attributes which predict better survivorship of the offspring, good potential parenting by the male, or possession of resources by the male that will support the offspring during their growth and development. Additionally, in most species, females are more likely to provide parental care. Females that carefully select their mates are at a lower risk of losing their reproductive investment. Males may be under strong selection for certain traits that are favoured by females. Most females look at these traits as indicators of their partner's fitness. Selection favours females that choose males that enhance the likelihood of her offspring's success.

Males with more elaborate ornamentation, or that are more colourful, can be displaying a good indicator of value as a mate, and may win the chance to mate with a particular female (Fig. 21.10). Although mating is important, it can be a costly event—females are predicted to be choosier about selecting their mates than males because of risks during mating, such as aggression or disease transmission, which may negatively impact the female's reproductive output.

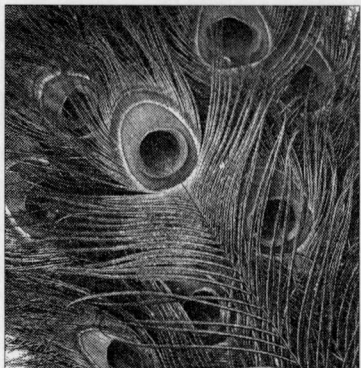

Fig. 21.10: Eyespots from peacock tail feathers. Elaborate ornamentation usually evolves in intrasexual selection and is used in mate choice.

Male Mate Choice

The importance of male mate choice is controversial. Older theory predicts that male mate choice should be less common in animals. However it plays an important role in many mating systems, and the cost of mating for males may have been underestimated in earlier studies. Male mate choice occurs most often when males are substantially involved in caring for their offspring, or when there is great variation in the quality of the females as mates within a population. If males are choosy about their mate, then over time females may evolve ornamentation or colouration that is subject to sexual selection.

Types of Mating Systems

Monogamy

Social monogamy is the behavioral pairing of a single male with a single female. It is most common in birds and rare in other animals. Theoretically, individuals in monogamous pairs will both contribute to the defense and parental care of offspring. Choosing an inappropriate mate could have a high fitness cost (see the sections above for more on mate choice). Because the costs of poor mate choice in monogamous species can be so high, in some instances organisms engage in strategies of either serial monogamy or extra-pair copulations. Extra-pair copulations are very common in birds. Monogamy reduces the potential for genetic variation among a female's offspring. By mating with more than one male over the course of her lifetime, a female gains higher genetic variation among her offspring. The benefits of monogamy, which are shared parental care and territorial resources, are maintained by having only one mate at a time, or by concealing extra-pair partnerships.

Polygyny

Polygyny is the association of one male with multiple females. This mating system is found in a few birds and insects, but is most common in mammals. Polygyny is a strategy used by males to increase their reproductive fitness.

Resource defense polygyny

In resource defense polygyny, groups of females are attracted to a resource—males then compete for territorial possession of the resource, and, by extension, mating priority with females at the resource.

Harems

Another common type of polygyny is membership in a harem, a defended group of females associated with one male. Females may initially associate in a harem for group defense, or they may be herded together by a male. Males compete for control of the groups. Harems typically exhibit a dominance hierarchy among the females in the group.

Leks

A lek is an aggregation of males that are each seeking to attract a mate. Within a lek, males typically perform sexual displays. Unlike most other mating systems, leks are not associated with resources. Aggregations of males may be near particularly attractive females or in areas where females are likely to travel. It is thought that males form leks because they attract more females than do isolated males. Attracting more females is a strategy used by males to help increase their reproductive success.

Polyandry

Polyandry is a group with one female and many males. Polyandry is a reproductive strategy that helps a female ensure reproductive success by providing her with multiple mating options.

Resource defense polyandry

In the Spotted Sandpiper, females control resources, which in turn controls male mating associations.

Cooperative polyandry

The Galapagos hawk exhibits cooperative polyandry. In this case all males in the group copulate with the female and all participate in brood provisioning.

Polygynandry

Some mating systems have looser male-female bonds within groups. In polygynandrous groups, multiple females and males mate with each other, and males may care for the broods of several females. Chimpanzees and bonobos rely on this strategy—it allows groups of males and females to live together and spend less time being concerned with mate competition. Polygynandry may be advantageous from the female's perspective because it causes paternity confusion, which decreases infanticide and allows her to have multiple males care for her brood.

Promiscuity

In promiscuity there are no pair bonds, and males and females, although sometimes choosy, often seem to mate randomly. As it is typically more advantageous for one or both sexes to pick their mate, promiscuity may occur in species for which the environment is unpredictable.

Sperm competition

Although sperm competition is not a type of mating system *per se*, it is a form of male-male competition that plays an important role in mating systems. If more than one male mates with a female in a short time period, competition can occur after the males have released their sperm. In other words, once a male has released sperm, its sperm must be the first to reach an egg. This is often apparent in animals that use external fertilisation. In aquatic animals that release their gametes into the water, animals that release the largest amount of sperm, and sperm that are highly capable of swimming, are likely to produce the most offspring. Animals with internal fertilisation also experience sperm competition. Several mechanisms have evolved to facilitate a male's reproductive success with females that have multiple mates. For example, in one species of damselfly, males physically remove any sperm present from the female before it mates. Sperm competition adds to the difficulty of obtaining a successful reproductive event by males. Thus, to transfer their genes to the next generation successfully, animals need to choose a suitable mate. Failure to do so leads to low or no reproductive success—that is, poor fitness. But reproductive success can also hinge on the number of mates, and on social interactions that extend beyond mating. By classifying social interactions, scientists have been able to identify different types of mating systems, such as monogamy and polygyny. The mating systems described in this article represent a variety of strategies to achieve reproductive success. The diversity of mating systems in animals is a fascinating example of the incredible variety of solutions that a complex evolutionary problem can yield.

EVOLUTION OF PLANT MATING SYSTEM

Diversity is the rule in living organisms. While this diversity is manifest at the various levels of the life tree, the diversity in the vegetable kingdom is probably the most apparent form, as revealed by the high diversity of plant morphologies and life histories even at small spatial scale. Since the first investigations in plant biology, botanists have always focused on the high variation of reproductive systems in plants and the floral diversity (forms and colours) in higher plants is one of the most obvious forms of variation. This has provided the basis for discriminating and classifying plants. In the 18th century, variation in sexual structures of plants has thus provided the basis for the Linnaean classification. Interestingly, such variation reveals variation and adaptation of the mating system and results from evolutionary processes in the phylogeny. Moreover, mating systems are central in population biology first because it ensures the maintenance (and eventually the growth) of populations and second because it shapes the transmission of phenotypic traits via the transmission of the hereditary material, thus conditioning evolutionary processes.

If the diversity of plant reproductive systems and floral morphologies have intrigued naturalists for a long time, botanic studies have long been only descriptive, without any evolutionary interpretation for the rise of such diversity. The first evolutionary interpretation has been proposed by Darwin who devoted three volumes on plants reproductive biology. Pollination processes and the dependence to pollen vectors was the central selective force in Darwin's view. The rise of mendelian laws and more recently population genetics, particularly Sir Ronald Fisher's work in the 1940's, have laid the foundation for a solid theoretical framework, based on gene dynamics. In contrast, the botanical tradition has been developed in a more empirical way. These two historical traditions have given birth to two different approaches that have remained relatively separated until recently. In the last ten years, the rapprochement is however perceptible. Interestingly, plant mating system studies is good example of fruitfull interaction between field data, theory and experiments. Field observations of flowering plants, interactions with pollinators have provided an important corpus of data. Also, mating system theory is an active field of research addressing major issues in evolutionary biology such as kin selection, the effect of deleterious mutations or mutual interactions. Finally, plant mating system is an area where the experimental approach to test specific hypotheses has been succesful thanks to suitable tools and techniques. As a matter of example, self-fertilisation can be precisely measured under natural conditions thanks to genetic markers, it can also be manipulated in laboratory thus allowing to test adaptive hypotheses.

In this section techniques and empirical data developed in plant mating system is discussed. Plant mating system encompasses various subfields such as the evolution of separate sexes, asexuality, the maintenance of sexual polymorphism in populations and the evolution in inbreeding regime. Because the evolution of selffertilisation has been intensively studied and because hermaphroditism is widespread in plants, my chapter will focus mainly on the evolution of self-fertilisation in hermaphroditic plants.

Inbreeders and Outbreeders in Plants

Diversity of flowering plants

In higher plants, the flower is the fundamental unit for sexual reproduction. While the perfect flower is hermaphroditic, bearing both male (stamen) and female (pistil) functions, variations around the perfect type are theoretically possible. Some individuals may bear only female flower while other individuals bear male flower. Also, different type of flowers can coexist within individuals. These variations may be predicted by various combinations and it is important to note that most of them have been found in nature. For example, dioecy corresponds to two types of individuals within populations: male bearing male flowers and female bearing female flowers. On this basis, up to seven types of sexual systems have been found in natural populations. Among them, hermaphroditism where a single sexual type occurs in populations is by far the most widespread sexual types in higher plants representing more than 70%. It is worth noting that hermaphroditism also exists in many animal phyla though it has mostly been studied in plants. The evolution of separate sexes has often been considered as a way to avoid inbreeding but Charnov has provided another important argument based on resource allocation. Even in absence of self-fertilisation in hermaphrodites, Charnov showed that dioecy may be selectively advantageous depending on ressource trade-offs between male and female functions.

PANMIXIA

Panmixia (or panmixis) means random mating. A panmictic population is one where all individuals are potential partners. This assumes that there are no mating restrictions, neither genetic nor behavioural, upon the population, and that therefore all recombination is possible. The Wahlund effect assumes that the overall population is panmictic. It has recently been reported that a panmictic population of Monostroma latissimum, a marine green algae, shows sympatric speciation in southwest Japanese islands. Although panmictic, molecular phylogenetics using nuclear introns revealed staggering diversification of the population. In genetics, random mating involves the mating of individuals regardless of any physical, genetic, or social preference. In other words, the mating between two organisms is not influenced by any environmental, hereditary, or social interaction. Hence, potential mates have an equal chance of being selected. Random mating is a factor assumed in the Hardy-Weinberg principle and is distinct from lack of natural selection: in viability selection for instance, selection occurs before mating.

In simpler terms, it is the ability of individuals in a population to move about freely within their habitat, possibly over a range of hundreds to thousands of miles, and thus breed with other members of the population that defines panmixia (or panmicticism).

To signify the importance of this, imagine several different finite populations of the same species (for example: a grazing herbivore), isolated from each other by some physical characteristic of the environment (dense forest areas separating grazing lands). As time progresses, natural selection and genetic drift will slowly move each population toward genetic differentiation that would make each population genetically unique (that could eventually lead to speciation events or extirpation). However, if the separating factor is removed before this happens (ex. a road is cut through the forest), and the individuals are allowed to move about freely, the individual populations will still be able to interbreed. As the species populations interbreed over time, they become more genetically uniform, functioning again as a single panmictic population.

In attempting to describe the mathematical properties of structured populations, Sewall Wright proposed a 'factor of Panmixia' (P) to include in the equations describing the gene frequencies in a population, and accounting for a population's tendency towards panmixia, while a 'factor of Fixation' (F) would account for a population's departure from the Hardy-Weinberg expectation, due to less than panmictic mating. In this formulation, the two quantities are complementary, i.e. P = 1 − F. From this factor of fixation, he later developed the F statistics.

HARDY–WEINBERG PRINCIPLE

The Hardy–Weinberg principle (also known as the Hardy–Weinberg equilibrium, model, theorem, or law) states that allele and genotype frequencies in a population will remain constant from generation to generation in the absence of other evolutionary influences. These influences include mate choice, mutation, selection, genetic drift, gene flow and meiotic drive. Because one or more of these influences are typically present in real populations, the Hardy–Weinberg principle describes an ideal condition against which the effects of these influences can be analysed (Fig. 21.11).

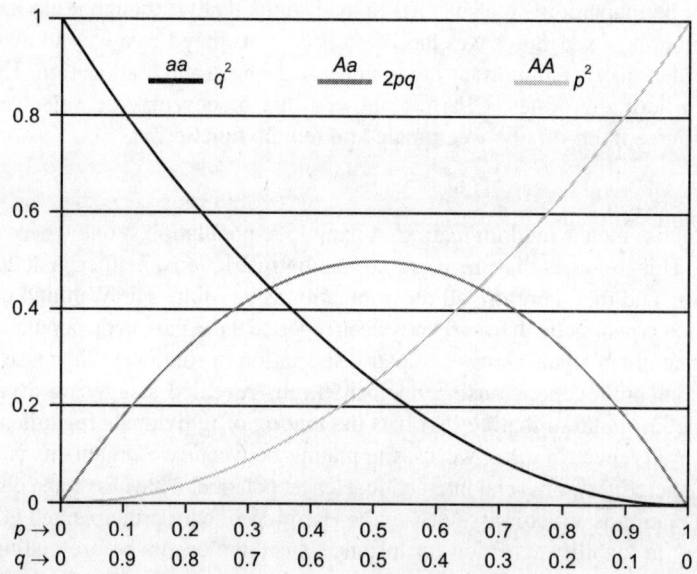

Fig. 21.11: Hardy–Weinberg proportions for two alleles: the horizontal axis shows the two allele frequencies *p* and *q* and the vertical axis shows the expected genotype frequencies. Each line shows one of the three possible genotypes.

In the simplest case of a single locus with two alleles denoted A and a with frequencies $f(A) = p$ and $f(a) = q$, respectively, the expected genotype frequencies are $f(AA) = p2$ for the AA homozygotes, $f(aa) = q^2$ for the aa homozygotes, and $f(Aa) = 2pq$ for the heterozygotes. The genotype proportions p^2, $2pq$, and q^2 are called the Hardy-Weinberg proportions. [Note that the sum of all genotype frequencies of this case is the binomial expansion of the square of the sum of p and q, and such a sum, as it represents the total of all possibilities, must be equal to 1. Therefore $(p + q)^2 = p^2 + 2pq + q^2 = 1$. The solution of this equation is $q = 1 - p$.

If union of gametes to produce the next generation is random, it can be shown that the new frequency f' satisfies $f'(A) = f(A)$ and $f'(a) = f(a)$. That is, allele frequencies are constant between generations.

This principle was named after G. H. Hardy and Wilhelm Weinberg, who first demonstrated it mathematically.

Consider a population of monoecious diploids, where each organism produces male and female gametes at equal frequency, and has two alleles at each gene locus. Organisms reproduce by random union of gametes (the 'gene pool' population model). A locus in this population has two alleles, A and a, that occur with initial frequencies $f_0(A) = p$ and $f_0(a) = q$, respectively. The allele frequencies at each generation are obtained by pooling together the alleles from each genotype of the same generation according to the expected contribution from the homozygote and heterozygote genotypes, which are 1 and 1/2, respectively:

$$f_t(A) = f_t(AA) + \frac{1}{2} f_t(Aa) \qquad \qquad \ldots(21.1)$$

$$f_t(a) = f_t(aa) + \frac{1}{2} f_t(aa) \qquad \qquad \ldots(21.2)$$

The different ways to form genotypes for the next generation can be shown in a Punnett square, where the proportion of each genotype is equal to the product of the row and column allele frequencies from the current generation.

The sum of the entries is $p^2 + 2pq + q^2 = 1$, as the genotype frequencies must sum to one. Note again that as $p + q = 1$, the binomial expansion of $(p + q)^2 = p^2 + 2pq + q^2 = 1$ gives the same relationships.

Summing the elements of the Punnett square or the binomial expansion, we obtain the expected genotype proportions among the offspring after a single generation:

$$f_1(AA) = p^2 = f_0(A)^2 \qquad \qquad \ldots(21.3)$$

$$f_1(Aa) = pq + qp = 2\,pq = 2\,f_0(A)\,f_0(a) \qquad \qquad \ldots(21.4)$$

$$f_1(aa) = q^2 = f_0(a)^2 \qquad \qquad \ldots(21.5)$$

These frequencies define the Hardy–Weinberg equilibrium. It should be mentioned that the genotype frequencies after the first generation need not equal the genotype frequencies from the initial generation, e.g. $f_1(AA)\,f_0(AA)$. However, the genotype frequencies for all future times will equal the Hardy-Weinberg frequencies, e.g. $f_t(AA) = f_1(AA)$ for $t > 1$. This follows since the genotype frequencies of the next generation depend only on the allele frequencies of the current generation which, as calculated by Eqs 21.1 and 21.2, are preserved from the initial generation:

$$f_t(A) = f_1(AA) + \frac{1}{2} f_1(Aa) = p^2 + pq = p(p+q) = p = f_0(A)$$

$$f_t(a) = f_1(aa) + \frac{1}{2} f_1(Aa) = q^2 + pq = q(p+q) = q = f_0(a)$$

For the more general case of dioecious diploids [organisms are either male or female] that reproduce by random mating of individuals, it is necessary to calculate the genotype frequencies from the nine possible matings between each parental genotype (AA, Aa, and aa) in either sex, weighted by the expected genotype contributions of each such mating.

Equivalently, one considers the six unique diploid-diploid combinations:

$$[(AA, AA), (AA, Aa), (AA, aa), (Aa, Aa), (Aa, aa), (aa, aa)]$$

and constructs a Punnett square for each, so as to calculate its contribution to the next generation's genotypes. These contributions are weighted according to the probability of each diploid-diploid combination, which follows a Multinomial distribution with $k = 3$. For example, the probability of the mating combination (AA, aa) is $2 f_t(AA) f_t(aa)$ and it can only result in the Aa genotype: $[0,1,0]$. Overall, the resulting genotype frequencies are calculated as:

$$[f_{t+1}(AA), f_{t+1}(Aa), f_{t+1}(aa)]$$

$$= f_t(AA) f_t(AA) [1,0,0] + 2 f_t(AA) f_t(Aa) [1/2, 1/2, 0] + 2 f_t(AA) f_t(aa) [0, 1, 0]$$

$$+ f_t(Aa) f_t(Aa) [1/4, 1/2, 1/4] + 2 f_t(Aa) f_t(aa) [0, 1/2, 1/2] + f_t(aa) f_t(aa) [0, 0, 1]$$

$$= \left[\left(f_t(AA) + \frac{f_t(Aa)}{2} \right)^2, 2\left(f_t(AA) + \frac{f_t(Aa)}{2} \right)\left(f_t(aa) + \frac{f_t(Aa)}{2} \right), \left(f_t(aa) + \frac{f_t(Aa)}{2} \right)^2 \right]$$

$$= [f_t(A)^2, 2f_t(A) f_t(a), f_t(a)^2]$$

As before, one can show that the allele frequencies at time $t + 1$ equal those at time t, and so, are constant in time. Similarly, the genotype frequencies depend only on the allele frequencies, and so, after time $t = 1$ are also constant in time.

If in either monoecious or dioecious organisms, either the allele or genotype proportions are initially unequal in either sex, it can be shown that constant proportions are obtained after one generation of random mating. If dioecious organisms are heterogametic and the gene locus is located on the X chromosome, it can be shown that if the allele frequencies are initially unequal in the two sexes [e.g. XX females and XY males, as in humans], $f'(a)$ in the heterogametic sex 'chases' $f(a)$ in the homogametic sex of the previous generation, until an equilibrium is reached at the weighted average of the two initial frequencies.

Deviations from Hardy–Weinberg Equilibrium

The seven assumptions underlying Hardy–Weinberg equilibrium are as follows:

- Organisms are diploid.
- Only sexual reproduction occurs.
- Generations are non overlapping.
- Mating is random.
- Population size is infinitely large.
- Allele frequencies are equal in the sexes.
- There is no migration, mutation or selection.

Violations of the Hardy–Weinberg assumptions can cause deviations from expectation. How this affects the population depends on the assumptions that are violated.

- Random mating: The HWP states the population will have the given genotypic frequencies (called Hardy–Weinberg proportions) after a single generation of random mating within the population. When the random mating assumption is violated, the population will not have Hardy–Weinberg proportions. A common cause of non-random mating is inbreeding, which causes an increase in homozygosity for all genes.

If a population violates one of the following four assumptions, the population may continue to have Hardy–Weinberg proportions each generation, but the allele frequencies will change over time.

- Selection, in general, causes allele frequencies to change, often quite rapidly. While directional selection eventually leads to the loss of all alleles except the favoured one, some forms of selection, such as balancing selection, lead to equilibrium without loss of alleles.

- Mutation will have a very subtle effect on allele frequencies. Mutation rates are of the order 10^{-4} to 10^{-8}, and the change in allele frequency will be, at most, the same order. Recurrent mutation will maintain alleles in the population, even if there is strong selection against them.

- Migration genetically links two or more populations together. In general, allele frequencies will become more homogeneous among the populations. Some models for migration inherently include nonrandom mating (Wahlund effect, for example). For those models, the Hardy–Weinberg proportions will normally not be valid.

- Small population size can cause a random change in allele frequencies. This is due to a sampling effect, and is called genetic drift. Sampling effects are most important when the allele is present in a small number of copies.

Sex linkage

Where the A gene is sex linked, the heterogametic sex (e.g. mammalian males, avian females) have only one copy of the gene (and are termed hemizygous), while the homogametic sex (e.g. human females) have two copies. The genotype frequencies at equilibrium are p and q for the heterogametic sex but p^2, $2pq$ and q^2 for the homogametic sex. For example, in humans red–green colourblindness is an X-linked recessive trait. In western European males, the trait affects about 1 in 12, ($q = 0.083$) whereas it affects about 1 in 200 females (0.005, compared to $q^2 = 0.007$), very close to Hardy–Weinberg proportions. If a population is brought together with males and females with a different allele frequency in each subpopulation (males or females), the allele frequency of the male population in the next generation will follow that of the female population because each son receives its X chromosome from its mother. The population converges on equilibrium very quickly.

NON-RANDOM MATING, INBREEDING AND POPULATION STRUCTURE

Jewelweed, *Impatiens capensis* (Fig. 21.12), is a common woodland flower in the Eastern US. You may have seen the swollen seed pods that explosively pop when you touch time, which is the source of an alternative name for this plant, 'touch-me-not'. Another interesting thing is that it produces two kinds of flowers. Many of the flowers are orange and conspicuous. Those flowers have various features to attract pollinators, primarily nectar that is secreted at the base of the curved spur in the back of the flower. Bees and hummingbirds visit the flower to feed on the nectar and in the process transfer some of the pollen from one flower to another.

Most plant species produce both pollen and ovules in the same flower so there is a potential for self-fertilisation to occur. That can happen either when pollen is transferred to the stigma of the same flower, or when pollen is transferred between flowers on the same plant. The showy flowers have evolved various mechanisms to limit self-fertilisation within a flower. They typically produce pollen for one day, after which the anther falls off to reveal the stigma. Therefore pollen receipt (female function) is separated in time from pollen donation (male function). Within flower selfing is minimal because pollen and stigma are not functional at the same time. In addition to the showy orange flowers, the plant produces another set of flowers that never even open. Those tiny green *cleistogamous* (meaning 'closed

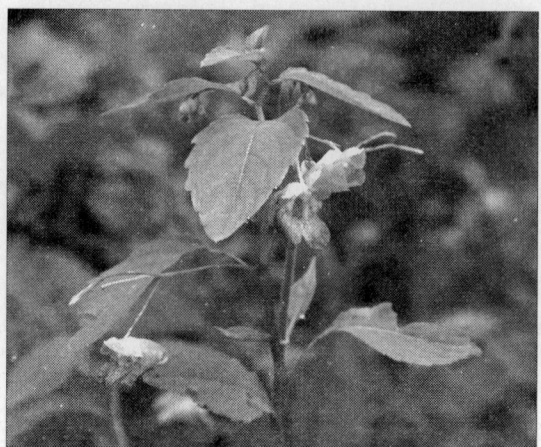

Fig. 21.12: *Impatiens capensis.*

mating') flowers look more like buds. Pollen is shed inside the unopened flower directly onto its stigma, so all of the seeds are produced by self-fertilisation. Presumably the cleistogamous flowers have a reproductive assurance advantage, since they are able to produce seeds even in the absence of pollinators. Thus Impatiens shows two extremes of mating: 100% self-fertilisation in the tiny cleistogamous flowers, and normal crossing between plants in the showy (*'chasmogamous'*) flowers.

HETEROZYGOTE ADVANTAGE

A heterozygote advantage (heterozygous advantage) describes the case in which the heterozygote genotype has a higher relative fitness than either the homozygote dominant or homozygote recessive genotype. The specific case of heterozygote advantage due to a single locus is known as overdominance. In more general terms, overdominance is a condition in genetics where the phenotype of the heterozygote lies outside of the phenotypical range of both homozygote parents, and heterozygous individuals have a higher fitness than homozygous individuals.

Polymorphism can be maintained by selection favouring the heterozygote, and this mechanism is used to explain the occurrence of some kinds of genetic variability. A common example is the case where the heterozygote conveys both advantages and disadvantages, while both homozygotes convey a disadvantage. A well-established case of heterozygote advantage is that of the gene involved in sickle cell anaemia. Often, the advantages and disadvantages conveyed are rather complicated, because more than one gene may influence a given trait or morph.

Major genes almost always have multiple effects (pleiotropism), which can simultaneously convey separate advantageous traits and disadvantageous traits upon the same organism. In this instance, the state of the organisms environment will provide selection, with a net effect either favouring or working in opposition to the gene, until an environmentally determined equilibrium is reached. Heterozygote advantage is a major underlying mechanism for heterosis, or 'hybrid vigor', which is the improved or increased function of any biological quality in a hybrid offspring. Previous research, comparing measures of dominance, overdominance and epistasis (mostly in plants), found that the majority of cases of heterozygote advantage were due to complementation (or dominance), the masking of deleterious recessive alleles by wild-type alleles, as discussed in the section Heterosis and Complementation (genetics), but there were also findings of overdominance, especially in rice. More recent research, however, has established that there is also an epigenetic contribution to heterozygote advantage, primarily as determined in plants, though also reported in mice.

Heterozygote Advantage in Theory

When two populations of any sexual organism are separated and kept isolated from each other, the frequencies of deleterious mutations in the two populations will differ over time, by genetic drift. It is highly unlikely, however, that the same deleterious mutations will be prevalent in both populations after a long period of separation. Since loss-of-function mutations tend to be recessive (given that dominant mutations of this type generally prevent the organism from reproducing and thereby passing the gene on to the next generation), the result of any cross between the two populations will be fitter than the parent. This section deals with the specific case of fitness overdominance, where the fitness advantage of the cross is caused by being heterozygous at one specific locus alone.

Experimental confirmation

Cases of heterozygote advantage have been demonstrated in several organisms, including humans. The first experimental confirmation of heterozygote advantage was with *Drosophila melanogaster*, a fruit fly that has been a model organism for genetic research. In a classic study, Kalmus demonstrated how polymorphism can persist in a population through heterozygote advantage.

If weakness were the only effect of the mutant allele, so it conveyed only disadvantages, natural selection would weed out this version of the gene until it became extinct from the population. However, the same mutation also conveyed advantages, providing improved viability for heterozygous individuals. The heterozygote expressed none of the disadvantages of homozygotes, yet gained improved viability. The homozygote wild type was perfectly healthy, but did not possess the improved viability of the heterozygote, and was thus at a disadvantage compared to the heterozygote in survival and reproduction.

This mutation, which at first glance appeared to be harmful, conferred enough of an advantage to heterozygotes to make it beneficial, so that it remained at dynamic equilibrium in the gene pool. Kalmus introduced flies with the ebony mutation to a wild-type population. The ebony allele persisted through many generations of flies in the study, at genotype frequencies that varied from 8 to 30%. In experimental populations, the ebony allele was more prevalent and therefore advantageous when flies were raised at low, dry temperatures, but less so in warm, moist environments.

Heterozygote Advantage in Human Genetics

Sickle-cell anemia

Sickle-cell anemia (SCA) is a genetic disorder caused by the presence of two incompletely recessive alleles. When a sufferer's red blood cells are exposed to low-oxygen conditions, the cells lose their healthy round shape and become sickle-shaped. This deformation of the cells can cause them to become lodged in capillaries, depriving other parts of the body of sufficient oxygen. When untreated, a person with SCA may suffer from painful periodic bouts, often causing damage to internal organs, strokes, or anemia. Typically, the disease results in premature death.

Because the genetic disorder is incompletely recessive, a person with only one SCA allele and one unaffected allele will have a 'mixed' phenotype: The sufferer will not experience the ill effects of the disease, yet will still possess a sickle cell trait, whereby some of the red blood cells undergo benign effects of SCA, but nothing severe enough to be harmful. Those afflicted with sickle-cell trait are also known as carriers: If two carriers have a child, there is a 25% chance their child will have SCA, a 50% chance their child will be a carrier, and a 25% chance that the child will neither have SCA nor be a carrier. Were the presence of the SCA allele to confer only negative traits, its allele frequency would be expected to decrease generation after generation, until its presence were completely eliminated by selection and by chance.

However, convincing evidence indicates, in areas with persistent malaria outbreaks, individuals with the heterozygous state have a distinct advantage (and this is why individuals with heterozygous alleles are far more common in these areas). Those with the benign sickle trait possess a resistance to malarial infection. The pathogen that causes the disease spends part of its cycle in the red blood cells and triggers an abnormal drop in oxygen levels in the cell. In carriers, this drop is sufficient to trigger the full sickle-cell reaction, which leads to infected cells being rapidly removed from circulation and strongly limiting the infection's progress. These individuals have a great resistance to infection and have a greater chance of surviving outbreaks. However, those with two alleles for SCA may survive malaria, but will typically die from their genetic disease unless they have access to advanced medical care. Those of the homozygous 'normal' or wild-type case will have a greater chance of passing on their genes successfully, in that there is no chance of their offspring's suffering from SCA, yet, they are more susceptible to dying from malarial infection before they have a chance to pass on their genes.

This resistance to infection is the main reason the SCA allele and SCA disease still exist. It is found in greatest frequency in populations where malaria was and often still is a serious problem. Approximately one in 375 African Americans is a carrier, as their recent ancestry is from malaria-stricken regions, far fewer than in Central Africa. Other populations in Africa, India, the Mediterranean and the Middle East have higher allele frequencies, as well. As effective antimalarial treatment becomes increasingly available to malaria-stricken populations, the allele frequency for SCA is expected to decrease, so long as SCA treatments are unavailable or only partially effective. If effective sickle-cell anemia treatments become available to the same degree, allele frequencies should remain at their present levels in these populations.

In this context, 'treatment effectiveness' refers to the reproductive fitness it grants, rather than the degree of suffering alleviation.

Cystic fibrosis

Cystic fibrosis (CF) is an autosomal recessive hereditary monogenic disease of the lungs, sweat glands and digestive system. The disorder is caused by the malfunction of the CFTR protein, which controls intermembrane transport of chloride ions, which is vital to maintaining equilibrium of water in the body. The malfunctioning protein causes viscous mucus to form in the lungs and intestinal tract. Before modern times, children born with CF would have a life expectancy of only a few years, but modern medicine has made it possible for these people to live into adulthood. However, even in these individuals, CF typically causes male infertility. It is the most common genetic disease among people of European descent. The presence of a single CF mutation may influence survival of people affected by diseases involving loss of body fluid, typically due to diarrhea. The most common of these maladies is cholera, which throughout history has killed many Europeans. Those with cholera would often die of dehydration due to intestinal water losses. A mouse model of CF was used to study resistance to cholera, and the results were published in Science in 1994. The heterozygote (carrier) mouse had less secretory diarrhea than normal, noncarrier mice.

Thus, it appeared for a time that resistance to cholera explained the selective advantage to being a carrier for CF and why the carrier state was so frequent.

This theory has been called into question. Hogenauer, and others have challenged this popular theory with a human study. Prior data were based solely on mouse experiments. These authors found the heterozygote state was indistinguishable from the noncarrier state. Another theory for the prevalence of the CF mutation is that it provides resistance to tuberculosis. Tuberculosis was responsible for 20% of all European deaths between 1600 and 1900, so even partial protection against the disease could account for the current gene frequency. As of 2007, the selective pressure for the high gene prevalence of CF mutations is still uncertain. Approximately one in 25 persons of European descent is a carrier of the disease, and one in 2500 to 3000 children born is affected by Cystic fibrosis.

Triosephosphate isomerase

Triosephosphate isomerase (TPI) is a central enzyme of glycolysis, the main pathway for cells to obtain energy by metabolising sugars. In humans, certain mutations within this enzyme, which affect the dimerisation of this protein, are causal for a rare disease, triosephosphate isomerase deficiency. Other mutations, which inactivate the enzyme (= null alleles) are lethal when inherited homozygously (two defective copies of the TPI gene), but have no obvious effect in heterozygotes (one defective and one normal copy). However, the frequency of heterozygous null alleles is much higher than expected, indicating a heterozygous advantage for TPI null alleles. The reason is unknown, however, new scientific results are suggesting cells having reduced TPI activity are more resistant against oxidative stress.

Resistance to hepatitis C virus infection

There is evidence that genetic heterozygosity in humans provides increased resistance to certain viral infections. A significantly lower proportion of HLA-DRB1 heterozygosity exists among HCV-infected cases than uninfected cases. The differences were more pronounced with alleles represented as functional supertypes ($P = 1.05 \times 10^{-6}$) than those represented as low-resolution genotypes ($P = 1.99 \times 10^{-3}$). These findings constitute evidence that heterozygosity provides an advantage among carriers of different supertype HLA-DRB1 alleles against HCV infection progression to end-stage liver disease in a large-scale, long-term study population.

MHC heterozygosity and human scent preferences

Multiple studies have shown, in double-blind experiments, females prefer the scent of males who are heterozygous at all three MHC loci. The reasons proposed for these findings are speculative, however, it has been argued that heterozygosity at MHC loci results in more alleles to fight against a wider variety of diseases, possibly increasing survival rates against a wider range of infectious diseases. The latter claim has been tested in an experiment, which showed outbreeding mice to exhibit MHC heterozygosity enhanced their health and survival rates against multiple-strain infections.

SEX LINKAGE

Sex linkage is the phenotypic expression of an allele related to the chromosomal sex of the individual. This mode of inheritance is in contrast to the inheritance of traits on autosomal chromosomes, where both sexes have the same probability of inheritance. Since humans have many more genes on the X than the Y, there are many more X-linked traits than Y-linked traits.

In mammals, the female is the homogametic sex, with two X chromosomes (XX), while the male is heterogametic, with one X and one Y chromosome (XY). Genes on the X or Y chromosome are called sex-linked.

In birds, the opposite is true: the male is the homogametic sex, having two Z chromosomes (ZZ), and the female (hen) is heterogametic, having one Z and one W chromosome (ZW).

X-linked recessive traits are expressed in all heterogametics, but are only expressed in those homogametics that are homozygous for the recessive allele. For example, an X-linked recessive allele in humans causes haemophilia. Haemophilia is much more common in males than females because males are hemizygous they only have one copy of the gene in question and therefore express the trait when they inherit one mutant allele. In contrast, a female must inherit two mutant alleles, a less frequent event since the mutant allele is rare in the population. Tsarevich Alexei of Russia was the most famous sufferer of X-linked haemophilia.

The incidence of recessive X-linked phenotypes in females is the square of that in males (squaring a proportion less than one gives an outcome closer to 0 than the original). If 1 in 20 males in a human population are red-green colour blind, then 1 in 400 females in the population are expected to be colour-blind (1/20)*(1/20). (The term 'colour-blind' is not completely accurate. There are degrees of weakness in colour vision and it is now called 'colour vision deficiency'.)

X-linked traits are maternally inherited from carrier mothers or from an affected father. Each son born to a carrier mother has a 50% probability of inheriting the X-chromosome carrying the mutant allele. There are a few Y-linked traits, these are inherited from father.

X-linked Dominant Inheritance

Each child of a mother affected with an X-linked dominant trait has a 50% chance of inheriting the mutation and thus being affected with the disorder. If only the father is affected, 100% of the daughters will be affected, since they inherit their father's X-chromosome, and 0% of the sons will be affected, since they inherit their father's Y-chromosome.

X-linked Recessive Inheritance

Females possessing one X-linked recessive mutation are considered carriers and will generally not manifest clinical symptoms of the disorder. All males possessing an X-linked recessive mutation will be affected, since males have only a single X-chromosome and therefore have only one copy of X-linked genes. All offspring of a carrier female have a 50% chance of inheriting the mutation if the father does not carry the recessive allele. All female children of an affected father will be carriers (assuming the mother is not affected or a carrier), as daughters possess their father's X-chromosome. No male children of an affected father will be affected, as males only inherit their father's Y-chromosome.

Y-linked

Various failures in the SRY genes.

Sex-linked traits in other animals

- Fur colour in domestic cats: The gene that causes orange pigment is on the X chromosome, thus a Calico or tortoiseshell cat, with both black (or gray) and orange pigment, is nearly always female.
- White eyes in *Drosophila melanogaster* flies—the first sex-linked gene discovered in *Drosophila*.
- The first sex-linked gene ever discovered was the 'lacticolour' X-linked recessive gene in the moth Abraxas grossulariata by Leonard Doncaster.

DNA PROFILING

DNA profiling (also called DNA fingerprinting, DNA testing, or DNA typing) is a forensic technique used to identify individuals by characteristics of their DNA. A DNA profile is a small set of DNA variations that is very likely to be different in all unrelated individuals, thereby being as unique to individuals as are fingerprints (hence the alternate name for the technique). DNA profiling should not be confused with full genome sequencing. First developed and used in 1985, DNA profiling is used in, for example, parentage testing and criminal investigation, to identify a person or to place a person at a crime scene, techniques which are now employed globally in forensic science to facilitate police detective work and help clarify paternity and immigration disputes.

Although 99.9% of human DNA sequences are the same in every person, enough of the DNA is different that it is possible to distinguish one individual from another, unless they are monozygotic ('identical') twins. DNA profiling uses repetitive ('repeat') sequences that are highly variable, called variable number tandem repeats (VNTRs), in particular short tandem repeats (STRs). VNTR loci are very similar between closely related humans, but are so variable that unrelated individuals are extremely unlikely to have the same VNTRs.

DNA Profiling Process

Developed by Professor of Genetics Sir Alec Jeffreys, the process begins with a sample of an individual's DNA (typically called a 'reference sample'). The most desirable method of collecting a reference sample is the use of a buccal swab, as this reduces the possibility of contamination. When this is not available (e.g. because a court order is needed but not obtainable) other methods may need to be used to collect a sample of blood, saliva, semen, or other appropriate fluid or tissue from personal items (e.g. a toothbrush, razor) or from stored samples (e.g. banked sperm or biopsy tissue). Samples obtained from blood relatives (related by birth, not marriage) can provide an indication of an individual's profile, as could human remains that had been previously profiled.

A reference sample is then analysed to create the individual's DNA profile using one of a number of techniques, discussed below. The DNA profile is then compared against another sample to determine whether there is a genetic match.

RFLP analysis

The first methods for finding out genetics used for DNA profiling involved RFLP analysis. DNA is collected from cells, such as a blood sample, and cut into small pieces using a restriction enzyme (a restriction digest). This generates thousands of DNA fragments of differing sizes as a consequence of variations between DNA sequences of different individuals. The fragments are then separated on the basis of size using gel electrophoresis. The separated fragments are then transferred to a nitrocellulose or nylon filter, this procedure is called a Southern blot. The DNA fragments within the blot are permanently fixed to the filter, and the DNA strands are denatured. Radiolabeled probe molecules are then added that are complementary to sequences in the genome that contain repeat sequences. These repeat sequences tend to vary in length among different individuals and are called variable number tandem repeat sequences or VNTRs. The probe molecules hybridise to DNA fragments containing the repeat sequences and excess probe molecules are washed away. The blot is then exposed to an X-ray film. Fragments of DNA that have bound to the probe molecules appear as dark bands on the film.

PCR analysis

Developed by Kary Mullis in 1983, a process was reported by which specific portions of the sample DNA can be amplified almost indefinitely. This has revolutionised the whole field of DNA study. The process, the polymerase chain reaction (PCR), mimics the biological process of DNA replication, but confines it to specific DNA sequences of interest. With the invention of the PCR technique, DNA profiling took huge strides forward in both discriminating power and the ability to recover information from very small (or degraded) starting samples.

STR analysis

The system of DNA profiling used today is based on PCR and uses simple sequences or short tandem repeats (STR). This method uses highly polymorphic regions that have short repeated sequences of DNA (the most common is 4 bases repeated, but there are other lengths in use, including 3 and 5 bases). Because unrelated people almost certainly have different numbers of repeat units, STRs can be used to discriminate between unrelated individuals. These STR loci (locations on a chromosome) are targeted with sequence-specific primers and amplified using PCR. The DNA fragments that result are then separated and detected using electrophoresis. There are two common methods of separation and detection, capillary electrophoresis (CE) and gel electrophoresis.

AmpFLP

Another technique, AmpFLP, or amplified fragment length polymorphism was also put into practice during the early 1990s. This technique was also faster than RFLP analysis and used PCR to amplify DNA samples. It relied on variable number tandem repeat (VNTR) polymorphisms to distinguish various alleles, which were separated on a polyacrylamide gel using an allelic ladder (as opposed to a molecular weight ladder).

DNA family relationship analysis

Using PCR technology, DNA analysis is widely applied to determine genetic family relationships such as paternity, maternity, siblingship and other kinships. During conception, the father's sperm cell and the mother's egg cell, each containing half the amount of DNA found in other body cells, meet and fuse to form a fertilised egg, called a zygote. The zygote contains a complete set of DNA molecules, a unique combination of DNA from both parents. This zygote divides and multiplies into an embryo and later, a full human being.

Y-chromosome analysis

Recent innovations have included the creation of primers targeting polymorphic regions on the Y-chromosome (Y-STR), which allows resolution of a mixed DNA sample from a male and female or cases in which a differential extraction is not possible. Y-chromosomes are paternally inherited, so Y-STR analysis can help in the identification of paternally related males. Y-STR analysis was performed in the Sally Hemings controversy to determine if Thomas Jefferson had sired a son with one of his slaves. The analysis of the Y-chromosome yields weaker results than autosomal chromosome analysis. The Y male sex-determining chromosome, as it is inherited only by males from their fathers, is almost identical along the patrilineal line. This leads to a less precise analysis than if autosomal chromosomes were testing, because of the random matching that occurs between pairs of chromosomes as zygotes are being made.

Mitochondrial analysis

For highly degraded samples, it is sometimes impossible to get a complete profile of the 13 CODIS STRs. In these situations, mitochondrial DNA (mtDNA) is sometimes typed due to there being many copies of mtDNA in a cell, while there may only be 1–2 copies of the nuclear DNA. Forensic scientists amplify the HV1 and HV2 regions of the mtDNA, and then sequence each region and compare single-nucleotide differences to a reference. Because mtDNA is maternally inherited, directly linked maternal relatives can be used as match references, such as one's maternal grandmother's daughter's son. In general, a difference of two or more nucleotides is considered to be an exclusion. Heteroplasmy and poly-C differences may throw off straight sequence comparisons, so some expertise on the part of the analyst is required. mtDNA is useful in determining clear identities, such as those of missing people when a maternally linked relative can be found. mtDNA testing was used in determining that Anna Anderson was not the Russian princess she had claimed to be, Anastasia Romanov.

DNA databases

An early application of a DNA database was the compilation of A Mitochondrial DNA Concordance, prepared by Kevin W. P. Miller and John L. Dawson at the University of Cambridge from 1996 to 1998 from data collected as part of Miller's PhD thesis. There are now several DNA databases in existence around the world. Some are private, but most of the largest databases are government controlled.

Fake DNA evidence

In one case, a criminal even planted fake DNA evidence in his own body: John Schneeberger raped one of his sedated patients in 1992 and left semen on her underwear. Police drew what they believed to be Schneeberger's blood and compared its DNA against the crime scene semen DNA on three occasions, never showing a match. It turned out that he had surgically inserted a Penrose drain into his arm and filled it with foreign blood and anticoagulants.

Development of artificial DNA

In August 2009, scientists in Israel raised serious doubts concerning the use of DNA by law enforcement as the ultimate method of identification. In a paper published in the journal Forensic Science International: Genetics, the Israeli researchers demonstrated that it is possible to manufacture DNA in a laboratory, thus falsifying DNA evidence. The scientists fabricated saliva and blood samples, which originally contained DNA from a person other than the supposed donor of the blood and saliva.

INBREEDING

Inbreeding is the sexual reproduction of offspring from the mating or breeding of individuals or organisms that are closely related genetically. By analogy, the term is used in human reproduction, but more commonly refers to the genetic disorders and other consequences that arise from incestuous sexual relationships and consanguinity. Inbreeding results in homozygosity, which can increase the chances of offspring being affected by recessive or deleterious traits. This generally leads to a decreased biological fitness of a population (called inbreeding depression), which is its ability to survive and reproduce. An individual who inherits such deleterious traits is referred to as inbred. The avoidance of such deleterious recessive alleles caused by inbreeding, via inbreeding avoidance mechanisms, is the main selective reason for outcrossing. Crossbreeding between populations also often has positive effects on fitness-related traits. Inbreeding is a technique used in selective breeding. In livestock breeding, breeders may use inbreeding when, for example, trying to establish a new and desirable trait in the stock, but will need to watch for undesirable characteristics in offspring, which can then be eliminated through further selective breeding or culling. Inbreeding is used to reveal deleterious recessive alleles, which can then be eliminated through assortative breeding or through culling. In plant breeding, inbred lines are used as stocks for the creation of hybrid lines to make use of the effects of heterosis. Inbreeding in plants also occurs naturally in the form of self-pollination.

Offspring of biologically related persons are subject to the possible effect of inbreeding, such as congenital birth defects. The chances of such disorders is increased the closer the relationship of the biological parents. This is because such pairings increase the proportion of homozygous zygotes in the offspring, in particular deleterious recessive alleles, which produce such disorders. Because most recessive alleles are rare in populations, it is unlikely that two unrelated marriage partners will both be carriers of the alleles. However, because close relatives share a large fraction of their alleles, the probability that any such deleterious allele is inherited from the common ancestor through both parents is increased dramatically. Contrary to common belief, inbreeding does not in itself alter allele frequencies, but rather increases the relative proportion of homozygotes to heterozygotes. However, because the increased proportion of deleterious homozygotes exposes the allele to natural selection, in the long run its frequency decreases more rapidly in inbred population. In the short term, incestuous reproduction is expected to produce increases in spontaneous abortions of zygotes, perinatal deaths, and postnatal offspring with birth defects. The advantages of inbreeding may be the result of a tendency to preserve the structures of alleles interacting at different loci that have been adapted together by a common selective history.

Malformations or harmful traits can stay within a population due to a high homozygosity rate and it will cause a population to become fixed for certain traits, like having too many bones in an area, like the vertebral column in wolves on Isle Royale or having cranial abnormalities in Northern elephant seals, where their cranial bone length in the lower mandibular tooth row has changed. Having a high homozygosity rate is bad for a population because it will unmask recessive deleterious alleles generated by mutations, reduce heterozygote advantage, and it is detrimental to the survival of small, endangered animal populations. When there are deleterious recessive alleles in a population it can cause inbreeding depression. The authors think that it is possible that the severity of inbreeding depression can be diminished if natural selection can purge such alleles from populations during inbreeding. If inbreeding depression can be diminished by natural selection than some traits, harmful or not, can be reduced and change the future outlook on a small, endangered populations. There may also be other deleterious effects besides those caused by recessive diseases. Thus, similar immune systems may be more vulnerable to infectious diseases.

COEFFICIENT OF RELATIONSHIP

The coefficient of relationship is a measure of the degree of consanguinity (or biological relationship) between two individuals. A coefficient of inbreeding can be calculated for an individual, as a measure for the amount of pedigree collapse within that individual's genealogy. The term coefficient of relationship was defined by Sewall Wright and was derived from his definition of the coefficient of inbreeding. The measure is most commonly used in genetics and genealogy.

Coefficient of Inbreeding

The coefficient of inbreeding (f) is a measure of the likelihood of genetic effects due to inbreeding to be expected based on a known pedigree (a fully documented genealogy, e.g. due to a fixed system of breeding). The measure expresses the expected percentage of homozygosity arising from a given system of breeding.

HUMAN RELATIONSHIPS

The coefficient of relationship is sometimes used to express degrees of kinship in numerical terms in human genealogy. In human relationships, the value of the coefficient of relationship is usually calculated based on the knowledge of a full family tree extending to a comparatively small number of generations, perhaps of the order of three or four. As explained above, the value for the coefficient of relationship so calculated is thus a lower bound, with an actual value that may be up to a few percent higher. The value is accurate to within 1% if the full family tree of both individuals is known to a depth of seven generations.

IDENTITY BY DESCENT

A DNA segment is identical by state (IBS) in two or more individuals if they have identical nucleotide sequences in this segment. An IBS segment is identical by descent (IBD) in two or more individuals if they have inherited it from a common ancestor without recombination, that is, the segment has the same ancestral origin in these individuals. DNA segments that are IBD are IBS per definition, but segments that are not IBD can still be IBS due to the same mutations in different individuals or recombinations that do not alter the segment. All individuals in a finite population are related if traced back long enough and will, therefore, share segments of their genomes IBD. During meiosis segments of IBD are broken up by recombination. Therefore, the expected length of an IBD segment depends on the number of generations since the most recent common ancestor at the locus of the segment. The length of IBD segments that result from a common ancestor n generations in the past (therefore involving $2n$ meiosis) is exponentially distributed with mean $1/(2n)$ Morgans (M). The expected number of IBD segments decreases with the number of generations since the common ancestor at this locus. For a specific DNA segment, the probability of being IBD decreases as $2-2n$ since in each meiosis the probability of transmitting this segment is $1/2$.

Applications

Identified IBD segments can be used for a wide range of purposes. As noted above the amount (length and number) of IBD sharing depends on the familial relationships between the tested individuals. Therefore one application of IBD segment detection is to quantify relatedness. Measurement of relatedness can be used in forensic genetics, but can also increase information in genetic linkage mapping and help to decrease bias by undocumented relationships in standard association studies. Another application of IBD is genotype imputation and haplotype phase inference. Long shared segments of IBD, which are broken up by short regions may be indicative for phasing errors.

Pedigree chart

A pedigree chart is a diagram that shows the occurrence and appearance or phenotypes of a particular gene or organism and its ancestors from one generation to the next, most commonly humans, show dogs, and race horses. The word pedigree is a corruption of the French 'pied de grue' or crane's foot, because the typical lines and split lines (each split leading to different offspring of the one parent line) resemble the thin leg and foot of a crane.

Properties

A Pedigree results in the presentation of family information in the form of an easily readable chart. Pedigrees use a standardised set of symbols, squares represent males and circles represent females. It should be noted that pedigree construction is a family history, and as such details about an earlier generation may be uncertain as memories fade. If the sex of the person is unknown a diamond is used. Someone with the phenotype in question is represented by a filled-in (darker) symbol. Heterozygotes, when identifiable, are indicated by a shade dot inside a symbol or a half-filled symbol.

Relationships in a pedigree are shown as a series of lines. Parents are connected by a horizontal line and a vertical line leads to their offspring. The offspring are connected by a horizontal sibship line and listed in birth order from left to right. If the offspring are twins then they will be connected by a triangle. If an offspring dies then its symbol will be crossed by a line. If the offspring is still born or aborted it is represented by a small triangle. Each generation is identified by a Roman numeral (I, II, III, and so on), and each individual within the same generation is identified by an Arabic number (1, 2, 3, and so on). Analysis of the pedigree using the principles of Mendelian inheritance can determine whether a trait has a dominant or recessive pattern of inheritance. Pedigrees are often constructed after a family member afflicted with a genetic disorder has been identified. This individual, known as the proband, is indicated on the pedigree by an arrow.

In human use

In England and Wales pedigrees are officially recorded in the College of Arms, which has records going back to the Middle Ages, including pedigrees collected during roving inquiries by its heralds during the sixteenth and seventeenth centuries. The purpose of these heraldic visitations was to register and regulate the use of coats of arms. Those who claimed the right to bear arms had to provide proof either of a grant of arms to them by the College, or of descent from an ancestor entitled to arms. It was for this reason that pedigrees were recorded by the visitations. Pedigrees continue to be registered at the College of Arms and kept up to date on a voluntary basis but they are not accessible to the general public without payment of a fee.

Pedigrees are commonly used in families to find out the probability of a child having a disorder in a particular family. its two most prominent goals are to discover where the genes in question are located (X, Y, or autosome chromosome), and to determine whether a trait is dominant or reccessive. Pedigrees show an autosomal disease when it is a 50/50 ratio between men and women the disorder is autosomal. it is considered an X-linked disease when most of the males in the pedigree are affected the disorder is X-linked. Another use of the pedigrees is to determine whether the disorder is dominant or recessive. if the disorder is dominant, one of the parent must have said disorder. however, if it is recessive, then neither parent has to have it. Some examples of Dominant traits include: Baldness (male), astigmatism, and dwarfism. Some examples of Recessive traits include: small eyes, little body hair, and tall stature.

In animal husbandry

In the practice of selective breeding of animals, particularly in animal fancy and livestock, including horses, pedigree charts are used to track the ancestry of animals and assist in the planning of suitable breeding programmes to enhance desirable traits. Breed registries are formed and are dedicated to the accurate tracking of pedigrees and maintaining accurate records of birth, death and identifying characteristics of each registered animal.

HUMAN EVOLUTIONARY GENETICS

Human evolutionary genetics studies show one human genome differs from another human genome, the evolutionary past that gave rise to it, and its current effects. Differences between genomes have anthropological, medical and forensic implications and applications. Genetic data can provide important insight into human evolution. Biologists classify humans, along with only a few other species, as great apes (species in the family Hominidae). The Hominidae include two distinct species of chimpanzee (the bonobo, *Pan paniscus*, and the common chimpanzee, *Pan troglodytes*), two species of gorilla (the western gorilla, *Gorilla gorilla*, and the eastern gorilla, *Gorilla graueri*), and two species of orangutan (the Bornean orangutan, *Pongo pygmaeus*, and the Sumatran orangutan, *Pongo abelii*). Apes, in turn, belong to the primates order (>400 species). Data from both mitochondrial DNA (mtDNA) and nuclear DNA (nDNA) indicate that primates belong to the group of Euarchontoglires, together with Rodentia, Lagomorpha, Dermoptera, and Scandentia. This is further supported by Alu-like short interspersed nuclear elements (SINEs) which have been found only in members of the Euarchontoglires.

Cladistics

A phylogenetic tree is usually derived from DNA or protein sequences from populations. Often, mitochondrial DNA or Y chromosome sequences are used to study ancient human demographics. These single-locus sources of DNA do not recombine and are almost always inherited from a single parent, with only one known exception in mtDNA. Individuals from closer geographic regions generally tend to be more similar than individuals from regions farther away. Distance on a phylogenetic tree can be used approximately to indicate:

- Genetic distance: The genetic difference between humans and chimps is less than 2%, or twenty times larger than the variation among modern humans.
- Temporal remoteness of the most recent common ancestor: The mitochondrial most recent common ancestor of modern humans lived roughly 200000 years ago, latest common ancestors of humans and chimps between four and seven million years ago.

Speciation of Humans and the African Apes

The separation of humans from their closest relatives, the non-human apes (chimpanzees and gorillas), has been studied extensively for more than a century.

Five major questions have been addressed:

1. Which apes are our closest ancestors?
2. When did the separations occur?
3. What was the effective population size of the common ancestor before the split?
4. Are there traces of population structure (subpopulations) preceding the speciation or partial admixture succeeding it?
5. What were the specific events prior to and subsequent to the separation?

General observations

As discussed before, different parts of the genome show different sequence divergence between different hominoids. It has also been shown that the sequence divergence between DNA from humans and chimpanzees varies greatly. For example, the sequence divergence varies between 0% to 2.66% between non-coding, non-repetitive genomic regions of humans and chimpanzees. Additionally gene trees, generated by comparative analysis of DNA segments, do not always fit the species tree.

Summing up:

- The sequence divergence varies significantly between humans, chimpanzees and gorillas.
- For most DNA sequences, humans and chimpanzees appear to be most closely related, but some point to a human-gorilla or chimpanzee-gorilla clade.

- The human genome has been sequenced, as well as the chimpanzee genome. Humans have 23 pairs of chromosomes, while chimpanzees, gorillas, and orangutans have 24. Human chromosome 2 is a fusion of two chromosomes 2a and 2b that remained separate in the other primates.

Divergence times

The divergence time of humans from other apes is of great interest. One of the first molecular studies, published in 1967 measured immunological distances (IDs) between different primates. Basically the study measured the strength of immunological response that an antigen from one species (human albumin) induces in the immune system of another species (human, chimpanzee, gorilla and Old World monkeys). Closely related species should have similar antigens and therefore weaker immunological response to each others antigens. The immunological response of a species to its own antigens (e.g. human to human) was set to be 1.

The ID between humans and gorillas was determined to be 1.09, that between humans and chimpanzees was determined as 1.14. However the distance to six different Old World monkeys was on average 2.46, indicating that the African apes are more closely related to humans than to monkeys. The authors consider the divergence time between Old World monkeys and hominoids to be 30 million years ago (MYA), based on fossil data, and the immunological distance was considered to grow at a constant rate. They concluded that divergence time of humans and the African apes to be roughly ~5 MYA. That was a surprising result. Most scientists at that time thought that humans and great apes diverged much earlier (>15 MYA). The gorilla was, in ID terms, closer to human than to chimpanzees, however, the difference was so slight that the trichotomy could not be resolved with certainty. Later studies based on molecular genetics were able to resolve the trichotomy: chimpanzees are phylogenetically closer to humans than to gorillas. However, some divergence times estimated later (using much more sophisticated methods in molecular genetics) do not substantially differ from the very first estimate in 1967, but a recent paper puts it at 11–14 MYA.

Divergence times and ancestral effective population size

Current methods to determine divergence times use DNA sequence alignments and molecular clocks. Usually the molecular clock is calibrated assuming that the orangutan split from the African apes (including humans) 12–16 MYA. Some studies also include some old world monkeys and set the divergence time of them from hominoids to 25–30 MYA. Both calibration points are based on very little fossil data and have been criticised. If these dates are revised, the divergence times estimated from molecular data will change as well. However, the relative divergence times are unlikely to change. Even if we can't tell absolute divergence times exactly, we can be pretty sure that the divergence time between chimpanzees and humans is about sixfold shorter than between chimpanzees (or humans) and monkeys. One study used 15 DNA sequences from different regions of the genome from human and chimpanzee and 7 DNA sequences from human, chimpanzee and gorilla.

They determined that chimpanzees are more closely related to humans than gorillas. Using various statistical methods, they estimated the divergence time human-chimp to be 4.7 MYA and the divergence time between gorillas and humans (and chimps) to be 7.2 MYA. Additionally they estimated the effective population size of the common ancestor of humans and chimpanzees to be ~100000. This was somewhat surprising since the present day effective population size of humans is estimated to be only ~10000. If true that means that the human lineage would have experienced an immense decrease of its effective population size (and thus genetic diversity) in its evolution.

Another study sequenced 53 non-repetitive, intergenic DNA segments from a human, a chimpanzee, a gorilla, and orangutan. When the DNA sequences were concatenated to a single long sequence, the generated neighbour-joining tree supported the *Homo-Pan* clade with 100% bootstrap (that is that humans and chimpanzees are the closest related species of the four). When three species are fairly closely related to each other (like human, chimpanzee and gorilla), the trees obtained from DNA sequence data may not be congruent with the tree that represents the speciation (species tree).

The shorter internodal time span (T_{IN}) the more common are incongruent gene trees. The effective population size (N_e) of the internodal population determines how long genetic lineages are preserved in the population. A higher effective population size causes more incongruent gene trees. Therefore, if the internodal time span is known, the ancestral effective population size of the common ancestor of humans and chimpanzees can be calculated. When each segment was analysed individually, 31 supported the *Homo-Pan* clade, 10 supported the *Homo-Gorilla* clade, and 12 supported the *Pan-Gorilla* clade. Using the molecular clock the authors estimated that gorillas split up first 6.2–8.4 MYA and chimpanzees and humans split up 1.6–2.2 million years later (internodal time span) 4.6–6.2 MYA. The internodal time span is useful to estimate the ancestral effective population size of the common ancestor of humans and chimpanzees.

A parsimonious analysis revealed that 24 loci supported the *Homo-Pan* clade, 7 supported the *Homo-Gorilla* clade, 2 supported the *Pan-Gorilla* clade and 20 gave no resolution. Additionally they took 35 protein coding loci from databases. Of these 12 supported the *Homo-Pan* clade, 3 the *Homo-Gorilla* clade, 4 the *Pan-Gorilla* clade and 16 gave no resolution. Therefore, only ~70% of the 52 loci that gave a resolution (33 intergenic, 19 protein coding) support the 'correct' species tree. From the fraction of loci which did not support the species tree and the internodal time span they estimated previously, the effective population of the common ancestor of humans and chimpanzees was estimated to be ~52 000 to 96 000. This value is not as high as that from the first study (Takahata), but still much higher than present day effective population size of humans.

A third study used the same dataset that Chen and Li used but estimated the ancestral effective population of only ~12000 to 21000, using a different statistical method.

Genetic Differences between Humans and Other Great Apes

The alignable sequences within genomes of humans and chimpanzees differ by about 35 million single-nucleotide substitutions. Additionally about 3% of the complete genomes differ by deletions, insertions and duplications. Since mutation rate is relatively constant, roughly one half of these changes occurred in the human lineage. Only a very tiny fraction of those fixed differences gave rise to the different phenotypes of humans and chimpanzees and finding those is a great challenge.

The vast majority of the differences are neutral and do not affect the phenotype. Molecular evolution may act in different ways, through protein evolution, gene loss, differential gene regulation and RNA evolution. All are thought to have played some part in human evolution.

Gene loss

Many different mutations can inactivate a gene, but few will change its function in a specific way. Inactivation mutations will therefore be readily available for selection to act on. Gene loss could thus be a common mechanism of evolutionary adaptation (the 'less-is-more' hypothesis). 80 genes were lost in the human lineage after separation from the last common ancestor with the chimpanzee. 36 of those were for olfactory receptors. Genes involved in chemoreception and immune response are over represented. Another study estimated that 86 genes had been lost.

Hair keratin gene KRTHAP1

A gene for type I hair keratin was lost in the human lineage. Keratins are a major component of hairs. Humans still have nine functional type I hair keratin genes, but the loss of that particular gene may have caused the thinning of human body hair. The gene loss occurred relatively recently in human evolution— less than 240000 years ago.

Myosin gene MYH16

Stedman and others stated that the loss of the sarcomeric myosin gene MYH16 in the human lineage led to smaller masticatory muscles. They estimated that the mutation that led to the inactivation (a two base pair deletion) occurred 2.4 million years ago, predating the appearance of Homo ergaster/erectus in Africa. The period that followed was marked by a strong increase in cranial capacity, promoting speculation that the loss of the gene may have removed an evolutionary constraint on brain size in the genus Homo. Another estimate for the loss of the MYH16 gene is 5.3 million years ago, long before Homo appeared.

Other

CASPASE12, a cysteinyl aspartate proteinase. The loss of this gene is speculated to have reduced the lethality of bacterial infection in humans.

Gene addition

Segmental duplications (SDs or LCRs) have had roles in creating new primate genes and shaping human genetic variation.

Human-specific DNA insertions

When the human genome was compared to the genomes of five comparison primate species, including the chimpanzee, gorilla, orangutan, gibbon, and macaque, it was found that there are approximately 20000 human-specific insertions believed to be regulatory. While most insertions appear to be fitness neutral, a small amount have been identified in positively selected genes showing associations to neural phenotypes and some relating to dental and sensory perception-related phenotypes. These findings hint at the seemingly important role of human-specific insertions in the recent evolution of humans.

Selection pressures

Human accelerated regions are areas of the genome that differ between humans and chimpanzees to a greater extent than can be explained by genetic drift over the time since the two species shared a common ancestor. These regions show signs of being subject to natural selection, leading to the evolution of distinctly human traits. Two examples are HAR1F, which is believed to be related to brain development and HAR2 (a.k.a. HACNS1) that may have played a role in the development of the opposable thumb. It has also been hypothesised that much of the difference between humans and chimpanzees is attributable to the regulation of gene expression rather than differences in the genes themselves. Analyses of conserved non-coding sequences, which often contain functional and thus positively selected regulatory regions, address this possibility.

Sequence divergence between humans and apes

When the draft sequence of the common chimpanzee (Pan troglodytes) genome was published in the summer 2005, 2400 million bases (of ~3160 million bases) were sequenced and assembled well enough to be compared to the human genome. 1.23% of this sequenced differed by single-base substitutions. Of this, 1.06% or less was thought to represent fixed differences between the species, with the rest being variant sites in humans or chimpanzees. Another type of difference, called indels (insertions/deletions) accounted for many fewer differences (15% as many), but contributed ~1.5% of unique sequence to each genome, since each insertion or deletion can involve anywhere from one base to millions of bases.

A companion paper examined segmental duplications in the two genomes, whose insertion and deletion into the genome account for much of the indel sequence. They found that a total of 2.7% of euchromatic sequence had been differentially duplicated in one or the other lineage.

The sequence divergence has generally the following pattern: Human-Chimp < Human-Gorilla << Human-Orangutan, highlighting the close kinship between humans and the African apes. Alu elements diverge quickly due to their high frequency of CpG dinucleotides which mutate roughly 10 times more often than the average nucleotide in the genome. The mutation rate is higher in the male germ line, therefore the divergence in the Y chromosome—which is inherited solely from the father—is higher than in autosomes. The X chromosome is inherited twice as often through the female germ line as through the male germ line and therefore shows slightly lower sequence divergence. The sequence divergence of the Xq13.3 region is surprisingly low between humans and chimpanzees.

Mutations altering the amino acid sequence of proteins (K_a) are the least common. In fact ~29% of all orthologous proteins are identical between human and chimpanzee. The typical protein differs by only two amino acids. DNA sequences may however also differ by insertions and deletions (indels) of bases. These are usually stripped from the alignments before the calculation of sequence divergence is performed.

Genetic Differences between Modern Humans and Neanderthals

An international group of scientists completed a draft sequence of the Neanderthal genome in May 2010. The results indicate some breeding between modern humans (*Homo sapiens*) and Neanderthals (*Homo neanderthalensis*), as the genomes of non-African humans have 1–4% more in common with Neanderthals than do the genomes of subsaharan Africans. Neanderthals and most modern humans share a lactose-intolerant variant of the lactase gene that encodes an enzyme that is unable to break down lactose in milk after weaning. Modern humans and Neanderthals also share the FOXP2 gene variant associated with brain development and with speech in modern humans, indicating that Neanderthals may have been able to speak. Chimps have two amino acid differences in FOXP2 compared with human and Neanderthal FOXP2.

Genetic Differences among Modern Humans

H. sapiens is thought to have emerged about 300,000 years ago. It dispersed throughout Africa, and after 70000 years ago throughout Eurasia and Oceania. A 2009 study identified 14 'ancestral population clusters', the most remote being the San people of Southern Africa. With their rapid expansion throughout different climate zones, and especially with the availability of new food sources with the domestication of cattle and the development of agriculture, human populations have been exposed to significant selective pressures since their dispersal. For example, East Asians have been found to be separated from Europids by a number of concentrated alleles suggestive of selection pressures, including variants of the EDAR, ADH1B, ABCC1, and ALDH2genes. The East Asian types of ADH1B in particular are associated with rice domestication and would thus have arisen after the development of rice cultivation roughly 10,000 years ago. Several phenotypical traits of characteristic of East Asians are due to a single mutation of the EDAR gene, dated to c. 35000 years ago.

As of 2017, the Single Nucleotide Polymorphism Database (dbSNP), which lists SNP and other variants, listed a total of 324 million variants found in sequenced human genomes. Nucleotide diversity, the average proportion of nucleotides that differ between two individuals, is estimated at between 0.1% and 0.4% for contemporary humans (compared to 2% between humans and chimpanzees). This corresponds to genome differences at a few million sites, the 1000 Genomes Project similarly found that 'a typical [individual] genome differs from the reference human genome at 4.1 million to 5.0 million sites affecting 20 million bases of sequence.'

MUTATION–SELECTION BALANCE

Mutation–selection balance is an equilibrium in the number of deleterious alleles in a population that occurs when the rate at which deleterious alleles are created by mutation equals the rate at which deleterious alleles are eliminated by selection. The majority of genetic mutations are neutral or deleterious, beneficial mutations are relatively rare. The resulting influx of deleterious mutations into a population over time is counteracted by negative selection, which acts to purge deleterious mutations. Setting aside other factors (e.g. balancing selection and genetic drift), the equilibrium number of deleterious alleles is then determined by a balance between the deleterious mutation rate and the rate at which selection purges those mutations.

Mutation–selection balance was originally proposed to explain how genetic variation is maintained in populations, although several other ways for deleterious mutations to persist are now recognised, notably balancing selection. Nevertheless, the concept is still widely used in evolutionary genetics, e.g. to explain the persistence of deleterious alleles in actual populations as in the case of spinal muscular atrophy, or, in theoretical models, mutation-selection balance can appear in a variety of ways and has even been applied to beneficial mutations (i.e. balance between selective loss of variation and creation of variation by beneficial mutations).

Natural selection results in the reduction of genetic variation through the elimination of maladapted individuals and consequently of the mutations that caused the maladaptation. At the same time, new mutations occur, resulting in a Mutation–selection balance. The exact outcome of the two processes depends both on the rate at which new mutations occur and on the strength of the natural selection, which is a function of how unfavourable the mutation proves to be. Consequently, changes in the mutation rate or the selection pressure will result in a different Mutation–selection balance.

SECTION IX

Evolutionary and Conservation Genetics

Chapter 22

Evolutionary Genetics

INTRODUCTION

Evolution is the cornerstone of modern biology. It unites all the fields of biology under one theoretical umbrella. Evolution is a change in the gene pool of a population over time. A gene is a hereditary unit that can be passed on unaltered for many generations. The gene pool is the set of all genes in a species or population. The English moth, *Biston betularia*, is a frequently cited example of observed evolution. Evolution is a change in the gene pool. In this moth there are two colour morphs, light and dark. H. B. D. Kettlewell found that dark moths constituted less than 2% of the population prior to 1848. The frequency of the dark morph increased in the years following. By 1898, the 95% of the moths in Manchester and other highly industrialised areas were of the dark type. Their frequency was less in rural areas. The moth population changed from mostly light coloured moths to mostly dark coloured moths. The moths' colour was primarily determined by a single gene. [gene: a hereditary unit] So, the change in frequency of dark coloured moths represented a change in the gene pool. [gene pool: the set all of genes in a population]. This change was, by definition, evolution.

The increase in relative abundance of the dark type was due to natural selection. The late eighteen hundreds was the time of England's industrial revolution. Soot from factories darkened the birch trees the moths landed on. Against a sooty background, birds could see the lighter coloured moths better and ate more of them. As a result, more dark moths survived until reproductive age and left offspring. The greater number of offspring left by dark moths is what caused their increase in frequency. This is an example of natural selection.

Populations evolve: [Evolution: a change in the gene pool] In order to understand evolution, it is necessary to view populations as a collection of individuals, each harboring a different set of traits. A single organism is never typical of an entire population unless there is no variation within that population. Individual organisms do not evolve, they retain the same genes throughout their life. When a population is evolving, the ratio of different genetic types is changing — each individual organism within a population does not change. For example, in the previous example, the frequency of black moths increased, the moths did not turn from light to gray to dark in concert. The process of evolution can be summarised in three sentences: Genes mutate. [gene: a hereditary unit] Individuals are selected.

Evolution can be divided into microevolution and macroevolution. The kind of evolution documented above is microevolution. Larger changes, such as when a new species is formed, are called macroevolution. Some biologists feel the mechanisms of macroevolution are different from those of microevolutionary change. Others think the distinction between the two is arbitrary — macroevolution is cumulative microevolution.

The word evolution has a variety of meanings. The fact that all organisms are linked via descent to a common ancestor is often called evolution. The theory of how the first living organisms appeared is often called evolution. This should be called abiogenesis. And frequently, people use the word evolution when they really mean natural selection — one of the many mechanisms of evolution.

IMPORTANCE OF EVOLUTION

Evolution can occur without morphological change, and morphological change can occur without evolution. Humans are larger now than in the recent past, a result of better diet and medicine. Phenotypic changes, like this, induced solely by changes in environment do not count as evolution because they are not heritable, in other words the change is not passed on to the organism's offspring. Phenotype is the morphological, physiological, biochemical, behavioral and other properties exhibited by a living organism. An organism's phenotype is determined by its genes and its environment. Most changes due to environment are fairly subtle, for example size differences. Large scale phenotypic changes are obviously due to genetic changes, and therefore are evolution.

Evolution is not progress: Populations simply adapt to their current surroundings. They do not necessarily become better in any absolute sense over time. A trait or strategy that is successful at one time may be unsuccessful at another. Paquin and Adams demonstrated this experimentally. They founded a yeast culture and maintained it for many generations. Occasionally, a mutation would arise that allowed its bearer to reproduce better than its contemporaries. These mutant strains would crowd out the formerly dominant strains. Samples of the most successful strains from the culture were taken at a variety of times. In later competition experiments, each strain would outcompete the immediately previously dominant type in a culture. However, some earlier isolates could outcompete strains that arose late in the experiment. Competitive ability of a strain was always better than its previous type, but competitiveness in a general sense was not increasing. Any organism's success depends on the behavior of its contemporaries. For most traits or behaviors there is likely no optimal design or strategy, only contingent ones. Evolution can be like a game of paper/scissors/rock.

Organisms are not passive targets of their environment. Each species modifies its own environment. At the least, organisms remove nutrients from and add waste to their surroundings. Often, waste products benefit other species. Animal dung is fertiliser for plants. Conversely, the oxygen we breathe is a waste product of plants. Species do not simply change to fit their environment, they modify their environment to suit them as well. Beavers build a dam to create a pond suitable to sustain them and raise young. Alternately, when the environment changes, species can migrate to suitable climes or seek out microenvironments to which they are adapted.

GENETIC VARIATION

Evolution requires genetic variation: If there were no dark moths, the population could not have evolved from mostly light to mostly dark. In order for continuing evolution there must be mechanisms to increase or create genetic variation and mechanisms to decrease it. Mutation is a change in a gene. These changes are the source of new genetic variation. Natural selection operates on this variation.

Genetic variation has two components: allelic diversity and non- random associations of alleles. Alleles are different versions of the same gene. For example, humans can have A, B or O alleles that determine one aspect of their blood type. Most animals, including humans, are diploid — they contain two alleles for every gene at every locus, one inherited from their mother and one inherited from their father. Locus is the location of a gene on a chromosome.

Humans can be AA, AB, AO, BB, BO or OO at the blood group locus. If the two alleles at a locus are the same type (for instance two A alleles) the individual would be called homozygous. An individual with two different alleles at a locus (for example, an AB individual) is called heterozygous. At any locus there can be many different alleles in a population, more alleles than any single organism can possess. For example, no single human can have an A, B and an O allele.

Considerable variation is present in natural populations. At 45 per cent of loci in plants there is more than one allele in the gene pool. [allele: alternate version of a gene (created by mutation)] Any given plant is likely to be heterozygous at about 15 per cent of its loci. Levels of genetic variation in animals range from roughly 15% of loci having more than one allele (polymorphic) in birds, to over 50% of loci being polymorphic in insects.

Mammals and reptiles are polymorphic at about 20% of their loci- amphibians and fish are polymorphic at around 30% of their loci. In most populations, there are enough loci and enough different alleles that every individual, identical twins excepted, has a unique combination of alleles.

Linkage disequilibrium is a measure of association between alleles of two different genes. [Allele: alternate version of a gene] If two alleles were found together in organisms more often than would be expected, the alleles are in linkage disequilibrium. If there two loci in an organism (A and B) and two alleles at each of these loci (A1, A2, B1 and B2) linkage disequilibrium (D) is calculated as D = f(A1B1) f(A2B2) − f(A1B2) f(A2B1) (where f(X) is the frequency of X in the population). [Loci (plural of locus): location of a gene on a chromosome] D varies between -1/4 and 1/4, the greater the deviation from zero, the greater the linkage. The sign is simply a consequence of how the alleles are numbered. Linkage disequilibrium can be the result of physical proximity of the genes. Or, it can be maintained by natural selection if some combinations of alleles work better as a team.

Natural selection maintains the linkage disequilibrium between colour and pattern alleles in *Papilio memnon*. [Linkage disequilibrium: association between alleles at different loci] In this moth species, there is a gene that determines wing morphology. One allele at this locus leads to a moth that has a tail, the other allele codes for a untailed moth. There is another gene that determines if the wing is brightly or darkly coloured. There are thus four possible types of moths: brightly coloured moths with and without tails, and dark moths with and without tails. All four can be produced when moths are brought into the lab and bred. However, only two of these types of moths are found in the wild: brightly coloured moths with tails and darkly coloured moths without tails. The non-random association is maintained by natural selection. Bright, tailed moths mimic the pattern of an unpalatable species. The dark morph is cryptic. The other two combinations are neither mimetic nor cryptic and are quickly eaten by birds.

Assortative mating causes a non-random distribution of alleles at a single locus. [Locus: location of a gene on a chromosome] If there are two alleles (A and a) at a locus with frequencies p and q, the frequency of the three possible genotypes (AA, Aa and aa) will be p2, 2pq and q2, respectively. For example, if the frequency of A is 0.9 and the frequency of a is 0.1, the frequencies of AA, Aa and aa individuals are: 0.81, 0.18 and 0.01. This distribution is called the Hardy-Weinberg equilibrium.

Non-random mating results in a deviation from the Hardy-Weinberg distribution. In populations that mate this way, fewer heterozygotes are found than would be predicted under random mating.

[heterozygote: an organism that has two different alleles at a locus] A decrease in heterozygotes can be the result of mate choice, or simply the result of population subdivision. Most organisms have a limited dispersal capability, so their mate will be chosen from the local population.

EVOLUTION WITHIN A LINEAGE

In order for continuing evolution there must be mechanisms to increase or create genetic variation and mechanisms to decrease it. The mechanisms of evolution are mutation, natural selection, genetic drift, recombination and gene flow. This can grouped into two classes — those that decrease genetic variation and those that increase it.

Mechanisms that Decrease Genetic Variation

Natural selection

Some types of organisms within a population leave more offspring than others. Over time, the frequency of the more prolific type will increase. The difference in reproductive capability is called natural selection. Natural selection is the only mechanism of adaptive evolution, it is defined as differential reproductive success of preexisting classes of genetic variants in the gene pool.

The most common action of natural selection is to remove unfit variants as they arise via mutation. [natural selection: differential reproductive success of genotypes] In other words, natural selection usually prevents new alleles from increasing in frequency. This led a famous evolutionist, George Williams, to say 'Evolution proceeds in spite of natural selection.' Natural selection can maintain or deplete genetic variation depending on how it acts. When selection acts to weed out deleterious alleles, or causes an allele to sweep to fixation, it depletes genetic variation. When heterozygotes are more fit than either of the homozygotes, however, selection causes genetic variation to be maintained. [Heterozygote: an organism that has two different alleles at a locus homozygote: an organism that has two identical alleles at a locus] This is called balancing selection. An example of this is the maintenance of sickle-cell alleles in human populations subject to malaria. Variation at a single locus determines whether red blood cells are shaped normally or sickled. If a human has two alleles for sickle-cell, he/she develops anemia — the shape of sickle-cells precludes them carrying normal levels of oxygen. However, heterozygotes who have one copy of the sickle-cell allele, coupled with one normal allele enjoy some resistance to malaria — the shape of sickled cells make it harder for the plasmodia (malaria causing agents) to enter the cell. Thus, individuals homozygous for the normal allele suffer more malaria than heterozygotes. Individuals homozygous for the sickle- cell are anemic. Heterozygotes have the highest fitness of these three types. Heterozygotes pass on both sickle-cell and normal alleles to the next generation. Thus, neither allele can be eliminated from the gene pool. The sickle-cell allele is at its highest frequency in regions of Africa where malaria is most pervasive.

Balancing selection is rare in natural populations. [balancing selection: selection favouring heterozygotes] Only a handful of other cases beside the sickle-cell example have been found. At one time population geneticists thought balancing selection could be a general explanation for the levels of genetic variation found in natural populations. That is no longer the case. Balancing selection is only rarely found in natural populations. And, there are theoretical reasons why natural selection cannot maintain polymorphisms at several loci via balancing selection.

Individuals are selected: Dark coloured moths had a higher reproductive success because light coloured moths suffered a higher predation rate. The decline of light coloured alleles was caused by light coloured individuals being removed from the gene pool (selected against). Individual organisms either reproduce or fail to reproduce and are hence the unit of selection. One way alleles can change in frequency is to be housed in organisms with different reproductive rates. Genes are not the unit of selection (because their success depends on the organism's other genes as well), neither are groups of organisms a unit of selection. There are some exceptions to this 'rule,' but it is a good generalisation.

Organisms do not perform any behaviors that are for the good of their species. An individual organism competes primarily with others of it own species for its reproductive success. Natural selection favours selfish behavior because any truly altruistic act increases the recipient's reproductive success while lowering the donors. Altruists would disappear from a population as the non- altruists would reap the benefits, but not pay the costs, of altruistic acts. Many behaviors appear altruistic. Biologists, however, can demonstrate that these behaviors are only apparently altruistic. Cooperating with or helping other organisms is often the most selfish strategy for an animal. This is called reciprocal altruism. A good example of this is blood sharing in vampire bats. In these bats, those lucky enough to find a meal will often share part of it with an unsuccessful bat by regurgitating some blood into the other's mouth. Biologists have found that these bats form bonds with partners and help each other out when the other is needy. If a bat is found to be a 'cheater,' (he accepts blood when starving, but does not donate when his partner is) his partner will abandon him. The bats are thus not helping each other altruistically, they form pacts that are mutually beneficial.

Helping closely related organisms can appear altruistic, but this is also a selfish behavior. Reproductive success (fitness) has two components, direct fitness and indirect fitness. Direct fitness is a measure of how many alleles, on average, a genotype contributes to the subsequent generation's gene pool by reproducing. Indirect fitness is a measure of how many alleles identical to its own it helps to enter the gene pool. Direct fitness plus indirect fitness is inclusive fitness. J. B. S. Haldane once remarked he would gladly drown, if by doing so he saved two siblings or eight cousins. Each of his siblings would share one half his alleles, his cousins, one eighth. They could potentially add as many of his alleles to the gene pool as he could. Natural selection favours traits or behaviors that increase a genotype's inclusive fitness. Closely related organisms share many of the same alleles. In diploid species, siblings share on average at least 50% of their alleles. The percentage is higher if the parents are related. So, helping close relatives to reproduce gets an organism's own alleles better represented in the gene pool. The benefit of helping relatives increases dramatically in highly inbred species. In some cases, organisms will completely forgo reproducing and only help their relatives reproduce. Ants, and other eusocial insects, have sterile castes that only serve the queen and assist her reproductive efforts. The sterile workers are reproducing by proxy.

The words selfish and altruistic have connotations in everyday use that biologists do not intend. Selfish simply means behaving in such a way that one's own inclusive fitness is maximised, altruistic means behaving in such a way that another's fitness is increased at the expense of ones' own. Use of the words selfish and altruistic is not meant to imply that organisms consciously understand their motives.

The opportunity for natural selection to operate does not induce genetic variation to appear — selection only distinguishes between existing variants. Variation is not possible along every imaginable axis, so all possible adaptive solutions are not open to populations. To pick a somewhat ridiculous example, a steel shelled turtle might be an improvement over regular turtles. Turtles are killed quite a bit by cars these days because when confronted with danger, they retreat into their shells — this is not a great strategy against a two ton automobile. However, there is no variation in metal content of shells, so it would not be possible to select for a steel shelled turtle. Here is a second example of natural selection. Geospiza fortis lives on the Galapagos islands along with fourteen other finch species. It feeds on the seeds of the plant Tribulus cistoides, specialising on the smaller seeds. Another species, G. Magnirostris, has a larger beak and specialises on the larger seeds. The health of these bird populations depends on seed production. Seed production, in turn, depends on the arrival of wet season. In 1977, there was a drought. Rainfall was well below normal and fewer seeds were produced. As the season progressed, the G. fortis population depleted the supply of small seeds. Eventually, only larger seeds remained. Most of the finches starved, the population plummeted from about twelve hundred birds to less than two hundred. Peter Grant, who had been studying these finches, noted that larger beaked birds fared better than smaller beaked ones. These larger birds had offspring with correspondingly large beaks. Thus, there was an increase in the proportion of large beaked birds in the population the next generation. To prove that the change in bill size in Geospiza fortis was an evolutionary change, Grant had to show that differences in bill size were at least partially genetically based. He did so by crossing finches of various beak sizes and showing that a finch's beak size was influenced by its parent's genes. Large beaked birds had large beaked offspring, beak size was not due to environmental differences (in parental care, for example).

Natural selection may not lead a population to have the optimal set of traits. In any population, there would be a certain combination of possible alleles that would produce the optimal set of traits (the global optimum), but there are other sets of alleles that would yield a population almost as adapted (local optima). Transition from a local optimum to the global optimum may be hindered or forbidden because the population would have to pass through less adaptive states to make the transition. Natural selection only works to bring populations to the nearest optimal point. This idea is Sewall Wright's adaptive landscape. This is one of the most influential models that shape how evolutionary biologists view evolution. Natural selection does not have any foresight. It only allows organisms to adapt to their current environment. Structures or behaviors do not evolve for future utility. An organism adapts to its environment at each stage of its evolution. As the environment changes, new traits may be selected for. Large changes in populations are the result of cumulative natural selection. Changes are introduced into the population by mutation, the small minority of these changes that result in a greater reproductive output of their bearers are amplified in frequency by selection.

Complex traits must evolve through viable intermediates. For many traits, it initially seems unlikely that intermediates would be viable. What good is half a wing? Half a wing may be no good for flying, but it may be useful in other ways. Feathers are thought to have evolved as insulation (ever worn a down jacket?) and/or as a way to trap insects. Later, proto-birds may have learned to glide when leaping from tree to tree. Eventually, the feathers that originally served as insulation now became co-opted for use in flight. A trait's current utility is not always indicative of its past utility. It can evolve for one purpose, and be used later for another. A trait evolved for its current utility is an adaptation, one that evolved for another utility is an exaptation. An example of an exaptation is a penguin's wing. Penguins evolved from flying ancestors, now they are flightless and use their wings for swimming.

Common misconceptions about selection

Selection is not a force in the sense that gravity or the strong nuclear force is. However, for the sake of brevity, biologists sometimes refer to it that way. This often leads to some confusion when biologists speak of selection 'pressures.' This implies that the environment 'pushes' a population to more adapted state. This is not the case. Selection merely favours beneficial genetic changes when they occur by chance — it does not contribute to their appearance. The potential for selection to act may long precede the appearance of selectable genetic variation. When selection is spoken of as a force, it often seems that it is has a mind of its own, or as if it was nature personified. This most often occurs when biologists are waxing poetic about selection. This has no place in scientific discussions of evolution. Selection is not a guided or cognizant entity, it is simply an effect. A related pitfall in discussing selection is anthropomorphising on behalf of living things. Often conscious motives are seemingly imputed to organisms, or even genes, when discussing evolution. This happens most frequently when discussing animal behavior. Animals are often said to perform some behavior because selection will favour it. This could more accurately worded as 'animals that, due to their genetic composition, perform this behavior tend to be favoured by natural selection relative to those who, due to their genetic composition, don't.' Such wording is cumbersome. To avoid this, biologists often anthropomorphize. This is unfortunate because it often makes evolutionary arguments sound silly. Keep in mind this is only for convenience of expression.

The phrase 'survival of the fittest' is often used synonymously with natural selection. The phrase is both incomplete and misleading. For one thing, survival is only one component of selection — and perhaps one of the less important ones in many populations. For example, in polygynous species, a number of males survive to reproductive age, but only a few ever mate. Males may differ little in their ability to survive, but greatly in their ability to attract mates — the difference in reproductive success stems mainly from the latter consideration. Also, the word fit is often confused with physically fit. Fitness, in an evolutionary sense, is the average reproductive output of a class of genetic variants in a gene pool. Fit does not necessarily mean biggest, fastest or strongest.

Sexual selection

In many species, males develop prominent secondary sexual characteristics. A few oft cited examples are the peacock's tail, colouring and patterns in male birds in general, voice calls in frogs and flashes in fireflies. Many of these traits are a liability from the standpoint of survival. Any ostentatious trait or noisy, attention getting behavior will alert predators as well as potential mates. How then could natural selection favour these traits?

Natural selection can be broken down into many components, of which survival is only one. Sexual attractiveness is a very important component of selection, so much so that biologists use the term sexual selection when they talk about this subset of natural selection.

Sexual selection is natural selection operating on factors that contribute to an organism's mating success. Traits that are a liability to survival can evolve when the sexual attractiveness of a trait outweighs the liability incurred for survival. A male who lives a short time, but produces many offspring is much more successful than a long lived one that produces few. The former's genes will eventually dominate the gene pool of his species. In many species, especially polygynous species where only a few males monopolise all the females, sexual selection has caused pronounced sexual dimorphism. In these species males compete against other males for mates. The competition can be either direct or mediated by female choice. In species where females choose, males compete by displaying striking phenotypic characteristics and/or performing elaborate courtship behaviors. The females then mate with the males that most interest them, usually the ones with the most outlandish displays. There are many competing theories as to why females are attracted to these displays.

The good genes model states that the display indicates some component of male fitness. A good genes advocate would say that bright colouring in male birds indicates a lack of parasites. The females are cueing on some signal that is correlated with some other component of viability. Selection for good genes can be seen in sticklebacks. In these fish, males have red colouration on their sides. Milinski and Bakker showed that intensity of colour was correlated to both parasite load and sexual attractiveness. Females preferred redder males. The redness indicated that he was carrying fewer parasites.

Evolution can get stuck in a positive feedback loop. Another model to explain secondary sexual characteristics is called the runaway sexual selection model. R. A. Fisher proposed that females may have an innate preference for some male trait before it appears in a population. Females would then mate with male carriers when the trait appears. The offspring of these matings have the genes for both the trait and the preference for the trait. As a result, the process snowballs until natural selection brings it into check. Suppose that female birds prefer males with longer than average tail feathers. Mutant males with longer than average feathers will produce more offspring than the short feathered males. In the next generation, average tail length will increase. As the generations progress, feather length will increase because females do not prefer a specific length tail, but a longer than average tail. Eventually tail length will increase to the point were the liability to survival is matched by the sexual attractiveness of the trait and an equilibrium will be established. Note that in many exotic birds male plumage is often very showy and many species do in fact have males with greatly elongated feathers. In some cases these feathers are shed after the breeding season.

None of the above models are mutually exclusive. There are millions of sexually dimorphic species on this planet and the forms of sexual selection probably vary amongst them.

Genetic drift

Allele frequencies can change due to chance alone. This is called genetic drift. Drift is a binomial sampling error of the gene pool. What this means is, the alleles that form the next generation's gene pool are a sample of the alleles from the current generation. When sampled from a population, the frequency of alleles differs slightly due to chance alone. Alleles can increase or decrease in frequency due to drift. The average expected change in allele frequency is zero, since increasing or decreasing in frequency is equally probable. A small percentage of alleles may continually change frequency in a single direction for several generations just as flipping a fair coin may, on occasion, result in a string of heads or tails. A very few new mutant alleles can drift to fixation in this manner.

In small populations, the variance in the rate of change of allele frequencies is greater than in large populations. However, the overall rate of genetic drift (measured in substitutions per generation) is independent of population size. [genetic drift: a random change in allele frequencies] If the mutation rate is constant, large and small populations lose alleles to drift at the same rate. This is because large populations will have more alleles in the gene pool, but they will lose them more slowly. Smaller populations will have fewer alleles, but these will quickly cycle through. This assumes that mutation is constantly adding new alleles to the gene pool and selection is not operating on any of these alleles.

Sharp drops in population size can change allele frequencies substantially. When a population crashes, the alleles in the surviving sample may not be representative of the precrash gene pool. This change in the gene pool is called the founder effect, because small populations of organisms that invade a new territory (founders) are subject to this. Many biologists feel the genetic changes brought about by founder effects may contribute to isolated populations developing reproductive isolation from their parent populations. In sufficiently small populations, genetic drift can counteract selection. [genetic drift: a random change in allele frequencies] Mildly deleterious alleles may drift to fixation.

Wright and Fisher disagreed on the importance of drift. Fisher thought populations were sufficiently large that drift could be neglected. Wright argued that populations were often divided into smaller subpopulations. Drift could cause allele frequency differences between subpopulations if gene flow was small enough. If a subpopulation was small enough, the population could even drift through fitness valleys in the adaptive landscape. Then, the subpopulation could climb a larger fitness hill. Gene flow out of this subpopulation could contribute to the population as a whole adapting. This is Wright's Shifting Balance theory of evolution. Both natural selection and genetic drift decrease genetic variation. If they were the only mechanisms of evolution, populations would eventually become homogeneous and further evolution would be impossible. There are, however, mechanisms that replace variation depleted by selection and drift. These are discussed below.

Mechanisms that Increase Genetic Variation

Mutation

The cellular machinery that copies DNA sometimes makes mistakes. These mistakes alter the sequence of a gene. This is called a mutation. There are many kinds of mutations. A point mutation is a mutation in which one 'letter' of the genetic code is changed to another. Lengths of DNA can also be deleted or inserted in a gene, these are also mutations. Finally, genes or parts of genes can become inverted or duplicated. Typical rates of mutation are between 10^{-10} and 10^{-12} mutations per base pair of DNA per generation. Most mutations are thought to be neutral with regards to fitness. (Kimura defines neutral as $|s| < \frac{1}{2} Ne$, where s is the selective coefficient and Ne is the effective population size.) Only a small portion of the genome of eukaryotes contains coding segments. And, although some non-coding DNA is involved in gene regulation or other cellular functions, it is probable that most base changes would have no fitness consequence.

Most mutations that have any phenotypic effect are deleterious. Mutations that result in amino acid substitutions can change the shape of a protein, potentially changing or eliminating its function. This can lead to inadequacies in biochemical pathways or interfere with the process of development. Organisms are sufficiently integrated that most random changes will not produce a fitness benefit. Only a very small percentage of mutations are beneficial. The ratio of neutral to deleterious to beneficial mutations is unknown and probably varies with respect to details of the locus in question and environment.

Mutation limits the rate of evolution. The rate of evolution can be expressed in terms of nucleotide substitutions in a lineage per generation. Substitution is the replacement of an allele by another in a population. This is a two step process: First a mutation occurs in an individual, creating a new allele. This allele subsequently increases in frequency to fixation in the population. Thus, the rate of evolution is $k = 2 Nvu$ (in diploids) where k is nucleotide substitutions, N is the effective population size, v is the rate of mutation and u is the proportion of mutants that eventually fix in the population.

Mutation need not be limiting over short time spans. The rate of evolution expressed above is given as a steady state equation, it assumes the system is at equilibrium. Given the time frames for a single mutant to fix, it is unclear if populations are ever at equilibrium. A change in environment can cause previously neutral alleles to have selective values, in the short term evolution can run on 'stored' variation and thus is independent of mutation rate. Other mechanisms can also contribute selectable variation. Recombination creates new combinations of alleles (or new alleles) by joining sequences with separate microevolutionary histories within a population. Gene flow can also supply the gene pool with variants. Of course, the ultimate source of these variants is mutation.

Fate of Mutant Alleles

Mutation creates new alleles. Each new allele enters the gene pool as a single copy amongst many. Most are lost from the gene pool, the organism carrying them fails to reproduce, or reproduces but does not pass on that particular allele. A mutant's fate is shared with the genetic background it appears in. A new allele will initially be linked to other loci in its genetic background, even loci on other chromosomes. If the allele increases in frequency in the population, initially it will be paired with other alleles at that locus — the new allele will primarily be carried in individuals heterozygous for that locus. The chance of it being paired with itself is low until it reaches intermediate frequency. If the allele is recessive, its effect won't be seen in any individual until a homozygote is formed. The eventual fate of the allele depends on whether it is neutral, deleterious or beneficial.

Neutral alleles

Most neutral alleles are lost soon after they appear. The average time (in generations) until loss of a neutral allele is $2(Ne/N) \ln(2N)$ where N is the effective population size (the number of individuals contributing to the next generation's gene pool) and N is the total population size. Only a small percentage of alleles fix. Fixation is the process of an allele increasing to a frequency at or near one. The probability of a neutral allele fixing in a population is equal to its frequency. For a new mutant in a diploid population, this frequency is $1/2N$.

If mutations are neutral with respect to fitness, the rate of substitution (k) is equal to the rate of mutation(v). This does not mean every new mutant eventually reaches fixation. Alleles are added to the gene pool by mutation at the same rate they are lost to drift. For neutral alleles that do fix, it takes an average of 4N generations to do so. However, at equilibrium there are multiple alleles segregating in the population. In small populations, few mutations appear each generation.

The ones that fix do so quickly relative to large populations. In large populations, more mutants appear over the generations. But, the ones that fix take much longer to do so. Thus, the rate of neutral evolution (in substitutions per generation) is independent of population size. The rate of mutation determines the level of heterozygosity at a locus according to the neutral theory. Heterozygosity is simply the proportion of the population that is heterozygous. Equilibrium heterozygosity is given as $H = 4Nv/[4Nv+1]$ (for diploid populations). H can vary from a very small number to almost one. In small populations, H is small (because the equation is approximately a very small number divided by one). In (biologically unrealistically) large populations, heterozygosity approaches one (because the equation is approximately a large number divided by itself). Directly testing this model is difficult because N and v can only be estimated for most natural populations. But, heterozygosities are believed to be too low to be described by a strictly neutral model. Solutions offered by neutralists for this discrepancy include hypothesising that natural populations may not be at equilibrium. At equilibrium there should be a few alleles at intermediate frequency and many at very low frequencies. This is the Ewens-Watterson distribution. New alleles enter a population every generation, most remain at low frequency until they are lost. A few drift to intermediate frequencies, a very few drift all the way to fixation. In *Drosophila pseudoobscura*, the protein Xanthine dehydrogenase (Xdh) has many variants. In a single population, Keith, and others found that 59 of 96 proteins were of one type, two others were represented ten and nine times and nine other types were present singly or in low numbers.

Deleterious alleles

Deleterious mutants are selected against but remain at low frequency in the gene pool. In diploids, a deleterious recessive mutant may increase in frequency due to drift. Selection cannot see it when it is masked by a dominant allele. Many disease causing alleles remain at low frequency for this reason. People who are carriers do not suffer the negative effect of the allele. Unless they mate with another carrier, the allele may simply continue to be passed on. Deleterious alleles also remain in populations at a low frequency due to a balance between recurrent mutation and selection. This is called the mutation load.

Beneficial alleles

Most new mutants are lost, even beneficial ones. Wright calculated that the probability of fixation of a beneficial allele is 2s. (This assumes a large population size, a small fitness benefit, and that heterozygotes have an intermediate fitness. A benefit of 2s yields an overall rate of evolution: k=4Nvs where v is the mutation rate to beneficial alleles) An allele that conferred a one per cent increase in fitness only has a two per cent chance of fixing. The probability of fixation of beneficial type of mutant is boosted by recurrent mutation. The beneficial mutant may be lost several times, but eventually it will arise and stick in a population. (Recall that even deleterious mutants recur in a population.)

Directional selection depletes genetic variation at the selected locus as the fitter allele sweeps to fixation. Sequences linked to the selected allele also increase in frequency due to hitchhiking. The lower the rate of recombination, the larger the window of sequence that hitchhikes. Begun and Aquadro compared the level of nucleotide polymorphism within and between species with the rate of recombination at a locus. Low levels of nucleotide polymorphism within species coincided with low rates of recombination. This could be explained by molecular mechanisms if recombination itself was mutagenic.

In this case, recombination with also be correlated with nucleotide divergence between species. But, the level of sequence divergence did not correlate with the rate of recombination. Thus, they inferred that selection was the cause. The correlation between recombination and nucleotide polymorphism leaves the conclusion that selective sweeps occur often enough to leave an imprint on the level of genetic variation in natural populations.

One example of a beneficial mutation comes from the mosquito *Culex pipiens*. In this organism, a gene that was involved with breaking down organophosphates - common insecticide ingredients -became duplicated. Progeny of the organism with this mutation quickly swept across the worldwide mosquito population. There are numerous examples of insects developing resistance to chemicals, especially DDT which was once heavily used in this country. And, most importantly, even though 'good' mutations happen much less frequently than 'bad' ones, organisms with 'good' mutations thrive while organisms with 'bad' ones die out. If beneficial mutants arise infrequently, the only fitness differences in a population will be due to new deleterious mutants and the deleterious recessives.

Selection will simply be weeding out unfit variants. Only occasionally will a beneficial allele be sweeping through a population. The general lack of large fitness differences segregating in natural populations argues that beneficial mutants do indeed arise infrequently. However, the impact of a beneficial mutant on the level of variation at a locus can be large and lasting. It takes many generations for a locus to regain appreciable levels of heterozygosity following a selective sweep.

Recombination

Each chromosome in our sperm or egg cells is a mixture of genes from our mother and our father. Recombination can be thought of as gene shuffling. Most organisms have linear chromosomes and their genes lie at specific location (loci) along them. Bacteria have circular chromosomes. In most sexually reproducing organisms, there are two of each chromosome type in every cell. For instance in humans, every chromosome is paired, one inherited from the mother, the other inherited from the father. When an organism produces gametes, the gametes end up with only one of each chromosome per cell. Haploid gametes are produced from diploid cells by a process called meiosis. In meiosis, homologous chromosomes line up. The DNA of the chromosome is broken on both chromosomes in several places and rejoined with the other strand. Later, the two homologous chromosomes are split into two separate cells that divide and become gametes. But, because of recombination, both of the chromosomes are a mix of alleles from the mother and father. Recombination creates new combinations of alleles. Alleles that arose at different times and different places can be brought together. Recombination can occur not only between genes, but within genes as well. Recombination within a gene can form a new allele. Recombination is a mechanism of evolution because it adds new alleles and combinations of alleles to the gene pool.

Gene flow

New organisms may enter a population by migration from another population. If they mate within the population, they can bring new alleles to the local gene pool. This is called gene flow. In some closely related species, fertile hybrids can result from interspecific matings. These hybrids can vector genes from species to species. Gene flow between more distantly related species occurs infrequently. This is called horizontal transfer. One interesting case of this involves genetic elements called P elements. Margaret Kidwell found that P elements were transferred from some species in the *Drosophila willistoni* group to *Drosophila melanogaster*. These two species of fruit flies are distantly related and hybrids do not form. Their ranges do, however, overlap.

The P elements were vectored into *D. melanogaster* via a parasitic mite that targets both these species. This mite punctures the exoskeleton of the flies and feeds on the 'juices'. Material, including DNA, from one fly can be transferred to another when the mite feeds. Since P elements actively move in the genome (they are themselves parasites of DNA), one incorporated itself into the genome of a *melanogaster* fly and subsequently spread through the species. Laboratory stocks of *melanogaster* caught prior to the 1940's lack of P elements. All natural populations today harbor them.

Overview of Evolution within a Lineage

Evolution is a change in the gene pool of a population over time, it can occur due to several factors. Three mechanisms add new alleles to the gene pool: mutation, recombination and gene flow. Two mechanisms remove alleles, genetic drift and natural selection. Drift removes alleles randomly from the gene pool. Selection removes deleterious alleles from the gene pool. The amount of genetic variation found in a population is the balance between the actions of these mechanisms.

Natural selection can also increase the frequency of an allele. Selection that weeds out harmful alleles is called negative selection. Selection that increases the frequency of helpful alleles is called positive, or sometimes positive Darwinian, selection. A new allele can also drift to high frequency. But, since the change in frequency of an allele each generation is random, nobody speaks of positive or negative drift.

Except in rare cases of high gene flow, new alleles enter the gene pool as a single copy. Most new alleles added to the gene pool are lost almost immediately due to drift or selection, only a small per cent ever reach a high frequency in the population. Even most moderately beneficial alleles are lost due to drift when they appear. But, a mutation can reappear numerous times.

The fate of any new allele depends a great deal on the organism it appears in. This allele will be linked to the other alleles near it for many generations. A mutant allele can increase in frequency simply because it is linked to a beneficial allele at a nearby locus. This can occur even if the mutant allele is deleterious, although it must not be so deleterious as to offset the benefit of the other allele. Likewise a potentially beneficial new allele can be eliminated from the gene pool because it was linked to deleterious alleles when it first arose. An allele 'riding on the coat tails' of a beneficial allele is called a hitchhiker. Eventually, recombination will bring the two loci to linkage equilibrium. But, the more closely linked two alleles are, the longer the hitchhiking will last. The effects of selection and drift are coupled. Drift is intensified as selection pressures increase. This is because increased selection (i.e. a greater difference in reproductive success among organisms in a population) reduces the effective population size, the number of individuals contributing alleles to the next generation. Adaptation is brought about by cumulative natural selection, the repeated sifting of mutations by natural selection. Small changes, favoured by selection, can be the stepping-stone to further changes. The summation of large numbers of these changes is macroevolution.

DEVELOPMENT OF EVOLUTIONARY THEORY

Biology came of age as a science when Charles Darwin published 'On the Origin of Species.' But, the idea of evolution wasn't new to Darwin. Lamarck published a theory of evolution in 1809. Lamarck thought that species arose continually from nonliving sources. These species were initially very primitive, but increased in complexity over time due to some inherent tendency. This type of evolution is called orthogenesis. Lamarck proposed that an organism's acclimation to the environment could be passed on to its offspring. For example, he thought proto-giraffes stretched their necks to reach higher twigs. This caused their offspring to be born with longer necks. This proposed mechanism of evolution is called the inheritance of acquired characteristics. Lamarck also believed species never went extinct, although they may change into newer forms. All three of these ideas are now known to be wrong.

Darwin's contributions include hypothesising the pattern of common descent and proposing a mechanism for evolution — natural selection. In Darwin's theory of natural selection, new variants arise continually within populations. A small percentage of these variants cause their bearers to produce more offspring than others. These variants thrive and supplant their less productive competitors. The effect of numerous instances of selection would lead to a species being modified over time.

Darwin's theory did not accord with older theories of genetics. In Darwin's time, biologists held to the theory of blending inheritance — an offspring was an average of its parents. If an individual had one short parent and one tall parent, it would be of medium height. And, the offspring would pass on genes for medium sized offspring. If this was the case, new genetic variations would quickly be diluted out of a population. They could not accumulate as the theory of evolution required. We now know that the idea of blending inheritance is wrong. Darwin didn't know that the true mode of inheritance was discovered in his lifetime. Gregor Mendel, in his experiments on hybrid peas, showed that genes from a mother and father do not blend. An offspring from a short and a tall parent may be medium sized, but it carries genes for shortness and tallness. The genes remain distinct and can be passed on to subsequent generations. Mendel mailed his paper to Darwin, but Darwin never opened it.

It was a long time until Mendel's ideas were accepted. One group of biologists, called biometricians, thought Mendel's laws only held for a few traits. Most traits, they claimed, were governed by blending inheritance. Mendel studied discrete traits. Two of the traits in his famous experiments were smooth versus wrinkled coat on peas. This trait did not vary continuously. In other words, peas are either wrinkled or smooth — intermediates are not found. Biometricians considered these traits aberrations. They studied continuously varying traits like size and believed most traits showed blending inheritance.

Incorporating Genetics into Evolutionary Theory

The discrete genes Mendel discovered would exist at some frequency in natural populations. Biologists wondered how and if these frequencies would change. Many thought that the more common versions of genes would increase in frequency simply because they were already at high frequency.

Hardy and Weinberg independently showed that the frequency of an allele would not change over time simply due to its being rare or common. Their model had several assumptions — that all alleles reproduced at the same rate, that the population size was very large and that alleles did not change in form. Later, R. A. Fisher showed that Mendel's laws could explain continuous traits if the expression of these traits were due to the action of many genes. After this, geneticists accepted Mendel's Laws as the basic rules of genetics. From this basis, Fisher, Sewall Wright and J. B. S. Haldane founded the field of population genetics. Population genetics is a field of biology that attempts to measure and explain the levels of genetic variation in populations.

R. A. Fisher studied the effect of natural selection on large populations. He demonstrated that even very small selective differences amongst alleles could cause appreciable changes in allele frequencies over time. He also showed that the rate of adaptive change in a population is proportional to the amount of genetic variation present. This is called Fisher's Fundamental Theorem of Natural Selection. Although it is called the fundamental theorem, it does not hold in all cases. The rate at which natural selection brings about adaptation depends on the details of how selection is working. In some rare cases, natural selection can actually cause a decline in the mean relative fitness of a population.

Sewall Wright was more concerned with drift. He stressed that large populations are often subdivided into many subpopulations. In his theory, genetic drift played a more important role compared to selection. Differentiation between subpopulations, followed by migration among them, could contribute to adaptations amongst populations. Wright also came up with the idea of the adaptive landscape — an idea that remains influential to this day. Its influence remains even though P. A. P. Moran has shown that, mathematically, adaptive landscapes don't exist as Wright envisioned them. Wright extended his results of one-locus models to a two-locus case in proposing the adaptive landscape. But, unbeknownst to him, the general conclusions of the one-locus model don't extend to the two-locus case.

J. B. S. Haldane developed many of the mathematical models of natural and artificial selection. He showed that selection and mutation could oppose each other, that deleterious mutations could remain in a population due to recurrent mutation. He also demonstrated that there was a cost to natural selection, placing a limit on the amount of adaptive substitutions a population could undergo in a given time frame. For a long time, population genetics developed as a theoretical field. But, gathering the data needed to test the theories was nearly impossible. Prior to the advent of molecular biology, estimates of genetic variability could only be inferred from levels of morphological differences in populations. Lewontin and Hubby were the first to get a good estimate of genetic variation in a population. Using the then new technique of protein electrophoresis, they showed that 30% of the loci in a population of *Drosophila pseudoobscura* were polymorphic. They also showed that it was likely that they could not detect all the variation that was present. Upon finding this level of variation, the question became — was this maintained by natural selection, or simply the result of genetic drift? This level of variation was too high to be explained by balancing selection. Motoo Kimura theorised that most variation found in populations was selectively equivalent (neutral). Multiple alleles at a locus differed in sequence, but their fitnesses were the same. Kimura's neutral theory described rates of evolution and levels of polymorphism solely in terms of mutation and genetic drift. The neutral theory did not deny that natural selection acted on natural populations, but it claimed that the majority of natural variation was transient polymorphisms of neutral alleles. Selection did not act frequently or strongly enough to influence rates of evolution or levels of polymorphism.

Initially, a wide variety of observations seemed to be consistent with the neutral theory. Eventually, however, several lines of evidence toppled it. There is less variation in natural populations than the neutral theory predicts. Also, there is too much variance in rates of substitutions in different lineages to be explained by mutation and drift alone. Finally, selection itself has been shown to have an impact on levels of nucleotide variation. Currently, there is no comprehensive mathematical theory of evolution that accurately predicts rates of evolution and levels of heterozygosity in natural populations.

EVOLUTION AMONG LINEAGES

Pattern of Macroevolution

Evolution is not progress. The popular notion that evolution can be represented as a series of improvements from simple cells, through more complex life forms, to humans (the pinnacle of evolution), can be traced to the concept of the scale of nature. This view is incorrect. All species have descended from a common ancestor. As time went on, different lineages of organisms were modified with descent to adapt to their environments. Thus, evolution is best viewed as a branching tree or bush, with the tips of each branch representing currently living species. No living organisms today are our ancestors. Every living species is as fully modern as we are with its own unique evolutionary history. No extant species are 'lower life forms,' atavistic stepping stones paving the road to humanity.

A related, and common, fallacy about evolution is that humans evolved from some living species of ape. This is not the case — humans and apes share a common ancestor. Both humans and living apes are fully modern species, the ancestor we evolved from was an ape, but it is now extinct and was not the same as present day apes (or humans for that matter). If it were not for the vanity of human beings, we would be classified as an ape. Our closest relatives are, collectively, the chimpanzee and the pygmy chimp. Thus, the next nearest relative is the gorilla.

Evidence for Common Descent and Macroevolution

Microevolution can be studied directly. Macroevolution cannot. Macroevolution is studied by examining patterns in biological populations and groups of related organisms and inferring process from pattern. Given the observation of microevolution and the knowledge that the earth is billions of years old — macroevolution could be postulated. But this extrapolation, in and of itself, does not provide a compelling explanation of the patterns of biological diversity we see today. Evidence for macroevolution, or common ancestry and modification with descent, comes from several other fields of study. These include: comparative biochemical and genetic studies, comparative developmental biology, patterns of biogeography, comparative morphology and anatomy and the fossil record.

Closely related species (as determined by morphologists) have similar gene sequences. Overall sequence similarity is not the whole story, however. The pattern of differences we see in closely related genomes is worth examining.

All living organisms use DNA as their genetic material, although some viruses use RNA. DNA is composed of strings of nucleotides. There are four different kinds of nucleotides: adenine (A), guanine (G), cytosine (C) and thymine (T). Genes are sequences of nucleotides that code for proteins. Within a gene, each block of three nucleotides is called a codon. Each codon designates an amino acid (the subunits of proteins). The three letter code is the same for all organisms (with a few exceptions). There are 64 codons, but only 20 amino acids to code for, so, most amino acids are coded for by several codons. In many cases the first two nucleotides in the codon designate the amino acid. The third position can have any of the four nucleotides and not effect how the code is translated.

A gene, when in use, is transcribed into RNA — a nucleic acid similar to DNA. (RNA, like DNA, is made up of nucleotides although the nucleotide uracil (U) is used in place of thymine (T).) The RNA transcribed from a gene is called messenger RNA. Messenger RNA is then translated via cellular machinery called ribosomes into a string of amino acids — a protein. Some proteins function as enzymes, catalysts that speed the chemical reactions in cells. Others are structural or involved in regulating development. Gene sequences in closely related species are very similar. Often, the same codon specifies a given amino acid in two related species, even though alternate codons could serve functionally as well. But, some differences do exist in gene sequences. Most often, differences are in third codon positions, where changes in the DNA sequence would not disrupt the sequence of the protein.

There are other sites in the genome where nucleotide differences do not effect protein sequences. The genome of eukaryotes is loaded with 'dead genes' called pseudogenes. Pseudogenes are copies of working genes that have been inactivated by mutation. Most pseudogenes do not produce full proteins. They may be transcribed, but not translated. Or, they may be translated, but only a truncated protein is produced. Pseudogenes evolve much faster than their working counterparts. Mutations in them do not get incorporated into proteins, so they have no effect on the fitness of an organism.

Introns are sequences of DNA that interrupt a gene, but do not code for anything. The coding portions of a gene are called exons. Introns are spliced out of the messenger RNA prior to translation, so they do not contribute information needed to make the protein. They are sometimes, however, involved in regulation of the gene. Like pseudogenes, introns (in general) evolve faster than coding portions of a gene.

Nucleotide positions that can be changed without changing the sequence of a protein are called silent sites. Sites where changes result in an amino acid substitution are called replacement sites. Silent sites are expected to be more polymorphic within a population and show more differences between populations. Although both silent and replacement sites receive the same amount of mutations, natural selection only infrequently allows changes at replacement sites. Silent sites, however, are not as constrained.

Kreitman was the first to demonstrate that silent sites were more variable than coding sites. Shortly after the methods of DNA sequencing were discovered, he sequenced 11 alleles of the enzyme alcohol dehydrogenase (AdH). Of the 43 polymorphic nucleotide sites he found, only one resulted in a change in the amino acid sequence of the protein. Silent sites may not be entirely selectively neutral. Some DNA sequences are involved with regulation of genes, changes in these sites may be deleterious. Likewise, although several codons code for a single amino acid, an organism may have a preferred codon for each amino acid. This is called codon bias.

If two species shared a recent common ancestor one would expect genetic information, even information such as redundant nucleotides and the position of introns or pseudogenes, to be similar. Both species would have inherited this information from their common ancestor.

The degree of similarity in nucleotide sequence is a function of divergence time. If two populations had recently separated, few differences would have built up between them. If they separated long ago, each population would have evolved numerous differences from their common ancestor (and each other). The degree of similarity would also be a function of silent versus replacement sites. Li and Graur, in their molecular evolution text, give the rates of evolution for silent vs. replacement rates. The rates were estimated from sequence comparisons of 30 genes from humans and rodents, which diverged about 80 million years ago. Silent sites evolved at an average rate of 4.61 nucleotide substitution per 10^9 years. Replacement sites evolved much slower at an average rate of 0.85 nucleotide substitutions per 10^9 years.

Groups of related organisms are 'variations on a theme' — the same set of bones are used to construct all vertebrates. The bones of the human hand grow out of the same tissue as the bones of a bat's wing or a whale's flipper, and, they share many identifying features such as muscle insertion points and ridges. The only difference is that they are scaled differently. Evolutionary biologists say this indicates that all mammals are modified descendants of a common ancestor which had the same set of bones.

Closely related organisms share similar developmental pathways. The differences in development are most evident at the end. As organisms evolve, their developmental pathway gets modified. An alteration near the end of a developmental pathway is less likely to be deleterious than changes in early development. Changes early on may have a cascading effect. Thus most evolutionary changes in development are expected to take place at the periphery of development, or in early aspects of development that have no later repercussions. For a change in early development to be propagated, the benefit of the early alteration must outweigh the consequences to later development.

Because they have evolved this way, organisms pass through the early stages of development that their ancestors passed through up to the point of divergence. So, an organism's development mimics its ancestors although it doesn't recreate it exactly. Development of the flatfish, Pleuronectes, illustrates this point. Early on, Pleuronectes develops a tail that comes to a point. In the next developmental stage, the top lobe of the tail is larger than the bottom lobe (as in sharks). When development is complete, the upper and lower lobes are equally sized. This developmental pattern mirrors the evolutionary transitions it has undergone.

Natural selection can modify any stage of a life cycle, so some differences are seen in early development. Thus, evolution does not always recapitulate ancestral forms — butterflies did not evolve from ancestral caterpillars, for example. There are differences in the appearance of early vertebrate embryos. Amphibians rapidly form a ball of cells in early development. Birds, reptiles and mammals form a disk. The shape of the early embryo is a result of different yolk concentrations in the eggs. Birds' and reptiles' eggs are heavily yolked. Their eggs develop similarly to amphibians except the yolk has deformed the shape of the embryo. The ball is stretched out and lying atop the yolk. Mammals have no yolk, but still form a disk early. This is because they have descended from reptiles. Mammals lost their yolky eggs, but retained the early pattern of development. In all these vertebrates, the pattern of cell movements is similar despite superficial differences in appearance. In addition, all types quickly converge upon a primitive, fish-like stage within a few days. From there, development diverges.

Traces of an organism's ancestry sometimes remain even when an organism's development is complete. These are called vestigial structures. Many snakes have rudimentary pelvic bones retained from their walking ancestors. Vestigial does not mean useless, it means the structure is clearly a vestige of an structure inherited from ancestral organisms. Vestigial structures may acquire new functions. In humans, the appendix now houses some immune system cells.

Closely related organisms are usually found in close geographic proximity, this is especially true of organisms with limited dispersal opportunities. The mammalian fauna of Australia is often cited as an example of this, marsupial mammals fill most of the equivalent niches that placentals fill in other ecosystems. If all organisms descended from a common ancestor, species distribution across the planet would be a function of site of origination, potential for dispersal, distribution of suitable habitat, and time since origination. In the case of Australian mammals, their physical separation from sources of placentals means potential niches were filled by a marsupial radiation rather than a placental radiation or invasion.

Natural selection can only mold available genetically based variation. In addition, natural selection provides no mechanism for advance planning. If selection can only tinker with the available genetic variation, we should expect to see examples of jury-rigged design in living species. This is indeed the case. In lizards of the genus *Cnemodophorus* (Fig. 22.1), females reproduce parthenogenetically. Fertility in these lizards is increased when a female mounts another female and simulates copulation. These lizards evolved from sexual lizards whose hormones were aroused by sexual behavior. Now, although the sexual mode of reproduction has been lost, the means of getting aroused (and hence fertile) has been retained.

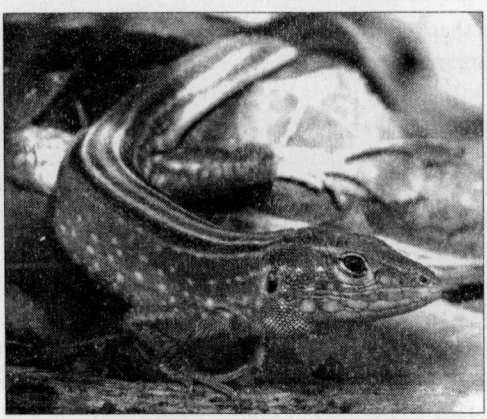

Fig. 22.1: *Cnemodophorus.*

Fossils show hard structures of organisms less and less similar to modern organisms in progressively older rocks. In addition, patterns of biogeography apply to fossils as well as extant organisms. When combined with plate tectonics, fossils provide evidence of distributions and dispersals of ancient species. For example, South America had a very distinct marsupial mammalian fauna until the land bridge formed between North and South America. After that marsupials started disappearing and placentals took their place. This is commonly interpreted as the placentals wiping out the marsupials, but this may be an over simplification.

Transitional fossils between groups have been found. One of the most impressive transitional series is the ancient reptile to modern mammal transition. Mammals and reptiles differ in skeletal details, especially in their skulls. Reptilian jaws have four bones. The foremost is called the dentary. In mammals, the dentary bone is the only bone in the lower jaw. The other bones are part of the middle ear. Reptiles have a weak jaw and a mouthful of undifferentiated teeth. Their jaw is closed by three muscles: the external, posterior and internal adductor. Each reptile tooth is single cusped. Mammals have powerful jaws with differentiated teeth. Many of these teeth, such as the molars, are multi-cusped. The temporalis and masseter muscles, derived from the external adductor, close the mammalian jaw. Mammals have a secondary palate, a bony structure separating their nostril passages and throat, so most can swallow and breathe simultaneously. Reptiles lack this.

The evolution of these traits can be seen in a series of fossils. *Procynosuchus* shows an increase in size of the dentary bone and the beginnings of a palate (Fig. 22.2). *Thrinaxodon* has a reduced number of incisors, a precursor to tooth differentiation. *Cynognathus* (a doglike carnivore) shows a further increase in size of the dentary bone. The other three bones are located inside the back portion of the jaw. Some teeth are multicusped and the teeth fit together tightly. *Diademodon* (a plant eater) shows a more advanced degree of occlusion (teeth fitting tightly). *Probelesodon* has developed a double joint in the jaw. The jaw could hinge off two points with the upper skull. The front hinge was probably the actual hinge while the rear hinge was an alignment guide. The forward movement of a hinge point allowed for the precursor to the modern masseter muscle to anchor further forward in the jaw. This allowed for a more powerful bite. The first true mammal was *Morgonucudon*, a rodent-like insectivore from the late Triassic. It had all the traits common to modern mammals. These species were not from a single, unbranched lineage. Each is an example from a group of organisms along the main line of mammalian

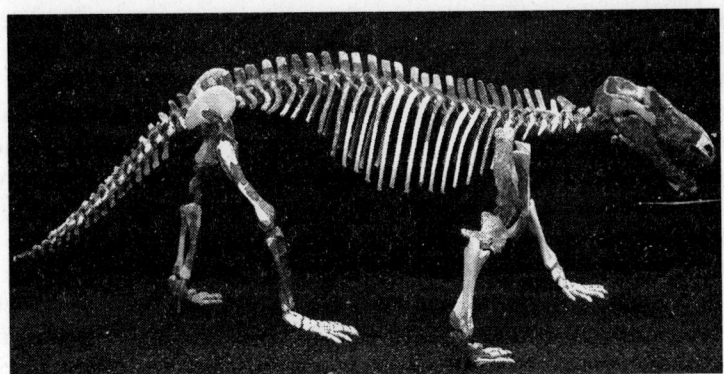

Fig. 22.2: *Procynosuchus.*

ancestry. The strongest evidence for macroevolution comes from the fact that suites of traits in biological entities fall into a nested pattern. For example, plants can be divided into two broad categories, non-vascular (ex. mosses) and vascular. Vascular plants can be divided into seedless (ex. ferns) and seeded. Vascular seeded plants can be divided into gymnosperms (ex. pines) and flowering plants (angiosperms). Angiosperms can be divided into monocots and dicots. Each of these types of plants have several characters that distinguish them from other plants. Traits are not mixed and matched in groups of organisms. For example, flowers are only seen in plants that carry several other characters that distinguish them as angiosperms. This is the expected pattern of common descent. All the species in a group will share traits they inherited from their common ancestor. But, each subgroup will have evolved unique traits of its own. Similarities bind groups together. Differences show how they are subdivided.

The real test of any scientific theory is its ability to generate testable predictions and, of course, have the predictions borne out. Evolution easily meets this criterion. If two organisms share a similar anatomy, one would then predict that their gene sequences would be more similar than a morphologically distinct organism. This has been spectacularly borne out by the recent flood of gene sequences — the correspondence to trees drawn by morphological data is very high. The discrepancies are never too great and usually confined to cases where the pattern of relationship was debated.

Mechanisms of Macroevolution

Speciation — increasing biological diversity

Speciation is the process of a single species becoming two or more species. Many biologists think speciation is key to understanding evolution. Some would argue that certain evolutionary phenomena apply only at speciation and macroevolutionary change cannot occur without speciation. Other biologists think major evolutionary change can occur without speciation. Changes between lineages are only an extension of the changes within each lineage. In general, paleontologists fall into the former category and geneticists in the latter.

Modes of speciation

Biologists recognise two types of speciation: allopatric and sympatric speciation. The two differ in geographical distribution of the populations in question. Allopatric speciation is thought to be the most common form of speciation. It occurs when a population is split into two (or more) geographically isolated subdivisions that organisms cannot bridge. Eventually, the two populations' gene pools change independently until they could not interbreed even if they were brought back together. In other words, they have speciated.

Sympatric speciation occurs when two subpopulations become reproductively isolated without first becoming geographically isolated. Insects that live on a single host plant provide a model for sympatric speciation. If a group of insects switched host plants they would not breed with other members of their species still living on their former host plant. The two subpopulations could diverge and speciate. Agricultural records show that a strain of the apple maggot fly *Rhagolettis pomenella* began infesting apples in the 1860's. Formerly it had only infested hawthorn fruit. Feder, Chilcote and Bush have shown that two races of *Rhagolettis pomenella* have become behaviorally isolated. Allele frequencies at six loci (aconitase 2, malic enzyme, mannose phosphate isomerase, aspartate amino-transferase, NADH-diaphorase-2, and beta-hydroxy acid dehydrogenase) are diverging. Significant amounts of linkage disequilibrium have been found at these loci, indicating that they may all be hitchhiking on some allele under selection. Some biologists call sympatric speciation microallopatric speciation to emphasise that the subpopulations are still physically separate at an ecological level.

Biologists know little about the genetic mechanisms of speciation. Some think a series of small changes in each subdivision gradually lead to speciation. The founder effect could set the stage for relatively rapid speciation, a genetic revolution in Ernst Mayr's terms. Alan Templeton hypothesised that a few key genes could change and confer reproductive isolation. He called this a genetic transilience. Lynn Margulis thinks most speciation events are caused by changes in internal symbionts. Populations of organisms are very complicated. It is likely that there are many ways speciation can occur. Thus, all of the above ideas may be correct, each in different circumstances.

Observed speciations

Speciation has been observed. In the plant genus *Tragopogon*, two new species have evolved within the past 50–60 years. They are *T. mirus* and *T. miscellus*. The new species were formed when one diploid species fertilised a different diploid species and produced a tetraploid offspring. This tetraploid offspring could not fertilise or be fertilised by either of its two parent species types. It is reproductively isolated, the definition of a species.

Extinction — Decreasing Biological Diversity

Ordinary extinction

Extinction is the ultimate fate of all species. The reasons for extinction are numerous. A species can be competitively excluded by a closely related species, the habitat a species lives in can disappear and/or the organisms that the species exploits could come up with an unbeatable defense.

Some species enjoy a long tenure on the planet while others are short- lived. Some biologists believe species are programmed to go extinct in a manner analogous to organisms being destined to die. The majority, however, believe that if the environment stays fairly constant, a well adapted species could continue to survive indefinitely.

Mass extinction

Mass extinctions shape the overall pattern of macroevolution. If you view evolution as a branching tree, it's best to picture it as one that has been severely pruned a few times in its life. The history of life on this earth includes many episodes of mass extinction in which many groups of organisms were wiped off the face of the planet. Mass extinctions are followed by periods of radiation where new species evolve to fill the empty niches left behind. It is probable that surviving a mass extinction is largely a function of luck. Thus, contingency plays a large role in patterns of macroevolution.

The largest mass extinction came at the end of the Permian, about 250 million years ago. This coincides with the formation of Pangaea II, when all the world's continents were brought together by plate tectonics. A worldwide drop in sea level also occurred at this time.

The most well-known extinction occurred at the boundary between the Cretaceous and Tertiary Periods. This called the K/T Boundary and is dated at around 65 million years ago. This extinction eradicated the dinosaurs. The K/T event was probably caused by environmental disruption brought on by a large impact of an asteroid with the earth. Following this extinction the mammalian radiation occurred. Mammals coexisted for a long time with the dinosaurs but were confined mostly to nocturnal insectivore niches. With the eradication of the dinosaurs, mammals radiated to fill the vacant niches. Currently, human alteration of the ecosphere is causing a global mass extinction.

Punctuated Equilibrium

The theory of punctuated equilibrium is an inference about the process of macroevolution from the pattern of species documented in the fossil record. In the fossil record, transition from one species to another is usually abrupt in most geographic locales — no transitional forms are found. In short, it appears that species remain unchanged for long stretches of time and then are quickly replaced by new species. However, if wide ranges are searched, transitional forms that bridge the gap between the two species are sometimes found in small, localised areas. For example, in Jurassic brachiopods of the genus *Kutchithyris*, *K. acutiplicata* appears below another species, *K. euryptycha*. Both species were common and covered a wide geographical area. They differ enough that some have argued they should be in a different genera. In just one small locality an approximately 1.25m sedimentary layer with these fossils is found. In the narrow (10 cm) layer that separates the two species, both species are found along with transitional forms. In other localities there is a sharp transition.

Eldredge and Gould proposed that most major morphological change occurs (relatively) quickly in small peripheral population at the time of speciation. New forms will then invade the range of their ancestral species. Thus, at most locations that fossils are found, transition from one species to another will be abrupt. This abrupt change will reflect replacement by migration however, not evolution. In order to find the transitional fossils, the area of speciation must be found.

There has been considerable confusion about the theory. Some popular accounts give the impression that abrupt changes in the fossil record are due to blindingly fast evolution, this is not a part of the theory. Punctuated equilibrium has been presented as a hierarchical theory of evolution. Proponents of punctuated equilibrium see speciation as analogous to mutation and the replacement of one species by another as analogous to natural selection. This is called species selection. Speciation adds new species to the species pool just as mutation adds new alleles to the gene pool. Species selection favours one species over another just as natural selection can favour one allele over another. Evolutionary trends within a group would be the result of selection among species, not natural selection acting within species. This is the most controversial part of the theory. Many biologists agree with the pattern of macroevolution these paleontologists posit, but believe species selection is not even theoretically likely to occur.

Critics would argue that species selection is not analogous to natural selection and therefore evolution is not hierarchical. Also, the number of species produced over time is far less than the amount of different alleles that enter gene pools over time. So, the amount of adaptive evolution produced by species selection (if it did occur) would have to be orders of magnitude less than adaptive evolution within populations by natural selection. Tests of punctuated equilibrium have been equivocal. It has been known for a long time that rates of evolution vary over time, that is not controversial. However, phylogenetic studies conflict as to whether there is a clear association between speciation and morphological change. In addition, there are major polymorphisms within some species. For example, bluegill sunfish have two male morphs. One is a large, long-lived, mate-protecting male, the other is a smaller, shorter-lived male who sneaks matings from females guarded by large males. The existence of within species polymorphisms demonstrates that speciation is not a requirement for major morphological change.

Importance of Evolution in Biology

'Nothing in biology makes sense except in the light of evolution.' — Theodosius Dobzhansky Evolution has been called the cornerstone of biology, and for good reasons. It is possible to do research in biology with little or no knowledge of evolution. Most biologists do. But, without evolution biology becomes a disparate set of fields. Evolutionary explanations pervade all fields in biology and brings them together under one theoretical umbrella.

We know from microevolutionary theory that natural selection should optimise the existing genetic variation in a population to maximise reproductive success. This provides a framework for interpreting a variety of biological traits and their relative importance. For example, a signal intended to attract a mate could be intercepted by predators. Natural selection has caused a trade- off between attracting mates and getting preyed upon. If you assume something other than reproductive success is optimised, many things in biology would make little sense. Without the theory of evolution, life history strategies would be poorly understood. Macroevolutionary theory also helps explain many things about how living things work. Organisms are modified over time by cumulative natural selection. The numerous examples of jury- rigged design in nature are a direct result of this. The distribution of genetically based traits across groups is explained by splitting of lineages and the continued production of new traits by mutation. The traits are restricted to the lineages they arise in.

Details of the past also hold explanatory power in biology. Plants obtain their carbon by joining carbon dioxide gas to an organic molecule within their cells. This is called carbon fixation. The enzyme that fixes carbon is RuBP carboxlyase. Plants using C3 photosynthesis lose 1/3 to 1/2 of the carbon dioxide they originally fix. RuBP carboxlyase works well in the absence of oxygen, but poorly in its presence. This is because photosynthesis evolved when there was little gaseous oxygen present. Later, when oxygen became more abundant, the efficiency of photosynthesis decreased. Photosynthetic organisms compensated by making more of the enzyme. RuBP carboxylase is the most abundant protein on the planet partially because it is one of the least efficient.

Ecosystems, species, organisms and their genes all have long histories. A complete explanation of any biological trait must have two components. First, a proximal explanation — how does it work? And second, an ultimate explanation — what was it modified from? For centuries humans have asked, 'Why are we here?' The answer to that question lies outside the realm of science. Biologists, however, can provide an elegant answer to the question, 'How did we get here?'

Chapter 23

Conservation Genetics

INTRODUCTION

Conservation genetics is concerned with population genetic variation, population viability, and the future evolution of species. Conservation genetics, ecology, and habitat management together provide the technical underpinnings of conservation biology, a crisis oriented science of biodiversity management. Still in its infancy, conservation genetics focuses on the characterisation of variation in populations and species and on the management of innate levels of variation in evolutionary significant units in nature and in their captive or managed analogs. Conservation genetic methods are borrowed from evolutionary biology and molecular genetics and are under development. Although some genetic management principles flow directly from current evolutionary theory, several key scientific problems remain to be solved before we can effectively deal with the issues presented by the biodiversity crisis. Although single species ecological methods have dominated conservation management practice, it is clear that maintaining the future evolvability of species will require greater genetic intervention in the future. Conservation genetics is thus a cornerstone of biodiversity conservation.

GENETIC VARIATION AND ITS SIGNIFICANCE

Until the 1960s, it was widely thought that genetic variation was unusual. Biologists regarded populations as being composed of many very similar 'wild type' individuals and a few rare mutant individuals. Following the introduction of allozyme electrophoresis it quickly became clear that most plant and animal populations were highly variable. Subsequently, it has become possible to examine DNA sequences directly and large numbers of base pair mutations have been discovered in functional genes of most living organisms studied. Even higher levels of variation occur in the introns and highly repetitive stretches of non-coding 'junk DNA' that lie between eukaryote genes. High levels of variability characterise most natural populations of plants and animals and this variability is thought to be both a product of evolutionary agents and a determinant of the future evolvability of a population. Genetics became a cornerstone of conservation science in 1981 with the publication of Frankel and Soules Conservation and Evolution. Since then, geneticists have studied the effects of the ongoing global reduction of genetic variability on population viability and species persistence.

Estimates of variability in a population vary with the feature examined and analytical method used. Karyotypic variation is usually low within a species, allozyme variation is high, and DNA sequence variation may be very high in some parts of the genome. The principle of high natural variability is perhaps best illustrated by the published surveys of allozyme patterns in plants and animals. Geneticists typically sample a population of 20 individuals and determine each individuals genotype at 10–20 loci. This allows them to calculate the mean number of alleles per locus (A), the mean individual heterozygosity (H), and the proportion of loci in the population that are polymorphic (P). A few thousand species have been examined to date and variation is typically in the following range: $H = 0.05–0.15$ and $P = 0.20–0.50$.

Still higher levels of natural variation are found at the DNA sequence level, especially in areas of the genome which are apparently free to mutate. Short repeat sequences (microsatellites) of nuclear DNA, for example, are often 10 times more variable than allozyme loci. A polymorphic allozyme may have 2 or 3 alleles segregating in a population, whereas a dinucleotide repeat microsatellite may have 10–15 alleles (differing in the number of times the motif is repeated) in the same individuals. Biochemical and molecular genetics have shown that most living organisms are richly variable. Much of the cryptic variation in natural populations that has been discovered in the past 30 years appears to be selectively neutral or near neutral in its effect on the phenotype. That is, the individuals carrying these various allelic variants appear perfectly healthy. It is rare to find a single locus genetic trait in which a deleterious condition such as albinism is controlled by a single allelic variant. In fact, there is strong circumstantial evidence that much of this genetic variation is actually beneficial. Although the relationship between genetic variability and individual fitness is not well understood, it is clear that variability is associated with viability. Experiments and field observations with a few species have shown that there is a positive relationship between genetic variability and individual growth rate, size at maturity, symmetry of body parts, fecundity, and health as measured by parasite load. Extrapolating from the individual level to the population level, it is a fundamental maxim of evolutionary biology that genetic variation is positively related to adaptability or evolvability. Fisher's fundamental theorem holds that additive genetic variation in fitness is positively related to a population's ability to respond to natural selection. Evolutionary success, the ability of a species to persist despite changes in climate and exposure to new diseases, predators, and competitors, is somehow related to innate genetic variability. In a world of unpredictable change, alleles that are selectively neutral for thousands of generations may suddenly become lifesavers for the individuals that carry them. If evolution is largely dependent on genetic variability, then the conservation of species will sooner or later depend on the conservation of their innate genetic variability.

Of course, there are many apparently successful genetically invariant plants and animals. There are many known clonal organisms whose descendents are genetically identical to their mothers. Such clonal plants, snails, fish, and lizards are genetically invariant even though they may exhibit great ecological success. However, they are more likely to go extinct when their environment changes than are closely related sexually reproducing species. Although meiosis ensures the maintenance of high variability in the sexual species, their asexually reproducing daughter species gradually lose their initial low variability and over time become evolutionary dead ends.

There are many different ways of measuring genetic variability, including the examination of karyotypes and singlelocus markers (allozymes, mitochondrial and chloroplast DNA restriction fragment length polymorphisms), DNA minisatellite fingerprints, random amplified polymorphic DNA, mtDNA sequences, nuclear DNA sequences, and nDNA microsatellites (simple sequence repeats). Benirschke and Kumamoto and Smith and Wayne provide numerous examples of the application of karyotypes and molecular genetic markers, respectively, to conservation. The various methods differ in their resolution of pedigree, population, and species level questions and there is no single correct technique. One method, allozyme electrophoresis, is informative with mammals but frustratingly uninformative for birds. The methods also differ greatly in their cost and technical difficulty. Some relatively inexpensive methods are satisfactory for one time analyses but the results cannot be built on in subsequent studies. Other methods, in contrast, provide genotypes which can be archived in expandable permanent databases such as GenBank for future comparative study of samples collected at other times or places. Although a given method will give comparable results in a study of closely related populations or species, results across unrelated taxa may not be comparable.

Currently, nuclear and mitochondrial sequence data are the most informative methods for characterising variability at or above the level of populations. For studies of variation within populations, hyper variable nuclear microsatellite loci are ideal markers. Sequence data and microsatellite genotypes can now be deter—mined directly from minute DNA samples amplified many times by the polymerase chain reaction. Boti methods require fully equipped laboratories, trained personnel, and considerable time and money for developing the synthetic DNA primers to amplify the gene sequences of interest in species that have never been studied before. Noninvasive genotyping methods involving the extraction of DNA from shed hair and feathers were introduced in 1989 and are now widely used. Noninvasive (shed tissues, feces, urine, and scent markings) and nondestructive (toe, tail, and ear clips and fish scales) genotyping permits the study of wildlife populations that previously were almost impossible to sample. Not surprisingly, the DNA extracted from some types of samples may be degraded and very difficult to work with. Nevertheless, with technical care and patience it is possible to genotype some animals without actually seeing or handling them.

Conservation geneticists can also genotype museum specimens and determine patterns of variability over periods of decades and sometimes centuries. Several species that have gone extinct recently, including the dodo, moa, thylacine, and quagga, have been characterised genetically. DNA can also be extracted and sequenced from some fossil remains, but DNA degradation rates are such that fossils more than a few million years old are unlikely to yield reliable sequences. Although enormously interesting to evolutionary biologists, such ancient DNA cannot be used to recreate extinct organisms. Conservation geneticists must concentrate on saving existing biodiversity, they cannot fall back on the idea of being able to recreate extinct species from the tiny fragments of DNA (typically less than 0.00001% of an organism's genome) currently under scrutiny.

Genetic data, once acquired, are used by conservation geneticists to quantify within and between population variability. Variability within populations is used to establish pedigree relations, mating system, sex ratio, and genetic effective population size (N_e). Inter population comparisons reveal spatial structuring and historical patterns of gene flow. Geographic variation is normal within a species and the new field of phylogeography uses genetic information to infer the historical relationships among populations. Single and multilocus genetic differences between kin, populations, subspecies, and species are expressed as genetic distances. These metrics and their interpretations are beyond the scope of this review, but it is important to note that the absolute values of genetic distances will vary between different groups of plants and animals and increase over geological time. Within a group of related species a major difference in the genetic distances observed within and between taxa can be used to define species and other evolutionarily significant units for conservation management purposes. Although the previous discussion focused on molecular genetic variation, the growing field of quantitative trait genetics promises to provide a new means of measuring evolutionarily significant population variables. Quantitative genetics is concerned with characters such as morphology, behaviour, parasite resistance, and physiology that are controlled by several to many genes that work additively, in dominance/recessive relationships, or epistatically. Such oligogenic and polygenic control, involving quantitative trait loci (QTL), is characteristic of many traits of interest to conservationists—those that effect longterm population persistence and evolvability. QTLs affecting body size, hatching date, and predator avoidance behaviour (escape speed), for example, are ecologically important and are arguably of greater significance to conservationists than allozyme polymorphism. Conservationists are therefore interested in the heritability of such traits that have a direct impact on fitness.

High heritabilities of a QTL indicate that a population has great potential for trait evolution and low heritabilities indicate a more limited ability to respond to environmental change. Unfortunately, such heritability is difficult to measure because it requires pedigreelevel studies conducted over several generations or longterm manipulative experiments such as controlled garden plots. Heritability (h^2) is the ratio of the variance of the genetically inherited proportion of a trait (the additive genetic variance, V_A) to the total phenotypic variance V_p measured in the population. VA is one component of genetic variance (V_G) which also includes nonadditive genetic variance due to dominance (VD) and epistasis (V_i), only V_A responds to directional selection. Estimating V_A is further complicated by the need to estimate variance due to the environment (V_E) as well as the other genetic components.

Nevertheless, the preparation of studbooks for captive populations of endangered animals and the comparison of laboratory raised seedlings of rare plants to their parents in the wild have provided opportunities for the first limited applications of QTL analyses to conservation. Future technical advances may permit the inclusion of QTL in the conservation geneticist's tool kit of predictors of a population's risk of extinction.

A major issue requiring resolution is the validity of the widely held relationship between molecular genetic variation and ecological viability and evolutionary potential. Are single gene markers (those typically surveyed by geneticists) useful indicators of variation at quantitative traits? Are multilocus allozyme surveys unreliable as predictors of a population's viability since heterozygosity may be only weakly correlated with the additive genetic variation associated with QTLs? In desert topminnows of the genus Poeciliopsis, Vrijenhoek found that rapid losses of heterozygosity in small, isolated populations were associated with a decline in fitness that was manifested as poor competitive ability, growth rate, developmental stability, and resistance to parasites. O'Brien, in a remarkable series of genetic studies of captive and wild cheetahs (Acynonyx jubatus), demonstrated a powerful association between low levels of genetic variability and susceptibility to viral diseases.

There is no 'normal' level of variation for a population—even as determined with a specific method. Cheetah, northern elephant seal (Mirounga angustirostris), and European badger (Meles meles) are ecologically successful despite low absolute levels of genetic variation. Different types of genetic variability will respond differently to natural selection, inbreeding, population collapse, and range fragmentation. Conservation geneticists can identify cases in which variation has or is being lost, establish the causes of the loss, and make recommendations to counter its ultimate effects.

Because currently available genetic markers are only proxies for fitness determinants, this underscores the importance of using different markers. It is not the purpose of this review to discuss the technical problems associated with each method or the applicability of the different methods to different groups of plants and animals, but it is important to emphasise that each method has unresolved technical problems (e.g. null alleles, allelic dropout, pseudogenes, and nonreplicable patterns). Until molecular and QTL genotyping become routine, conservation geneticists must guard against the natural tendency to overstate the statistical power of their results.

LEVELS OF INTEREST TO CONSERVATION GENETICISTS

Genes

Long before the term conservation genetics was coined, the phrase 'genetic conservation' was introduced to describe the science of managing specific genes or phenotypic traits in crop plants, land races and cultivars, bacteria and fungi used in food production, and domes ticated animals. Genetically modified organisms (GMOs) are simply special cases that require even more intensive management for their perpetuation. The methods of gene discovery and artificial selection developed for managing micro-organisms, plants, and animals are relevant to the far more broadly focused field of conservation genetics, but very few wild species have received such intensive effort.

Discussions of the need to save this or that desired gene in a population are in fact arguments for saving a particular allelic form (variant) of a gene and not the gene itself. Some alleles are common and others are rare. Deleterious alleles (e.g. alleles responsible for albinism or other genetic 'defects') are typically very rare and have frequencies of less than 0.0001. Conservation geneticists are often asked to devise breeding plans that will further reduce or even eliminate such alleles from a population. On the other hand, it has been argued that conservation geneticists should strive to save rare alleles in threatened populations because they may provevital for a populations adaptation to future environmental changes. Although this argument is reasonable, the maintenance of desirable rare alleles, even if they were identifiable, requires very large population sizes ($N_e > 5000$) and is simply not possible in most management programs. Rarealleles contribute very little to variation in fitness among individuals and are less likely than alleles at relatively high frequency to be the basis of adaptive response to environmental change. It has been suggested that conservationists should focus on saving diversity at major histocompatibility complex (MHC) genes because they play a role in recognition of infectious agents, disease susceptibility, and defense. This recommendation was well intended but rejected because the functional (fitness related) significance of the large number of alleles at each of the many MHC genes is unknown. Managing them as a single linkage group would require very large populations or the inevitable loss of variation at other potentially important loci.

Populations

Interest in the concept of minimum viable populations spawned the development of new methods of pedigree analysis and population viability analysis. Populations have both a census size (N) and a genetic effective population size (N_e), the latter is one of the most important concepts in theoretical conservation biology and is deffrred in Section III,G and by Lande and Barrow clough. The characterisation of genetic variation within and among populations enables geneticists to help set conservation priorities. Comparative levels of variation and gene flow (or lack of either) provide clues to a population's viability and extinction proneness. Data on genetic relationships among populations guide translocation decisions and identify well-defined clusters of populations for management as separate entities.

Pedigree analysis refers to a suite of genetic models for understanding processes in small populations. First developed for assessing management practices in captive populations, pedigree analysis is also applicable to wild populations of individually monitored organisms. It is used to establish kinship and individual founder contributions, to identify genetically desirable and undesirable individuals and their descendents, to minimise inbreeding, to describe population structure and mating system, and to choose individuals for reintroduction or translocation. Examples of pedigree analysis with the Gene Drop computer program include Haig's study of the redcockaded woodpecker, Picoides borealis. Pedigree management programs based on meankinship or equalising founder contributions seek to minimise inbreeding in local subpopulations and in the metapopulation as a whole. Captive breeding programs have been successful in slowing the loss of genetic variation and preventing inbreeding depression.

Population viability analysis (PVA) is the methodology used to assess the ecological and genetic risks facing a wild or captive population and to develop a conservation management plan. PVA refers to a suite of mathematical models that seek to predict the probability of a population's extinction by some time in the future, e.g. 20 or 100 years. Early models considered demography (growth rate, present population size, and birth rate) and environmental stochasticity, but Gilpin and Soulé broadened the definition to include genetic factors. Genetic factors, including genetic drift and fixation of deleterious mutations, are expressed through demographic factors that affect population dynamics. The genetic factors thus contribute to extinction probabilities through a very complex and little understood series of interactions affecting fitness. Geneticists can use population variation to provide estimates of the various parameters of interest to modelers and managers. Unfortunately, genetic models with linkages to ecological factors are still insufficiently developed to yield the type of statistically powerful PVAs managers seek. Most PVAs, in fact, have not included genetic parameters, but this is changing as the significance of genetics in the longterm survival of small populations becomes more widely appreciated.

Metapopulations are populations of subpopulations within some defined area, in which dispersal from one local population (subpopulation) to at least some other habitat patchesis possible. There is significant turnover of local populations, local extinction, and recolonisation bydispersal. The metapopulation concept is central to much ecology and conservation theory and single and multiple species metapopulation dynamics are reviewed by Hanski and Gilpin. The genetic effective size of a metapopulation is affected by the carrying capacity of the habitat patches, the rates of extirpation and recolonisation, the number and source of the founders, the number of local populations, and the rate of gene flow between patches. It is difficult to establish metapopulation effective size using genetic data because it is strongly affected by extirpation and recolonisation dynamics. As in the case of genetic effective population size of single populations, the metapopulation effective size is 10–100 times less than the census size in many species. Metapopulation dynamics, with frequent local extinction and recolonisation of habitat patches by few founders, can reduce N, to a small fraction of N, with a resulting loss of genetic variability like that associated with a demographic bottleneck. Detailed studies of metapopulations are reviewed by Hanski and Gilpin and include the Glanville fritillary butterfly (*Melitaea cinxia*) and the red bladder campion (*Silene dioica*), both in Sweden, the checkerspot butterfly (*Euphydryas editha*) restricted to serpentine outcrops in California, and the pikas (*Ochotona principes*), a small mammal restricted to isolated talus slopes in alpine areas. Although the theory of metapopulations is well developed, and the relevance of metapopulation theory to the management of small, semi isolated populations of threatened species is clear, the empirical testing of the ecological and genetic predictigngis only just beginning.

Using molecular markers to characterise mating system, population structure, and phylogeography permits recognition of management units (MUs, sets of populations with shared distinctive alleles frequencies) and evolutionarily significant units (ESUs, sets of populations distinguished by strong phylogenetic structure based on multilocus mtDNA or nDNA variation). Moritz describes Australian examples of MUS (the yellow footed wallaby, Petrogale xanthopus, which is patchily distributed on isolated rock outcrops in southwest Queensland) and ESUs (four ghost bat ESUs previously treated as a single widespread species, Macroderma gigas, whose evolutionary divergence was not apparent until genetic methods were applied). Although the criteria used to define these two categories are not agreed upon, ESUs represent deep phylogenetic subdivisions typically within a species or occasionally, as in the case of local endemics, the entire species, and MUs reflect shallower subdivisions within a species which for practical reasons become the focus of management activities. Translocations between ESUs are typically undesirable.

Subspecies

Subspeciesor local geographic races have been the focus of intense conservation efforts. Genetics is useful in establishing whether such groups of populations are sufficiently different to warrant separate conservation efforts. The conservation of every local race or subspecies is difficult to justify if they are genetically almost identical. Although we may recommend trying to preserve every variety of wild tomato or maize in a seed bank, it is difficult to use the same justification to try to conserve all local variants of geographical'y widespread organisms.

Many biologists have abandoned the subspecies concept and the associated trinomial nomenclature. To them, the subspecies is an evolutionarily insignificant artificial taxon typically based on a few superficial morphological features. There are numerous cases in which genetic studies provide no support for the traditional subspecific taxonomy. Nevertheless, there is much to be learned from the geographic patterns of variation in nature. Subspecies were typically defined as geographical races with allopatric or parapatric distributions. The observation of significant hybridisation without introgression, in the latter cases, led to the development of the semispecies concept which is of relevance to conservation. Semispecies are typically parapatrically distributed and hybridise where their ranges meet, but they show very limited introgression. They are effectively isolated groups of populations evolving independently of one another. Collectively, a group of semispecies comprise a superspecies and each semispecies is treated taxonomically as a full species. In this case, geographically defined taxa that used to betreated as subspecies are actually independent evolutionary lineages and therefore as worthy of conservation as other 'good' species.

Conservation geneticists are often asked to advise on proposals to pool individuals from allopatric populations on the argument that it is better to save a generic species than no species. Although poorly differentiated subspecies may often be mixed without genetic harm, the pooling of individuals of well differentiated semispecies or species is likely to have negative genetic consequences.

Geneticists are often involved in two other situations involving subspecies and local variants. The first involves populations on either side of national or state boundaries that may be assigned to different subspecies and can receive radically different levels of protection, a species wide conservation plan may allocate resources differently and be biologically preferable. The second situation occurs when peripheral populations of a widespread species become the focus of conservation activities. Although such peripheral populations may be at high risk of local extinction, their conservation may not be warranted, especially in cases in which reintroduction is practical. On the other hand, someperipheral populations may be critical to a species' longterm survival. Some peripheral populations may be better adapted to changing climatic conditions than central populations even though the latter may be more genetically variable. At a time of global warming, poleward peripheral populations of a species may be more important than those closest to the equator.

Species

As it is thought that half the species of larger vertebrates are at risk of extinction in the next 100 years, most discussions of the conservation of biodiversity focus on species. Species are fundamental units of evolution and classification (taxonomy). However, despite their centrality to the field, conservation geneticists rarely work at the level of whole species and concentrate instead on infraspecific levels of organisation. Ernst Mayr introduced the biological species concept in 1942, species were defined as groups of actually or potentially interbreeding natural populations that are reproductively isolated from other such groups. This concept stimulated an enormous amount of research in the second half of the twentieth century. Despite its impact, problems with Mayr's original definition, with its overemphasis on reproductive isolation and its focus on sexually reproducing out crossing populations over short time spans, led to the development of atleast 18 alternative concepts by the end of the century. Although some of these have limited operational utility, three newer biological species concepts are of particular relevance to conservation geneticists. All seek to recognise discrete groups of populations with a shared evolutionary future. All three concepts, like Mayr's, seek to capture the essential genetic relatedness within, and the genetic distance between, biological species. All allow that the absolute values of observed relatedness and distance will vary with the geological age of a species and will vary in different groups of plants and animals.

Mayr's biological species concept forced researchers to search for reproductive isolating mechanisms between species in nature and to investigate their potential significance in laboratory and greenhouse hybridisation experiments. Such work typically took years and the results were often compromised by methodological limitations. It became clear that morphology was not always a good indicator of species boundaries and not surprisingly that traditional taxonomy was often a poor guide for conservation decision making. The introduction of protein electrophoresis and molecular genetic methods of measuring genetic variation has dramatically changed the approach to defining species. It is now possible to quickly establish whether populations exchange genes or whether they are effectively reproductively isolated. It is possible to estimate genetic distances between groups of populations and gauge their significance in comparison to within population variation. It is possible to estimate the time since a speciation event and the historical patterns of gene flow within and between taxa. Our newly foundability to characterise and recognise species genetically does not diminish the value of field and laboratory studies of behavioural ecology, but it does permit geneticists to make powerful contributions to the practice of conservation. Although it is fortunately still unusual for geneticists to work on the conservation of entire species, there are an increasing number of cases in which every individual in a species has been genotyped to some degree for management purposes. Such cases include Przewalski's horse (*Equus przewalski*), San Clemente loggerhead shrike (*Lanius ludovicianus mearnsi*), whooping crane (*Grus americana*), and Catalina mahogany (*Cerocarpus traskiae*).

Communities

Although it is unusual to think of geneticists working at higher levels of organisation than species, regional multispecies phylogeographic surveys are useful in defining the historical interactions of whole communities of organisms. Studies of regional phylogeographic structure, as for example in the southeastern United States or savanna ecosystems of Tanzania, are relevant to the design and maintenance of biodiversity sanctuaries. Elsewhere, populations in ecotonal regions have been found to have higher genediversity and are thus recommended for higher conservation priority.

EVOLUTIONARY PROCESSES OF INTEREST TO CONSERVATION GENETICISTS

Mutation

Mutations, the occurrence of heritable changes in the genetic material, are typically very rare processes that ultimately provide the raw material of genetic variation upon which the other agents of evolution operate. Mutations span a wide array of phenomena, from single base pair changes in the genetic code to accidental doublings of the number of chromosomes in a gamete. Many mutations are deleterious or lethal, some are near neutral, and a few may be beneficial to the carrier. The vast majority of mutations are completely invisible in the phenotype and can only be detected with an array of genetic techniques.

Mutations become of concern to conservationists in a couple of circumstances. First, the presence of a normally very rare allele of major effect in a remnant or closed captive population can have serious consequences. Deleterious traits discussed by Ryder and Fleischer include hairlessness in redruffed lemurs (*Varecia variegata ruber*), funnel chest in black and white ruffed lemurs (*Varecia variegata variegata*), and congenital diaphragmatic hernia in golden lion tamarin (*Leontopithecus rosalia*). Second, artificial selection for rare alleles is sometimes the goal of captive breeding programs. White tigers (*Pantheratigris*), homozygous for a recessive allele, are beautiful but suffer genetic disease with metabolic, nervous, and developmental consequences. Selection for such traits in the context of the conservation of an endangered species is unjustified.

As most populations of conservation concern lose genetic variability, the question arises as to whether new mutations will replace variability lost by population extirpation and genetic erosion. The answer is yes and no. Given that mutation rates are typically on the order of one per 10^9 cell divisions, the time for the accumulation of new variants in a population is on the order of tens of thousands of years. Therefore, conservation geneticists are more concerned with the deleterious effects of mutations in small populations than with their very longterm benefits.

Extinction due to genetic causes is almost unknown, but their contribution to the process should not be ignored. Although natural selection purges deleterious alleles from populations almost immediately, mildly deleterious, near neutral mutations will gradually increase in frequency and become serious problems when their frequencies exceed 0.05 or $1/(2N_e)$. Fortunately, this process takes hundreds of generations in all but the smallest isolated populations. Therefore, although such mildlydeleterious mutations are rarely considered by wildlife conservationists, they will ultimately diminish the longterm viability of many threatened taxa. On the other hand, managers of captive populations have to recognise this threat from the outset. If the goal of a breeding program is to return a captive population to the wild, then managers should maximise genetic variation including mildly deleterious mutants. Alternatively, if a population cannot be returned to the wild and must be sustained in captivity for many generations, then managers will need to purge deleterious mutations as they are identified.

Mutation rates at near neutral genes controlling quantitative characters set a lower limit on the population size necessary for future evolution. Harmful mutation rates set lower limits for population sizes for avoiding inbreeding depression and for preventing genetic erosion of fitness by the accumulation of mildly deleterious mutations. The suggestion that small populations ($N_e < 100$) may decline in fitness with the accumulation of mildly deleterious mutations, termed mutational meltdown, is under theoretical and experimental study.

Mating System

Although much population genetic theory is premised on 'random mating,' such behaviour is rarely observed in nature. Even related species may have very different mating systems with very different genetic consequences. Self fertilisation in hermaphroditic organisms and obligate out breeding in dioecious organisms are the two extreme modes. Conservation managers have to be aware of these differences if they are to mimic a species' natural history. The most extreme examples of conservation problems involving mating systems involve cases in which the last surviving individuals in a sexually reproducing population all belong to the same sex. The last passenger pigeon (*Ectopistes migratorius* Fig. 23.1) was a female, the last member of one of the 11 surviving subspecies of Galapagostortoise (Geochelone elephantopsus) is a male, Lonesome George. It is likely that cloning technologies currently under development will be applicable to saving such lineages in the future.

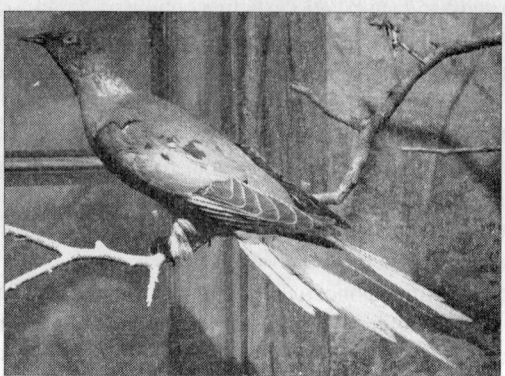

Fig. 23.1: *Ectopistes migratorius.*

Inbreeding

Inbreeding refers to the mating of close relatives in species that are normally outbreeding. Matings between father and daughter, brother and sister, or first cousins are examples of inbreeding. Many species of plants and animals have evolved devices to minimise close inbreeding. Species vary greatly in their tolerance of inbreeding, some trees and dioecious plants are obligate outcrossers. The genetic underpinnings of inbreeding depression are best understood in *Drosophila*, in which recessive lethal mutations and mildly deleterious mutations are major causes. Gradual inbreeding permits natural selection to purge the former but the partially recessive near neutral mutations continue to increase in frequency and significance. Outcrossing populations that suddenly decline in numbers usually experience reduced viability and fecundity known as inbreeding depression. Inbreeding produces increased homozygosity of recessive partially deleterious mutants and by chancein small populations these alleles become fixed. In the simplest genetic situation of a trait under the control of a lethal recessive allele, there is an increased risk that the offspring of two related healthy but heterozygous individuals will inherit the harmful allele from each parent and die. Although the risk in this case is only one in four, this amounts to a powerfully strong fitness differential on which natural selection will act. Generalising from this simplest singlelocus case, geneticists speak of inbreeding depression as the manifestation of the whole genomic effects of mating of close relatives. These effects may involve outright genetic disease (congenital abnormalities) but are more often subtle and appear as decreased growth rate, behavioural abnormalities, and reduced fertility and fecundity. Therefore, inbreeding is rare in typically outbreeding populations but becomes a serious problem in small isolated populations. In small fragmented populations in nature and in captive populations, inbreeding depression can threaten population viability. Animal breeders learned these lessons from centuries of experience with artificial selection, and they limit inbreeding rates to less than 2% per generation. The consequences of very close inbreeding are well illustrated by experience with establishing 'inbred' strains of laboratory mice, the majority of inbred lines die out within 10 generations. There is abundant evidence that captive wildlife populations suffer inbreeding depression. Ralls was the first to show that even well intended captive breeding programs subjected small populations to inbreeding depression. Smith and others empirical records for 40 species, mainly ungulates, in zoos and found inbreeding to be a problem in most cases. Inbreeding is also associated with decreased growth rate and blindness in a captive wolf population in Sweden. In the wild, the final decline of the heath hen (*Tympanuchus cupido* Fig. 23.2) on Martha's Vineyard island in 1932 involved inbreeding effects. Other better documented cases involving declining or threatened wild populations involve the middle spotted woodpecker (*Dendrocopos medius*) in Sweden, the Florida panther (*Puma concolor coryi*), Barrow Island populations of the black footed rock wallaby (*Petrogale lateralis*), common shrews (Sorex ananeus) in England, deer mice (*Peromyscus polionotus*), and Glanville fritillary butterfly (*Melitaea cinxia*) in the Aland Islands, Finland.

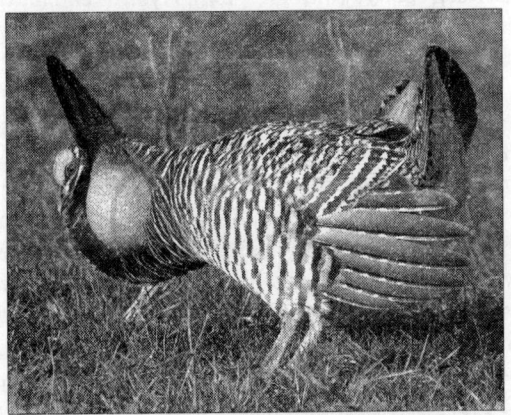

Fig. 23.2: *Tympanuchus cupido.*

In 1980, Franklin and Soulé independently showed, based on theory and experiments, that inbreeding depression can be avoided in the short term if $N_e > 50$. The inbreeding coefficient F increases by ½N, per generation and centuries of animal breeding experience shows that a 1% increase in F per generation is tolerable, thus, an $N_e = 50$ is necessary to avoid inbreeding depression. Franklin and Soulé further concluded that an $N_e > 500$ was necessary to enable a population to continue to evolve in the long term. Although this 500 number has been revised upwards, the simplicity of the FranklinSoulé numbers caught the attention of managers and legitimised the role of genetics in conservation. The theory behind the 50 number is still accepted, but it is important to realise that its derivation was based on controlled laboratory experiments, larger N_e are required in nature, where environmental fluctuations are more severe and stressful.

Outbreeding

Outbreeding, or the crossing of unrelated individuals, is widespread in nature. It is widely believed that sexual reproduction evolved in part because chromosomal crossing over and recombination facilitated by outbreeding produces more genetic variability than do other mating systems. Many species of plants and animals have effective immunological and behavioural mechanisms to favour outbreeding. The latter include sexbiased dispersal of young adults from their natal population and elaborate courtship behaviours. Even in plants with both male and female flowers, outbreeding is ensured by asynchronous maturation of male and female gametes and the evolution of various self incompatibility systems.

Outbreeding depression occurs when very distantly related conspecific individuals are mated or when members of two different but related species hybridise. The male and female genomes are sufficiently different to produce a hybrid with genetic disorders. Conservation geneticists encounter outbreeding depression in inadvertently mixed captive populations. Sterility, or partial sterility in one sex, and high neonate mortality are commonly observed manifestations.

Hybridisation

Outbreeding depression occurs in nature in some hybrid zones between semispecies and species of plants and animals. Hybrids are interesting because they show that the evolution of many groups of plant and animal species involves both lineage splitting and lineage anastamosis. Fertile inter specific hybrids permit gene flow between species (introgression). Hybrids call into question species definitions that overemphasise reproductive isolation. The notion that 'species' are somehow 'purebred' and always reproductively isolated from their close relatives is not borne out by observations of some animal groups and many plants, in which low rates of hybridisation between congeners often occur in nature.

In the past, it was argued that hybrid populations did not qualify for legal protection under the US Endangered Species Act. However, hybrids are very much a normal part of nature. Rare or very rare in some groups, and more common in others, they present conservationists with a dilemma because their occurrence appears to diminish the value of a taxon. Should one save Florida panthers if they are known to harbour genes of introduced South American panthers, a different subspecies? Do Texas red wolves (Canis rufus) merit conservation if they are gray wolf—coyote hybrids? Should one save the remaining Przewalski's horses if it is shown that historical mismanagement resulted in a large fraction of the surviving animals being tainted by the genes of domestic horses, a karyologically distinct species? Whether hybrids should be afforded the samepriority as nonintrogressed populations or species will remain controversial, in the previous cases, the answer was yes and geneticists contributed to pedigree management.

Habitat disturbance can result in increased opportunities for hybridisation between species that would not normally interbreed. Fragmentation of the recently continuous Pacific Northwest old growth forest has led to hybridisation between the declining northern spotted owl (Strix occidentalis) and the barred owl (S. varia), which favours disturbed sites. Hybridisation is more common in plants than in animals, therefore, not surprisingly it is in plants that there are numerous examples of rare species being hybridised into extinction (genetic assimilation) by hybridisation with a more common sympatric congener. This is the case for the Catalina Island mahogany, in which 5 of the remaining 11 adult trees are actually hybrids with the more common mountain mahogany. Other cases involve plants (Asteracea: Argyranthemum) in the Canary Islands. The Simien jackal (Canis simensis) of Ethiopia is at risk of being introgressed into extinction by hybridisation with domestic dogs. It is now recognised that restocking rivers with genetically uniform hatcherybred salmon has contributed to the collapse of the Pacific Northwest salmonruns. Hatchery fish show reduced fitngss in the wild (they are not locally adapted) and compete and hybridise harmfully with the remaining wild salmon.

Gene Flow

Gene flow is a fundamental agent of evolution based on the dispersal of genes between populations of a species. It involves the active or passive movement of individual plants, animals, gametes, or seeds. Gene flow involves not just dispersal but also the successful establishment of the immigrant genotypes in the new population. Geneflow is often confusingly referred to as migration, but the latter term is best reserved to describe dispersal behaviours involving a seasonal or longer term round trip. Gene flow tends to homogenise linked populations and lack of gene flow permits interpopulation differentiation. It is of interest to geneticists and managers in that to conserve a population one needs to establish the historical patterns and rates of gene flow. This is typically estimated from allele frequency data and reported in terms of the number of 'migrants' per generation. In theory, one migrant per generation between two populations will ensure that they remain genetically homogeneous. Inbreeding depression can be ameliorated by the artificial translocation of one reproducing migrant per generation between populations.

Geneflow is often gender biased and limited to certain phases of the life cycle. It may be accelerated under certain climatic conditions that occur at frequencies of many years or at irregular intervals many years apart. Inter specific gene flow results in introgressive hybridisation. The translocation of individual organisms results in gene flow if they reproduce at the release site. In the future, genetically depauperate populations will be enhanced by translocation of individuals from more secure areas. Unfortunately, such genetic enhancement carries risks associated with the introduction of pathogens that could harm the target population or completely unrelated species. Furthermore, the introduction of individuals from genetically well differentiated source populations may result in outbreeding depression in the threatened population of conservation concern. Geneflow can thuserode the genetic basis of adaptation to local conditions.

If previously continuous populations become fragmented, historical patterns of dispersal and gene flow may be disrupted with potentially serious consequences for population viability. For example, if young female chimpanzees can no longer emigrate from their natal social group because of habitat destruction in the surrounding countryside, their isolated natal population will experience increased inbreeding.

Genetic Drift

Genetic drift involves the loss of alleles from a population by chance. Random fluctuations in allele frequencies in small populations reduce genetic variation, leading to increased homozygosity and loss of evolutionary adaptability to change. The rate at which alleles are lost from a sexually reproducing population by genetic drift can be predicted. Sewall Wright developed the basic theoretical model in 1931 and showedanalytically how the rate varies with population size. Actually, it is not the census size (N) that is important but rather the genetic effective population size (N_e). This parameter takes into account the fact that closely related individuals will share alleles by common descent. Monozygotic twins are genetically identical and~ therefore should be counted as one individual rather than two. Sibs share half their genes with each other and half with each of their parents and are therefore not equivalent to two genetically unrelated individuals. The genetic effective number of individuals in a population is therefore almost always less than the number of individuals counted by an ecologist. N_e can, under some breeding systems, be one or two orders efmagnitudeless than N. Consider, for example, the fuimber of adults in a sexually reproducing population. In a monogamous species the census count of adults is useful, but in a harem species only 1 of the 10 males may be contributing to N_e. N_e can be variously defined in terms of unequal sex ratios among breeders, fluctuations in population size over several generations, and variance in family size. Wright defined the variance effective population size (N_e) as the number of individuals in an ideal population that would experience genetic drift at the same rate as the actual population. N_e can be defined and estimated in various ways using temporal ecological data, DNA sequences, and various methods of estimating migration rate. Some methods of estimation have theoretical value but little operational utility—it is almost impossible to determine the values that some algorithms require. Nevertheless, by estimating N, one can assess the effects of different population management strategies. Unequal numbers of males and females, increased variance in family size, and temporal fluctuations in

N all cause N_e to be much less than the census size, N_e. In many endangered populations N_e is only 1030, and at such levels genetic variation becomes significant for a population's viability.

Population Bottlenecks

Sudden population declines followed by recovery in numbers are referred to as population or demographic bottlenecks. They can have an immediate impact on variability at molecular genetic loci as genetic drift robs the population of its innate variation. The evidence of a bottleneck may persist for hundreds of thousands to millions of generations in low levels of variation at allozyme and molecular genetic marker loci. However, large populations that are almost isogenic at such loci may maintain high heritable variance in QTL, low inbreeding depression, and high heterozygosity for simple repetitive microsatellite DNA because variation at QTL may return to out bred various levels. Furthermore, bottlenecks can actually result in a short term increase in population variation because epistatic variation (due to interactions among genes controlling a trait) is converted into additive variation. Whether such release of previously hidden variation is beneficial or harmful to population viability is unknown. Sudden reduction in N results in a loss of fitness unless there is a rapid and sustained recovery. Gradual reduction, on the other hand, permits natural selection to purge recessive lethal mutations and avoid a substantial part of inbreeding depression. The best advice a geneticist can give the manager of a collapsed population is to increase N as fast as possible and then worry about genetics. Very low variability is known for many sexually reproducing species whose currently large populations have recovered from one or repeated brushes with extinction. If a large variable population collapses, then the few individuals that survive the catastrophe carry only a fraction of the original population's genetic variability through the demographic bottleneck. By chance, some individuals and the alleles they carried are lost to genetic drift. Only one of six mtDNA haplotypes survived the severe bottleneck ($N = 14$) in the whooping crane in 1938. Genetic drift becomes a significant agent of evolutionary change in small populations.

Drift may account for the very low levels of variability observed in African cheetahs and northern elephant seals. Cheetahs were not known to begenetically less variable than other cats or at genetic risk until half of a large captive breeding colony died soon after being exposed to a common domestic cat coronavirus (feline infectious peritonitis virus). Although the northern elephant seals are known to have recovered after having been over hunted to near extinction in the late nineteenth century, the low levels of variation in the cheetah may beat tributable to metapopulation dynamics rather than a classic population collapse. Metapopulation structure, with frequent extirpation and recolonisation of subpopulations, can reduce metapopulation N_e orders of magnitude below the census population size and mimics the genetic effects of a demographic bottleneck.

Genetic Erosion

Genetic erosion, the decrease in population variation due to random genetic drift and inbreeding, is both a symptom and a cause of endangerment of small isolated populations. Population genetic theory shows that variation will be lost by genetic drift with an almost clock like regularity. In closed populations, in the absence of factors promoting genetic variation (mutation and gene flow), the expectedrate of loss of heterozygosity, or rate of loss of genetic variance in quantitative characters or selectively neutral variation, is ½N, per generation. Little variation is lost in any one generation but small N sustained for several generations can severely deplete variability. Most variability is lost within 2N, generations. An effective population of 10 is predicted to lose heterozygotes five times faster than a population of effective size 100, 50% of its heterozygosity will be lost in approximately 20 generations. Therefore, in theory, small isolated populations have a higher rate of loss of heterozygosity and are expected to have lower levels of genetic variation than large continuously distributed populations. Because variability is inherently related to evolvability, genetic erosion in small, recently fragmented populations may contribute to their endangerment.

Barrett and Kohn and Young and others review the growing literature of the population genetic consequences of habitat fragmentation for plants. There are numerous examples of a positive relationship between N, and population genetic variation at allozyme loci for remnant populations. Ouberg and colleagues conducted experimental investigations of genetic erosion with Scabiosa columbaria and Salvia pratensis plants under common garden conditions and found positive correlations between variance for adaptive traits related to growth rates and population size. Recently, others studied Clarkia pulchella and found an increased probability of extinction associated with decreased N_e. Such experimental studies indicate the potential significance of genetic erosion in natural populations.

The phenomenon of genetic erosion has long been understood in terms of population genetic theory, but the critical early stages of the process in nature have gone undocumented because the changes are rapid and difficult to monitor. During years 58 post fragmentation, the demographic collapse of these communities and genetic erosion in three common species [a forest rat (*Maxomys surifer*), a tree mouse (*Chiropodomys gliroides*), and a tree shrew (*Tupia glis*)] whose populations were effectively isolated on some islands were monitored. Nuclear microsatellite markers are sufficiently variable to be used to monitor the process of genetic erosion in nature. As expected, small populations lost variability by genetic drift faster than large populations, and allelic variability is a better indicator of the onset of genetic erosion than heterozygosity. Interestingly, in one of the three species studied, genetic erosion commenced before detectable demographic decline.

This demonstration that the process of genetic erosion can be monitored in free ranging natural populations provides numerous research opportunities because habitat fragmentation is a very ubiquitous phenomenon. Furthermore, the method can easily be upscaled to larger mammals of conventional concern to conservationists. Although monitoring genetic erosion in long lived species may not be practical, much can be learned immediately by comparing isolated populations to those still more continuously distributed.

The importance of such rapid genetic erosion on population viability remains unclear because there are so few studies of the process in nature. Two larger questions remain to be answered: At what point (in terms of N and N_e) does genetic erosion threaten a population's viability? and What level of natural or artificial gene flow can protect a population from the negative effects of genetic erosion? Answers to such questions may emerge from the 35 year study of the decline and assisted recovery of an isolated population of greater prairie chicken, Tympanuchus cupido. Unfortunately, there are very few studies of this duration. Genetic enhancement, the introduction of selected individuals into a threatened population with the intent of maintaining or increasing its genetic variability and hence viability, is a conservation method inits infancy. Although the genetics may seem straightforward, the translocation of new individuals carries a significant risk of introducing diseases into the threatened population. Furthermore, illplanned genetic enhancement maylead to a breakdown of local adaptation (outbreeding depression) and actually decrease a threatened population's viability.

Natural Selection and Adaptation

Natural selection, the differential survival and reproduction of some genotypes over others, is the major agent of microevolutionary change. It is of interest to conservation geneticists for two reasons. First, human activities can radically alter selection coefficients in both natural populations and managed ones. Such human influenced evolutionary change is termedartificial selection whether or not it is intentional. Intense harvesting based on size or gender can cause rapid changes in behaviour and natural history and reduce fitness. Examples include reduced body size in game fish and the impact of hunting only male horned or tusked mammals on social behaviour. Second, one of the major challenges facing geneticists this century will be assisting species to adapt to ongoing global climatic changes. In the past, in the absence of humans, natural selection favoured individuals adapted to change and many species shifted their ranges to accommodate major changes. Unfortunately, in the twenty first century, the pace of environmental alteration and destruction is too fast for many species to respond. Conservation managers will have to intervene on behalf of many species if they are to survive.

Quantitative characters are typically under stabilising selection and show some optimum phenotype from which they can evolve in response to environmental changes. This optimum balances current fitness with the need for future flexibility or adaptability. The maintenance of this variability imposes a fitness cost or genetic load on a population—the price for longterm evolvability.

The rate of directional selection that a population can manage, in response to some environmental change, is determined in part by its innate variability. Rapid anthropogenic changes, such as those associated with global warming, place a premium on genetic variation and adaptability, especially in fragmented populations. To maintain variability in quantitative characters (longterm adaptability), the Franklin—Soulé number for an effective population size of at least $N_e = 500$ is often cited. Revisionary work by Lande has shown, however, that an upward revision to $N_e = 5000$ is required. Such numbers are larger than those found in many endangered and threatened populations and underscore the need for genetic vigilance in their management and the importance of keeping numbers as high as possible.

The risk of extinction due to fixation of mildly deleterious mutations is comparable in importance to environmental stochasticity and could substantially decrease the longterm viability of populations with N_e of less than a few thousand. The current recovery goals for many threatened species are inadequate to ensure their longterm viability if this requires $N = 10,000$ individuals. Genetic and demographic factors, acting synergistically, require that minimum viable populations be $>10^4$.

GENETIC MANAGEMENT: EXAMPLES

Until a textbook on conservation genetics is written, the reader must consult conference proceedings and the primary literature for examples of the application of genetics to conservation management. The journals Conservation Biology and Molecular Ecology are especially useful in this regard. Without making reference to the specific methods employed (because these continuously change), the following examples, in addition to those mentioned previously, are illustrative of the type of contributions conservation geneticists have made.

Pedigree Management in Very Small Populations

Olney and others describe examples of multiinstitutional breeding plans with genetic components for numerous species, including Przewalski's horse, Pere David's deer (Elaphurus davidianus), Hawaiian goose (*Branta sandvicensis*), California condor (*Gymnogyps californianus*), and Tahitian Partula tree snails, all of which wereextirpated in the wild. Cases of more intensive genetic management, including the establishment of relationships, founder representation, and breeding to maximise N_e, include captive populations of liontailed macaque (*Macaca silenus*) (*San Diego Zoo*), Speke's gazelle (*Gazella spekei*) (*St. Louis Zoo*), Waldrapp ibis (*Geronticus eremita*) (*Zurich Zoo*), Guam rail (*Rallus owstoni*), Micronesian kingfisher (*Halcyon cinnamomina*), and Mauritius pink pigeon (*Nesoenas mayeri*). Genetic sex determination of juvenile California condors enabled recovery program managersto pair birds efficiently. Geneticists have identified low genetic variability as a concern in wild and captive populations of many species, including cheetah, Californian Channel Island fox (*Urocyonlittoralis*), Newfoundland black bear (*Ursus americanus*), Gir Forest Asian lions (*Panthera leo*), southern koalas (*Phascolarctus cinereus*), European bison (*Bison bonasus*), Arabian oryx (*Oryx leucoryx*), Pere David's deer, and Torrey pine (*Pinus torreyana*). A loss of self incompatibility alleles may pose a threat to reproduction in plants with genetically determined self incompatibility systems such as the rare lake side daisy (Hymenoxys acaulis) in Illinois. Geneticists identified inbreeding as a probable cause of reproductive failures in populations of Ngorongoro lions (*Panthera leo*), Florida panther (*Puma concolor coryi*), Barrow Island black footed rock wallaby (*Petrogale lateralis*), bighorn sheep (*Ovis canadensis*), Puerto Rican parrot (*Amazonvittata*), and the Isle Royale gray wolf (*Canis lupus*).

Matifig System

Geneticists have discovered that the mating systems of many species differ from expectations based on direct observations, often with profound implications for captive management and for management of 'wild' populations. In some species, females preferentially mate with males outside their social group, e.g. Atlantic salmon (*Salmo salar*), blue tits (*Parus caeruleus*), and pilot whales (*Globicephala* sp.). Preferential interpod mating in long finned pilot whales indicates the importance of conserving as many pods as possible. Genetics shows that highly gregarious black vultures (*Coragypsatratus*) are in fact monogamous and that Galapagos hawks (*Buteo galapagoensis*) are polyandrous. Despite behavioural observations suggesting a high frequency of matings between sibs in Australian splendid fairy wrens (*Malurus splendens*), genetics shows that outcrossingis the norm. In other birds, including stripe backed wrens (Campylorhynchus nuchalis), geneticists found that subordinate males reproduce. The mating system of wild gray wolf, chimpanzees, and other species have been established and used to improve captive breeding programs or management in reserves. Establishing the mating system of the redcockaded woodpecker led to improved estimates of N_e and changes in the recovery program for a small population in South Carolina.

Problems of Hybrids

Geneticists have elucidated the hybridity of some taxa in both the wild and in captivity, including Przewalski's horses (many of which are domestic horse hybrids), Asian lions (most animals in Western zoos were hybrids between Asian and African lions and were removed from the breeding program), and the red wolf of Texas [shown to be primarily a natural coyote (*Canis latrans*) X gray wolf hybrid]. Genetic data revealed the threat by hybridisation to indigenous Scottish deer (*Cervus elaphus scoticus*) by introduced Japanese sika deer (*C. nippon*). Genetics was used to identify hybrids among the remaining Catalina Island mahogany and establish seedlings of pure Cercocarpus trashiae at several sites to protect the species from extinction by introgression. Genetic markers are being used to conserve remnant cut throat trout populations by identifying and removing populations introgressed by hybridisation with non native species.

Genetic Censusing

Because every individual in most species is genetically distinct, it is possible to census populations by counting unique multilocus genotypes in an area. Geneticists have censused very difficult to count animals such as African forest elephants and the largelyfossorial northern hairynosed wombats

(*Lasiorhinus krefftii*) by individually genotyping dung samples. Fecal genotyping (including sexing) has also been used to provide more accurate census data of animals such as coyotes and bears than could be obtained from longterm ecological surveys. The genetic data also provided information on home ranges and pedigree relatedness without requiring that the animals be seen or disturbed.

Phylogeography, Gene Flow, and Population Structure

Avise reviews many examples of phylogeographic studies that provide managers with essential data on population structure and on the characterisation of MUs and ESUs. Geneticists have also provided estimates of historical gene flow between populations that would be impossible to obtain by direct observation (e.g. chimpanzees, humpback whales, and green turtles). Comparative phylogeographic studies of four sympatric species of East African bovids underscore the dangers of extrapolating results from one species to another and support conservation efforts that take species specific differences into account.

Defining Species, ESUs, and MUs

Karyological differences distinguish Bornean and Sumatran orangutans (Pongo pygmaeus) and captive breeding programs are now managed to prevent hybridisation of the two. Dikdik species (Madoqua) canalso be distinguished karyologically and neonate mortality in captive populations has been reduced following the sorting of animals by karyotype. MtDNA sequences have been used to sort sibling species and subspecies of gibbons (*Hylobates* sp.) of unknown geographic origin into correct ESUs, to distinguish sibling species of chimpanzees (*Pan troglodytes and P. verus*) that have been mixed in captivity, and to identify subspecies of black rhinoceros, Diceros bicornis. Genetics was used to show that the conservation of the living fossil tuatara (*Sphenodon*) of New Zealand depends on the management of not one but two genetically recognizable species. There are many cases in which genetic data justify conservation efforts for isolated subspeciesor varieties that are shown to be genetically well differentiated—for example, Darwin's fox (*Dusicyon fulvipes*) of Chile, Kemp's ridley turtle (*Lepidochelys kempi*), San Clemente Island loggerhead shrike, and several 'subspecies' of Hawaiian Amakilu honey creeper (*Hemignathus virens*). The Mexican wolf (*Canis lupus baileyi*) was found to be a genetically distinct ESU, untainted by hybridisation with gray wolf, coyote, or dog.

The endangered San Clemente Island shrikeis illustrative of several of the points made previously because it is technically a subspecies of a widespread mainland bird and might accordingly be written off as a peripheral population, local variant, or 'just a subspecies.' Taxonomic practice and field observations notwithstanding, my genetic survey revealed no evidence that it has hybridised with the neighbouring mainland subspecies since 1915 despite repeated opportunities. It is genetically differentiated and apparently reproductively isolated and merits management as a separate ESU.

Geneticists have also provided data questioning the justification of other taxon focused conservation efforts. The 27 original subspecies of leopard (*Panthera pardus*) were foundto bereferable to only 8 genetically defined subspecies or ESUs. Similarly, genetic variation provides no justification for conserving all 30 described subspecies of puma (*Pumaconcolor*). The dusky seaside sparrow (*Ammodramus maritimus nigriscens*), after considerable and unsuccessful efforts to save it, was shown to be only a marginallydistinct local race of a common widespread species.

Taxonomic status (species or subspecies) does not automatically lead to the justification of conservation efforts. Proposals to reduce the eastern Pacific black sea turtle, Chelonia agassizii, to a subspecies of the wide spread green turtle, *C. mydas*, are supported genetically but do not justify the abandonment of this taxon as a high conservation priority. A phylogeographic survey of 14 subspecies of the songbird banana quit (*Ceoreba* sp.) from 15 West Indian islands and the mainland of South and Central America showed that if it were necessary to restock the small and vulnerable populations on the northern Lesser Antilles Islands, the birds from nearby Puerto Rico or from Jamaica would be genetically inappropriate. Similar studies of orioles (*Icterus* sp.) are relevant to the conservation of the Montserrat oriole, I. oberi, which is under threat of catastrophic (volcanic) extinction. Phylogeographic analyses have also helped to define natal homing patterns in marine turtles on foraging grounds. It was found that both green turtle and loggerhead turtle rookeries are demographically autonomous and that low levels of interrookery matrilineal exchange suggest that extirpated colonies are unlikely to recover by natural recruitment of nonindigenous females. Similar methods have been used to define stocks in whales and dolphin and elucidate the migratory strategies of different groups of humpback whales intermingled at the breeding ground near Hawaii.

Hierarchical phylogenetic analyses have been used to suggest conservation priorities among species of cranes. Within a group of related species the evolutionarily oldest monophyletic clades are considered to represent a greater genetic heritage than recently originated clades. Similarly, it has been argued that areas with a disproportionate number of evolutionary ancient genotypes are more valuable than areas populated by recent colonists.

Reintroductions, Translocations, and Genetic Enhancement

Two genetic generalisations complicate the prospects for successfully moving organisms around in the wild or for returning them to the wild after a period in captivity. First, the chances for successful reintroduction are diminished by evidence for rapid genetic adaptation to captivity in fish, plants, and *Drosophila*. The same problem applies to wildlife brought into captivity for reintroduction at some future time. Second, in plants, cryptic local adaptation results in the fitness of transplants being about half that of residents even when environments are apparently similar. This makes it difficult to re-establish populations once they are extirpated. Genetic criteria were used to chose founders for a new population of the extirpated Guam rail on the island of Rota, for sea otters (*Enhydra lutris*), and for a Western Australian shrub (*Corrigan grevillea*) reduced to 27 plants. Genetic data were also used to influence the choice of source population for a Gila topminnow reintroduction program. Fish from a population with high allozymic diversity were selected to successfully replenish the diversity and viability of a declining and nearly monomorphic population rather than fish from a less variable but adjacent population. Genetic study of redcockaded woodpeckers in the southeastern United States led to the recommendation that translocations be made between nearby populations rather moving birds over great distances. In another study, it was shown to begenetically appropriate to use gray wolves from British Columbia as a source of animals for reintroduction into Yellow stone National Park. Genetic variation and multilocus genetic similarity were used to justify the introduction of panthers from Texas (traditionally regarded as a different subspecies) to counter severe inbreeding depression (low heterozygosity, poor sperm quality, and cryptorchidism) in the remnant Florida panther population.

Genetic criteria have also been used to argue against certain types of translocations. For example, it was found that Tasmanian eastern barred bandicoots (*Parmeles gunnii*) should not be used as a source population for enhancing the endangered mainland Australian population. South African wild dogs (*Lycaon pictus*) were genetically inappropriate for reintroduction into Kenya. Isolated northern and southern populations of Brazilian muriqui (*Brachyteles arachnoides*) are well differentiated genetically, so threatened northern populations should perhaps not be translocated to larger southern reserves. An example of the hazards of implementing a transplantation program without first considering genetic factors involves the endangered Hawaiian silvers word. In this case, the outplanted individuals were all descendents of only one or two maternal plants and therefore retained only a small fraction of the genetic diversity of the remaining populations of the species they represented.

Furthermore, because they were so closely related to one another, they had significant reproductive problems associated with self incompatibility and a seed set of <20%. H.

Conservation Management

Genetic methods are used in forensic identification of tissues of endangered species in illegal or mis-represented trade (e.g. abalone, 'caviar,' cage birds, and primates including chimpanzees). Misrepresentation occurs when a wild caught parrot or falcon is claimed to belegally captive bred. Geneticists showed that some whale meat legally on sale in Japan was actually meat of endangered and allegedly protected species including humpback whale. Sequence data revealed that loggerhead turtles from Caribbean nesting beaches are threatened by a Mediterraneanfishery off Spain.

Geneticists are playing an increasingly important role in the management of mixed stocks of threatened and commercially harvested fish. Consider the conservation management of salmon (Oncorhynchus) in the U.S. Pacific Northwest. Salmon with their precise homing behaviour present a major problem because each local spawning population should be managed as a genetically distinct taxon. Should managers give every natal stream adapted salmon stock equal priority? Geneticists have developed allelic frequency marker systems for stock identification that are sufficiently sensitive to permit real time regulation of mixed stock fisheries involving both hatchery and wild salmon. The latter can be partially protected because they return from the sea to the rivers a few weeks later than the former and the fishery can be terminated when they are detected. Using the same approach, geneticists developed markers to identify endangered and protected winter run chinook salmon in the Sacramento River in California. Fall (hatchery) and spring run chinook salmon do not enjoy protection, but the fishery could not be managed from a conservation perspective until the different races could be identified during the downstream migration of smolts to the ocean.

Genetic tracking of movements of migratory birds permits sorting arctic and Mexicanfalcons (*Falco perigrinus*) that mix when the former reach their wintering grounds. Similar genetic tracking permitted the identification of the wintering grounds of several species of declining arctic shorebirds andled to changes in conservation focus from the breeding grounds to the wintering grounds. Finally, geneticists have been able to monitor the loss of variability in translocated populations of wild turkey (*Meleagris gallopavo*), whitetail deer (*Odocoileus virginianus*), and alpine ibex (*Capra ibex*).

Other Applications

Space does not permit presentation of all the caveats, corrections, and revised recommendations made in most of the previous cases as more data becameavailable and as various tests were repeated. Many of the classic examples are less clear-cut than originally proposed. Space does also not permit mention of all the examples in which genetics showed populations were not genetically depauperate or sufficiently distinct to warrant priority conservation efforts. Such contributions are of equal importance to biodiversity conservation because they free up limited resources for other investigations.

Although most of the previous examples involved captive or wild populations of threatened species, much useful conservation genetics can be done using laboratory animals as model organisms. Valuable experimental tests of conservation genetic principles have been completed using *Drosophila*, Tribolium, mosquitofish (*Gambusia holbrooki*), the butterfly (*Bicyclus anynana*), Mus, and Peromyscus For example, using laboratory populations of *Drosaphila* it has been shown that equalising family size can double N, and more intensive pedigree management can increase the N./N ratio 40 fold. Similarly, in most of the examples discussed previously, investigators also examined the genetics of a close relative of the taxon of interest. It is standard practice to develop genetic methods using a common relative as a surrogate before commencing work on a highly endangered taxon. This approach also has the advantage of providing comparative data useful in interpreting the results of a study of an endangered taxon.

GENETICS, EVOLVABILITY, AND THE FUTURE OF BIODIVERSITY

The magnitude of the task facing conservation geneticists is daunting. There are on the order of 10 million species living on the planet today and about 2 million of these are recognised and namedin a formal taxonomic sense. Describing a new species requires little more than that a scientist know what it looks like and where it is found, unfortunately, this constitutes our state of knowledge for most of biodiversity. Closer to 10 than to $10°$ species have been characterised ecobehaviorally, and only on the order of $10°$ species have been examined by geneticists. If sound conservation is based on a knowledge of ecology, behaviour, and genetics, then we must admit that we are currently capable of scientifically managing the evolution of less than 1000 species. However, the number of species requiring individual management to prevent their extinction in the next 100 years is in excess of 10000.

Conservation geneticists have devoted their efforts disproportionately toward the charismatic mega vertebrates. Whales and cats have received more attention than bats and rats. Given the enormous number of species requiring attention, one might inquire as to how Priorities are set. First, most research has gone into species that were favoured for utilitarian reasons, they provide us with food, clothing, medicines, recreation, or companionship. Most of this research has been aimed at stock improvement rather than whole genome or species conservation. Second, as already noted, the charismatic mega vertebrates and a few groups of flowering plants have received inordinate attention. Perhaps not surprisingly, rare species have also been studied more than common ones. The same applies to phylogenetically unique species, living fossils, and evolutionary relics. However, because the real goal is to save functional ecosystems, conservation geneticists are rethinking their priorities. Although some rare species clearly merit genetic management, it would be better to focus more attention on ecological keystone species whose activities are critical to the maintenance of entire communities.

We also need to know more about the genetics of ecologically successful colonising species and of clades of species that have evolved very recently (the cichlid flocks of Rift Valley lakes) because their study may teach us how to manage apparently less successful taxa.

Conservation geneticists rarely advocate bringing plants and animals into captivity 'to save them.' Species are typically better managed in their natural communities than in isolation. Existing institutions concerned with conservation, however, are not equipped to deal with the magnitude of the task they face. Parks and wildlife reserves are the preferred approach to both species and community conservation. Zoos and botanic gardens are extremely limited in what they can accomplish and can at best serve only to shelter a few critical cases that require intensive care. Germplasm frozen storage systems are valuable adjuncts for researchers, but no credible geneticist has yet proposed that we will be able to awaken these frozen tissues and recreate the animals from which they were derived. Although frozen tissue banks are extremely valuable for geneticists, the revitalisation of mammoths, quaggas, thylocenes, and dodosis still science fiction. In its first two decades, conservation genetics was perceived by some wild life ecologists as an unnecessary intrusion into their field. It was argued that demography and behaviour are far more important than genetics in saving endangered species. Others have argued that the genetic threat to population viability has been overstated. Genetics was viewed as too theoretical and contributing too little and too slowly to the day today efforts to save populations in nature. Furthermore, molecular genetics studies, which are relatively expensive, compete for the limited funds available to the traditional conservationists. Some of the criticisms were justified and some were not. It is easy to disparage the potential contribution of genetics to saving a particular population or species if genetics is defined very narrowly as, for example, the determination of heterozygosity in a remnant population. In the case of cheetahs in Africa, it is clear that predation by lions and humans is more significant today than low variability. Similarly, in captivity, different husbandry practices in different zoos are more significant than poor sperm quality.

Although there are clearly times when genetic studies will be lower priority in a multifaceted conservation strategy, it is undeniable that increasingly more populations will need genetic management. Genetics, ecology, and behaviour are all necessary parts of biodiversity conservation. Although conservation geneticists focus on populations and species, their ultimate goal is the conservation not of things but of a process, evolution, that produced them. The ultimate goal of conservation biology is to preserve the processes of organic evolution—to maintain the ability of populations and species to evolve and communities to function and provide ecosystem services. The basic science is still not equal to the task conservation geneticists are expected to perform.

The relationship between genetic variation and genetic health is illusive and needs clarification. Society's expectations of conservation geneticists also need to be specified or we will forever be accused of treating the symptoms and not the causes of the biodiversity crisis. Typically, species are not afforded legal protection until their populations have fallen into the hundreds, 10–100 times below the level at which their genetic integrity and viability are reasonably secure. Geneticists need to point out that current standards of endangerment are far too low, that recovery from previous mass extinctions took on the order of 10 million years, and that we have not thought through the global implications of a 50% decrease in the number of remaining larger plant and vertebrate species.

SECTION X

Ethical Issues and Intellectual Property Rights of Genetic Engineering

Chapter 24

Ethical Issues of Genetics

INTRODUCTION

In the past 35 years, the rapid progression of genetic research has been a source of increasing tension between research ethics in genetics and traditional medical ethics. Evolving from research on single gene disorders to population genomics and now personal genomics, new ethical challenges have emerged. With funding priorities shifting toward translational research initiatives and technology transfer, as well as the advent of commercial direct-to-consumer (DTC) companies, the genetic genie is getting ever closer to health-care management and clinical practice. It is becoming clear that the ethical frameworks developed following the Nuremberg Trials, and other abusive experimentation involving humans, inadequately address the distinct context of twenty-first century genetics.

Traditional ethical duties to obtain an informed consent and protect the confidentiality of medical data have taken new contours, while the level of physical risk to research participants is almost non-existent in genetic research. Adapting ethical guidelines and educating ethics committees (also called independent review board) about the benefits and ethical challenges of contemporary genetic research should be a priority in the coming years.

A realistic look at the ethical issues raised by genetics at the start of the twenty-first century reveals a wide spectrum of possibilities, potential benefits, and ethical issues, as well as numerous efforts to devise policy structures that will ensure that newly acquired genetic knowledge is used ethically. This chapter discusses some of the more current, recurring issues related to ethical aspects.

GENETIC INFORMATION BE TREATED DIFFERENTLY FROM OTHER MEDICAL INFORMATION

With the beginning of the Human Genome Project in the 1990s, genetic information was considered special and therefore to be treated differently from other types of medical information. This current of thought was later coined as 'genetic exceptionalism'. Certain authors claimed that genetic information is a particularly sensitive form of personal information because of its familial and probabilistic nature. They also pointed out that genetic information can be easily stored and shared via Internet databases. Opponents of genetic exceptionalism, however, argued that the issues raised by genetic information are actually quite similar to those raised by other types of sensitive personal or health information. According to these experts, numerous types of health data, quite apart from genetic information, have familial implications and can be just as predictive of future health outcomes (e.g. cholesterol test or HIV status). In their opinion, genetic exceptionalism is a self-fulfilling approach. Genetic information is perceived as unique and stigmatising by community members because genetic-specific legislation and exaggerated coverage in popular and academic media reinforce that view.

Genetics and Privacy

In the coming years, genomic research and personalised medicine will increasingly rely on international data sharing and large-scale biobanking to generate the kind of robust, reliable findings that are needed for regulatory approval and translational research. However, because of recent technological and statistical advances, it has become increasingly difficult to protect the identity of patients and research participants. A small amount of genetic information is now sufficient to reidentify an individual in a genetic database. The value of data anonymisation, once thought to be a sufficient safeguard for all genetic privacy issues, has recently been put into question.

Solutions proposed to address these new challenges include greater transparency about the limits of applicable privacy protection mechanisms in consent forms; developing elaborate, independent governance structures for biobanks; using state-of-the-art information technology security mechanisms; and moving toward more coherent national and international privacy frameworks. In clinical practice, given the advent of computerised medical files and the fact that a growing number of health workers (e.g. doctors, genetic counselors, nurses, pharmacists, etc.) will have access to genetic information from patients, privacy protection will also become an important factor.

Given the popular anxiety generated by risk of confidentiality breaches and misuse of genetic information by third parties (e.g. genetic discrimination), it would be beneficial to gather additional empirical data about the frequency and real impact of these types of events on patients and research participants. Greater knowledge about actual genetic discrimination might both appease unjustified concerns and help better address undesirable scenarios.

GENETICS AND MEDICAL CARE

Given the potential of genetics for health care, its progressive integration into clinical practice should be favourably viewed. The ethical issues arising in clinical genetics are so far quite similar to those arising in other areas of medicine. Typical problems include those of conveying difficult information to patients and their families, including the potential duty to warn at-risk relatives of participants receiving positive test results in specific circumstances and to recontact patients if new meaningful genomic findings surface. As is usually the case in a clinical context, one will need to ensure that genuinely informed consent to tests and treatments is obtained and that the confidentiality of genetic information is protected.

Physicians will need to be informed about new genetic clinical tools, medical products, and guidelines and educated on how to properly integrate them into their daily practice. Health-care payers will have to make difficult choices relating to access and reimbursement of new medical devices and therapeutic products, which will likely be expensive. It will also be important to develop thorough legal and ethical frameworks to ensure that genetics is not misused in the clinic to promote eugenic practices or the commodification of human beings, or to provide patients with complex, indecipherable information that simply does not meet clinical utility standards.

NONMEDICAL USE OF GENETIC INFORMATION

Because of its predictive and identifying properties, genetic information may also be used outside of the medical context. In the insurance and employment fields, the concern is that genetic information could be used by private entities to discriminate and exclude at-risk individuals in order to save costs. A sample scenario could be an insurer requiring insurance candidates to pass a genetic test and refusing life insurance applications from those highly predisposed to developing a condition that would result in early death or offering lower premiums to those presumed to be 'healthy'. As previously discussed, the true extent of genetic discrimination in developed countries remains unknown, but existing data point to a modest incidence.

The fact that only a few genetic tests are currently truly useful to predict future health, coupled with the still relatively high cost associated with genetic testing and interpretation of results, will hopefully convince stakeholders to avoid widespread use of genetic discrimination in the near future.

The highly identifying nature of genetic information also explains why it is now increasingly used for criminal enquiries (for profiling (genetic or DNA profiling) and evidence purposes), paternity testing, and immigration proceedings (to verify the existence of a biological link between presumed family members). To prevent abuses and over reliance on genetic data compared to more traditional sources of information (e.g. birth certificates, fingerprints, photographic evidence, oral testimony), clear limits will need to be determined by society and integrated into administrative policies, statutes, and case law.

DTC GENETIC TESTING

Technical and scientific advancements in genomics have raised expectations among members of the public who would like to see promising research findings translated more quickly into medical practice. Companies, eager to capitalise on this opportunity, have begun offering genetic services directly to consumers via the Internet. They justify their practice by pointing out the need to increase access to valuable new genetic tests and to empower individuals to take charge of their health. However, the practice of DTC genetic testing also raises serious ethical concerns. One of the chief concerns is the questionable validity and clinical utility of many of the tests currently offered. Also troubling is the fact that DTC services are usually provided without adequate genetic counselling, making it difficult for consumers to truly understand the various implications of their results. It should be noted that some of these DTC companies also have commercial research agendas. The high incidence of false or misleading advertising by DTC companies also deserves mention. Efficiently regulating DTC companies is a huge undertaking and a more positive impact might be achieved through the development of simple, easily accessible education programmes for the general public.

POPULATION BIOBANKS

Since 2000, large national population studies that build longitudinal databases and biobanks have emerged. These ongoing studies serve as infrastructures for more specific disease research. Concentrating on the role of the environment on gene expression over time, these resources contain extensive amounts of personal and socio-demographic data, in addition to blood and urine samples. Since the biobanks can go back to their participants for updates, the data and samples are both historical and contemporary. Participants in such resources derive no personal benefit, are usually asymptomatic (i.e., presumably healthy), and receive no individual results. Overall general results are made available, as well as information on what research has been granted access to the samples and data and for what purpose. A broad consent to future unspecified research is obtained, but in counterbalance, there is a higher degree of data security and ethics oversight and governance. With the advent of whole-genome sequencing technologies that will no doubt be used by researchers accessing the biobank, it remains to be seen whether the 'no return of results' policy will survive, considering that a plethora of health data, including incidental findings (some clinically significant), will become available.

ETHICAL ISSUES IN HUMAN GENETICS AND GENOMICS

Genetic information is often considered exceptional when compared to other medical information about an individual for a number of reasons. Genetic conditions are family health problems. A diagnosis or a finding of inherited predisposition in a family member has implications for other family members. Health professionals have an ethical responsibility to prevent harm or avoid seriously jeopardising the health of others (the duty of care). Similarly, individuals undergoing genetic testing have a responsibility to consider not only what it means for their own health, but also what the information may mean for their relatives, and their responsibilities towards those relatives.

Geographic distance or discord in families can sometimes lead to difficulties in revealing genetic test results that may be important for other family members. Responsibility and obligation however needs to be balanced with the right of an individual to choose to know their personal genetic information or, equally, not to know. The emphasis needs to be on the right of the person to choose. Genetic counselling is essential both before and after genetic testing so that all the implications of undertaking testing including having information which might be of interest to others can be understood.

Limitations of Genetic Testing

While in some cases, genetic tests provide reliable and accurate information on which people can make decisions, in other cases it may not be possible to obtain a definitive result. An individual is much more than the sum of their genes: the individual's environment can modify the expression of genetic messages to the body and many health factors are not genetic.

The discovery of a variation in a particular gene may provide some information about the nature of the condition that the person has, will develop or for which they may be at increased risk, but can rarely predict the severity of the condition or the age at which symptoms will first onset. This lack of precision in relating the expression of the condition (called the phenotype) to an individual's genetic make-up (called the genotype) can make the decision-making process in regard to acting on the information very challenging. This is particularly so when the genetic testing is done for prenatal testing of a condition. Genetic counselling is essential to assist families in that decision making process and ensure that the decision is as informed as possible.

Predictive/Pre-symptomatic testing – generally for adult-onset conditions

This type of genetic testing applies to families in which an underlying genetic cause for their condition has been identified and can be used to identify currently healthy family members that are at-risk, if they wish to do so. Pre-test counselling is important in these cases and aims to provide accurate information so that the individual can make an informed decision about whether or not to have testing.

This is called informed consent and means that the person undergoing the test should only do so on a voluntary basis and with a full understanding of all the implications. There can be a danger of coercion, for example, an enthusiastic researcher or a member of a family may try to persuade others in the family to undergo testing about which they feel uncomfortable.

Discussion of the potential emotional impact on family members of finding out test results should also be undertaken before testing. This can be substantial whether the results are bad or good, for example the feelings of guilt often felt by 'survivors' who have not inherited the gene fault. Discussion of implications for other family members and obligations to inform, as well as the potential interest of third parties in genetic information revealed by testing such as insurance and employment, are also important.

Potential for discrimination

Genetic testing may impact an individual's ability to obtain life insurance and employment in certain professions. This is especially the case with predictive/presymptomatic testing which provide information about an individual's future health.

Reproductive choices/Prenatal testing

Whether or not to have children is a major decision for any individual. It is even more difficult where one or both of the prospective parents knows or suspects that they may carry a faulty gene associated with a health problem which could affect their children.

The decision to have a baby may lead to a number of further decisions to be made in regards to the possible genetic testing of the embryo/fetus during the pregnancy. Limitations of such testing are the same as those discussed previously, in particular detection of a faulty gene or a chromosomal change may not provide all the information about the potential or quality of life for the child or the severity of a particular condition When a problem with a developing baby is detected, support is essential for whatever difficult decision is made. Some expectant parents will decide to continue the pregnancy and try to put in place the professional, medical and social support that will be required. Others may choose to terminate the pregnancy. This decision may conflict with moral, religious and cultural beliefs. Different individuals, communities, cultures and religions have different perceptions of disability and this may raise additional issues.

Inappropriate applications of genetic testing

Genetic testing has many potential applications, however some of these are in conflict with what may be considered ethical. These include the use of genetic testing to confirm paternity without the informed consent of all individuals involved and sex selection of a fetus for family balancing reasons.

Setting boundaries in applications of the genetics technology

Philosophers on science have put the view that science is morally neutral. It is the uses to which the science is put that might be good or bad. With the new advances in genetics, as with any powerful new scientific tool, there is a potential for abuse. Controversial applications of genetic testing such as reproductive cloning and genetic testing for enhancement create a huge challenge worldwide and require implementation of international regulations on the boundaries within which these applications can be applied. Moral, religious and cultural beliefs underpin decision-making by individuals, couples, families and communities and may challenge such boundaries.

Forensic DNA Databanks

The use of fingerprints (more accurately known as dermatoglyphic fingerprints) for forensic identification purposes has been in place since the 1890s. One hundred years later, DNA fingerprinting is being used to complement the traditional system, or is being used in isolation for identification. The public has also contributed to investigations of unsolved crimes by volunteering genetic samples. Overall there is a need to ensure that samples are used for the purpose for which they were collected and protected from misuse.

Patenting of Genes

The issue of patenting genes as recognition of the intellectual achievement required to isolate a single gene from the 20000 or so genes in the cell is contentious.

The Federal Government issued a response in 2011 confirming that the government does not support the absolute prohibition of gene patenting, however will aim to ensure that gene patents do not lead to patients being denied 'reasonable access to healthcare'.

Chapter 25

Genetic Inventions and Intellectual Property Rights

INTRODUCTION

Biotechnology is a fast-moving field in which new products and services are developed from an increasingly complex and cumulative set of underlying technologies. The ability to sequence genes, identify their functions and mutations, create systems to selectively express, regulate or silence genes, predict protein structures and expression, map the influence of genetic make-up on metabolism and otherwise analyse the vast amounts of genetic data has been dubbed the genomics revolution. These many technologies contribute to the rapid pace of advancement in the life sciences and offer tremendous promise for improving human health and furthering economic development.

The genomics revolution, however, has reopened debate about intellectual property rights (IPR). OECD member countries are trying to balance the need to keep information and access to genetic data open in order to encourage the diffusion of research results with the commercial need to protect inventions in order to create revenue from investments in research and development (R&D). From the start, advances in biotechnology have tested the boundaries of the intellectual property rights system.

In many OECD countries, patent protection for biotechnological inventions has been available and expanding for close to 20 years. The existing patent system's adaptability to innovations in biotechnology has contributed to the rapid development of a new and dynamic industry.

A subset of these biotechnology patents covers 'genetic inventions'. These gene – or DNA – patents have claims that cover nucleotide (DNA or RNA) sequences that may encode genes or fragments of genes. The number of gene patents granted has risen dramatically since the second half of the 1990s.

The rise in the number of patents for genetic inventions can be a sign of dynamism in a new technological sector. Questions have been raised, however, about the potential impact of the growing web of gene patents on: (i) the research environment, (ii) the market dynamics for new product development, and (iii) the clinical uptake of new tests and treatments. Since gene patents have existed for several years, the concerns they raise are increasingly about the way the patents are used and licensed (or not licensed) by their owners.

Unfortunately, policy debate about gene patenting has generally not benefited from reliable information on the licensing practices of title holders to genetic inventions.

PATENTING OF GENETIC INVENTIONS

This chapter provides a brief factual overview of the patenting of genetic inventions. It relates the basic principles of intellectual property protection, summarises the key issues in patent protection, and describes how patent protection for genetic inventions currently works. It also provides a brief review of the types of reform proposals being debated which would influence the patenting and licensing of genetic inventions.

Basic Principles of IP Protection

The essential principle of all forms of IPR is to recognise and reward the work of inventors, designers and authors because society deems that it benefits from the promotion of the useful and cultural arts. This recognition is achieved by the granting of a measure of legal protection, of a specified duration, against unauthorised use and reproduction by others of the invention, design or protected work.

When technological innovations lead to new processes and products, as is often the case with genetic inventions, patents are the form of IPR most often used to protect the invention. The laws on copyright and database rights may also apply to certain aspects of the disclosure of information in the field of gene sequences. Indeed, the rise of genomic databases, and the algorithms to analyse them, may make other forms of protection increasingly valuable in the near future.

Objectives of the patent system

The patent system has many objectives. As mentioned above, it aims to protect inventors and those who fund their work. It also promotes the disclosure of inventions, as against secrecy, through the publication of patent applications. One condition for granting a patent is that the inventor must disclose the invention in a written description (the patent specification) which gives a skilled person adequate instructions for putting the invention to practical use. A third objective has a more implicit purpose, namely, to stimulate others to 'invent around' patents. Inventions may be viewed as new solutions to technical problems. Therefore, in-so-far as a patent gives its holder the exclusive right to benefit from his/her particular solution, others may be induced to find alternative solutions which can be used without infringing the patent in question. The necessity to 'design around' or 'work outside' the patent is often the mother of further invention.

The patent system is designed to diffuse technical knowledge rather than maintain secrecy, while industrial or trade secrecy is the main alternative to patents for avoiding piracy or the imitation of inventions. In most countries, patent applications are published long before a decision is made to grant or refuse a patent (in many countries, this only occurs 18 months after application). For certain technologies for which secrecy might be attractive, it may be possible to exploit the invention by limiting the availability of crucial biological materials or information to one's potential partners or licensees. Examples might be genetically modified cell lines which produce monoclonal antibodies for diagnosis and therapy, or genomic databases which combine sequence data with protein structure and possible function. When secrecy is used to protect intellectual property, access to materials and information relies on the negotiation of private contracts between the parties. Those who make use of the patent system, and those who work in it professionally, see it as one form of regulating competition in a liberal economy by striking a balance between the legal protection of innovators and the freedom of other parties to operate commercially without undue limitation. The patent system, as the term is used here, means not only the laws governing the granting of patent rights but also the ways in which patent holders may exercise these rights.

Understanding Patent Protection

To start the discussion about the effects of patent protection on genetic inventions, it is necessary to look at the sorts of rights a patent grants, as well as how those rights are limited and enforced. The fundamental principles of the patent system are frequently misunderstood. This section therefore reviews the basic features of the patent system, before moving to a discussion about patents for genetic inventions.

Nature of patents

A patent is a property right granted by a state authority which excludes others from the use or benefit of the patented invention without the consent of the patent holder. A patent does not confer the positive right to use an invention. Freedom of use may, for example, be dependent on the existence of prior rights or on regulatory approval. Not infrequently, a patent for an improvement on a basic product or process will be subject to, or dependent on, a prior patent for the basic product or process.

Patent application

To obtain a patent, an application must be filed with the relevant national authority (e.g. patent office) and will be examined for compliance with legal requirements. Separate patent applications are usually necessary in each country where protection is required, though a single application at the European Patent Office covers a number of European countries.

Patentability

The principal legal requirements for patentability are that the invention is: (i) new, (ii) involves an inventive step, and iii) has an industrial or other useful capability. In addition, the patent application must include a specification of the invention which contains instructions that are adequate to enable a skilled person to produce or perform the invention. In other words, the specification must be 'enabling'.

The invention itself is defined in the 'claims' which form part of the specification. In biotechnology applications, common forms of claims involve an apparatus or device, a process or product of manufacture, and a method of treatment, testing or use. The claims are a guide to the scope of protection conferred by the granted patent.

Identifying the scope of a patent

In considering any patent, the most important task is to decide what it covers, i.e. the extent of the protection it gives to its owner. Identifying the 'scope of the claims' (alternatively, the "breadth of the claims") will help determine whether one is working within or outside the legal scope of a particular patent. The claims constitute the legal part of the patent – as distinct from the technical description – as they define in words what is protected by the patent. Frequently, several types of claims are made. For genetic inventions, claims are usually a combination of definitions of new products, processes, methods, compositions and uses. Claims can also be directed to devices for use in genetic testing. Identifying the 'scope of the claims' is a crucial issue in litigation or in any preliminary assessment of the likelihood of potential litigation and its outcome.

Official examination

The patent office will carry out a search of previously published documents, including the scientific and patent literature, to determine the relevant prior art. The prior art is therefore a continuously expanding corpus of knowledge which has to be taken into account when assessing patentability.

The application is examined in the light of these search results. In the examination process, there are usually arguments about the specification, and especially about the scope of the claims, which may take several years to settle.

Opposition or re-examination

Even after acceptance by the patent office, a patent application or patent can in most countries be opposed by third parties who may raise objections and prior art similar or in addition to those already overcome by the applicant. This process is termed 'opposition' or 'revocation', depending on the country, and involves argument between the applicant/patentee and the opponent.

Both have equal status as contending parties. In the United States, patent law does not provide for opposition in this sense but allows a third party to request official re-examination of the patent in the light of prior art not already considered. If this succeeds, it may result in limitation of the scope of the claims or outright revocation of the patent.

Conflicting patent applications

In some cases, two or more inventors independently seek a patent for the same invention (i.e. their claims cover the same ground). Most countries operate a 'first-to-file' system, according to which the application with the earliest filing date usually prevails, assuming that it is effective as a proper 'enabling disclosure' of the invention. The United States, however, has a 'first-to-invent' system, and in the case of conflicting patent applications, the USPTO has to decide which application has priority. Provided the dates of filing their respective applications are close to one another, the USPTO will declare an 'interference', a procedure based on examining laboratory notebook records and other evidence to determine the dates on which each party made the invention, and thus which was 'first to invent'.

Duration of a patent

The term during which a patent is valid differs from country to country. In the United States, Japan and most European countries, the term is 20 years from the application date. The payment of annual official renewal fees is required in most countries to avoid lapsing of the protection.

Enforcing patent rights

For the limited period in which a patent is in force, a patent holder is allowed to exclude others from the use of the patented invention. However, a patent is not self-enforcing. When there is infringement, it is up to the patent holder to take action to bring unauthorised use of the invention to an end. While the patent holder can seek remedy in a court of law, litigation is a last resort because it is risky and costly. In the course of litigation, for example, the validity of the patent may be challenged by the alleged infringer. While the patent may be upheld by the court, a patent holder faces the real possibility that court might revoke the patent or narrow the permissible claims. Instead of going to court, a patent holder often chooses to resolve the problem by licensing the patent to the other party on reasonable terms.

Licensing patents

The patent holder may wish to be the sole provider of the product or service covered by the patent and, subject to certain safeguards, this is permitted. Alternatively, the patent holder may license the patent to others for appropriate payment, either to one other party only (an exclusive licence) or to more than one party (a non-exclusive licence). Where the patent holder is not an industrial or commercial organisation and does not wish to create a start-up company to commercialise the invention, licensing the patent to an industrial partner is the most effective way of securing a financial return on the investment in research.

Patent Protection for Genetic Inventions

The economic value of patent protection in the life sciences, and especially in the pharmaceutical and agrochemical industries, is widely recognised. In no other fields is the relationship between patent protection and the incentives to innovate so strong. In biotechnology, where a wide variety of inventions originate in basic and applied research, the relationship between patents and research is very important. Even public research scientists and administrators, steeped as they may be in a culture of open science, have come to value the importance of patent protection in the past decades.

Legal situation

Here the focus is on patents for 'genetic inventions' which are defined as all uses of new discoveries of the role of genes and related DNA or RNA molecules. Of interest in this report are genetic inventions in the health field – inventions relevant to the diagnosis and therapeutic treatment of diseases. Genetic inventions more broadly understood also encompass agricultural, environmental and industrial uses. Claims in gene patent applications pertain, among other things, to:

- Genes or partial DNA sequences such as cDNAs, ESTs, SNPs, promoters and enhancers.
- Proteins encoded by these genes and their functions in the organism.
- Vectors used for the transfer of genes from one organism to another.
- Genetically modified micro-organisms, cells, plants and animals.
- Processes used for the making of a genetically modified product.
- Uses of genetic sequences or proteins which include: genetic tests for specific genetic diseases or predisposition to such diseases, drugs developed on the basis of the knowledge of proteins and their biological activity, industrial applications of protein functions.

In this particular field, the question is whether the patent system is achieving its objectives in ways that best serve the public interest. It is useful first to summarise what sort of protection is permitted for genetic inventions under the present law as interpreted by patent offices and courts of law across OECD countries.

Although the appropriateness of granting patents on DNA and other nucleotide sequences continues to be publicly debated, the position of the official patent authorities in OECD countries has been more or less stable for some time. Assuming that a DNA sequence is novel (not previously publicly known or used in a public manner) and that the other criteria of patentability are also met (utility, inventiveness/non-obviousness), the substance of the DNA itself can be patented. To be precise, the claims concern not the sequence as abstract information, but a molecule which has the defined sequence and function. This type of product claim will often be qualified in some respect, especially if the substance exists in nature. For example, in the European Community a directive of the European Council and European Parliament establishes that no patent can cover a substance *in situ* in the human body but only when isolated from its natural source. The policy of the USPTO is similar in intent since it requires product claims for genetic materials to be limited to the 'purified' or 'isolated' material.

Apart from the above restriction, a DNA sequence can be claimed as the substance *per se*, without limitation to any particular process of purification or isolation and without any limitation as to its intended use. In patent parlance this is known as a 'product *per se*' claim and it confers 'absolute product protection'. The potential scope of such a claim can be broad.

Granting "product *per se*" patents for genetic inventions is consistent with the established practice for new pharmaceuticals and other chemical compounds. The trend in many countries over the years has been to allow such product claims, as against previous more restrictive policies of allowing claims only to the particular chemical processes described in the patent application for making end products. In fact, the World Trade Organisation (WTO) Trade Related Intellectual Property Rights (TRIPS) Agreement requires patent protection to be available for process and product claims in all branches of technology, without discrimination. Nevertheless, whether product *per se* claims should continue to be allowed for genetic inventions is a source of continuing debate. In its 2001 Guidelines, the USPTO addressed many of the arguments against the patenting of genes as products *per se*. The USPTO rejected the contentions that: (i) genes are discoveries and not inventions, (ii) genes are products of nature and therefore not 'new', (iii) Congress should be consulted on this question, (iv) genes are the basic core of humanity and should not be 'owned' as property, (v) gene patents should be limited to specific disclosed uses, (vi) gene sequencing is routine and obvious. Likewise, the EPO much earlier stated its position as follows:

'An initial question to be considered is the protection which is conferred by a claim to a physical entity such as a compound *per se*. It is generally accepted as a principle underlying the EPC that a patent which claims a physical entity *per se* confers absolute protection upon such physical entity, that is, wherever it exists and whatever its context (and therefore for all uses of such physical entity, whether known or unknown).'

For most national patent authorities and courts of OECD member countries, product patents for genetic inventions are standard provided that they meet the requirements for patentability. The scope of such product patents can, in full legality, be quite broad and extend to areas which the inventor neither stipulated nor contemplated. Nevertheless, because genetic inventions have been among the most challenging areas of technology for patent offices, efforts have been made through the trilateral co-operation of the US, European and Japanese patent offices to harmonise their approach to the examination of patent applications in biotechnology. Much common ground has already been found for applying the main criteria of patentability to the examination of biotechnology patent applications (novelty, inventive step, adequate disclosure of the making and using of the claimed DNA and proteins for which they code). Patent authorities have also tried to clarify the circumstances under which genetic inventions such as SNPs, ESTs and cDNA are patentable.

The appropriate scope of claims has been one of the most contentious issues. While some differences among national patent offices remain, inventors are now more aware of what is required to justify their claims internationally. Through administrative reforms, patent offices have tried to temper over-ambitious patent applicants who seek much wider protection than is justified by the contribution made in their patent disclosure. Whether patent office efforts alone are sufficient is hotly debated.

Reforming the System of IP Protection for Genetic Inventions

In discussing possible reforms to the present system of IP protection for genetic inventions various researchers and authors stressed the enormous challenge of striking a new balance between the protection of inventions and the promotion of greater legal access to information and technology. Achieving this balance is the essence of all negotiations between patent attorneys and patent examiners and is at the core of most IP disputes. The arbiters of these debates are frequently the patent offices and the law courts, which decide on a case-by-case basis whether patents are valid and the extent of the claims allowed. For many users of the patent system, the slow and intermittent interpretation of statutes and precedence is perhaps costly and imperfect but adequate to the task of finding a just reward for genetic inventions that does not unduly hamper research or commerce.

However, the patent offices and the courts are simply the executors of the existing patent system. They usually do not take into account and are not competent to judge the economic repercussions of their decisions. If indeed DNA patents are found to lead to systematic and serious access problems, final authority about whether the patent system functions for the greatest public good rests with the government. A number of proposals for reform have been put forward in an effort to 'rebalance' the protection afforded genetic inventions. Some of these proposed changes are directed at the IP regime itself, and involve new legislation, while others suggest measures outside the IP regime.

The proposals under discussion can be classified into legislation (usually to amend the patent regime), regulations and regulatory bodies that would act as a check on either the patent offices or the patent holders themselves, administrative reforms to change the behaviour of public bodies (e.g. patent offices, funding agencies, public laboratories), and efforts to encourage more self-regulation by patent holders. Examples of each type of intervention includes:

- Judicial decisions and case law: Legal action involving both public and private sectors which results in binding decisions by courts on such issues as the validity of patents, clarification of dependency, acceptable patent scope, research exemptions.
- Legislation: To alter patent laws, for example: the introduction of grace periods, clarification of research, experimental and diagnostic use exemptions, the expansion of exclusions to patentable subject matter, and/or the addition and use of public order (order public) and morality clauses.
- Regulation: (i) expanded use of compulsory licences and/or antitrust procedures, (ii) creation of new regulatory bodies, or the granting of regulatory powers to existing bodies, for example to stipulate how the criteria of patentability should be interpreted for genetic inventions, or to decide on the criteria for public order and morality.
- Administration: (i) reforming the administration of patents, for example by raising the criteria for patentability of genetic inventions (e.g. requiring greater proof of utility or inventive step) and how to apply these criteria, (ii) licensing guidelines (e.g. for the licensing of technologies developed in public research bodies).
- Self-regulation: (i) public funding of research with the explicit aim of putting results into the public domain (e.g. HUGO, the SNPs Consortium), (ii) private-sector access initiatives (e.g. consortia, patent pools, or collective licensing organisations), (iii) educational or public relation initiatives.

Each of these reform suggestions has its advantages and disadvantages. Legislative changes are enacted very slowly and are not always based on the level of expertise or subtlety needed in crafting effective policies for a fast-moving field like biotechnology. Judicial decisions can also take time, and their outcome is not directed by policy imperatives or based on economic or social analysis. Creating new regulatory authorities is costly and may be cumbersome, but in theory these could have the advantage of being insulated from interest group politics and better informed about the social and economic impact of proposed changes to IPR policies. Administrative reforms of patent offices may be quicker, and perhaps more targeted at particular problems, but they suffer from a lack of wider public legitimacy. The development of best practice guidelines through a consultative process might be able to help with the problem of legitimacy. Self-regulation and efforts to promote self-regulation are attractive because they are less likely to distort incentives to innovation, but they are less likely to garner public trust and their effectiveness in changing behaviour has yet to be proven.

Thus, in the development of genetics, authorities made it clear that nonhuman life forms, otherwise meeting the legal patent requirements, would generally be patentable. More recently, following a few high profile controversies, the application of the patent system to genetic research had to face an increasing amount of criticism. The criticism, based on a number of moral (e.g. the impact of gene patenting on human dignity and humanness), scientific, legal, and economic arguments, eventually convinced authorities to adopt a more restrictive approach to the granting of genetic patents. Today, the thresholds that must be met to obtain genetic patents and the exceptions to patentability vary from one country to another. This creates much uncertainty. For example, patenting an embryonic stem cell is currently not possible in most European countries for reasons of morality, while a recent judgment from a United States Court of Appeals for the Federal Circuit invalidated patent applications on a diagnostic test method to detect hereditary breast cancer because they claimed unpatentable subject matter. It is presently difficult to assess the economic and social impact of gene patents. However, if genetic research is to proceed with some support from the private sector, reward mechanisms will always remain necessary due to the uncertainties as well as the high cost associated with research and development in this field.

References

Allen, M.G., *Introduction to Genetics*, CRC Press, USA.

Bergeron, R.S, *Principles of Genetics,* Harper & Row, New York.

Brazma, K.D., *Population Genetics*, Elsevier Applied Science, London.

Bryan, M.E., *Molecular Genetics.* Cambridge University Press, Cambridge, England.

Close, K.W., *Genetics and Molecular Biology*, Prentice Hall, New York.

Coffee, L. *Human Genetic Diseases*, Academic Press, USA.

Craig, T.H., *The Wonder of Genetics*, Tata-Mcgraw-Hill, New York.

De Jong, K.A., *Basic Concepts of Genetics*, Elsevier, New York.

Dorian, L., *Quantitative Genetics*, Harper & Row, New York.

Duncan, M.E., *Human Molecular Genetics*, Cambridge University Press, New Delhi.

Freund, R.D., *Forensic Genetics*, Marcel Dekker, Inc., New York.

Godfrey, D.I., *Genetics of Bacteria*, Tata-Mcgraw-Hill, New York.

Gold, K.W., *Molecular Genetics*, Oxford University Press, New Delhi.

Gregor Mendle, *Mendle's Principles of Heredity*, Cambridge University Press, London.

Hampel, T.F., *Conservation Genetics*, Academic Press, Inc., London.

Harper, L.J., *Molecular Genetics.* Harvard University Press, Cambridge.

Henikoff, S., *Genetics Disorder*, Wiley, New York.

Ian, R.L., *Fundamentals or Genetics*, Marcel Dekker, Inc., New York.

James, C.W., *Genetic Analysis,* McGraw-Hill, New York

Jenni, P.R., *Principles of Genetics*, Plenum, New York.

Johnson, V.K., *Behavioural Genetics,* Elsevier, Philadelphia.

Kimbrell, D.A., *Genetics and Genomes*, CRC Press, USA.

Leinster Murray, *Human Heredity*, Pergamon Press, Oxford, London.

Lewis, L.J., *Human Genetics*, Academic Press, Inc., London.

Maalouf Amin, *Viral Genetics,* Academic Press, New York.

MacLeod, I.R., *Population Genetics*. Macmillan, New York.

Marrett Damian, *Principles of Cancer Genetics*, Springer, USA.

Mount, D.W., *Genetics of Genomics*, University of Hertfordshire Press, UK.

Munn, R.F., *Bacteria and Genetics*, Elsevier, New York.

Painter, D.E., *Reproductive Genetics*, Lippincott Williams & Wilkins, Philadelphia.

Pevzner, P.A., *Population Genetics*, John Wiley and Sons, Inc, New Jersey.

Ricci, F.G., *Molecular Genetics*, Saunders Elsevier, Philadelphia.

Richard M. Twyman, *Genetics of Bacteria*, John Wiley and Sons, Inc, New Jersey.

Schrowebel, J., *Genomes*, Pergamon Press, Oxford, London.

Smith, T.F., Anthony J. Murgo, *Fundamentals of Genetics,* CRC Press, USA.

Snell, I.D., *Genetic Engineering,* Saunders Elsevier, Philadelphia.

Waterman, M.S., *Genetics and Molecular Biology*, CRC Press, USA.

Wilbur, W.J., *Genetics*, McGraw Hill, New York.

Willam Bateston, Problems of Genetics, Cambridge University Press, London.

Willam S. Klug, *Essential of Genetics*, Pearson, India.

Index